Terri Lannigan

W9-ALT-720

Terri Lannigan

Wound Healing

Evidence-Based Management

4th Edition

Contemporary Perspectives in Rehabilitation

CPR *Contemporary Perspectives in Rehabilitation*

Steven L. Wolf, PT, PhD, FAPTA, Editor-in-Chief

Spinal Cord Injury Rehabilitation
Edelle C. Field-Fote, PT, PhD

Fundamentals of Musculoskeletal Imaging, 3rd Edition
Lynn N. McKinnis, PT, OCS

Vestibular Rehabilitation, 3rd Edition
Susan J. Herdman, PT, PhD, FAPTA

Pharmacology in Rehabilitation, 4th Edition
Charles D. Ciccone, PT, PhD

Modalities for Therapeutic Intervention, 4th Edition
Susan L. Michlovitz, PT, PhD, CHT and Thomas P. Nolan, Jr., PT, MS, OCS

Evaluation and Treatment of the Shoulder:
An Integration of the Guide to Physical Therapist Practice
Brian J. Tovin, PT, MMSc, SCS, ATC, FAAOMPT and Bruce H. Greenfield, PT, MMSc, OCS

Cardiopulmonary Rehabilitation: Basic Theory and Application, 3rd Edition
Frances J. Brannon, PhD, Margaret W. Foley, RN, MN, Julie Ann Starr, PT, MS, CCS, and
Lauren M. Saul, MSN, CCRN

For more information on each title in the Contemporary Perspectives in Rehabilitation series, go to www.fadavis.com.

Wound Healing

Evidence-Based Management

4th Edition

Joseph M. McCulloch, PhD, PT, CWS, FACCWS, FAPTA
Professor and Dean
School of Allied Health Professions
Louisiana State University Health Sciences Center
Shreveport, Louisiana

Luther C. Kloth, MS, PT, CWS, FACCWS, FAPTA
Professor Emeritus
Physical Therapy Department
Marquette University
Milwaukee, Wisconsin

F.A. Davis Company • Philadelphia

F. A. Davis Company
1915 Arch Street
Philadelphia, PA 19103
www.fadavis.com

Copyright © 2010 by F. A. Davis Company

Copyright © 2010 by F. A. Davis Company. All rights reserved. This product is protected by copyright. No part of it may be reproduced, stored in a retrieval system, or transmitted in any form or by any means, electronic, mechanical, photocopying, recording, or otherwise, without written permission from the publisher.

Printed in the United States of America

Last digit indicates print number: 10 9 8 7 6 5 4 3 2 1

Acquisitions Editor: Melissa Duffield
Manager of Content Development: George W. Lang
Developmental Editor: Karen Carter
Art and Design Manager: Carolyn O'Brien

As new scientific information becomes available through basic and clinical research, recommended treatments and drug therapies undergo changes. The author(s) and publisher have done everything possible to make this book accurate, up to date, and in accord with accepted standards at the time of publication. The author(s), editors, and publisher are not responsible for errors or omissions or for consequences from application of the book, and make no warranty, expressed or implied, in regard to the contents of the book. Any practice described in this book should be applied by the reader in accordance with professional standards of care used in regard to the unique circumstances that may apply in each situation. The reader is advised always to check product information (package inserts) for changes and new information regarding dose and contraindications before administering any drug. Caution is especially urged when using new or infrequently ordered drugs.

Library of Congress Cataloging-in-Publication Data

Wound healing: evidence-based management/[edited by] Joseph M. McCulloch, Luther C. Kloth.—4th ed.
    p. ; cm.—(Contemporary perspectives in rehabilitation)
 Prev. ed. has subtitle: alternatives in management.
 Includes bibliographical references and index.
 ISBN-13: 978-0-8036-1904-3
 ISBN-10: 0-8036-1904-9
 1. Wound healing. I. McCulloch, Joseph M. II. Kloth, Luther. III. Series: Contemporary perspectives in rehabilitation (Unnumbered)
 [DNLM: 1. Wound Healing. 2. Wounds and Injuries—rehabilitation. WO 185 W93827 2010]
 RD94.W67 2010
 617.1—dc22

                                    2009053478

Authorization to photocopy items for internal or personal use, or the internal or personal use of specific clients, is granted by F. A. Davis Company for users registered with the Copyright Clearance Center (CCC) Transactional Reporting Service, provided that the fee of $.25 per copy is paid directly to CCC, 222 Rosewood Drive, Danvers, MA 01923. For those organizations that have been granted a photocopy license by CCC, a separate system of payment has been arranged. The fee code for users of the Transactional Reporting Service is: 8036-1904-3/10 + $.25.

To my wife, Gail; my sons, Bowen and Brett; other family members; and my friends and professional colleagues at Louisiana State University Health Sciences Center who provided support and encouragement. – *JMM*

To my wife, Doris, who in my semiretirement has been very patient and understanding regarding my commitment to this fourth edition; my sons, Eric and Dana; my daughter, Diane, and her husband, Bob, and daughters, Katelyn and Lauren. Also, to other family members, friends, colleagues, and students at Marquette University for their support and encouragement. – *LCK*

The preface written by Joe McCulloch and Lu Kloth to the fourth edition of what is now most appropriately called *Wound Healing: Evidence Based Management*, has made my job remarkably easy. In their Preface to this edition, they have nicely highlighted the wonderful additions in content and authorship since the third edition was published in 2002. This text is truly an international masterpiece on a subject that has now drawn attention from multidisciplinary clinicians and students facing the need to demonstrate treatment efficacy for any traumatically or metabolically-induced pathology of the integument and underlying structures. Dr. McCulloch and Prof. Kloth have accomplished this goal through fine tuning of a process begun over 20 years ago. They have watched this field grow with diligence, and, in the process, have attracted a cadre of colleagues who recognize the value residing in their contributions to arguably the most comprehensive text on this subject. More importantly, the willingness of this diverse team of contributors to spend the time and resources to offer contemporary information is tempered by the realization that their efforts required comprehensive documentation to support many contentions made regarding treatment approaches and modality/technique utilization. Such a requirement forms the cornerstone of all texts comprising the *Contemporary Perspectives in Rehabilitation* series. Each text must provide information based on evidence while challenging the student or clinician through thought-provoking case histories or other unique vehicles. In that context, Dr. McCulloch and Prof. Kloth become the first to insert the notion of "pearls (of wisdom)" within chapters comprising this volume. Such pearls can be used to extract essential points of information, or, more comprehensively, to guide readers' thinking as they absorb information within most chapters.

So why is all the attention to detail and the expansion of evidence-based information about the anatomy, pathology, and treatment of wounds so important? If we recognize that health-care insurers continue to seek ways to reduce reimbursement for rehabilitative efforts, virtually every aspect of patient care for which physical or occupational therapists might be engaged has become scrutinized more carefully. Our currency for communication in our efforts to engage these enterprises as we fight for our patients has now become "evidence." In this regard, the facts are that the presence of a serious wound is most apparent to the naked eye, can evoke sympathy or empathy from even the least dispassionate decision maker, and brings to a level of conscientiousness the implications for failed treatment as measured by further medical costs as well as reduced quality of life. Such visibly obvious signs of immobility or disfigurement afford, in a most curious way, an opportunity to relate evidence for effective treatment approaches to obvious indicators of functional and aesthetic restoration. For example, such visible cues for impairment can draw the focus in a way often unattended by those who do not see the implications for functional imitation seen in the patient with a hemiparetic arm, a rigid gait, or with persistent low back pain. The contents of this book and utilization of information herein, whether impacting the patient with ulcerative lesions caused by uncontrolled diabetes, or subsequent to sustaining a serious burn, can potentially make the difference in the number of treatments provided to these patients and the concomitant but often unappreciated impact on health-related quality of life.

So, to all student or clinician users of the magnificent effort housed within these pages, we hope that your ability to extract the abundance of evidence reflected in each chapter will serve you and your patients well and help to reduce an emergent atrophy in rehabilitation care.

Steven L. Wolf, PhD, PT, FAPTA
Atlanta, Georgia
Editor-in-Chief,
Contemporary Perspectives in Rehabilitation Series

When the first edition of *Wound Healing: Alternatives in Management* premiered in 1990, little did we know that we would find ourselves 20 years later bringing to market a fourth edition that far exceeded any of our expectations. The field of wound management has grown over the past two decades into a medical subspecialty with board-certified practitioners. The growth in subject matter content has been documented in the first three editions of our text and is readily evident in this edition, which we have renamed *Wound Healing: Evidence-Based Management,* 4th edition. Working on these editions over the years has been much like parents watching their first child being born, mature through adolescence, and head off to college. Here we find ourselves with a fully "grown up" edition that presents a broad overview of present-day wound management. Of course, just as we all aspire to be life-long learners, we know that this text will continue to change and improve, as will practice.

In the preface to the third edition, we commented on the addition of a 50-picture color insert along with 13 new authors and topics divided into four sections. This seems to pale in comparison to the fourth edition, which offers fully integrated color and features 35 chapters by 45 nationally and internationally acclaimed authors. These chapters offer case studies and "pearls" that help the reader scan the chapter and locate major points of interest. Another unique addition to the text is an appendix with annotated multiple choice questions that summarize major content in each chapter and help readers see if they understand key concepts.

The fourth edition is divided into six logically organized categories that take the reader from anatomy and physiology into patient assessment, general wound management principles, wound etiologies, and physical technologies, and concludes with practical information on managing a wound care practice.

The first part, entitled "The Wound Healing Environment," contains five chapters that integrate the basic science aspects of wound management. The section begins with an introduction to integumentary anatomy and follows with an overview of the wound healing process and how growth factors and the extracellular matrix influence repair. The section concludes with a discussion of the role of nutrition in wound healing and how other complications delay healing.

Part II, "Assessing the Patient," takes the reader through a general wound examination, addressing techniques applicable to a variety of patient types. This is followed by a chapter that focuses on tests and measures useful in assessing the circulatory and neurological systems. Several new chapters are included that provide information on assessing and controlling bioburden and identifying and managing atypical wounds. A new chapter on the role of imaging in wound care highlights some of the more commonly encountered radiographic assessments used to evaluate individuals with wounds.

Part III, "General Management Principles in Patients with Wounds," addresses wound bed preparation and how débridement, dressings, and skin substitutes facilitate repair. A new chapter in this section focuses on topical agents used for débridement, bacterial control, and facilitation of healing.

Part IV examines etiological factors contributing to some of the more common wounds seen in clinical practice. New chapters in this section discuss causative factors leading to ulceration of the feet in individuals with diabetes. This is complemented by another new chapter addressing diabetes in general and how the disease process negatively impacts healing. Principles of venous ulcer development and treatment are discussed, then followed next by new chapters covering ischemic ulcers and lymphatic disease. The chapter on pressure ulcers and management has been completely revised and addresses both bedbound individuals as well as those who are functional users of wheelchairs. Additional new chapters have been included to address burn management from both the medical and rehabilitative perspectives. This is then followed by discussions on the management of wound pain, surgical considerations in wound management, and neonatal and pediatric issues.

Part V looks at biophysical technologies. The change in name from physical modalities or agents to biophysical technologies demonstrates the broadened perspective addressed in this section. Included are discussions on electrical stimulation, ultrasound, and ultraviolet therapies, but distinctions are made between endogenous and exogenous electrical fields and the role of electromagnetic stimulation in wound repair. The section concludes with a review of compression therapies and two new chapters that address the rapidly expanding fields of negative-pressure wound therapy and oxygen therapy.

Part VI concludes the text with an overview of issues pertinent to practice administration. The first chapter speaks to the proper means of documenting wound management and properly coding bills to meet third-party payment requirements. A new chapter provides information on developing an effective clinical wound care program. The text then concludes with helpful advice from the legal arena and discusses contemporary issues being addressed in the courts.

All in all, we feel we have provided the wound care clinician with an evidenced-based text that should prove of great value in the daily management of patients who present with challenging wounds and increasingly complex medical problems.

Joseph M. McCulloch
Luther C. Kloth

Shannon Abney, LOTR
Occupational Therapist
Department of Rehabilitation Services
LSU Health Sciences Center
Shreveport, Louisiana

Karen Albaugh, PT, DPT, MPH, CWS
Assistant Professor
Physical Therapy Program
Neumann University
Aston, Pennsylvania
and
Clinical Coordinator of Research and Hyperbaric
    Medicine
The Center for Advanced Wound Care™
Wyomissing, Pennsylvania

**Mona Mylene Baharestani,
    PhD, APN, CWOCN, CWS, FACCWS**
Clinical Associate Professor
East Tennessee State University Quillen College of Medicine
Department of Surgery
and
Associate Professor
East Tennessee State University
Center for Nursing Research
and
James H. Quillen Veterans Affairs Medical Center
Johnson City, Tennessee

**Sharon Baranoski,
    MSN, RN, CWOCN, APN, FAPWCA, FAAN**
Administrative Director of Clinical Programs and
    Development
Administrator of Home Health
Silver Cross Hospital
Joliet, Illinois

Teresa Conner-Kerr, PT, PhD, CWS
Professor and Chair, Department of Physical Therapy
Winston-Salem State University
Winston-Salem, North Carolina

Marie K. Hoeger Bement, PT, PhD
Assistant Professor
Physical Therapy Department
College of Health Sciences
Marquette University
Milwaukee, Wisconsin

Amy M. Brogle, MSPT, CWS
Physical Therapist—Outpatient Rehabilitation
Greenwich Hospital
Greenwich, Connecticut

Jeffrey M. Davidson, PhD
Professor of Pathology
Director, Phenotype Core, Skin Diseases Research Center
Vanderbilt University School of Medicine
Nashville, Tennessee

Sharon L. Dunn, PT, PhD, OCS
Director, Program in Physical Therapy
Department of Rehabilitation Sciences
School of Allied Health Professions
LSU Health Sciences Center
Shreveport, Louisiana

William J. Ennis, DO, CWS, FACCWS, MBA, FACOS
Comprehensive Center for Wound and Disease Management
St. James Hospital—Olympia Fields Campus
Olympic Fields, Illinois

Jason Hanft, DPM, FACFAS
The Foot and Ankle Institute of South Florida
South Miami, Florida

Maureen Heldmann, MD
Clinical Professor, Department of Radiology
LSU Health Sciences Center
Shreveport, Louisiana

Heather Hettrick, PT, PhD, CWS, MLT, FACCWS
Director of Clinical Education
American Medical Technologies
Irvine, California

Eric P. Kindwall, MD
Medical Director Emeritus
Hyperbaric Medicine, St. Luke's Medical Center
Executive Director, American College of Hyperbaric
    Medicine
Milwaukee, Wisconsin

Robert S. Kirsner, MD, PhD
Professor, Department of Dermatology and Cutaneous
    Surgery
University of Miami
Miami, Florida

Katherine E. Lampe, PT, MPT, CWS, FACCWS
Assistant Professor
DPT Program
St. Ambrose University
Davenport, Iowa

Renee Trahan Lane, PT, ATP
Seating and Staffing Solutions, LLC
Lafayette, Louisiana

Joyce Stamp Lilly, RN, JD, PC
Law Offices of Joyce Stamp Lilly
Houston, Texas

Harriett B. Loehne, PT, DPT, CWS, FACCWS
Clinical Educator, Archbold Center for Wound Management
    and Hyperbaric Medicine
Thomasville, Georgia

David E. Mahon, MD, CWS, FACCWS, FACS
Advanced Surgical Associates
Arlington Heights, Illinois

Edward Mahoney, MSPT, DPT, CWS
Assistant Professor of Physical Therapy
Department of Rehabilitation Sciences
School of Allied Health Professions
LSU Health Sciences Center
Shreveport, Louisiana

Abbie Kemper-Martin, MD, PhD, CWS, MLT, FACCWS
Associate Professor, Department of Radiology
LSU Health Sciences Center
Shreveport, Louisiana

Robert G. Martindale, MD, PhD, FACS
Director of Nutrition, Division of General Surgery
Oregon Health Sciences University
Portland, Oregon

Stanley Keith McCallon, MPT, DPT, CWS, FACCWS
Assistant Professor and Director, Physical Therapy
    Post-graduate Wound Management Residency
Department of Rehabilitation Sciences
School of Allied Health Professions
LSU Health Sciences Center
Shreveport, Louisiana

Patricio Meneses, PhD
Comprehensive Center for Wound and Disease
    Management
St. James Hospital—Olympic Fields Campus
Olympic Fields, Illinois

Jeffrey Niezgoda, MD, FACHM, FAPWCA, FACEP
Medical Director
The Centers for Comprehensive Wound Care
    and Hyperbaric Oxygen Therapy
St. Luke's Medical Center, Aurora Health Care Hyperbaric
    and Wound Care Associates
Milwaukee, Wisconsin

Liza G. Ovington, PhD, CWS, FACCWS
Medical Director
Johnson and Johnson Wound Management
A division of Ethicon, Inc.
Somerville, New Jersey

Asha R. Patel, MD
Dermatology Resident
Columbia University
New York, New York

Gregory Patterson, MD, CWS, FACS, FASA
Medical Director, Archbold Center for Wound
    Management and the John D. Archbold Level II
    Trauma Center
Thomasville, Georgia

Howard B. Petusevsky, DPM, FACFAOM
South Florida Podiatry Associates
Lauderhill, Florida

Arthur A. Pilla, PhD
Adjunct Professor, Department of Orthopedics
Mount Sinai School of Medicine and Department of
    Biomedical Engineering
Columbia University
New York, New York

Laurie Rappl, PT, CWS
Cytomedix, Inc.
Rockville, Maryland

Kathryn Richardson, MD
Assistant Professor of Clinical Surgery, Department of
    Surgery
LSU Health Sciences Center
Shreveport, Louisiana

Carla Saulsbery, LOTR, CHT
Chief, Occupational Therapy
Department of Rehabilitation Services
LSU Health Sciences Center
Shreveport, Louisiana

Pamela Scarborough, PT, MS, CDE, CWS, FACCWS
Director of Clinical Development
American Medical Technologies
Austin, Texas

Pamela Sheffield, RN, CDE
Carrollton, Texas

**Gary Sibbald,
    BS, MD, FRCPC (MED), FRCPC (DERM), Med**
Women's College Hospital
Toronto, Ontario
Canada

Kevin Sittig, MD
Professor of Surgery and Director, Regional Burn Center
Medical Director, University Hospital
LSU Health Sciences Center
Shreveport, Louisiana

Kathleen A. Sluka, PT, PhD
Professor
Physical Therapy and Rehabilitation Science Graduate
    Program
Neuroscience Graduate Program
Pain Research Program
College of Medicine
University of Iowa
Iowa City, Iowa

Robert Snyder, DPM, FACFAS, CWS, FACCWS
Doctor of Podiatric Medicine
Tamarac, Florida

Stephen Sprigle, PT, PhD
Center for Assistive Technology and Environmental Access
Atlanta, Georgia

Pamela G. Unger, PT, CWS, FAPWCA
Vice President of Clinical Research and
    Reimbursement
Celleration MIST Therapy
Eden Prairie, Minnesota

Carol G.T. Vance, PT, MA
Associate
Physical Therapy and Rehabilitation Science Graduate
    Program
College of Medicine
University of Iowa
Iowa City, Iowa

Dot Weir, RN, CWON, CWS
Program Director
The Wound Healing Center
Osceola Regional Medical Center
Kissimmee, Florida

Stephanie Woelfel, PT, MPT, CWS, FACCWS
Director of Patient Care Services
Greater Peoria Specialty Hospital
Peoria, Illinois

Kevin Woo, RN, MSc, PhD(C), ACNP, GNC(C), FAPWCA
Clinical Scientist/Nurse Practitioner
Wound Healing Clinic
Women's College Hospital
Toronto, Ontario
Canada

Min Zhao, MD, PhD
Professor
Department of Dermatology and Department of
    Ophthalmology
School of Medicine
University of California at Davis
Davis, California

Cathy S. Elrod, PhD, PT
Assistant Professor of Physical Therapy
School of Health Professions
Marymount University
Arlington, Virginia

Beverly Fein, PT, EdD
Associate Professor of Physical Therapy
Coordinator of Clinical Education
Sacred Heart University
Fairfield, Connecticut

Ellen Wruble Hakim, PT, DScPT, MS, CWS, FACCWS
Vice Chair for Professional Programs
Director of Entry-Level DPT Program
Department of Physical Therapy and Rehabilitation Science
University of Maryland School of Medicine
Baltimore, Maryland

Heather Hettrick, PT, PhD, CWS, MLT, FACCWS
Director of Clinical Education
American Medical Technologies
Irvine, California

Christine J. Kasinskas, DPT, MS, BA, BS
Assistant Professor of Physical Therapy
Quinnipiac University
Hamden, Connecticut

Harriett B. Loehne, PT, DPT, CWS, FACCWS
Clinical Educator Archbold Center for Wound Management
    & Hyperbaric Medicine
Thomasville, Georgia

Deborah M. Michael, PT, DPT, CPed
Clinical Assistant Professor
Division of Physical Therapy
Georgia State University
Atlanta, Georgia

Janet L. Mutschler, PT, MHS
Instructor
Department of Physical Therapy
University of Maryland, Eastern Shore
Princess Anne, Maryland

Emily Karwacki Sheff, MS, CMSRN, FNP-BC
Lecturer, Clinical Instructor
Nursing
Massachusetts General Hospital Institute of Health
    Professions
Boston, Massachusetts

We wish to thank the following individuals, without whom the publication of this fourth edition would not have been achievable:

Our contributors, who graciously endured our critical assessments and editing of their manuscripts.

The reviewers and copyeditors for their comments and suggestions for improving the book.

The F.A. Davis Company staff, including Karen Carter, Melissa Duffield, Kimberly Harris, and Margaret Biblis; and Marsha Hall, Project Manager, Progressive Publishing Alternatives.

The students we have taught in the program in physical therapy at Louisiana State University Health Sciences Center and the Department of Physical Therapy Marquette University College of Health Sciences for their opinions and constructive comments on this fourth edition.

The thousands of physical therapists, nurses, and physicians from clinical and academic settings who provided us with their useful suggestions for improving this fourth edition.

The patients and our colleagues affiliated with the LSU Health Sciences Center and the Department of Physical Therapy, Marquette University, College of Health Sciences.

Integumentary Anatomy: Skin—The Largest Organ

Sharon Baranoski, MSN, RN, CWOCN, APN, FAPWCA, FAAN

Our knowledge of the integumentary system (skin) has evolved over the last 20 years. A true biological universe, the skin incorporates all major support systems: blood, muscle, and innervation as well as roles in immunocompetence, psycho-emotional, ultraviolet radiation sensing, and endocrine functions.[1]

The integumentary system is the external covering of the human body. The name is derived from the Latin *integumentum,* which means "a covering." The integumentary system includes the skin, hair, nails, and sweat glands and their products. It is often referred to as is the largest organ of the body. It is composed of two main layers: the epidermis, known as the outermost layer, and the dermis, the innermost layer. The dermal-epidermal junction, commonly referred to as the basement membrane zone (BMZ), separates the two layers. Under the dermis lies a layer of loose connective tissue, called subcutis (subcutaneous) tissue, or hypodermis. (Fig. 1.1)

Epidermis

The epidermis is a thin outer layer of skin. It is an avascular layer that regenerates itself every 4 to 6 weeks. It contains melanin, which gives skin its color and allows the skin to tan. Carotene and oxygen-rich hemoglobin also contribute to the color of skin.[2] The epidermis is divided into five sublayers, or strata, composed of keratin-producing cells called *keratinocytes.*[1-5] (Fig. 1.2):

- *Stratum corneum:* top layer, consists of dead keratinocyte cells
- *Stratum lucidum:* packed translucent line of cells; not seen in thin skin; found only on the palms and soles

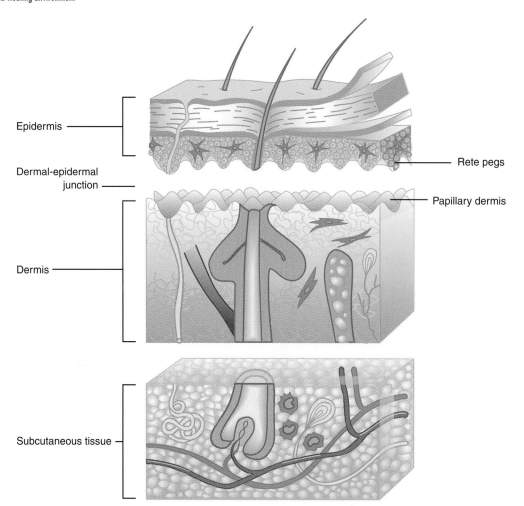

Figure 1•1 *Layers of the skin.*

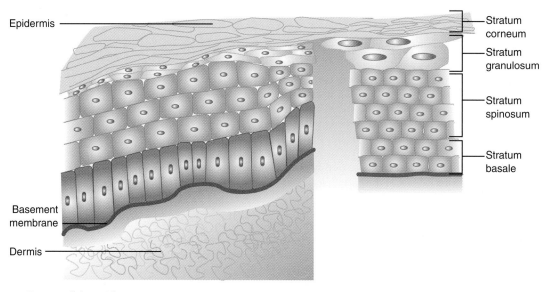

Figure 1•2 *Layers of the epidermis.*

- *Stratum granulosum*: contains keratinocytes and Langerhans cells
- *Stratum spinosum*: "spiny" layer, contains keratinocytes and Langerhans cells
- *Stratum basale or germinativum*: single layer of epidermal cells; contains melanocytes and Merkel cells

The epidermis is composed of hard, horny keratinocyte cells that migrate up from the bottom single layer of cells, the stratum basale, to the stratum corneum. Epidermal cell differentiation usually takes 28 days and is affected by aging and chemotherapy.

▶ **PEARL 1•1** The primary functions of the epidermis are protection from epidermal water loss and maintaining skin integrity against bacterial invasion and physical barriers, such as shear, friction, and toxic irritants.[6-8]

The BMZ divides the epidermis from the dermis. It contains fibronectin (an adhesive glycoprotein), type IV collagen (a non-fiber-forming collagen), heparin sulfate proteoglycan, and glycosaminoglycan.[8,9] The BMZ has an irregular surface—called rete ridges or pegs—projecting downward from the epidermis that interlocks with the upward projections of the dermis. This structure anchors the epidermis to the dermis, preventing it from sliding back and forth. (Fig. 1.3)

▶ **PEARL 1•2** As skin ages, the basement membrane flattens and the area of contact between the epidermis and dermis is decreased by 50%, thus increasing the risk of skin injury by traumatic, accidental separation of the epidermis from the dermis.[8]

Dermis

The dermis, or corium, is the thickest layer of skin. It is often referred to as the "true skin." Variation in thickness occurs throughout the body. For example, the dermis of the back is thicker than the dermal covering of the scalp, forehead, abdomen, thigh, wrist, and palm. The average thickness measures 2 mm but can vary from 2 to 4 mm.[8] In contrast to the epidermal layer, the dermis is sparsely populated, primarily by fibroblasts. Despite its great volume, the dermis contains far fewer cells and gets its bulk from fibrous and amorphous extracellular matrix (ECM).[1] Fibroblasts are migratory cells that make and degrade ECM. There is significant research regarding the factors that control the "differentiation" of the dermal fibroblast, especially in relationship to wound healing. Other cell types present in the dermis include macrophages, lymphocytes, and mast cells, the latter of which can trigger allergic reactions by secreting bioactive mediators such as histamine.[1] The major proteins found in this layer are collagen and elastin, which are synthesized and secreted by fibroblasts.

Collagen

Collagen forms up to 75% of the skin's total dry weight.[1,9-11] Collagen can function in many ways, such as by providing tissue integrity (tissue repair, migration, and adhesion) to facilitating tissue morphogenesis and even platelet aggregation.[1,8,9]

▶ **PEARL 1•3** Collagen is essential for epidermal adherence to the dermis.

It provides the anchoring fibrils and filaments that link the basal keratinocytes with the basement membrane. It is a structural protein that gives skin its tensile strength.[12]

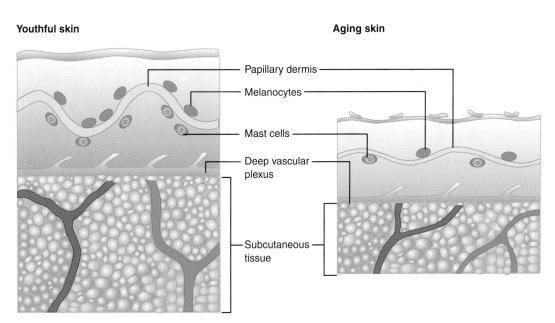

Youthful skin

Aging skin

Papillary dermis

Melanocytes

Mast cells

Deep vascular plexus

Subcutaneous tissue

Figure 1•3 *The effects of aging on the BMZ.*

Elastin

Another major ECM protein is elastin, which provides the skin its elasticity.[1] Elastin fibers form structures similar to a spring or coil that allows this protein to stretch and, when released, to return to its inherent configuration.[12]

The "shock absorber" dermis is divided into an upper papillary and a lower reticular portion, both representing their respective composition of connective tissue components, cell number, and supply of blood vessels and nerves.[1]

Papillary Dermis

The papillary dermis is composed of collagen and reticular fibers. The papillary layer is very thin, lies next to the epidermis, and is highly vascular. It contains a higher level of water than does the reticular layer. Its fingerlike projections called *papillae* project into the epidermis. Its distinct, unique pattern allows fingerprint identification for each individual. It contains capillaries for skin nourishment and pain and touch receptors (pacinian corpuscles and Meissner's corpuscles).[9-11]

Reticular Dermis

The reticular dermis (deep layer) is composed of collagen bundles that anchor the skin to the subcutaneous tissue. This layer makes up about 80% of the dermis. Collagen fibers are arranged and entwined, thus providing strength and flexibility. Sweat glands, hair follicles, nerves, and blood vessels are found in this layer.[11]

▸ **PEARL 1•4** Providing tensile strength, support, moisture retention, and blood and oxygen to the skin is the main role or function of the dermis.[10]

The reticular dermis protects the underlying muscles, bones, and organs. The dermis also contains the sebaceous glands, which secrete sebum, a substance rich in oil that lubricates the skin. Furthermore, it also contains hair follicles that are the source of multipotent stem cells, which have the capacity to restore the epidermis.[8]

The subcutaneous tissue, or hypodermis, attaches the dermis to underlying structures. Its function is to promote an ongoing blood supply to the dermis to aid in regeneration. It comprises primarily adipose tissue, which provides a cushion between skin layers, muscles, and bones. It promotes skin mobility, molds body contours, and insulates the body.[12]

Skin Appendages

Skin appendages are the eccrine and apocrine sweat glands, hair follicles, sebaceous glands, and the nails. Except for the nails, all skin appendages are located in the dermis.[13]

Eccrine Sweat Glands

Sweat is produced in a coiled tubule in the dermis and is transported by a sweat duct through the epidermis and is secreted. The release of sweat from the eccrine glands is the body's cooling process. The entire body surface has 2 million to 3 million eccrine sweat glands and can produce up to 10 liters of sweat per day.[13]

Apocrine Sweat Glands

Like the eccrine glands, apocrine sweat is also produced in coiled tubules in the dermis, but the apocrine duct drains sweat into a hair follicle from which it reaches the skin's surface.[13,14] These glands are situated in specific areas of the body: the armpits, eyelids, pubic area, and the genitals. They remain inactive until puberty.[14] The action of normal skin bacteria on excreted apocrine sweat is responsible for body odor.[13]

Hair Follicles

Hair is made of keratin, the same substance that forms nails and the top layer of the epidermis (stratum corneum).[13] Hair is located everywhere on the body except the palms and soles. Humans have two types of hair: vellus (light and fine) and terminal (dark and thick).[1,13] Cells located in the root of the hair produce keratin and melanin, which gives hair its color.[13] Attached to each hair of the body is a sebaceous gland, which secretes *sebum*, an oily substance that drains into the canal of a hair follicle to reach the surface of the skin.[1,13,14]

Sebaceous Glands

Sebum is produced by the sebaceous glands. They are found in the scalp, face, and upper trunk and are absent from the palms and soles of the feet. These glands increase in size and produce more sebum in response to increased hormone levels, specifically androgen, during adolescence.[13,14]

Nails

Nails are the only skin appendage not located in the dermis, but instead at the ends of fingers and toes. The nail plate is made of dead keratin, which forms a hard, protective structure. The nail bed is the epidermal layer that is tightly attached to the bottom of the nail plate. The blood vessels of the nail bed give nails their pink color.[13]

Skin Function

Skin is an important organ with diverse functions that are not readily understood. The development of subspecialities in cutaneous biology will undoubtedly provide a greater understanding of skin and its true function. Dubbed the largest external organ, in adults the skin weighs about 6 pounds and covers over 20 feet (up to 15% of total adult body weight).[12] Skin thickness varies from 0.5 mm to 6 mm, according to its location on the body; for example, skin can be as thin as 1/50 of an inch on the eyelids and as thick as 1/3 of an inch on the palms and soles, where greater protection is needed.

▸ **PEARL 1•5** The skin receives one third of the body's circulating blood volume—an oversupply of blood compared to its metabolic needs.

The skin's major functions are protection, temperature regulation, sensation, metabolism, and communication. See Table 1.1 for a detailed list. Skin protects the body by serving as a barrier from invasion by organisms such as bacteria.

Table 1•1 Skin Layer Functions

Skin Layer	Characteristics	General Function
Epidermis	Makes up the outer layer of skin Consists of five layers (or strata): corneum, lucidum, granulosum, spinosum, and basale (or germinativum) Repairs and regenerates itself every 28 days	Provides protective barrier Supplies organization of cell content Synthesizes vitamin D and cytokines Divides and mobilizes cells Maintains contact with dermis Provides pigmentation (contains melanocytes) Recognizes allergen (contains Langerhans cells) Differentiates into hair, nails, sweat glands, and sebaceous glands
Dermis	Consists of two layers—papillary dermis and reticular dermis—and is composed of collagen, reticulum, and elastin fibers Contains a network of nerve endings, blood vessels, lymphatics, capillaries, sweat and sebaceous glands, and hair follicles.	Supports structure Provides mechanical strength Supplies nutrition Resists shearing forces Supplies inflammatory response
Subcutaneous tissue (hypodermis)	Comprises adipose and connective tissue Contains major blood vessels, nerves, and lymphatic vessels	Attaches to underlying structure Provides thermal insulation Stores calories (energy) Controls body shape Serves as mechanical "shock absorber"

Reprinted with permission from Baranoski, S, Ayello, EA: Wound Care Essentials, Practice Principles, ed. 2. Philadelphia, Lippincott Williams & Wilkins, 2007, Chap. 4.

Protection

Sebum, a lipid-rich, oily substance secreted by sebaceous glands provides an acidic covering that supports and assists in maintaining a protective skin barrier function. The normal acidic range of skin pH is 4 to 6.5 in healthy people.[12,15,16] The mean pH is 5.5. This "acid mantle" has a protective advantage and helps maintain a normal skin flora. The acid mantle protects the skin from bacterial and fungal infections. It also provides indirect protection against invasion by microorganisms and against alkaline substances.[15] If the acid mantle loses its acidity, the skin can become more prone to damage and infection. Frequent use of soap products and overwashing can alter the stratum corneum and its ability to serve as a protective barrier.

▶ **PEARL 1•6** Several skin conditions can cause an increase in skin surface pH: eczema, contact dermatitis, atopic dermatitis, and dry skin.[17,18]

Systemic diseases such as diabetes, chronic renal failure, and cerebrovascular disease can also increase skin surface pH.[19] Staphylococcal species (such as *Staphylococcus aureus* or *Staphylococcus epidermis*) tolerate salt and are present in

large numbers as resident bacteria on the skin.[20,21] Another organism found on the skin is yeast, which is commonly found on the trunk and ear and as fungus between the toes.[20,21]

Sensation

Sensation is a well-known and key function of the skin. Areas that are most sensitive to touch have a greater number of nerve endings.[21] These areas include the lips, nipples, and fingertips. In humans, the fingertips are the most sensitive touch organ and enable us to correctly identify objects by touch rather than by sight. Many tactile corpuscles lie at the base of hair follicles, and shaving reduces the tactile sensibility of that skin area. In hairless body regions, the tactile corpuscles are called Meissner's corpuscles.[21] Pleasurable, firm touching sensations, such as from a massage or hugs of affection, are transmitted via the skin to the brain as they generate nerve transmissions through these tactile corpuscles.

Somatic pain (from the outer body surfaces and framework) is also communicated through the skin. Superficial (acute) pain is usually transmitted to a local area via very rapid nerve impulses by A-delta nerve fibers.[21] Such pain tends to be sharp and ceases when the pain stimulus stops. Deep (chronic) pain impulses are transmitted slowly over the smaller, thinly myelinated C fibers. In contrast, this type of pain tends to be felt over a more diffuse area, lasts for longer periods of time, and remains even after the pain stimulus is gone.[21]

Temperature Regulation

Temperature regulation and fluid and electrolyte balance are achieved in part by the skin. Thermoregulation is controlled by the hypothalamus in response to internal core body temperature.[22-25] Peripheral temperature receptors in the skin assist in this process of temperature homeostasis. By sweating and insensible loss of water through the skin, lungs, and buccal mucosa, homeostasis of body temperature is maintained. Skin temperature is controlled by the dilatation or constriction of skin blood vessels. When the body core temperature rises, the body will attempt to reduce the temperature by releasing heat from the skin. This is accomplished by sending a chemical signal to increase blood flow in the skin by vasodilation, which will raise skin temperature.[25]

Metabolism

The skin plays an important role in the regulation of vitamin D within our body.

▶ **PEARL 1•7** Synthesis of vitamin D occurs in the skin in the presence of sunlight.[12]

Ultraviolet radiation converts a sterol found in sebum to a cholecalciferol (vitamin D).[26]

The skin also aids in the excretion of the end products of cell metabolism and prevents excessive loss of fluid. Other important functions of the skin include its manufacturing ability and immune functions.[26] While the skin's hypersensitivity responses in allergic reactions are commonly seen, the skin's role in immune function is not always fully appreciated. Present in the skin are Langerhans cells and tissue macrophages, which play an important role in digesting bacteria, as well as mast cells, which are needed to provide proper immune system functioning.[26,27]

Psychosocial/Communication

Skin is very important to all human beings. The television and magazine industries use skin to sell many products: we are lead to believe that perfect skin is something everyone wants. From birth to old age, our skin and its appearance play an important role in our relationship with others as well as how we see ourselves. As an organ of communication, facial skin, along with underlying muscles, is capable of expressions such as smiling, frowning, and pouting.[12] The sensation of touch can also convey feelings of comfort, concern, friendship, and love.[12]

The Aging Process

Normal skin changes occur with aging, but elderly skin is especially vulnerable to insult. As skin ages, the epidermis gradually thins. The dermal-epidermal junction flattens, and dermal papillae and epidermal rete pegs are effaced,

making the skin more susceptible to mild mechanical trauma. Decreases in the number of sweat glands and their output explains some of the dry skin seen in elderly people.[28-30] The ability to retain moisture is decreased in aging skin due to diminished amounts of dermal proteins, which cause oncotic pressure shifts and diminished fluid homeostasis, thereby putting elderly patients at risk for dehydration.[29,30]

▶ **PEARL 1•8** Because soap increases skin pH to an alkaline level, using emollient soap and bathing every other day instead of every day can decrease the incidence of skin injury, such as skin tears, in elderly patients.[15]

An elderly person's skin is more easily stretched due to a decrease in elastin fibers.[29] The skin becomes a less-effective barrier against water loss, bruising, and infection, as well as having impaired thermal regulation, decreased tactile sensitivity, and decreased pain perception.[29,31] Due to a decreased amount of dermal proteins, the blood vessels become thinner and more fragile, thereby leading to a type of hemorrhaging known as senile purpura. According to Selden and colleagues, the pathophysiology of skin tears parallels that of senile purpura.[32]

Many dermal changes occur with aging, but the most prominent is the approximately 20% loss in dermal thickness, which probably accounts for the paper-thin appearance of aging skin.[29]

▶ **PEARL 1•9** This decrease in dermal cells, blood vessels, nerve endings, and collagen leads to altered or reduced sensation, thermoregulation, rigidity, moisture retention, and sagging skin.[30]

The decrease of subcutaneous fat during aging results in a loss of protective functions. Subcutaneous tissue undergoes site-specific atrophy in such areas as the face, dorsal aspect of the hands, shins, and plantar aspects of the foot, increasing the energy absorbed by the skin when trauma occurs to these areas.[32] Aging skin is less able to manufacture vitamin D when exposed to ultraviolet sunlight.[29] The decline in the number of Langerhans cells and mast cells in aging skin translates into diminished immune functioning of the skin.[29,32]

Skin aging appears to be the result of both scheduled and continuous wear-and-tear processes that damage cellular DNA and proteins.[33] Skin aging can be due to either a chronological process or to photoaging. An expected chronological aging process occurs to us all. The physiological alteration in skin functions affects all of us if we live long enough. Our skin becomes thin, pale, and dry, with fine wrinkles appearing. Photoaging results from exposure to the ultraviolet radiation (UVR) of sunlight, and the damage thus becomes apparent in sun-exposed skin.[33]

▶ **PEARL 1•10** The use of protective sunscreens will decrease the UVR effects when properly applied. The best defense is to avoid the sun as much as possible and use protection on exposed areas.

Skin Assessment

The skin, or integumentary system, should be part of the routine head-to-toe assessment of all patients. A skin assessment should include an actual observation of the entire body. It differs from a wound assessment in that a skin assessment looks at intact skin and not just open wounds.[34]

What constitutes a minimal skin assessment? The usual practice includes a minimum of the following five parameters: temperature, color, moisture, turgor, and intact skin or presence of open areas.[34] Due to lack of consensus in the literature, the Centers for Medicare and Medicaid Services (CMS) recommend the five parameters as stated above as a minimal skin assessment in long-term care settings.[35] This author strongly recommends that a basic skin assessment be done across the continuum of care. Some patients may require a more comprehensive assessment after completion of the basic assessment. This should include looking for and documenting any lesions, scars, bruising, or hemosiderin deposits or pressure points.

Summary

Skin, the largest human body organ, protects individuals from heat, light, injury, and infection and serves to (1) help regulate body temperature; (2) store water, vitamin D, and fat; (3) help sense pain and other stimuli; and (4) prevent the entry of bacteria.[36] Our skin is exposed daily to environmental irritants and chemicals as well as physical and mechanical injury, any of which may lead to impaired skin integrity. It is essential that health-care providers realize that the skin is an organ that can fail, the same as any other organ.

References

1. Tobin, DJ: Biochemistry of human skin—Our brain on the outside. Chem Soc Rev 2006; 35:52–67.
2. Wikipedia. Available at: http://en.wikipedia.org/wiki/Integumentary-system. Accessed 10-16-09.
3. Koch, S, Kohl, K, Klein, E, et al: Skin homing of Langerhans cell precursors: Adhesion, chemotaxis, and migration. J Allergy Clin Immunol 2006; 117:163–168.
4. Blumenberg, M, Tomic-Canic, M: Human epidermal keratinocyte: Kertinization processes. EXS 1997; 78:1–29.
5. Freed, IM, Tomic-Canic, M, Komine, M, et al: Keratins and the keratinocyte activation cycle. J Invest Dermatol 2001; 116:633–640.
6. Tomic-Canic, M, Magnus, SA, Oscar, MA: Epidermal repair and the chronic wound. In: Rovee, DT, Maibach, HL (eds): Epidermis in Wound Healing. Boca Raton, FL, CRC Press, 2003, pp. 25–57.
7. Tomic-Canic, M: Keratinocyte cross-talks in wounds. Wounds 2005; 17:S3–6.
8. Morasso, MI, Tomic-Canic, M: Epidermal stem cells: The cradle of epidermal determination, differentiation and wound healing. Biol Cell 2005; 97:173–183.
9. Habif, TP: Clinical Dermatology: A Color Guide to Diagnosis and Therapy, 4th ed. Philadephia, Mosby, 2004.
10. Kanitakis, J: Anatomy, histology and immunohistochemistry of normal human skin. Eur J Dermatol 2002; 12:390–399, quiz 400.
11. Eckes, B, Krieg, T: Regulation of connective tissue homeostasis in the skin by mechanical forces. Clin Exp Rheumatol 2004; 22:S73–S76.
12. Wysocki, AB: Anatomy and Physiology of Skin and Soft Tissue. In Bryant R, Nix, D (eds.): Acute and Chronic Wounds, 3rd ed. Philadelphia, Mosby, 2007.
13. Choi, CM: Anatomy of the skin. Wounds1.com. Available at: http://www.wounds1.com/news/mainstory_pf.cfm?newsarticle=13. Accessed 10/03/09.
14. Available from: http://www.skin-science.com In Skin appendages (no author) Accessed 10-16-09.
15. Yosipovitch, G, Hu, J: The importance of skin pH. Skin & Aging 2003; 11:88–93.
16. Waller, JM, Maivach, HI: Age and skin structure and function, a quantitative approach (I): Blood flow, pH, thickness, and ultrasound echogenicity. Skin Res Technol 2005; 11:221–235.
17. Rippke, F, Schreiner, V, Doering, T, et al: Stratum corneum pH in atopic dermatitis: Impact on skin barrier function and colonization with *Staphylococcus aureus.* Am J Clin Dermatol 2004; 5:217–223.
18. Yilmaz, E, Borchert, HH: Effect of lipid-containing, positively charged nanoemulsions on skin hydration, elasticity and erythema—An in vivo study. Int J Pharm 2006; 307:232–238.
19. Kurabayashi, H, Tamura, K, Machida, HI, et al: Inhibiting bacteria and skin pH in hemiplegis: Effects of washing hands with acidic mineral water. Am J Phys Med Rehabil 2002; 81:40–46.
20. Damjanov, I: Pathology for the health-related professions. Philadelphia, W.B. Saunders, 2000.
21. Hughes, E, Van Onselen, J: Dermatology nursing: A practical guide. London, Churchill Livingston, 2001.
22. Barden, A, Nizet, V, Gallo, RL: Antimicrobial peptides and the skin. Expert Opin Biol Ther 2004; 4:543–549.
23. Niyonsaba, F, Ogawa, H: Protective roles of the skin against infection: Implications of naturally occurring human antimicrobial agents beta-defensins, cathelicidin LL-37 and lysozyme. J Dermatol Sci 2005; 40:157–168.
24. Charkoudian, N: Skin blood flow in adult human thermoregulation: How it works, when it does not, and why. Mayo Clin Proc 2003; 78:603–612.
25. Minson, CT: Hypoxic regulation of blood flow in humans. Skin blood flow and temperature regulation. Adv Exp Med Biol 2003; 543:249–262.
26. Wolpowitz, D, Gilchrest, BA: The vitamin D questions: How much do you need and how should you get it? J Am Acad Dermatol 2006; 54:301–317.
27. Kupper, TS, Fuhlbrigge, RC: Immune surveillance in the skin: Mechanisms and clincial consequences. Nat Rev Immunol 2004; 4:211–222.
28. Fisher, GJ: The pathophysiology of photoaging of the skin. Cutis 2005; 75:5–8, discussion 8–9.
29. Venna, SSG, BA: Skin aging and photoaging. Skin & Aging 2004; 12:56–59.
30. Gilhar, A, Ullmann, Y, Karry, R, et al: Ageing of human epidermis: The role of apoptosis, Fas and telomerase. Br J Dermatol 2004; 150:56–63.
31. Baranoski, S, Ayello, EA, Tomic-Canic, M. Skin an essential organ. In Baranoski, S, Ayello, EA (eds.): Wound Care Essentials: Practice Principles. Philadelphia, Lippincott, Williams, Wilkins, Ambler, 2008; pp. 4–63.
32. Selden, ST, Cowell, B, Fenno, J, et al: Skin tears: Recognizing and treating this growing problem. Skin & Aging 2002; 10:55–60.
33. Hashizume, H: Skin aging and dry skin. J Dermatol 2004; 31:603–609.

34. Baranoski, S: Skin tears: Staying on guard against the enemy of frail skin. Nursing 2003; 33:S14–20.

35. Centers for Medicare and Medicaid Services (CMS). Revised Nov. 2004 (p 144). Guidance to Surveyors for Long Term Care Facilities. Revised Tag F 314 Pressure Sores. www.cms.hhs.gov/medicaid/survey-cert/siqhome.asp

36. University of Virginia Health System. Dermatology: Anatomy of the skin. Available at: http://www.healthsystem.virginia.edu/uvahealth/adult_derm/anatomy.cfm. Accessed 10/04/09.

chapter 2

The Wound Healing Process

Sharon L. Dunn, PT, PhD, OCS

Introduction

Wound healing consists of a symphony of events that, when well orchestrated, results in reepithelialization of the skin and restoration of its barrier function. The first event after wounding is the establishment of hemostasis by plugging the defect with a fibrin clot. This is followed by overlapping stages of inflammation, repair (proliferation), and remodeling (Fig. 2.1). Cellular and humoral mediators conduct the symphony and consist of inflammatory cells (neutrophils, lymphocytes, mast cells, and monocytes/macrophages); repair cells (fibroblasts, myofibroblasts, and fibrocytes); epithelial cells (keratinocytes); and soluble proteins (cytokines, chemokines, enzymes, and growth factors). The extracellular matrix (ECM) provides the stage on which these mediators play, serving as a physical scaffold for repair and presenting a milieu of protein intermediates.

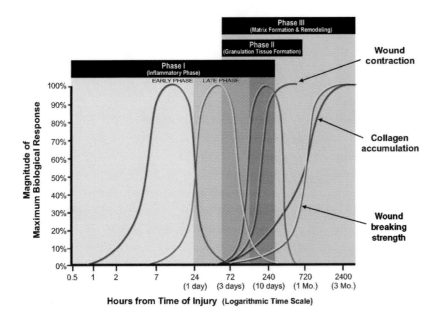

Figure 2•1 *Phases of healing and relative time. The overlapping phases of healing identified by the relative time from injury.*

9

Stage Recognition by Gross Inspection

The stages of healing may be identified by gross inspection of the wound. (Fig. 2.2) Hemostasis is identified by clot formation and cessation of active bleeding. Inflammation is recognized by the cardinal signs of dolor (pain), rubor (erythema), calor (increased temperature), tumor (swelling—drainage or pus in this case), and loss of function. During the early part of the repair stage, the wound bed is covered by granulation tissue, which is marked by robust proliferation of fibroblasts and neovascularization, giving the wound a red and granular appearance. Granulation tissue serves as a welcoming surface for keratinocyte migration (epithelialization) during the latter part of repair. Keratinocytes may migrate from the periphery of the wound edges, or in the case of partial-thickness wounds in which the hair follicles are spared, epithelialization may arise and spread from the hair follicles. The repair stage is also identified by wound margin contraction, in which the wound edges approach the center of the wound. The repair stage culminates in the complete covering of the wound with epithelium, recognized by the cessation of drainage and a thin, pink layer of skin. Following closure, the scar continues to reorganize and gain strength through the remodeling or maturation stage. During this phase, the scar will increase in type I collagen content and vascularization will be reduced to normal, resulting in strengthening of the scar and reduction in erythema over time.

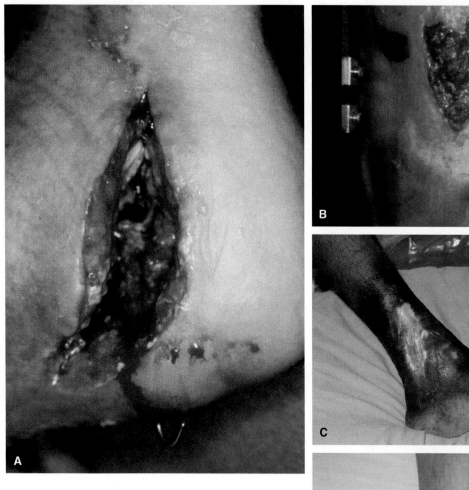

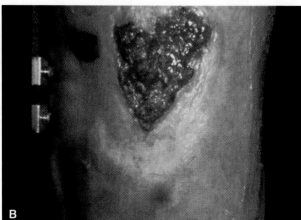

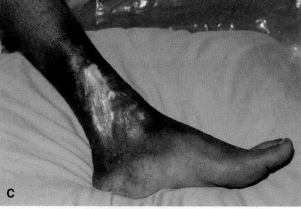

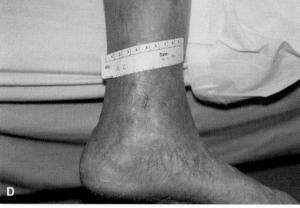

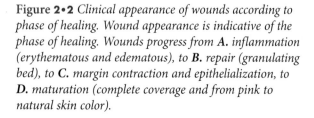

Figure 2•2 *Clinical appearance of wounds according to phase of healing. Wound appearance is indicative of the phase of healing. Wounds progress from **A.** inflammation (erythematous and edematous), to **B.** repair (granulating bed), to **C.** margin contraction and epithelialization, to **D.** maturation (complete coverage and from pink to natural skin color).*

▶ **PEARL 2•1** There are three stages of healing: *inflammation*—cardinal signs of dolor, rubor, calor, tumor, and loss of function; *repair*—granulation, epithelialization, and contraction; and *remodeling*—scar strength and reduction of erythema.

For successful healing, the initiation, duration, and resolution of each stage of healing are all dependent on the severity of the wound, exposure to microbes, and the health and nutrition of the patient.

Types of Wound Healing

Wounds heal by either primary or secondary intention. Primary healing occurs as a result of surgical closure, and secondary intention occurs when the wound is left open to heal by regenerating tissue that has been destroyed by trauma or cell death.[1] Surgical closure brings the wound edges in close proximity and is accomplished by direct side-to-side closure, flaps, or grafts, each reducing the gap necessary for tissue healing.[2] Depth, location, and geometry of the wound affect the rate of closure by secondary intention.[3] Wounds in anatomic areas with limited blood supply, or areas affected by pressure, tend to heal slower. Regardless of type of healing, all wounds progress through the phases of inflammation, repair, and maturation.[2]

Impact of Wound Severity (Depth)

Wound depth is defined by determining which layers of the skin are involved in the insult. Partial-thickness wounds involve only the epidermis and varying depths of the dermis, whereas full-thickness wounds involve the epidermis, entire dermis, and subdermal structures. Full-thickness wounds and partial-thickness wounds heal differently. Partial-thickness wounds undergo minimal contraction and reepithelialize from the wound margin and from epidermal stem cell populations around sweat glands and hair follicles.[4,5] Full-thickness wounds depend fully on epithelialization from the wound edges due to the destruction of these additional epidermal stem cell populations associated with a full-thickness wound. Additionally, full-thickness wounds are more likely to undergo contraction during healing, possibly resulting in a cosmetically or functionally undesirable contracture.

Biology Review

In order to better understand the biology of wound healing, it is necessary to briefly review the basics of cellular biology. Recent advances in molecular biology, experimental techniques, and the Human Genome Project[6,7] have resulted in scientific advances toward genetic manipulation, proteomics, and biological materials engineering. As a result, our understanding of wound healing has improved along with our potential to enhance the clinical care of wounds.

Human cells interact with their environment (adjacent cells, soluble proteins, or extracellular matrix) through cell surface receptors, which are proteins either embedded in the cell membrane or linked by lipid intermediates. (Fig. 2.3) These receptors are matched and bind to extracellular proteins

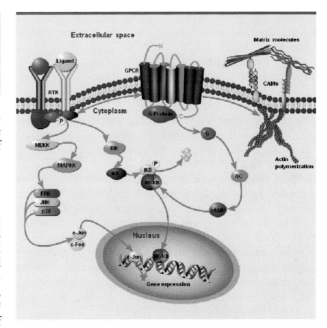

Figure 2•3 *Review of cell biology. Cells interact with their environment through cell surface receptors (RTK, receptor tyrosine kinase, and GPCRs, G protein–coupled receptors, represented here) or cell adhesion molecules (CAMS). Receptor binding of ligand (protein such as cytokine, growth factor, or hormone) initiates a signaling cascade within the cell, ultimately influencing gene expression and protein production. Cellular expression and extracellular binding of CAMS influence cell shape, adhesion, and migration. Figure developed with* Pathway BuilderTool v. 2.0, Protein Lounge.

(ligands). Binding of ligand to receptor initiates a sequence of intracellular events described as signal transduction, which ultimately influences gene expression and cellular behavior. The intracellular events are often mediated by secondary messengers (proteins) in the cytoplasm that can translocate into the nucleus of the cell and influence the genetic expression by either upregulating or downregulating mRNA production (transcription), thereby regulating the protein production (translation) of the cell. Intracellular signal transduction pathways commonly involved in wounding and repair include the mitogen-activated protein kinase (MAPK) pathway and the nuclear factor κB (NFκB) pathway through receptor tyrosine kinase (RTK) receptors or G protein–coupled receptors (GPCRs). (Fig. 2.3) Signal transduction via these receptors and pathways can alter cellular migration, proliferation, protein production and secretion, and cell cycle events.

Soluble proteins that act as ligands for these receptors and that are involved in wound healing include proinflammatory and anti-inflammatory cytokines, growth factors, hormones, and chemokines. Chemokines are small proteins that specialize in cell recruitment by chemoattraction and chemotaxis (migration). They produce a gradient attraction to numerous cell types, which causes them to migrate toward the concentrated attractant. Cytokines are also small proteins that have profound effects on cellular behavior by directing the inflammatory response. Growth factors signal for cellular proliferation and direct cell cycle activities.

These soluble protein mediators are secreted into the wound from a variety of sources; they are covered in more detail in Chapter 3.

Cells also interact with their environment through cell adhesion molecules (CAMs), which include five principle classes of proteins: cadherins, immunoglobulin superfamily, mucins, integrins, and selectins.[8] (Fig. 2.3) These molecules recognize and bind similar proteins on adjacent cells or extracellular matrix components and are critical to leukocyte extravasation and cellular migration in wound healing. Integrins mediate cell-matrix interactions, and cadherins mediate cell-cell interactions; selectins and integrins are both important to extravasation.[8] CAMs are frequently linked through the cell membrane to intracellular cytoskeletal proteins and are able to direct actin polymerization into filamentous projections such as lamellipodia and ruffles to influence cellular migration and adhesion. The production, expression, and activation of these adhesion molecules on the cell surface is regulated by the cellular environment and can be upregulated or downregulated according to the signals received by the cell.

Cells are influenced directly or indirectly through three mechanisms, either autocrine, whereby a cell influences its own behavior; paracrine, when the cell is influenced by something in the immediate environment; or endocrine, when the cell is influenced by a mediator at some distance through vascular or hormonal effects. All of these mechanisms influence the cell through signal transduction pathways to invoke cellular responses. The messages may be synergistic to provide additive effects or they may be antagonistic for a regulatory or control effect.

▶ **PEARL 2•2** Cells respond to their environment through signal transduction, which results in the stimulation or inhibition of gene expression; protein production; and cellular migration, adhesion, or death.

Ultimately, cellular responses lead to wound healing, and our challenge is to influence those responses to get the best clinical outcome for our patients with wounds.

Hemostasis (Immediately Upon Injury)

The initial step in the wound healing process is to prevent additional hemorrhage at the damaged blood vessels. Key to this step is the development of a fibrin clot, which first stops the bleeding by plugging the injured vessels via platelet aggregation, then serves as a provisional matrix for wound healing.

Platelet Activation

Platelets are anucleated cytoplasmic fragments of bone marrow-derived megakaryocytes.[9] They circulate in blood, numbering 150,000 to 400,000/mL, and under normal conditions do not adhere to the endothelium of blood vessels.[10,11] However, once activated by endothelial injury or exposure to extracellular matrix components,[12] they adhere promptly to the vascular lesion, recruit additional platelets,

and initiate the coagulation cascade. Activated platelets mediate these functions through their granular release of serotonin, adenosine diphosphate (ADP), thromboxane A2, fibrinogen, fibronectin, von Willebrand factor, and thrombospondin.[13] The coagulation cascade has long been documented as a sequential series of events in which activation of one clotting factor leads to the stepwise activation of the subsequent pro-factor, ultimately leading to a burst of thrombin generation and propagation of coagulation.[14,15] These models have been used clinically as predictors of bleeding and are known by the screening tests prothrombin time (PT) and activated partial thromboplastin time (aPTT).

More recently, the coagulation cascade has been determined to be influenced by cellular presentation of clotting cofactors.[16-18] The initial adhesive interactions of platelets are determined by the expression pattern of receptors on the activated platelet surface and their interaction with various ligands found on extracellular matrix components and other cells, which results in the variability of thrombin generation on the platelet surface.[11,19] For example, a platelet population with a heightened coagulation potential has been identified and referred to as collagen- and thrombin-stimulated (COAT) platelets.[20] These platelets are primed with enhanced thrombin-generating ability through binding to collagen and prior exposure to thrombin.[21,22] Ultimately, this burst of thrombin production on the surface of activated platelets leads to the formation and stabilization of the fibrin clot.

Activated platelets also secrete several growth factors into the wound milieu, including platelet-derived growth factor (PDGF), transforming growth factors-α and -ß (TGF-α and TGF-ß), and epidermal growth factor (EGF). These growth factors stimulate fibroblasts to produce collagen, proteoglycans, and glycosaminoglycans,[23,24] which contribute to the provisional matrix of the fibrin clot.

Fibrin Clot

The platelet aggregate (plug) is initially unstable and requires stabilization through fibrin matrix production. Thrombin converts platelet-derived fibrinogen to fibrin during the final steps of the coagulation cascade. Thrombin, accumulated on the surface of platelets, cleaves soluble fibrinogen propeptide, converting fibrinogen into fibrin monomers that form insoluble fibrin polymers. Fibrin polymerization is then activated by thrombin, resulting in a stable cross-linked fibrin matrix.[25]

The structure of the fibrin matrix determines its biological capabilities and ultimately the quality of wound healing, and it can be defined by such terms as *porosity, permeability, fiber diameter,* and *branching.*[26] These parameters are affected by the rates of clotting, polymerization, and lateral branching, which are influenced by local concentrations of thrombin, salt, clotting factors, chloride, and heparin.[27-30] Larger diameter, course fibrin matrices are more susceptible to plasmin fibrinolysis and therefore are more rapidly infiltrated by tube-forming endothelial cells (neovascularization) than are their thinner fiber matrix counterparts.[30-32]

The fibrin matrix serves as a scaffold for attachment of infiltrating cells and extracellular matrix components. Many cell types, including leukocytes, endothelial cells, fibroblasts, and smooth muscle cells, have been reported to bind fibrin matrices, either through their integrin receptors or adhesion molecules.[33–43] Thus, the fibrin matrix serves as a depot for propagation and eventual resolution of the local inflammatory process, the in-growth of new vessels, and fibroblast migration and proliferation into the defect. (Fig. 2.4)

▶ **PEARL 2•3** The fibrin clot serves as a provisional extracellular matrix for early repair, and its structure and composition determine the quality of wound healing.

Endothelial cells restructure the architecture of the fibrin matrix through the production of matrix metalloproteases (MMPs) and plasmin, performing the necessary fibrinolysis to make way for angiogenesis.[44,45] Subsequent to remodeling, the endothelial cells proliferate and elongate, forming tubular structures (neovascularization or angiogenesis) on the substrate of the fibrin matrix[46,47] guided by the presence of growth factors such as vascular endothelial growth factor (VEGF) and fibroblast growth factor-2 (FGF-2) contained within the matrix milieu.

At about 5 days postinjury, fibroblasts migrate into the matrix and, upon stimulation by PDGF, TGF-β, and fibrin, they proliferate, express their integrin receptors, and continue migration into the wound bed.[48,49] Here, the fibroblasts begin producing extracellular matrix components, eventually replacing the provisional fibrin matrix. Keratinocytes do not express fibrin-binding receptors, making them adept at dissecting through the adherent fibrin matrix at the dermal interface as they migrate across the wound during the repair phase of healing.[50]

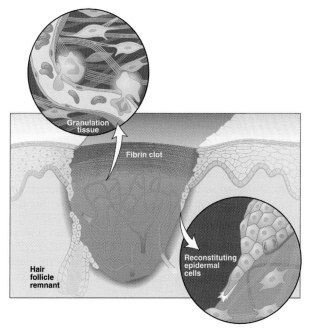

Figure **2•4** *Fibrin clot and infiltrating cells. The fibrin matrix serves as a depot for propagation and eventual resolution of the local inflammatory process, the in-growth of new vessels, and fibroblast migration and proliferation into the defect. From Martin, P: Wound healing—Aiming for perfect skin regeneration. Science 1997; 276:75–78. Used with permission from AAAS.*

Fibrinolysis

As important as the fibrin clot is to hemostasis and provisional matrix formation, its removal is just as important to a favorable outcome. The fibrinolytic system disrupts the fibrin clot through the action of plasmin, an enzyme that cleaves fibrin into soluble degradation products. Plasmin is activated from its inactive precursor form, plasminogen, by two activators, tissue type (tPA) and urokinase type (uPA) plasminogen activators. The presence of these activators in plasma regulates the extent of plasmin formation and thereby regulates the rate of clot removal.[19,51]

Inflammation (Days 4 Through 6)

The inflammatory process is initiated immediately upon wounding and is characterized by the infiltration of leukocytes into the local environment. A few of these cells are present in the local tissue (resident cells); however, the vast majority are recruited into the wound from the circulating leukocyte population, and therefore must migrate, or diapedesis, from the vessel into the extravascular space.

Leukocyte Extravasation

Extravasation is a three-step process that begins with leukocyte tethering and rolling on the endothelial luminal surface (Fig. 2.5), continues with firm adhesion, and concludes with diapedesis, which is the migration of leukocytes either through endothelial cells or between endothelial cell junctions.[52–60] (Fig. 2.6) Inflammatory stimuli, such as mast cell–produced and platelet-produced cytokines, transiently activate leukocytes and endothelial cells to express their cell surface molecular machinery required for leukocyte capture and migration. (Fig. 2.7) This machinery includes selectins, integrins, hyaluronan receptor CD44, additional cell adhesion molecules (CAMs), and proteases for endothelial junction and basement membrane rearrangement.[8,52,59,61]

▶ **PEARL 2•4** Three sequential steps of leukocyte extravasation are (1) tethering/rolling, (2) firm adhesion, (3) diapedesis.

Leukocyte rolling begins with a low-affinity binding of transiently expressed P-selectin on the endothelial surface to a carbohydrate ligand specific to P-selectin expressed on the leukocyte surface. While P-selectin is responsible for the initial tethering of leukocytes, E-selectin stabilizes the rolling to slow it down.[62–64] Another mechanism for leukocyte rolling involves the transient binding of CD44 expressed on some subpopulations of lymphocytes to hyaluronan on the endothelial surface.[65] These low-affinity contacts are temporary, allowing leukocytes the opportunity to slow down to a roll in the rapidly flowing bloodstream in order to sense the chemoattractant environment.[8,59]

Rolling is arrested to a firm adhesion as chemokines on the endothelial surface bind G protein–coupled receptors on the leukocyte surface, signaling the leukocyte to activate surface integrins.[59,61] Integrins are also activated by platelet-activating

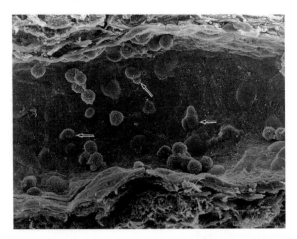

Figure 2•5 *Neutrophils on the endothelial surface. Captured with scanning electron microscopy at 1000×, neutrophils adhere to the luminal portion of a postcapillary venule. Arrows indicate transendothelial migration of neutrophils. From Hoshi, O, Ushiki, T: Scanning electron microscopic studies on the route of neutrophil extravasation in the mouse after exposure to the chemotactic peptide N-formyl-methionyl-leucyl-phenylalanine (fMLP). Arch Histol Cytol 1999; 62:253–260. Used with permission.*

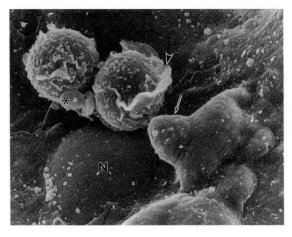

Figure 2•6 *Adherent and migrating neutrophils. Captured with scanning electron microscopy at 5000×, two neutrophils are adherent and one is polarized with a membranous trailing edge (arrowhead). The other neutrophil (arrow) is transmigrating by piercing the endothelial cell. The arrow indicates the portion of the neutrophil within the vessel lumen and the remainder is beneath the endothelial sheet. Also apparent are the nucleus of the endothelial cell (N) and a neutrophil-bound platelet (*). From Hoshi, O, Ushiki, T: Scanning electron microscopic studies on the route of neutrophil extravasation in the mouse after exposure to the chemotactic peptide N-formyl-methionyl-leucyl-phenylalanine (fMLP). Arch Histol Cytol 1999; 62:253–260. Used with permission.*

factor expressed by endothelial cells.[8] The fully activated integrins, containing either an α4 or β2 subunit, then bind endothelial surface proteins such as intercellular adhesion molecule-1 (ICAM-1) or vascular cell adhesion molecule-1 (VCAM-1), resulting in high-affinity, shear-resistant interactions that arrest the leukocyte on the endothelial surface.[8,52,59,61] These firm interactions are dependent on the integrity of the actin cytoskeleton that anchors the integrins within the leukocyte to establish firm adhesion under shear flow conditions.[61]

Firm adhesion leads to leukocyte polarization in preparation for transendothelial migration. Polarization is stimulated by a chemokine gradient that gives the leukocyte a directional stimulus. A polarized leukocyte has a redistribution of surface molecules, establishing a leading edge and a trailing edge with an extended rear projection, called a *uropod*, poised for directional movement.[61,66] Chemokine receptors are distributed toward the leading edge, and integrins form clusters at both the leading edge and uropod.[67,68] Integrins generate dynamic interactions depending on environmental cues, integrating chemical and mechanical stimuli to appropriately increase or decrease affinity for external ligands.[69–71] This polarization and contact integration produces directional movement of the leukocyte toward the chemokine gradient.

Once the leukocyte becomes polarized, it can then transmigrate or move by diapedesis through the endothelial cell layer and underlying basement membrane into the perivascular ECM. Debate continues as to whether leukocytes migrate through pores in endothelial cells or between endothelial cells through their junctional proteins. Evidence exists for both pathways and may represent two mechanisms that may be specific to cell type, stimulus, or condition.[58,60,72–75]

When leukocytes migrate through endothelial cell junctions, they must reversibly modify endothelial tight junctions at the apical surface and adherens junctions at the lateral surfaces of endothelial cells to be able to get through.[52,59,61] This modification is carried out by specialized interactions between CAMs expressed on the surface of leukocytes and endothelial cells. Platelet endothelial cell adhesion molecule-1 (PECAM-1) is expressed on endothelial cells, platelets, neutrophils, monocytes, and some T cells and mediates homophilic interactions.[59] PECAM-1 acts at two steps of diapedesis: initiation of transmigration at the luminal or apical surface of the endothelial cell junction and assistance of leukocytes through the basement membrane of the vessel.[76–79] Junctional adhesion molecule-A (JAM-A) is found in the tight junctions of endothelial cells and on platelets and leukocytes.[80–83] It forms homophilic interactions to assist diapedesis but also regulates leukocyte motility through cellular signaling properties.[84,85] Endothelial selective adhesion molecule (ESAM) is expressed only on endothelial cells and platelets, and participates in opening endothelial junctions during neutrophil extravasation, but not on activated T cells.[86]

Adherens junctions maintain integrity of the lateral surfaces of endothelial cells, and vascular endothelial-cadherin is an essential CAM that represents a barrier to extravasating leukocytes. The mechanism for VE-cadherin dissociation is not known but is hypothesized to be regulated by intracellular signaling during migration that decreases affinity of the adhesions.[59] Additional CAMs involved in diapedesis include

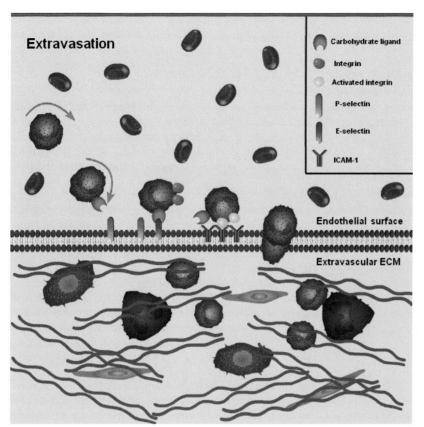

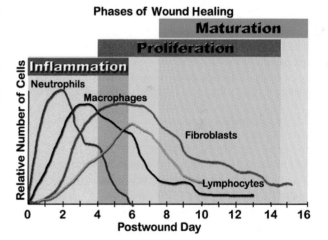

Figure 2•7 *Leukocyte extravasation. Leukocyte rolling begins with low-affinity tethering to P-selectin expressed on the endothelial surface. Rolling is stabilized by binding E-selectin, and finally firm adhesion is accomplished as activated surface integrins bind endothelial surface ICAMs or VCAMs. The leukocyte becomes polarized and transmigrates between or through endothelial cells into the perivascular extracellular matrix according to a chemokine gradient. Figure developed with* Pathway BuilderTool v. 2.0, Protein Lounge.

ICAM-1 and CD99, which function downstream of the PECAM-1 step at the basement membrane, assisting leukocytes to the collagen ECM.

Matrix metalloproteases (MMPs) are also involved in diapedesis and have been shown to cleave VE-cadherin in adherens junctions.[87] Membrane-bound or associated MMPs, such as MMP-2 and MMP-9, are likely responsible for degradation of endothelial cell junctions at the site of leukocyte migration. Endothelial cell–associated MMPs are immediately activated by superoxides, available in the environment by adjacent neutrophil degranulation, but lymphocyte-associated MMPs take several hours for activation. Therefore, diapedesis is probably regulated by endothelial MMP activity, and leukocyte MMP activity is likely used for subsequent migration through extravascular ECM.[52]

Inflammatory Cells

Leukocytes are recruited locally by specific receptors on the surface of activated platelets and adhesion molecules expressed on the provisional fibrin matrix. Activated platelets interact with neutrophils through selectins and integrins to promote a secondary capture of additional leukocytes to the wound. Adherent platelets serve as a link between hemostasis and inflammation through the secretion of cytokines, which stimulate neutrophils and endothelial cells to amplify the inflammatory response.[88] Subsets of leukocytes are also recruited to the wound by chemokines in phase-specific sequence.[89] (Fig. 2.8)

The first leukocytes to arrive on the scene are the neutrophils, whose primary role is to kill microbes through

Figure 2•8 *Cellular arrival according to phase of healing. Cellular migration into the wound bed is sequentially ordered according to cellular function and the phase of healing. From Witte, MB, Barbul, A: General principles of wound healing. Surg Clin North Am 1997; 77:510–528. ©Elsevier, 1997.*

phagocytosis and lysosomal degradation. In doing so, neutrophils produce reactive oxygen species (free radicals), eicosanoids (prostaglandins, thromboxanes, and leukotrienes), and proteases,[90–92] which wreak havoc on the local tissue, as well. Neutrophils are the predominant infiltrating cells for the first 3 days of inflammation, peaking in number at 48 hours postwounding.[93] Macrophages, the "professional" phagocytes, arrive next, peaking at 72 to 84 hours, and enhance debridement through phagocytosis of the matrix and cellular debris left in the wake of neutrophils. Macrophages also produce and secrete cytokines and growth factors in preparation for repair.[94,95] Resident mast cells degranulate early (within the first hours), producing an initial source of histamine, cytokines, and chemokines, then are recruited at a later time as repair proceeds.[96] T lymphocytes arrive last, around day 5, during the proliferative phase, peak at day 7, and participate in both downregulation of excessive inflammation and control of proliferation.[97,98] The arrival and function of the leukocyte populations involved in the inflammatory process are overlapping, sequenced by design, and result in the temporal and spatial release of cytokines and growth factors critical to effective microbial defense, resolution of inflammation, and repair.

▸ **PEARL 2•5** The sequence of leukocyte arrival is ordered: First, neutrophils kill bacteria; second, macrophages clean the debris and prepare the stage; and finally, lymphocytes monitor for infection and control inflammation and proliferation.

Neutrophils (Polymorphonuclear Leukocytes)

Neutrophils serve as the first line of innate immune defense and are recruited in bulk to the wound site within a few hours. Chemokines, produced by resident mast cells and bacterial products, enhance their recruitment. Chemokines most critical to neutrophil migration are IL-8, growth-related oncogene-α (GRO-α), and monocyte chemoattractant protein-1 (MCP-1).[89] Once on site, polymorphonuclear leukocytes (PMNs) initiate bacterial killing through the release of toxic substances such as free radicals, promote the inflammatory cascade through the release of proteases and eicosanoids, phagocytose bacterial debris, and stimulate the repair response.[92]

Neutrophils are the most abundant white blood cells in circulation under normal conditions, constituting 45% to 70% of circulating leukocytes. They are recognized microscopically by their highly lobulated nuclei. They contain three types of cytoplasmic granules. (Table 2.1) The primary granules, also known as peroxidase-positive or azurophilic granules, are lysosomes that contain acidic hydrolases and peroxidases useful in bacterial killing and digestion. Upon bacterial ingestion, these lysosomal enzymes generate hydrogen peroxide and superoxides, which are effective antimicrobials, but they also destroy surrounding tissues when leaked into the extracellular environment. The secondary (specific) and tertiary (gelatinase) granules (both known as peroxidase-negative granules) store inflammatory cytokines and proteolytic enzymes used in the amplification of the inflammatory cascade and the initiation of repair.[10] The production of the mediators in these granules is induced by a large transcriptional activation program activated upon PMN migration to the wound site.[99] This activation program requires tight regulation; otherwise, it results in overproduction of toxins that negatively affect the surrounding

tissues and may underlie the persistent tissue-destroying nature of chronic wound inflammation.[100] Indeed, some of the proteins produced by activated neutrophils are inhibitors of their own proteases, indicating a programmed autoregulatory mechanism that could restrict tissue destruction.[101]

The steps of neutrophil degranulation are ordered. Released first are the peroxidase-negative granules that contain MMP-8, -9, and -25, with enzymatic specificity to laminin, proteoglycan, fibronectin, and collagen. The twofold purpose of local matrix breakdown is to (1) enhance antimicrobial access and (2) increase pressure on adjacent lymphatics and capillaries, leading to local vascular collapse. This traps the bacteria from nearby escape routes, perhaps preventing systemic infection. The peroxidase-negative granules also contain lactoferrin, lipocalin, lysozyme, and LL37, a chemotactic antimicrobial. Next, the primary or peroxidase-positive granules are released. These contain α-defensins, myeloperoxidase (MPO), lipopolysaccharide-binding bactericidal permeability-increasing protein (BPI), and serprocidins. The α-defensins are an abundant source of broad-spectrum antimicrobials.[102] MPO is an iron-containing enzyme that converts hydrogen peroxide to the potent antiseptics: hypochlorous acid, the active ingredient in bleach, hypobromous acid, and hypoidous acid, with reactions that give pus a green tint. BPI targets gram-negative bacteria. The serprocidins include the serine proteases cathepsin-G, protease 3, and neutrophil elastase and serve as broad-spectrum antibiotics. This staged release of granules furnishes neutrophils with the capacity to create a favorable environment for bacterial killing prior to the release of their bactericidal agents.[103]

During degranulation, neutrophils develop a phagocytic vacuole at the cell membrane that engulfs and degrades bacteria and debris. Phagocyte oxidases, or phox proteins, at the phagocytic vacuole surface produce reactive oxygen intermediates (ROI), also known as free radicals, which are pumped into the vacuole to complete the bacterial killing.[104] In addition, both types of cytosolic granules fuse with the phagocytic vacuole, and within 20 seconds of particle uptake their contents are released into the phagocytic vacuole, thus providing additional bactericidal and degradation capacity as antimicrobial insurance.[105] Neutrophils also contain secretory vesicles packed with proteins and membrane components that serve as a reservoir of replacement products to replenish the cell membrane after phagocytosis. These products include serum albumin and cell receptor proteins.[101,104]

Mature PMNs have a limited capacity for protein synthesis and are therefore unable to generate a response after their initial rapid burst of activity. They undergo apoptosis (programmed death) soon after bacterial phagocytosis and killing, and they constitute the primary cellular component of pus, sometimes referred to as pus cells.[10] Apoptotic neutrophils are marked for safe disposal by phosphatidylserine, a lipid marker on the outer membrane that promotes phagocytosis through the attraction of macrophages.[106]

Macrophages (Tissue Monocytes)

Monocytes are recruited to the wound through the selective homing mechanisms of chemokines, cytokines, microbes, and apoptotic neutrophils to destroy and phagocytose infectious

Table 2•1 Neutrophil Granules, Contents, Actions

Granules	Contents	Actions
Primary (azurophilic, peroxidase positive)	α-Defensins Myeloperoxidase BPI Seprocidins	Broad-spectrum antibiotic Antiseptic Gram-negative bactericidal Protease and antibiotic
Secondary (specific, peroxidase negative)	MMP-8, MMP-25 Lysozyme Lactoferrin and LL37	Local matrix (collagen) breakdown Bacterial cell wall lysis Antibiotic
Tertiary (gelatinase, peroxidase negative)	Gelatinase (MMP-9) Glycoproteins	Collagen depolymerization Phagocytosis enhanced

agents, clear ECM fragments, and revascularize the area.[107] They are the largest of the leukocytes (up to 20 μm in diameter), constitute 2% to 10% of circulating white blood cells (WBCs) in normal conditions, and are identified microscopically by a large, often bilobed, eccentrically placed nucleus. Monocytes respond to inflammatory or necrotic conditions by migrating from blood to the resident tissue, where they differentiate into macrophages. Macrophages are known as the professional phagocytes because of their ability to engulf and destroy debris with continual lysosomal activity and regeneration.[10] Macrophages become the predominant cell population in the wound until fibroblast migration and replication occurs during the repair phase.[97]

Macrophages serve as the transitional marker between the inflammatory and reparative phases of healing, shifting phenotypes from a proinflammatory secreting phagocyte while clearing debris to an anti-inflammatory initiator of repair. Historically, doctrine has classified macrophage responses into two generalized groups according to their cytokine stimulation: interferon gamma–activated (IFN-γ–activated) or tumor necrosis factor alpha–activated (TNF-α–activated) macrophages or IL-4– or IL-10–inhibited macrophages.[108,109] This dichotomy has been further classified as either a type 1 proinflammatory/cytotoxic "classical response," or type 2 anti-inflammatory/humoral "alternative response."[110-113] Recently, however, the concept of "functional adaptivity" has been proposed[114] due to mounting evidence suggesting that macrophages progress through multiple diverse functional phenotypes and adapt according to the changing cytokine microenvironment.[111,115-117] Not only do they express different functional patterns, but they display different progressions through functional patterns in response to common stimuli.[118] Given the changing microenvironment after successful wound debridement, macrophages may progress from a proinflammatory phenotype to a phenotype that suppresses inflammation, then supports repair.[114]

Macrophages' major contribution to wound healing is the production and secretion of cytokines, complement components, reactive oxygen species, proteases, protease inhibitors, and growth factors (which act to recruit other cells

and stimulate them to migrate, proliferate, and secrete their proteins), and ECM products.[107,119,120] (Table 2.2) Through these functions, macrophages influence angiogenesis, fibroplasia, and matrix synthesis.[97] Among the cytokines and growth factors that macrophages produce are TNF-α, IL-1 and IL-6, TGF-α and TGF-β, PDGF and insulin-like growth factor-1 (IGF-1), VEGF, FGF-2, prostaglandin E2 (PGE₂), oxygen-related protein 150 (ORP 150), and MMP-1.[121-132] They also produce nitric oxide (NO) in the early phase of inflammation through their increase in inducible nitric oxide synthase (iNOS) expression.[133-135]

Macrophages also have a role in angiogenesis through the production of angiogenic cytokines, growth factors, and proteolytic enzymes.[136,137] Macrophages respond to hypoxia through altered gene expression controlled by the upregulation of transcription factors known as hypoxia-inducible factors (HIF). Wounds exhibit hypoxia in areas of vascular compromise, either by vessel damage or intense cellular metabolic activity.[138] Immediately postinjury, oxygen tension is reduced from 150 mm Hg to 20 to 30 mm Hg within the wound, and by day 4 this is further reduced to 5 to 7 mm Hg.[139] These HIFs translocate to the nucleus and bind the DNA response elements of hypoxia-inducible genes.[140-142] This genetic influence creates an increase in production of proteins required for macrophage survival, tissue revascularization, and recruitment and activation of more macrophages and inflammatory cells.[143] These hypoxia-inducible proteins include iNOS, TNF-α, and IL-6.[144] Following the repair phase, macrophages respond to IFNs by producing thrombospondin (TSP) and ELR-CXC chemokines such as platelet factor-4, which correspond to the inhibition of angiogenesis through a decrease in endothelial cell proliferation.[145-147] Therefore, macrophages are able to sense the environment and, in response, produce either go or stop signals for both inflammation and angiogenesis.

> ▶ **PEARL 2•6** Macrophages serve a dual role in wound vascularity: Early, they respond to hypoxia by promoting angiogenesis, and later, they respond to interferons by inhibiting angiogenesis.

Table 2•2 **Macrophage Contents and Actions**

Contents	Actions
TNF-α	Proinflammatory
IL-1	Proinflammatory and enhances endothelial adhesion
IL-6	Proinflammatory and anti-inflammatory
TGF-α, TGF-β	Promotes cell proliferation, migration, differentiation, and apoptosis
PDGF	Promotes cell proliferation, migration, and angiogenesis; required for fibroblast proliferation
IGF-1	Stimulates cell growth and proliferation and inhibits apoptosis
VEGF	Angiogenesis
FGF-2	Endothelial cell proliferation
PGE$_2$	Mediates inflammatory response and vessel diameter
ORP-150	Proangiogenic
MMP-1	Collagen breakdown and ECM remodeling
iNOS	NO production and vasodilation
Thrombospondin	Antiangiogenic
ELR-CXC	Antiangiogenic

Resident Macrophages (Langerhans Cells)

In the epidermis, along with recruited macrophages, there are resident macrophages called Langerhans cells. These cells are derived from bone marrow as immunocompetent dendritic cells, and upon migration to the epidermis they differentiate and mature through exposure to epidermal cytokines. Langerhans cells serve as sentinels of the immune system, recognizing antigens in the skin and transporting them to the lymph nodes, where antigen is presented to responsive T lymphocytes.[148]

Langerhans cells are influenced by the microenvironment through cytokine stimulation. Cutaneous trauma-induced IL-1β and TNF-α, from adjacent keratinocytes and from Langerhans cells themselves, act in paracrine and autocrine fashion to signal detachment from the ECM and migration to the lymph, antigen in tow.[149,150] Besides transport and presentation of antigen to T cells, Langerhans cells are also equipped to internalize and process antigen molecules, making them effective in ensuring an appropriate immune response to microbial threats to the skin.[148]

T Lymphocytes

Lymphocytes are recruited in later phases of healing and are apparent during the maturation phase. They are the smallest of WBCs, constitute 20% to 50% of circulating leukocytes in normal conditions, and are recognized microscopically by their large, round nucleus that occupies most of the cell. Lymphocytes are subdivided into categories according to their maturation and function. T lymphocytes migrate from bone marrow to the thymus (hence the "T"), where they mature while acquiring surface proteins marked for specific antigens. When released into circulation, T lymphocytes can either directly target and kill antigen-bearing cells or activate macrophages and B lymphocytes. B lymphocytes mature in the bone marrow (hence the "B") and function primarily in the synthesis and secretion of antibodies toward specific antigens.[10]

T lymphocytes are further categorized into helper T cells, suppressor T cells, and cytotoxic T cells. The helpers secrete cytokines that stimulate activation of B cells and macrophages, the suppressors regulate the immune response once the initiating stimulus has been removed, and the cytotoxic cells kill virus-infected and malignant cells.[10] The suppressor cells play an inhibitory role in wound healing, downregulating inflammation and proliferation as the wound approaches maturity,[97] perhaps preventing inflammatory chronicity and/or keloid formation.

There is a population of resident T cells in epithelium, the γδ T cell, which plays unique roles in maintenance of homeostasis and response to tissue injury or malignancy.[151] The γδ T cells monitor neighboring epithelial cells through intimate contact and are able to sense cellular distress, lyse damaged cells, and participate in tissue repair through recruitment of inflammatory cells and secretion of growth factors. The γδ T cells have also been shown to be required for effective keratinocyte proliferation and wound reepithelialization,[152] macrophage recruitment,[153] and hyaluronan synthase and hyaluronan expression by keratinocytes during wound repair.[151]

Mast Cells

Mast cells are resident defense cells localized within the tissues; higher densities of mast cells are found in skin, GI lining, peritoneum, and perivascular areas, indicating their function against microbe invasion at vulnerable locations, their role in sustained cellular recruitment, and influence over local vasculature.[10,154] Two types of mast cells have been identified: connective tissue type, localized in skin, perivascular areas and in the peritoneal cavity, and mucosal type, localized in the gut and respiratory system.[155]

Mast cells are characterized by an extensive cytoplasm packed with large granules, containing the proteoglycans heparin and chondroitin sulphate, which, through their matrix-binding capacities, may serve as a local depot for cytokines and growth factors within the ECM.[154,156,157] (Table 2.3) Mast cell granules also contain histamine, serotonin, and other vasoactive mediators such as smooth muscle spasmogens and vasopermeability agents.[155] Mast cells immediately respond to tissue damage by releasing histamine, eicosanoids, and vasoactive proteins, so they are responsible for the immediate vasospasm and subsequent vasodilation and leakiness of vessels at the wound site.[10,154] Proteolytic enzymes, including tryptases, chymases, and carboxypeptidases, are also found in granules and have roles in tissue remodeling, cellular recruitment, and activation of endothelial cells and neutrophils through G protein–coupled receptors.[158] Activated endothelial cells express their adhesion molecules and become sticky for leukocytes and leaky to fluid. Activated neutrophils bind endothelium and express increased platelet-activating factor, which reinforces the firm adhesion of leukocytes and platelets to the leaky vessel. Granule-associated growth factors include FGF-2 and VEGF, which also have roles in cellular recruitment and angiogenesis.[154]

Table 2•3 Mast Cell Contents and Actions

Contents	Actions
Heparin	Anticoagulant, matrix-binding capacity, serves as depot for cytokines and growth factors
Chondroitin sulfate	Matrix-binding capacity, serves as depot for cytokines and growth factors
Histamine	Vasodilation, leukocyte chemotaxis
Serotonin	Vasoconstriction
Tryptases	Serine protease, allergenic response
Chymases	Serine protease, proinflammatory
Carboxypeptidases	Protein activation
FGF-2	Endothelial cell proliferation
VEGF	Angiogenesis
Leukotrienes (LTC_4, LTB_4)	Proinflammatory, increase neutrophil chemotaxis and vascular permeability
Prostaglandins (PGD_2, PGE_2)	Mediate inflammatory response and vessel diameter
Platelet-activating factor	Vasodilation and platelet aggregation
TNF-α	Inflammatory response
IL-1α, IL-1β	Inflammatory response and enhance endothelial adhesion
IL-6	Proinflammatory and anti-inflammatory
IL-18	Proinflammatory and stimulates production of IFN-γ
GM-CSF	Proliferation of leukocytes
LIF	Promotes cell growth and differentiation
IFN-α, IFN-β, IFN-γ	Antiviral, activation of macrophages and natural killer cells, and presentation of microbes to T cells
IL-10	Anti-inflammatory, inhibits proinflammatory cytokine production
TGF-β	Apoptosis
Chemokines	Induction of leukocyte chemotaxis

Besides the granule-associated mediators, mast cells also produce lipid mediators, leukotrienes LTC-4 and LTB-4, prostaglandins PGD_2 and PGE_2, and platelet-activating factor. The lipid-mediated responses of mast cells are responsible for rapid initiation of vascular changes and cellular recruitment and activation.[154] Mast cells also produce and secrete proinflammatory cytokines TNF, IL-1α and IL-1β, IL-6, IL-18; granulocyte macrophage-colony stimulating factor (GM-CSF); leukemia inhibitory factor (LIF); IFN-α, -β, and -γ; anti-inflammatory cytokines IL-10 and TGF-β; and chemokines.[154]

Mast cells can be activated directly by pathogen binding or indirectly through receptor-mediated responses. These varied mechanisms of activation give mast cells the capacity to selectively respond according to the stimulus. Specific profiles of cytokines and chemokines may be released without inducing degranulation,[159] or a full granular response may be elicited if necessary. Therefore, mast cells sense the environment and conduct the recruitment of specific cell populations from the vasculature and surrounding tissue according to the potential threats, phase of inflammation, or phase of healing.

To summarize the inflammatory phase of wound healing, the body responds to trauma and potential infection by summoning a vascular and cellular response. (Fig. 2.9) The vasculature reacts to the insult by initial vasoconstriction, then vasodilation with increased permeability in response to vasoactive mediators released by local mast cells. Platelets are activated to form a clot and make the endothelium sticky to circulating neutrophils. The traumatized mast cells degranulate, thereby recruiting and activating more neutrophils to the local tissue. Neutrophils respond with a respiratory burst of activity, degranulate, activate MMPs, and make an initial attempt to engulf invading bacteria, while leaving a path of ECM destruction and cellular suicide in their wake. Macrophages are then recruited to clear the remaining debris, alert the immune system (lymphocytes) to any remaining antigen, amplify the inflammatory cascade if necessary, and finally, once the area is cleared, transform the inflamed tissue into a repair zone.

Repair—Proliferative Phase (Day 4 Through 14)

The hallmark observation of the proliferative phase of healing is the appearance of granulation tissue, a robust, beefy-red, granular-appearing tissue (Fig. 2.10) that consists of macrophages, fibroblasts, developing blood vessels, immature collagen, and newly forming ECM. Fibroblasts are the predominant cellular mediator during the repair phase, assisting with endothelial angiogenesis and participating in wound contraction and matrix production. Epithelialization also occurs near the end of the repair phase and is apparent with keratinocyte migration from the wound margins, eventually covering the wound with a thin cellular layer.

Neovascularization

An essential step in wound healing is the formation of new blood vessels within the granulation tissue of the developing matrix. Neovascularization refers to new vessel growth and includes both vasculogenesis and angiogenesis.

▶ **PEARL 2•7** Vasculogenesis is new vessel development. Angiogenesis is proliferation and migration of adjacent mature endothelium.

It was formerly believed that vasculogenesis occurred only during development and embryonic life; however, the discovery of bone marrow–derived endothelial progenitor cells (BMD EPCs) in adult blood and their contribution to new vessel formation has clarified that these cells can differentiate in tissue and give rise to a replacement vascular network, or *vasculogenesis*.[160–163] Interestingly, BMD EPCs are found in significantly higher numbers in granulation tissue of rapidly healing wounds as compared to delayed-healing wounds.[164] Angiogenesis is defined as the process of proliferation and migration of the adjacent mature endothelial

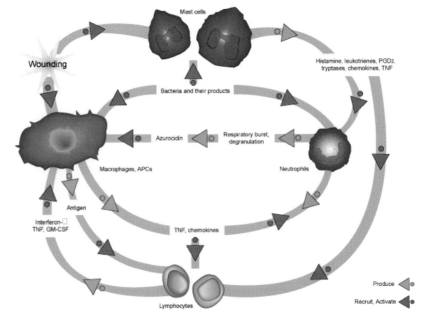

Figure 2•9 *Review of inflammatory response to trauma. Trauma triggers a sequence of cellular and humoral events. The initial steps are necessary to clear bacterial products and debris through recruitment of specific cell types whose products sequentially recruit additional cells. Ultimately, the area is cleared and transformed from one of inflammation to that of repair.*

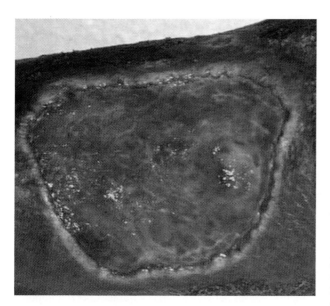

Figure 2•10 *Granulating wound. The beefy, red, granular appearance of granulation tissue is due to a robust proliferation of fibroblasts and neovascularization during the repair phase of healing.*

cells. Neovascularization remodels the initially avascular provisional matrix, providing blood to the new tissue.[165–170] Both processes are enhanced and assisted by fibroblasts and their local secretion of growth factors and proteases, which help to remodel ECM for endothelial tubular formation.

Many of the signals for neovascularization are produced during the inflammatory phase of healing. Hypoxia at the wound site stimulates vasculogenesis, angiogenesis, fibroblast proliferation, and collagen deposition. Macrophages respond to hypoxia by the production of iNOS, TNF-α, and IL-6.[144] Nitric oxide (NO) produced by nitric oxide synthase (NOS) plays a central role in the mobilization and release of BMD EPCs from bone marrow, and they are homed to the hypoxic wound by the chemokine SDF-1α.[171,172] New vessel growth also requires additional chemotactic factors from neighboring cells and matrix, a matrix upon which to grow, and the "free edge effect," which means an absence of a neighboring endothelial cell in the direction of growth.[173] Mature adjacent endothelial cells begin to form pseudopodia in the direction of the wound, secrete collagenase, and migrate into the perivascular space on the second wound day.[174] Upon migration, endothelial cells begin to proliferate and develop tube structures in response to exposure to fibronectin, heparin, and growth factors sequestered in the provisional matrix.[175]

▶ **PEARL 2•8** VEGF is produced by fibroblasts, endothelial cells, keratinocytes, mast cells, and macrophages.

The primary angiogenic growth factors include VEGF, angiopoietins, FGF, and TGF-β.[176–179] VEGF influences endothelial cells through specific tyrosine kinase receptors and is a potent mitogen, inducing proliferation, migration, sprouting, upregulation of integrin receptors, and endothelial cell survival through upregulation of the antiapoptotic protein Bcl-2.[180–184] VEGF is produced by fibroblasts, endothelial cells,

keratinocytes, mast cells, and macrophages.[185] Angiopoietins (Ang-1 to Ang-4) signal endothelial cells through specific tyrosine kinase receptors and produce additive effects with VEGF on angiogenesis. Angiopoietins are involved in maintaining vascular stability through securing endothelial contacts with neighboring cells, endothelial cell survival, and induction of sprouting and tube formation.[177,186–188] FGF-1 and FGF-2 (basic FGF or bFGF) are also potent mitogens for endothelial cells promoting proliferation, differentiation, and migration through interaction with specific FGF tyrosine kinase receptors on the endothelial cell surface.[189–191] FGF is produced by inflammatory cells, endothelial cells, and fibroblasts.[192–194] Migration of endothelial cells in early wound healing is induced by FGF through an upregulation of uPA secretion, which facilitates their migration through the fibrin clot by stimulating protease activity.[195] During the repair phase, FGF stimulates endothelial cell integrin activation and MMP-2 localization, both of which facilitate migration into the granulation tissue.[196,197] TFG-β acts on endothelial cells through specific serine/threonine kinase receptors, stimulating migration, differentiation, tubule formation, integrin upregulation, and ECM deposition.[179,198–203] In addition to these direct effects, TGF-β exhibits strong multipotent indirect effects on angiogenesis through the stimulation of fibroblasts to produce VEGF and the recruitment of inflammatory cells and their subsequent local release of VEGF, PDGF, and FGF for an additive effect on angiogenesis.[204–207]

Growth factors, cytokines, and chemokines are sequestered in the ECM, and as vessel growth proceeds, the secretion of protease remodels the ECM and frees these soluble mediators. In addition, the ECM presents a scaffold on which the new vessels develop, and the presence of fibronectin, collagen, vitronectin, tenascin, and laminin in the matrix milieu present binding sites for activated integrins on the endothelial cell surface.[208–210] These matrix-integrin interactions provide both traction and tension for the migrating endothelial cells, but also produce intracellular signaling cascades that add to the proliferation and migration of vessel cells along with the deposition of new matrix components to support the vessel in the developing granulation tissue.[175]

Fibroblasts

A robust fibroblast invasion into the fibrin clot marks the initiation of repair as macrophages sense the clearance of debris and release chemotactic signals. Fibroblasts arise from two sources: migration from adjacent intact dermis, or from fibrocytes, a subpopulation of bone marrow–derived leukocyte progenitor cells that rapidly enter sites of tissue injury by extravasation and differentiate into fibroblasts.[211,212] Fibroblasts derived from fibrocytes are in greater numbers in full-thickness wounds and differentiate into myofibroblasts at higher rates than their dermal fibroblast counterparts.[213] Fibroblasts are attracted to the wound environment by PDGF, a potent chemoattractant and mitogen for fibroblasts, secreted by platelets and macrophages.[214,215] Fibroblast migration is mediated by binding of surface integrins to cell adhesion molecules in the ECM. In early repair, they bind fibronectin in the provisional matrix, and as collagen and proteoglycans are secreted by fibroblasts, they bind and migrate on these substrates as well.[43,216–218] The

ECM components influence fibroblast proliferation and migration by regulating integrin expression and activation and signaling through these surface contacts.[218] Fibroblasts are able to remodel the ECM through production and secretion of multiple proteases, including a variety of MMPs, seprase, uPA, and tissue inhibitors of MMPs (TIMPs). Seprase is a membrane-bound serine protease that localizes to filopodia and lamellipodia in migrating fibroblasts, participating in release of focal adhesions from ECM components and allowing the fibroblast freedom to migrate.[219] Secretion of uPA by fibroblasts activates adjacent MMPs and assists in degrading fibrin and fibronectin of the provisional matrix.[220,221] The variety of MMPs secreted by fibroblasts provides the capacity to selectively degrade any ECM component encountered, but their expression and activation is tightly regulated spatially and temporally by TIMPs, chemotactic signals, and the sensing of the molecular composition of the ECM.[222,223]

> ▸ **PEARL 2•9** Protease activity determines direction and rate of migration of endothelial cells, fibroblasts, and keratinocytes during repair. Matrix composition influences protease activity.

Upon arrival in the provisional matrix, fibroblasts begin to proliferate and deposit a new collagen-rich matrix. Fibroblast proliferation is stimulated by multiple growth factors, including PDGF, EGF, FGF, and hypoxia at the wound center.[224–229] As neovascularization proceeds, the hypoxic stimulus for fibroblast proliferation decreases.[230] Fibroblasts play a key role in matrix deposition; molecular components of the new matrix include collagen, elastin, reticulin, proteoglycans, and glycosaminoglycans (GAGs).[231,232] (Fig. 2.11)

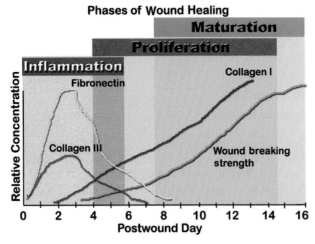

Phases of Wound Healing

Figure **2•11** *Matrix deposition according to phase of healing. In the early stages of repair, the fibrin clot provides a provisional matrix of fibronectin. As fibroblasts invade the fibrin clot, they begin to produce collagen. Initially, type III collagen predominates, but is replaced by stronger type I collagen during the proliferative and maturation phases. From Witte, MB, Barbul, A: General principles of wound healing. Surg Clin North Am 1997; 77:510–528. ©Elsevier, 1997.*

Extracellular Matrix Deposition

TGF-β is a potent stimulator of collagen production, stimulating the production of both types I and III collagen in the wound.[233] Type III is the predominant form of collagen in early granulation tissue; it appears at day 2 and is maximally secreted for 5 to 7 days.[233] Collagen synthesis occurs within the cell and results in the secretion of procollagen, a triple helix that must be processed by proteases outside the cell to develop insoluble fibrillar collagen. Fibrillar collagen is the principal protein lending strength and structure to the extracellular matrix. The diameter of type III collagen is about 30% that of type I collagen, yielding poor strength to the immature matrix, but over time, during the maturation phase, type I collagen is the predominant form synthesized, eventually replacing the type III.[234,235] Elastin and reticulin give additional support to the developing ECM. Elastin surrounds collagen fibers and by virtue of its wavy network, provides extensibility and elasticity to the matrix.[236,237] Reticulin develops a very thin, fine fibrous network and lays a framework for additional collagen deposition.[238,239]

Besides these fibrous components of the ECM, fibroblasts also secrete an amorphous, viscous ground substance consisting of proteoglycans and GAGs, which are composed of highly hydrophilic proteins and carbohydrates, lending form, compliance, and integrity to the developing matrix. Hyaluronic acid (HA), a nonsulfated GAG, is the most abundantly produced GAG from days 4 to 5, and its production by fibroblasts is stimulated by TGF-β, FGF, PDGF, and EGF.[240–242] HA's negative charge attracts large amounts of water, producing tissue edema, which allows enhanced migration and proliferation of cells. Chondroitin-4-sulfate and dermatan sulfate become the major GAGs produced on days 5 to 7. These sulfated GAGs are more stiff than HA, providing a more stable and resilient matrix that inhibits cellular migration and proliferation.[240] Proteoglycans, synthesized by fibroblasts concomitantly with collagen, assist with collagen assembly by accelerating polymerization of monomers and developing cross-links between collagen fibrils.[243] Proteoglycans in the ECM include aggrecan, syndecan, and decorin. Besides offering structural support, they participate in growth factor sequestration and presentation during proteolysis and matrix remodeling.[8]

Myofibroblasts and Wound Contraction

Some fibroblasts in granulation tissue differentiate into a tension-producing phenotype known as myofibroblasts. These cells have contractile properties, express α-smooth muscle actin (α-SMA), and secrete type I collagen; their transformation is dependent on TGF-β.[244,245] Fibroblasts appear to go through a two-step progression from fibroblast to fully differentiated myofibroblast. (Fig. 2.12) An intermediate form, the proto-myofibroblast, develops contractile features upon sensing mechanical tension in the ECM.[245] In addition to tension, PDGF is important to this progressive step but does not induce the expression of α-SMA evident in the differentiated phenotype.[246, 247] The initial tensile stimulus occurs as a traction force that develops during fibroblast migration as collagen fibers and fibroblasts orient parallel to the wound bed.[248,249] Transforming fibroblasts develop focal adhesions to

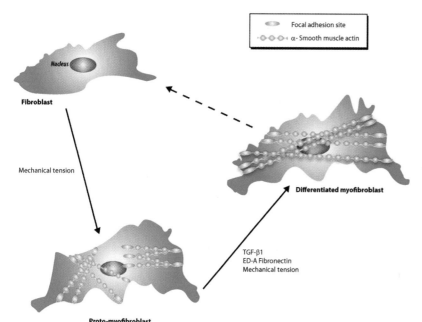

Figure 2•12 *Myofibroblast differentiation. Fibroblasts go through a two-step progression from fibroblast to fully differentiated myofibroblast. An intermediate form, the proto-myofibroblast, develops contractile features upon sensing mechanical tension along with the addition PDGF. These proto-myofibroblasts can be stimulated to progress to differentiated myofibroblasts by the addition of TGF-β and ED-A fibronectin. Differentiated myofibroblasts express α-SMA, which dramatically enhances force generation and serves as the hallmark of the contraction phase of wound healing.*

the ECM, stress fibers (filamentous actin and associated proteins) arise within the cell, and they begin to express a fibronectin splice variant, ED-A fibronectin.[245,250] Cells of this phenotype are apparent in granulation tissue of wounds at days 3 to 5.[249] These proto-myofibroblasts can be stimulated to progress to differentiated myofibroblasts by TGF-β, which is initially secreted into the wound by platelets and macrophages and by fibroblasts, keratinocytes, and injured epithelial cells after the inflammatory phase.[179,251–259] In addition to TGF-β, ED-A fibronectin is necessary for terminal differentiation. Differentiated myofibroblasts express α-SMA and have increased expression of ED-A fibronectin, increased stress fibers, and supermature focal adhesions.[245,260] The expression of α-SMA correlates with dramatically enhanced force generation by myofibroblasts and serves as the hallmark of the contraction phase of wound healing.[252,261–263] (Fig. 2.13)

> ▶ **PEARL 2•10** Wound contraction requires a tensile stimulus, PDGF, TGF-β, and ED-A fibronectin.

Myofibroblast differentiation is greatly influenced by the mechanical stiffness of the ECM. As matrix rigidity increases, the expression of α-SMA increases.[264,265] In uninjured tissue, fibroblasts are "stress shielded" by the intact ECM, but when the protective matrix is injured, fibroblasts encounter a dramatically different mechanical microenvironment.[245,266,267] Soft tissues typically have an elastic modulus between 100 and 20,000 pascals (Pa), but in the provisional matrix of the fibrin clot, the elastic modulus is decreased to about 10 to 100 Pa.[268–270] In experimental wounds, fibroblasts begin to develop stress fibers at 3000 to 6000 Pa, and α-SMA is expressed at 20,000 Pa.[269,271,272] As ECM is established in granulation tissue, matrix stiffness increases to greater than 50,000 Pa, providing ample stimulus for α-SMA expression.[272]

Myofibroblasts participate in wound contraction through their extensive cell-matrix contacts, called supermature focal adhesions. These specialized focal adhesions contain high

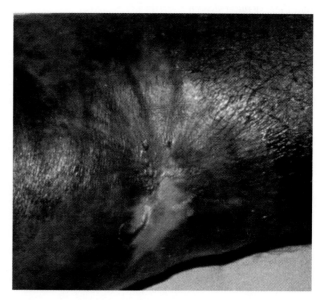

Figure 2•13 *Wound contraction. Wound margin closure is facilitated by myofibroblast contraction as evidenced in this healed wound by the tension-generated striations of the regenerated epithelial layer.*

levels of integrins, vinculin, paxillin, and tensin, which are linked to their intracellular stress fibers.[260,265] These complexes bind collagen fibers in the granulation bed, resulting in local matrix contraction and incremental shortening events.[245] (Fig. 2.14) As matrix deposition continues on the shortened construct, the myofibroblasts can either contract again to continue ECM shortening or become stress shielded by the load-bearing ECM and subsequent apoptosis.[273,274]

Besides stress shielding, additional factors that suppress myofibroblast differentiation and α-SMA expression include IL-1 secretion by keratinocytes and T-cell secretion of IFN-γ, both stimuli present during the later stages of repair and

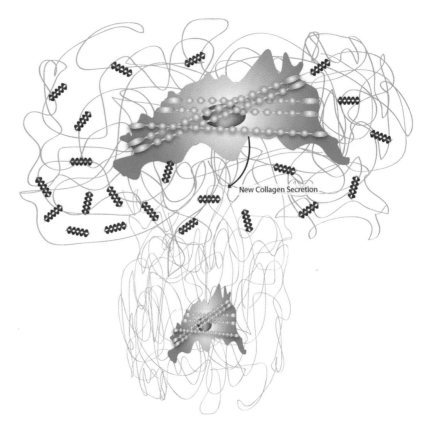

New Collagen Secretion

Figure 2•14 *Mechanism of matrix contraction. Differentiated myofibroblasts have extensive matrix contacts that bind and thereby pull collagen fibers in the extracellular matrix into a shorter construct. As matrix deposition continues, the myofibroblasts proceed with incremental shortening.*

remodeling.[275,276] Cell density also downregulates α-SMA expression. A massive myofibroblast apoptosis occurs after wound healing and reepithelialization.[273] However, in pathologic wound healing with hypertrophic scarring, myofibroblast activity persists, leading to tissue deformation and severe contracture.[277] (Fig. 2.15) In these wounds a positive-feedback loop may promote a vicious cycle of tension, facilitating TGF-β production, which activates α-SMA expression and subsequent production of additional tension.

Keratinocyte Migration

Coverage by keratinocytes marks the final step of the repair phase as these cornified epithelial cells provide the outermost cellular barrier to the environment. Within 24 hours of wounding, fibroblasts secrete keratinocyte growth factors (KGF-1 and KGF-2) and IL-6, stimulating keratinocyte migration, proliferation, and differentiation.[278] In a symbiotic relationship, keratinocytes enhance fibroblast differentiation into myofibroblasts through the release of TGF-β. In addition, keratinocyte-derived IL-1 inhibits α-SMA expression, thereby limiting myofibroblast contraction.[251] Through this paracrine signaling relationship, fibroblasts and keratinocytes synergistically control the rate of wound contraction and cellular coverage.

Keratinocytes migrate from two layers of the adjacent uninjured epidermis, the basal cell layer and the suprabasal cell layer. (Fig. 2.16) Basal cells are normally bound to the basement membrane by hemidesmosomes and to each other by desmosomes, both of which are junctional complexes made of cell adhesion molecules that "spot weld" cells in organized epithelial tissues.[279–281] In order for basal cells to migrate, they reorganize these contacts by detaching, withdrawing, and internalizing them to a perinuclear location.[282] They then undergo a dramatic

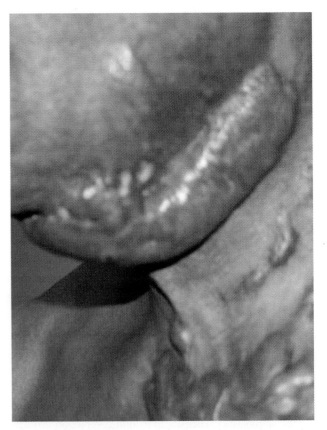

Figure 2•15 *Hypertrophic keloid scar. Severe contracture and scarring of a cervical and chest wound as a result of persistent, pathological myofibroblast activity.*

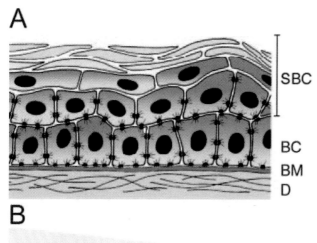

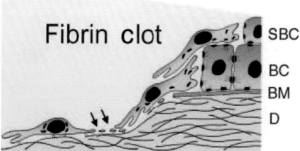

Figure 2•16 *Keratinocyte layers and migration.* **A.** *Keratinocytes migrate from two layers of the adjacent uninjured epidermis, the basal cell layer (BC) and the suprabasal cell layer (SBC).* **B.** *They undergo a dramatic change in shape from an organized columnar phenotype to flattened elongated cells with lamellipodia and membrane ruffles at their leading edges. While the basal cells migrate along the dermal (D) ECM, cells from the suprabasal layer enhance migration by leapfrogging the basal cells at the wound perimeter. Reproduced with permission from Kirfel, G, Herzog, V: Migration of epidermal keratinocytes: mechanisms, regulation, and biological significance.* Protoplasma *2004; 223:67–78.*

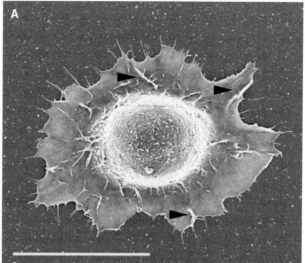

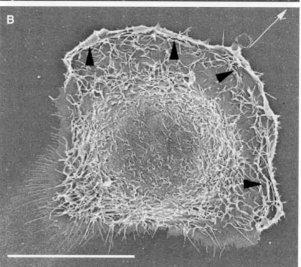

Figure 2•17 *Induction of keratinocyte polarity.* **A.** *Few ruffles (arrow heads) are present in an inactivated, non-polarized keratinocyte.* **B.** *A polarized keratinocyte has lamellipodia and membrane ruffles (arrowheads) at its leading edge. (White arrow represents the direction of migration.) Numerous growth factors stimulate keratinocyte migration through tyrosine kinase receptors, which convey polarity to the cell through actin cytoskeletal polymerization and reorganization. Reproduced with permission from Kirfel, G, Herzog, V: Migration of epidermal keratinocytes: mechanisms, regulation, and biological significance.* Protoplasma *2004; 223:67–78.*

change in shape from an organized columnar phenotype to flattened elongated cells, with lamellipodia and membrane ruffles at their leading edges.[283] (Fig. 2.17) While the basal cells migrate along the dermal ECM of granulation tissue, creating a migrating epidermal tongue, cells from the suprabasal layer enhance migration by leapfrogging the basal cells at the wound perimeter.[284]

Numerous growth factors stimulate keratinocyte migration and signal mobility through tyrosine kinase receptors, which convey polarity to the cell through actin cytoskeletal polymerization and reorganization. Focal adhesions are also assembled in response to the stimulus and contribute to the cells' ability to crawl across the matrix.[285,286] Keratinocyte growth factor (KGF) is a principle regulator of keratinocyte migration and proliferation and is secreted into the wound by dermal fibroblasts, which increase secretion of KGF 100-fold within 24 hours of wounding.[287] Additional growth factors that stimulate keratinocyte migration include epidermal growth factor (EGF), heparin-binding EGF (HB-EGF), insulin-like growth

factor (IGF), transforming growth factor-β (TGF-β), and the secretory form of the Alzheimer amyloid precursor protein (sAPP). These factors come from a variety of local cellular sources, which include platelets, macrophages, dermal fibroblasts, and keratinocytes themselves.[288–294]

The leading edge of migrating keratinocytes display protease activity that degrades and remodels the ECM in their path. Plasmin activators, uPA and tPA, along with their receptors and MMPs, are upregulated in the leading edge of keratinocytes.[295–299] MMP-9 cleaves collagens IV and VII, which are components of the basement membrane; plasmin degrades the fibrin of the provisional matrix; and MMP-1 degrades collagens I and III of the new dermal ECM. These proteases are temporally and spatially expressed simultaneously with the expression of specific integrin receptors, suggesting a cooperative effort for efficient matrix reorganization and migration.[300]

Migrating keratinocytes contact the ECM through integrins on their surface. The expression profile of these adhesion molecules is specifically induced upon contact with certain matrix components.[301] Migrating keratinocytes do not express the fibrin-specific integrin αvβ3, therefore they do not go through the fibrin clot. Instead keratinocytes migrate beneath it, contacting the dermal matrix while dissecting the clot from the wound bed, thereby participating in liquification of progressive eschar to slough.[50]

> **PEARL 2•11** Keratinocytes do not bind to the fibrin matrix, but do bind to the dermal matrix, thereby providing an efficient debridement of eschar from the dermal layer while reepithelializing.

As keratinocytes move, contacts develop at their integrin-rich lamellipodia, while other contacts at the rear of the cell are freed so that the cell may move toward the chemotactic gradient.[300] This requires a dynamic sensing of the matrix and reorganization of integrins at the cell surface along with a local release of proteases.[302,303] As a result of these contacts, "outside-in" signaling promotes the development of lamellipodia, filopodia, and actin polymerization within the keratinocyte.[304] "Inside-out" signaling regulates the activation of integrins and matrix-binding capacity.[305]

While migrating across the dermal ECM, keratinocytes produce and deposit a variety of ECM components for a provisional basement membrane. These include laminin, fibronectin, and collagen IV.[306–309] In addition, keratinocytes leave a track of integrins and membrane components called *microaggregates* in their wake.[310] (Fig. 2.18) These microaggregates result from membrane ripping that occurs during rapid migration, and they provide a provisional basement membrane and adhesion sites as a path for additional cells to follow.[300,311,312] As keratinocytes close in on each other from the wound perimeter, cell-cell contact signals reepithelialization and migration is discontinued.

Remodeling (Day 8 Through 1 Year)

Remodeling, the final phase of wound healing, consists of collagen maturation and reorganization, orchestrated by fibroblasts, growth factors, MMPs, and their TIMPs. Initially, the immature collagen is deposited in a random fashion, but through selective degradation, secretion, and reorganization, the structure and composition of the matrix is eventually normalized in the remodeling phase.[222] Growth factors and tensile forces through integrin-mediated signaling participate in this reorganization.[313–315]

Over time, the immature dermal matrix is reorganized to a stronger, more organized mature scar. At 1 week postwound, the scar has 3% of its ultimate strength; at 3 weeks, 30%; and at

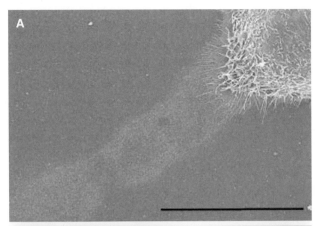

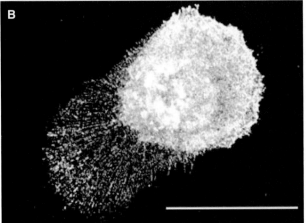

Figure 2•18 *Keratinocyte leaving tracks.* **A.** *Scanning Electron Microscopy and* **B.** *Immunofluorescense for β1-integrin. While migrating across the dermal ECM, keratinocytes produce and deposit a variety of ECM components along with a track of integrins and membrane components called microaggregates. These provide a provisional basement membrane and adhesion sites as a path for additional cells to follow. Reproduced with permission from Kirfel, G, Herzog, V: Migration of epidermal keratinocytes: mechanisms, regulation, and biological significance.* Protoplasma *2004; 223:67–78.*

3 months and thereafter, the scar is 80% of the original strength of uninjured skin.[316] This change in strength correlates to the composition and alignment of collagen in the matrix. The smaller diameter type III collagen deposited in granulation tissue comprises 30% of collagen in the new matrix. This is gradually replaced by thicker type I collagen during maturation to the normal levels of 10% type III and 90% type I.[317]

As the immature scar is utilized during functional activities, integrin signaling triggered by tension participates in realignment of the collagen fibers from a random orientation to one of structure according to function.[313–315] This is orchestrated by tightly controlled synthesis and degradation of matrix components by fibroblast production and secretion of proteases (MMPs and TIMPs) balanced by growth factor–stimulated deposition of collagen and other matrix proteins. Production of MMP-2, MMP-7, and TIMP-2 is elevated in the early remodeling phase and is coordinated with a decrease in production of MMP-1, MMP-9, and TIMP-1.[318] Growth factors involved in the regulation of proteases and their inhibitors include TGF-β, PDGF, and IL-1.[319–321] Net collagen deposition by fibroblasts increases until about 21 days postwound, at which time the rate of collagen synthesis decreases as collagen alignment and strength increases.[322,323]

Vascularity to the tissue also is reduced to baseline during the remodeling phase. The enhanced capillary density established during granulation through neovascularization gradually decreases in response to antiangiogenic mediators, including thrombospondin-1.[324–326] This is evidenced as the scar gradually goes from pink to white at terminal maturation. Mature epidermal scars also lack hair follicles and sweat glands, probably secondary to an absence of stem cell populations for these appendages in the regenerated dermis.[327–329] Aside from the epidermal cellular covering, the mature scar is relatively acellular. Once the cellular mediators of wound healing complete their tasks, they either undergo apoptosis, as is the case with myofibroblasts, or migrate out of the scar to prepare for another area of need, as is the case with some inflammatory cells.

Implications for the Future

Although not perfect, nature has provided the opportunity for skin to heal with an adequate replacement material that ultimately provides barrier protection. As scientific technology improves, the goal for optimal wound recovery is to mimic the process of fetal wound healing. Fetal healing is fast, efficient, and results in near-perfect skin regeneration and matrix alignment without scar formation.[330] Some of the clues to perfect healing have been unveiled. Full-thickness fetal wounds are able to regenerate hair follicles and sweat glands.[331] Genetic expression of lymphoid-enhancer factor, sonic hedgehog, bone morphogenic protein-2, and FGF-4 appear to participate in the development of these cutaneous appendages in embryos.[332] Adult wounds are able to respond to these hair-inducing signals, but do not typically receive them from their wounded dermis.[333] Fetal keratinocytes also migrate in a sweeping fashion, without having to reorganize their actin cytoskeleton in order to crawl across the matrix. An actin cable promptly develops at the fetal wound margin and pulls the epidermal cells together in a purse-string mechanism.[334,335] (Fig. 2.19) Some small adult gut wounds heal in a similar fashion, so perhaps adult keratinocytes could be induced to do the same.[330,336] Fetal wounds also heal with very little transiently expressed TGF-β, the absence of which may prevent scarring.[330,337,338] Embryonic wounds contract but do not convert fibroblasts to myofibroblasts, a process that requires TGF-β in adult healing.[244,245,334–339] In addition, excessive scarring in adult wounds is neutralized by blocking the action of TGF-β.[340,341] Studies using genetic knockout animals and continued research with the use of novel approaches will continue to provide more clues to the ultimate goal of rapid, perfect regeneration of the skin.

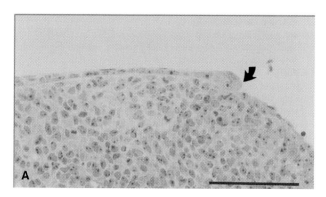 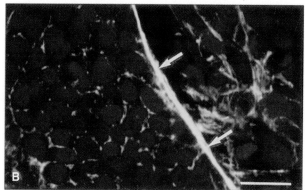

Figure 2•19 *Embryologic repair—sweeping keratinocytes.* **A.** *Fetal keratinocytes migrate in a sweeping fashion, without having to reorganize their actin cytoskeleton in order to crawl across the matrix (arrow at leading edge).* **B.** *An actin cable (arrows) promptly develops at the fetal wound margin and pulls the epidermal cells together in a purse-string mechanism. From Martin, P: Wound healing—Aiming for perfect skin regeneration.* Science *1997; 276: 75–81. Used with permission from AAAS.*

References

1. Kirsner, RS, Eaglstein, WH, Kerdel, FA, et al: Split-thickness skin grafts for lower extremity ulcerations. Dermatol Surg 1997; 25:85.
2. Kirsner, RS, Bogensberger, G: The normal healing process. In: Kloth, LC, McCulloch, JM. (eds): Wound Healing: Alternatives in Management. Philadelphia, FA Davis, 2001, pp. 3–34.
3. Zitelli, J: Wound healing for the clinician. Adv Dermatol 1987; 2:243.
4. Kirsner, RS, Eaglstein, WH: The wound healing process. Dermatol Clin 1993; 11:629
5. Krawczyk, WS: A pattern of epidermal cell migration during wound healing. J Cell Biol 1971; 49:247.
6. Venter, JC, Adams, MD, Myers, EW, et. al: The sequence of the human genome. Science 2001; 291.
7. The International Human Genome Mapping Consortium: A physical map of the human genome. Nature 2001; 409: 934–941.
8. Lodish, HF, Berk, A, Zipursky, SL, et al: Integrating cells into tissues. In Molecular Cell Biology. New York, WH Freeman, 1999, pp. 968–1002.
9. Schulze, H, Shivdasani, RA: Mechanisms of thrompopoiesis. J Thromb Haemost 2005; 3:1717–1724.

10. Burkitt, HG, Young, B, Heath, JW: Blood. In: Wheater's Functional Histology: A Text and Colour Atlas. Churchill Livingstone, Hong Kong, 1993, pp. 42–60.

11. Ruggeri, ZM, Mendolicchio, GL: Adhesion mechanisms in platelet function. Circ Res 2007; 100:1673–1685.

12. Ruggeri, ZM: Platelets in atherothrombosis. Nat Med 8: 1227–1234, 2002.

13. Plow, EF, Pierschbacher, MD, Ruoslahti, E, et al: Related binding mechanisms for fibrinogen, fibronectin, von Willebrand factor, and thrombospondin on thrombin-stimulated human platelets. Blood 1985; 66:724-727.

14. Macfarlane, RG: An enzyme cascade in the blood clotting mechanism and its function as a biological amplifier. Nature 1964; 202:498–499.

15. Davie, EW, Ratnoff, OD: Waterfall sequence for intrinsic blood clotting. Science 1964; 145:1310–1312.

16. Monroe, DM, Roberts, HR, Hoffman, M: Platelet procoagulant complex assembly in a tissue factor-initiated system. Br J Haematol 1994; 88:364–371.

17. Monroe, DM, Hoffman, M, Roberts, HR: Transmission of a procoagulant signal from tissue factor-bearing cell to platelets. Blood Coagul Fibrinolysis 1996; 7:459–464.

18. Hoffman, M, Monroe, DM, Oliver, JA, et. al: Factors IXa and Xa play distinct roles in tissue factor-dependent initiation of coagulation. Blood 1995; 86:1794–1801.

19. Hoffman, M, Monroe, DM: Coagulation 2006: A modern view of hemostasis. Hematol Oncol Clin N Am 2007; 21:1–11.

20. Alberio, L, Safa, O, Clemetson, KJ, et. al: Surface expression and functional characterization of alpha-granule factor V in human platelets: Effects of ionophore A23187, thrombin, collagen, and convulxin. Blood 2000; 95:1694–1702.

21. Dale, GL: Stimulated platelets use seratonin to enhance their retention of procoagulant proteins on the cell surface. Nature 2002; 415:175–179.

22. Kempton, CL, Hoffman, M, Roberts, HR, et al: Platelet heterogeneity: Variation in coagulation complexes on platelet subpopulations. Arterioscler Thromb Vasc Biol 2005; 25:861–866.

23. Bauer, EA, Cooper, TW, Huang, JS, et al: Stimulation of in vitro human skin collagenase expression by platelet-derived growth factor. Proc Natl Acad Sci USA 1985; 82:4132–4136.

24. Brissett, AE, Hom, DB: The effects of tissue sealants, platelet gels, and growth factors on wound healing. Curr Opin Otolaryngol Head Neck Surg 2003; 11:245–250.

25. Weisel, JW, Francis, CW, Nagaswami, C, et al: Determination of the topology of factor XIIIa-induced fibrin gamma-chain cross-links by electron microscopy of ligated fragments. J Biol Chem1993; 268:26618–26624.

26. Mosesson, MW, Siebenlist, KR, Meh, DA: The structure and biological features of fibrinogen and fibrin. Ann N Y Acad Sci 2001; 936:11–30.

27. DiStasio, E, Nagaswami, C, Weisel, JW, et al: Cl- regulates the structure of the fibrin clot. Biophys J 1998; 75:1973–1979.

28. Standeven, KF, Ariens, RA, Grant, PJ: The molecular physiology and pathology of fibrin structure/function. Blood Rev 2005; 19:275–288.

29. Parise, P, Morini, M, Agnelli, G, et al: Effects of low molecular weight heparins on fibrin polymerization and clot sensitivity to tPA-induced lysis. Blood Coagul Fibrinolysis 1993; 4:721–727.

30. Collen, A, Smorenburg, SM, Peters, E, et al: Unfractionated and low molecular weight heparin affect fibrin structure and angiogenesis in vitro. Cancer Res 2000; 60:6196–6200.

31. Collet, JP, Allali, Y, Lesty, C, et al: Influence of fibrin network conformation and fibrin fiber diameter on fibrinolysis speed: Dynamic and structural approaches by confocal microscopy. Arterioscler Thromb Vasc Biol 2000; 20:1354–1361.

32. Collen, A, Koolwijk, P, Kroon, ME, et al: Influence of fibrin structure on the formation and maintenance of capillary-like tubules by human microvascular endothelial cells. Angiogenesis 1998; 2:153–165.

33. Bennett, JS: Platelet-fibrinogen interactions. Ann N Y Acad Sci 2001; 936:340–354.

34. Martinez, J, Ferber, A, Bach, TL.,et al: Interaction of fibrin with VE-cadherin. Ann N Y Acad Sci 2001; 936:386–405.

35. Ugarova, TP, Yakubenko, VP: Recognition of fibrinogen by leukocyte integrins. Ann N Y Acad Sci 2001; 936:368–385.

36. Yakovlev, S, Zhang, L, Ugarova, T, et al: Interaction of fibrin(ogen) with leukocyte receptor alpha M beta 2 (Mac-1): Further characterization and identification of a novel binding region within the central domain of the fibrinogen gamma-module. Biochemistry 2005; 44:617–626.

37. Rybarczyk, BJ, Lawrence, SO, Simpson-Haidaris, PJ: Matrix-fibrinogen enhances wound closure by increasing both cell proliferation and migration. Blood 2003; 102:4035–4043.

38. Nisato, RE, Tille, JC, Jonczyk, A, et al: Alpha-v-beta-3 and alpha-v-beta-5 integrin antagonists inhibit angiogenesis in vitro. Angiogenesis 2003; 6:105–119.

39. Sahni, A, Francis, CW: Stimulation of endothelial cell proliferation by FGF-2 in the presence of fibrinogen requires alpha-v-beta-3. Blood 2004; 104:3635–3641.

40. Suehiro, K, Gailit, J, Plow, EF: Fibrinogen is a ligand for integrin alpha-5-beta-1 on endothelial cells. J Biol Chem 1997; 272:5360–5366.

41. Farrell, DH, al Mondhiry, HA: Human fibroblast adhesion to fibrinogen. Biochemistry 1997; 36:1123–1128.

42. Gailit, J, Clarke, C, Newman, D, et al: Human fibroblasts bind directly to fibrinogen at RGD sites through integrin alpha(v)beta3. Exp Cell Res 1997; 232:118–126.

43. Gailit, J, Clark, RAF: Studies in vitro on the role of alpha-v and beta-1 integrins in the adhesion of human dermal fibroblasts to provisional matrix proteins fibronectin, vitronectin, and fibrinogen. J Invest Dermatol 1996; 106: 102–108.

44. Collen, A, Hanemaaijer R, Lupu F, et al: Membrane-type matrix metalloproteinase-mediated angiogenesis in a fibrin-collagen matrix. Blood 2003; 101:1810–1817.

45. Marx, G: Immunological monitoring of fenton fragmentation of fibrinogen. Free Radic Res Commun 1991; 12-13:517–520.

46. Carmeliet, P: Angiogenesis in health and disease. Nat Med 2003; 9:653–660.

47. Folkman, J: Fundamental concepts of the angiogenic process. Curr Mol Med 2003; 3:643–651.

48. Becker, JC, Domschke, W, Pohle, T: Biological in vitro effects of fibrin glue: Fibroblast proliferation, expression, and binding of growth factors. Scand J Gastroenterol 2004; 39:927–932.

49. Kilarski, WW, Jura, N, Gerwins, P An ex vivo model for functional studies of myofibroblasts. Lab Invest 2005; 85:643–654.

50. Kubo, M, Van De Water, L, Plantefaber, LC, et al: Fibrinogen and fibrin are anti-adhesive for keratinocytes: A mechanism for fibrin eschar slough during wound repair. J Invest Dermatol 2001; 117:1369–1381.

51. Szymanski, LM, Pate, RR, Durstine, JL: Effects of maximal exercise and venous occlusion on fibrinolytic activity in physically active and inactive men. J Appl Physiol 1994; 77:2305–2310.

52. Cook-Mills, JM, Deem, TL: Active participation of endothelial cells in inflammation. J Leukoc Biol 2005; 77:487–495.

53. Luscinskas, FW, Cybulsky, MI, Kiely, JM, et al: The role of endothelial cell lateral junctions during leukocyte trafficking. Immunol Rev 2002; 186:57–67.

54. Gopalan, PK, Burns, AR, Simon, SI, et al: Preferential sites for stationary adhesion of neutrophils to cytokine-stimulated HUVEC under flow conditions. J Leukoc Biol 2000; 68:7–57.

55. Mamdouh, Z, Chen, X, Pierini, LM, et al: Targeted recycling of PECAM from endothelial surface-connected compartments during diapedesis. Nature 2003; 421:748–753.

56. Muller, WA: Migration of leukocytes across endothelial junctions: Some concepts and controversies. Microcirculation 2001; 8:181–193.

57. Shaw, SK, Bamba, PS, Perkins, BN, et al: Real-time imaging of vascular endothelial-cadherin during leukocyte transmigration across endothelium. J Immunol 2001; 167:2323–2330.

58. Feng, D, Nagy, JA, Hipp, J, et al: Neutrophils emigrate from venules by a transendothelial cell pathway in response to fMLP. J Exp Med 1998; 187:903–915.

59. Vestweber, D: Adhesion and signaling molecules controlling the transmigration of leukocytes through endothelium. Immunol Rev 2007; 218:178–196.

60. Hoshi, O, Ushiki, T: Scanning electron microscopic studies on the route of neutrophil extravasation in the mouse after exposure to the chemotactic peptide N-formyl-methionyl-leucyl-phenylalanine (fMLP). Arch Histol Cytol 1999; 62:253–260.

61. Rose, DM, Alon, R, Ginsberg, MH: Integrin modulation and signaling in leukocyte adhesion and migration. Immunol Rev 2007; 218:126–134.

62. McEver, RP: Role of PSGL-1 binding to selectins in leukocyte recruitment. J Clin Invest 1997; 100:485–491.

63. Kunkel, EJ, Ley, K: Distinct phenotype of E-selectin-deficient mice: E-selectin is required for slow leukocyte rolling in vivo. Circ Res, 1996; 79:1196–1204.

64. Smith, ML, Olson, TS, Ley, K: CXCR2- and E-selectin-induced neutrophil arrest during inflammation in vivo. J Exp Med 2004; 200:935–939.

65. DeGrendele, HC, Estess, P, Picker, LJ, et al: CD44 and its ligand hyaluronate mediate rollng under physiological flow: A novel lymphocyte-endothelial cell primary adhesion pathway. J Exp Med 1996; 183:1119–1130.

66. Sanchez-Madrid, F, Angel delPozo, M: Leukocyte polarization in cell migration and immune interactions. EMBO J 1999; 18:501–511.

67. Shimonaka, M, Katagiri, K, Nakayama, T, et al: Rap1 translates chemokine signals to integrin activation, cell polarization, and motility across vascular endothelium under flow. J Cell Biol 2003; 161:417–427.

68. Green, GE, Schaff, UY, Sarantos, MR, et al: Dynamic shifts in LFA-1 affinity regulate neutrophil rolling, arrest, and transmigration on inflamed endothelium. Blood 2006; 107:2101–2111.

69. Alon, R, Dustin, M: Force as a facilitator of integrin conformation changes during leukocyte arrest on blood vessels and antigen-presenting cells. Immunity 2007; 26:17–27.

70. Schwartz, MA, Horwitz, AR: Integrating adhesion, protrusion, and contraction during cell migration. Cell 2006; 125:1223–1225.

71. Gupton, SL, Waterman-Storer, CM: Spatiotemporal feedback between actomyosin and focal adhesion systems optimizes rapid cell migration. Cell 2006; 125:1361–1374.

72. Marchesi, VT, Florey, HW: Electron micrographic observations on the emigration of leukocytes. Q J Exp Physiol Cogn Med Sci 1960; 45:343–348.

73. Williamson, J, Grisham, J: Electron microscopy of leukocytic margination and emigration in acute inflammation in dog pancreas. Am J Pathol 1961; 39:239–256.

74. Marchesi, VT: The site of leukocyte emigration during inflammation. Q J Exp Physiol Cogn Med Sci 1961; 46:115–118.

75. Hurley, J, Xeros, N: Electron microscopic observation on the emigration of leukocytes. Aust J Exp Biol Med Sci 1961; 39:609–624.

76. Liao, F, Huynh, HK, Eiroa, A, et al: Soluble domain 1 of platelet-endothelial cell adhesion molecule (PECAM) is sufficient to block transendothelial migration in vitro and in vivo. J Exp Med 1997; 185:1349–1357.

77. Duncan, GS, Andrew, DP, Takimoto, H, et al: Genetic evidence for functional redundancy of platelet/endothelial cell adhesion molecule-1 (PECAM-1): CD31-deficient mice reveal PECAM-1-independent functions. J Immunol 1999; 162:3022–3030.

78. Liao, F, Huynh, HK, Eiroa, A, et al: Migration of monocytes across endothelium and passage through extracellular matrix involve separate molecular domains of PECAM-1. J Exp Med 1995; 182:1337–1343.

79. Wakelin, MW, Sanz, MJ, Dewar, A, et al: An anti-platelet-endothelial cell adhesion molecule-1 antibody inhibits leukocyte extravasation from mesenteric microvessels in vivo by blocking the passage through the basement membrane. J Exp Med 1996; 184:229–239.

80. Martin-Padura, I, Lostaglio, S, Schneemann, M, et al: Junctional adhesion molecule, a novel member of the immunoglobulin superfamily that distributes at intercellular junctions and modulates monocyte transmigration. J Cell Biol 1998; 142:117–127.

81. Malergue, F, Galland, F, Martin, F, et al: A novel immunoglobulin superfamily junctional molecule expressed by antigen presenting cells, endothelial cells, and platelets. Mol Immunol 1998; 35:1111–1119.

82. Liu, Y, Nusrat, A, Schnell, F, et al: Human junction adhesion molecule regulates tight junction resealing in epithelia. J Cell Sci 2000; 113:2363–2374.

83. Itoh, M, Sasaki, H, Furuse, M, et al: Junctional adhesion molecule (JAM) binds to PAR-3: A possible mechanism for the recruitment of PAR-3 to tight junctions. J Cell Biol 2001; 154:491–497.

84. Cera, MR, Del Prete, A, Vecchi, A, et al: Increased DC trafficking to lymph nodes and contact hypersensitivity in junctional adhesion molecule-A-deficient mice. J Clin Invest 2004; 114:729–738.

85. Corada, M, Chimenti, S, Cera, MR, et al: Junctional adhesion molecule-A-deficient polymorphonuclear cells show reduced diapedesis in peritonitis and heart ischemia-reperfusion injury. Proc Natl Acad Sci USA 2005; 102:10634–10639.

86. Wegmann, F, Petri, B, Khandoga, AG, et al: ESAM supports neutrophil extravasation, activation of Rho and VEGF-induced vascular permeability. J Exp Med 2006; 203:1671–1677.

87. Herren, B, Levkau, B, Raines, EW, et al: Cleavage of beta-catenin and plakoglobin and shedding of VE-cadherin during endothelial apoptosis: Evidence for a role for caspases and metalloproteinases. Mol Biol Cell 1998; 9:1589–1601.

88. Zarbock, A, Polanowska-Grabowska, RK, Ley, K: Platelet-neutrophil-interactions: Linking hemostasis and inflammation. Blood Rev 2007; 21:99–111.

89. Engelhardt, E, Toksoy, A, Goebeler, M, et al: Chemokines IL-8, GRO-alpha, MCP-1, IP-10, and Mig are sequentially and differentially expressed during phase-specific infiltration of leukocyte subsets in human wound healing. Am J Pathol 1998; 153:1849–1860.

90. Clark, RA: The Molecular and Cellular Biology of Wound Repair. New York, Plenum Press, 1996.

91. Weiss, SJ: Tissue destruction by neutrophils. N Engl J Med 1989; 320:365–376.

92. Eming, SA, Krieg, T, Davidson, JM: Inflammation in wound repair: Molecular and cellular mechanisms. J Invest Dermatol 2007; 127:514–525.

93. Tsirogianni, AK, Moutsopoulos, NM, Moutsopoulos, HM: Wound healing: Immunological aspects. Injury 2006; 37S:S5–S12.

94. Leibovich, SJ, Ross, R: A macrophage-dependent factor that stimulates the proliferation of fibroblasts in vitro. Am J Pathol 1976; 84:501–514.

95. Rappolee, DA, Mark, D, Banda, MJ, et al: Wound macrophages express TGF-alpha and other growth factors in vivo: Analysis by mRNA phenotyping. Science 1988; 241:708–712.

96. Trautmann, A, Toksoy, A, Engelhardt, E, et al: Mast cell involvement in normal human skin wound healing: Expression of MCP-1 is correlated with recruitment of mast cells which synthesize IL-4 in vivo. J Pathol 2000; 190:100–106.

97. Park, JE, Barbul, A: Understanding the role of immune regulation in wound healing. Am J Surg 2004; 187:11S–16S.

98. Fishel, RS, Barbul, A, Beschorner, WE, et al: Lymphocyte participation in wound healing: Morphologic assessment using monoclonal antibodies. Ann Surg 1987; 2006:25–29.

99. Theilgaard-Monch, K, Knudsen, S, Follin, P, et al: The transcriptional activation program of human neutrophils in skin lesions supports their important role in wound healing. J Immunol 2004; 172:7684–7693.

100. Martin, P, Leibovich, SJ: Inflammatory cells during wound repair: The good, the bad and the ugly. Trends Cell Biol 2005; 15:599–607.

101. Borregaard, N, Sorensen, OE, Theilgaard-Monch, K: Neutrophil granules: A library of innate immunity proteins. Trends Immunol 2007; 28:340–345.

102. Selsted, ME, Ouellette, AJ: Mammalian defensins in the antimicrobial immune response. Nat Immunol 2005; 6:551–557.

103. Nathan, C: Neutrophils and immunity: Challenges and opportunities. Nat Rev Immunol 2006; 6:173–182.

104. Segal, AW: How neutrophils kill microbes. Ann Rev Immunol 2005; 23:197–223.

105. Segal, AW, Dorling, J, Coade, S: Kinetics of fusion of the cytoplasmic granules with phagocytic vacuoles in human polymorphonuclear

leukocytes: Biochemical and morphological studies. J Cell Biol 1980; 85:42–59.

106. Saville, J, Haslett, C: Granulocyte clearance by apoptosis in the resolution of inflammation. Semin Cell Biol 1995; 6:385–393.

107. Crowther, M, Brown, NJ, Bishop, ET, et al: Microenvironmental influence on macrophage regulation of angiogenesis in wounds and malignant tumors. J Leukoc Biol 2001; 70:478–490.

108. Stout, RD, Suttles, J: T-cell signaling of macrophage function in inflammatory disease. Frontiers Biosci 1997; 2:d197–d206.

109. Stout, RD, Suttles, J: T-cell signaling of macrophage activation. In: Landes, RG. (ed.): Cell Contact-dependent and Cytokine Signals. Austin, TX, Springer-Verlag, 1995.

110. Gordon, S: Alternative action of macrophages. Nat Rev Immunol 2003; 3:23–35.

111. Mosser, DM: The many faces of macrophage activation. J Leukoc Biol 2003; 73:209–212.

112. Goerdt, S, Orfanos, CE: Other functions, other genes: Alternative activation of antigen-presenting cells. Immunity 1999; 10:137–142.

113. Mills, CD, Kincaid, K, Alt, JM, et al: M-1/M-2 macrophages and the Th1/Th2 paradigm. J Immunol 2000; 164:6166–6173.

114. Stout, RD, Jiang, C, Matta, B, et al: Macrophages sequentially change their functional phenotype in response to changes in microenvironmental influences. J Immunol 2005; 175:342–349.

115. Wells, CA, Ravasi, T, Sultana, R, et al: Genetic control of the innate immune response. BMC Immunol 2003; 4:5–23.

116. Williams, L, Jarai, G, Smith, A, et al: IL-10 expression profiling in human monocytes. J Leukoc Biol 2002; 72:800–809.

117. Lang, R, Patel, D, Morris, JJ, et al: Shaping gene expression in activated and resting primary macrophages by IL-10. J Immunol 2002; 169:2253–2263.

118. Stout, RD, Suttles, J: Functional plasticity of macrophages: Reversible adaptation to changing microenvironments. J Leukoc Biol 2004; 76:509–513.

119. Wahl, SM: Host immune factors regulating fibrosis. In: Evered, D, Whelan, J (eds.) Fibrosis. Ciba Foundation Symposium Series, No. 114, Pitman, London, 1985.

120. Barbul, A: Immune aspects of wound care. Clin Plast Surg 1990; 17:433–442

121. Kovacs, EJ, DiPietro, LA: Fibrogenic cytokines and connective tissue production. FASEB J 1994; 8:854–861.

122. Wei, LH, Kuo, ML, Chen, CA, et al: Interleukin-6 in cervical cancer: The relationship with vascular endothelial growth factor. Gynecol Oncol 2001; 82:49–56.

123. Wang, Z, Castresana, MR, Newman, WH: Reactive oxygen and NF-kappa B in VEGF-induced migration of human vascular smooth muscle cells. Biochem Biophys Res Commun 2001; 285:669–674.

124. Roesel, JF, Nanney, LB: Assessment of differential cytokine effects on angiogenesis using an in vivo model of cutaneous wound repair. J Surg Res 1995; 58:449–459.

125. Galluchi, RM, Sugawara, T, Yucesoy, B, et al: Interleukin-6 treatment augments cutaneous wound healing in immunosuppressed mice. J Interferon Cytokine Res 2001; 21:603–609.

126. Malecaze, F, Simorre, P, Chollet, JL, et al: Interleukin-6 in tear fluid after photorefractive keratectomy and its effects on keratocytes in culture. Cornea 1997; 16:580–587.

127. Hankenson, KD, Watkins, BA, Schoenlein, IA, et al: Omega-3 fatty acids enhance ligament fibroblast collagen formation in association with changes in interleukin-6 production. Proc Soc Exp Biol Med 2000; 223:88–95.

128. Swift, ME, Kleinman, HK, DiPietro, LA. Impaired wound repair and delayed angiogenesis in aged mice. Lab Invest 1999; 79:1479–1487.

129. Kibe, Y, Takenaka, H, Kishimoto, S: Spatial and temporal expression of basic fibroblast growth factor protein during wound healing of rat skin. Br J Dermatol 2000; 143:720–727.

130. Kelley, CJ, Gallagher, H, Wolf, BA, et al: Alterations in macrophage signal transduction pathways mediate post-traumatic changes in macrophage function. J Surg Res 1994; 57:221–226.

131. Ozawa, K, Kondo, T, Hori, O, et al: Expression of the oxygen-regulated protein ORP 150 accelerates wound healing by modulating intracellular VEGF transport. J Clin Invest 2001; 108:41–50.

132. Gu, Q, Wang, D, Gao, Y, et al: Expression of MMP 1 in surgical and radiation-impaired wound healing and its effects on the healing process. J Environ Pathol Toxicol Oncol 2002; 21:71–78.

133. Schaffer, MR, Tantry, U, van Wesep, RA, et al: Nitric oxide metabolism in wounds. J Surg Res 1997; 71:25–31.

134. Reichner, JS, Meszaros, AJ, Louis, CA, et al: Molecular and metabolic evidence for the restricted expression of inducible nitric oxide synthase in healing wounds. Am J Pathol 1999; 154:1097–1104.

135. Lee, RH, Efron, D, Tantry, U, et al: Nitric oxide in the healing wound: A time-course study. J Surg Res 2001; 101:104–108.

136. Sunderkotter, C, Goebeler, M, Schulze-Osthoff, K, et al: Macrophage-derived angiogenesis factors. Pharmacol Ther 1991; 51:195–216.

137. Shapiro, SD, Campbell, EJ, Senior, RM, et al: Proteinases secreted by human mononuclear phagocytes. J Rheumatol Suppl 1991; 27:95–98.

138. Allen, DB, Maguire, JJ, Mahdavian, M, et al: Wound hypoxia and acidosis limit neutrophil bacterial killing mechanisms. Arch Surg 1997; 132:991–996.

139. Niinikoski, JC, Heughan, C, Hunt, TK. Oxygen and carbon dioxide tensions in experimental wounds. Surg Gynecol Obstet 1971; 133:1003–1007.

140. Burke, B, Giannoudis, A, Corke, KP, et al: Hypoxia-induced gene expression in human macrophages: Implications for ischemic tissues and hypoxia-regulated gene therapy. Am J Pathol 2003; 163:1233–1243.

141. Talks, KL, Turley, H, Gatter, KC, et al: The expression and distribution of the hypoxia-inducible factors HIF-1a and HIF-2a in normal human tissues, cancers, and tumor-associated macrophages. Am J Pathol 2000; 157:411–421.

142. Semenza, GL: Signal transduction to hypoxia-inducible factor 1. Biochem Pharmacol 2002; 64:993–998.

143. Lewis, CE, Murdoch, C Macrophage responses to hypoxia: Implications for tumor progression. Am J Pathol 2005; 167:627–635.

144. Albina, JE, Henry, W, Mastrofrancesco, B, et al: Macrophage activation by culture in an anoxic environment. J Immunol 1995; 155:4391–4396.

145. Jaffe, EA, Ruggiero, JT, Falcone, DJ: Monocytes and macrophages synthesize and secrete thrombospondin. Blood 1985; 65:79–84.

146. Belperio, JA, Keane, MP, Douglas, AA, et al: CXC chemokines in angiogenesis. J Leukoc Biol 2000; 68:1–8.

147. Fivenson, DP, Faria, DT, Nickoloff, BJ, et al: Chemokine and inflammatory cytokine changes during chronic wound healing. Wound Repair Regen 1997; 5:310–322.

148. Cumberbatch, M, Dearman, RJ, Griffiths, CE, et al: Langerhans cell migration. Clin Exp Dermatol 2000; 25:413–418.

149. Schuler, G, Steinman, R M: Murine epidermal Langerhans cells mature into potent immunostimulatory dendritic cells in vitro. J Exp Med 1985; 161:526–546.

150. Heufler, C, Koch, F, Schuler, G: Granulocyte/macrophage colony-stimulating factor and interleukin 1 mediate the maturation of murine epidermal Langerhans cells into potent immunostimulatory dendritic cells. J Exp Med 1988; 167:700–705.

151. Havran, WL, Jameson, JM, Witherden, DA: Epithelial cells and their neighbors III: Interactions between intraepithelial lymphocytes and neighboring epithelial cells. Am J Physiol Gastrointest Liver Physiol 2005; 289:627–630.

152. Jameson, JM, Cauvi, G, Witherden, DA, et al: A role for skin γδ T cells in wound repair. Science 2002; 296:747–749.

153. Jameson, JM, Cauvi, G, Sharp, LL, et al: γδ-T cell-induced hyaluronan production by epithelial cells regulates inflammation. J Exp Med 2005; 201:1269–1279.

154. Marshall, JS: Mast-cell response to pathogens. Nat Rev Immunol 2004; 4:787–799.

155. Weller, CL, Collington, SJ, Brown, JK, et al: Leukotriene B₄, an activation product of mast cells, is a chemoattractant for their progenitors. J Exp Med 2005; 201:1961–1971.

156. Davidson, S, Gilead, L, Amira, M, et al: Synthesis of chondroitin sulfate D and heparin proteoglycans in murine lymph node-derived mast cells: The dependence on fibroblasts. J Biol Chem 1990; 265:12324–12330.

157. Gilead, L, Livni, N, Eliakim, R, et al: Human gastric mucosal mast cells are chondroitin sulfate E-containing cells. Immunology 1987; 62:23–28.

158. Nathan, C: Points of control in inflammation. Nature 2002; 420:846–852.

159. Mellor, EA, Frank, N, Soler, D, et al: Expression of the type 2 receptor for cysteinyl leukotrienes (CysLT2R) by human mast cells: Functional distinction from CysLT1R. Proc Natl Acad Sci USA 2003; 100:11589–11593.

160. Tepper, OM, Capla, JM, Galiano, RD, et al: Adult vasculogenesis occurs through the in situ recruitment, proliferation, and tubulization of circulating bone marrow derived cells. Blood 2005; 105:1068–1077.

161. Reyes, M, Dudek, A, Jahagirdar, B, et al: Origin of endothelial progenitors in human postnatal bone marrow. J Clin Invest 2002; 109:337–346.

162. Takahashi, T, Kalka, C, Masuda, H, et al: Ischemia- and cytokine-induced mobilization of bone marrow-derived endothelial progenitor cells for neovascularization. Nat Med 1999; 5:434–438.

163. Asahara, T, Murohara, T, Sullivan, A, et al: VEGF contributes to postnatal neovascularization by mobilizing bone marrow-derived endothelial cells. EMBO J 1999; 18:3964–3972.

164. Bauer, SM, Goldstein, LJ, Bauer, RJ, et al: The bone marrow-derived endothelial progenitor cell response is impaired in delayed wound healing from ischemia. J Vasc Surg 2006; 43:134–141.

165. Bauer, SM, Bauer, RJ, Velazquez, OC: Angiogenesis, vasculogenesis, and induction of healing in chronic wounds. Vasc Endovascular Surg 2005; 39: 293–306.

166. Bauer, SM, Bauer, RJ, Liu, ZJ, et al: Vascular endothelial growth factor-C promotes vasculogenesis, angiogenesis, and collagen constriction in three-dimensional collagen gels. J Vasc Surg 2005; 41:699–707.

167. Hanahan, D: Signaling vascular morphogenesis and maintenance. Science 1997; 277:48–50.

168. Carmeliet, P: Mechanism of angiogenesis and arteriogenesis. Nat Med 2000; 6:389–395.

169. Velazquez, OC, Snyder, R, Liu, ZJ, et al: Fibroblast-dependent differentiation of human microvascular endothelial cells into capillary-like 3-dimensional networks. FASEB J 2002; 16:1316–1318.

170. Liu, ZJ, Snyder, R, Souma, A, et al: VEGF-A and alphaVbeta3 integrin synergistically rescue angiogenesis via N-Ras and PI3-K signaling in human microvascular endothelial cells. FASEB J 2003; 17:1931–1933.

171. Ceradini, DJ, Kulkarni, AR, Callaghan, MJ, et al: Progenitor cell trafficking is regulated by hypoxic gradients through HIF-1 induction of SDF-1. Nat Med 2004; 10:858–864.

172. Aicher, A, Heeschen, C, Mildner-Rihm, C, et al: Essential role of endothelial nitric oxide synthase for mobilization of stem and progenitor cells. Nat Med 2003; 9:1370–1376.

173. Arnold, F, West, D, Kumar, S: Wound healing: The effect of macrophage and tumor derived angiogenesis factors on skin graft vascularization. Bri J Exp Pathol 1987; 68:569–574.

174. Kalebic, T, Garbisa, S, Glaser, B, et al: Basement membrane collagen: Degradation by migrating endothelial cells. Science 1983; 221:281.

175. Li, J, Zhang, Y, Kirsner, RS. Angiogenesis in wound repair: Angiogenic growth factors and the extracellular matrix. Microsc Res Tech 2003; 60:107–114.

176. Keck, PJ, Hauser, SD, Krivi, G, et al: Vascular permeability factor, an endothelial cell mitogen related to PDGF. Science 1989; 246:1309–1313.

177. Suri, C, Jones, P, Patan, S, et al: Requisite role of angiopoietin-1, a ligand for the TIE2 receptor, during embryonic angiogenesis. Cell 1996; 87:1171–1180.

178. Folkman, J, Klagsbrun, M: Angiogenic factors. Science 1987; 235: 442–448.

179. Yang, EY, Moses, HL: Transforming growth factor beta 1-induced migration, proliferation, and angiogenesis in the chicken chorioallantoic membrane. J Cell Biol 1990; 111:731–741.

180. de Vries, C, Escobedo, JA, Ueno, H, et al: The fms-like tyrosine kinase, a receptor for vascular endothelial growth factor. Science 1992; 255:989–991.

181. Conn, G, Bayne, ML, Soderman, DD, et al: Amino acid and cDNA sequences of a vascular endothelial cell mitogen that is homologous to platelet-derived growth factor. Proc Natl Acad Sci USA 1990; 87:2628–2632.

182. Senger, DR, Ledbetter, SR, Claffey, KP, et al: Stimulation of endothelial cell migration by vascular permeability factor/vascular endothelial growth factor through cooperative mechanisms involving the alphavbeta3 integrin, osteopontin, and thrombin. Am J Pathol 1996; 149:293–305.

183. Senger, DR, Claffey, KP, Benes, JE, et al: Angiogenesis promoted by vascular endothelial growth factor: Regulation through alpha1beta1 and alpha2beta1 integrins. Proc Natl Acad Sci USA 1997; 94:13612–13617.

184. Gerber, HP, Dixit, V, Ferrara, N: Vascular endothelial growth factor induces expression of the antiapoptotic proteins Bcl-2 and A1 in vascular endothelial cells. J Biol Chem 1998; 237:13313–13316.

185. Berse, B, Brown, LF, Van de Water, L, et al: Vascular permeability factor (vascular endothelial growth factor) gene is expressed differentially in normal tissues, macrophages, and tumors. Mol Biol Cell 1992; 3:211–220.

186. Papapetropoulos, A, Fulton, D, Mahboubi, K, et al: Angiopoietin-1 inhibits endothelial cell apoptosis via the Akt/survivin pathway. J Biol Chem 2000; 275:9102–9105.

187. Fujikawa, K, de Aos, Scherpenseel, I, Jain, SK, et al: Role of PI 3-kinase in angiopoietin-1-mediated migration and attachment-dependent survival of endothelial cells. Exp Cell Res 1999; 253:663–672.

188. Hayes, AJ, Huang, WQ, Mallah, J, et al: Angiopoietin-1 and its receptor Tie-2 participate in the regulation of capillary-like tubule formation and survival of endothelial cells. Microvasc Res 1999; 58:224–237.

189. Peters, KG, Werner, S, Chen, G, et al: Two FGF receptor genes are differentially expressed in epithelial and mesenchymal tissues during limb formation and organogenesis in the mouse. Development 1992; 114:233–243.

190. Brown, KJ, Maynes, SF, Bezos, A, et al: A novel in vitro assay for human angiogenesis. Lab Invest 1996; 75:539–555.

191. Kanda, S, Landgren, E, Ljungstrom, M, et al: Fibroblast growth factor receptor 1 induced differentiation of endothelial cell line established from tsA58 large T transgenic mice. Cell Growth Differ 1996; 7:383–395.

192. Baird, A, Mormede, P, Bohlen, P: Immunoreactive fibroblast growth factor in cells of peritoneal exudate suggests its identity with macrophage-derived growth factor. Biochem Biophys Res Commun 1985; 126:358–364.

193. Schweigerer, L, Neufeld, G, Friedman, J, et al: Capillary endothelial cells express basic fibroblast growth factor, a mitogen that promotes their own growth. Nature 1987; 325:257–259.

194. Kandel, J, Bossy-Wetzel, E, Radvanyi, F, et al: Neovascularization is associated with a switch to the export of bFGF in the multistep development of fibrosarcoma. Cell 1991; 66:1095–1104.

195. Gualandris, A, Presta, M: Transcriptional and posttranscriptional regulation of urokinase-type plasminogen activator expression in endothelial cells by basic fibroblast growth factor. J Cell Physiol 1995; 162:400–409.

196. Sepp, NT, Li, LJ, Lee, KH, et al: Basic fibroblast growth factor increases expression of the alpha v beta 3 integrin complex on human microvascular endothelial cells. J Invest Dermatol 1994; 103:295–299.

197. Brooks, PC, Stromblad, S, Sanders, LC, et al: Localization of matrix metalloproteinase MMP-2 to the surface of invasive cells by interaction with integrin alpha v beta 3. Cell 1996; 85:683–693.

198. Franzen, P, ten Dijke, P, Ichijo, H, et al: Cloning of a TGF-beta type I receptor that forms a heteromeric complex with the TGF beta type II receptor. Cell 1993; 75:681–692.

199. Lin, HY, Wang, XF, Ng-Eaton, E, et al: Expression cloning of the TGF-beta type II receptor, a functional transmembrane serine/threonine kinase. Cell 1992; 68:775–785.

200. Merwin, JR, Anderson, JM, Kocher, O, et al: Transforming growth factor beta 1 modulates extracellular matrix organization and cell-cell junctional complex formation during in vitro angiogenesis. J Cell Physiol 1990; 142:117–128.

201. Enenstein, J, Waleh, NS, Kramer, RH: Basic FGF and TGF-beta differentially modulate integrin expression of human microvascular endothelial cells. Exp Cell Res 1992; 203:499–503.

202. Collo, G, Pepper, MS: Endothelial cell integin alpha5beta1 expression is modulated by cytokines and during migration in vitro. J Cell Sci 1999; 112:569–578.

203. Sankar, S, Mahooti-Brooks, N, Bensen, L, et al: Modulation of transforming growth factor beta receptor levels on microvascular endothelial cells during in vitro angiogenesis. J Clin Invest 1996; 97:1436–1446.

204. Falcone, DJ, McCaffrey, TA, Haimovitz-Friedman, A, et al: Transforming growth factor-beta 1 stimulates macrophage urokinase expression and release of matrix-bound basic fibroblast growth factor. J Cell Physiol 1993; 155:595–605.

205. Kim, KY, Jeong, SY, Won, J, et al: Induction of angiogenesis by expression of soluble type II transforming growth factor-beta receptor in mouse hepatoma. J Biol Chem 2001; 276:38781–38786.

206. Trompezinski, S, Pernet, I, Mayoux, C, et al: Transforming growth factor beta-1 and ultraviolet A1 radiation increase production of vascular endothelial growth factor but not endothelin-1 in human dermal fibroblasts. Br J Dermatol 2000; 143:539–545.

207. Sanchez-Elsner, T, Botella, LM, Velasco, B, et al: Synergistic cooperation between hypoxia and transforming growth factor-beta pathways on human vascular endothelial growth factor gene expression. J Biol Chem 2001; 276:38527–38535.

208. Ruoslahti, E, Yamaguchi, Y: Proteoglycans as modulators of growth factor activities. Cell 1991; 64:867–869.

209. Witt, DP, Lander, AD: Differential binding of chemokines to glycosaminoglycan subpopulations. Curr Biol, 1994; 4:394–400.

210. Feng, X, Clark, RAF, Galanakis, D, et al: Fibrin and collagen differentially regulate human dermal microvascular endothelial cell integrins: Stabilization of alphav/beta3 mRNA by fibrin 1. J Invest Dermatol 1999; 113:913–919.

211. Abe, R, Donnelly, SC, Peng, T, et al: Peripheral blood fibrocytes: Differentiation pathway and migration to wound sites. J Immunol 2001; 166:7556–7562.

212. Bucala, R, Spiegel, LA, Chesney, M, et al: Circulating fibrocytes define a new leukocyte subpopulation that mediates tissue repair. Mol Med 1994; 1:71–81.

213. Metz, CN: Fibrocytes: A unique cell population implicated in wound healing. Cell Mol Life Sci 2003; 60:1342–1350.

214. Deuel, TF, Kawahara, RS, Mustoe, TA, et al: Growth factors and wound healing: Platelet-derived growth factor as a model cytokine. Ann Rev Med 1991; 42:567–584.

215. Heldin, CH, Westermark, B: Mechanism of action and in vivo role of platelet-derived growth factor. Physiol Rev 1999; 79:1283–1316.

216. Welch, MP, Odland, GF, Clark, RA: Temporal relationships of F-actin bundle formation, collagen and fibronectin matrix assembly, and fibronectin receptor expression to wound contraction. J Cell Biol 1990; 110:133–145.

217. Greiling, D, Clark, RA: Fibronectin provides a conduit for fibroblast transmigration from collagenous stroma into fibrin clot provisional matrix. J Cell Sci 1997; 110:861–870.

218. Xu, J, Clark, RA: Extracellular matrix alters PDGF regulation of fibroblast integrins. J Cell Biol 1996; 132:239–249.

219. Chen, WT: Proteases associated with invadopodia, and their role in degradation of extracellular matrix. Enzyme Protein 1996; 49:59–71.

220. Birkedal-Hansen, H, Moore, WG, Bodden, MK, et al: Matrix metalloproteinases: A review. Crit Rev Oral Biol Med 1993; 4:197–250.

221. Schafer, BM, Katharina, M, Eickhoff, U, et al: Plasminogen activation in healing human wounds. Am J Pathol 1994; 144:1269–1280.

222. Steffensen, B, Hakkinen, L, Larjava, H: Proteolytic events of wound healing: Coordinated interactions among matrix metalloproteinases, integrins, and extracellular matrix molecules. Crit Rev Oral Biol Med 2001; 12:373–398.

223. Schneider, IC, Haugh, JM: Quantitative elucidation of a distinct spatial gradient-sensing mechanism in fibroblasts. J Cell Biol 2005; 171:883–892.

224. Grotendorst, GR: Alteration of the chemotactic response of NIH/3T3 cells to PDGF by growth factors, transformation, and tumor promoters. Cell 1984; 36:279.

225. Ross, R, Bowen-Pope, DF, Raines, EW: Platelet-derived growth factor: Its potential roles in wound healing, atherosclerosis, neoplasia, and growth and development. Ciba Found Symp 1985; 116:98.

226. Buckley, A, Davidson, JM, Kamerath, CD, et al: Epidermal growth factor increases granulation tissue formation dose dependently. J Surg Res 1987; 43:322.

227. Franklin, TJ, Gregory, H, Morris, WP: Acceleration of wound healing by recombinant human urogastrone (epidermal growth factor). J Lab Clin Med 1986; 108:103.

228. Roberts, AB, Sporn, MB: Transforming growth factor-beta: Potential common mechanisms mediating its effects on embryogenesis, inflammation-repair, and carcinogenesis. Int J Rad Appl Instrum B 1987; 14:435.

229. Kanzler, MH, Gorsulowsky, DC, Swanson, NA: Basic mechanisms in the healing cutaneous wounds. J Dermatol Surg Oncol 1986; 12:1156.

230. McGrath, MH, Hundahl, SA: The spatial and temporal quantification of myofibroblasts. Plast Reconstr Surg 1982; 69:975.

231. Pierce, G, Mustoe, T, Altrock, B: Role of platelet-derived growth factor in wound healing. J Cell Biochem 1991; 45:319–326.

232. Woodley, DT, O'Keefe, EJ, Prunieras, J: Cutaneous wound healing: A model for cell-matrix interactions. J Am Acad Dermatol 1985; 12:420.

233. Varga, J, Jimenez, SA: Stimulation of normal human fibroblast collagen production and processing by transforming growth factor-beta. Biochem Biophys Res Commun 1986; 138:974.

234. Burgeson, RE: The collagens of skin. Curr Probl Dermatol 1987; 17:61.

235. Fleischmajer, R: Collagen fibrillogenesis: A mechanism of structural biology. J Invest Dermatol 1986; 5:553.

236. Braveman, IM, Fonferko, E: Studies in cutaneous aging I: The elastic fiber network. J Invest Dermatol 1982; 78:434.

237. Mier, PD, Cotton, DWK: The Molecular Biology of Skin. Blackwell Scientific, London, 1976.

238. Stewart, WD, Danto, JL, Maddin, S: Dermatology.; St. Louis, CV Mosby, 1974.

239. Lever, WF, Schaumberg-Lever, G: Histopathology of Skin, ed. 6. Philadelphia, Lippincott Williams & Wilkins, 1983.

240. Anseth, A: Glycosaminoglycans in corneal regeneration. Exp Eye Res 1961; 1:122.

241. Price, RD, Myers, S, Leigh, IM, et al: The role of hyaluronic acid in wound healing. Am J Clin Dermatol 2005; 6:393–402.

242. Heldin, P, Laurent, TC, Heldin, CH: Effect of growth factors on hyaluronan synthesis in cultured human fibroblasts. Biochem J 1989; 258:919–922.

243. Wood, GC: The formation of fibrils from collagen solutions: Effect of chondroitin sulfate and other naturally occurring polyanions on the rate of formation. Biochem J 1960; 75:605.

244. Hinz, B: Formation and function of the myofibroblast during tissue repair. J Invest Dermatol 2007; 127:526–537.

245. Tomasek, JJ, Gabbiani, G, Hinz, B, et al: Myofibroblasts and mechanoregulation of connective tissue remodelling. Nat Rev Mol Cell Biol 2002; 3:349–363.

246. Desmouliere, A, Rubbia-Brandt, L, Grau, G, et al: Heparin induces α-smooth muscle actin expression in cultured fibroblasts and in granulation tissue myofibroblasts. Lab Invest 1992; 67:716–726.

247. Rubbia-Brandt, L, Sappino, AP, Gabbiani, G: Locally applied GM-CSF induces the accumulation of α-smooth muscle actin

containing myofibroblasts. Virchows Arch B Cell Pathol Incl Mol Pathol 1991; 60:73–82.

248. Gabbiani, G, Ryan, GB, Majno, G Presence of modified fibroblasts in granulation tissue and their possible role in wound contraction. Experientia 1971; 27:549–550.

249. Hinz, B, Mastrangelo, D, Iselin, CE, et al: Mechanical tension controls granulation tissue contractile activity and myofibroblast differentiation. Am J Pathol 2001; 159:1009–1020.

250. Serini, G, Bochaton-Piallat, ML, Ropraz, P, et al, The fibronectin domain ED-A is crucial for myofibroblastic phenotype induction by transforming growth factor-beta1. J Cell Biol 1998; 142:873–881.

251. Werner, S, Krieg, T, Smola, H: Keratinocyte-fibroblast interactions in wound healing. J Invest Dermatol 2007; 127:998–1008.

252. Vaughan, MB, Howard, EW, Tomasek, JJ: Transforming growth factor-beta1 promotes the morphological and functional differentiation of the myofibroblast. Exp Cell Res 2000; 257:180–189.

253. Ronnov-Jessen, L, Petersen, OW: Induction of alpha-smooth muscle actin by transforming growth factor-beta1 in quiescent human breast gland fibroblasts: Implications for myofibroblast generation in breast neoplasia. Lab Invest 1993; 68:696–707.

254. Roberts, AB, Sporn, MB: Transforming growth factor-β. In: Clark, RA, (ed.): The Molecular and Cellular Biology of Wound Repair. Plenum Press, New York, 1996, pp. 275–308.

255. O'Kane, S, Ferguson, MW: Transforming growth factor-betas and wound healing. Int J Biochem Cell Biol 1997; 29:63–78.

256. Massague, J: The transforming growth factor-beta family. Ann Rev Cell Biol 1990; 6:597–641.

257. Border, WA, Noble, NA: Transforming growth factor-beta in tissue fibrosis. N Engl J Med 1994; 331:1286–1292.

258. Schmid, P, Itin, P, Cherry, G, et al: Enhanced expression of transforming growth factor-beta type I and type II receptors in wound granulation tissue and hypertrophic scar. Am J Pathol 1998; 152:485–493.

259. Kim, SJ, Angel, P, Lafyatis, R, et al: Autoinduction of transforming growth factor-beta1 is mediated by the AP-1 complex. Mol Cell Biol 1990; 10:1492–1497.

260. Dugina, V, Fontao, L, Chaponnier, C, et al: Focal adhesion features during myofibroblastic differentiation are controlled by intracellular and extracellular factors. J Cell Sci 2001; 114:3285–3296.

261. Bostrom, H, Willets, K, Penky, M, et al: PDGF-A signaling is a critical event in lung alveolar mofibroblast development and alveogenesis. Cell 1996; 85:863–873.

262. Hinz, B, Celetta, G, Tomasek, JJ, et al: Alpha-smooth muscle actin expression upregulates fibroblast contractile activity. Mol Biol Cell 2001; 12:2730–2741.

263. Arora, PD, McCulloch, CA: Dependence of collagen remodelling on α-smooth muscle actin expression by fibroblasts. J Cell Physiol 1994; 159:161–175.

264. Aurora, PD, Narani, N, McCulloch, CA: The compliance of collagen gels regulates transforming growth factor-beta induction of alpha-smooth muscle actin in fibroblasts. Am J Pathol 1999; 154:871–882.

265. Hinz, B, Pittet, P, Smith-Clerc, J, et al: Alpha-smooth muscle actin is crucial for focal adhesion maturation in myofibroblasts. Mol Biol Cell 2003; 14:2508–2519.

266. Eckes, B, Kreig, T: Regulation of connective tissue homeostasis in the skin by mechanical forces. Clin Exp Rheumatol 2004; 22:S73–S76.

267. Marenzana, M, Wilson-Jones, N, Mudera, V, et al: The origins and regulation of tissue tension: Identification of collagen tension-fixation process in vitro. Exp Cell Res 2006; 312:423–433.

268. Fung, YC: Mechanical Properties of Living Tissues, ed. 2. Springer Verlag, New York, 1993.

269. Discher, DE, Janmey, P, Wang, YL: Tissue cells feel and respond to the stiffness of their substrate. Science 2005; 310:1139–1143.

270. Kaufman, LJ, Brangwynne, CP, Kasza, KE, et al: Glioma expansion in collagen I matrices: Analyzing collagen concentration-dependent growth and motility patterns. Biophys J 2005; 89:635–650.

271. Yeung, T, Georges, PC, Flanagan, LA, et al: Effects of substrate stiffness on cell morphology, cytoskeletal structure, and adhesion. Cell Motil Cytoskeleton 2005; 60:24–34.

272. Goffin, JM, Pittet, P, Csucs, G, et al: Focal adhesion size controls tension-dependent recruitment of alpha-smooth muscle actin to stress fibers. J Cell Biol 2006; 172:259–268.

273. Desmouliere, A, Redard, M, Darby, I, et al: Apoptosis mediates the decrease in cellularity during the transition between granulation tissue and scar. Am J Pathol 1995; 146:56–66.

274. Grinnell, F, Zhu, M, Carlson, MA, et al: Release of mechanical tension triggers apoptosis of human fibroblasts in a model of regressing granulation tissue. Exp Cell Res 1999; 248:608–619.

275. Shephard, P, Martin, G, Smola-Hess, S, et al: Myofibroblast differentiation is induced in keratinocyte fibroblast co-cultures and is antagonistically regulated by endogenous transforming growth factor-beta and interleukin-1. Am J Pathol 2004; 164:2055–2066.

276. Higashi, K, Inagaki, Y, Fujimori, K, et al: Interferon-gamma interferes with transforming growth factor-beta signaling through direct interaction of YB-1 with Smad3. J Biol Chem 2003; 278:43470–43479.

277. Schurch, W, Seemayer, TA, Hinz, B, et al: The myofibroblast. In: Mills, SE. (ed.): Histology for Pathologists. Philadelphia, Lippincott Williams & Wilkins, 2006.

278. Jimenez, P, Rampy, M: Keratinocyte growth factor-2 accelerates wound healing in incisional wounds. J Surg Res 1999; 81:238–242.

279. Green, KJ, Jones, JC: Desmosomes and hemidesmosomes: Structure and function of molecular components. FASEB J 1996; 10:871–881.

280. Green, KJ, Gaudry, CA: Are desmosomes more than tethers for intermediate filaments? Nat Rev Mol Cell Biol 2000; 1:208–216.

281. Borradori, L, Sonneberg, A: Structure and function of hemidesmosomes: More than simple adhesion complexes. J Invest Dermatol 1999; 112:411–418.

282. Krawczyk, WS, Wilgram, GF: Hemidesmosome and desmosome morphogenesis during epidermal wound healing. J Ultrastruct Res 1973; 45:93–101.

283. Ortonne, JP, Löning, T, Schmitt, D, et al: Immunomorphological and ultrastructural aspects of keratinocyte migration in epidermal wound healing. Virchows Arch A Pathol Anat Histol 1981. 392:217–230.

284. Garlick, JA, Taichman, LB: Fate of human keratinocytes during reepithelialization in an organotypic culture model. Lab Invest 1994; 70:916–924.

285. Manske, M, Bade, EG: Growth factor-induced cell migration: Biology and methods of analysis. Int Rev Cytol 1994; 155:49–96.

286. Felsenfeld, DP, Schwartzberg, PL, Venegas, A, et al: Selective regulation of integrin-cytoskeletal interactions by the tyrosine kinase. Src. Nat Cell Biol 1999; 1:200–206.

287. Werner, S, Peters, KG, Longaker, MT, et al: Large induction of keratinocyte growth factor expression in the dermis during wound healing. Proc Natl Acad Sci USA 1992; 89:6896–6900.

288. Carpenter, G: EGF: New tricks for an old growth factor. Curr Opin in Cell Biol 1993; 5:261–264.

289. Iwamoto, R, Mekada, E: Heparin-binding EGF-like growth factor: A juxtacrine growth factor. Cytokine Growth Factor Rev 2000; 11:335–344.

290. Derynk, R: Transforming growth factor alpha. Cell 1988; 54:593–595.

291. Stracke, ML, Kohn, EC, Aznavoorian, SA, et al: Insulin-like growth factors stimulate chemotaxis in human melanoma cells. Biochem Biophys Res Commun 1988; 30:1076–1083.

292. Yue, J, Mulder, KM: Transforming growth factor-beta signal transduction in epithelial cells. Pharmacol Ther 2001; 91:1–34.

293. Hoffmann, J, Twiesselmann, C, Kummer, MP, et al: A possible role for the Alzheimer amyloid precursor protein in the regulation of epidermal basal cell proliferation. Eur J Cell Biol 2000; 79:905–914.

294. Kirfel, G, Borm, B, Rigort, A, et al: The secretory b-amyloid precursor protein is a motogen for human epidermal keratinocytes. Eur J Cell Biol 2002; 81:664–676.

295. Ossowski, L, Aguirre-Ghiso, JA: Urokinase receptor and integrin partnership: Coordination of signaling for cell adhesion, migration and growth. Curr Opin Cell Biol 2000; 12:613–620.

296. McCawley, LJ, Matrisian, LM: Matrix metalloproteinases: They're not just for matrix anymore! Curr Opin Cell Biol 2001; 13:534–540.

297. Seiki, M: The cell surface: The stage for matrix metalloproteinase regulation of migration. Curr Opin Cell Biol 2002; 14:624–632.

298. Grondahl-Hansen, J, Lund, LR, Ralfkiaer, E, et al: Urokinase- and tissue-type plasminogen activators in keratinocytes during wound reepithelialization in vivo. J Invest Dermatol 1988; 90:790–795.

299. Romer, J, Lund, LR, Eriksen, J, et al: The receptor for urokinase-type plasminogen activator is expressed by keratinocytes at the leading edge during reepithelialization of mouse skin wounds. J Invest Dermatol 1994; 102:519–522.

300. Kirfel, G, Herzog, V: Migration of epidermal keratinocytes: Mechanisms, regulation, and biological significance. Protoplasma 2004; 223:67–78.

301. Grinnell, F: Wound repair, keratinocyte activation and integrin modulation. J Cell Sci 1992; 101:1–5.

302. Werb, Z: ECM and cell surface proteolysis: Regulating cellular ecology. Cell 1997; 91:439–442.

303. Murphy, G, Gravrilovic, J: Proteolysis and cell migration: Creating a path? Curr Opin Cell Biol 1999; 11:614–621.

304. Larjava, H, Salo, T, Haapasalmi, K, et al: Keratinocyte integrins in wound healing and chronic inflammation of the human periodontium. Oral Dis 1996; 2:77–86.

305. Giancotti, FG, Ruoslahti, E: Integrin signaling. Science 1999; 285:1028–1032.

306. Clark, RA: Fibronectin matrix deposition and fibronectin receptor expression in healing and normal skin. J Invest Dermatol 1990; 94:128S–134S.

307. Caviani, A, Zambruno, G, Marconi, A, et al: Distinctive integrin expression in the newly forming epidermis during wound healing in humans. J Invest Dermatol 1993; 101:600–604.

308. Larjava, H, Salo, T, Haapasalmi, K, et al: Expression of integrins and basement membrane components by wound keratinocytes. J Clin Invest 1993; 92:1425–1435.

309. Gailit, J, Clark, RA: Wound repair in the context of extracellular matrix. Curr Opin in Cell Biol 1994; 6:717–725.

310. Regen, CM, Horwitz, AF: Dynamics of beta 1 integrin-mediated adhesive contacts in motile fibroblasts. J Cell Biol 1992; 119:1347–1359.

311. Bard, JBL, Hay, ED: The behaviour of fibroblasts from the developing avian cornea: Morphology and movement in situ and in vitro. Cell Biol 1975; 67:400–418.

312. Chen, WT: Mechanisms of retraction of the trailing edge during fibroblast movement. J Cell Biol 1981; 90:187–200.

313. Juliano, R: Cooperation between soluble factors and integrin-mediated cell anchorage in the control of cell growth and differentiation. Bioessays 1996; 18:911–917.

314. Shyy, JY, Chien, S: Role of integrins in cellular responses to mechanical stress and adhesion. Curr Opin Cell Biol 1997; 9:707–713.

315. Rosenfeldt, H, Lee, DJ, Grinnell, F: Increased c-fos mRNA expression by human fibroblasts contracting stressed collagen matrices. Mol Cell Biol 1998; 18:2659–2667.

316. Sabiston, D: Textbook of Surgery: The Biologic Basis of Modern Surgical Practice, ed. 15. St. Louis, Saunders, 1997.

317. Ehrlich, H, Krummel, T: Regulation of wound healing from a connective tissue perspective. Wound Repair Regen 1996; 4:203.

318. Soo, C, Shaw, WW, Zhang, X, et al: Differential expression of matrix metalloproteinases and their tissue-derived inhibitors in cutaneous wound repair. Plast Reconstr Surg 2000; 105:638–647.

319. Werner, S, Grose, R: Regulation of wound healing by growth factors and cytokines. Physiol Rev 2003; 83:835–870.

320. Werb, Z, Tremble, P, Damsky, CH: Regulation of extracellular matrix degradation by cell-extracellular matrix interactions. Cell Differ Dev 1990; 32:299–306.

321. Circolo, A, Welgus, HG, Pierce, GF, et al: Differential regulation of the expression of proteinases/antiproteinases in fibroblasts: Effects of interleukin-1 and platelet-derived growth factor. J Biol Chem 1991; 266:12283–12288.

322. Monaco, JL, Lawrence, WT: Acute wound healing: An overview. Clin Plast Surg 2003; 30:1–12.

323. Lawrence, WT: Physiology of the acute wound. Clin Plast Surg, 1998; 25:321–340.

324. DiPietro, LA, Nissen, NN, Gamelli, RL, et al: Thrombospondin 1 synthesis and function in wound repair. Am J Pathol 1996; 148:1851–1860.

325. Raugi, GJ, Olerud, JE, Gown, AM: Thrombospondin in early human wound tissue. J Invest Dermatol 1987; 89:551–552.

326. Reed, MJ, Puolakkainen, P, Lane, TF, et al: Differential expression of SPARC and thrombospondin1 in wound repair: Immunolocalization and in situ hybridization. J Histochem Cytochem 1993; 41:1467–1477.

327. Esser, S, Wolburg, K, Wolburg, H, et al: Vascular endothelial growth factor induces endothelial fenestrations in vitro. J Cell Biol 1998; 140:947–959.

328. Watt, FM, Hogan, BL: Out of Eden: Stem cells and their niches. Science 2000; 287:1427–1430.

329. Spradling, A, Drummond-Barbarosa, D, Kai, T: Stem cells find their niche. Nature 2001; 414:98–104.

330. Martin, P, Wound healing–Aiming for perfect skin regeneration. Science 1997; 276:75–81.

331. Sengel, P: Epidermal-dermal interactions. In: Bereiter-Hahn, J, Matolsty, G, Richards, KS. (eds): Biology of the Integument. Berlin, Verlag-Springer, 1986.

332. Nohno, T, Kawakami, Y, Ohuchi, H, et al: Involvement of the sonic hedgehog gene in chick feather formation. Biochem Biophys Res Commun 1995; 206:33–39.

333. Jahoda, CA: Induction of follicle formation and hair growth by vibrissa dermal papillae implanted into rat ear wounds: Vibrissa-type fibres are specified. Development 1992; 115:110–1109.

334. McCluskey, J, Martin, P: Analysis of the tissue movements of embryonic wound healing—diI studies in the limb bud stage mouse embryo. Dev Biol 1995; 170:102–114.

335. Martin, P, Lewis, J: Actin cables and epidermal movement in embryonic wound healing. Nature 1992; 360: 179–183.

336. Heath, JP: Epithelial cell migration in the intestine. Cell Biol Int 1996; 20:139–146.

337. Whitby, DJ, Ferguson, MWJ: Immunohistochemical localization of growth factors in fetal wound healing. Dev Biol 1991; 147:207–215.

338. Martin, P, Dickson, MC, Millan, FA, et al: Rapid induction and clearance of TGF1 is an early response to wounding in the mouse embryo. Dev Gen 1993; 14:225–238.

339. Estes, JM, VandeBerg, JS, Adzick, NS, et al: Phenotypic and functional features of myofibroblasts in sheep fetal wounds. Differentiation 1994; 56:173–181.

340. Shah, M, Foreman, DM, Ferguson, MW: Control of scarring in adult wounds by neutralising antibody to transforming growth factor β. Lancet 1992; 339:213–214.

341. Shah, M, Foreman, DM, Ferguson, MW: Neutralisation of TGF-beta 1 and TGF-beta 2 or exogenous addition of TGF-beta 3 to cutaneous rat wounds reduces scarring. J Cell Sci 1995; 108:985–1002.

Growth Factors and Extracellular Matrix in Wound Repair

Jeffrey M. Davidson, PhD

Introduction

A wound site begins as a void or zone of destruction that must be reorganized by adjacent and circulating cells into a tissue that has both mechanical integrity and proper architecture. This reorganization is determined by the progressive construction and remodeling of an extracellular matrix (ECM) that serves as a scaffold for cell migration and growth. In the absence of a matrix, cells cannot move or carry out their normal duties. The matrix around cells defines a microenvironment that provides both mechanical and biochemical information to cells through specific receptors, and it also acts as a biological buffer for the cell-derived signals that drive wound healing.

The orchestrated process of wound healing is carried out by a characteristic progression of cellular performers that communicate by using hormone-like signal proteins: growth factors and cytokines. Each of these signals is recognized on the target cell surface by specific receptors, which then convert the binding interaction into a chemical signal within the cell. The term *cytokines* is used to describe a collection of small protein signal molecules that are principally derived from cells of the inflammatory system.[1] Perhaps the best-known cytokines are the *interleukins,*[2] leukocyte intercellular signaling molecules; however, a wide variety of other secreted cytokines interact with their receptors to induce responses such as cell movement, cell differentiation, or even cell death. In contrast to cytokines, which are frequently involved in regulating inflammation, the cellular *growth factors* are a distinct group of proteins crucial to the repair process.[3] As implied by their name, the principal function of these protein molecules is to promote cell and tissue growth, although these molecules often stimulate cell movement, migration, and differentiation. Some of the growth factors also affect the processes of extracellular matrix accumulation and remodeling. All these signal molecules are regarded as hormones that act at the local tissue level to bring about specific tissue responses. As such, they act in autocrine, paracrine, or juxtacrine fashion, depending on the nature of the target cell. (Fig. 3.1) Growth factors are also stored and released by the extracellular matrix, and many of the signals generated by these factors will occur only if the cell is also bound to an extracellular matrix. (Fig. 3.2)

The removal of damaged extracellular matrix and the remodeling of newly formed ECM is carried out by *proteinases*, which are protein-degrading enzymes produced by both inflammatory and connective tissue cells.[4,5] Proteinases inside the cell deal with the processing of proteins before secretion or the complete degradation of partially digested fragments of matrix or foreign material that is engulfed by the cell. Proteinases acting outside the cell are crucial for degrading foreign material, for promoting cell movement through tissue spaces, and for tightly regulating the abundance and distribution of

Principles of Growth Factor Interaction

Autocrine

Paracrine

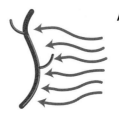

Mobilization

Extracellular matrix

Juxtacrine

Figure 3•1 *Principles of growth factor interaction. Cells both secrete and react to growth factors as a form of intercellular communication. There are three basic modes of signal transmission.* Autocrine *signaling is a mode in which a cell can drive an internal feedback loop by secreting factors (proteins in the case of growth factors) that are bound to and recognized by receptors on the same cell. Receptor binding then signals to the cell interior. In* paracrine *signaling, two different cell types communicate, and there is often an extracellular matrix between them. This matrix often contains highly charged, sulfated sugars bound to proteins (heparan sulfate proteoglycans) that can trap the growth factors in the matrix and act as a buffer. Degradation of these sugars or the matrix is one way to release these stored growth factors. Once released, growth factors can interact directly with their receptors or in a partnership between the receptors and other sulfated sugars chains on the cell surface. In* juxtacrine *signaling, communication is between similar cell types.*

various molecules in the extracellular space. Some proteinases are also important catalysts in biochemical reactions such as blood coagulation.

Extracellular Matrix

Traumatic or surgical wounds cause the destruction of the resident cells and their surrounding extracellular matrix. During the initial healing phase of hemostasis, this void is rapidly filled by blood and plasma to form a fibrin clot with the assistance of blood platelets. The fibrin scaffold, together with the molecules that are discharged from the platelet, forms the first *provisional*

Cell Division

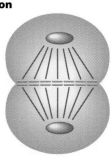

Epidermal growth factor

Platelet derived growth factor

Insulin-like growth factor

Keratinocyte growth factor

Angiogenesis

Fibroblast growth factor

Vascular endothelial growth factor

Matrix Modification

Transforming growth factor-β
Connective tissue growth factor

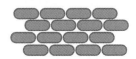

Figure 3•2 *Properties of growth factors. This figure illustrates the predominant, but not exclusive, modes of action of some of the more familiar growth factors that have significant effects in wound healing. Factors with a predominant action on cell division tend to produce a highly cellular response. Angiogenic factors promote the formation of new blood vessels. Transforming growth factor-ß and connective tissue growth factor have more striking effects on extracellular matrix accumulation in wound tissue. Proper wound healing requires the orchestration of all these types of signals.*

matrix at the wound site.[6] The two key plasma proteins involved in fibrin formation are fibrinogen and thrombin, which is converted from prothrombin by the clotting cascade. Platelets also aggregate and discharge their stored granule contents in response to their exposure to collagen outside of damaged blood vessels. Activated platelets release many factors, but two platelet-derived matrix molecules are significant to the provisional matrix: fibronectin and thrombospondin. Fibronectin is also present in the plasma, but the form found in platelets is a variant that is produced during embryonic development and by the connective tissue cells that subsequently repopulate the wound. Connective tissue cells such as fibroblasts and endothelial cells can migrate into the fibrin clot only if the adhesive protein fibronectin is present. This interaction depends on the presence of a fibronectin-binding integrin called 5ß1 on the cell surface, as discussed below.

Structural Proteins

The extracellular matrix (ECM) governs the integrity and mechanical properties of every tissue. ECM consists of a complex mixture of fibrous, space-filling, and adhesive macromolecules that determine such physical characteristics as tensile strength, elasticity, hydration, and compressibility.[7,8] The best-known and most abundant component of the ECM is *collagen,* which is an ancient family of fiber-forming proteins characterized by a ropelike arrangement of three individual polypeptide chains (triple helix) that confers to the collagen molecule a high degree of tensile strength, resistance to proteolytic degradation, and a highly defined, rigid structure. The very stable triple helix will begin to unfold (melt) above 45°C, leading to the formation of gelatin. The thermal stability of the helix is absolutely dependent on the presence of the amino acid hydroxyproline, which is a modified form of proline that is produced during the synthesis of each chain of the collagen molecule. Ascorbic acid is required for this critical enzymatic step. Cells synthesize and secrete collagen as a larger, soluble precursor, procollagen, which is converted to collagen by enzymatically clipping off non-triple-helical regions at each end of the protein. After secretion and processing has taken place, the collagen molecules can then assemble into fibrils and thence fibers whose organization is stabilized by covalent, chemical cross-links between individual molecules to produce the predominant fibrous component of tendons, ligaments, and skin. Many members of the large collagen family of proteins are specialized to serve more particular functions, such as determining overall fibril diameter or promoting interactions with other components in the extracellular matrix. In addition, several of the collagen types (presently types I to XXVII) have very restricted distributions in either the basement membrane underlying epithelial surfaces or in structures that attach epithelium to underlying connective tissue.[9,10] The stiff, helical regions of several of these "minor" collagens are interrupted by flexible sections that allow the molecules to assume different geometric arrangements, with less emphasis on the pure tensile properties of linear fibers.

Collagen fibers in the skin and elsewhere are composite structures in which the presence of other minor collagen types determines the overall form and function of the arrays of collagen fibers that are seen at the electron microscopic level. For example, the presence of type III and type V collagens in the type I collagen fibers has major effects on fiber diameter and hence extensibility. Type III collagen tends to be relatively more enriched in early wounds, in prenatal development, and in more extensible connective tissues. Type IX collagen, which has a short, non-helical hinge region that likely adds to the flexibility of the collagen chain, seems to use this property to allow part of the helix to align with the fibril while the remainder can project at an angle from the fibril surface. In addition, type IX collagen can be decorated with highly charged, sulfated glycosaminoglycans.

Under physiological conditions, the triple helical part of collagen is degraded only by highly specialized proteolytic enzymes known as *collagenases.*[11] The principal collagenase in humans is matrix metalloproteinase-1 (MMP-1), and this enzyme's unique ability to cleave native, intact (type I to III) collagen molecules at a single site in the helical region causes a significant shift in the thermal stability (melting temperature) of the collagen helix, making it possible for other MMPs, known as gelatinases (MMP-2, MMP-9) to complete the process of collagen degradation. The MMP

family consists of a large number of members, some of which have selective cleavage activity, such as MMP-12 (metalloelastase), MMP-3 (stromelysin, proteoglycans), and MMP-14 (a surface-bound MMP that activates other soluble MMPs by enzymatic cleavage.

Elastin is, as the name implies, a rubberlike protein that is often found in association with collagen in skin, blood vessels, and other elastic tissues.[12] Unlike collagen, elastin does not form highly organized fibers, perhaps because this would interfere with its function as a rubbery, cross-linked network. The unique cross-links in elastin render the protein extremely durable and resistant to degradation. The principal role of elastin appears to be the development of elastic properties in tissues. The elastic fiber, like collagen, is also a composite, in which elastin is deposited on a microfibrillar framework that largely consists of the protein *fibrillin.*[13] Fibrillin is noteworthy because mutations in the protein can lead to Marfan syndrome. In addition, fibrillin is structurally related to a group of proteins known as the large transforming growth factor-ß (TGF-ß) binding proteins.[14] TGF-ß is a growth factor that plays a central role in regulation of matrix synthesis and degradation (see below). Elastin is noteworthy in wound healing because, at least in the skin, it is one of the last components to be replaced during the repair sequence. Cutaneous scars lack elastic fibers for years.

Proteoglycans are composite molecules, as the name implies. They consist of a core protein to which are attached acidic sugar chains (glycosaminoglycans) distinctively built up by a complex enzymatic system in cells that directs the addition of disaccharide subunits and then adds charged groups such as sulfates.[15] Hyaluronic acid is an extremely long, unsulfated glycosaminoglycan chain that is particularly important for cell movement, lubrication of joints, and hydration of tissues.[16,17] These highly charged molecules bind water molecules, and they also interact strongly with many other components in the ECM, including connective tissue proteins and growth factors.

▶ **PEARL 3•1** The extracellular matrix is a dynamic scaffold that both permits and instructs wound reorganization.

Adhesive Proteins

Whether cells are moving about in tissue or fixed in place, they require adhesive interactions with their surroundings in order to give them traction and to react to changes in the mechanical environment. This interaction is accomplished by the pairing of specific cell surface receptors with matrix molecules in the extracellular environment. The classic example of this system of cell-matrix interactions can be seen in the family of *integrin* molecules.[18] Integrins are the principal interface between fibrous structures on the inside and outside of the cell. These matrix receptors each consist of two subunits that are mainly external to the cell but that span the cell membrane. The smaller, interior portion of the protein is closely associated with many elements of the *cytoskeleton* on the cell interior. Thus, the engagement of an integrin with a matrix molecule can transmit a signal to intracellular machinery. On the outer cell surface, these integrins interact with specific sites in extracellular matrix components to provide adhesion and even some recognition functions. Integrins can bind to a number of different collagen types. They are most closely associated with a group of molecules known as cellular *attachment factors,* most of which are glycoproteins, large protein molecules with branched sugar chains attached to the protein backbone. The best known of these adhesive glycoproteins is the molecule fibronectin, a component of plasma that is also produced in a variant form by embryos during development and cells during wound repair.[19] This molecule has many different interactive regions. Fibronectin may form a bridging link from cells (via integrins) to collagen, to heparin or heparin-containing proteoglycans, and to fibrin. Thus, this glycoprotein is a prototype for the intercellular cement that links many of the elements of the matrix together with its constituent cells. Another prominent attachment factor is the plasma protein, vitronectin.[20] Cells themselves produce many other attachment and migration factors, including osteopontin, osteonectin, tenascin, and thrombospondin. These latter two molecules, depending on the cell type and other circumstances, can have anti-adhesive properties.[21]

Collagen has important integrin-mediated interactions. Two distinct platelet integrins react with exposed collagen and newly formed fibrin after vessel injury to initiate the process of degranulation and thrombus formation.[22] A separate set of integrins on fibroblasts recognizes the major collagens in the ECM and utilizes the integrin-collagen interaction for traction and biomechanical feedback.[23,24] As epithelial cells migrate to resurface a wound, they move their collagen-binding integrins to the basal surface in order to permit efficient cell movement.

▸ **PEARL 3•2** Cells need adhesion to the matrix to move and differentiate.

Basement Membranes

Epithelial cells, which cover the body surface and line cavities, are polarized cells with an upper and lower (inner and outer) surface, and they are tightly connected to each other to form continuous sheets. A highly specialized extracellular matrix organization is found in the *basement membrane* (basal lamina) underlying epithelial cells and separating them from connective tissue. This structure also acts as a physical barrier to large molecular complexes and cells. Basement membranes lie under the vascular endothelium of all blood vessels, and they underlie epidermal surfaces. Although basement membranes are usually microscopically thin and evanescent, they serve an important function in maintaining the polar organization of the epithelium, assuring its appropriate attachment to and communication with underlying connective tissue. When tissue injury destroys the basement membrane, an important scaffold for epithelial reorganization is lost. Basement membranes characteristically contain some unique members of each of the extracellular matrix classes already discussed: type IV collagen, which tends to form lattices rather than extended fibers; laminin, a multifunctional, cross-shaped attachment factor; and perlecan, a proteoglycan that is particularly rich in heparan sulfate side chains.[25] Because of the high content of highly charged proteoglycans, basement membranes can bind and store many growth factors. Keratinocytes are connected into the epidermal basement membrane by yet another collagen, type XVIII, which is anchored through the keratinocyte cell membrane and inserted into the ECM of the basement membrane. The epidermal basement membrane is in turn tethered to the underlying ECM by type VII collagen, which forms *anchoring fibrils.* Genetic defects in type VII collagen produce a severe form of the blistering disease, epidermolysis bullosa.

Cytokines, Growth Factors, and Their Receptors

Many growth factors have most significant, positive actions during the wound healing process. There are several common features of growth factors. They are all proteins that are secreted by cells. Growth factors are distinguished from other peptide hormones such as insulin by their *local* action in the cellular environment. (Fig. 3.1) As the name implies, one of the principal actions of these secreted molecules is the ability to stimulate cell division. A few of the factors have important effects on the accumulation of extracellular matrix. (Fig. 3.2) One of the major reasons for this concentrated action is due to the fact that many growth factors are strongly bound to the extracellular matrix, which thus serves as a reservoir for storage and buffering of growth factor action.[26] Growth factor binding to the extracellular matrix can protect these proteins from degradation, but it can also limit their bioavailability as therapeutic agents. Like other peptide hormones, there are very specific, tight interactions between each growth factor and its receptor. When these factors bind to their receptors, changes in the shape of the receptor trigger an amplified chemical cascade in the interior of the cell, leading to biochemical reactions that can stimulate cell movement, cell growth, and the activation of other genes. Excess growth factor activity can produce pathological changes in tissues, and several growth factor-receptor genes can undergo genetic or epigenetic alterations in cancer. The major growth factor categories and their properties are listed in Table 3.1.

▸ **PEARL 3•3** Growth factors signal among and between cells to drive forward the healing process.

Mitogenic Factors

Epidermal growth factor (EGF) is the prototypical growth factor. EGF and its related proteins predominantly stimulate wound healing by promoting cell migration and cell division. This small protein was originally discovered in the salivary gland of male mice, where it was noteworthy for stimulating the premature opening of eyelids in the neonatal mouse. EGF is actually part of a family of related proteins that include epidermal growth factor, transforming growth factor-β, betacellulin, heparin-binding EGF, and amphiregulin. As is true of all the growth factors, these proteins bind to very specific and selective cellular receptors that transmit a set of signals within the cell to stimulate cell growth and division.[27] An unusual feature of the EGF family is that many members actually start out as larger cell surface proteins, with "tails" penetrating into

Table 3•1 Growth Factors, Sources, and Actions

Growth Factor Family	Cell Source	Actions
Transforming Growth Factor β		
TGF-β1	Platelets	Chemotatic for fibroblast
TGF-β2	Fibroblasts	Promotes extracellular matrix formation
TGF-β3	Macrophages	↑Collagen and TIMP synthesis
		↓MMP synthesis
		Reduces scarring
		↓Collagen, ↓Fibronectin
Platelet-Derived Growth Factor		
PDGF-AA, PDGF-BB	Platelets	Activates immune cells and fibroblasts
VEGF	Macrophages	Promotes ECM formation
	Keratinocytes	↑Collagen and TIMP synthesis
	Fibroblasts	↓MMP synthesis
		↑Angiogenesis
Fibroblast Growth Factor		
Acidic FGF, basic FGF	Macrophages	↑Angiogenesis
KGF	Endothelial cells	↑Keratinocyte proliferation and migration
	Fibroblasts	↑ECM deposition
Insulin-like Growth Factor		
IGF-I, IGF-II	Liver	↑Keratinocyte and fibroblast proliferation
Insulin	Skeletal muscle	↑Angiogenesis
	Fibroblasts	↑Collagen synthesis
	Macrophages	↑ECM formation
	Neutrophils	↑Cell metabolism
Epidermal Growth Factor		
EGF, HB-EGF, TGF-α	Keratinocytes	↑Keratinocyte proliferation and migration
Amphiregulin, betacellulin	Macrophages	↑ECM formation
Connective Tissue Growth Factor		
CTGF	Fibroblasts	↑Collagen synthesis
	Endothelial cells	Mediates action of TGF-βs on collagen synthesis
	Epithelial cells	

the cell interior. The active forms are then enzymatically cleaved from the exterior of the cell surface. EGF is extensively processed before being released in its final, soluble form. EGF itself is not stored in cells or the extracellular matrix, and significant amounts are excreted in the urine. However, some members of the EGF family do stick to the matrix. EGF family members are stored on the cell surface, but higher levels of production require activation of gene expression. EGF has been shown in a number of studies to stimulate wound repair in many animal models by accelerating the growth of fibroblasts and epidermal cells[28]; however, this group of proteins has not achieved much clinical success, although EGF is presently used in some formulations for corneal lubrication. EGF, if delivered appropriately, could improve wound filling and resurfacing.

A second important class of growth-stimulating molecules is platelet-derived growth factor (PDGF). This molecule is contained in platelet granules, and the release of PDGF at sites of injury during clot formation is certainly an important aspect of the repair process.[29] As with EGF, the cellular response to this stimulus is dictated by the presence of specific PDGF receptors. PDGF is produced in two isoforms (A and B), and PDGF molecules exist as AA, AB, or BB dimers that are selectively recognized by two different kinds of PDGF receptors. PDGF does have some ability to bind to the extracellular matrix. Based on the knowledge that platelets contain and release a number of growth factors and other proteins involved in cell migration, commercial preparations of platelet lysates have been used in the clinic, their activity being most likely due to the presence of PDGF and other growth factors. Purified PDGF as well as transfected PDGF cDNA can accelerate repair. Recombinant PDGF-BB is the only economically successful growth factor, with significant effects on the improvement of the time taken to complete closure in diabetic foot ulcers.[30,31] PDGF is also associated with pathology. This molecule has been widely implicated in the pathological growth of vascular smooth muscle cells during atherosclerosis, and one of the two peptide chains of PDGF is closely related to a viral (V-SIS) oncogene. Thus, growth factor–like molecules are involved in growth control of transformed cells. PDGFs predominantly stimulate wound healing by stimulating fibroblast migration and division; however, the extracellular matrix initially produced with PDGF tends to have more proteoglycan and less collagen, and there is frequently evidence of greater vascularity. This may be due to the action of PDGF to help generate vascular smooth muscle cells and pericytes that surround venules, arterioles, and capillaries.[32]

The insulin-like growth factors IGF-1 and IGF-2 are small proteins structurally related to insulin. They each have their own cell receptor. Insulin itself can interact with the IGF-1 receptor but at about 100-fold higher concentrations. IGF-1 is a growth factor often associated with bone development as an important downstream target of the action of growth hormone. There are significant circulating levels of IGF-1, but it also can be produced locally. IGF-2 binds to a receptor also known as the mannose-6-phosphate receptor. IGF-2 expression is more closely associated with development than with tissue repair. IGF-1 bioavailability and action is thought to be tightly regulated by a group of molecules known as the

IGF-binding proteins (IGF-BPs). Various members of this group can either facilitate the activity of IGF on its receptor or act as sequestering agents to prevent action. Much of the regulation of IGF could thus be at the level of IGF-BP control. IGF-1, in combination with PDGF, has also had favorable results in cartilage, bone, and periodontal repair.[33]

Hepatocyte growth factor (HGF; scatter factor) has a number of properties that are consistent with a role in wound healing.[34,35] HGF is able to induce cell movement, cell division, and cell rearrangements, all of which are critical elements of the repair process. HGF activity can be controlled by the expression of the gene; the activation of its precursor, proHGF; the level of HGF inhibitors; and the local concentration of its receptor, c-MET. In contrast to some of the other growth factors, some HGF may reach the wound site from the liver as an inactive form. HGF may be particularly influential in the transformation of sedentary epidermal keratinocytes into a migratory phenotype during wound resurfacing.

Angiogenic Growth Factors

Two growth factor classes are significant for their ability to stimulate angiogenesis, the growth of new blood vessels. *Fibroblast growth factor* (FGF) refers to a family of proteins that interact with one or more of four related receptors on a variety of cell types. FGF-1 and FGF-2 (acidic and basic FGF) are particularly noteworthy for their ability to stimulate endothelial cell growth and capillary cell invasion in a variety of models. FGF-2 in particular has shown efficacy in many preclinical wound models. Although it has not achieved acceptance in the United States or European Union, FGF-2 is widely used at present in Japan and China for wound healing in the clinic setting.[36,37] The angiogenic properties of FGF-2 have also lead to a number of clinical trials designed to develop collateral blood supply in ischemic heart muscle. Most forms of FGF have growth effects on many cell populations, although endothelial cells appear to have a greater sensitivity to FGF; however, there are two novel forms of FGF, FGF-7 and FGF-10 (keratinocyte growth factor-1 and -2 [KGF-1 and -2]), that specifically stimulate the proliferation and differentiation of epithelial cells because of unique receptors present on epithelium.[38] Keratinocyte growth factors have a classical *paracrine* mode of action because they are produced by fibroblasts in the dermis and act upon keratinocytes in the epidermis. Although neither KGF has achieved remarkable results in cutaneous wound healing, FGF-10/KGF-2 appears to be helpful in treatment of oral mucositis, a frequent, painful side effect of chemotherapy.

Vascular endothelial growth factor (VEGF), or vascular permeability factor (VPF), is the most selective of the growth factors for endothelial action. VEGF-A to VEGF-D are members of a family of genes with similar activity. Placental growth factor is another member of the VEGF family with activity in wound healing. As the name implies, VEGF acts to stimulate both endothelial cell growth and migration. It is a very potent stimulus for the outgrowth of new capillary microvessels. The name *vascular permeability factor* refers to an important property of VEGF, the ability to increase capillary permeability and leakage of plasma into tissue space. VEGF has received much notoriety for its apparent ability to stimulate the revascularization of ischemic limbs and cardiac muscle.[39] It is very likely that this molecule will assume an important role in the therapy of wound repair, particularly where blood supply is compromised. VEGF alone is able to stimulate neovascularization, but the blood vessels are leaky and hemorrhagic in the absence of surrounding pericytes. The principal growth factor for pericyte stabilization is angiopoietin,[40] although, as previously mentioned, PDGF appears to contribute to the stabilization of capillaries. VEGF has also become a major pharmacological target for the control or suppression of tumor vascularization.[41]

Fibrogenic Factors

TGF-ß is part of a very large superfamily of proteins that are involved in development, growth, and differentiation.[42] Besides TGF-ß itself (there are three different forms in humans), other well-known members of this family are the bone morphogenic proteins, activin, inhibin, and Mullerian inhibitory substance. TGF-ß plays two very prominent, diverse roles in inflammation and repair. TGF-ß is a very potent inhibitor of immune reactivity, and it can modulate the immune system.[43] Indeed, when mice have been created lacking the TGF-ß1 gene, offspring die early in postnatal life from a massive inflammatory reaction. The second major role of TGF-ß is in matrix formation and wound healing, where TGF-ß strongly induces—directly or indirectly—the expression of many connective tissue molecules, including collagen, elastin, fibronectin, and some proteoglycans, while it suppresses the expression of connective tissue–degrading enzymes such as collagenase and related matrix metalloproteinases. TGF-ß also increases the expression of proteinase inhibitors that act on both the metalloenzyme class of proteinases (TIMPs) and the serine proteinase, plasminogen activator inhibitor-1. Thus, it is no surprise that TGF-ß expression is often associated with fibrosis and excessive scarring.[44,45] Administration of TGF-ß has been shown to accelerate repair in many wound models, and clinical trials have been run with TGF-ß isoforms (TGF-ß1, TGF-β2, and TGF-β3) as a treatment for chronic wounds.

Connective tissue growth factor (CTGF) is a newer growth factor introduced in the literature. It is chemically distinct from other growth factors, and it is a member of the CCN cytokine family.[46] Unlike many of the other growth factors, CTGF appears to be highly specific for connective tissue cells such as fibroblasts and chondrocytes. Its expression is associated with sites of tissue repair. CTGF is distinctively able to stimulate selectively connective tissue formation as well. CTGF synthesis is strongly induced by treatment of cells and tissues with TGF-ß, but other factors such as VEGF, mechanical stress, and metabolic stress may also trigger its expression. Recent findings suggest that CTGF may be the downstream signal molecule that actually carries out the matrix-forming activities of TGF-ß. CTGF is considered an important target for fibrosis, since it has relatively selective effects on fibroblasts and their ECM.

All of these growth factors are proteins, and therefore their production is dictated by the activity of distinct genes. However, regulation occurs at many levels of growth factor action. First, many of these growth factors are synthesized as larger precursor molecules that are biologically inactive until cleared or released. Second, a number of them are expressed in various isoforms whose structure is regulated by alternative splicing. Third, alternative splicing also generates receptor diversity, particularly in the case of FGF. Fourth, unlike endocrine hormones, these proteins are not generally found freely circulating in tissue fluid or plasma. Instead, they are frequently associated with other molecules, including those of the ECM, by either electrostatic interactions or more specific protein-protein interactions. Specific examples include the very tight binding of FGF family members to positively charged proteoglycans such as the heparan sulfate proteoglycans. TGF-ß binds to a cell surface proteoglycan, betaglycan, and has also been reported to interact with a small matrix proteoglycan, decorin, and fibrillin-1, a component of the elastic fiber microfibril. Fibrillin is in turn a member of a larger family of molecules known as the large TGF-ß binding proteins (LTBPs). The implication of these observations is that the presence of a growth factor or the activity of its gene is not equivalent to bioavailable, active material. In addition, simple supplementing of a factor to a wound site does not ensure that the biologically active molecule will reach its appropriate receptor and evoke a tissue response.

Growth factor efficacy can be severely limited by ECM sequestration and proteinase activity. A large number of preclinical experiments have shown the power of gene delivery to overcome these limitations. Clinical trials of growth factors have been limited by the need to evaluate a single growth factor, whereas the wound environment is a constantly shifting mixture of signals that cells use to determine their fate.

Pathobiology of Wound Repair

There are three highly significant pathologies that occur in the area of wound healing: nonhealing wounds, excessive healing, and the specialized response of tissues to burns. Nonhealing wounds or ulcers can arise from a variety of sources. Nevertheless, they share some important common features. First, ulcers all fail to develop an underlying connective tissue structure. Second, the lack of this important groundwork for cell organization results in impaired overgrowth of epithelium. Third, there is often reduced angiogenesis and reduced fibroplasia. Fourth, there is the persistent presence of inflammatory cells: neutrophils or macrophages. Fifth, because of this persistent failure to restore tissue integrity, the chronic wound is often a site of persistent bacterial infection, which in itself can stimulate inappropriate inflammatory cell responses. In each of these elements, growth factors and ECM play a significant role.

> ▶ **PEARL 3•4** Growth factors can help healing, but their imbalance can lead to wound pathology.

Many clinical subtypes of nonhealing wounds are not distinguished precisely enough at the biochemical level to allow classification. Many of these conditions arise as a result of transient or chronically impaired vascular supply. In the former case, local ischemia caused by pressure or other kinds of physical or even chemical injury can lead to the loss of oxygen and tissue perfusion, leading to local cell necrosis and tissue death. Reperfusion may exacerbate the injury. Under many circumstances, ischemia leads to the progressive replacement of damaged tissue by scar tissue, with loss of important mechanical and physiological properties.

In the skin, nonhealing wounds classically form on the extremities and over bony processes as the result of either unrelieved pressure or repeated trauma. There is frequently a failure of both granulation tissue formation and epithelial overgrowth. Currently, there is insufficient information about levels of active growth factors at sites of chronic nonhealing wounds. It is likely that either growth factor abundance, bioavailability, or responsiveness is severely reduced in chronic wounds. Growth factor expression is reduced in diabetic wounds. For this reason, a number of growth factors are being used in clinical trials in an attempt to remedy nonhealing wounds.

The present evidence points to an imbalance between ECM accumulation and proteolytic degradation as a major cause of wound healing failure. Many proteinases, including elastase and some of the metalloproteinases, are capable of degrading not only adhesive substrates for cell migration and other components of the extracellular matrix but also signaling molecules such as growth factors and cytokines. In addition, excess proteolysis may cause a release of high levels of connective tissue breakdown products that inappropriately activate inflammatory cell processes. Thus, much attention is being given to the development of appropriate proteinase inhibitors and devices that can neutralize or adsorb proteinases for control of certain forms of nonhealing wounds. It should be noted, however, that necrotic tissue is an important negative factor in prolonging nonhealing wound, particularly in the second- and third-degree burn. It is well recognized that extensive and aggressive débridement of such wounds is essential to stimulate healing. For this reason a number of manufacturers have developed protease formulations that discriminate between necrotic and living tissue to various degrees.

Excessive Healing

Uncontrolled overgrowth at various phases of the repair process is an important aspect of wound repair pathobiology. An example of wounds locked in the earliest phases of repair are pyogenic granuloma/pyoderma granulosum and other chronic inflammatory conditions of skin and other organs. Little is known about the mechanism that brings about these conditions, but certainly many of the inflammatory states are due to immunologic stimuli.

Uncontrolled growth of scar tissue can take two forms. In hypertrophic scarring there is an excess growth of scar tissue within the wound margins that may project well above the plane of the skin. These sites usually contain overabundant collagen and may be hypervascularized. Hypertrophic scars are commonly associated with second- and third-degree burns, for which their lateral extent may provoke the formation of excessive contractures. Physical forces seem to play an important role in generating these types of scars, since coverage of injured areas with skin substitutes or splinting of the wound with a variety of films can often moderate the effects. Hypertrophic scars are known to contain fibroblasts that have abnormal growth factor responses and growth factor production profiles. It is quite likely that fibroblasts within the hypertrophic scar represent a subpopulation that has excess fibrotic tendencies due to the overproduction of molecules such as TGF-ß and a higher sensitivity to fibrogenic stimulation by this molecule. Presently, the only antagonist being evaluated in clinical trials is interferon-α. It is likely that further studies will attempt to address the problem more directly with TGF-β antagonists or perhaps molecules that block the action of the downstream effector, CTGF.

The other well-known cutaneous scar pathology is the keloid.[47] This is an intriguing condition in which cutaneous injury results in scar formation that takes on the appearance of a benign tumor. Keloids grow beyond the lateral margins of the wound, and they are usually restricted to the upper trunk, face, neck, and ears. This regional variation emphasizes the heterogeneity of skin cell populations. There is also a predilection to keloid formation in many darker-skinned races. There is anecdotal evidence of familial inheritance of the keloid tendency. Current studies are underway to map the keloid gene.

The consequences of excessive healing in organs other than skin can be far more life threatening. Pulmonary, renal, and hepatic fibrosis have marked effects on appropriate mechanical or secretory function in these tissues. The formation of surgical adhesions is also an excess response to injury. Scarring occurs subsequent to ischemic injury of various organs, and it leads to major health complications in coronary artery insufficiency and in stroke.

Summary

The movement and support of cells and tissue within the wound site is critically dependent on the correct arrangement of the ECM. The wound site is one of the most dynamic examples of ECM accumulation and remodeling. Insufficient or poorly organized ECM will lead to wound healing defects. The ECM is also an important reservoir and buffer for the actions of the dozens of short-range signals provided by growth factors and cytokines. The earliest signals come from the damaged tissue itself, as well as platelets in the fibrin clot; however, the entry of inflammatory cells rapidly augments the level of orchestration. Eventually, newly recruited tissue cells will assume the coordination of vascularization and remodeling. Many of the growth factors have beneficial effects on cells and wound models, but the appropriate delivery of these proteins in the context of the ECM and the proteinases of the wound environment can significantly compromise growth factor effectiveness. Gene delivery or microencapsulation methods may prove to be critical to further successes in advanced wound therapy.

Knowledge of the importance of nutritional status in healing requires an examination of how patients become nutritionally deficient. We know that the metabolic response to injury is much different from that of overall starvation. In starvation, there is a general decrease in metabolic rate within 24 hours after the onset of starvation. During these first 24 hours, glycogen stores in the liver are exhausted as they are used as an early form of nutrition. At this point, new glucose formation, the process of gluconeogenesis, will utilize amino acids as its primary substrate. These amino acids come from protein intake. Once this occurs, the body knows to increase mobilization of fatty acids from fat stores to preserve overall muscle mass. In the process of starvation, the brain, which normally uses glucose, can actually use products from fatty acid metabolism known as *ketone bodies*. In the presence of starvation, ketone bodies, mobilized from fatty acids, can provide up to 70% of the body's normal energy requirements. This starvation adaption is an evolutionary process that ensures human preservation by maintaining lean body mass and overall muscle protein. This causes a decrease in overall amino acid demand due to starvation and decreasing overall protein turnover, thus preserving lean body mass.

In the stress response, which usually follows an injury or severe stress such as a septic event, there is an overall change in the cardiac and vascular physiology, with a decreased systemic vascular resistance that causes lower blood pressures. This, in turn, causes elevated cardiac output, increasing the metabolic demands of the heart. This is usually accompanied by fever and an overall inability to use glucose normally, which leads to hyperglycemia. Additionally, muscle is sacrificed to power the body in this time of stress. This sacrifice leads to significant loss of lean body mass, which can ultimately negatively impact wound healing and, in turn, provide significant problems with pressure ulcer formation and other wound issues.

> **PEARL 4•1** Protein energy malnutrition has been shown to increase mortality and morbidity, and negatively effect wound healing.

Many of the patients, both young and old, seen in the acute care hospital experience malnutrition from stress or a septic event rather than from starvation, as is seen in older individuals who cannot maintain normal intake in either an acute or chronic setting. Bistrain et al, in a landmark article in the *Journal of the American Medical Association*, proposed a type of malnutrition known as *protein calorie* or *protein energy malnutrition*.[13] This type of malnutrition is characterized by a depletion of muscle visceral protein stores and overall body fat. This so-called protein energy malnutrition has been shown to increase mortality and morbidity as well as impair wound healing, increase length of stay in an acute care setting, and compromise the overall immune status of a patient.

What is surprising is that even mild protein energy malnutrition affects overall wound healing, and there is really no overall difference between levels of malnutrition and the effect on overall wound healing. This is extremely important because we know that severe protein calorie malnourishment causes a major effect on wound healing, but we also know that mild protein energy malnutrition may also affect overall wound healing, thus leading eventually to nonhealing wounds and, ultimately, death. The question should then be asked, why don't we assume all wounded patients have some type of protein energy malnutrition and treat it? Of course, the cost of such supplementation becomes an issue. Other factors include problems with invasive forms of supplementation, such as parenteral nutrition, problems with hyperglycemia and resultant excess supplementation in some of these patients, and the fact that overfeeding can cause immune suppression.

As previously mentioned, obesity is actually a form of malnutrition, and there may be excessive nutrition in one area and not enough in another. In patients with morbid obesity, that lack is most frequently protein. Often, these patients are put on protein-sparing diets or supplemented with protein while carbohydrates and other nutrients such as fats are withheld so that the patient will lose fats through fatty acid metabolism. The wounds may still heal with the increased protein requirements.

Traditionally, protein energy malnutrition has three forms: marasmus, kwashiorkor, and marasmus kwashiorkor. Marasmus is essentially wasting, with overall severe calorie deprivation or severe impaired absorption of calories. Patients with marasmus often have concomitant vitamin and mineral deficiencies and may sometimes have normal visceral protein levels, but they have had significant weight loss. Common causes of marasmus include cancer and chronic obstructive pulmonary disease (COPD).[14,15]

Kwashiorkor is hypoalbuminemic malnutrition, which is normal to excessive calorie input with inadequate protein input. Kwashiorkor may be difficult to detect because there is sometimes early sparing of the patient's overall muscle mass. With this eventual loss of overall protein, there is loss of oncotic pressure in the vascular system, which leads to increased edema. This can masquerade the overall usual wasting look that is typical of malnutrition. In kwashiorkor there is also decreased albumin and eventually cellular immunity, both of which require protein for maintenance. Infection, skin breakdown, and pressure ulcers are common in these patients.

Marasmus kwashiorkor, a combination of the two types of malnutrition, is usually a late-stage finding in severe to profound malnutrition. This type of malnutrition has the highest associated mortality and morbidity.[16]

> **PEARL 4•2** Diabetes mellitus is the most common form of malnutrition secondary to excess nutrients other than obesity.

The most common form of malnutrition due to excess nutrients, besides obesity, is diabetes mellitus (DM). Individuals with DM show a significant problem with abnormal carbohydrate metabolism and overall malnutrition. Even if a patient does not have diabetes, a significant stress such as sepsis may often result in hypoglycemia. Typically with hypoglycemia we see diuresis, which can lead to overall dehydration. Additionally, at blood sugars above 180 mg/dL, neutrophils cannot undergo chemotaxis in response to an infection, and at over 200 mg/dL, the effect of the neutrophils' ability to carry out oxidative bursts within their phagosomes is lost, thus leading to intracellular live bacteria and neutrophilic death. This in turn leads to increased abscess formation. Goodson and Hunt showed that diabetes also produces some true wound healing abnormalities, that of microvascular and macrovascular changes that affect not only wound healing but also the tensile strength of wounds and epithelialization.[17] They also demonstrated decreased collagen deposition, decreased or inhibited epithelial cell activity, and direct inhibition of fibroblasts. Mann showed that hyperglycemia interfered with the cellular transport of vitamin C into fibroblasts and leukocytes.[18] Vitamin C is an important cofactor in collagen synthesis, as is known from the disease scurvy. Often, vitamin C is supplemented to overcome these transport issues. This is one of the few clinical areas in which supplementation of vitamins can affect wound healing.[19]

One might think that the overall correction of hyperglycemia would alleviate some of the abnormalities mentioned above, but this has not been the case. Barr and Joyce showed that there was decreased re-endothelialization of microarterial anastomoses in a mouse model even when insulin was given.[20] Goodson and Hunt, however, did show that early insulin administration in the presence of hyperglycemia can facilitate normal wound healing despite sometimes decreasing wound tensile strength.[21] Hanam et al have shown that topical insulin has also been demonstrated to improve overall wound healing in a mouse model.[22]

Assessment

Every patient should be screened for nutritional abnormalities. The Joint Commission on Accreditation in Healthcare Organizations (JCAHO) has stressed the need for screening to identify any patient who is at either moderate or high risk for malnutrition. JCAHO also requires that nutritional interventions, just as any other intervention, be monitored for effectiveness and appropriateness. The Clinical Practice Guideline on treatment of pressure ulcers from the U.S. Public Health Service also says that patients should have nutritional assessments performed.[6] After establishing that nutritional assessments need to be done, how does one go about performing nutritional screenings in wound care settings. Screenings may include everything from utilizing weight, such as ideal body weight or usual body weight or a comparison of the two, to anthropometric skin fold measurements, questionnaires, and assessment of visceral proteins.

Ideal body weight (IBW) is the recommended body weight or desired body weight. Instead of evaluating IBW alone, it is usually more reliable to look at the percentage of change in body weight. The percentage of ideal weight is computed by multiplying the actual weight times 100 and dividing by the usual body weight. Severity of weight loss should also be evaluated; 2% loss in 1 week or 10% in 6 months is considered a significant weight loss. Unfortunately, ideal body weight allows for very little body weight to be accounted for as fat. Also, ideal body weight may fluctuate significantly in certain patients who have problems with fluid status, that is, congestive heart failure (CHF) or end-stage renal disease (ESRD) on dialysis.

Skinfold, or anthropometric, measurements are often done in healthy populations to look at overall nutritional parameters. This is an excellent tool for population-based studies, but

not good for use in patients who have significant skin turgor issues. This is often the case in the elderly or in patients with excess body fat but protein energy malnutrition issues.

Questionnaires are often used in both acute and chronic settings and are good for identifying medical conditions that may predispose an individual to malnutrition. Unfortunately, there is no one best survey or questionnaire, and they often need to be administered to patients who have little or no education or who have psychosocial issues that make it difficult for them to understand the survey.

▶ **PEARL 4•3** Indirect calorimetry is the most accurate means of assessing the use of nutritional therapy.

The most accurate method for assessing the use of nutritional therapy is by using indirect calorimetry. This method uses oxygen consumption and CO_2 production to give the resting energy expenditure (REE), which is measured on inspired and expired gas analysis. Unfortunately, this has certain limitations, including a prolonged calibration time of more than 30 minutes before measurements can be obtained. This often requires a wound patient to be on a ventilator. Air leaks in the ventilator circuit or lung abnormalities that require high inspired concentrations of oxygen, such as adult respiratory distress syndrome (ARDS), may also affect metabolic measurements.

Multiple other laboratory assessments of nutritional therapy have been used. Previously mentioned is the assessment of glucose, with the optimal control being less than 150 mg/dL. Other measurements are also important, such as levels of phosphorus and magnesium, overall renal function, or 24-hour urea nitrogen excretion with a calculation of overall nitrogen balance. Additionally, assessments of total lymphocyte count and visceral proteins should be made. The normal total lymphocyte count is typically 2000 to 2500 per microliter but may increase due to infection or leukemia. Decreased lymphocyte counts may be seen in chemotherapy, chronic steroid use, acute surgery, and radiation therapy treatments for cancer. The degree of depletion is mild at 1500 to 1800 per microliter, moderate at 900 to 1500 per microliter, and severe at less than 900 per microliter.

The classic visceral protein measurement is the level of albumin. Unfortunately, albumin has a long half-life, more than 20 days, and can be very sensitive to hydration status, which may be problematic in hepatic or renal disease. Albumin has a large body pool, but because of its long half-life, this measurement can underestimate protein energy malnutrition or even fail to identify it at all. Other more accurate measures of visceral protein are levels of transferrin and retinal binding protein. These measurements are not widely available, however, and are expensive to use. Prealbumin level has been the most widely used measure of protein over the last 10 to 15 years. It has a short, reasonable half-life of 48 to 72 hours, which when monitored twice weekly, will allow for intervention and follow-up to be made in the same week, if necessary. Prealbumin is not affected by dehydration or overall hydration status, has a relatively small body pool, and in modern tests is not affected by renal failure. Prealbumin is also not an acute-phase reactant that increases in times of stress. When a patient has a septic event or some type of body stress, the prealbumin level will decrease correspondingly and not show any false elevation that would lead the clinical provider to think that the patient's nutritional status was normal.

Table 4•1 Harris-Benedict Equation

Men	Women
EER (kcal) = 66.5 + 13.75W + 5.00H – 6.77A	EER (kcal) = 655.1 + 9.56W + 1.85H – 4.67A
EER (kJ) = 278 + 57.7W + 20.93H – 28.35A	EER (kJ) = 2741 + 40.0W + 7.74H – 19.56A

EER, estimated energy requirement; W, weight (kg); H, height (cm); A, age (years)

Table 4•2 Schofield Equation to Determine Energy Requirements

Age (years)	Male	Female
15–18	BMR = 17.6 × weight (kg) + 656	BMR = 13.3 × weight (kg) + 690
18–30	BMR = 15.0 × weight (kg) + 690	BMR = 14.8 × weight (kg) + 485
30–60	BMR = 11.4 × weight (kg) + 870	BMR = 8.1 × weight (kg) + 842
>60	BMR = 11.7 × weight (kg) + 585	BMR = 9.0 × weight (kg) + 656

To the calculated BMR:

A. Add stress factor: severe sepsis = 10%–30%, extensive surgery = 10%–30%, fracture/trauma = 10%–30%, burns/wound = 50%–150%.

B. Add a combined factor for activity and diet-induced thermogenesis:

Bedbound immobile	+10%
Bedbound mobile/sitting	+15%–20%
Mobile on ward	+25%

C. Add or subtract 400–1000 kcal/day if weight gain/loss required.

D. Add up to 10% for each 1°C rise in temperature.

BMR, basal metabolic rate

Once the nutritional assessment has been performed, the clinician can then determine nutritional requirements. The classic Harris-Benedict equation is most commonly used to predict nutritional requirements. The equation factors in sex, weight, height, and age differences to calculate a basal energy expenditure (BEE). (Table 4.1) Once the BEE is calculated, a stress factor is added to account for the increase in metabolic rate, as well as an activity factor that addresses other energy expenditures related to movement. (Table 4.2)

The Harris-Benedict equation can be used to calculate specific needs for obese patients as well. One must figure the overall body mass index (BMI) using the formula of BMI = weight (kg)/height (m²). If the BMI is between 25 and 30, the patient is considered overweight. If the individual has a BMI greater than 30, the clinician should use 75% of the calculated BEE while providing normal or increased protein requirements. For adults, recommendations for overall caloric need can be made through an estimate of between 25 and 30 kilocalories per kilogram per day as nonprotein calories (carbohydrates and lipids). This nonprotein calorie concept is very important. The normal calories required for daily body function, such as activity and stress, come from carbohydrates and lipids. This keeps protein in reserve to use for wound healing as well as protection of the immune system; 1.5 g/kg of protein per day is the general requirement. This may be increased to 2 to 3 g/kg per day in burns or other high metabolic states. Lipids or fats should provide approximately 20% to 30% of total calories. This percentage may be much higher in neonates and early infancy. Too much lipid can cause immune suppression, whereas lipid deficiencies can indirectly affect wound healing secondary to a decreased production of phospholipids. Phospholipids are an important part of the basement membrane of cells, and deficiency can lead to decreased production of prostaglandins, which are important in the inflammatory phase of wound healing. Without the inflammatory phase, otherwise normal wound healing does not occur. Also, excessive administration of omega-3 fatty acids can have an anti-inflammatory effect via the eicosanoid pathway. This leads to inhibition of platelet-activating factor IL-1 and TNF-α. Animals whose diets are enriched with omega-3 fatty acids have weaker wounds than do controls at 30 days postwounding. Omega-3 fatty acids do not cause a decrease in collagen. The weakness is instead thought to be related to the cross-linking of collagen, as well as to its overall maturation.[23]

Multiple theories exist to explain how much protein should be provided, depending on the stress response. In general, approximately 20% of the calorie requirements should come from protein. This is typically about 1.5 g/kg per day. If protein is used for basal energy needs, 1 g of protein provides approximately 4 calories. But one must remember that not all calories are created equal. Protein calories should be used for wound healing and for immune functions rather than nonprotein calories such as carbohydrates and lipids, which should be used for overall energy needs. This is fairly obvious when one considers the exudates from wounds or burns, which tend to be very rich in protein. This causes a protein "sink" and therefore may require increased protein supplementation because of increased stress.

Nutritional Administration

Oral administration of nutrition is the preferred method. This should remain true throughout all areas of medicine and nutritional administration. The philosophy should be: if the gut works, use it. Clinical data have demonstrated that severely compromised patients fed enterally had reduced septic complications, better immune function, and possibly less incidence of multiorgan failure than did patients who were fed parenterally. Typical routes of administration for enteral feeding may be available through the mouth (PO), but also can be provided through tubes inserted into the stomach and small intestines. Parenteral nutrition ("around the gut") usually uses the venous system, either through peripheral or central access.

▶ **PEARL 4•4** When considering nutritional supplementations, the rule of thumb should be, if the gut works, use it.

Enteral nutrition supplements consist of commercially available products or homemade products such as shakes using anything from whole milk to instant breakfast and whey proteins. Enteric formulas may be specialized to treat certain nutritional deficiencies and gut abnormalities for absorptive purposes. Effective strategies for enteral feeding include a variety of access mechanisms. These mechanisms include short-term nasal access, fluoroscopically guided placement of tubes, needle catheters applied surgically, and long-term access via percutaneous endoscopic gastrostomy (PEG) tubes or open gastrostomies and jejunostomies.

Parenteral nutrition, or hyperalimentation, can be given either peripherally through a regular IV to a central line or through a peripherally inserted central catheter (PICC line). Once the insult to the GI tract is addressed or normal GI function is achieved, the patient should convert from parenteral to enteral feeds when possible.

Overfeeding, which has been previously mentioned, can cause immune suppression and can lead to other problems such as hyperglycemia, increased CO_2 production, and hepatic steatosis. Hyperlipidemia, azotemia, and immune suppression can also occur.

Certain agents can be used to increase recovery from wounds, burns, and overall injuries. Growth hormones, insulin-like growth factor-1 (IGF-1), and anabolic steroids have all been used. The most commonly used anabolic steroid is oxandrolone. It has been shown by Demling to cause less weight loss associated with burns as well as to allow for faster donor site turnaround in burn patients.[24] Oxandrolone has a low occurrence of overall side effects but is costly, and often wound care providers are afraid to provide steroids for fear that they may actually interfere with overall wound healing.

It makes sense to administer certain amino acids to increase or enhance wound healing. Glutamine is the most abundant amino acid in the body, making up approximately 20% of the overall circulating pool of the 22 known amino acids.[22] It is the main fuel source for enteral sites of the small intestines and is often the critical substrate, along with alanine, for hepatic gluconeogenesis. Glutamine has been shown to be a primary fuel source for lymphocytes and is essential for lymphocyte proliferation.[25,26] It has also been shown to be a precursor for nucleotide production in fibroblasts and macrophages.[27,28] Demling demonstrated that glutamine stimulates the inflammatory response in wound healing.[24] It is also known that glutamine levels fall in both muscle and plasma after trauma.[29,30] Supplementation of glutamine in the diet can be beneficial in certain clinical situations, but no clear-cut benefit has been demonstrated in wound healing.[31,32]

Arginine is one of the two semiessential amino acids that becomes critical in times of stress when the body cannot provide enough. The role of arginine in wound healing was first described in the 1970s.[33,34] Seifter showed in an adult rat model that rats fed an arginine-deficient diet showed a decrease in wound-breaking strength, a decrease in collagen deposition, and an overall increase in mortality to 50% when compared with controls.[34] Barbul demonstrated that rats fed a high dose of arginine showed increased wound-breaking strength, increased collagen deposition, and improved immune function as well.[35] Chyun confirmed this by using a mature, or older, rat.[36] Goodson and Hunt evaluated the effects of arginine on humans by implanting polytetrafluoroethylene grafts in subcutaneous tissue and feeding patients arginine.[37] The implants were later removed and evaluated for collagen deposition. An increase in fibroblast activity and collagen deposition was noted in the experimental subjects. Barbul gave young patients a high-dose regular diet and one deficient in arginine.[38] With arginine supplementation there was an increase in hydroxyproline content and an overall total protein deposition. This was also confirmed in an adult model by Kirk et al.[39] Additional supplementation with hydroxy-methylbutyrate (HMB) has been shown to help support immune function and decrease muscle breakdown, but it needs to be given with arginine and glutamine supplementation.[40]

With regard to vitamins and trace minerals, the major question is who should receive supplements and how much should they receive? One should supplement patients who are obviously malnourished or have been unable to eat orally for at least 1 week and who, in turn, have not been given any other form of nutritional supplementation through alternative routes. Also, patients who have documented vitamin or trace mineral deficiencies may require supplementation. Supplementation may be carried out PO with medications, liquids, or replacements, or intravenously. As a general rule, the U.S. Department of Agriculture's (USDA's) recommended dosages should be followed and superphysiological doses or megadoses avoided. One should especially watch for fat-soluble vitamins such as vitamin A and vitamin E, which may lead to toxicity with high doses and increased storage in overall fat tissues.

Vitamin A was originally discovered in the early 1900s. Brandaleone noted deficiencies in wound healing in the 1940s.[41] Ehrlich and Hunt showed the benefit of supplementation on nondeficient patients in the 1960s.[42] True vitamin A deficiencies will affect wound healing at all stages by impacting function of macrophages, monocytes, fibronectin deposition, and overall cellular adhesion. The end result is decreased wound strength. Vitamin A supplementation by an oral dose may be as high as 25,000 units per day, which is five times the recommended daily requirement. This dose is typically given in severely injured patients and has been used without overall side effects. Often in a superficial wound, topical application may be just as effective, using more than 200,000 units up to three times per day. One should be cautious in excessive supplementation in patients on steroids as it can decrease the overall effectiveness of steroids and complicate a disease process. When vitamin A is supplemented, one sees an increase in the inflammatory response in wounds, which is possibly secondary to enhanced lysosomal membrane permeability. In vitro studies have demonstrated an increase in epidermal growth factor (in the work of Jetten), as well as an increase in collagen synthesis of fibroblastic cell cultures (in work by Demetriou et al).[43,44]

Vitamin C, or ascorbic acid, is a known essential cofactor in the hydroxylation of lysine and proline in collagen synthesis and the overall cross-linking and maturation of collagen. Supplementation can increase a patient's ability to resist infection and is often used as a classic treatment of the common cold. Vitamin C facilitates leukocyte migration into a wound. Classic deficiency has been reported to result in scurvy; some overall impairment of wound healing may occur without any systemic signs or symptoms of scurvy, even though it may be present. Standard supplementation with vitamin C is 100 to 1000 mg per day.

Vitamin E, one of the fat-soluble vitamins, is an antioxidant and also has excellent anti-inflammatory properties. Deficiencies of vitamin E are rare, as in all fat-soluble vitamins, and standard supplementation in the form of a multivitamin preparation is usually sufficient. One can have problems in wound healing with excess vitamin E administration. Vitamin E, with its antioxidant properties, is often taken for antiaging therapy, and excessive administration can decrease collagen production, decrease inflammatory response, and can affect overall wound healing. Patients taking large doses of vitamin E can have significant problems in surgery, and often physicians will insist on the patient stopping vitamin E prior to elective surgery.

Trace Element Deficiencies

Deficiencies of trace elements often are not a problem in patients who have wound healing difficulties. Standard supplementation at USDA dosing is often adequate, and excessive administration has not been shown to accelerate wound healing.

Zinc is an important cofactor in over 100 enzymatic reactions in the body and is an essential cofactor for normal cellular growth and replication. Zinc directly influences the processes of epithelialization, fibroblast proliferation, and many immunologic responses such as phagocytosis and bactericidal activities of white cells. The etiology of zinc deficiencies is typically due to chronic alcoholism, severe surgical trauma, large body surface area burns, psoriasis, and gastrointestinal fistulas. Therefore, it makes sense that supplementation with approximately 220 mg of zinc per day is usually adequate in wound healing since often wound care providers encounter multiple primary causes of zinc deficiency. One must remember, though, that excess zinc administration can lead to problems with patients who are septic and should be limited to just a few days at a time.

Iron is required not only for heme molecules in the form of hemoglobin- and oxygen-carrying capacities but also is important in DNA production. It is also an important cofactor required for the conversion of hydroxyproline to proline and collagen maturation. Therefore, iron is very important in wound healing. The most common iron deficiency is anemia, but clinical studies have shown that wound healing is rarely affected by any acute or chronic iron deficiency. In fact, if tissue perfusion is adequate, tissue oxygenation can be maintained even with very low hemoglobin levels.

Summary

Does nutrition really make a difference in wound healing? Some say it is very important, and others say it is not. Multiple animal studies have been performed showing that nutrition clearly makes a difference if it is severely deficient. Human studies support the value of protein supplementation but are not as clear about the benefits of other forms of supplementation. While additional studies need to be performed, clinicians should still ensure that patients receive a proper nutritional assessment and that basal energy needs are addressed, with particular attention to the increased needs caused by stress and wound healing.

▶ **Case Study 4•1** | **65-Year-Old Male with CVA, large Sacral Ulcer, and Nutritional Deficiency**

A 65-year-old male with multiple medical problems had a major stroke, leaving him with a major neurological deficit, paralyzed on the right side of his body, and with complete aphasia. He was placed in a local nursing home for several weeks, but his family eventually took him back home where he developed a large sacral ulcer. He was eventually hospitalized. Initial nutritional evaluation took place on admission. Initial prealbumin levels were 8.3 mg/dL (normal 20 to 38 mg/dL). Nutritional support was started parenterally because the patient had some evidence of aspiration secondary to his stroke. Twice weekly, prealbumin levels were ordered and débridement of the ulcer was performed. Because of the need for long-term nutritional support, a percutaneous endoscopic gastrostomy tube was inserted, and the patient was converted to enteral feeds. Prealbumin levels slowly improved, and advanced wound therapies were started, with some improvement in the wound noted. The patient was transferred to a long-term care facility, where wound care and nutritional support were continued.

References

1. Levenson, SM, Pirani, CL, Brasch, JW, et al: The effect of thermal burns on wound healing. Surg Gynecol Obstet 1954; 99:74–82.

2. Levenson, SM, Upjohn, HL, Preston, JA: Effect of thermal burns on wound healing. Ann Surg 1957; 146:357–367.

3 Levenson, SM, Crowley, LV, Oates, JF, et al: Effect of severe burn on liver regeneration. Surg Forum 1959; 9:493–500.

4. Crowley, LV, Seifter, E, Kriss, P, et al: Effects of environmental temperature and femoral fracture on wound healing. J Trauma 1977; 17:436–445.

5. Albina, JE: Nutrition and Wound Healing. JPEN J Parenter Enteral Nutr 1994; 18:367–376.

6. Bergstrom, N, Bennett, MA, Carlson, CE, et al: Pressure Ulcer Treatment. Clinical Practice Guideline. Quick Reference Guide for Clinicians. No. 15, Pub. No. 95-0653. Rockville, MD, US Department of Health and Human Services, Public Health Service, Agency for Health Care Policy and Research, 1994.

7. Ferguson, M, Cook, A, Rimmasch, H, et al: Pressure ulcer management: The importance of nutrition. Medsurg Nurs 2000; 9:163–177.

8. Spanheimer, RG, Peterkossky, B: A specific decrease in collagen synthesis in acutely fasted, vitamin C supplemented guinea pigs. J Biol Chem 1985; 260:3955–3962.

9. Yue, DK, McLennan, S, Marcdh, M, et al: Abnormalities of granulation tissue and collagen formation in experimental diabetes, uremia and malnutrition. Diabet Med 1986; 3:221–225.

10. Windsor, JA, Knight G.S, Hill, GL: Wound healing responses surgical patients: Recent food intake is more important than nutritional status. Br J Surg 1988; 75:135–137.

11. Haydock, DA, Hill, GL: Wound healing response in surgical patients receiving intravenous nutrition. Br J Surg 1987; 74:320–323.

12. Schroeder, D, Gillanders, L, Mahr, K, et al: Effects of immediate post-operative nutrition in body composition, muscle function and wound healing. JPEN J Parenter Enteral Nutr 1991, 15:376–383.

13. Bistrain, BR, Blackburn, GL, Hallowell, E, et al: Protein status of general surgical patients JAMA 1974; 230:858.

14. Haydock, DA, Hill, GL: Impaired wound healing in surgical patients with varying degrees of malnutrition. JPEN J Parenter Enteral Nutr 1986; 10:550–554.

15. Windsor, JA, Knight, GS, Hill, GL: Wound healing response in surgical patients: Recent food intake is more important than nutritional status. Br J Surg 1988; 75:135–137.

16. Curtas, S, et al: Evaluation of nutritional status. Nurs Clin North Am 1989; 2:301–311.

17. Goodson, WH, Hunt, TK: Wound collagen accumulation in obese hyperglycemic mice. Diabetes 1986; 35:491–495.

18. Mann, GV: The membrane transport of ascorbic acid. Ann N Y Acad Sci 1974; 258:243.

19. Schneir, M, Rettura, G, et al: Dietary ascorbic acid increases collagen production in skin of streptozotocin-induced diabetic rats by normalizing ribosomal efficiency. Ann N Y Acad Sci 1987; 194:42.

20. Barr, LC, Joyce, AD: Microvascular anastomoses in diabetes: An experimental study. Br J Plast Surg 1989; 42:50–53.

21. Goodson, WH, Hunt, TK: Studies of wound healing in experimental diabetes mellitus. J Surg Res 1977; 22:221–227.

22. Hanam, SR, Singleton, CE, Rudek, W, et al: The effect of topical insulin on infected cutaneous ulcerations in diabetic and nondiabetic mice. J Foot Surg 1983; 22:298–301.

23. Albina, JE, Gladden, P, Walsh, WR: Detrimental effects of an omega-3 enriched diet on wound healing. JPEN J Parenter Enteral Nutr 1993; 17:519–521.

24. Demling, RH, DeSanti, L: Involuntary weight loss and the nonhealing wound: The role of anabolic agents. Adv Wound Care 1999; 12(suppl): 1–14.

25. Ardawi, MS.M, Newsholme, P, et al: Glutamine metabolism in lymphocytes of the rat. Biochemistry 1983; 12:855.

26. Newsholme, EA, Newsholme, P: A role for muscle in the immune system and its importance in surgery, trauma, sepsis and burns. Nutrition 1988; 4:261.

27. Zetterberg, A, Engstrom, W: Glutamine and the regulation of DNA replication and cell multiplication in fibroblasts. J Cell Physiol 1981; 108:365–373.

28. Zielke, HR, Ozand, PT, Tidon, JT, et al: Growth of human diploid fibroblasts in the absence of glucose utilization. Proc Natl Acad Sci 1976; 73:4110–4114.

29. Roth, E, Funovics, J: Metabolic disorders in severe abdominal sepsis: Glutamine deficiency in skeletal muscle. Clin Nutr 1982; 1:25.

30. Askanazi, J, Carpentier, YA, Michelsen, CB, et al: Muscle and plasma amino acids following injury: Influence of intercurrent infection. Ann Surg 1980; 192:78–85.

31. Ziegler, TR, Young, LS, Benfell, K, et al: Clinical and metabolic efficacy of glutamine-supplemented parenteral nutrition after bone marrow transplant. A randomized double blind controlled study. Ann Intern Med 1992; 116:821–828.

32. McCauley, R, Platell, C, Hall, J, et al: Effects of glutamine on colonic strength anastomosis in the rat. JPEN J Parenter Enteral Nutr 1991; 15:437–439.

33. Rose, WC: Amino acid requirements of man. Fed Proc 1949; 8:546.

34. Seifter, E, Rettura, G, Barbul, A, et al: Arginine: An essential amino acid for injured rats. Surgery 1978; 84:224–230.

35 Barbul, A, Fichel, RS: Intravenous hyperalimentation with high arginine levels improves wound healing and immune function. J Surg Res 1985; 39:328–334.

36. Chyun, J, Griminger, P: Improvement of nitrogen retention by arginine and glycine supplementation and its relation to collagen synthesis. J Nutr 1984; 114:1697–1704.

37. Goodson, WH, Hunt, TK: Development of a new miniature method for the study of wound healing in human subjects. J Surg Res 1982; 33:394–401.

38. Barbul, A, Lazarou, S: Arginine enhances wound healing in humans. Surgery 1983; 108:331.

39. Kirk, SJ, Hurston, M, Regan, MC, et al: Arginine stimulates wound healing and immune function in elderly humans. Surgery 1994; 114:155.

40. Williams, JZ, Abumrad, N, Barbul, A: Effect of a specialized amino acid mixture on human collagen deposition. Ann Surg 2002; 236:369–375.

41. Brandaleone, H, Papper, E: The effect of the local and oral administration of cod liver oil on the rate of wound healing in vitamin A deficient and normal animals. Ann Surg 1941; 114:791.

42. Ehrlich, HP, Hunt, TK: Effects of cortisone and vitamin A on wound healing. Ann Surg 1968; 167:324–328.

43. Jetten, AM: Modulation of cell growth by retinoids and their possible mechanisms of action. Fed Proc 1984; 43:134–139.

44. Demetriou, AA, Levenson, SM, Rettura, G, et al: Vitamin A and retinoic acids: Induced fibroblast differentiation in vitro. Surgery 1985; 98:931–934.

chapter 5

Complications in Repair

William J. Ennis, DO, CWS, FCCWS, MBA, FACOS

Patricio Meneses, PhD

Introduction
Evidence-Based Outcomes

The normal process of wound healing has been described in Chapter 2 of this book. Unfortunately, many patients fail to proceed through the sequential phases of healing and end up with chronic, nonhealing wounds. The term *chronic wound* implies a temporal relationship with defined, fixed time points. In fact, the terms *acute* and *chronic* carry a slightly different meaning for wound care compared to other areas of medicine. A chronic wound is one that fails to heal within the expected time frame for the underlying wound etiology.[1] This definition implies there are evidenced-based wound healing time frames for various wound etiologies. The clinical reality is that there is rather a continuum of healing, with physiological steps that require completion before healing can proceed. If these time frames were known and accepted, then a clinician could turn to more advanced therapeutic options when the healing process fails to proceed.[2] Does a 70-year-old patient with ischemia and a diabetic foot ulcer heal within the same time frame as a 48-year-old patient with a venous ulcer and severe lipodermatosclerosis? The answer to these questions must be obtained before we can classify any wound as acute or chronic. We hope that in the future genetic and biochemical markers will be available to guide our therapy and to classify acute and chronic wounds.[3,4] Despite the well-accepted theory that a wound healing trajectory is dependent on the underlying wound etiology, a review of our own data failed to reveal any statistically significant differences in Kaplan-Meier–derived survival time plots.[5]

This exemplifies the importance of taking an evidence-based approach to practice. Since a universal diagnostic and therapeutic approach known as the Comprehensive Wound Assessment and Treatment System (CWATS), which includes the least common denominator (LCD) model, was used in the treatment of all wounds, it is not surprising that similar healing rates were achieved.[6] (Table 5.1 and Box 5.1) These findings raise the question of whether there are truly significant wound healing rate variations or simply wide practice variations. This also makes meta-analysis techniques difficult in wound care.

Another important factor to consider when reviewing wound healing outcome reports is the site of care (i.e., nursing home vs outpatient clinic) and the professional makeup of the clinical team performing the therapy.[7] There is some agreement on the core set of principles that make up the standard of care for wound healing and some knowledge of healing percentages that can be expected.[8] For example, Margolis described the healing percentages for the control groups from a number of randomized controlled trials (RCT) that focused on diabetic foot ulcers as a useful benchmark to follow.[9] Using an evidence-based approach as noted above is useful for the clinician to establish a target for healing, but it is important to note that often there is a poor correlation between the efficacy results from an RCT compared with the effectiveness results obtained in a real-world clinical setting.[10]

Factors Impeding Healing Process—Local, Systemic, and Clinician Induced

Classically, factors impeding healing are divided into three distinct categories. Local factors include conditions that impede healing at the wound bed. These include, but are not limited to, the presence of bacteria, perfusion defects, the presence of a foreign body or nonviable tissue, moisture, nutrients, and oxygen levels. Systemic factors are those that affect the individual as a whole and therefore impact the wound secondarily. Comorbid disease, nutritional status,

Table 5•1	Kaplan-Meier Mean and Median of Wound Healing Duration (weeks) by Type of Wound				
Wound Type	*n*	*n* Healed	% Healed	Mean ± SE	Median ± SE
Venous	74	57	77	13 ± 2	9 ± 1
Arterial	17	8	47	27 ± 6	13 ±16
Diabetic	56	44	78	13 ± 3	7 ± 1
Pressure	36	23	64	11 ± 1	10 ± 2
Postoperative	33	23	70	11 ± 3	10 ± 2
Traumatic	77	55	71	8 ± 1	7 ± 1
Collagen	15	11	73	18 ± 5	16 ± 6
Other	4	2	50	8 ± 1	1
Arterial mix	1	1	100	10	10
Total	313	224	72	14 ± 1	9 ± 1

n, number of patients; SE, standard error. No significant difference was detected.

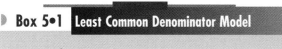

▶ **Box 5•1** **Least Common Denominator Model**

- Tissue Perfusion Oxygenation
- Infection
- Nutrition/Immune Status
- Wound Bed
- Psychosocial
- Pressure/Neuropathy

©William J. Ennis

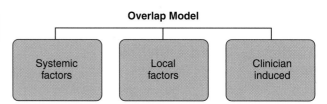

Figure 5•1 *An overlap model showing the factors that impact healing.*

obesity, and advancing age are cited as examples. The third category includes those factors that are iatrogenic or clinician induced, such as medications, dressings, and some physical energy treatments that impact the healing process.

Overlap Theory

The authors have proposed an "overlap model" that more accurately describes the factors that impact healing.[11] (Fig. 5.1) While it is helpful to use traditional categories for educational purposes, it does not reflect a clinical reality. A 70-year-old diabetic patient with vascular disease and a leg ulcer obviously has systemic factors, including age and diabetes, impacting healing. Ischemia, at the macrocirculatory level, translates into a microcirculatory defect with its associated paucity of nutrients and cellular oxygen. The use of insulin and medications such as pentoxifylline are clinician-induced factors, which have specific effects on the healing process both systemically and locally. The overlap model attempts to break down each of the three "traditional categories" into their least common denominator at the cellular and biochemical level. This theory is in alignment with our diagnostic and therapeutic approach to wound care and eliminates the need for complicated wound-specific diagnostic and treatment algorithms. We will attempt to tie in the "overlap" model concepts as we explore the factors impeding wound healing. We will use the traditional categories for ease of explanation and because most readers are familiar with the approach. What follows is not an exhaustive review of all possible factors impeding healing, but merely an overview. Emphasis on certain factors reflects the authors' expertise, lack of expertise, and the body of available literature and is not intended to assign clinical significance or rate the importance of the factors.

Local Factors
Bioburden Continuum

Bacteria are present in all chronic wounds. There is a natural balance between the quantity of bacteria present (bioburden) and the host's immune status. When equilibrium is reached, there is no clinical infection. If the inoculum of bacteria is increased ($>10^5$ organism per gram of tissue) or the host suffers a decrease in immunity, clinical infection occurs.[12] Many examples are cited in the literature describing the failure of skin grafts, delayed surgical closures, and overall wound healing problems when the bacterial bioburden exceeds 10^5.[13] This value is accepted by many as the quantitative definition of infection, except in the presence of β-hemolytic streptococcus where the value is somewhat lower (10^3).[14] Recent wound protocols have recommended using more than 10^6 bacteria as a cutoff for the definition of infection in a chronic wound.[15]

Bacteria compete with host cells for nutrients and oxygen in the wound bed. Bacterial by-products of metabolism can be toxic to normal cellular functioning. The presence of necrotic debris, a foreign body, and the desiccation of the wound bed will lead to enhanced bacterial growth. The concept of colonization (the presence of nonreplicating organisms) and infection (the invasion of organisms into the surrounding host tissue) can usually be determined by the physical exam.[16] The cardinal signs of inflammation, erythema, pain, swelling, and increased temperature, may be clues to impending infection. There are numerous ways to obtain cultures of a wound, but the quantitative biopsy remains the gold standard.[17] Unfortunately, this technique is not available in many institutions. Alternative rapid techniques are available but not widely used.[18,19]

Wound bioburden and infection must be thought of as a continuum and not a point in time when a specific number of organisms are present. The generation of granulation tissue actually depends on the presence of low levels of bacteria.[20] Certain bacteria enhance the initial inflammatory phase of healing.[21-23] It is frequently taught that the presence of granulation tissue (proud flesh) indicates a healing, healthy wound bed. Further analysis of granulation tissue, however, may reveal heavy colonization and possibly a subclinical infection.[24] Easy bleeding, friable tissue, and a deep red color are indications that granulating tissue is heavily colonized and could be infected subclinically.[25] This discussion of bioburden should alert practitioners to the concept that bacteria are always present in chronic wounds, and there is no evidence for the use of antibiotics in all cases. The authors have previously published data on the potential negative impact of using antibiotics without a definitive diagnosis of wound infection.[26] A more recent report identified the use of antibiotics as a negative predictor in the healing of pressure ulcers.[27]

Mertz and Ovington described the importance of both the quantity and identity of the organisms as they relate to an individual host.[28] A relatively new concept considers a point on the continuum at which there is multiplication of organisms, an absence of local invasion, but impaired healing. This concept has been termed *critical colonization*.[29,30] Although clinical signs of infection and standard laboratory results fail to detect a "critically colonized" wound, a healing wound that plateaus or becomes a "stunned wound" could be a surrogate marker.[31] Bacteria might negatively affect healing without creating a clinical host response through biochemical pathways. Many organisms are now known to form biofilms that are highly resistant to antimicrobial action.[32] Other organisms can express chemicals that impact immunity and cellular healing responses.[33,34] In these clinical cases, it might be beneficial to use either a dressing or modality that is capable of lowering the bioburden and thereby tipping the balance back toward healing.[30] There has been an explosion in the use of silver-impregnated dressings over the past several years.[35] Initially, this approach was thought to be beneficial because of the absence of resistance. However, recent reports indicate that

resistance might become a problem in the future.[36] More importantly, from a biochemical perspective, it does not make any more sense to use local bioburden-controlling products on all cases than it does to use antibiotics for all wound care cases. Nonetheless, the wound clinician needs to think of bacterial presence on a continuum and recognize that the quantity, quality, and host factors all overlap at the biochemical level.

▶ **PEARL 5•1** Consider both the quantity of bacteria present in the wound as well as the overall flora. The host's response to the bacteria will result in the ultimate clinical outcome, such as infection, a stunned wound, or unimpeded wound healing.

Tissue Perfusion

Macrocirculatory Issues

The circulatory system can be divided into two distinctive vascular beds. The *macrocirculation* refers to all vessels large enough to be seen by the unaided eye. Much clinical attention has been focused on the macrovasculature because of the large number of innovative therapeutic procedures that have been developed to treat these vessels (balloon angioplasty, atherectomy, laser, etc.).[37] The use of these less-invasive procedures has greatly improved limb salvage and wound healing options.[38] Since the macrovascular and microvascular beds are connected in series, a reduction in macrovascular flow will lead to a decrease in microvascular flow unless compensatory mechanisms are stimulated. The presence of an adequate macrovascular supply, however, does not always translate into adequate microcirculatory flow and the tissue perfusion required for wound healing.[39] The ankle-brachial index (ABI) is a standard noninvasive examination used by clinicians to assess the macrovascular status in an extremity.[40] Abnormalities in the ABI would lead the clinician to order additional studies that "map" out the anatomy of the macrovascular system and prepare for possible revascularization. The results of the ankle-brachial index should be interpreted cautiously in patients with diabetes and renal failure due to the presence of falsely elevated values.[40] Recently, the use of computerized tomographic angiography and magnetic resonance angiography has allowed a detailed evaluation of the arterial tree in a less-invasive manner than the use of standard angiography.[41]

Microcirculatory Issues

The microcirculation refers to a "web" of tiny vessels located throughout the body. The skin and chronic wounds are dependent on the microcirculation for oxygen, nutrients, and the elimination of metabolic wastes. Oxygen travels in the bloodstream both bound to hemoglobin and dissolved in the plasma. Decreased quantities of oxygen lead to decreased bacterial killing by leukocytes, decreased collagen production, and decreased epithelialization.[42,43] There are, however, some beneficial effects of low oxygen, such as stimulating the release of proangiogenic factors from macrophages.[44] A patient with a nonhealing wound should be assessed on both the macrovascular and microvascular levels.[45] A patient may have compromised macrovascular flow but due to compensatory mechanisms such as the development of collateral flow be able to heal a wound. In a study of 111 patients with nonreconstructible vascular disease, the microcirculatory assessment was predictive of ultimate limb salvage.[46] The clinician can treat the microcirculation through the use of various modalities that increase angiogenesis and local blood flow to the wound bed.[47] A concept known as the *push-pull theory* has been presented by the authors as a working theoretical construct.[48] The push is achieved by the macrovascular-based arterial reconstruction. The pull component is achieved through the use of mechanical energy-based technologies that lead to vasodilation and subsequent angiogenesis.[47,49] These therapies, such as noncontact, low-frequency ultrasound, pull the blood flow toward the microcirculation in a bimodal pattern that has been demonstrated by scanning laser Doppler results.[50] Initial increases in flow are due to vasodilation and capillary recruitment, and later-stage increases are secondary to angiogenesis. Local microcirculatory perfusion can also be influenced by both vasoconstriction and adequate volume status. Noxious stimuli such as hypothermia, stress, pain, and depression can all lead to increased sympathetic tone and subsequent decreased tissue perfusion.[51] Smoking, through the action of nicotine, can also result in decreased microcirculatory flow.[52] Several medications, including beta-blockers, have been thought in the past to negatively impact the microcirculation, but improved imaging techniques indicate that they are safe.[53,54] Other medications (pentoxifylline) can be used to augment microcirculation and tissue perfusion.[55] These multiple factors help explain why local, systemic, and clinician-induced factors all combine to potentially affect the wound healing process at the cellular level. It is incumbent on the wound care practitioner to evaluate the oxygen status from the macrocirculatory to the microcirculatory level in order to maximize wound healing.

▸ **PEARL 5•2** During the workup of a patient with a non-healing wound, the clinician should assess tissue perfusion at both the macrovascular and microvascular level. Adequate flow at the macrovascular level is important but doesn't always predict overall healing.

Dessication and Eschar

Another local factor affecting wound healing is the state of the wound bed's hydration. Historically, the purpose of dressings was to cover and protect the wound. Left to its own design, the body will create an eschar (scab) to cover the dermal defect. For years the scab was considered the "body's natural dressing" and thought to be highly effective. Many people felt compelled to "let the air get at it" and allow the scab to form. Gauze dressings applied either dry or "wet to dry" became the mainstay of wound care from the early 1800s, and they are still frequently used today in wound care.[27] As investigators began to analyze the qualities of the ideal dressing, the concept of moist healing evolved. In 1948 a taping procedure was advocated that allowed a moist wound dressing to remain in place for 2 to 3 days.[56] In 1962 George Winter published his landmark article in the journal *Nature* describing the benefits of moist healing under a polyurethane film dressing. He used a pig model to show that epithelialization was two times faster with moist healing versus scab formation.[57] In a 1963 follow-up article, Winter again used the pig model and demonstrated a faster epithelialization rate in moist healing when compared to air-dried wounds.[58] In the article, the authors stated it would be impractical to use moist healing in the human model for fear of developing infection under occlusive dressings. Hinman and Maibach confirmed Winter's earlier work, but used a human model.[59] Despite literature to the contrary, many clinicians today still fear the development of infection under occlusive dressings.[60] Products began to arrive on the scene in the late 1970s and early 1980s that used the moist healing concepts. Wound desiccation and eschar formation interfere with the healing process and should be prevented if possible. That mechanism involves death of cells, inactivation of growth factors, a hostile local milieu for cellular functioning, and decreased epithelial migration under the eschar. One exception is the presence of a heel eschar (pressure ulcer) in an ischemic limb. These eschars are better treated with dry protective dressings and with frequent monitoring.[61] The vast majority of wounds, however, should be treated with moist healing.

Foreign Body

There are several types of foreign body materials that can be found in chronic wounds. Some items are surgically placed (mesh, sutures), and others appear naturally (eschar, necrotic slough). Wound healing can be adversely impacted by the presence of these foreign bodies.

The presence of necrotic tissue in a wound can significantly impair healing. Necrotic slough can provide a fertile environment for bacterial growth. Depending on the chemical composition of the debris, toxic metabolites can be released from the action of the bacteria on the slough material. For example, pyocyanin, released from pseudomonas, can have a proapoptotic effect on neutrophils.[62] The presence of necrotic debris in a wound bed slows the process of granulation tissue formation and wound contraction. If the debris is allowed to desiccate, then the newly formed, hardened eschar further impedes contraction by "stenting" the wound edges apart. Débridement should be performed to remove all necrotic slough, fibrin, debris, and eschar. Débriding techniques include sharp (nonsurgical), sharp (surgical), autolytic (moist wound dressings), enzymatic (topical chemical enzymes), mechanical (wet-to-dry dressings, whirlpool, abrasion, kilohertz frequency ultrasound), and biological (maggot therapy) techniques.[63] Since all the factors mentioned in this chapter "overlap," it is imperative to assess the circulatory status prior to deciding when and how to proceed with débridement. In the presence of significant local infection, the necrotic slough should be removed rapidly with wide excision (surgically). In a chronic situation, without infection, sharp (nonsurgical), autolytic, or enzymatic débridement may be appropriate. In the severely dysvascular patient, cautious débridement is necessary so as to avoid creating a larger nonhealing defect. Thus, as for many other impediments to healing mentioned in this chapter, a global assessment of the patient must precede any decision on how to deal with the presence of necrotic debris.

The choice of sutures for primary or delayed secondary closure can impact wound healing. The amount of inflammation, incidence of infection, and cosmetic appearance of a wound are all, to a degree, determined by the choice of suture material used.[64] Specific surgical techniques, including choice of closure, knot security, suture tension, tissue bite, and the placement of sutures outside the healing zone of a wound, all impact healing.[65]

The presence of a synthetic mesh in an open wound can be problematic for the wound care clinician. Surgical cases in which the abdominal fascia is weak or when massive edema prevents primary closure are situations in which synthetic products are used to assist in wound closure. In addition, there are now several known medical indications that require leaving the abdomen open postoperatively.[66] As wound clinicians become integrated with inpatient wound care programs, complex abdominal wounds are more frequently encountered. Historically, the two most commonly used synthetic products were polytetrafluoroethylene (PTFE) and polypropylene mesh (PPM). Articles have been published describing infectious postoperative complications due to the use of these synthetic mesh products.[67] When using PTFE for abdominal wall reconstruction in the face of infection, it showed less bacterial adherence than did PPM in an animal model.[68] Secondary to the increased risk of infection, fistulae formation, and chronic pain syndromes, surgeons have increasingly turned to the use of xenogeneic and allogeneic materials for abdominal wall repair.[67,69]

There is very little published literature concerning the treatment of chronic wounds with exposed synthetic mesh. Should the mesh be removed in a wound with a high bioburden? If the clinician elects to allow granulation tissue to grow over the mesh, should antibiotics be used? If they are used, for how long? There is an increased inflammatory response as measured in wound effluent when synthetic grafts are used.[70] Wound clinicians are using negative-pressure wound therapy as a method to help granulate and cover wounds with underlying dermal substitutes.[71]

Systemic Factors
Stress

The biochemical outcomes from various sources of stress are known to impede wound healing. This topic is included in the category of systemic factors but clearly impacts the wound healing process at a local level. Clinicians play a major role in trying to alleviate stressful situations and environments in order to maximize healing potential. Psychological stress, noise, and pain will be discussed below.

The sympathetic nervous system and the adrenal axis play major roles in the hormonal response to stress. Catecholamines, norepinephrine, and epinephrine are released in response to stress with the ultimate result being vasoconstriction and decreased tissue perfusion. Tissue perfusion has already been discussed in this chapter as a critical issue in wound healing. In addition to decreased perfusion, evidence exists that elevation in stress hormones inhibit fibroblast growth, which results in decreased granulation tissue formation.[72] The magnitude of the hormonal response is directly related to the severity of stress.

Laparoscopic cholecystectomy, for example, results in less stress as measured by cortisol and catecholamine levels than does the standard open surgical procedure.[73]

Psychological Stress

Psychological stress, much like surgical stress, can result in cellular dysfunctions.[74] These interactions are frequently reported in the field of psychoneuroimmunology.[75] The concept that stress would lead to abnormal healing was described in a report by Christian et al.[76] In an earlier experiment by Kiekolt-Glaser et al, caregivers who were under stress underwent punch biopsies and received standard moist wound care. The caregivers demonstrated slower healing than matched controls who were not under stress.[77] Several researchers have extensively studied the connection between depression and healing through biochemical analysis and impaired wound healing models.[78-81] The stress of having a chronic disease, such as a nonhealing wound, therefore may factor into the clinical response to various treatment regimens and should be considered when treating a patient with such a wound. The wound clinician should also consider screening patients for underlying depression as part of the comprehensive workup.

> ▶ **PEARL 5•3** Patients presenting to a wound clinic should be questioned about their mood and affect. Depression is a common finding among patients with chronic illness, and failure to diagnose and treat it can impede healing.

Noise

Noise has been shown to increase plasma cortisol and adrenocorticotropic hormone levels.[82,83] Wysocki demonstrated a significant reduction in wound healing in an animal model after it was exposed to standard doses of white noise.[84] Hospitals are known to provide noisy environments in excess of normal levels.[85] Since many patients are treated in hospital-based clinics or as inpatients, it should not be surprising that this stressor may also impede wound healing at the point of care.

Pain

Pain management received appropriate recognition only after the Joint Commission (Joint Commission on Accreditation of Healthcare Organizations; JCAHO) released mandatory guidelines.[86] Most clinicians lack understanding of the physiology of pain and the multiple pain management options. Health-care providers tend to underdose patients suffering with pain. This problem is further compounded by the fact that many elderly patients are unable to adequately express their level of pain. Débridement at the bedside is frequently performed in the hospital without any analgesia. Krasner has contributed several articles that help identify the different types of pain experienced by a patient with a nonhealing wound.[87,88] For a more thorough coverage of wound-related pain and its treatment, please see Chapter 22.

Obesity and Wound Healing

There is a growing epidemic of obesity worldwide.[89] Surgical complications are more common in the morbidly obese patient; in particular, wound infections and disruptions are more common.[90] Factors include prolonged operations, greater blood loss, and wound healing problems. One study found an increased incidence of infections, bacteremia, sepsis, and increased number of days on mechanical ventilation for burn patients who were obese versus controls.[91] In another study focused on major reconstructive vascular surgery, wound infections were significantly more common in obese than nonobese patients.[92]

There are several conditions that prolong wound healing as a consequence of obesity, including decreased tissue perfusion and oxygenation, increased intra-abdominal pressure, immobility, and prolonged hospitalization. Obese patients that remain bedbound have an increased chance of developing pressure ulcers and should be monitored actively to ensure surgical site healing.[93,94]

Nutrition

The topic of nutrition and its impact on wound healing has been covered in Chapter 4 of this book. However, because of the impact of poor nutrition on wound healing, a few general comments are presented here.

In general, protein calorie malnutrition is a more common problem in chronic wound care than are isolated nutrient or vitamin deficiencies.[95] A patient with a wound has physiological stress with a subsequent neurohormonal response not unlike that of the many other stressors already mentioned in this chapter. The hypermetabolic state that results from malnutrition is an adaptive response that results in a significant increase in basal energy expenditure. The body has to meet these increased energy demands through an adequate intake of protein and calories. Clinicians underestimate the total protein needs for patients with chronic wounds.[96] The elderly can be at a significant disadvantage secondary to physiological changes (decreased appetite, physical difficulties with eating and swallowing) and many social issues that limit access to food and water. The goal of nutritional planning for patients with nonhealing wounds begins with an intensive history and estimation of daily caloric needs. Many formulas and clinical measurement techniques are available for this purpose.[97] After somatic and visceral protein stores have been determined and protein calorie needs calculated, the method of replacement must be determined (enteral vs parenteral). Estimation of the hydration status must accompany the evaluation as well as a plan to replenish vitamins and trace elements.

Nutritional issues are equally important when reviewing patients who are at risk for wounds as when planning therapy for a patient who already has a wound. Studies have been conducted on nursing home patients that demonstrate a correlation between the presence of pressure ulcers and malnutrition.[98] There are many studies that show a relationship between the presence of ulcers and malnutrition, and however limited the cause and effect, prospective data exist.[99]

Temperature

Temperature can affect wound healing on both a systemic and local level. Hypothermia, which occurs frequently in the perioperative period, has a negative impact on healing. The hypothermic stress causes thermoregulatory vasoconstriction, which in turn leads to decreased cutaneous blood flow and subcutaneous oxygen tension.[100] In addition to the altered flow, there is also an impact on immune function. Hypothermia can impair chemotaxis, phagocytosis, and the motility of macrophages.[100] Coagulation can also be negatively impacted with a higher recorded surgical blood loss.[101]

Kurz et al noted a significant increased infection rate and hospital length of stay for a hypothermic control group compared to an actively warmed treatment group.[100] Despite this knowledge, most surgical procedures are performed in cold operating rooms, and few institutions mandate policies for warming patients. Additionally, investigators have reported that keeping wounds warm maintains elevation of tissue oxygen tension, which impacts collagen deposition,[102] and other studies have conveyed positive clinical outcomes after chronic wounds were warmed with radiant heat.[103,104] These findings suggest that cell activities and healing processes may be delayed during extended dressing changes that allow the wound to cool significantly.

Comorbidities

Poorly controlled systemic illness can have a negative effect on the healing process in patients with chronic or acute wounds. It is of vital importance that a wound care clinician conduct a thorough history, physical examination, and appropriate laboratory testing prior to initiating wound care to ensure an accurate diagnosis for the wound etiology. Frequently, systemic therapy must be used in parallel with local wound care in order to achieve healing. Almost all medical conditions can impact some aspect of healing, and there are obviously too many to review in this chapter. A helpful approach to this overwhelming challenge is the LCD model (least common denominator). (Box 5.1) After establishing the diagnosis, the clinician must evaluate the potential impact of the disease on each of the six components noted in the LCD model. This approach helps to strategize the treatment plan without overlooking the impact of the various comorbid illnesses at the local level. Specific therapeutic protocols can be applied to improve the status in all six categories

Diabetes

The current worldwide epidemic of diabetes will impact over 260 million people by 2025.[105] As the most common cause of lower extremity amputation in the United States, diabetes is a relevant clinical condition that is used to exemplify how a systemic disorder impacts the various factors noted in the LCD model.[106] Diabetes has a known impact on the macrocirculation, in particular impacting the infrapopliteal arterial tree with atherosclerosis.[107] It is also widely known that diabetic patients suffer from endothelial dysfunction, inadequate nitric oxide release, and an inappropriate venoarteriolar reflux, leading to dependent edema and insufficient microcirculation for healing.[108] These microcirculatory defects sometimes persist despite adequate revascularization procedures.[109] The diabetic patient is more prone to infection secondary to both the decreased microcirculatory perfusion and defective leukocyte functioning.[110] The diabetic patient can also have nutritional difficulties secondary to diet restrictions, and as previously described, immune function is not optimal, increasing the risk for infections. The combination of motor and sensory neuropathy can lead to abnormal bone deformities of the foot secondary to high peak plantar pressure, callus formation, and ultimately diabetic foot ulcerations for many patients.[111] Amputation is frequently preceded by the presence of a diabetic foot ulcer, and ulceration is the leading cause of hospital admission for diabetic patients.[112] Overall quality of life is significantly impacted for these patients, and the presence of reactive depression can further complicate the medical care for these patients.[113] In essence, all of the components from the LCD model are impacted at the cellular/biochemical level by the presence of diabetes. The same approach should be taken when considering any and all medical conditions noted in the history of a patient with a nonhealing ulcer.

Peripheral Vascular Disease
Arterial Insufficiency
The presence of peripheral arterial disease (PAD) is a major complicating condition that impairs wound healing. PAD can be present alone or in combination with any other disease state. It is therefore imperative to assess the arterial circulation in all patients with wounds. It is often difficult to assign a primary wound etiology in cases where multiple conditions coexist. For example, a diabetic patient with a foot ulcer may have severe ischemia in addition to the neuropathic condition that resulted in the ulceration. A physical examination that includes palpation of pulses, ulcer location, wound bed characteristics, and a handheld Doppler examination should confirm the suspicions raised in the history.[114]

Treatment needs to be directed to both the systemic and local level. The priority is to reestablish arterial flow in the most expeditious and effective way possible. It is also important to collaborate with the vascular team so that they are aware of the wound location and the overall condition of the patient. Correcting an anterior tibial stenosis in a patient with a calcaneal ulcer and an incomplete pedal arch will not likely lead to healing. Prior to establishing flow, the wound should be protected and carefully observed for signs of infection. In wounds presenting with an active infection, débridement should be limited prior to revascularization. Débridement prior to adequate revascularization can lead to a larger defect that becomes recalcitrant to treatment. After adequate flow is established, appropriate moist dressings and débridement, as required, can be carried out.

The absence of macrovascular flow often results in poor microcirculatory flow, however the converse is not always true.[115] For example, a patient may have bounding palpable pulses but severe lipodermatosclerosis surrounding a venous ulcer, which results in a decreased microcirculatory flow despite the normal peripheral vascular exam. Therefore, the presence of pulses, while helpful, does not ensure adequate tissue perfusion for wound healing. Transcutaneous oxygen monitoring, Doppler image analysis, and, more recently, hyperspectral frequency analysis of the tissue might be required in these cases.[45,116] LoGerfo et al dispelled the myth of "small vessel" disease in diabetic patients with a landmark paper in 1984.[115] Many surgeons were previously under the impression that diabetic patients could not undergo bypass procedures because of the presence of atherosclerosis in the small vessels of the foot. Subsequently, others have shown that the problem resides within the microcirculation in these patients.[117] The endothelium (inner lining of the blood vessel) plays a significant role in regulating biochemical pathways that can either increase or decrease flow to the tissue level. Insulin resistance may have an effect at the endothelial cell surface through insulin receptors.[108] The wound clinician needs to be comfortable ordering, interpreting, and referring patients for both macrovascular and microvascular testing when working up a patient with a nonhealing wound. (Table 5.2)

Venous Insufficiency
Valvular insufficiency, outflow obstruction, and a hostile biochemical microenvironment all lead to the formation of venous leg ulcerations.[118] Specific mechanisms describing the pathogenesis of venous leg ulcerations include fibrin cuffing of venules, white blood cell trapping, growth factor trapping, reperfusion injury, incompetent venous valves, and outflow obstruction.[119-122] Venous leg ulcerations (VLUs) are the most common lower extremity ulcer treated in U.S. outpatient hospital-based wound centers, affecting an estimated 1 million patients at a cost of $1 billion per year to the health-care system.[123]

Table 5•2 Tissue Perfusion—Techniques for Assessment

Macrovascular Flow	Macrovascular Oxygen	Microvascular Flow	Microvascular Oxygen
Ankle-brachial index	Arterial blood gas	Laser Doppler image analysis	Transcutaneous oxygen monitor
Arterial duplex		Isotope washout techniques	^{31}P-NMR spectroscopy
Magnetic resonance angiography		Remittance spectroscopy	Positron emission tomography
Angiography		Near-infrared scanning	Hyperspectral frequency analysis
Computerized tomographic angiography			

P-NMR, phosphorus-31 nuclear magnetic resonance.

The evaluation of a patient with a suspected venous ulcer should always begin with an ankle-brachial index to rule out underlying concomitant arterial disease. The presence of a mixed arterial-venous ulcer significantly alters the treatment protocol (modified compression, revascularization prior to compression, etc.). There are numerous methods for evaluating the venous system, including anatomic and functional evaluations. For anatomic functions, the duplex ultrasound evaluation can rule out deep venous thrombosis, identify perforator veins, and measure valvular incompetence.[124] Air and impedance plethysmography can evaluate the overall function of the venous system and help predict ulcer risk.[125] New surgical options are available to correct abnormal venous hemodynamics and help prevent ulcer recurrence.[126]

▷ **PEARL 5•4** Patients with suspected venous ulcers should undergo noninvasive studies to identify potential surgically correctable defects that can help lower ulcer recurrence rates.

Age and Wound Healing

Fetal Skin

During fetal development, the skin undergoes maturation. The constitution of fetal skin varies considerably from that of the adult. By the 28th week of gestation, fetal skin is well equipped with blood vessels, dermal lymphatics, nerves, and supporting structures; however, many of the tissues are not fully functional. Vascular plexuses are developed in the skin after birth. Sweat glands begin basic functioning a few days after birth. These glands become fully functional after 1 or 2 years of age. Before the eighth fetal month, keratinocytes are scarce in the skin, and the stratum corneum is formed toward the end of intrauterine life. Consequently, the permeability of fetal skin is diminished over time, ultimately becoming impermeable at the time of birth. Collagen content increases from 2.4 g/kg (grams of collagen per kilogram of wet skin tissue) in early fetal development, to 16.8 g/kg in the newborn, 39 g/kg in the infant, and finally, 45 g/kg in the adult. The epidermal water content, on the contrary, diminishes from 917 meq/kg (milliequivalent of water per kilogram of wet skin tissue) in the fetus to 694 meq/kg in the adult.[127] Fetal wound healing is rapid and proceeds with a limited inflammatory phase.[128] The fetus lives in a sterile environment rich in hyaluronic acid and growth factors.[129] In addition, the fetal immune system is immature and underdeveloped.[130] Fetal tissue is relatively hypoxic, but this does not seem to have the adverse effect noted in the adult.[131] The fetus has a low collagen concentration and undetectable levels of TGF-β (transforming growth factor-β). A high level of steroids and low quantity of neutrophils are factors that give rise to a diminished inflammatory response in fetal wound healing.

Skin Changes with Age

Changes in human skin related to aging have been reported in the literature for many years. The obvious visible skin changes of the aging process help to reinforce the notion that aging is a negative factor for wound healing. These changes are summarized in Table 5.3. Several skin properties, however, do not change with aging, including epidermal thickness, the number of epidermal cell layers, the ability of the stratum corneum to prevent water loss, collagen IV, laminin B1 and B2 expression, production of collagen VII, hyaluronan, and cellular infiltration.[127-129]

Table 5•3 Changes in Skin Related to Age

Structure or Function	Phenomenon	Clinical Effect
Corneocyte	Cells become smaller. Cells from sun-exposed areas retain nuclear remnants, loss of lines of overlap, and roughening of border edges.	Unknown
Microvasculature	Regression and disorganization on capillaries and small vessels is present. There is about a 30% reduction in the number of venular cross-sections per 3 mm of skin surface. Blood flow is reduced.	Thinning hair and pallor is present. Skin surface temperature is reduced. Sweat production is diminished. Insulating subcutaneous fat is reduced. Rate of substance diffusion across the skin is reduced.
Integumental reactivity	Mast cells are reduced. Resistance to degranulation is increased.	Inflammatory response is diminished. This response can be missing entirely in aged individuals.
Perception of pain	Pain sensitivity is progressive, diminishing as age increases after age 50.	Elderly are less capable of sensing danger and reacting appropriately. Burns tend to be more serious.

Morphological changes, such as increased roughness, wrinkling, loss of elasticity, and uneven pigmentation, are not the necessary results of cutaneous senescence. They may be the response of a cumulative environmental stress.

Three factors have been poorly controlled for when assessing the impact of aging on wound healing. They include the nutritional status of the patient, the nature and site of the wound, and the presence of any comorbid states. Reports in the literature have identified changes related to the cellular microenvironment of the skin independent from any macroenvironmental changes.[130] Thrombospondin, a major component of the matrix produced by newborn cells, is secreted, but is absent from the matrix in an adult cell.[131] This may explain the absence of angiogenesis noted in adult tissue compared with the fetus.[131]

Studies from both an outpatient wound clinic and a subacute wound unit have identified only the over-90-year-old age group as having any statistically significant differences in healing.[7]

Clinician-Induced Factors

There are factors under the control of a clinician that impede healing. Clinicians need to accept that any and all therapies prescribed for the patient with a nonhealing wound carry the potential for a negative systemic side effect or impact on healing. Patients frequently forget to mention medications they are using, especially over-the-counter topical preparations, birth control pills, vitamin supplements, and antibiotics prescribed for reasons other than the wound under treatment.

Medications

The prophylactic use of antibiotics for the treatment of leg ulcers has not resulted in an improvement in healing rates.[132] The resulting increase in resistant organisms has already been mentioned, and it has been shown that systemic antibiotics do not reach adequate levels in chronic granulation tissue, providing further questions regarding the role of systemic antibiotics in wound care.[133] Surgical management of bioburden (débridement, curettage) may be more effective, but tissue destruction and bleeding are possible negative outcomes of the surgical approach.

Steroids are known to impede the inflammatory phase of healing, which can delay the healing cascade through a decrease in collagen production and fibroblast dysfunction.[134] Both systemic and topical steroids can have negative effects on healing.[135] Several papers have addressed the positive use of systemic and topical vitamin A to reverse the negative effects of steroids on healing while others challenge the concept.[136-138] The clinician needs to obtain a drug history to check for current or prior use of steroids. In addition, when topical steroids are required for periwound conditions, care must be taken to avoid exposing the wound to the steroid cream.

NSAID medications can also have a negative impact on healing by reducing the inflammatory response. The effect is greatest if the medication is used shortly after injury. It is unclear how important this effect is in the chronic wound.[139]

Immunosuppressive agents are used frequently today for a host of indications, including but not limited to cancer, connective tissue diseases, transplantation, and hematologic disorders. These medications alter wound healing by their effect on duplicating cells. One study revealed that chemotherapeutic agents did not increase the incidence of wound complications, and the authors encouraged early use of chemotherapy postoperatively after observing an increase in survival with this approach.[140] More recently, antiangiogenesis therapy is being used for a number of oncological and inflammatory disorders.[141] There is concern that wound healing will be delayed in patients taking this form of therapy.[142] The individual clinical needs of the patient must again be balanced against the impact on wound healing potential.

Another category of medications that has been shown to impact wound healing are the cox-2 inhibitors.[143] These medications can retard the healing process through a combination of anti-inflammation and antiangiogenesis. Angiotensin-converting enzyme inhibitors (ACEs) and calcium channel blockers can also alter the biochemical processes necessary for normal wound healing.[144,145]

> ▶ **PEARL 5•5** A detailed medication history should be obtained from patients because many medications can impact the healing process. Many patients take over-the-counter (OTC) medications and supplements that they do not consider "medications"; therefore, the clinician should specifically ask about OTC medications and any alternative therapeutics that the patient may be using.

Topical Agents

There are numerous topical agents that are used in clinical wound care that may have possible toxic effects. This practical point applies to any cleanser, antibiotic, antiseptic, analgesic, or disinfectant that has been recommended for use in an open wound. Most of the most commonly used agents do not even have an FDA-approved indication for use in open wounds. Many agents have been used for the process of wound cleansing, but many of these solutions have been shown to have a toxic effect on fibroblasts and polymorphonuclear cells (PMNs).[146] Normal saline and sterile water should be used for the overwhelming majority of wound-cleansing needs. There are now nonionic surfactants that are specifically designed for wound bed cleansing that are also safe for topical use on open wounds. Antiseptic agents such as Dakin's solution, iodine solutions, and numerous others have little use in wound care except for infected wounds that either cannot undergo surgical débridement or are awaiting surgery and where the goal is moisture and cytotoxicity to control the infection. Disinfectants should not be routinely used in wound care and have documented toxicity to numerous cells and the healing process overall.[147,148]

Controversy surrounds the use of topical antimicrobials, including silver, despite some reports indicating benefits.[149]

Controversy also surrounds the use of topical anesthetics. Topical lidocaine has been shown to decrease leukocyte migration into a wound bed.[150] Conflicting reports are present in the literature concerning the impact of EMLA Cream (lidocaine/prilocaine) in open wounds.[151,152] A recent report demonstrated an antibacterial effect of EMLA Cream when used as a topical anesthetic.[153]

Wound Modalities

Whirlpool and Pulsed Lavage

As most wound modalities have been covered elsewhere in this book, what follows is a brief review of several modalities used by wound care clinicians that impact the healing process.

The whirlpool is a frequently misused modality in wound care. The whirlpool cleanses and removes debris through mechanical débridement. Once a wound is clean, with a healthy granulating wound bed, this modality should be discontinued. Toxic disinfectives are frequently added to the whirlpool bath, and these can retard healing as mentioned above. Irrigation forces greater than 8 to 12 pounds per square inch can lead to damage of healthy tissue. Lower extremity edema can actually be worsened by keeping the leg in a dependent, knee-bent seated position for this procedure. The temperature of the bath needs to be carefully monitored in a neuropathic patient to avoid burn injury. Finally, the whirlpool tank itself needs to be aggressively cleaned so as not to cross-contaminate patients with resistant, virulent organisms. The use of pulse lavage has increased in part because of the problems noted with the whirlpool. Although pulse lavage uses sterile, disposable equipment, has the benefit of negative suction, and is more site specific, there have been increasing reports of infection spread through the aerosolization of microorganisms.[154]

Dressings

It is now widely accepted that wet-to-dry traditional gauze dressings are to be used as a means for mechanical débridement and do not play a significant role in a healthy, healing wound. The most user-friendly, cost-effective, safest, and clinically beneficial dressing should be selected. The dressings should be changed according to the patient's needs and wound conditions. The dressing choice should be altered as the wound moves through the phases of healing. There are many moisture-retentive, modern wound dressings available with various benefits and potential complications, but reviews of the published literature have failed to demonstrate statistically improved healing with any one category of dressing compared to another.[155] It is therefore incumbent on the clinician to assess the local tissue conditions and match dressing characteristics with those of the wound. Using a moisture-retentive dressing in a case with excessive exudation will lead to maceration and potentially worsening of the wound. At the opposite extreme, using a dressing with a high moisture vapor transmission rate when there is a relatively dry wound bed can lead to desiccation and impede keratinocyte migration.

Summary

In this chapter we have reviewed some of the factors that impede wound healing. The traditional categories of local, systemic, and clinician-induced factors were described as well as a newer approach, the overlap model. Taken together, the factors that impede wound healing constitute a brief overview of wound healing in general. An emphasis has been stressed in this chapter on the importance of a thorough history and physical examination in addition to a wound bed analysis. A standardized approach should be taken to all wound patients in order to obtain a consistent approach to both the diagnosis and treatment. Wound care practitioners need to stay current on all recent developments in the field and to constantly question their own practice habits. As this field continues to grow, the importance of organizing multidisciplinary teams will become paramount to master the scope and variety of wound etiologies and treatments.

▶ **Case Study 5•1** **Mixed Etiology Wound—Popliteal Entrapment**

MJ is a 36-year-old white male with a history of claudication since he was 15 years old. He is currently a police officer and is having a problem maintaining his position because of the limitations he experiences when trying to run any distance greater than 2 blocks. As well, he is currently suffering with a nonhealing wound located at the medial malleoli of the right leg. The wound is 1.8 cm², 0.1 cm deep, surrounded by a zone of hyperpigmentation, and completely filled with healthy-appearing granulation tissue. The wound has opened and closed several times over the past 5 years. The history is also positive for a prior interventional vascular procedure (balloon angioplasty) with concurrent use of urokinase (clot-dissolving medicine). A physical examination reveals a well-developed male with normal physical examination results. Pulses were present, with biphasic signals in both the dorsalis pedis and the posterior tibial vessels. When the pulses were examined after the patient exercised for 5 minutes, they were noted to be absent. A CAT scan performed on the legs revealed the presence of an abnormally located medial head of the gastrocnemius muscle. The muscle in effect "traps" the popliteal artery and vein during active motion. The condition is known as *popliteal entrapment syndrome.* This finding was confirmed with an angiogram. As the patient's foot was actively plantar flexed, one could see the cut off of contrast flowing down the vessel. The treatment for this was the surgical removal of the medial head of the muscle, which freed up both the artery and vein. The ulcer was then treated as a standard venous ulcer with local moist wound care and compression. The patient went on to heal and was able to resume normal activities again.

Clinical Points

1. The presence of a pulse does not preclude further investigation if the symptoms warrant. As well, we have demonstrated in this chapter that the presence of macrovascular flow does not always imply adequate microcirculation.
2. Consider evaluating both the ABI and the pulses after exercise in a patient with a history compatible with vascular disease and palpable pulses at rest.
3. A venous investigation should be performed when recurrent or recalcitrant venous ulcers are encountered.

▶ Case Study 5•2 | Venous Ulcer: Rule Out Malignancy First

SC is a 68-year-old white female with a history of lower extremity radiation therapy for a malignancy when she was 8 years old. She has a history of a nonhealing wound on this leg measuring 40 cm², with dense fibrin and subcutaneous calcification throughout. Angiography reveals a paucity of vessels within the entire region of the wound. An above-knee amputation was recommended by another physician before she arrived at the wound center. A surgical débridement down to muscle was carried out to remove all subcutaneous calcium and fibrinous debris. Small areas of hyperpigmentation were noted in several locations on the leg without a known diagnosis. Prior to the use of electrical stimulation, a biopsy of these pigmented areas was performed and the tissue was found to contain basal cell carcinoma, thereby contraindicating the use of electrical stimulation. Vacuum-assisted closure was used to develop a granulating bed, along with IV antibiotics. Subsequently, split-skin grafting was carried out, and the patient achieved a 95% graft take. She was discharged home with PO antibiotics for lifetime suppression of a methicillin-resistant *Staphylococcus aureus* (MRSA) infection and has been able to resume ambulation after physical therapy for gait training and strengthening.

Clinical Points

1. Always diagnosis suspicious lesions prior to initiating electrical stimulation.

2. Although the radical nature of the débridement required in this case is not common, it is always necessary to remove all nonviable tissue in order for normal healing to proceed.

3. If macrovascular flow can not be reestablished, then consider techniques that enhance local flow, such as electrical stimulation, vacuum-assisted closure, or techniques to enhance tissue oxygenation (i.e., hyperbaric oxygen) before resorting to amputation. In some instances primary amputation is clinically appropriate, but always consider the psychosocial, rehabilitation, and clinical (i.e., cardiac status) factors before making this decision.

4. Amputation should be considered when all the factors that impede healing have been identified and either corrected or, at a minimum, addressed.

References

1. Lazarus, GS, Cooper, DM, Knighton, D: Definitions and guidelines for assessment of wounds and evaluation of healing. Arch Dermatol 1994; 130:489–493.
2. Mulder, G, Armstrong, D, Seaman, S: Standard, appropriate, and advanced care and medical-legal considerations: Diabetic foot ulcerations. Wounds 2003; 15(Pt 1):92–106.
3. Tarnuzzer, RW, Schultz, GS: Biochemical analysis of acute and chronic wound environments. Wound Repair Regen 1996; 4:321–325.
4. Brem, H, Stojadinovic, O, Diegelmann, RF: Molecular markers in patients with chronic wounds to guide surgical debridement. Mol Med 2007; 13:30–39.
5. Ennis, WJ, Vargas, VM, Lee, C, et al: Wound outcomes from a single practice at a sub-acute wound care unit and 2 hospital based, outpatient settings. Wounds 2004; 16:165–172.
6. Ennis, WJ, Meneses, P: Comprehensive wound assessment and treatment system. In: Falabella, A, Kirsner, R (eds.): Wound Healing. Boca Raton, FL, Taylor & Francis, 2005, pp 59–68.
7. Ennis, WJ, Fiberger, E, Messner, K, Meneses, P: Wound healing outcomes: The impact of site of care and patient stratification. Wounds 2007;19(11) 286-293
8. Tatsioni, A, Balk, E, O'Donnell, T, et al: Usual care in the management of chronic wounds: A review of the recent literature. J Am Coll Surg 2007; 205:617–624. <A.
9. Margolis, DJ, Kantor, J, Berlin, A: Healing of diabetic neuropathic foot ulcers receiving standard treatment. A meta-analysis. Diabetes Care 1999; 22:692–695.
10. Margolis, DJ: The swings and roundabouts of randomized controlled studies in wound healing. Int J Low Extrem Wounds 2004; 3:4–6.
11. Ennis, WJ, Meneses, P: Factors impeding wound healing. In: Kloth, LC, McCulloch, J. (eds): Wound Healing: Alternatives in Management. Philadelphia, FA Davis, 2001, pp 68–96.
12. Robson, MC: Infection in the surgical patient: An imbalance in the normal equilibrium. Clin Plast Surg 1979; 6:493–503.
13. Robson, MC: Wound infection. A failure of wound healing caused by an imbalance of bacteria. Surg Clin North Am 1997; 77:637–650.
14. Robson, MC, Stenberg, BD, Heggers, JP: Wound healing alterations caused by infection. Clin Plast Surg 1990; 17:485–492.
15. Whitney, J, Phillips, L, Aslam, R: Guidelines for the treatment of pressure ulcers. Wound Repair Regen 2006; 14:663–679.
16. Field, FK, Kerstein, MD: Overview of wound healing in a moist environment. Am J Surg 1994; 167:2S–6S.
17. Stotts, NA: Determination of bacterial burden in wounds. Adv Wound Care 1995; 8(suppl):46–52.
18. Kim, SH, Hubbard, GB, Whorley, BL: A rapid section technique for burn wound biopsy. J Burn Care Rehabil 1985; 6:433–435.
19. Heggers, JP, Robson, MC, Doran, ET: Quantitative assessment of bacterial contamination of open wounds by a slide technique. Trans R Soc Trop Med Hyg 1969; 63:532–534.
20. Burke, JF: Effects of inflammation on wound repair. J Dent Res 1971; 50:296–303.
21. Laato, M, Lehtonen, OP, Niinikoski, J: Granulation tissue formation in experimental wounds inoculated with *Staphylococcus aureus*. Acta Chir Scand 1985; 151:313–318.
22. Tenorio, A, Jindrak, K, Weiner, M: Accelerated healing in infected wounds. Surg Gynecol Obstet 1976; 142:537–543.
23. Levenson, SM, Kan-Gruber, D, Gruber, C: Wound healing accelerated by *Staphylococcus aureus*. Arch Surg 1983; 118:310–320.
24. Cutting, KF, White, RJ: Criteria for identifying wound infection—revisited. Ostomy Wound Manage 2005; 51:28–34.
25. Cutting, KF: Identification of infection in granulating wounds by registered nurses. J Clin Nurs 1998; 7:539–546.
26. Ennis, WJ, Meneses, P: Clinical evaluation: Outcomes, benchmarking, introspection, and quality improvement. Ostomy Wound Manage 1996; 42(suppl):40S–47S.
27. Jones, KR, Fennie, K: Factors influencing pressure ulcer healing in adults over 50: An exploratory study. J Am Med Dir Assoc 2007; 8:378–387.
28. Mertz, PM, Ovington, LG: Wound healing microbiology. Dermatol Clin 1993; 11:739–747.
29. Ayton, M: Wound care: Wounds that won't heal. Nurs Times 1985; 81(suppl):16–19.

30. White, RJ, Cutting, KF: Critical colonization—The concept under scrutiny. Ostomy Wound Manage 2006; 52:550–556.

31. Ennis, WJ, Meneses, P: Wound healing at the local level: The stunned wound. Ostomy Wound Manage 2000; 46(suppl):39S–48S; quiz 49S–50S.

32. Costerton, JW: Cystic fibrosis pathogenesis and the role of biofilms in persistent infection. Trends Microbiol 2001; 9:50–52.

33. Allen, L, Dockrell, DH, Pattery, T: Pyocyanin production by *Pseudomonas aeruginosa* induces neutrophil apoptosis and impairs neutrophil-mediated host defenses in vivo. J Immunol 2005; 174:3643–3649.

34. Stephens, P, Wall, IB, Wilson, MJ: Anaerobic cocci populating the deep tissues of chronic wounds impair cellular wound healing responses in vitro. Br J Dermatol 2003; 148:456–466.

35. Cutting, K, White, R, Edmonds, M: The safety and efficacy of dressings with silver—Addressing clinical concerns. Int Wound J 2007; 4:177–184.

36. Landsdown, AB, Williams, A: Bacterial resistance to silver in wound care and medical devices. J Wound Care 2007; 16:15–19.

37. Perera, GB, Lyden, SP: Current trends in lower extremity revascularization. Surg Clin North Am 2007; 87:1135–1147.

38. DeRubertis, BG, Faries, PL, McKinsey, JF: Shifting paradigms in the treatment of lower extremity vascular disease: A report of 1000 percutaneous interventions. Ann Surg 2007; 246:415–422; discussion 422–424.

39. Arora, S, LoGerfo, FW: Lower extremity macrovascular disease in diabetes. J Am Podiatr Med Assoc 1997; 87:327–331.

40. Holland-Letz, T, Endres, HG, Biedermann, S: Reproducibility and reliability of the ankle-brachial index as assessed by vascular experts, family physicians and nurses. Vasc Med 2007; 12:105–112.

41. Perry, JT, Statler, JD: Advances in vascular imaging. Surg Clin North Am 2007; 87:975–993.

42. Allen, DB, Majuire, JJ, Mahdavian, M: Wound hypoxia and acidosis limit neutrophil bacterial killing mechanisms. Arch Surg 1997; 132:991–996.

43. Hunt, TK, Pai, MP: The effect of varying ambient oxygen tensions on wound metabolism and collagen synthesis. Surg Gynecol Obstet 1972; 135:561–567.

44. Knighton, DR, Hunt, TK, Scheuenstuhl, H: Oxygen tension regulates the expression of angiogenesis factor by macrophages. Science 1983; 221:1283–1285.

45. Ennis, WJ, Meneses, P: Technologies for assessment of wound microcirculation. In: Krasner, DL, Sibbald, RG, Rodeheaver, G (eds.): Chronic Wound Care: A Clinical Source Book for Healthcare Professionals, ed 4. Malverne, PA, HMP Communications, 2007, pp. 417–426.

46. Ubbink, DT, Spincemaille, GH, Reneman, RS: Prediction of imminent amputation in patients with non-reconstructible leg ischemia by means of microcirculatory investigations. J Vasc Surg 1999; 30:114–121.

47. Ennis, WJ, Lee, C, Meneses, P: A biochemical approach to wound healing through the use of modalities. Clin Dermatol 2007; 25:63–72.

48. Ennis, WJ: Microcirculation: The push-pull theory. Gynecological Oncology 2008;111:S81–S86.

49. Hightower, CM, Intaglietta, M: The use of diagnostic frequency continuous ultrasound to improve microcirculatory function after ischemia-reperfusion injury. Microcirculation 2007; 14:571–582.

50. Ennis, WJ, Valdes, W, Gainer M, et al: Evaluation of clinical effectiveness of MIST ultrasound therapy for the healing of chronic wounds. Adv Skin Wound Care 2006; 19:437–446.

51. Coulling, S: Fundamentals of pain management in wound care. Br J Nurs 2007; 16:S4–S6, S8, S10.

52. Arrick, DM, Mayhan, WG: Acute infusion of nicotine impairs nNOS-dependent reactivity of cerebral arterioles via an increase in oxidative stress. J Appl Physiol 2007;103(6):2062–2067.

53. Pullar, CE, Zhao, M, Song, G, et al: Beta-adrenergic receptor agonists delay while antagonists accelerate epithelial wound healing: Evidence of an endogenous adrenergic network within the corneal epithelium. J Cell Physiol 2007; 211:261–272.

54. Ubbink, DT, Verhaar, EE, Lie, HK, et al: Effect of beta-blockers on peripheral skin microcirculation in hypertension and peripheral vascular disease. J Vasc Surg 2003; 38:535–540.

55. Wollina, U, Abdel-Naser, MB, Mani, R: A review of the microcirculation in skin in patients with chronic venous insufficiency: The problem and the evidence available for therapeutic options. Int J Low Extrem Wounds 2006; 5:169–180.

56. Gilje, O: On taping (adhesive tape treatment) of leg ulcers. Acta Dermaol Venereol 1948; 28:454.

57. Winter, GD: Formation of the scab and the rate of epithelization of superficial wounds in the skin of the young domestic pig. Nature 1962; 193:293–294.

58. Winter, GD, Scales JT: Effect of air drying and dressings on the surface of a wound. Nature 1963; 197:91–92.

59. Hinman, CD, Maibach, H: Effect of air exposure and occlusion on experimental human skin wounds. Nature 1963; 200:377–378.

60. Hutchinson, JJ, Lawrence, JC: Wound infection under occlusive dressings. J Hosp Infect 1991; 17:83–94.

61. Agency for Healthcare Policy and Research Guidelines: Treatment of Pressure Ulcers. No. 15. Rockville, MD, U.S. Department of Health and Human Services, 1994.

62. Lau, GW, Hasset, DJ, Ran, H, et al: The role of pyocyanin in *Pseudomonas aeruginosa* infection. Trends Mol Med 2004; 10:599–606.

63. Ayello, EA, Cuddigan, JE: Debridement: Controlling the necrotic/cellular burden. Adv Skin Wound Care 2004; 17:66–75; quiz 76–78.

64. Spotnitz, WD, Falstrom, JK, Rodeheaver, GT: The role of sutures and fibrin sealant in wound healing. Surg Clin North Am 1997; 77:651–669.

65. Carlson, MA: Acute wound failure. Surg Clin North Am 1997; 77:607–636.

66. Schecter, WP, Ivatury, RR, Rotondo, MF, et al: Open abdomen after trauma and abdominal sepsis: A strategy for management. J Am Coll Surg 2006; 203:390–396.

67. Bellows, CF, Alder, A, Helton, WS: Abdominal wall reconstruction using biological tissue grafts: Present status and future opportunities. Expert Rev Med Devices 2006; 3:657–675.

68. Brown, GL, Richardson, JD, Malangoni, MA, et al: Comparison of prosthetic materials for abdominal wall reconstruction in the presence of contamination and infection. Ann Surg 1985; 201:705–711.

69. Bellows, CF, Alder, A, Helton, WS: Abdominal wall repair using human acellular dermis. Am J Surg 2007; 194:192–198.

70. Di Vita, G, Patti, R, Vetra, G, et al: Production of cytokines at the operation site. G Chir 2005; 26:241–245.

71. Chuo, CB, Thomas, SS: Absorbable mesh and topical negative pressure therapy for closure of abdominal dehiscence with exposed bowel. J Plast Reconstr Aesthet Surg 2007;61(11):1378–1381.

72. Saito, T, Tazawa, K, Yokoyam, Y, et al: Surgical stress inhibits the growth of fibroblasts through the elevation of plasma catecholamine and cortisol concentrations. Surg Today 1997; 27:627–631.

73. Karayiannakis, AJ, Makri, G, Mantzioka, A, et al: Systemic stress response after laparoscopic or open cholecystectomy: A randomized trial. Br J Surg 1997; 84:467–471.

74. Esterling, BA, Kiecolt-Glaser, KJ, Bodnar, JC, et al: Chronic stress, social support, and persistent alterations in the natural killer cell response to cytokines in older adults. Health Psychol 1994; 13:291–298.

75. Irwin, MR: Human psychoneuroimmunology: 20 Years of discovery. Brain Behav Immun 2007;22(2):129–139.

76. Christian, LM, Graham, JE, Padgett, DA, et al: Stress and wound healing. Neuroimmunomodulation 2006; 13:337–346.

77. Kiecolt-Glaser, JK, Marucha, PT, Malarkey, WB, et al: Slowing of wound healing by psychological stress. Lancet 1995; 346:1194–1196.

78. Engeland, CG, Bosch, JA, Cacioppo, JT, et al: Mucosal wound healing: The roles of age and sex. Arch Surg 2006; 141:1193–1197; discussion 1198.

79. Horan, MP, Quan, N, Subramanian, SV, et al: Impaired wound contraction and delayed myofibroblast differentiation in restraint-stressed mice. Brain Behav Immun 2005; 19:207–216.

80. Sheridan, JF, Padgett, DA, Avitsur, R, et al: Experimental models of stress and wound healing. World J Surg 2004; 28:327–330.

81. Bosch, JA, Engeleand, CG, Cacioppo, JT, et al: Depressive symptoms predict mucosal wound healing. Psychosom Med 2007; 69:597–605.

82. Cantrell, RW: Physiological effects of noise. Otolaryngol Clin North Am 1979; 12:537–549.

83. Morrison, WE, Haas, EC, Schaffner, DH, et al: Noise, stress, and annoyance in a pediatric intensive care unit. Crit Care Med 2003; 31:113–119.

84. Wysocki, AB: The effect of intermittent noise exposure on wound healing. Adv Wound Care 1996; 9:35–39.

85. Christensen, M: Noise levels in a general intensive care unit: A descriptive study. Nurs Crit Care 2007; 12:188–197.

86. Sandrick, K: Gearing up for the JCAHO's new pain management standards: Some hospitals are ahead of the game. Strateg Healthcare Excell 2000; 13:1–8.

87. Price, P, Fogh, K, Glynn, C, et al: Managing painful chronic wounds: The Wound Pain Management Model. Int Wound J 2007; 4(suppl):4–15.

88. Krasner, D: The chronic wound pain experience: A conceptual model. Ostomy Wound Manage 1995; 41:20–25.

89. Karam, JG, El-Sayegh, S, Nessim, F, et al: Medical management of obesity: An update. Minerva Endocrinol 2007; 32:185–207.

90. Gendall, KA, Raninga, S, Kennedy, R, et al: The impact of obesity on outcome after major colorectal surgery. Dis Colon Rectum 2007;50(12):2223–2237.

91. Gottschlich, MM, Mayes, T, Khoury, JC, et al: Significance of obesity on nutritional, immunologic, hormonal, and clinical outcome parameters in burns. J Am Diet Assoc 1993; 93:1261–1268.

92. Nicholson, ML, Dennis, MJ, Makin, DS, et al: Obesity as a risk factor in major reconstructive vascular surgery. Eur J Vasc Surg 1994; 8:209–213.

93. Baugh, N, Zuelzer, H, Meador, J, et al: Wound wise: Wounds in surgical patients who are obese. Am J Nurs 2007; 107:40–50; quiz 51.

94. Knudsen, AM, Gallagher, S: Care of the obese patient with pressure ulcers. J Wound Ostomy Continence Nurs 2003; 30:111–118.

95. Harris, CL, Fraser, C: Malnutrition in the institutionalized elderly: The effects on wound healing. Ostomy Wound Manage 2004; 50:54–63.

96. Pompeo, M: Misconceptions about protein requirements for wound healing: Results of a prospective study. Ostomy Wound Manage 2007; 53:30–32, 34, 36–38.

97. Zulkowski, K: Nutrition and aging: A transdisciplinary approach. Ostomy Wound Manage 2006; 52:53–57.

98. Pinchcofsky-Devin, GD, Kaminski, MV: Correlation of pressure sores and nutritional status. J Am Geriatr Soc 1986; 34:435–430.

99. Thomas, DR: Improving outcome of pressure ulcers with nutritional interventions: A review of the evidence. Nutrition 2001; 17:121–125.

100. Kurz, A, Sessler, DI, Lenhardt, R: Perioperative normothermia to reduce the incidence of surgical-wound infection and shorten hospitalization. Study of Wound Infection and Temperature Group. N Engl J Med 1996; 334:1209–1215.

101. Ying, CL, Tsang, SF, Ng, KF: The potential use of desmopressin to correct hypothermia-induced impairment of primary haemostasis— An in vitro study using PFA-100((R)). Resuscitation 2008; 76(1): 129–133.

102. Hunt, TK: The effect of varying ambient oxygen tensions on wound metabolism and collagen synthesis. Surg Gynecol Obstet 1972; 135:561–567.

103. Price, P, Bale, S, Crook, H, et al: The effect of a radiant heat dressing on pressure ulcers. J Wound Care 2000; 9:203–205.

104. Kloth, LC, Berman, JE, Dumit-Minkel, S, et al: Effects of a normothermic dressing on pressure ulcer healing. Adv Skin Wound Care 2000; 13:69–74.

105. Diamant, AL, Babey, SH, Hastert, TA, et al: Diabetes: the growing epidemic. Policy Brief UCLA Cent Health Policy Res 2007; Aug-PB 2007-9:1–12.

106. Krishnan, S, Nash, F, Baker, N, et al: Reduction in diabetic amputations over eleven years in a defined UK population—Benefits of multidisciplinary team working and prospective audit. Diabetes Care 2008;31(1):99–101.

107. Danese, C, Vestri, AR, D'Alfonso, V, et al: Do hypertension and diabetes mellitus influence the site of atherosclerotic plaques? Clin Ter 2006; 157:9–13.

108. Kearney, M, Duncan, E, Kahn, M, et al: Insulin resistance and endothelial cell dysfunction. Exp Physiol 2008;93(1):158–163.

109. Arora, S, Pomposelli, F, LoGerfo, FW, et al: Cutaneous microcirculation in the neuropathic diabetic foot improves significantly but not completely after successful lower extremity revascularization. J Vasc Surg 2002; 35:501–505.

110. Delamaire, M, Maugendre, D, Moreno, M, et al: Impaired leucocyte functions in diabetic patients. Diabet Med 1997; 14:29–34.

111. Kiziltan, ME, Gunduz, A, Kiziltan, G, et al: Peripheral neuropathy in patients with diabetic foot ulcers: Clinical and nerve conduction study. J Neurol Sci 2007; 258:75–79.

112. Andersen, CA, Roukis, TA: The diabetic foot. Surg Clin North Am 2007; 87:1149–1177.

113. Debono, M, Cachia, E: The impact of diabetes on psychological well being and quality of life. The role of patient education. Psychol Health Med 2007; 12:545–555.

114. Ennis, WJ, Meneses, P: Leg ulcers: A practical approach to the leg ulcer patient. Ostomy Wound Manage 1995; 41(suppl):52S–62S; discussion 63S.

115. LoGerfo, FW, Coffman, JD: Current concepts. Vascular and microvascular disease of the foot in diabetes. Implications for foot care. N Engl J Med 1984; 311:1615–1619.

116. Khaodhiar, L, Dinh, T, Schmoaker, KT, et al: The use of medical hyperspectral technology to evaluate microcirculatory changes in diabetic foot ulcers and to predict clinical outcomes. Diabetes Care 2007; 30:903–910.

117. De Mattia, G, Bravi, MC, Laurenti, O, et al: Endothelial dysfunction and oxidative stress in type 1 and type 2 diabetic patients without clinical macrovascular complications. Diabetes Res Clin Pract 2008;79(2):337–342.

118. Ennis, WJ, Meneses, P: Standard, appropriate and advanced care and medicolegal considerations: Venous ulcerations. Wounds 2003; 15(Pt 2):107–122.

119. Browse, NL, Burnand, KG: The cause of venous ulceration. Lancet 1982; 2:243–245.

120. Falanga, V, Eaglstein, WH: The "trap" hypothesis of venous ulceration. Lancet 1993; 341:1006–1008.

121. Coleridge Smith, PD, Thomas, P, Scurr, JH, et al: Causes of venous ulceration: A new hypothesis. Br Med J (Clin Res Ed) 1988; 296:1726–1727.

122. Coleridge Smith, PD: From skin disorders to venous leg ulcers: Pathophysiology and efficacy of Daflon 500 mg in ulcer healing. Angiology 2003; 54(suppl):S45–S50.

123. Abbade, LP, Lastoria, S: Venous ulcer: Epidemiology, physiopathology, diagnosis and treatment. Int J Dermatol 2005; 44:449–456.

124. Whiddon, LL: The treatment of venous ulcers of the lower extremities. Proc (Bayl Univ Med Cent) 2007; 20:363–366.

125. Marston, WA: PPG, APG, duplex: Which noninvasive tests are most appropriate for the management of patients with chronic venous insufficiency? Semin Vasc Surg 2002; 15:13–20.

126. Barwell, JR, Davies, CE, Deacon, JU, et al: Comparison of surgery and compression with compression alone in chronic venous ulceration (ESCHAR study): Randomised controlled trial. Lancet 2004; 363:1854–1859.

127. Leyden, JJ: Clinical features of ageing skin. Br J Dermatol 1990; 122(suppl):1–3.

128. Meyer, LJ, Stern, R: Age-dependent changes of hyaluronan in human skin. J Invest Dermatol 1994; 102:385–389.

129. Holt, DR, Kirk, SJ, Reagan, MC, et al: Effect of age on wound healing in healthy human beings. Surgery 1992; 112:293–297; discussion 297–298.

130. Fenske, NA, Lober, CW: Structural and functional changes of normal aging skin. J Am Acad Dermatol 1986; 15(Pt 1):571–585.

131. Kramer, RH, Fuh, GM, Bensch, KG, et al: Synthesis of extracellular matrix glycoproteins by cultured microvascular endothelial cells isolated from the dermis of neonatal and adult skin. J Cell Physiol 1985; 123:1–9.

132. Ennis, WJ, Meneses, P: Strategic planning for the wound care clinic in a managed care environment. Ostomy Wound Manage 1996; 42:54–56, 58, 60.

133. Robson, MC, Edstrom, LE, Krizek, TJ, et al: The efficacy of systemic antibiotics in the treatment of granulating wounds. J Surg Res 1974; 16:299–306.

134. Ehrlich, HP, Hunt, TK: Effects of cortisone and vitamin A on wound healing. Ann Surg 1968; 167:324–328.

135. Ponec, M, de Haas, C, Bachra, BN, et al: Effects of glucocorticosteroids on primary human skin fibroblasts. I. Inhibition of the proliferation of cultured primary human skin and mouse L929 fibroblasts. Arch Dermatol Res 1977; 259:117–123.

136. Hunt, TK, Ehrlich, HP, Garcia, JA, et al: Effect of vitamin A on reversing the inhibitory effect of cortisone on healing of open wounds in animals and man. Ann Surg 1969; 170:633–641.

137. Haws, M, Brown, RE, Suchy, H, et al: Vitamin A-soaked gel foam sponges and wound healing in steroid-treated animals. Ann Plast Surg 1994; 32:418–422.

138. Golan, J, Mitelman, S, Baruchin, A, et al: Vitamin A and corticosteroid interaction in wound healing in rats. Isr J Med Sci 1980; 16:572–575.

139. Krischak, GD, Augat, P, Claes, L, et al: The effects of non-steroidal anti-inflammatory drug application on incisional wound healing in rats. J Wound Care 2007; 16:76–78.

140. Kolb, BA, Buller, RE, Conner, JP, et al: Effects of early postoperative chemotherapy on wound healing. Obstet Gynecol 1992; 79:988–992.

141. Folkman, J: Is angiogenesis an organizing principle in biology and medicine? J Pediatr Surg 2007; 42:1–11.

142. Haroon, ZA, Amin, K, Saito, W, et al: SU5416 delays wound healing through inhibition of TGF-beta 1 activation. Cancer Biol Ther 2002; 1:121–126.

143. Busti, AJ, Hooper, JS, Amaya, CJ, et al: Effects of perioperative anti-inflammatory and immunomodulating therapy on surgical wound healing. Pharmacotherapy 2005; 25:1566–1591.

144. Ugurlu, L, Turan, M, Canbay, E, et al: Effect of nifedipine on the healing of left colonic anastomoses in rats. Surg Today 2003; 33:902–908.

145. Ilhan, YS, Bulbuller, N, Kirkil, C, et al: The effect of an angiotensin converting enzyme inhibitor on intestinal wound healing. J Surg Res 2005; 128:61–65.

146. Scanton, E, Stubbs, N: To use or not to use? The debate on the use of antiseptics in wound care. Br J Community Nurs 2002;sept 8,10(12) passim.

147. Brown, CD, Zitelli, JA: A review of topical agents for wounds and methods of wounding. Guidelines for wound management. J Dermatol Surg Oncol 1993; 19:732–737.

148. Smith, RG: A critical discussion of the use of antiseptics in acute traumatic wounds. J Am Podiatr Med Assoc 2005; 95:148–153.

149. Chambers, H, Dumville, JC, Cullum, N: Silver treatments for leg ulcers: A systematic review. Wound Repair Regen 2007; 15:165–173.

150. Eriksson, AS, Sinclair, R, Cassuto, J, et al: Influence of lidocaine on leukocyte function in the surgical wound. Anesthesiology 1992; 77:74–78.

151. Powell, DM, Rodeheaver, GT, Foresman, PA, et al: Damage to tissue defenses by EMLA cream. J Emerg Med 1991; 9:205–209.

152. Hansson, C, Holm, J, Lillieborg, S, et al: Repeated treatment with lidocaine/prilocaine cream (EMLA) as a topical anaesthetic for the cleansing of venous leg ulcers. A controlled study. Acta Derm Venereol 1993; 73:231–233.

153. Berg, JO, Mossner, BK, Skov, MN, et al: Antibacterial properties of EMLA and lidocaine in wound tissue biopsies for culturing. Wound Repair Regen 2006; 14:581–585.

154. Maragakis, LL, Cosgrove, SE, Song, X, et al: An outbreak of multidrug-resistant *Acinetobacter baumannii* associated with pulsatile lavage wound treatment. JAMA 2004; 292:3006–3011.

155. Palfreyman, S, Nelson, EA, Michaels, JA: Dressings for venous leg ulcers: Systematic review and meta-analysis. BMJ 2007; 335:244.

chapter 6

The General Evaluation

Katherine E. Lampe, PT, MPT, CWS, FACCWS

Wound evaluation is the foundation upon which appropriate wound interventions are based. Evaluation may include specific measurements and tests to assess the wound, periwound skin, limb, or adjacent anatomical regions. Physiological and anatomical systems, general health, functional status, and other factors that affect an individual should also be evaluated. The next step in the evaluation process entails making a judgment about or placing a value on test and measurement data. These clinical judgments drive the plan of care for the patient with a wound. Continuous and timely reevaluation of the individual and his or her wound aids the clinician in monitoring healing. Evaluation of wound and patient responses to treatment allows the clinician to determine treatment effectiveness. If the examination and evaluation reveal negative outcomes, adjustments in the intervention are necessary to augment healing. Consequently, wound evaluation will influence which interventions are chosen to produce or enhance the best outcome for the patient.

Evaluation also serves additional purposes besides directing the decision-making process in wound management. Wound evaluation provides vital information for communication between members of the interdisciplinary wound management team. Communication is essential for ensuring consistency and quality of care provided by the team. The documentation of wound evaluation also plays a role in communication with reimbursement agencies because agencies require this documentation in order to make decisions for payment. Documentation of wound evaluation should include tools, tests, and measures used in the evaluation process. Please see Chapter 33 for more details on documentation and reimbursement. Accurate, valid, reliable, and practical evaluation tools and measures are needed to further the knowledge base regarding all aspects of wound management. Communication, quality patient care, reimbursement, research, and clinical decision making are all factors that will influence selection and utilization of appropriate wound and patient evaluation procedures.

This chapter begins by focusing on aspects of a patient's history that influence evaluation and clinical decision making in wound management. Before considering objective aspects, a review of risk assessment, along with its objective aspects, is appropriate. Knowledge of patient history and possible risk factors for wound development enables clinicians to implement wound prevention tactics. Evaluation of a person with a wound should be based on practical, efficient, reliable, and valid evaluation tools and measures. Also included is a brief discussion of devices, equipment, and other miscellaneous factors to consider when completing a thorough evaluation. Finally, a discussion of wound reevaluation, outcome prediction, and a patient case are presented. Overall, this chapter presents the building blocks needed to lay the solid foundation for a complete wound evaluation, which is the foundation of clinical decision making.

Patient History

The patient's history, often part of a subjective examination, plays a crucial role in evaluation and subsequent treatment of the patient with a wound. While collecting the history, a clinician simultaneously formulates strategies for essential evaluation. This concurrent decision-making process includes gathering information for determination of the diagnosis and prognosis, as well as for planning interventions and predicting possible outcomes. Another aspect of the subjective evaluation, which should not be taken for granted, is the establishment of rapport. Rapport is vital for the growth of the therapeutic relationship. The first encounter with the patient, family, or caregiver will set the stage for development of a trusting, productive relationship with the clinician.

Patient evaluation entails data collection, interpretation, treatment implementation, and continuous reevaluation. Patient management is best served by assessing all factors that impact patient outcomes. Various guidelines, publications, and agencies exist to provide a framework for patient management. One tool, developed by the American Physical Therapy Association (APTA), is the *Guide to Physical Therapist Practice* (referred to here as *The Guide*).[1] This APTA publication has six components: examination, evaluation, diagnosis, prognosis, intervention, and management of outcomes. Table 6.1 provides an expanded description of these components. The Agency for Healthcare Research and Quality (AHRQ) has made recommendations regarding patient history to ensure a comprehensive, accurate assessment of the individual with a wound. Two AHRQ publications relevant to wound management are *Pressure Ulcers in Adults: Prediction and Prevention: Clinical Practice Guidelines*,[2] and *Treatment of Pressure Ulcers: Clinical Practice Guidelines*.[3] The latter addresses a comprehensive approach to the patient population with pressure ulcers. Although this guideline is for pressure ulcer treatment, it is the only guideline by the AHRQ to actually address the evaluation and treatment of any type of wound. Consequently, a brief review of what the document recommends for inclusion in a patient history is prudent here. The guideline recommends a complete history and physical examination, including complications and comorbidities, nutritional status, wound-related pain, psychosocial issues, and risk for development of other ulcers. Many of the items in the patient history section of this chapter will reflect the recommendations of both the APTA and the AHRQ guidelines. These documents make similar statements emphasizing the necessity of addressing the entire patient when completing a wound evaluation, including the procurement of the patient history. Certainly, few would disagree that knowledge of the entire patient is vital for the appropriate clinical judgments that result from the evaluation.

Patient Demographics

Typically, the first data gathered from a patient include demographic information. The individual may be required to fill out a form detailing demographics, past and present history, and other health information. Although this may be a more efficient use of the clinician's time, the burden is on the clinician to review the information during the evaluation and analyze it adequately. Demographic information pertinent to wound evaluation may include age, gender, race, ethnicity, and preferred language. Age, a factor discussed in Chapter 5, may affect wound healing. Age, gender, and race are informational items that aid the clinician in differential diagnosis. The primary language of the patient, family, and caregiver is important to ensure adequate information gathering and subsequent communication during treatment.

Occupation/Employment

How the patient occupies his or her time provides an indication of the patient's functional needs and goals. Occupation or employment includes not only the requirements or functions of a job but also community activities or responsibilities, including school and educational needs. This information is essential for the collaboration of the clinician and patient, family, and caregivers in development of meaningful goals. The occupation or employment of the patient may also provide insight into causes of wounds. For example, do the job, schooling, and other community activities require excessive standing or sitting, which may impact lower extremity circulation? Issues related to tissue trauma, repetitive activities, and many other areas might need to be identified to gain an accurate picture of all concerns related to wound management.

Social Information

Patients often have social factors that affect their care. Social information will aid the clinician in designing a realistic plan of care that will mesh with the patient and family lifestyle and

Table 6•1	Guide to Physical Therapy Practice: Patient Management Components[1]	
Components	**Description**	
Examination	History, systems review, tests, measures	
Evaluation	Clinical judgment based on examination	
Diagnosis	Information grouped in syndromes/categories; determines interventions	
Prognosis	Determination of optimal improvement level/time needed to reach this level	
Intervention	Therapist, patient, family collaboration resulting in methods to produce results	
Management outcomes	Limitation/disability remediation, patient satisfaction, prevention	

value system. Often, treatment adherence issues for the patient, family, or caregiver may be disclosed by factors identified in the social history. Social roles held by the patient or members of the family, along with the patient's personal goals and needs, should be taken into consideration. Other social background elements to review may include cultural beliefs and behaviors; family and caregiver resources; various social interactions, activities, and support systems; lifestyle choices, and values and goals of the patient, family, and caregiver.[1,3] An understanding of the physical living situation and assistance available to the patient upon discharge allows the clinician to weigh this information in light of what is required for intervention. Social habits that impair tissue healing, such as the use of tobacco products, alcohol, and drugs, will be discussed in the section on general health. Clearly, social issues and concerns will impact wound management.

Past Medical Information

The past medical history of an individual with a wound contains information that will have repercussions for the expected outcomes. There are many diseases and disorders that can have a negative impact on the healing process. As an example, circulatory diseases will affect tissue oxygenation, nutrition, and health, as well as a person's function and mobility. Consequently, the peripheral vascular system deserves close scrutiny during the assessment of the patient's history. The clinician should question a patient about past history for peripheral vascular disease (arterial or venous insufficiency), arteriosclerosis, atherosclerosis, vein valvular incompetence, deep vein thrombosis, clotting disorders, hypertension, and congestive heart failure.

Diabetes often leads to circulatory, neuropathic, and metabolic changes that affect wound healing. The chronicity of diabetes and the maintenance of blood sugar control affect the rate of onset and severity of development of sensory, motor, and autonomic neuropathy. Diabetic neuropathy leads to biomechanical derangement of the foot secondary to loss of protective sensation, loss of proprioception in the foot, and hypermobility of tarsal and metatarsal joints. The ramifications of circulatory disease and diabetes on healing are examples of the importance of reviewing a patient's past medical history. Chapter 5 examines in greater depth how general health and other issues affect tissue repair.

A medical history review would not be complete without examining a patient's family history for disease and other comorbidities. Family history may provide clues to the extent of diagnosed problems. A family history of disease and patient risk factors may also lead the evaluation process into identifying undiagnosed conditions that may impact wound management.

Current Status

The patient's current health status must be completely reviewed. Items for discussion may include general health, functional abilities, psychological well-being, current medications, nutrition and hydration, recent tests or measures, current wound status, and wound-related pain. These issues need to be investigated in order to develop appropriate wound management interventions.[1]

The clinician should obtain all pertinent general health information from the patient. Much of this information is reflected in the review of past medical history. Specific questions should also be asked regarding medication or other agent allergies and intolerances in order to identify medications or chemical agents that have caused difficulties. Avoidance or alleviation of these agents is required if undesirable medication side effects or tissue irritation has occurred. Examples of such agents include whirlpool additives and cytotoxic topical wound agents.

The issue of adequate rest is also important to discuss. Patients with wounds may experience wound pain and discomfort that interrupts sleep at night and functioning during the day. This lack of sleep can affect general health, resulting in interrupted sleep patterns, complaints of low energy levels, and fatigue. Behavioral health risk factors and habits also need to be identified. Examples of habits or behavioral health risk factors that have a negative impact on wound repair include drug abuse, excessive alcohol consumption, and tobacco use.[4-6] Nicotine causes constriction of arteries, and long-term nicotine use can lead to arteriosclerosis.[5,6] Alcoholism has been linked to pressure ulcer development.[4] Inappropriate use of alcohol may also impact adequate nutritional intake. Current and past use of these substances should be noted, along with the frequency of drug, alcohol, and tobacco use.

Current and previous functional abilities of the patient must be determined for the formulation of appropriate patient- and family-centered goals. Functional capability information acquired from the patient, family, and caregiver should cover self-care, mobility, activities in the home, work, school, play, and leisure.[1] Every aspect of the patient's mobility, no matter how basic, should be examined. If the patient is bedbound, mobility must be ascertained. The ability to change positions in bed is a contributing factor in pressure ulcer development. Bed or wheelchair transfers and the ability to maintain a sitting posture require evaluation of sitting tolerance and skin interface pressures. This information will guide selection of seating systems or devices. When a patient can ambulate, the risk of pressure ulcers decreases; however, the clinician must check for protective sensation in the feet, foot deformities, proper fit of footwear, and provide care of the feet. See Chapter 19 for excellent information on pressure ulcer prevention and management.

Both APTA's *Guide to Physical Therapy Practice*[1] and AHRQ's *Treatment of Pressure Ulcers: Clinical Practice Guidelines*[3] encourage clinicians to assess the psychological status of the patient with a wound. *The Guide* suggests evaluation of the patient's psychological functioning, including memory, reasoning ability, anxiety, depression, and morale.[1] The AHRQ recommends the following for patients with pressure ulcers:

All individuals being treated for pressure ulcers should undergo a psychosocial assessment to determine their ability and motivation to comprehend and adhere to the treatment program. The assessment should include but not be limited to the following: mental status, learning ability, depression, goals, values, and lifestyle, social support, sexuality, polypharmacy or overmedication, culture and ethnicity, alcohol and/or drug abuse, stressors. Periodic reassessment is recommended.[3]

The clinician wishing to conduct a complete evaluation of the patient with a wound cannot overlook the psychosocial aspects that may influence wound management.

An understanding of medication effects on tissue healing is vital for optimal wound management and care of the patient. An accurate and complete listing of all patient medications must be obtained. Clinicians should be aware of the effects of polypharmacy on the elderly, medication interactions, side effects, and other pharmacological concerns. For example, steroids, used for their anti-inflammatory and immunosuppressive effects, may have a negative influence on healing. They may suppress the inflammatory process, increase the risk of infection, and over the long term could cause tissue catabolism.[7] Heavy metal residues found in various antimicrobials may cause irritation of viable tissue in some patients.[8] A thorough review of this topic is presented in Chapter 13. The reader is also referred to *Pharmacology in Rehabilitation*[7] for more information concerning medications and their implications in clinical practice.[9,10]

A review of nutrition and hydration is necessary to determine the need for a referral to a registered dietician. Poor nutrition can hamper the repair process. Although more detailed information on nutrition and hydration is presented in Chapter 4, some factors will be presented here regarding the need to identify problems associated with nutrition and hydration. Table 6.2 identifies a number of factors the clinician should consider when discussing the nutrition and hydration needs of a patient with a wound. Anthropometric measurements may reveal the amount of total body water, body fat, and protein stores of the patient. The water content of the adult body is approximately 73%.[11] Tissue hydration is needed for adequate tissue perfusion and healing. Caffeine and alcohol are diuretics and can lead to dehydration.[12] Items under the headings of biochemical data, clinical information, and dietary history in Table 6.2 can also assist in determining risk for wound development and ability to heal. For example, malnutrition has been indicated as a risk factor for pressure ulcer development in several studies.[13-17]

Recent tests and measures conducted by the therapist or other health-care provider may provide more insight into biochemical and clinical considerations for nutritional status. Table 6.3 contains information on nutrition and laboratory data. The significance of biochemical data is demonstrated by adequate protein levels required to produce collagen, wound contraction, and other aspects of wound repair. Dietary history should also be discussed with the patient, family, or caregiver. Table 6.2 includes areas to discuss in the dietary history. In light of nutrition, hydration, and other metabolic considerations, a review of the patient's needs in these areas is warranted. Patients with chronic wounds, or individuals who are at risk for developing wounds, should be evaluated by a registered dietician. Nutrition and wound healing are covered in greater detail in Chapter 4.

Often, the patient with a wound will have experienced prior testing or examination by other health professionals. The information gathered from these tests, measures, and examinations can be invaluable in the decision-making process for wound management. Previously, laboratory values were discussed in relationship to the health status and nutrition of the patient. Results from laboratory work and other tests performed on the patient may be accompanied by normal values or ranges for each test. It should be noted that these ranges or desirable laboratory values may vary somewhat from facility to facility. See *Pathology: Implications for the Physical Therapist* for more

Table 6•2 Partial Listing of ABCDs of Nutritional Assessment and Their Significance[11,12]

Anthropometric Data	Biochemical Data	Clinical Data	Dietary History
Skin Fold Measurement Body fat/density	Plasma Protein Protein	Increased Metabolic Needs Fever, infection, trauma, burns, wounds	Dietary Intake Basic food groups, alcohol consumption, caffeine, fad diets, vitamin/minerals
Near-Infrared Interactance Body fat	Serum Transferrin and Albumin Acute protein changes	Nutrient/Fluid Loss Wound drainage, kidney dialysis	Hydration Fluid intake and output
Bioelectrical Impedance Total body water, body fat, fat-free mass	Total Lymphocyte Count Protein levels and immunity	GI System Disease, surgery, diarrhea, malabsorption	Eating Difficulties Chew, swallow, smell, taste
Body Weight Status General health	Nitrogen Balance Protein levels and metabolic expenditure	Diseases Effecting Nutrition/Metabolism Diabetes, liver or kidney disease, hypertension, cancer	Cultural/Religious Considerations Foods to avoid
Body Mass Index (kg/m²) Body fat and weight status	Serum Cholesterol Malnutrition, infection, cardiovascular disease	Medical History General health	Economic Considerations Ability to buy groceries

analysis of laboratory results.[18] Table 6.3 contains a partial listing of laboratory and test results clinicians may find useful for wound evaluation and treatment intervention. Other nonlaboratory procedures that may provide helpful information may include biopsies, MRIs, CT scans, radiographs, bone scans, and other procedures. Results from these procedures may alert the clinician to conditions such as cancer, osteomyelitis, abscess, and other diseases or comorbidities.[19] Radiographic imaging is discussed in greater detail in Chapter 9.

The Guide urges the clinician to gather information on the integument and wound current history.[1] Wound-related information may include current interventions, mechanism of injury or disease, date of wound onset, date of disease onset or duration of disease, course of events, and symptom

Table 6•3 Laboratory Tests and Values[18,19,131-134]

Laboratory Test/Measure	Accepted/Normal Values*	Significance
Fasting glucose	70–115 mg/dL	Control of diabetes
Glycosylated hemoglobin	4%–6%	Previous 2–3 months blood sugar control
Protein status:		
Albumin	3.5–5.5 g/dL	Recent nutrition, protein levels
Transferrin	200–400 mg/dL	
Prealbumin	20–40 mg/dL	
Retinol binding protein	~0.8 mg/dL	
C-reactive protein	2.6–7.6 mg/dL	Retinol binding protein: increases due to infections and when low albumin/prealbumin
Hemoglobin	Male: 13–18 g/dL Female: 12–16 g/dL	Adequate levels needed for healing
Hematocrit	Male: 42%–52% Female: 37%–48%	Adequate levels needed for healing Elevated levels at risk for thrombi
Hematology profile:		
Erythrocytes (RBCs)	Adult male: 4.7–6.1 10^6/mm³ Adult female: 4.2–5.4 10^6/mm³	RBC/WBC: immune ability
Thrombocytes (platelets)	150,000–400,000/μL	Platelets: clotting and growth factors
Leukocytes (WBCs):		WBCs: infection
Neutrophils	4,300–10,000 cells/mm³	Neutrophils/monocytes: infection
Monocytes		
Lymphocytes	1,800–7,000 cells/mm³ (45%–74%)	Lymphocytes: malnutrition
Eosinophils		
Basophils	0–1,000 cells/mm³ (4%–10%) 688–4,860 (16%–45%) 0–756 (0%–7%) 0–216 (0%–2%)	
HIV-1/HIV-2 antibodies	Negative	Immune implications for healing
Prothrombin time (PT) Partial thromboplastin time (PTT)	Adult/elderly: 12–15 sec 25–40 sec	Ability to clot
Blood urea nitrogen (BUN)	8–25 mg/dL	Renal function, hydration state
Creatinine	0.6–1.5 mg/dL	Protein levels, muscle wasting, dehydration
Urinalysis	pH 4.5–8.0 Negative for ketones, bacteria, protein, glucose, bilirubin, blood	Kidney, pancreas, liver function Rule out trauma, bacterial growth
Blood or wound cultures/gram stains	Negative for bacteria, microorganisms	Presence of bacteria, microorganisms

*Laboratory values and ranges may vary depending on facility.

onset and patterns.[1] When taking a history of the current wound, it is often best to begin by asking the patient and family their perception of the problem. Their problems or concerns will inform the clinician about what needs to be addressed for patient-oriented goals. The clinician must also determine the time frame of wound development and the causative factors involved. The patient should be asked when the wound was first noticed and what the symptoms were. The clinician should also determine whether trauma was involved or if the wound began insidiously. If trauma, such as pressure, is a causative factor, determining the amount and location of pressure can provide information to determine what pressure-reducing interventions will be required. If wound onset was gradual, the medical history may provide clues to etiology. All disease states, comorbidities, and environmental factors involved in development of the wound must be identified and considered for prevention of future wounds. If the patient has a previous history of wounds, etiology must be ascertained. Past interventions, including treatment outcomes for previous wounds, must be identified. Past beneficial and nonbeneficial interventions will provide information on which to base the current interventions. The complete course of events that led to the current wound may alert the clinician to identify complicating factors or other relevant information that may assist in forming clinical judgments and decision making.

The location of symptoms and clinical manifestations such as wound-related edema, paresthesia, and pain must be evaluated. Symptom assessment will aid in wound diagnosis and in making clinical judgments for treatment. The patient should be asked to localize symptoms and indicate what causes them to increase or decrease. Knowledge of activities, positions, movement, and other considerations that change symptoms assist in wound type determination and possibly treatment. For example, pain behavior may distinguish wounds caused by venous insufficiency from those caused by arterial insufficiency. Arterial wounds tend to be painful with exercise and elevation; short-term dependent positioning may provide some degree of pain relief. On the other hand, venous wounds tend to exhibit discomfort with dependency and feel better when elevated. More information on the origins and symptoms of these types of wounds is presented in Chapters 16 and 17.

Many chronic wounds are painful, especially infected, inflamed, or ischemic wounds. Phillips et al found that 87% of patients with leg ulcers experienced pain.[20] Dallam and coworkers studied 132 hospitalized patients with pressure ulcers.[21] Pain evaluation instruments used in the study included the Visual Analog Scale[22] and Faces Pain Rating Scale.[23] One third of the subjects had the ability to respond to these tools. The other two thirds had difficulty responding due to difficulties in communication caused by conditions such as aphasia and intubation. Fifty-nine percent of those capable of responding reported they had pain. The authors stated it would be inappropriate to assume that the two thirds of the subjects that could not respond were pain free.[21] These two studies demonstrate that wound pain is a factor to be evaluated and effectively managed. Rook[24] recommends that a wound pain assessment should consider patient age, cognitive status, general health, and kidney/liver function when pain medications are used. He also encourages assessing pain caused by wound treatments such as débridement, dressing changes, and repositioning, as well as how wound pain affects sleep and functional activities. Rook advocates close observation of pain behavior and changes in vital signs when caring for the wounds of a noncommunicating patient.[24] The AHRQ[3] stipulates that all patients with pressure ulcers be assessed for wound-related pain as well as pain due to wound interventions. This document also mentions that clinicians should be aware that wound-related pain may exist for patients who are unresponsive or cannot communicate.[3] *The Guide* also includes pain evaluation in all six preferred practice patterns.[1] Wound-related pain has implications for quality of life, comfort, and the well-being of all patients. Consequently, a complete wound evaluation should contain a segment devoted to wound-related pain and the pain resulting from wound interventions. The reader will find more information on management of wound-related pain in Chapter 22 of this text.

▶ **PEARL 6•1** Information obtained from the patient history sets a firm foundation for a complete wound evaluation.

Risk Assessment

Wounds can be costly for both health-care and the patient. Cost containment is an obvious priority in health care. Costs for the patient and family go beyond actual financial costs of care. For example, patient and family costs may involve time spent in treatment, emotional costs of pain and suffering, as well as the multifaceted implications of functional limitations. Because of the far-reaching consequences of wounds, the ability to assess risks and implement prevention is worthwhile. There are a number of risk assessment tools available for various types of wounds.

There are numerous risk factors associated with pressure ulcers. Many of the factors can be classified under the general categories found in Table 6.4. Patients should at least be

Table 6•4 Risk Factors for Developing Pressure Ulcers[19,135,136]	
Inactivity/immobility: bedbound or chair bound	Frail elderly
Moisture: incontinence, perspiration, wound drainage	Poor physical condition
Nutritional issues: poor intake and hydration	Hypotension
Impaired mental status: consciousness, cognition	Obesity, low body weight
Skin status: dry, scaly, fragile	Cardiac failure
Mechanical forces: pressure, friction, shear	Joint contractures
Sensory deficit: pain, pressure	Diabetes
Increased body temperature	Cancer

assessed upon admission and when their status changes. Ayello and Braden[25] and Bergman-Evans et al[26] recommend reassessment as follows: every 2 days in the acute setting; weekly risk assessment in the first month of long-term care and then quarterly; in-home health-care reassessments at every visit.

Two risk assessment tools validated by research and recommended by the AHRQ[3] are the Braden Scale for Predicting Pressure Sore Risk[27] and Norton Risk Assessment Scale.[28] Other clinical risk assessment tools have been developed by Waterlow[29] and Gosnell.[30] (Table 6.5)

In summary, there are numerous factors to consider for the risk of pressure ulcer development. Tools for assessing the risk for developing pressure ulcers are available and should be used when appropriate. To date, the majority of wound risk assessment research has been done in an elderly population with

pressure ulcers. These pressure ulcer risk assessment tools are fairly well known and researched. However, current areas of research include development of assessment tools and identification of risk factors for other patient populations or wound types. For example, pressure ulcer risk assessment research is ongoing in individuals with spinal cord injuries,[4,31-33] children, and infants.[34-36]

Risk factors should also be assessed for wounds having other etiologies, such as those resulting from diabetes and vascular insufficiency. Diabetic ulcers of the lower extremity may have risk factors due to changes in the vascular status of the limb, from insensitivity associated with polyneuropathy, or other metabolic and tissue changes. See Table 6.6 for a listing of risk factors for wound development to consider when evaluating a patient with diabetes. While specific diabetic risk assessment tools do not appear in the literature, Boyko et al[37]

Table 6•5 Pressure Ulcer Risk Assessment Tools

Tool	Specificity	Sensitivity	Description
Braden Scale[7,137-140]	57%–100%	53%–100%	Assess: mobility, activity, sensation, moisture, nutrition, friction and shear High reliability Score range: 6–23; 18 and higher at risk
Norton Scale[28,137,139,140]	26%–100%	49%–100%	Assess: physical condition, mental status, activity, mobility, incontinence Reliability unknown Score range: 5–20; 16 or less at risk May overpredict risk
Gosnell Scale[30,137]	83%	85%	Assess: mental status, continence, mobility, activity, nutrition Reliability unknown Score range: 5–20; 16 or more at risk
Water low score[29,137]	82.5%	63%	Assess: weight/height, skin inspection, gender, age, continence, mobility, appetite, medications, other risk factors Reliability unknown Score range: 0–45; 16 or higher at risk

Table 6•6 Diabetic Ulcer Risk Factors[141-151]

Foot Issues	Diabetic Issues	Neuropathic Issues	Skin Issues	Miscellaneous Issues
Higher plantar temperature	Duration of diabetes	Absent Achilles tendon reflex	No extremity hair	Male
Elevated foot pressures	Poor glucose control	Insensate to 5.07 (10 g) Monofilament	Dryness	Taller height
Footwear rubbing more callosities	Needs insulin	Subjective neuropathic symptoms	Redness	History of amputation
Rigid foot deformities	Higher fasting glucose	Elevated vibration threshold	Previous ulcers	Alcohol/tobacco abuse
Trauma	Poor diabetes knowledge		Ulcer resulting from surgery	Divorced/living alone
			Occupational hazards	Immobile
			Trauma	$TcPo_2$ <30 mm Hg
				Poor vision
				Vascular disease
				Age
				Immunopathy
				Nephropathy

$TcPo_2$, transcutaneous partial pressure of oxygen.

devised a downloadable prediction model to determine risk of diabetic ulcers (www.eric.seattle.med.va.gov). The model, based upon common clinical diabetic information and tests, was used prospectively with 1285 diabetic veterans. The veterans were followed at 12- to 18-month intervals for up to 5 years to ascertain the first ulcer occurrence. The statistically significant predictors of diabetic ulcers in this study are listed in Table 6.7. The authors suggest that if a patient does not have a history of an amputation or a foot ulcer, impaired protective sensation, fungal nail infection, or poor eyesight, then the person has a low risk for developing an ulcer.

McGuckin[38] includes a review of the risk factors for wound development in venous disease. This guideline outlines the following as venous ulcer risk factors: history of varicose veins, venous hypertension, deep vein thrombophlebitis, pregnancy, previous vein surgery, lower extremity trauma, obesity, employment or other activities requiring lower extremity dependency, increasing age, and being male.[38] Other risk factors for venous disease include a family history and clotting disorders.[39] A review of the literature did not reveal any risk assessment tools designed specifically for predicting the risk of developing a venous ulcer.

Shai and Halevy[40] studied the histories and medical chart information of 64 patients with chronic venous insufficiency ulcers to determine ulcer cause. (Table 6.8) They found 26.3% had no direct trigger; however, approximately 33% of the wounds were the result of trauma: blunt or penetrating injury, intentional self-inflicted injury, burns, scratching, and insect bites. Thus, trauma may be a risk factor in ulcer development. Appropriate patient education in prevention of tissue trauma appears necessary.

With regard to arterial disease, the majority of risk factors appear to be associated with the diabetic population previously discussed. Some of the classical factors attributed to coronary artery disease also apply to risk for arterial insufficiency. These risk factors include age, family history of heart disease, atherosclerosis, arteriosclerosis, smoking, hypertension, hypercholesterolemia, diabetes, and a sedentary lifestyle.[41-47] Other risk factors may also include: elevated white blood cell count, elevated fibrinogen levels, and menopause in women.[48,49]

In summary, a complete history and review of pertinent risk factors allows the clinician to identify individuals who are

| Table 6•7 Boyko et al Diabetic Ulcer Risk[37] ||
Clinical Information	Hazard Ratio
History of amputation	2.57
History of foot ulcer	2.18
Monofilament insensate	2.03
Fungal nail infection	1.58
Poor vision	1.48
Increase in glycosylated hemoglobin	1.10
Tinea pedis	0.73

| Table 6•8 Shai and Halevy Venous Ulceration Triggers[40] ||
Trigger	Percent (%)
No trigger	26.3
Cellulitis	15.4
Penetrating injury	11.8
Contact dermatitis	10.9
Rapid edema increase	10.9
Burn	6.3
Scratching dry skin	5.4
Blunt trauma	4.5
Deliberate self-inflicted injury	4.5
Insect bite	1.8
Superficial vein bleed	1.8

at greater risk for developing a wound. When individuals are perceived to be at risk, a plan must be developed to address wound prevention.

▶ **PEARL 6•2** Wounds can have devastating costs for the patients, their loved ones, and society. Consequently, wound risk assessment is essential for providing the highest possible quality of care for patients.

Patient Assessment

Once patient history has been obtained and risk assessment conducted, the clinician can turn attention to wound and periwound issues as well as vascular and neurological assessment. Vascular and neurological assessments are presented in Chapter 7. Chapter 8 provides in-depth information on assessment of bioburden, and Chapter 9 rounds out the assessment information by detailing various imaging tests.

Before proceeding to the wound examination, the concept of wound bed preparation (WBP) and the mnemonics TIME and MEASURE will be reviewed. Sibbald et al[50] provide excellent recommendations for areas to assess for wound management, including ability to heal, causes of tissue damage, patient concerns and worries, the wound, bioburden, and the wound healing rate. See Table 6.9 for more detail on these issues. WBP allows the clinician to use the biology of healing to attain proper wound conditions to support healing and improve treatment effectiveness. Complete assessment and understanding of the wound status is of high priority in WBP.

The mnemonic TIME evolved from the wound bed preparation literature. TIME is as follows: T, tissue; I, infection/inflammation; M, moisture; and E, edge.[51-53] Table 6.10

Table 6•9 Sibbald et al Wound Bed Preparation Assessment[50]

Ability to heal: blood supply (pulses, Doppler/ABI, TcPo$_2$), medications, edema, anemia, comorbidities, etc

Causes of tissue damage: pressure, vascular issues, interventions (compression, offloading), blood sugar control, etc

Patient concerns: pain and quality of life

Wound: history and traits (MEASURE)

Bacterial load/infection:

Wound healing rate: to ascertain appropriate treatments

ABI, ankle-brachial index. TcPo$_2$, Transcutaneous partial pressure of oxygen.

Table 6•10 TIME: Wound Healing[51-53]

	Wound Trait	Possible Pathophysiology	Actions and Outcomes
T	Tissue	Nonviable tissue comprises defective extracellular matrix, and cellular debris impairs healing.	Débridement restores viable wound base and promotes healing and wound edge advancement.
I	Infection or inflammation	Bioburden or prolonged inflammation increases protease activity and inflammatory cytokines and decreases growth factor activity.	Control bioburden and inflammation with various topicals and other treatments. Goal is to reduce bacteria and inflammation to promote healing and wound edge advancement.
M	Moisture	Desiccation impairs epidermal advancement. Too much moisture leads to maceration.	Restore moisture balance with dressings and other interventions to promote healing and wound edge advancement.
E	Edge	Wound edge does not advance or there is undermining due to poor keratinocytes migration, extracellular matrix abnormalities, abnormal protease activity, nonresponsive wound cells. All impair healing.	Reassess wound etiology or explore other treatments: débridement, grafts, biological agents, other therapies. Goal is to stimulate appropriate healing and advancement of the wound edge.

provides more information on TIME for wound assessment and management.

Keast et al[54] developed a wound assessment framework: MEASURE. (Table 6.11) This guide for assessment is also cited in Sibbald.[50] The MEASURE mnemonic is a useful tool to remind clinicians to do or assess the following: M, measure; E, exudate; A, appearance; S, suffering; U, undermining; R, reevaluate regularly; and E, edge. Table 6.12 provides more details on the recommendations of MEASURE for wound assessment.

▶ **PEARL 6•3** Determination of wound etiology, current wound status, and all factors that impair healing are vital. Accurate patient and wound assessment is the cornerstone for developing the plan of care.

Wound Examination

Frequently, wound type may determine which characteristics require assessment, although it is ultimately up to the clinician to select the appropriate evaluative measures. Clinics will often devise their own form to speed the wound evaluation process; to ensure quality, accuracy, and consistent assessment; and to meet the needs for documentation and reimbursement. Wound location is often documented on a body diagram or described with appropriate terminology and use of anatomical landmarks: For instance, the wound is located 2 cm proximal to the right medial malleolus. Wound location may help the clinician to determine the type of wound. For instance, wounds secondary to venous insufficiency are often found on the distal, medial third of the lower extremity, and ischemic wounds are found on the toes, feet, and distal third of the leg. Neuropathic wounds are usually located on the plantar surface of the foot, and pressure ulcers are commonly found over bony prominences, such as the sacrum/coccyx, trochanter, ischium, malleoli, and heels. For an in-depth review of wound assessment, see the article by Keast et al.[54]

Dimensions

Wound Dimensions: Length, Width, Surface Area

Wound dimensions can be measured by a number of methods, including the recording of length, width, and wound surface

Table 6•11 MEASURE for Wound Assessment[54,89]

M	Measure	Assess wound depth with swab. If using length × width, have same person measure; use average of three measurements. Measure wound area with wound tracing and planimeter.
E	Exudate	Describe the quantity (none, small, moderate, large) and quality of exudate.
A	Appearance	Describe wound bed appearance: tissue type and amount (subjective estimate).
S	Suffering	Evaluate pain type and level with validated tools.
U	Undermining	Measure using the clock system if undermining is present.
R	Reevaluation	Reevaluate regularly (every 1–4 weeks). Monitor for infection, wound deterioration, or change in status.
E	Edge	Assess edge condition (attached vs unattached; presence of epithelium) and assess periwound for induration, inflammation, or maceration.

area. Regardless of the method used, accurate wound dimensions must be recorded at regular intervals. Healing progress or the lack of progress can be ascertained by comparisons with baseline measurements. Wound size reduction is a positive predictor of healing for venous, neuropathic, and pressure ulcers.[55-64]

Many measurement methods are available, ranging from quick, easy, and practical to time consuming, complicated, and costly to administer. The most simple, linear, two-dimensional measurements involve measuring the greatest length and the greatest width using a metric ruler or tape measure. (Fig. 6.1) The dimension orientation must be documented for consistent measurements in the future. For example, length is typically measured in the cephalad-caudal direction (vertical axis), and width is perpendicular to the length (horizontal axis). Clinicians may also use the image of a clock face superimposed over the wound. The patient's head is at 12 o'clock, and 6 o'clock is toward the feet. If the clock is not used with a cephalad-caudal measurement, then 12 o'clock must be defined in terms of an anatomical landmark. Dimensions are measured with reference to the numbers on the face of a clock, for example 12 o'clock to 6 o'clock measures 1.0 cm and 3 o'clock to 9 o'clock measures 2.3 cm. These direct measurements are quick, easy, reliable and inexpensive.[65-67] Two-dimensional measurements are not representative of actual wound size for irregular or circular

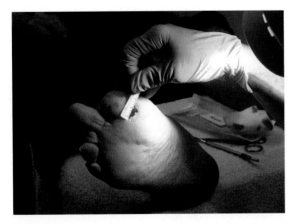

Figure 6•1 *Measurement of wound width with paper ruler.*

wounds. Because wounds are not rectangular or square, the product of the length and width does not accurately reflect the wound surface area. Multiplying wound length by width will give only a crude calculation of surface area. Table 6.12 presents dimension terminology definitions.

Wound dimensions can also be traced and measured on plastic transparencies. Wound tracings have the advantage of providing a permanent record of the wound dimensions. Tracings also provide a better visual record of the actual wound size and shape. The tracing procedure involves cleaning one side of a clear piece of plastic with alcohol. The clean side is placed over the wound, and a second piece of clear plastic is placed over the first. The wound borders are then very carefully traced with a fine-tipped, permanent marker. After the tracing procedure is complete, the plastic layer that came in contact with the wound is discarded and the tracing is kept for the patient's records. Plastic measuring tools or guides with grid markings, concentric circles or bull's-eye diameter calibrations may be purchased. Figure 6.2 demonstrates the use of E-Z Graph® for a wound tracing. Metric rulers may also be incorporated into the plastic sheet. A sheet of plastic without grid markings that has a wound tracing on it can be placed over a calibrated grid for measurement of wound area. Wound area may be approximated by counting the calibrated whole grid blocks in a wound tracing. Some clinicians count half blocks and bigger as whole blocks in their area calculations.[68] Counting these blocks can be time consuming in the clinic. Overall, tracing may be quick, easy to accomplish, and reliable.[69-72] Tracing area is more reliable than the length-width product.[69]

Lastly, the clinician must be aware of two sources of error with wound tracing: wound edge determination[73] and tracing accuracy.[68,74] Wound tracing combined with planimetry or digitization has been shown to have high intrarater and interrater reliability for determining wound surface area.[66,73,75] A planimeter is a mechanical or digital tool that measures the area of a two-dimensional shape. Planimeters can be expensive and time consuming to use. Both planimetry and digitization of the wound area are reliable.[67,70]

Another technique that provides measurement of wound area uses photography. Advantages of photography include the fact that nothing touches the wound bed and visual information on wound bed tissue is provided. Color pictures of the wound

Table 6•12 Terminology

Terminology	Definition
Clock positions	Clock hands used for wound measurement reference points. Head is 12 o'clock, feet are 6 o'clock, and 9 and 3 o'clock are lateral.
Length	Cephalad-caudal (vertical) measurement (12 to 6 o'clock).
Width	Perpendicular to length (horizontal) measurement (3 to 9 o'clock).
Depth	Deepest aspect of wound to horizontal plane of intact wound edge.
Tunnel	Linear channel extending beyond the open wound base. Use clock reference points for location; may have entrance and exit in same wound or two adjacent wounds.
Sinus tract	Dead end channel allowing an abscess to drain.
Undermining	Wound edge erosion where fascia separates from deeper tissue around wound edge. Use clock reference points for location.
Fistula	Vertical or oblique channel originating in a wound that penetrates a body cavity.

Adapted from Brown.[152]

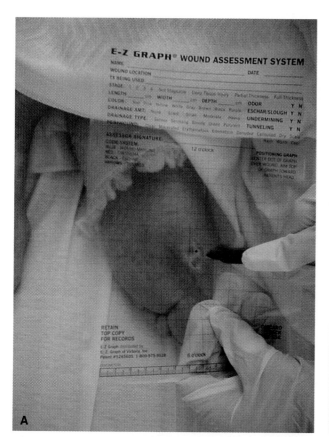
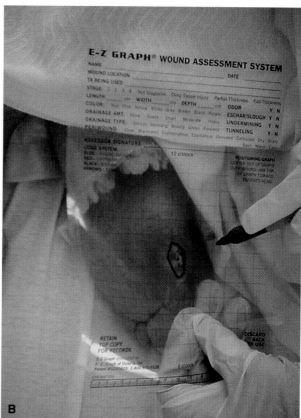

Figure 6•2 *(A, B) Wound tracing using the E-Z Graph®. Courtesy of EZ Graph of Victoria Inc., Victoria, TX.*

can be obtained with an instant camera, or color images from a digital camera or a video camera recording may be downloaded into a computer for surface area analysis. (Fig. 6.3) Polaroid® grid film will allow wound dimensions of length, width, and area to be determined from the photograph; however, this is less accurate than computer-digitized images downloaded into a computer from a digital or video camera. When using a camera to capture wound images, the clinician must follow the camera manufacturer's instructions. Certain factors must be standardized each time a wound image is captured, such as lighting,

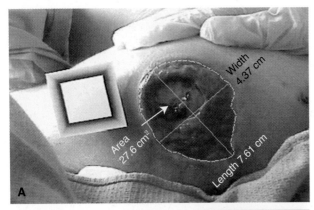

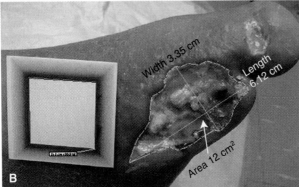

Figure **6•3** *(A, B) Computerized wound images downloaded from a digital camera. Courtesy of Vista Medical, Ltd., Winnipeg, MB, Canada.*

focal length or distance from the wound to the camera lens, and patient position. Standardizing all of these factors will result in a more accurate wound image. Also, wounds on convex surfaces may appear distorted on film and consequently will not be accurate for wound dimensions. Instant camera pictures are more expensive and less reliable than tracings for determining accurate wound dimensions. Area calculation from a photo can be influenced by angle of the camera and distance of camera from the wound bed. Consequently, photography may not be best method for calculating wound size.[71,76]

As stated previously, digital images can be downloaded into a computer. For example, digital wound measurement systems allow the clinician to determine wound length, width, depth, total wound area, percentage of change in wound size, and percentage of nonviable versus viable tissue. (Fig. 6.3) The Visitrak™ (Smith & Nephew, Largo, FL) system comprises a wound-tracing grid, depth probe, and the digital unit itself. Once the wound is traced, the image is placed on the digital unit and the wound border is retraced with a stylus.[77] There are disadvantages to the digitized wound images. The equipment is expensive, and digital images can be altered with various software packages.

Wound Dimensions: Vertical, Oblique and Horizontal

Although wound length, width, and area and wound imaging are important aspects of the wound evaluation, these characteristics may not always provide complete information regarding the extent of the wound. The wound depth, as well as the extent of sinus tracts, tunnels, fistulas, and undermining also provide vital information. See Table 6.12 for definitions used in this chapter for wound dimensions.

The terminology describing tissue erosion is not always consistent among clinicians and in the literature. Often, clinicians may use the terms *tract* and *tunnel* or *undermining* and *tunnel* interchangeably. However, a more precise explanation is that a tunnel is a channel that has an entrance and exit in the same wound or an entrance in one wound with an exit in an adjacent wound. Sinus tract is a channel from a draining abscess. These wound dimensions require other methods of measurement, which will be discussed in conjunction with measuring wound depth. The accepted technique for measurement of wound depth involves using a clean, gloved hand to insert a sterile swab to the depth of the wound base. The probe is placed at the deepest point in wound and a depth measurement taken to the horizontal wound edge.[65,69] The clinician then marks the depth of the wound on the shaft of the swab and removes the swab from the wound. The length of the mark to the tip of the swab is measured to the nearest millimeter. Depth cannot truly be assessed until the wound is completely débrided. Clinicians will also use this technique to measure the depth of sinus tracts, tunnels, undermining, and fistulas. See Figure 6.4 for wound tunnel measurement with a swab. Some commercial enterprises have calibrated the shaft of a swab or probe in millimeters, allowing easier depth measurement of tracts and undermining. The location(s) within the wound where depth is measured must be documented as well. Using the clock method for referencing the depth may be useful when measuring multiple depth locations.[78]

Wound Dimensions: Volume

Various techniques have been used to determine wound volume. One technique involves filling a wound completely with a measured amount of sterile saline. The accuracy of this technique is questionable due to spillage of the saline. Also, it may be inconvenient, difficult, or impractical to place the patient in position to prevent spillage. In this situation, an alternative approach involves placing an adhesive, transparent film securely over the wound. Using a syringe to puncture the film,

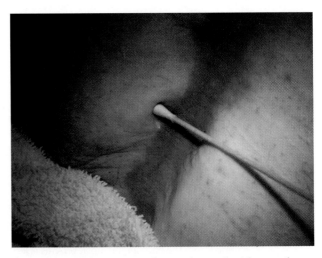

Figure **6•4** *Measurement of wound tunnel with a swab.*

the wound is filled completely with a measured amount of saline or amorphous hydrogel. If saline is used, care must be taken with the syringe to remove all air bubbles from under the film to ensure accurate volume measurement. Overfilling the wound, which causes spillage from under the film dressing, should be avoided, or measurement error will result. Determining wound volume using an amorphous gel can be accomplished more easily and with less spillage than using saline. Calibrated syringes containing 30 mL of viscous, amorphous gel are available commercially. Determining wound volume with these methods is time consuming and possibly inaccurate.[68] It is important to note that the clinical benefit of wound volume is not proven.[54,79]

Lastly, there are other more costly and highly technical volume determination methods that involve computers and various imaging techniques. Information is available related to these more infrequently used techniques, such as structured light and stereophotography,[68,80-86] interferometry,[87] and laser displacement.[88] Clinical wound measurement methods most frequently used are those that are quick, practical, and reliable. Reliability can be enhanced by choosing a measuring method and performing it precisely the same way each time the wound is reevaluated. Obtaining wound dimensions for reassessing the progress of wound healing will be discussed in more detail below. For additional information on wound measurement methodologies, please refer to Keast et al,[54,89] Culter et al,[75] Schubert and Zander,[79] and Xakellis and Frantz.[90] These references examine wound measurement methods in greater detail, including sensitivity to change, reliability, agreement between different measures, usage with appropriate types of wounds, and other relevant topics.

Classification

Wounds may be classified in a number of ways, including etiology, depth of tissue involvement, and tissue color. Wounds classified by etiology may include those due to venous and arterial insufficiency, pressure, neuropathology, diabetes, and surgery. Categorizing by wound etiology allows the clinician to develop a plan for evaluation and treatment tailored to the characteristics of the wound and needs of the patient.[91] Common terms used to describe wound depth include *partial thickness* and *full thickness*. The depth of a partial-thickness wound involves erosion through the epidermis and possibly the superficial dermis. A full-thickness wound extends through the epidermis, dermis, and subcutaneous tissues and may even erode into or through the muscle down to the bone.

Pressure ulcers have a unique staging system based on wound depth. Chapter 19 covers pressure ulcers in detail, but a review of the staging system is included here. In 1989, the National Pressure Ulcer Advisory Panel (NPUAP)[91,92] recommended a classification system based on the work of Shea.[93] This pressure ulcer staging system is advocated by the NPUAP[91] and the AHRQ ulcer guidelines.[19] Recently, the pressure ulcer staging system was revised.[94] The stages of pressure ulcers according to NPUAP are as follows.

(Suspected) Deep Tissue Injury: Purple or maroon localized area of discolored skin or blood-filled blister due to damage of underlying soft tissue from pressure and/or shear. The area may be preceded by tissue that is painful, firm, mushy, boggy, and warmer or cooler compared to adjacent tissue.

Further description: Deep tissue injury may be difficult to detect in individuals with dark skin tones. Evolution may include a thin blister over a dark wound bed. The wound may further evolve and become covered by thin eschar. Evolution may be rapid, exposing additional layers of tissue even with treatment.

Stage I: Intact skin with nonblanchable redness of a localized area, usually over a bony prominence. Darkly pigmented skin may not have visible blanching; its color may differ from the surrounding area.

Further description: The area may be painful, firm, soft, warmer or cooler as compared to adjacent tissue. Stage I may be difficult to detect in individuals with dark skin tones. May indicate at-risk persons (a heralding sign of risk).

Stage II: Partial-thickness loss of dermis presenting as a shallow open ulcer with a red-pink wound bed, without slough. May also present as an intact or open or ruptured serum-filled blister.

Further description: Presents as a shiny or dry shallow ulcer without slough or bruising. (Bruising indicates suspected deep tissue injury.) This stage should not be used to describe skin tears, tape burns, perineal dermatitis, maceration, or denudement.

Stage III: Full-thickness tissue loss. Subcutaneous fat may be visible, but bone, tendon, or muscle are not exposed. Slough may be present but does not obscure the depth of tissue loss. May include undermining and tunneling.

Further description: The depth of stage III pressure ulcer varies by anatomical location. The bridge of the nose, ear, occiput, and malleolus do not have subcutaneous tissue, and stage III ulcers can be shallow. In contrast, areas of significant adiposity can develop extremely deep stage III pressure ulcers. Bone/tendon is not directly visible or directly palpated.

Stage IV: Full-thickness tissue loss with exposed bone, tendon, or muscle. Slough or eschar may be present on some parts of the wound bed. Often includes undermining and tunneling.

Further description: The depth of stage IV pressure ulcer varies by anatomical location. The bridge of the nose, ear, occiput, and malleolus do not have subcutaneous tissue, and stage III ulcers can be shallow. Stage IV ulcers can extend into muscle and/or supporting structures (eg, fascia, tendon, or joint capsule) making osteomyelitis possible. Exposed bone/tendon is visible or directly palpable.

Unstageable: Full-thickness tissue loss in which the base of the ulcer is covered by slough (yellow, tan, gray, green, or brown) and/or eschar (tan, brown, or black) in the wound bed. Undermining and sinus tracts also may be associated with stage IV pressure ulcers.

Further description: Until enough slough and/or eschar is removed to expose the base of the wound, the true depth, and therefore the stage, cannot be determined. Stable (dry, adherent, intact without erythema or fluctuance) eschar on the heels serves as "the body's natural (biological) cover" and should not be removed.

This staging system should be used only to describe pressure ulcers. Wounds from other causes, such as arterial, venous, diabetic foot, skin tears, tape burns, perineal dermatitis, maceration, or denudement, should not be staged using this system. Other staging systems exist for some of these conditions and should be used instead.

In 1995 the NPUAP conference held a consensus session with the following recommendations regarding the staging system cited above: "(1) pressure ulcer staging is useful to evaluate the anatomic depth of an ulcer; (2) reversal of pressure ulcer staging is an inappropriate method to monitor healing; (3) pressure ulcer stage should only be used to identify the deepest layer of exposed tissue; and (4) pressure ulcer treatment should never be determined by stage alone."[95] Maklebust lists the following clinical uses for this staging system[96]: research studies, wound assessment and healing, reimbursement decisions, guide for assessing products, and marketing by manufacturers.

Burn injury information is presented in detail in Chapters 20 and 21. However, a brief summary of burn classification and assessment is presented here. Burns can be assessed by depth. (Table 6.13) Often, clinicians estimate how much of the body is burned using the rule of nines. The head and each individual upper extremity are designated as 9% of the body. Next, the anterior torso is 18%, the posterior torso is 18%, and each entire lower extremity is 18%. The genital area is 1%.[97] This estimation rubric can overestimate the extent of injury, and clinician experience is necessary for reliability.[98] Children's proportions are not the same as adults; that is, they have larger heads and smaller limbs. Taking this into account, the Lund-Browder classification, which uses percent estimation, may be more appropriate for children.[99] Lastly, the palmar method uses the palm of the hand to estimate burn size. The disadvantage with this method is the lack of agreement on what percentage the palm of the hand represents (0.5%–1%).[100,101]

Chapters 14 and 15 provide a wealth of information on the neuropathic ulcer and diabetes. Systems classifying diabetic wounds by depth and other characteristics will be presented briefly in this chapter. The Wagner scale[102] and the University of Texas Wound Classification System[103] are two such classifications systems. The University of Texas Wound Classification System for diabetic wounds places wounds in various grades and stages.[103] Please see Table 6.14 for more information on the University of Texas Wound Classification system. The Wagner classification for diabetic foot ulcers is often cited in the literature. It is as follows[102]:

0 = intact skin; precursor stage to ulcer formation, healed ulcer, or bony deformity
1 = superficial ulcer
2 = ulcer into subcutaneous layer
3 = infection present
4 = partial foot gangrene
5 = full foot gangrene

Wound Base and Edges

Assessment of a wound must include an evaluation of the wound base and edges. Examining wound tissue color and type, anatomical structures involved, and wound edge characteristics may aid in determining the extent of tissue damage, influence the choice of interventions, and assist in reevaluation of the healing progress. Ideally, granulation tissue will progressively develop in the wound base and ultimately fill in the wound cavity. This tissue should appear beefy red in color, indicating the tissue is well perfused and healthy. When the wound cavity is fully granulated, then the leading edge of epidermal cells should show evidence of migration onto the moist granulation tissue. (Figs. 6.1 and 6.5)

Wounds often have other types of tissue present. (Table 6.15) When necrotic tissue is present, débridement should be completed before estimating the type and amount of nonviable tissue. Necrotic tissue is not desirable in the wound bed. Dead tissue invites bacteria that impedes the healing process and increases the susceptibility of the wound to infection. Figure 6.3 (B) depicts slough in the wound bed and

Table 6•13	Burn Depth
Depth	**Description**
Superficial (first degree)	Epidermis only
Superficial partial thickness (superficial second degree)	Epidermis and papillary dermis
Deep partial thickness (deep second degree)	Epidermis and dermis
Full thickness (third degree)	Epidermis, dermis, and to the subcutaneous tissues
Subdermal (fourth degree)	Damage beyond the dermis into fat, muscle, tendon, bone

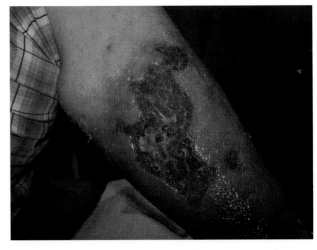

Figure 6•5 *Wound base with granulation tissue and slough. Note color and texture of periwound.*

Table 6•14 The University of Texas Wound Classification System for Diabetic Wounds[103]

	Grade 0	Grade I	Grade II	Grade III
Stage A	Preulcerative or postulcerative lesion completely epithelialized	Superficial wound not involving tendon, capsule, or bone	Wound penetrating to tendon or capsule	Wound penetrating to bone or joint
Stage B	Infection	Infection	Infection	Infection
Stage C	Ischemia	Ischemia	Ischemia	Ischemia
Stage D	Infection and ischemia	Infection and ischemia	Infection and ischemia	Infection and ischemia

Table 6•15 Description of Wound Base and Edges[112,152]

Wound Base Terminology	Description
Epithelial tissue	Translucent or white cell layer. Epithelial cells migrate onto granulation tissue from wound edge or epidermal appendages.
Granulation tissue	Pink/red, granular-looking, moist tissue containing new connective tissue, blood vessels, and cells necessary for wound repair.
Slough, fibrin, or necrotic fibrous tissue	Soft, moist, dead fibrous tissue. Appears white, yellow, tan, brown, or green. May be stringy, loose, or adherent to wound base.
Eschar	Brown or black necrotic tissue. May be adhered to wound edge or separated from edge. Texture can be hard, soft, or boggy.
Hypertrophic	Excessive granulation above horizontal wound edge plane.
Exposed structures	Bone is white, yellow, or gray in appearance. Tendon/ligament is white or yellow in appearance.
Wound Edge Terminology	**Description**
Complete epithelialization	Wound bed covered with epithelium.
Epithelializing	Epidermal cells advancing from wound edges and/or epidermal appendages.
Rolled or curled epithelium (epibole)	Curled wound edge due to excessive epidermal cell growth.
Callus or hyperkeratosis	Thick, hyperkeratotic tissue around part or all of wound edge.
Indistinct, diffuse	Cannot distinguish wound edges/boundaries from periwound.
Fibrotic, scarred	Immediate wound edge/periwound skin is scarred.

Figure 6.6 (A and B) demonstrates wound bases with black eschar. Wound drainage or exudate may be present and will be discussed later. An estimation of the types of tissue by percentage and color may be helpful in the assessment process and in planning interventions. The gradual replacement of the nonviable tissue with healthy granulation or epithelial tissue is a sign of progress toward healing.

When assessing the wound bed, the clinician should examine the wound for signs of increased bioburden (critical colonization) and infection. Chapter 8 covers wound bioburden; however, some information on infection will be presented here as well. All wounds contain bacteria. Concern lies, however, in the extent of bacterial replication and bacterial impact on the host and wound. See Table 6.16 for description of the spectrum of wound bacterial burden. Gardner et al[104,105] determined the validity and reliability of chronic wound infection signs using tissue biopsy cultures. Valid, reliable signs for chronic wound infection from these studies include increased pain, edema, wound breakdown, delayed healing, friable granulation tissue, and purulent or serous drainage.[104,105] If the patient presents with signs of infection (see Table 6.14) a wound culture should be performed. Please refer to Chapter 8 of this

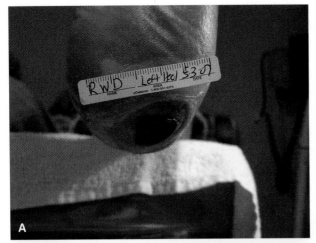

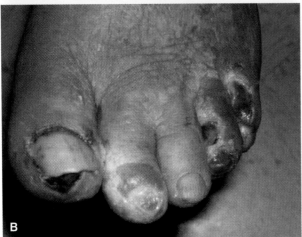

Figure 6•6 *(A, B) Wound bases with black eschar.*

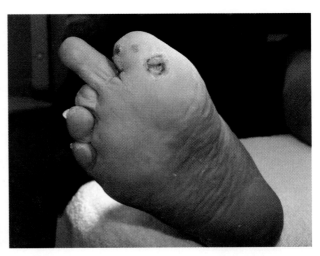

Figure 6•7 *Pale wound base with calloused wound edge. Note toe amputations.*

pale base of granulation tissue and callus around the wound edges. Wound edges and base can assist in differentiating venous, arterial, and neuropathic wounds. For example, venous wounds are often irregular in shape and have a red base. Arterial ulcers can also be irregular, but due to poor vascularization, the wound base is pale and dry. Neuropathic ulcers are often circular and deep.

Drainage and Odor

A wound may present with exudate or drainage. Drainage should not be confused with slough, which is a yellow-tan material consisting of solubilized fibrin or necrotic tissue. Research has confirmed that wound moisture is vital for appropriate and timely healing.[106-109] Acute damage to the skin will result in the production of exudate for 48 to 72 hours. However, chronic wounds that are inflamed or infected may also have exudate present. Venous wounds are characterized by heavy amounts of exudate due to edema and venous hypertension. The amount of wound exudate can be estimated for documentation and monitoring of progress. Accumulation of

text for details of the culturing procedure. Wound edges or boundaries also need to be examined. Descriptive terms such as indistinct, diffuse, flat, or attached edges may be used. Less desirable edges may be described as unattached, rolled, thick, fibrotic, or hyperkeratotic. Figure 6.7 shows a wound with a

Table 6•16 Spectrum of Wound Bioburden[50,153]

	Description	Signs/Symptoms
Contamination	Bacteria present in wound bed	None
Colonization	Replicating bacteria; no harm to the host	None
Critical colonization (occult or covert infection)	Replicating bacteria; immune response triggered, but no classical signs of an infection. Healing may be delayed or arrested.	Bright red granulation tissue, friable tissue, wound deterioration, increased exudate, foul odor.
Wound infection	Replicating bacteria in wound and surrounding tissue. Immune response triggered. Wound is not healing or is deteriorating.	Pain, swelling, induration, erythema, increased temperature, foul odor, undermining, wound breakdown.
Systemic infection	Replicating bacteria; systemic immune response.	Fever, chills, hypotension, rigors, organ failure.

wound exudate may depend on many factors, such as how long the current dressing has been in place, the type of dressing used, if there has been any application of topical medications or agents, and whether the wound is infected or inflamed. Descriptive terminology for exudate quantity may include none, small (light), moderate, or large (copious).

Another method for exudate assessment is demonstrated by the Pressure Ulcer Scale for Healing (PUSH).[110,111] The PUSH tool requires the clinician to estimate how much of the wound bed has exudate after the dressings are removed and before any cleansing or treatment. The tool instructs the clinician to estimate the amount of exudate using quadrants of the wound base (eg, less than one fourth, one fourth to one half, one half to three fourths, and more than three fourths). The exudate can also be assessed according to type as found in the Pressure Sore Status Tool (PSST): serous, serosanguinous, bloody, purulent, foul purulent.[112] Both the PUSH and PSST will be reviewed in the Reassessment and Prognosis section below. Wound exudate consistency may be described as watery or viscous. Exudate may also be categorized by color. (Table 6.17) Other descriptors encountered may include cloudy, white, opaque, yellow, green, tan, and brown. Wound and exudate odor may be described as sweet, fruity, fishy, ammonia-like, and foul.

Periwound Examination

The periwound skin surrounding a wound also requires periodic assessment and documentation. See Table 6.18 for periwound terminology. The following should be examined: the presence (or lack) of hair, callus, or hyperkeratosis (Fig. 6.7), blisters, and scarring. The clinical implications for these signs include the following examples. A lower extremity with arterial insufficiency will demonstrate shiny, thin, hairless skin. The presence of callus or blisters may denote areas of high pressure or bony deformity. Lastly, cutaneous scars may be the result of previous surgical attempts to restore perfusion or from musculocutaneous flap surgeries. Skin hydration must also be assessed. Maceration is excessive hydration and can lead to the breakdown of skin. Causes of maceration include persistent wound drainage onto the skin, incontinence, saturated dressings, and other sources of moisture. Examples of maceration

Table 6•18 Periwound Terminology[152]

Terminology	Definition
Ecchymotic or bruised	Blue, purple, black tissue from disrupted blood vessels.
Excoriated	Tissue injury from mechanical, chemical, or thermal injury.
Indurated	Tissue hardened from edema, inflammation, or granulation.
Inflamed	Tissue response to injury: redness, warmth, edema, pain, and loss of function.
Intact	Undamaged tissue.
Macerated	Tissue damage or softening from too much moisture.
Tape injury	Tape removal that damaged epidermis.

include excessive hydration of tissues around the wound perimeter or between the toes. Maceration must be prevented by appropriate use of skin barrier products and drying well between the toes after exposure to water. Patients may also present with skin that is too dry. An example of excessive dryness is the presence of fissures, especially on the feet. Skin dryness should be documented and addressed with appropriate moisture-enhancing interventions. Next, the color of the periwound skin may reveal bruising/ecchymosis or hemosiderin staining. Hemosiderin staining occurs when hemosiderin permanently discolors the skin purple-brown. (Fig. 6.5) This discoloration is a hallmark of venous insufficiency. Other skin pigmentations may also be present: light pigmentation for individuals with dark skin, dark pigmentation for people with intermediate skin tones, and erythema in light-colored skin. An example of a pigmentation change that signifies an early sign of tissue damage is nonblanchable redness. This skin is at risk for damage and needs immediate attention and protection. Erythema, another change in skin color, represents inflammation in light-colored skin and can be measured by including the reddened area on wound tracings. The periwound skin and tissue texture should be palpated to assess thickness, texture, turgor, and mobility. For example, the tissue of a patient who is elderly may be very thin and fragile, putting them at risk for pressure ulcers. Induration is another periwound attribute that must be assessed. Induration results from edema in the area, causing the tissue to feel hard to touch. Induration will impair the healing process. Venous insufficiency often causes edematous lower extremities with indurated, tender, hairless skin. If induration is noted, close monitoring is required, and the appropriate interventions must be started.

Edema

Edema will hamper the healing process of any wound. It is essential to obtain a baseline measurement of edema so that

Table 6•17 Wound Exudate Terminology[152,154]

Terminology	Definition
Serous	Clear, watery drainage found in inflammation and proliferation.
Sanguineous or bloody	Red, bloody-looking watery drainage due to damaged blood vessels.
Serosanguinous	Pink/reddish, watery drainage found in inflammation and proliferation.
Purulent or pus	Yellow, green, tan, blue drainage that is also cloudy; watery or viscous. Often due to infection. May have an odor.

the swelling reduction can be monitored. Interventions for reducing edema are addressed in Chapters 16 and 18. Soft and pitting edema is identified by digital pressure applied to the skin, which produces an indentation. This type of edema may be associated with congestive heart failure, early-stage venous insufficiency, lymphedema, and possibly pregnancy. Pitting edema may be rated using the following scale:

1+ There is a barely perceptible depression.
2+ Easily identified depression that takes ~15 seconds to rebound.
3+ Depression takes 15 to 30 seconds to rebound.
4+ Depression lasts for 30 seconds or more.

Induration, as mentioned previously, is periwound tissue that has hardened due to distended interstices from accumulated edema. Induration in the limb is easily identified by tissue that cannot be pinched upon manual palpation. Brawny edema is associated with longer-standing venous insufficiency. This edema is a result of high venous pressures in the limb, and when palpated, the edema in the limb feels taut and hard. The skin of individuals with lighter skin tones may also be ruddy in appearance. Objective measurements of edema are very important when monitoring and documenting interventions intended to reduce it. Examples of objective measures are discussed below.

Limb girth measurements are performed by measuring the circumference of the limb at various locations along the length. (Fig. 6.8) Measurements should be taken at locations on the limb where bony landmarks can be used as future references. Distances and directions from bony landmarks must be documented along with the girth measurements. For example, a lower extremity girth could be measured around the malleoli and then 3, 6, 9, and 12 cm proximal. To guard against obtaining invalid measurements, care must be taken to not pull the tape measure too taut against the skin when measuring the circumference. If the contralateral limb does not have edema, it may be used for comparison.

Volume measurements may also be used for an assessment of limb edema. This method relies on the principle that an object will displace water equal to the volume of the object. The limb is carefully placed in a volumeter containing tap water at room temperature, and the displaced water is collected and

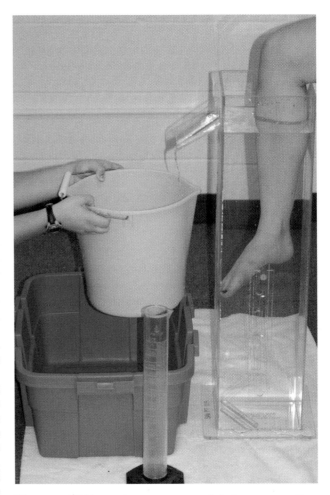

Figure 6•9 *Volumetric measurement of the lower extremity.*

measured with a graduated cylinder. The volume of the water displaced by the limb is measured in cubic centimeters and represents the volume of the limb. (Fig. 6.9) As stated previously, edema is an impediment to wound healing. To assess the efficacy of treatment intended to reduce swelling, edema must be accurately monitored by repeated measures of either girth or volume using the same procedure each time.

Other Tests, Measures, and Examinations

Beyond what has been presented thus far, clinicians may use other tests, measures, and examination tools. This section will briefly touch on these issues, as well as provide information on pressure ulcer assessment tools and emerging technology.

First, the circulatory status adjacent to the wound must be evaluated to aid in determination of wound etiology, to plan interventions, and to prevent further tissue destruction. Examination of the surrounding skin may assist in determining the vascular status. For example, loss of hair indicates poor circulation in the limb. Nail beds may be examined for perfusion by digital compression of the nail bed and timing the ability of capillaries to blanch and refill. Nails should be assessed for

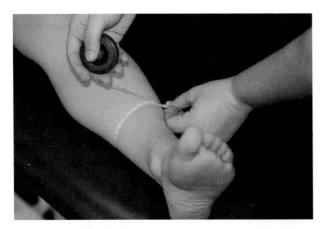

Figure 6•8 *Measurement of limb girth.*

fungal infection, thickness, ingrown nails, and any other condition that needs the attention of a clinician who specializes in foot care. Detailed information on vascular assessment is found in Chapter 7. Sensory deficits must be evaluated as well. Impaired sensation has implications for wound healing, as well as prevention of future wounds. Any disease or condition that involves the central or peripheral nervous system warrants an evaluation of sensation. The senses of touch, pressure, temperature, pain, vibration, and proprioception all provide the awareness required to prevent tissue injury. If a sensory deficit is suspected, the clinician must perform an appropriate evaluation to determine the extent of involvement. The neurological exam, including sensation, is discussed further in Chapter 7.

Skin temperature may reflect skin and subcutaneous perfusion, especially in the presence of inflammation or infection. Skin temperature can also be monitored to assess effects of treatments designed to increase tissue temperature. Interventions that may increase tissue temperature and perfusion include electrical stimulation, whirlpool, consensual heating with diathermy, and normothermia. Palpation is a quick, subjective method of evaluating skin temperature. Other methods that provide objective data include skin thermometer strips, thermistors, radiometers, thermographs, and infrared thermometers. Thermometer strips are inexpensive and can be applied to the skin to measure temperature above 95°F. Temperature is displayed in one-tenth-degree intervals. Normal skin temperature may range between 75°F and 80°F on the extremities and 92°F to 96°F on the torso, depending on circulation as well as the environmental temperature and duration of exposure in the room where it is tested.[113] A thermistor is relatively inexpensive and detects temperature by making contact with the skin, typically with a circular-shaped stainless steel disk or probe. A thermistor detects temperature by the changes in resistance in the semiconductor materials in the probe. The resistance in the probe decreases with increasing temperature.[114] An infrared thermometer measures skin temperature by detecting the infrared radiation emitted from the skin. This device does not require contact with the skin; therefore, it can be used over the wound surface and periwound area. Thermograms use liquid crystals to display skin temperature variation in a multicolor map or picture. This technique is infrequently used to assess wound-related temperatures. An infrared temperature scanner is a quick and efficient method for skin temperature detection. The scanner is used with or without skin contact. Regardless of the skin measurement methods used, the clinician should allow the limb or area to acclimate to room temperature prior to assessing skin temperature.

Next, the clinician may evaluate the patient's functional status and mobility needs. For example, range of motion, strength, transfers, balance, gait, or means of locomotion and any other functional activities must be examined and regularly monitored. The patient's medical condition, level of mobility, and type and location of wound dictate the types of devices or equipment used. For example, venous or lymphatic involvement may require compression bandages or garments (Chapters 16 and 18). Individuals at risk for pressure ulcers may need a pressure-mapping assessment (Chapter 19). Interventions will include pressure-reducing surfaces for the bed and wheelchair. Neuropathy may require orthotics, foot wear, or total contact casting to decrease plantar weight bearing (see Chapters 14 and 15). A comprehensive wound evaluation will always include an assessment of patient abilities, equipment, and devices.

A clinician may decide to use wound assessment tools designed specifically for a certain wound type. Assessment tools for pressure ulcers appear to be more common than for other types of wounds. See Table 6.19 for information on some

Table 6•19 Pressure Ulcer Assessment Tools

Pressure Ulcer Assessment Tool	Valid	Reliable	Responsive to Change
Sessing Scale[155-157] Assesses periwound edges, wound tissue, odor, sepsis. 0–6 Scale: as score increases, wound status worsens.	Yes	Yes	Possibly
Pressure Sore Status Tool[157-161] Assesses wound size, depth, undermining, necrosis, exudate, skin color, edema, induration, granulation, epithelialization. Score range: 13–65; increasing score means deterioration.	Yes	Yes	Unknown
Pressure Ulcer Scale for Healing[110,160-164] Assesses wound area, exudate, appearance. Score range: 8–34; increasing score means deterioration.	Yes	Yes	Possibly
Wound Healing Scale[157,165] Descriptive assessment for the following: unstageable, necrosis, infection, débrided, granulation, contraction, reepithelialization, healing.	Unknown	Unknown	Unknown
Sussman Wound Healing Tool[157,166] Assess wound tissue, location, healing, depth, undermining, tunneling. No scoring system.	Unknown	Unknown	Unknown

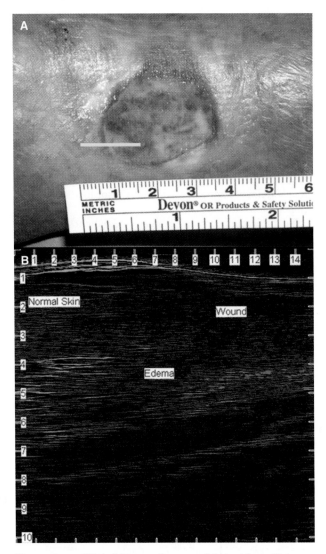

Figure 6•10 *Digital image of a wound (A) with an Episcan I-200 high-resolution ultrasound image below (B). Courtesy of Longport, Inc., Glen Mills, PA.*

of the common pressure ulcer assessment tools available. Clinicians should consider validity, reliability, and responsiveness to change when using formalized assessment tools. Lastly, the clinician will need to stay abreast of new assessment and evaluation technology as it is becomes available. For example, high-frequency, high-resolution ultrasound scanning is a new, noninvasive technique to assess deep tissue injury and monitor healing.[115-118] Please see Figure 6.10 for a visual example of high-frequency ultrasound of deeper tissues.

Practice Guidelines and Assessment

Various published wound care guidelines can be obtained by clinicians. Many of these guidelines entail extensive literature searches and wound expert consensus for wound evaluation and treatment. For example for the Wound Healing Society's *Guidelines for Best Care of Chronic Wounds*,[119]

Dr Adrian Barbul, principal investigator, and a panel of wound experts used evidence-based information to develop the guidelines.[119-123] The guidelines include well-controlled animal and human studies. The Canadian Association of Wound Care and the Registered Nurses' Association of Ontario guidelines (RNAO) have completed similar guideline projects. These guidelines are excellent efforts to elevate and standardize the level of wound care. Guidelines cover many aspects of wound care beyond examination and evaluation skills. The reader is encouraged to seek out these documents for further information. Two other guideline documents that are not primarily wound related are also presented. These documents are diabetic foot guidelines developed by Diabetes Committee of the American Orthopedic Foot and Ankle Society[124] and peripheral vascular disease (PAD) guidelines developed by the American College of Cardiology and the American Heart Association.[125] Both diabetes and PAD are some wound etiologies that complicate wound management. Please see Tables 6.20 to 6.23 for summaries of various guideline recommendations for diabetic, venous, pressure, and arterial insufficiency wounds. This guideline sampling steers the clinician toward assessing the following items: systemic disease, risk factors, other health issues impacting healing, vascular status, sensation, infection, wound healing rates, and other issues.

> ▶ **PEARL 6•4** Evidence-based, consensus-derived wound care guidelines enable the clinician to provide high-quality patient care.

Reassessment and Prognosis

Wound evaluation yields data needed to validate the effects of interventions used to enhance healing and recovery of function. Regular wound reassessment is also required so that appropriate changes may be made in the plan of care. The AHRQ *Treatment of Pressure Ulcers: Clinical Practice Guideline* recommends that the pressure ulcer be reassessed at least weekly or when wound deterioration is evident.[3] This document states, "A clean pressure ulcer should show evidence of some healing within 2 to 4 weeks. If no progress can be demonstrated, reevaluate the adequacy of the overall treatment plan as well as adherence to this plan, making modifications as necessary."[3] The *Venous Leg Ulcer Guideline* recommends the venous wound be assessed by the clinician at each visit.[38] Furthermore, this guideline recommends that if signs of healing are not evident after 2 to 4 weeks of treatment, other comorbidities may be contributing to the wound etiology. Examples of comorbid conditions to investigate are neoplasm, osteomyelitis, blood dyscrasias, silent infection, and other conditions that impair healing. The guideline also recommends referral to other health-care practitioners if healing is not proceeding as expected. In addition to recommendations regarding reevaluation, experienced clinicians must use their professional judgment as to how often reevaluation must occur.

If the clinician is to reevaluate a wound, it is critical to know what elements of the initial assessment will provide the data that will determine if healing or improvement in the patient condition is occurring. The various tests, measures, and

Table 6•20 Diabetic Ulcer Guideline Recommendations: Evaluation and Assessment

	WHS Guidelines for Best Care of Chronic Wounds[121]	Best Practice Recommendations for the Prevention and Treatment of Diabetic Foot Ulcers: Canadian Association of Wound Care/RNAO[167]	American Orthopedic Foot and Ankle Society: Diabetes Committee[124]
General issues and risk factors	Examine person as a whole: Systemic disease Medications Nutrition Tissue perfusion/oxygenation.	Classify patient into a risk category to aid in coordination of care (University of Texas treatment–based Diabetic Foot Classification System).	Screen at-risk patients for ulcers: Peripheral neuropathy Absent pulses One absent pulse and trophic changes Claudication Nontraumatic foot amputations History of diabetic foot ulcer Hospital admission for foot infection Bony deformities Peripheral edema Abnormal skin temperature.
Vascular	Check pedal pulses and/or ABI. Elderly or ABI over 1.2: Doppler waveform, toe-brachial index, TcPo$_2$, or color duplex ultrasonography scan.	Vascular status must be included in assessment.	Pedal pulses, skin temperature, capillary refill, dependant rubor, gangrene. Erythema (infection, inflammation, Charcot arthropathy). Swelling from infection, arterial and/or venous insufficiency, neuropathic fx/dislocations.
Sensation	5.07 Semmes-Weinstein monofilament.	Sensation should be assessed.	5.07 Semmes-Weinstein monofilament.
Infection	Biopsy or swab culture if at risk for infection or not healing with 2 weeks of treatment. Osteomyelitis: probe with swab, serial radiograph, MRI, CT scan or radionuclide scan.	Assess for infection: increased pain, wound breakdown, odor, friable, granulation tissue.	Assess for infection.
Wound/skin	Wound history. Wound traits: location, size, base, exudate, periwound, stage, and pain. Rate of healing.	Length/width: Measure using a consistent method. Depth.	Skin: dryness, keratoses, sensation. Wound: infection, necrosis, depth, bone involvement.
Healing rate	If wound size has not decreased by 40% at 4 or more weeks of treatment, then reassess and consider other interventions.		
Bony deformities		Bony and structural deformities must be assessed.	Check ankle, foot, and toes for deformities.
Footwear and foot issues		Assess footwear.	Shoe size, shape, inside shoe; toe box. Check wear patterns, insoles. Toe: check for ingrown nails, thickened nails. Toe web: check for maceration, cracks, wounds, infection.

ABI, ankle-brachial index; Registered Nurses' Association of Ontario, RNAO; TcPo$_2$, transcutaneous partial pressure of oxygen; WHS, Wound Healing Society.

Table 6•21 Venous Ulcer Guideline Recommendations: Evaluation and Assessment

	WHS Guidelines for Best Care of Chronic Wounds[120]	Best Practice Recommendations for the Prevention and Treatment of Venous Leg Ulcers: Canadian Association of Wound Care/RNAO[168]
General issues/risk factors	Examine patient as a whole: systemic disease, medications, nutrition, tissue perfusion/oxygenation. If at risk for sickle cell disease, conduct a sickle cell preparation and hemoglobin electrophoresis.	Take complete history: pain, systemic disease, local wound factors that impact healing. Rule out other diagnoses.
Vascular	Check pedal pulses and/or ABI to detect arterial disease. Use toe-brachial index or TcPo$_2$ for elderly, patients with diabetes, or when ABI is over 1.2. Perform color duplex ultrasonography scanning with proximal compression or Valsalva's maneuver to determine venous etiology.	Perform bilateral vascular assessment: ABI to rule out arterial disease. Determine cause of venous insufficiency: abnormal valves (reflux), obstruction, or calf muscle pump failure.
Infection	Perform tissue biopsy or swab culture with suspected infection or if wound not improving over 2 weeks of treatment.	
Wound	Consider wound history, recurrence. Identify wound traits: location, size, base, exudate, periwound, stage, pain.	Identify sound traits: location, borders, shape, wound bed, exudate, periwound, edema.
Healing rate	Assess rate of healing: increase in wound size after 6 weeks of treatment or if extremely painful; consider other pathologies (fungi, mycobacterium, pyoderma gangrenosum, systemic disease, etc). Biopsy: not healing for 3 months without treatment or if not healing with 6 weeks of intervention	After 3 months of nonhealing, assess for comorbidities and malignancy.

ABI, ankle-brachial index; Registered Nurses' Association of Ontario, RNAO; TcPo$_2$, transcutaneous partial pressure of oxygen; WHS, Wound Healing Society.

Table 6•22 Pressure Ulcer Guideline Recommendations: Evaluation and Assessment

	WHS Guidelines for Best Care of Chronic Wounds[122]	Best Practice Recommendations for the Prevention and Treatment of Venous Leg Ulcers: Canadian Association of Wound Care/RNAO[89]
General issues/risk factors	Assess all patients for risk of pressure ulcers. Examine patient as a whole: systemic disease, medications, nutrition, tissue perfusion/oxygenation. Perform nutritional assessment when patient enters health-care facility or when patient status changes may cause malnutrition.	Take complete history and perform physical exam: general health, risk factors, issues impacting pressure ulcer healing. Assess and modify situations that cause pressure. Assess and control pain. Assess and assist with psychological issues.
Infection	Perform biopsy or swab culture when infection suspected or if wound not improving in 2 weeks of treatment. Perform bone biopsy for suspected osteomyelitis.	Assess for infection.
Wound	Document location, stage, size, base, exudate, infection, pain.	Assess and stage the wound: NPUAP staging system, PSST, Sessing Scale, PWAT, PUSH Use the MEASURE mnemonic.
Healing rate	Monitor wound healing rate.	See above.

National Pressure Ulcer Advisory Panel, NPUAP; Pressure Sore Status Tool, PSST; Pressure Ulcer Scale for Healing, PUSH; Registered Nurses' Association of Ontario, RNAO; WHS, Wound Healing Society.

Table 6•23	Arterial Insufficiency Guideline Recommendations: Evaluation and Assessment	
	WHS Guidelines for Best Care of Chronic Wounds[123]	**ACC/AHA Guidelines for the Management of Patients with Peripheral Vascular Disease**[125]
General issues and risk factors	Examine patient as a whole: systemic disease, medications, nutrition, tissue perfusion/oxygenation. Complete workup by physician for atherosclerosis risk factors: smoking, diabetes, hypertension, hypercholesterolemia, advanced age, obesity, hypothyroidism. Consider other pathologies: thromboangiitis, vasculitis, Raynaud's disease, pyoderma gangrenosum, thalassemia, sickle cell disease.	Asymptomatic people: Screen for walking impairment, claudication, resting pain, nonhealing ulcers. Assess pulses/feet. Adults over 50 years at risk for atherosclerosis. For all adults over 70 years, assess walking impairment, claudication, ischemic resting pain, and/or nonhealing ulcers. Exercise ABI is useful for diagnosis of LE PAD for asymptomatic people at risk with normal ABI and no other symptoms. Toe-brachial index or pulse volume recording for LE PAD at risk with ABI over 1.3 and no symptoms/signs.
Vascular	Evaluate lower extremities: Pedal pulses Capillary refill Buerger's test (dependant rubor) ABI $TcPo_2$ Doppler waveforms Pulse volume recording	Suspected PAD: Resting ABI for the following: claudication, nonhealing wounds, over 70 years old or over 50 with history of smoking or diabetes. Use toe-brachial index when ABI not useful due to noncompressible vessels. Claudication: Should have a vascular exam and ABI. Exercise ABI if resting ABI is normal. Critical limb ischemia (CLI): Evaluate/treat factors that increase amputation risk: diabetes, severe renal failure, severe reduction in cardiac output, vasospastic disease, smoking/tobacco use, infection, skin break down, injury/trauma. If CLI history or if treated for CLI, vascular specialist evaluation twice a year. Regular foot inspections: people at risk for CLI; ABI less than 0.4 in nondiabetic; any person with diabetes with known LE PAD. Regular feet examination after successful treatment of CLI.

ABI, ankle-brachial index; American College of Cardiology/American Heart Association, ACC/AHA; LE, lower extremity; peripheral arterial disease, PAD; $TcPo_2$, transcutaneous partial pressure of oxygen; WHS, Wound Healing Society.

observations used for the initial assessment of the patient and wound should be selected to monitor improvement in outcome. For example, the clinician may examine changes in wound-related pain, limb volume, wound size, and wound appearance. A study by Eager surveyed 154 home health-care enterostomal therapy (ET) nurses to determine their methods for monitoring and documenting wound healing.[126] According to this study, 74% of the respondents performed weekly wound assessment. Over 96% of the ET nurses used wound length and width, characteristics of wound drainage, and wound bed changes to monitor healing.[126] Various tools or reassessment instruments that use a variety of measurements have been developed to monitor the healing of wounds.

Many of the wound characteristics mentioned earlier are difficult to quantify, such as exudate, percentage of devitalized and healthy tissue, odor, color, and maceration. (Refer back to the appropriate sections of this chapter for assessment of these wound attributes.) Wound length and width, area, perimeter, and edema are somewhat easier to measure. Wound closure rates may be calculated using wound dimension measurements such as changes in wound surface area. Wound area may also be determined from wound tracings and photography, as mentioned above. Wound area data can be used to calculate closure rates such as total area closed and percentage of area closed. Total area closed (or change in area) equals the initial wound area minus current wound area. Percentage of area healed can be determined by dividing the current wound area by the initial wound area and multiplying by 100. Both of these closure rates use a wound area that may be misleading, depending on whether the wound is large or small. The total area closed will overestimate the healing rate of large ulcers, and the percentage of area healed will overestimate the healing rate of a small wound. Jessup and other proponents[127-130] urge clinicians and researchers to use linear advancement of the wound edge to assess wound healing. These calculations may allow better comparisons of healing between studies. However, these calculations may be more time consuming and complicated for the typical clinician. The reader is encouraged to seek out information by these authors as to how to calculate linear wound edge advancement. A user-friendly software package using these calculations, along with digital images and other wound information, would be a great benefit to the clinician. Wound dimension changes are a factor to consider with wound prognosis. Researchers and clinicians are also focusing on wound assessment and its role in wound prognosis. The initial wound size, wound duration, and wound size change with intervention, as well as other issues, are being explored for wound prognosis. Wound prognosis is multifaceted. The clinician must take into account all the factors with each individual patient when developing a prognosis. Researchers are turning their efforts toward determining how the patient and what aspects of wound can aid in prognosis. See Table 6.24 for an example of wound-healing predictors. Clinicians must reassess the wounds in a timely manner to ascertain if interventions are facilitating healing. If the wound is not healing as expected, then the plan of care must be reassessed.

A complete wound reassessment should not focus solely on the wound, but should also include pertinent factors associated with the patient, family, and caregivers. For example, wound healing will definitely be affected by adherence of the patient, family, and caregivers to any instructions, recommendations, or treatments they have been asked to perform. Reassessment should encompass the following: assessment of risks for new wound development or deterioration of the current wound; any psychosocial-emotional issues affecting the patient; the status of any medical conditions and other medical issues that have implications for healing; the current wound condition, including all the previously mentioned items in the wound assessment section; as well as the patient's functional abilities and any devices or equipment currently in use. All of these elements of the wound evaluation puzzle must be examined so the clinician can determine the necessary interventions for obtaining optimal outcomes.

In summary, the wound evaluation process involves many aspects that the clinician must consider. Information from the patient, family, and caregivers is melded with data the clinician gathered from the objective evaluation. The clinician must weigh the importance and significance of all the information and develop a plan for intervention. The plan of care must balance risks and benefits of the interventions. It is obvious that a very complex decision-making process is part of the evaluation. Much is riding on the ability of the clinician to arrive at the appropriate decisions and implement the correct interventions. Once the management of the wound has begun, the clinician must be able to reassess the wound and patient. Wound healing is a dynamic process; consequently, regular reassessments are vital for determining the need for changes in interventions.

Table 6•24 Wound Prognosis

	Venous Ulcer		Neuropathic Ulcer		Pressure Ulcer	
	Healing	**Poor Healing**	**Healing**	**Poor Healing**	**Healing**	**Poor Healing**
Initial size/depth	Wound area <10 cm^2.[61]		Small/superficial: Wagner 1 or 2.[169-171]		With appropriate treatment; stage I and II heal quicker than stage III and IV.[172-174]	
Size change with treatment	Wound size decreases in first 2 to 3 weeks with treatment.[55-60]	Wound size increases with 4 weeks of treatment (see citations to right).	Wound size decreases after 4 weeks of treatment. Wound size decreases 54% in 4 weeks: 91% sensitive and 58% specific for healing Wagner 1 or 2 at 3 months.[62,63]		Decrease of 40%–50% in ulcer size in first 2 weeks of treatment.[56,64,175]	
Duration	Shorter wound duration.[61,176,177]	Wound present more than 3 months before medically treated.[177,178]	Duration of ulcer less than 2 months.[171]			
Miscellaneous issues	Deep veins uninvolved.[176] Patient using compression.[178]	Patient traits: older, higher body mass index, and lower extremity arterial disease.[176,177]		Infected ulcers: amputation is 154 times more likely to occur.[179]		Poor nutrition.[180]

▸ **PEARL 6•5** Valid, reliable wound assessments will enable the clinician to make appropriate wound prognoses, monitor wound healing, and implement appropriate wound interventions.

Summary

As stated at the outset, wound evaluation is the foundation upon which appropriate wound interventions are based. Wound evaluation should be comprehensive, and in addition to evaluating the wound and periwound skin or limb, it should include a systems review of general health, comorbidities, functional status, and many other factors. The clinician's professional judgment must be used to evaluate all of the data and information gathered prior to determining interventions. Timely reevaluation of the patient and his or her wound is essential for monitoring progress or lack of progress toward wound closure. The wound evaluation will influence the selection of interventions and the determination of treatment efficacy. Reimbursement agencies are focused on payment of efficacious and cost-effective treatments. Finally, evaluation has a vital role in wound management research. Randomized, well-controlled trials are needed to determine accurate, valid, reliable, cost-effective, and practical evaluation methods to aid in evaluating wound response to treatment. Wound evaluation will always have important implications for the quality of care provided to the patient with a wound.

▸ **Case Study 6•1** | **Evaluation of a Patient with a Complicated Venous Ulcer**

Case: A patient is referred with the following: open wounds on bilateral lower extremities—two wounds above the left lateral ankle, one wound above the right lateral ankle. What do you include in your wound evaluation?

Solution: The clinician must acquire more information on the background, history, and current status of this patient before developing the plan of care. The following information should be obtained.

Demographics: The patient is a 65-year-old male.

Occupation/Employment: He has retired from factory work, and he likes to garden.

Social Information: He is single, never married, and has no one to assist him at home.

Past Medical History and Current Health Status: He is relatively healthy except for heart disease. There is a history of alcohol abuse and poor nutrition. He takes no medications currently, and there are neither previous tests nor measurement information available.

Current Wound Status: He has had the wounds for 3 months. The wounds developed spontaneously with no apparent etiology, and the wounds became larger subsequent to self-treatment consisting of dry gauze dressings. He has had no previous medical interventions for the wounds. He experiences significant wound-related pain at night rated at 6 on a 0–10 scale and rated 3 during the day. Pain decreases with elevation and ambulation. He also presents with visible swelling in both legs.

Wound Assessment: Wounds are located above the ankles bilaterally. The clinician should measure wound dimensions such as length, width, depth, and wound surface area with techniques described earlier. The dimensions of each wound should be recorded independently. Each wound should be examined for the presence and extent of tunnels or undermining. In this case, no tunnels or undermining are noted. Wound edges are flat and attached to the periwound area. The wound bases for both wounds are covered completely with yellow slough material. There is a moderate amount of wound exudate that is slightly yellow in appearance, without odor.

The Periwound Area/Lower Extremities: Both legs are swollen, the skin is shiny, and hair is not present. The skin of both lower extremities below the knees is red-purple in color. The periwound area surrounding each wound is reddened and indurated.

Vascular Status: Arterial and venous circulation must be assessed. The patient has diagnosed heart disease that may also affect the arterial blood supply to the legs. He presents with possible signs and symptoms that suggest venous insufficiency. The edema may warrant compression. Consequently, the adequacy of arterial blood supply must be assessed prior to compression therapy. The venous circulation must be examined to determine the extent of venous insufficiency. The patient has palpable pulses and an ankle-brachial index (ABI) of 1.0.

Edema: Bilateral leg, ankle, and foot edema should be assessed by girth or volume measurement.

Sensation: Sensation testing reveals intact sensation in both lower extremities.

Miscellaneous: He has functional strength and range of motion without limitations in all extremities. He does not require any assistive devices or equipment at this time. He has stated that he is not sure about his tolerance for wearing compression garments.

Conclusion: The clinician should assess all the above information to formulate a plan for this patient who appears to have wounds due to venous insufficiency. His case is complicated by multiple factors: poor nutrition, alcohol abuse, possible arterial involvement related to a history of heart disease, ankle wounds for 3 months without treatment, and no sign of closure. In addition, there is nonviable tissue present in the wound, periwound erythema and induration, and bilateral lower extremity edema. The patient has indicated that he may not adhere to compression therapy. Having gathered this information, the clinician should design a plan of care to address the patient's needs. Goals should include facilitating edema reduction and wound closure. Treatment guidelines may be found in Chapter 16 on venous ulcers and Chapter 17 on ischemic ulcers.

References

1. American Physical Therapy Association. Guide to physical therapist practice. Phys Ther 2001; 81: 9–744.
2. U.S. Department of Health and Human Services: Pressure Ulcers in Adults: Prediction and Prevention. Clinical Practice Guideline. No. 3, Pub. No. 92-0047, Rockville, MD, U.S. Department of Health and Human Services, 1992.
3. Bergstrom, N, Bennet, M, Carlson, CE, et al: Treatment of Pressure Ulcers. Clinical Practice Guideline. No. 15. Rockville, MD, U.S. Department of Health and Human Services. Agency for Healthcare Research and Quality.
4. Vidal, J, Sarrias, M: An analysis of the diverse factors concerned with the development of pressure sores in spinal cord injured patients. Paraplegia 1991; 29:261–267.
5. Lakier, JB: Smoking and cardiovascular disease. Am J Med 1992; 93:8S–12S.
6. Corelli, F: Buerger's disease: Cigarette smoker disease may always be cured by medical therapy alone. Uselessness of operative treatment. J Cardiovasc Surg (Torino) 1973; 14:28–36.
7. Ciccone, CD: Pharmacology in Rehabilitation. Philadelphia, FA Davis, 2007.
8. Malone, T: Physical Therapy and Occupational Therapy: Drug Implications for Practice. Philadelphia, JB Lippincott, 1989.
9. Hunt, TK, Dunphy, JE: Fundamentals of Wound Management in Surgery. New York, Appleton-Century-Crofts, 1979.
10. Eddy, L: Physical Therapy Pharmacology. St. Louis, Mosby, 1992.
11. Heyward, VH, Stolarczyk, LM: Applied Body Composition Assessment. Champaign, IL, Human Kinetics, 1996.
12. Flanigan, KH: Nutritional aspects of wound healing. Adv Wound Care 1997; 10:48–52.
13. Bergstrom, N, Braden, B: A prospective study of pressure sore risk among institutionalized elderly. J Am Geriatr Soc 1992; 40:747–758.
14. Breslow, RA, Hallfrisch, J, Goldberg, AP: Malnutrition in tubefed nursing home patients with pressure sores. JPEN J Parenter Enteral Nutr 1991; 15:663–668.
15. Hanan, K, Scheele, L: Albumin vs weight as a predictor of nutritional status and pressure ulcer development. Ostomy Wound Manage 1991; 33:22–27.
16. Berlowitz, DR, Wilking, SV: Risk factors for pressure sores. A comparison of cross-sectional and cohort-derived data. J Am Geriatr Soc 1989; 37:1043–1050.
17. Pinchcofsky-Devin, GD, Kaminski, MV Jr.: Correlation of pressure sores and nutritional status. J Am Geriatr Soc 1986; 34:435–440.
18. Goodman, C, Boissonnault, WG, Fuller, KS: Laboratory test and values. In: Pathology: Implications for the Physical Therapist. Philadelphia, WB Saunders, 2003.
19. Marquez, RR: Wound evaluation. In: Clinical Wound Management. Thorofare, NJ, Slack, 1995.
20. Phillips, T, Stanton, B, Provan, A, et al: A study of the impact of leg ulcers on quality of life: Financial, social, and psychologic implications. J Am Acad Dermatol 1994; 31:49–53.
21. Dallam, L, Smyth, C, Jackson, BS, et al: Pressure ulcer pain: Assessment and quantification. J Wound Ostomy Continence Nurs 1995; 22:211–215; discussion 217–218.
22. Bond, MR, Pilowsky, I: Subjective assessment of pain and its relationship to the administration of analgesics in patients with advanced cancer. J Psychosom Res 1966; 10:203–208.
23. Bieri, D, Reeve, R, Champion, G, et al: The Faces Pain Scale for the self-assessment of the severity of pain experienced by children: Development, initial validation, and preliminary investigation for ratio scale properties. Pain 1990; 41:139–150.
24. Rook, JL: Wound care pain management. Adv Wound Care 1996; 9:24–31.
25. Ayello, EA, Braden, B: How and why to do pressure ulcer risk assessment. Adv Skin Wound Care 2002; 15:125–131; quiz 132–133.
26. Bergman-Evans, B, Cuddigan, J, Bergstrom, N: Clinical practice guidelines: Prediction and prevention of pressure ulcers. J Gerontol Nurs 1994; 20:19–26.
27. Braden, BJ, Bergstrom, N: Clinical utility of the Braden scale for predicting pressure sore risk. Decubitus 1989; 2:44–46, 50–51.
28. Norton, D: Calculating the risk: Reflections on the Norton Scale. 1989. Adv Wound Care 1996; 9:38–43.
29. Waterlow, JA: Reliability of the Waterlow score. J Wound Care 1995; 4:474–475.
30. Gosnell, DJ: Pressure sore risk assessment: A critique. The Gosnell scale. Decubitus 1989; 2(Pt 1):32–38.
31. Salzberg, CA, et al: A new pressure ulcer risk assessment scale for individuals with spinal cord injury. Am J Phys Med Rehabil 1996; 75:96–104.
32. Rochon, PA, et al: Risk assessment for pressure ulcers: An adaptation of the National Pressure Ulcer Advisory Panel risk factors to spinal cord injured patients. J Am Paraplegia Soc 1993; 16:169–177.
33. Lehman, CA: Risk factors for pressure ulcers in the spinal cord injured in the community. SCI Nurs 1995; 12:110–114.
34. Bedi, A: A tool to fill the gap. Developing a wound risk assessment chart for children. Prof Nurse 1993; 9:112–120.
35. Huffines, B, Logsdon, MC: The Neonatal Skin Risk Assessment Scale for predicting skin breakdown in neonates. Issues Compr Pediatr Nurs 1997; 20:103–114.
36. Waterlow, JA: Pressure sore risk assessment in children. Paediatr Nurs 1997; 9:21–24.
37. Boyko, EJ, et al: Prediction of diabetic foot ulcer occurrence using commonly available clinical information: The Seattle Diabetic Foot Study. Diabetes Care 2006; 29:1202–1207.
38. McGuckin, M: Venous Leg Ulcer Guideline. Wayne, PA, Health Management Publications, 1997.
39. Fahey, V: Vascular Nursing, ed 2. Philadelphia, WB Saunders, 1994.
40. Shai, A, Halevy, S: Direct triggers for ulceration in patients with venous insufficiency. Int J Dermatol 2005; 44:1006–1009.
41. Kannel, WB, McGee, DL: Update on some epidemiologic features of intermittent claudication: The Framingham Study. J Am Geriatr Soc 1985; 33:13–18.
42. Jonason, T, Ringqvist, I: Factors of prognostic importance for subsequent rest pain in patients with intermittent claudication. Acta Med Scand 1985; 218:27–33.
43. Hooi, JD, Stoffers, JE, Kester, AD, et al: Risk factors and cardiovascular diseases associated with asymptomatic peripheral arterial occlusive disease. The Limburg PAOD Study. Peripheral Arterial Occlusive Disease. Scand J Prim Health Care 1998; 16:177–182.
44. Cole, CW, Hill, GB, Fratad, E, et al: Cigarette smoking and peripheral arterial occlusive disease. Surgery 1993; 114:753–756; discussion 756–757.
45. Federman, DG, Trent, JT, Froelich, CW, et al: Epidemiology of peripheral vascular disease: A predictor of systemic vascular disease. Ostomy Wound Manage 1998; 44:58–62, 64, 66.
46. Bowlin, SJ, Medalie, JH, Flocke, SA, et al: Epidemiology of intermittent claudication in middle-aged men. Am J Epidemiol 1994; 140:418–430.
47. Fowkes, FG, Housley, E, Riemersma, RA, et al: Smoking, lipids, glucose intolerance, and blood pressure as risk factors for peripheral atherosclerosis compared with ischemic heart disease in the Edinburgh Artery Study. Am J Epidemiol 1992; 135:331–340.
48. Criqui, MH, Denenberg, JO, Langer, RD, et al: The epidemiology of peripheral arterial disease: Importance of identifying the population at risk. Vasc Med 1997; 2:221–226.
49. Gerhard, M, Baum, P, Raby, KE: Peripheral arterial-vascular disease in women: Prevalence, prognosis, and treatment. Cardiology 1995; 86:349–355.
50. Sibbald, RG, Orsted, HL, Coutts, PM, et al: Best practice recommendations for preparing the wound bed: Update 2006. Adv Skin Wound Care 2007; 20:390–405; quiz 406–407.
51. Schultz, GS, Barillo, DJ, Mozingo, DW, et al: Wound bed preparation and a brief history of TIME. Int Wound J 2004; 1:19–32.
52. Falanga, V: Classifications for wound bed preparation and stimulation of chronic wounds. Wound Repair Regen 2000; 8:347–352.

53. Schultz, GS, Sibbald, RTG, Falanga, V, et al: Wound bed preparation: A systematic approach to wound management. Wound Repair Regen 2003; 11(suppl):S1–S28.

54. Keast, DH, Bowering, K, Evans, W, et al: MEASURE: A proposed assessment framework for developing best practice recommendations for wound assessment. Wound Repair Regen 2004; 12(suppl):S1–S17.

55. Flanagan, M: Improving accuracy of wound measurement in clinical practice. Ostomy Wound Manage 2003; 49:28–40.

56. Flanagan, M: Wound measurement: Can it help us to monitor progression to healing? J Wound Care 2003; 12:189–194.

57. Hill, DP, Poore, S, Wilson, J, et al: Initial healing rates of venous ulcers: Are they useful as predictors of healing? Am J Surg 2004; 188(suppl):22–25.

58. Kantor, J, Margolis, DJ: A multicentre study of percentage change in venous leg ulcer area as a prognostic index of healing at 24 weeks. Br J Dermatol 2000; 142:960–964.

59. Arnold, TE, Stanley, JC, Fellows, EP, et al: Prospective, multicenter study of managing lower extremity venous ulcers. Ann Vasc Surg 1994; 8:356–362.

60. Margolis, DJ, Gross, EA, Wood, CR, et al: Planimetric rate of healing in venous ulcers of the leg treated with pressure bandage and hydrocolloid dressing. J Am Acad Dermatol 1993; 28:418–421.

61. Margolis, DJ, Allen-Taylor, L, Hoffstad, O, et al: The accuracy of venous leg ulcer prognostic models in a wound care system. Wound Repair Regen 2004; 12:163–168.

62. Sheehan, P, Jones, P, Caselli, A, et al: Percent change in wound area of diabetic foot ulcers over a 4-week period is a robust predictor of complete healing in a 12-week prospective trial. Diabetes Care 2003; 26:1879–1882.

63. Sheehan, P, Jones, P, Guirine, JM, et al: Percent change in wound area of diabetic foot ulcers over a 4-week period is a robust predictor of complete healing in a 12-week prospective trial. Plast Reconstr Surg 2006; 117(suppl):239S–244S.

64. Brown, GS: Reporting outcomes for stage IV pressure ulcer healing: A proposal. Adv Skin Wound Care 2000; 13:277–283.

65. Hess, CT: Care tips for chronic wounds: Pressure ulcers. Adv Skin Wound Care 2004; 17:477–479.

66. Majeske, C: Reliability of wound surface area measurements. Phys Ther 1992; 72:138–141.

67. Diamond, JE, Mueller, MJ, Delitto, A, et al: Reliability of a diabetic foot evaluation. Phys Ther 1989; 69:797–802.

68. Harding, KG: Methods for assessing change in ulcer status. Adv Wound Care 1995; 8(suppl):37–42.

69. Langemo, DK, Melland, J, Hanson, D, et al: Two-dimensional wound measurement: Comparison of 4 techniques. Adv Wound Care 1998; 11:337–343.

70. Samad, A, Hayes, S, French, L, et al: Digital imaging versus conventional contact tracing for the objective measurement of venous leg ulcers. J Wound Care 2002; 11:137–140.

71. Lagan, KM, Dusoir, AE, McDonough, SM, et al: Wound measurement: The comparative reliability of direct versus photographic tracings analyzed by planimetry versus digitizing techniques. Arch Phys Med Rehabil 2000; 81:1110–1116.

72. Thawer, HA, Houghton, PE, Woodbury, MG, et al: A comparison of computer-assisted and manual wound size measurement. Ostomy Wound Manage 2002; 48:46–53.

73. Griffin, JW, Tolley, EA, Tooms, RE, et al: A comparison of photographic and transparency-based methods for measuring wound surface area. Phys Ther 1993; 73:117–122.

74. Bohannon, RW, Pfaller, BA: Documentation of wound surface area from tracings of wound perimeters. Clinical report on three techniques. Phys Ther 1983; 63:1622–1624.

75. Cutler, NR, George, R, Seifert, RD, et al: Comparison of quantitative methodologies to define chronic pressure ulcer measurements. Decubitus 1993; 6:22–30.

76. Kutcher, J, Arnell, I: Documentation of skin using photography. Ostomy Wound Manage 1992; 38:23–24, 26–28.

77. Moore, K: Using wound area measurement to predict and monitor response to treatment of chronic wounds. J Wound Care 2005; 14:229–232.

78. Sussman, CASG: A uniform method to trace and measure chronic wounds. Poster presentation at: Symposium for Advanced Wound Care, San Francisco, CA, April 1991.

79. Schubert, V, Zander, M: Analysis of the measurement of four wound variables in elderly patients with pressure ulcers. Adv Wound Care 1996; 9:29–36.

80. Berg, W, Traneroth, C, Gunnarsson, A, et al: A method for measuring pressure sores. Lancet 1990; 335:1445–1446.

81. Bulstrode, CJ, Goode, AW, Scott, PJ: Stereophotogrammetry for measuring rates of cutaneous healing: A comparison with conventional techniques. Clin Sci (Lond) 1986; 71:437–443.

82. Frantz, RA, Johnson, DA: Stereophotography and computerized image analysis: A three-dimensional method of measuring wound healing. Wounds 1992; 4:58.

83. Ozturk, C, Nissannov, J, Dubin, S, et al: Measurement of wound healing by image analysis. Biomed Sci Instrum 1995; 31:189–193.

84. Plassmann, P, Jones, BF: Measuring leg ulcers by colour-coded structured light. J Wound Care 1992; 1:35.

85. Plassmann, P, Melhuish, JM, Harding, KG: Methods of measuring wound size: A comparative study. Ostomy Wound Manage 1994; 40:50–52, 54, 56–60.

86. Resch, CS, Kerner, E, Robson, MC, et al: Pressure sore volume measurement. A technique to document and record wound healing. J Am Geriatr Soc 1988; 36:444–446.

87. Altmeyer, P, Erbler, H, Kromer, T, et al: Interferometry: A new method for no-touch measurement of the surface and volume of ulcerous skin lesions. Acta Derm Venereol 1995; 75:193–197.

88. Ibbett, DA, et al: Measuring leg ulcers using a laser displacement sensor. Physiol Meas 1994; 15:325–332.

89. Keast, DH, Parslow, NE, Houghton, PE, et al: Best practice recommendations for the prevention and treatment of pressure ulcers: Update 2006. Adv Skin Wound Care 2007; 20:461–462.

90. Xakellis, GC Jr., Frantz, RA: Pressure ulcer healing: What is it? What influences it? How is it measured? Adv Wound Care 1997; 10:20–26.

91. The National Pressure Ulcer Advisory Panel: Pressure ulcers prevalence, cost and risk assessment: Consensus development conference statement—The National Pressure Ulcer Advisory Panel. Decubitus 1989; 2:24–28.

92. Henderson, CT, Ayello, EA, Sussman, C, et al: Draft definition of stage I pressure ulcers: Inclusion of persons with darkly pigmented skin. NPUAP Task Force on Stage I Definition and Darkly Pigmented Skin. Adv Wound Care 1997; 10:16–19.

93. Shea, JD: Pressure sores: Classification and management. Clin Orthop Relat Res 1975; 112:89–100.

94. Black, J, Baharestani, MM, Cuddigan, J, et al: National Pressure Ulcer Advisory Panel's updated pressure ulcer staging system. Adv Skin Wound Care 2007; 20:269–274.

95. NPUA Panel: Pressure ulcer healing: Controversy to consensus, assessment methods and outcomes. :8:1S.

96. Maklebust, J: Policy implications of using reverse staging to monitor pressure ulcer status. Adv Wound Care 1997; 10:32–35.

97. DeSanti, L: Pathophysiology and current management of burn injury. Adv Skin Wound Care 2005; 18:323–332; quiz 332–334.

98. Wachtel, TL, Berry, CC, Gillon, WC, et al: The inter-rater reliability of estimating the size of burns from various burn area chart drawings. Burns 2000; 26:156–170.

99. Rieg, LS, Jenkins, M: Burn injuries in children. Crit Care Nurs Clin North Am 1991; 3:457–470.

100. Hettiaratchy, S, Papini, R: Initial management of a major burn: Assessment and resuscitation. BMJ 2004; 329(Pt 2):101–103.

101. Richard, R: Assessment and diagnosis of burn wounds. Adv Wound Care 1999; 12:468–471.

102. Wagner, FW Jr.: The dysvascular foot: a system for diagnosis and treatment. Foot Ankle 1981; 2:64–122.

103. Armstrong, DG, Lavery, LA, Harkless, LB: Validation of a diabetic wound classification system. The contribution of depth, infection, and ischemia to risk of amputation. Diabetes Care 1998; 21:855–859.

104. Gardner, SE, Frantz, RA, Doebbeling, BN: The validity of the clinical signs and symptoms used to identify localized chronic wound infection. Wound Repair Regen 2001; 9:178–186.

105. Gardner, SE, et al: A tool to assess clinical signs and symptoms of localized infection in chronic wounds: development and reliability. Ostomy Wound Manage 2001; 47:40–47.

106. Kerstein, MD: Moist wound healing: The clinical perspective. Ostomy Wound Manage 1995; 41(suppl):37S–44S; discussion 45S.

107. Pollack, SV: The wound healing process. Clin Dermatol 1984; 2:8–16.

108. Winter, GD: Formation of the scab and reepithelialization of superficial wounds in the skin of the young domestic pig. Nature 1965; 193:293.

109. Wysocki, AB: Wound fluids and the pathogenesis of chronic wounds. J Wound Ostomy Continence Nurs 1996; 23:283–290.

110. Thomas, DR, et al: Pressure ulcer scale for healing: Derivation and validation of the PUSH tool. The PUSH Task Force. Adv Wound Care 1997; 10:96–101.

111. Maklebust, J: PUSH Tool reality check: audience response. Pressure Ulcer Scale for Healing. Adv Wound Care 1997; 10:102–106.

112. Bates-Jensen, BM: The Pressure Sore Status Tool a few thousand assessments later. Adv Wound Care 1997; 10:65–73.

113. Sussman, C: Assessment of the skin and wound. In: Wound Care. Gaithersburg, MD, Aspen Publications, 1998.

114. Wolf, S: Guide to Electronic Measurements and Laboratory Practice, ed 2. Englewood Cliffs, NJ, Prentice Hall, 1983, p 347.

115. Dyson, M, et al: Wound healing assessment using 20 MHz ultrasound and photography. Skin Res Technol 2003; 9:116–121.

116. Quintavalle, PR, et al: Use of high-resolution, high-frequency diagnostic ultrasound to investigate the pathogenesis of pressure ulcer development. Adv Skin Wound Care 2006; 19:498–505.

117. Fornage, BD, Deshayes, JL: Ultrasound of normal skin. J Clin Ultrasound 1986; 14:619–622.

118. Fornage, BD, et al: Imaging of the skin with 20-MHz US. Radiology 1993; 189:69–76.

119. Robson, MC, Barbul, A: Guidelines for the best care of chronic wounds. Wound Repair Regen 2006; 14:647–648.

120. Robson, MC, et al: Guidelines for the treatment of venous ulcers. Wound Repair Regen 2006; 14:649–662.

121. Steed, DL, et al: Guidelines for the treatment of diabetic ulcers. Wound Repair Regen 2006; 14:680–692.

122. Whitney, J, et al: Guidelines for the treatment of pressure ulcers. Wound Repair Regen 2006; 14:663–679.

123. Hopf, HW, et al: Guidelines for the treatment of arterial insufficiency ulcers. Wound Repair Regen 2006; 14:693–710.

124. Pinzur, MS, et al: Guidelines for diabetic foot care: Recommendations endorsed by the Diabetes Committee of the American Orthopaedic Foot and Ankle Society. Foot Ankle Int 2005; 26:113–119.

125. Hirsch, AT, et al: ACC/AHA Guidelines for the Management of Patients with Peripheral Arterial Disease (lower extremity, renal, mesenteric, and abdominal aortic): A collaborative report from the American Associations for Vascular Surgery/Society for Vascular Surgery, Society for Cardiovascular Angiography and Interventions, Society for Vascular Medicine and Biology, Society of Interventional Radiology, and the ACC/AHA Task Force on Practice Guidelines (Writing Committee to Develop Guidelines for the Management of Patients with Peripheral Arterial Disease)—Summary of recommendations. J Vasc Interv Radiol 2006; 17:1383–1397; quiz 1398.

126. Eager, CA: Monitoring wound healing in the home health arena. Adv Wound Care 1997; 10:54–57.

127. Jessup, RL: What is the best method for assessing the rate of wound healing? A comparison of 3 mathematical formulas. Adv Skin Wound Care 2006; 19:138–147.

128. Tallman, P, et al: Initial rate of healing predicts complete healing of venous ulcers. Arch Dermatol 1997; 133:1231–1234.

129. Gilman, T: Parameter for measurement of wound closure. Wounds 1990; 3:95–101.

130. Gorin, DR, et al: The influence of wound geometry on the measurement of wound healing rates in clinical trials. J Vasc Surg 1996; 23:524–528.

131. Rothstein, M, Roy, SH, Wolf, SL: The Rehabilitation Specialists Handbook, ed 2. Philadelphia, FA Davis, 1998.

132. Konstaninides, NN: Principles of nutritional support. In: Acute and Chronic Wounds. 1992, St. Louis, Mosby, 1992.

133. Panik, M, Paz, J: Vascular system and hematology. In: Acute Care Handbook for Physical Therapy. Boston, Butterworth-Heinemann, 1997.

134. Manum, K: Nutritional Aspects of Reducing the Risk for Integumentary Impairments. Presented to: American Physical Therapy Combined Sections Meeting, Seattle, WA, 1999.

135. Guralnik, JM: Occurrence and predictor of pressure sores in the national health and nutrition examination survey. J Am Geriatr Soc 1988; 36:807.

136. Feedar, J: Prevention and management of pressure ulcers. In: Wound Healing: Alternatives in Management. Philadelphia, FA Davis, 1995, p. 186.

137. Jalali, R, Rezaie, M: Predicting pressure ulcer risk: Comparing the predictive validity of 4 scales. Adv Skin Wound Care 2005; 18:92–97.

138. Pancorbo-Hidalgo, PL, et al: Risk assessment scales for pressure ulcer prevention: A systematic review. J Adv Nurs 2006; 54:94–110.

139. Lindgren, M, et al: A risk assessment scale for the prediction of pressure sore development: Reliability and validity. J Adv Nurs 2002; 38:190–199.

140. Bergstrom, N, Braden, BJ: Predictive validity of the Braden Scale among black and white subjects. Nurs Res 2002; 51:398–403.

141. Benbow, SJ, et al: The prediction of diabetic neuropathic plantar foot ulceration by liquid-crystal contact thermography. Diabetes Care 1994; 17:835–839.

142. Bresater, LE, Welin, L, Romanus, B: Foot pathology and risk factors for diabetic foot disease in elderly men. Diabetes Res Clin Pract 1996; 32:103–109.

143. Lavery, LA, et al: Practical criteria for screening patients at high risk for diabetic foot ulceration. Arch Intern Med 1998; 158:157–162.

144. Macfarlane, RM, Jeffcoate, WJ: Factors contributing to the presentation of diabetic foot ulcers. Diabet Med 1997; 14:867–870.

145. McNeely, MJ, et al: The independent contributions of diabetic neuropathy and vasculopathy in foot ulceration. How great are the risks? Diabetes Care 1995; 18:216–219.

146. Frykberg, RG: The team approach in diabetic foot management. Adv Wound Care 1998; 11:71–77.

147. Murray, HJ, et al: The association between callus formation, high pressures and neuropathy in diabetic foot ulceration. Diabet Med 1996; 13:979–982.

148. Abbott, CA, et al: Multicenter study of the incidence of and predictive risk factors for diabetic neuropathic foot ulceration. Diabetes Care 1998; 21:1071–1075.

149. Bennett, PJ, Stocks, AE, Whittam, DJ: Analysis of risk factors for neuropathic foot ulceration in diabetes mellitus. J Am Podiatr Med Assoc 1996; 86:112–116.

150. Young, MJ, et al: The prediction of diabetic neuropathic foot ulceration using vibration perception thresholds. A prospective study. Diabetes Care 1994; 17:557–560.

151. Abbott, CA, et al: The North-West Diabetes Foot Care Study: Incidence of, and risk factors for, new diabetic foot ulceration in a community-based patient cohort. Diabet Med 2002; 19:377–384.

152. Brown, G: Wound documentation: managing risk. Adv Skin Wound Care 2006; 19:155–165; quiz 165–167.

153. Fleck, CA: Identifying infection in chronic wounds. Adv Skin Wound Care 2006; 19:20–21.

154. Bates-Jensen, BM: Management of exudate and infection. In: Wound Care. Gaithersburg, MD, 1998, p 159.

155. Ferrell, BA, Artinian, BM, Sessing, D: The Sessing scale for assessment of pressure ulcer healing. J Am Geriatr Soc 1995; 43:37–40.

156. Ferrell, BA: The Sessing Scale for measurement of pressure ulcer healing. Adv Wound Care 1997; 10:78–80.

157. Woodbury, MG, et al: Pressure ulcer assessment instruments: A critical appraisal. Ostomy Wound Manage 1999; 45:42–45, 48–50, 53–55.

158. Bates-Jensen, BM, McNees, P: Toward an intelligent wound assessment system. Ostomy Wound Manage 1995; 41(suppl):80S–86S; discussion 87S.

159. Bates-Jensen, BM, Vredevoe, DL, Brecht, ML: Validity and reliability of the Pressure Sore Status Tool. Decubitus 1992; 5:20–28.

160. de Laat, EH, Scholte op Reimer, WJ, van Achterberg, T: Pressure ulcers: Diagnostics and interventions aimed at wound-related complaints: a review of the literature. J Clin Nurs 2005; 14:464–472.

161. Mullins, M, Thomason, SS, Legro, M: Monitoring pressure ulcer healing in persons with disabilities. Rehabil Nurs 2005; 30:92–99.

162. Gardner, SE, et al: A prospective study of the pressure ulcer scale for healing (PUSH). J Gerontol A Biol Sci Med Sci 2005; 60:93–97.

163. Berlowitz, DR, et al: The PUSH tool: A survey to determine its perceived usefulness. Adv Skin Wound Care 2005; 18:480–483.

164. Stotts, NA, et al: An instrument to measure healing in pressure ulcers: Development and validation of the pressure ulcer scale for healing (PUSH). J Gerontol A Biol Sci Med Sci 2001; 56:M795–M799.

165. Krasner, D: Wound Healing Scale, version 1.0: A proposal. Adv Wound Care 1997; 10:82–85.

166. Sussman, C, Swanson, G: Utility of the Sussman Wound Healing Tool in predicting wound healing outcomes in physical therapy. Adv Wound Care 1997; 10:74–77.

167. Orsted, H, et al: Best practice recommendations for the prevention, diagnosis and treatment of diabetic foot ulcers: Update 2006. Wound Care Canada 2006; 4:57.

168. Burrows, C, et al: Best recommendations for the prevention and treatment of venous leg ulcers: Update 2006. Wound Care Canada 2006; 4:

169. Margolis, DJ, et al: Risk factors for delayed healing of neuropathic diabetic foot ulcers: A pooled analysis. Arch Dermatol 2000; 136:1531–1535.

170. Margolis, DJ, et al: Diabetic neuropathic foot ulcers: The association of wound size, wound duration, and wound grade on healing. Diabetes Care 2002; 25:1835–1839.

171. Margolis, DJ, et al: Diabetic neuropathic foot ulcers: Predicting which ones will not heal. Am J Med 2003; 115:627–631.

172. Valdes, AM, Angderson, C, Giner, JJ: A multidisciplinary, therapy-based, team approach for efficient and effective wound healing: A retrospective study. Ostomy Wound Manage 1999; 45:30–36.

173. Narayanan, S, et al: Comparison of pressure ulcer treatments in long-term care facilities: Clinical outcomes and impact on cost. J Wound Ostomy Continence Nurs 2005; 32:163–170.

174. Bolton, L, et al: Wound-healing outcomes using standardized assessment and care in clinical practice. J Wound Ostomy Continence Nurs 2004; 31:65–71.

175. van Rijswijk, L, Polansky, M: Predictors of time to healing deep pressure ulcers. Ostomy Wound Manage 1994; 40:40–2, 44, 46–48.

176. Skene, AI, et al: Venous leg ulcers: a prognostic index to predict time to healing. BMJ 1992; 305:1119–1121.

177. Meaume, S, Couilliet, D, Vin, F: Prognostic factors for venous ulcer healing in a non-selected population of ambulatory patients. J Wound Care 2005; 14:31–34.

178. Phillips, TJ, et al: Prognostic indicators in venous ulcers. J Am Acad Dermatol 2000; 43:627–630.

179. Lavery, LA, et al: Home monitoring of foot skin temperatures to prevent ulceration. Diabetes Care 2004; 27:2642–2647.

180. van Rijswijk, L: Full-thickness pressure ulcers: patient and wound healing characteristics. Decubitus 1993; 6:16–21.

chapter 7

Assessing the Circulatory and Neurological Systems

Joseph McCulloch, PhD, PT, CWS, FACCWS, FAPTA

Just as surface area measurement can provide information on the rate of wound healing, observation and examination of the periwound skin may provide the clinician with information about circulatory and neurological status. For example, loss of hair over the toes or leg may suggest inadequate perfusion. Similarly, a diminished perception of light touch over the bottom of the foot could indicate that an individual is at risk of developing a plantar ulcer.

This chapter will address various components of the vascular and neurological examinations that may be useful adjuncts in evaluating individuals with ulcerations of the lower extremities. Key aspects of the neurovascular examination such as arterial perfusion, venous patency, valvular competence, and sensory testing will be discussed

Arterial Perfusion

It has been estimated that greater than 12 million people in the United States are affected by peripheral arterial disease (PAD), and more than half of these individuals present asymptomatically or with atypical findings.[1,2] Although PAD is discussed in greater detail in Chapter 17, we will look here at a variety of available tests that can provide information about the severity of arterial compromise. Many of these tests are sophisticated and invasive, and others are simple to perform, yet provide valuable clinical information.

The vascular examination should begin with a visual inspection of the extremity, with particular attention being paid to trophic changes. These include the skin taking on a dry, shiny, and hairless appearance. In addition, fissuring may be noted, particularly on the plantar aspect of the feet. Nails also tend to become dystrophic and brittle.

Pulses

Palpation of extremity pulses is likely one of the simplest, but in some cases the least definitive, methods of assessing peripheral blood flow. Despite this fact, no extremity examination is complete without a peripheral pulse palpation. Not only is the quality of the pulse important, but a comparison between sides can help detect problems that might otherwise go unnoticed.

The lower extremity arteries that should be tested are the iliac, femoral, popliteal, dorsalis pedis, and posterior tibial arteries. It is of note that the popliteal pulse is often more difficult to palpate due to its deeper location behind the knee. Palpation of the popliteal artery is more easily performed with the knee slightly flexed. In addition to noting the presence or absence of a pulse, the quality of the pulse can also be graded as follows:

0 = absence
1+ = pulse barely perceptible
2+ = diminished pulse
3+ = normal pulse
4+ = stronger than normal pulse; possible aneurysm.

It is quite common to find 3+ and 4+ pulses in the distal arteries in individuals with Charcot neuropathy, which is seen in more advanced forms of diabetes. This represents a loss of vasomotor control that results in the artery remaining in a dilated state.

▶ **PEARL 7•1** In Charcot arthropathy it is quite common to find that the patient has a bounding pedal pulse despite signs of advanced sensory neuropathy.

Rubor of Dependency

The rubor of dependency test evaluates the presence of lower extremity ischemia.[3] The patient is evaluated while lying supine. The examiner notes the color of the plantar aspect of the foot before testing. The extremity is then passively elevated to an angle of 45 degrees and held there for about 60 seconds. In the presence of arterial insufficiency, the foot will begin to blanch. The foot is then returned to a dependent position. In normal situations, foot color should return to pink within 15 seconds. In individuals with arterial disease, the color may take greater than 30 seconds to return, and the color will be a dark red (rubor). (See Fig. 7.1) This is a positive test for rubor of dependency.

Venous Filling Time

The venous filling time test provides another means to assess the arterial system, much like the test for rubor of dependency. Instead of examining the plantar aspect of the foot for color

change, the examiner looks at the dorsal veins of the foot. The patient is evaluated again by lying supine and having the leg passively elevated. As this is done, leg veins empty as they are raised above the level of the heart. The leg is then returned to a dependent position over the edge of the bed, and the examiner times how long it takes for the foot veins to distend. (Fig. 7.2) Again, this takes about 15 seconds in a normal state and greater than 30 seconds in the presence of arterial compromise. One caveat associated with this test is that the patient must have a normally functioning venous system. If venous valves are incompetent, blood will flow in a retrograde fashion with dependency, thus leading the examiner to think that arterial flow is normal in situations where this might not be the case.

▶ **PEARL 7•2** In the presence of incompetent venous valves, it is not possible to make an accurate assessment of arterial inflow status when performing a venous filling time test.

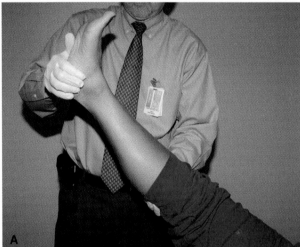

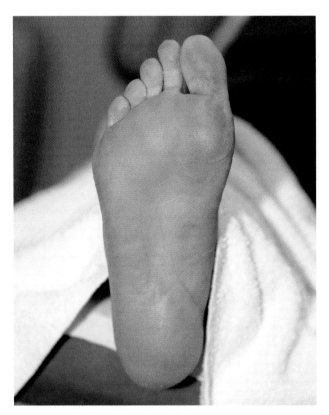

Figure 7•1 *Rubor of dependency. The sole of the right foot displays the bright red appearance that would result secondary to ischemia when performing a positive test for rubor of dependency in an individual with arterial disease.*

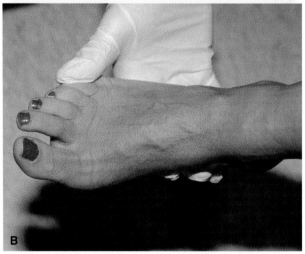

Figure 7•2 *Venous filling time test to assess arterial flow. (A) Leg elevated above the level of the heart to drain venous blood. (B) Extremity placed in a dependent position and the time to vein refilling is noted.*

Capillary Refill Test

The capillary refill test provides additional information related to arterial small vessel patency. The test is performed by applying light pressure over each of the digits of the lower extremity for 2 to 3 seconds. As the pressure is released, toe capillaries should refill quickly, causing the toes to flush with color. If perfusion is compromised, the digits will remain blanched for greater than 3 seconds.

Claudication Onset Time

One of the hallmarks of lower extremity arterial occlusive disease is ambulatory ischemic pain of the calf, termed intermittent claudication.[4] This painful phenomenon is produced by muscle cramping secondary to demand for blood and oxygen during activity. The cramping invariably stops ambulation and requires the patient to rest until the pain subsides, at which time the individual can resume activity until pain returns. Studies have reported improved ambulatory endurance in persons with intermittent claudication who have participated in a progressive ambulation program.[5,6]

Claudication onset time is used to objectify these symptoms and judge a participant's progress. The test is performed by having the patient walk on a treadmill at 1 mile per hour on level grade until claudication stops the test. The elapsed time is recorded and used as a gauge for a progressive walking program.

The American College of Sports Medicine also provides a scale to permit patients to subjectively grade claudication[7]:

Grade I: Pain, discomfort, cramping, or weakness with minimal exercise.
Grade II: Moderate pain, discomfort, cramping, or weakness with exercise.
Grade III: Severe or intense pain, discomfort, cramping, or weakness with exercise.
Grade IV: Excruciating or unbearable pain, discomfort, cramping, or weakness with exercise.

Ankle-Brachial Index

The ankle-brachial index (ABI) is a value obtained by dividing the greatest ankle systolic pressure by the greatest brachial systolic pressure.[8] The value obtained is often used to make clinical decisions regarding therapy and the possible need for referral to a vascular specialist. Table 7.1 provides commonly used interpretation of the various symptoms associated with specific ABI values. A Doppler ultrasound is used to obtain the systolic pressures of the brachial and posterior tibial or dorsalis pedis arteries in order to calculate the ABI. Typically, a Doppler ultrasound with a 5-MHz probe is used when assessing deeper vessels or when edema is present. An 8-MHz probe is useful for assessing more superficial vessels.

The test is performed by first placing a pressure cuff around the upper arm. A hydrogel coupling medium is then placed over the brachial vein in the antecubital fossa. The probe is angled at 45 degrees upstream so that the ultrasound beam will be directed head-on into the outflowing red blood cells in the vessel. Once an arterial signal is detected, the pressure cuff is inflated to obliterate flow in the vessel. The cuff is then slowly deflated and a notation made of the pressure at which the flow returns. This represents systolic pressure. The same process is then repeated in the lower extremity with the patient placed supine and a cuff placed around the ankle. Coupling medium is applied, and the ultrasonic probe is again placed at a 45-degree angle upstream over the dorsalis pedis or posterior tibial arteries. (Fig. 7.3) Once arterial flow is detected, the cuff is inflated in the same manner as performed on the upper extremity. After flow ceases, the cuff is slowly deflated, and the systolic pressure of the artery is recorded when the first sound is heard. The lower extremity systolic pressure is then divided by the upper extremity systolic pressure to obtain the ankle-brachial index.

The audible signal obtained with a Doppler ultrasound unit is produced by the Doppler effect, which occurs when the beam is reflected off the passing red blood cells.[11] This creates a shift in the frequency of the sound wave, which in turn is converted by the ultrasound device to an audible signal.

The accuracy of a Doppler examination can be affected by many factors, including poor cardiac output, calcification of the arteries, obesity, and edema. Additionally, patients with calcified arteries, as often seen in advanced stages of diabetes, may frequently have excessively high systolic pressure at the ankle.[12] This is due to the calcified vessels being uncompressible. In

Table 7•1 Ankle Brachial Index (ABI) Interpretation[9,10]	
ABI	**Clinical Significance**
1.2	Individuals with long-standing diabetes mellitus may have an ABI of this magnitude, indicating noncompressible, calcified large lower extremity arteries (ie, posterior tibial and/or popliteal arteries). In this case, an ABI provides no useful information.
1.0	Normal arterial blood flow. Compression therapy not contraindicated.
0.8–1.0	Mild arterial occlusive disease. May have no symptoms. Compression therapy with monitoring and caution.
0.5–0.8	Moderate arterial occlusive disease. Vascular specialist referral needed.
Below 0.5	Severe arterial occlusive disease. Vascular specialist referral needed. Compression therapy absolutely contraindicated. No débridement because of high risk for necrosis and infection.

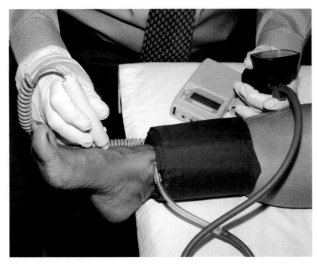

Figure 7•3 *Doppler ultrasound probe being used to assess ankle systolic pressure of the dorsalis pedis artery.*

such cases, the examiner could inaccurately report flow in the extremity as being normal. For this reason, an ABI greater than 1.2 should be regarded with suspicion, and further testing, such as digital pressures, should be performed. Toe systolic pressures can normally range from 60% to over 90% of the brachial systolic pressure. Toe pressures of less than 45 mm Hg may indicate that perfusion is inadequate to support wound healing.[13]

▶ **PEARL 7•3** A Doppler index greater than 1.2 is indicative of vessel calcification that prevents the artery from being effectively compressed.

Segmental Pressures

In addition to the standard examination for determining an ABI, it is often valuable to obtain segmental systolic pressures. Segmental pressures are typically assessed at the ankle, just below the knee, the low thigh, and the high thigh. Box 7.1 lists

the steps for performing the segmental exam. Indices can be computed at each level in the same manner as discussed regarding the ABI examination. A drop in the index value from one level to the next helps the clinician locate areas of occlusive involvement.

Segmental exams also permit the mapping of pulse waveforms. The damping of a waveform is indicative of arterial occlusive disease. Figure 7.4 provides an example of Doppler ultrasonic waveforms in a normal and abnormal state.[15]

Pulse Volume Recordings

Pulse volume recordings (PVR) are another assessment technique useful in evaluating arterial disease. PVR is similar to the Doppler waveform analysis, but pulsatile flow is detected through pressure cuffs placed around the extremity that measure changes in pressure during the cardiac cycle.[15] (Fig. 7.5) Tests are typically performed by injecting a standard volume of air into the pneumatic cuffs. The volume of air injected is enough to occlude venous, but not arterial, flow. The pulsatile arterial flow is then detected by the cuff and the signal transduced into a pressure contour waveform. In a normal test, the PVR produces a standard arterial waveform consisting of a systolic upstroke with a sharp peak, followed by a downstroke with a prominent dicrotic notch. Blunting of these signals is indicative of arterial disease.[14]

Transcutaneous Partial Pressure of Oxygen

Transcutaneous partial pressure of oxygen ($TcPo_2$) measurements are also useful in assessing arterial circulation. The test is performed by attaching an oxygen-sensitive probe over various points on the skin. The probe is secured with an adhesive ring that provides an airtight seal. The probe also contains a heating element that warms the skin to between 41° and 44°C. Heating causes cutaneous capillaries to dilate, thereby ensuring proper perfusion.

When toe ulcers are present, the probe is typically placed on the dorsum of the foot, proximal to the toes. Table 7.2 describes the significance of the $TcPo_2$ findings and how wound healing may be affected.

▶ **Box 7•1** | **Segmental Pressures Procedure: Doppler Ultrasound[10,14]**

1. Place the patient in a supine position; lower extremity with knee extended and hip externally rotated.
2. Obtain brachial systolic pressure using a blood pressure cuff and Doppler probe over the brachial artery at a 45- to 60-degree angle. Record highest brachial pressure.
3. Secure a blood pressure cuff above the ankle. For segmental pressures, cuffs will also need to be placed below knee, at midthigh, and higher on the thigh. Cuffs need to be about 20% larger in diameter than the limb for accuracy of measurement.
4. Place the Doppler probe over the vessel and hold it at a 45- to 60-degree angle. Record dorsalis pedis or posterior tibial artery pressure.
5. Inflate cuff at ankle to 20 to 30 mm Hg above last audible Doppler signal. Release pressure and monitor for first audible Doppler signal. Record ankle systolic pressure.
6. Repeat three times to ensure accuracy, and use highest value for ankle pressure. (Allow 1 minute between measurements with cuff deflated for artery to recover from pressure.)
7. Follow the same procedure for arteries above the ankle.
8. Determine the ankle-brachial index (ABI). ABI is the highest ankle pressure divided by the highest brachial pressure.

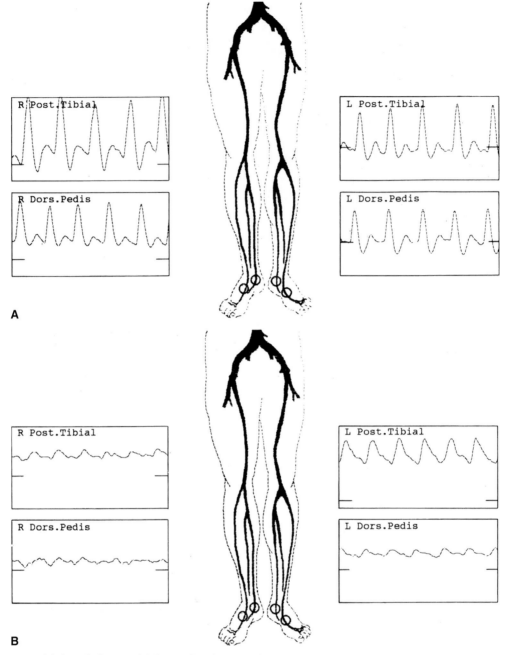

Figure 7•4 *Normal (A) and abnormal (B) Doppler ultrasound waveforms. (From Zink, M, Rousseau, P, Holloway, GA, et al: Lower extremity ulcers. In: Bryant, RA (ed): Acute and Chronic Wounds. St. Louis, Mosby, 1992, pp 176–177; used with permission.)*

Table 7•2 Transcutaneous Partial Pressure of Oxygen (TcPo$_2$)[15-17]	
TcPo$_2$	**Clinical Significance**
Less than 20 mm Hg	Impaired blood flow. Expect little to no healing. Do not débride foot ulcers if TcPo$_2$ less than 30 mm Hg proximal to toes. Vascular consult needed: vascular reconstruction or amputation very possible.
Above 30 mm Hg	Adequate or acceptable blood flow; potential to heal. Wounds managed in typical fashion including débridement. Minor amputations possible.
Above 40 mm Hg	Normal blood flow.

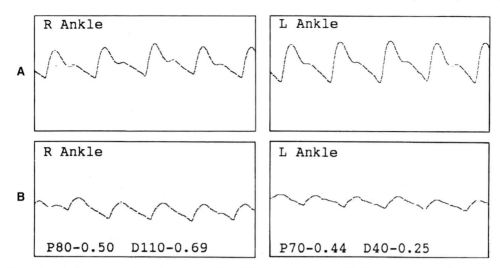

Figure 7•5 *Normal and abnormal pulse volume recording. (A) Normal tracing. (B) Abnormal tracing from arterial occlusive disease. (From Zink, M, Rousseau, P, Holloway, GA, et al: Lower extremity ulcers. In: Bryant, RA (ed): Acute and Chronic Wounds. St. Louis, Mosby, 1992, pp 176–177; used with permission.)*

Skin Perfusion Pressure

While prediction of wound healing outcomes by measurement of $TcPo_2$ has been used for years, skin perfusion pressure (SPP) has gained more recent popularity. Using laser Doppler flowmetry, SPP provides another noninvasive means of measuring microcirculatory flow. SPP is particularly good as an assessor of digital limb ischemia for patients whose ABIs cannot be accurately measured due to arterial calcification.[18] In a study by Sample et al, SPP was found to predict healing with 92% accuracy compared to 65% for $TcPo_2$ ($P<0.1$).[19]

Invasive Techniques

A variety of invasive techniques exist for assessing arterial, venous, and lymphatic patency. These tests often involve the injection of dyes or radioactive isotopes and the study the vessels radiographically. Included in this category are such tests as arteriography, venography, and lymphangiography. Several of these studies are presented in detail in Chapter 9.

Venous Patency and Valvular Competence

Prior to 1994, the field of chronic venous disorders lacked a way in which to precisely describe findings in venous disease. It was at this time that the CEAP classification was adopted worldwide to provide a means for communicating effectively between practitioners. The CEAP classification system, which stands for clinical, etiology, anatomy, and pathophysiology, was developed by an international ad hoc committee of the American Venous Forum and endorsed by the Society for Vascular Surgery. At the time of development, it was emphasized that the descriptive system should not be considered static, but rather would be refined as science and technology changed. Table 7.3 provides the classification system that existed as of 2004.[20]

As implied by the CEAP classification, much can be learned by a visual assessment of the venous system, with attention being paid to anatomy, etiology, and underlying pathophysiology. In a similar fashion, several simple physical assessment procedures can provide a wealth of information about the functional status of the system. Several such tests are presented here.

Percussion Test

The percussion test is a palpation examination that evaluates the functional status of the valves in the superficial venous system. When venous valves are working properly, they function much like baffles in a water bed that serve to dampen oscillatory signals. With the patient in the standing position, note that tapping of the saphenous vein with the fingers of one hand while simultaneously palpating a segment 15 to 20 cm away with fingers of the other hand should not produce any palpable signal. If, on the other hand, a pulsatile wave is palpated, this indicates that valvular incompetence exists between the two points and therefore permits the oscillation to be transmitted.

Trendelenburg Test

The Trendelenburg test measures the time required to refill the distal superficial veins on the dorsum of the foot and provides information about the competence of the valves in the superficial, perforator, and deep veins. The test is conducted with the patient supine and the patient's leg being passively raised. After about 60 seconds, a tourniquet is applied around the proximal thigh and the patient is assisted to the standing position. The examiner quickly notes any filling that might occur in the veins on the dorsum of the foot. Immediate filling is indicative of incompetence in the perforator system. The tourniquet is then released. If further distention of the dorsal foot veins occurs, or the veins distend for the first time, incompetence at the saphenofemoral junction is implicated. This test must be performed rather quickly because allowing too much time to elapse will allow the dorsal foot veins to fill

Table 7•3	Revised CEAP Classification 2004[20]

C – Clinical classification

C0 – No visible or palpable signs of venous disease

C1 – Telangiectases or reticular veins

C2 – Varicose veins

C3 – Edema

C4a – Pigmentation or eczema

C4b – Lipodermatosclerosis or atrophie blanche

C5 – Healed venous ulcer

C6 – Active venous ulcer

S – Symptomatic, including ache, pain, tightness, skin irritation, heaviness, muscle cramps, and other complaints attributable to venous dysfunction

A – Asymptomatic

Etiological Classification

Ec – Congenital

Ep – Primary

Es – Secondary (postthrombotic)

En – No venous cause identified

Anatomical Classification

As – Superficial veins

Ap – Perforator veins

Ad – Deep veins

An – No venous location identified

Pathophysiological Classification

Basic CEAP –

Pr – Reflux
Po – Obstruction
Pr,o – Reflux and obstruction
Pn – No venous pathophysiology identifiable

Advanced CEAP – In addition to the basic CEAP, 18 different named venous segments can be added to further clarify the location of the venous pathology.

on their own through the normal arterial pathway tested earlier in the venous filling time assessment.

Homan's Sign and Cuff Tests

Patients presenting with calf pain and unilateral edema are always suspect for a deep vein thrombosis (DVT). For years, a standard clinical examination technique for a DVT has been testing for Homan's sign, squeezing the calf to see if pain was elicited. The subjective nature of this test made it difficult to discriminate between a DVT and other musculoskeletal pathology. One attempt to provide a bit of objectivity to this test is to perform a cuff test. In a cuff test, a standard sphygmomanometer cuff is placed around the calf and carefully inflated. If calf pain is experienced, the cuff is rapidly deflated and the patient sent for more definitive testing. If cuff pressures can be tolerated up to 40 mm Hg, the suspicion of a DVT is lessened, but not absolutely ruled out. The test instead provides a means of semiquantitatively documenting the subjective symptoms since patients with a DVT would typically experience pain well before 40 mm Hg pressure is applied.

Doppler Assessment

When a patient presents with signs and symptoms of venous insufficiency, an ABI should also be performed to determine whether there is arterial insufficiency present because a significant number of patients have coexisting disease.[21] When an ABI of 0.8 is noted, many clinicians caution against any form of compression therapy. Of course, this is a clinical judgment call as compression has been used without difficulty in many patients with an ABI of 0.8.[22,23] Caution is certainly advised before considering any type of long stretch bandaging or aggressive vasopneumatic compression with ABIs below this level. Compression therapy for venous disease is discussed in greater detail in Chapter 30.

In addition to using the Doppler ultrasound to determine the ABI, the device can also be used to assess venous valvular competency and/or venous obstruction.[24] Frequency choices for Doppler evaluation of the veins include 8 MHz for the superficial veins and 5 MHz for the deeper veins. To assess valvular competency, the Doppler probe is placed over a vein and a venous signal obtained. The venous signal is significantly different from the brisk, staccato arterial signal and is described as a waxing and waning sound of wind. Once this signal is detected, the examiner manually compresses the vein 10 to 15 cm proximally. If valves between the Doppler probe and the site of compression are incompetent, the Doppler will produce a sound of increased frequency as the venous blood rushes in a retrograde fashion. If, on the other hand, the valves are competent and cusp when the blood tries to flow retrograde, there should be a sudden cessation in the auditory signal, which will then resume once the compression is released. Likewise, the Doppler probe can be used to evaluate occlusive venous disease by compressing the distal aspect of the vein in question while listening proximally. If the venous pathway is patent, there should be a sudden augmentation of the normal venous signal.

▶ **PEARL 7•4** Hearing an enhanced flow signal while listening with a Doppler probe placed distally on a vein and compressing the vein more proximally is indicative of reflux secondary to valvular incompetence.

Air Plethysmography

Air plethysmography (APG) is a test that provides quantitative information of ambulatory venous hypertension and is very useful in documenting the level of disease in patients who are prone to develop, or already have developed, venous ulceration.[25,26] APG uses a recorder system and a pressure cuff containing a pressure transducer and microprocessor to quantify volume changes in the lower extremity. With the patient supine, a specialized cuff is positioned along the calf and inflated to a pressure sufficient to prevent the cuff from slipping when the patient is upright. The first stage of the test involves an assessment of arterial inflow. A sphygmomanometer cuff is placed around the proximal thigh and inflated to a pressure of about 80 mm Hg. This pressure is substantial enough to occlude venous return while still permitting arterial inflow. The deep veins and venous sinusoids of the calf subsequently start to fill with blood since venous outflow is impeded. The recorder monitors the leg volume, and the speed of arterial inflow is noted. Once the blood volume plateaus, the proximal cuff is released. In a normal venous system, volume reduction of approximately 40% will occur in 1 second. If less than a 40% volume reduction is noted in the first second, venous patency may be compromised. The total time for the limb volume to return to baseline may also be determined and compared bilaterally. A few minutes are allowed before performing the second phase of the test because the patient's lower extremity circulation must be permitted to return to normal. In the second portion of the test, venous filling time may be determined by applying the cuff to the calf and immediately having the patient stand. The speed with which the calf refills with blood is noted. A rate of 2 mL/sec is a normal filling rate. A faster rate may signify incompetent valves that are permitting the venous blood to flow retrograde. Next, a calf ejection fraction is measured by having the patient rise up onto the toes. A normal calf ejection volume is a 60% reduction in calf volume. Residual volume is computed by measuring the calf volume after the patient does 10 toe rises. Ambulatory venous pressure corresponds with residual volume. An advantage of this relatively easy clinical test is that it can be completed before and after compression bandage garments are donned and doffed to analyze their effectiveness.

Photoplethysmography

Photoplethysmography provides another means of assessing the competence of venous valves by measuring venous refill time. During this procedure, the patient performs voluntary ankle pumps to remove venous blood from the calf. Next, the clinician uses infrared light to detect venous blood volume during vein refilling after the ankle pumps. Normally, veins take more than 24 seconds to refill. Veins with incompetent valves refill more quickly because of reflux.[27]

A variety of other tests to evaluate the venous system include venous Doppler ultrasonography, an imaging method that may be used to visualize veins for diagnosing incompetent valves, venous reflux, or DVT; impedance plethysmography, a method that uses electrical impedance to diagnose obstruction and changes in venous blood flow; duplex scanning with color flow imaging; radionuclide venography; and radiographs of veins. Some of these procedures are discussed in more detail in Chapter 9.

Assessing the Sensory System

Disordered sensation is one of the more common findings noted by clinicians who treat individuals with lower extremity wound. This is particularly evident when evaluating individuals with diabetes. The peripheral neuropathy associated with diabetes is insidious and chronic and, if left unchecked, leads to leg ulceration and amputation.[28] Early detection of sensory paresthesias is critical if clinicians are to intervene and prescribe appropriate footwear to protect against injury. While a variety of sophisticated sensory tests, such as nerve conduction studies, can provide valuable information about the status of the peripheral nervous system, they are not readily available to all clinicians and are outside of the scope of this chapter. We instead present a collection of reliable and valid sensory tests that can easily be performed by most practitioners.

The senses of touch, pressure, temperature, pain, vibration, and proprioception all provide the awareness required to prevent tissue injury. If a sensory deficit is suspected, the clinician must perform an appropriate evaluation to determine the extent of involvement.

Light Touch

Light touch can be assessed with a cotton ball or soft brush. Patients are asked to close their eyes or have their view of the testing area obstructed. They are then lightly touched over various areas of the extremity and asked to say "yes" or "now" when they perceive the touch. The examination should be performed slowly enough to allow the individual to perceive and respond to the stimulus, but touch should not be sustained and firm, as this would test perception of pressure instead of light touch.

Pinprick

Pain perception can be tested by pressing the sharp end of a pin or paper clip into the skin and asking the patient to both acknowledge perception of the stimulus and compare it to that felt on the opposite side. Doing such a comparison may aid the clinician in detecting early changes in an individual extremity. Both pinprick and light touch examinations carry with them the inherent problem of intertester variability in how the test is performed. Savic and colleagues noted, however, a very strong correlation between experienced clinicians on pinprick and light touch examinations and Pearson correlation coefficients and intraclass correlation coefficients exceeding 0.96, P <0.01.[29]

Position Sense

To assess position sense (proprioception), the clinician can passively move any joint; however, distal joints such as the toes, ankles, fingers, or wrists are often used. The clinician should use the least amount of physical contact to avoid providing other tactile cues that could bias the results and should ask the patient to close his or her eyes while being tested. For example, the clinician holds the medial and lateral sides of the great toe, slightly moves the joint and then holds it still, and prompts the subject to say "up" or "down." Testing for movement sense or kinesthesia is very similar to that of position sense. The test moves the joint through initial, mid-, or terminal range of motion. The patient must say "up" or "down" while the joint is moving. Any of the sensation-testing methods just described may reveal that the patient has intact, impaired, or absent sensation.

Two-Point Discrimination

Two-point discrimination testing is not commonly employed in evaluating lower extremity sensibility, but is instead frequently used in hand injuries. Both static and moving techniques are employed. In the static assessment, a tool that has prongs spaced at a fixed distance from 2 to 15 mm is employed. Only skin that has light-touch sensation intact should be tested. Starting with the prongs separated 10 to 15 mm, the examiner touches the area with a constant light force that is not great enough to blanch the skin. Either one or two prongs is used, and the patient is asked to state whether they feel one or two points of contact. Varying the number of prongs touching the individual helps to increase reliability of the patient's answers.[30]

Moving two-point discrimination is measured in a similar manner. The only difference is that instead of the prongs being placed on the skin in a stationary fashion, they are moved a short distance. Dellon and colleagues tested both static and moving discrimination in 20 nerve-injured patients.[31] They noted that interobserver variability was within 1 mm, or less, for moving two-point discrimination in 93.3% of the measurements and for 86.8% of the measurements in static discrimination.

Vibratory Testing

Vibratory testing is typically performed with a 128-Hz tuning fork. The fork is struck and the stem placed over the distal interphalangeal joint of the great toe. The patient is asked if he or she can feel the stimulus, and if so, to tell you when it can no longer be felt. The examiner should then see if he/she can still perceive the vibration. Dimitrakoudis and Bril note that perception is different between the dorsal and ventral aspects of the great toe.[32] Lower thresholds to stimulation are noted on the ventral surface, but fewer false-negative results are seen on the dorsal surface. The choice of testing site would therefore depend on whether higher sensitivity with more false positives or lower sensitivity with more false negatives is desired.

Recent studies by Juma and Mandal found a strong correlation between results obtained with a 128-Hz tuning fork and a 512-Hz tuning fork.[33] In light of these findings, they recommend using the 512-Hz fork as it is smaller and easier to carry.

In addition to the standard qualitative vibratory examination, quantitative techniques also exist. Pestronk and colleagues found strong correlations between quantitative measurements compared with sensory nerve action potentials in the sural nerve.[34] These findings were more strongly correlated than those of qualitative techniques. The tests were performed using a Rydel-Seiffer tuning fork (U.S. Neurologicals, Kirkland, WA). The device consists of a tuning fork with weighted ends that are scaled and convert the tuning from 128 to 64 Hz. As the intensity begins to diminish, two triangles on the fork move closer together, and their point of intersection moves upward. When the patient can no longer detect the vibration, the number adjacent to the intersected triangles is recorded.

Protective Sensation

In the presence of neuropathy, a single test may be used to see if patients have lost their protective sensation. Semmes-Weinstein monofilaments are used to assess for the presence or absence of protective sensation on the plantar aspect of the foot.[35-38] Monofilaments are graded on a scale from 1.65 to 6.65 for the

force required to slightly bow the filament when pressed against the plantar surface of the foot. The higher the monofilament number, the more force required to bow the monofilament.

The plantar surface of the foot is typically tested with a 5.07 monofilament. This monofilament requires that a force of 10 g be applied in order for the monofilament to bow. To perform the test, the clinician places the tip of the monofilament on the plantar surface of the patient's foot. Pressure is applied until the monofilament bows, and then the pressure is released. (See Fig. 7.6) With eyes closed, the patient indicates when and where the pressure is perceived. Patients who are not trying to feign illness generally wish to please their examiners. For this reason, they will often say they feel a stimulus when they actually do not. It is useful to ask the patient when and where they feel each stimulus while taking precautions to shield the test from their view.

The areas to be tested include those most vulnerable to ulceration. These include the first and fifth metatarsal heads and the great toe. A patient who cannot sense a 5.07 monofilament (10 g pressure) over the plantar bony prominences or the great toe has lost protective sensation and will be at risk for ulcer development. The repeated trauma of weight-bearing on the insensate foot leads to plantar soft tissue damage.

> ▶ **PEARL 7•5** Failure to detect 10 g of pressure on the plantar aspect of the foot in a patient with insensitivity places that person at high risk for developing a plantar ulceration.

Smieja and colleagues compared the reproducibility and accuracy of conventional sensory testing techniques such as ankle reflexes, pinprick, position sense, and vibration to monofilament testing.[39] They found that monofilament testing and ankle reflexes had the best reproducibility with moderate agreement (k statistic = 0.59). Pinprick, position, and vibration sense had fair agreement (k = 0.28–0.36). They further noted that a simplified monofilament examination that employed only four sites per foot detected 90% of patients with an abnormal complete exam. The four sites tested were the great toe and first, third,

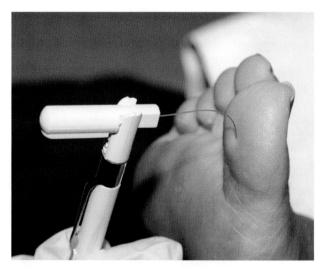

Figure 7•6 *Semmes-Weinstein test being performed to assess presence of protective sensation. Note the bowing of the filament indicating appropriate pressure has been applied.*

and fifth metatarsal heads. (See Chapter 14 for additional information on wounds that occur as a result of insensitivity.)

Summary

No wound examination, especially involving the lower extremity, is complete without an assessment of the circulatory and neurological systems. This is particularly true when dealing with individuals with neuropathic wounds secondary to diabetes. This chapter has presented an overview of various tests that are both reliable and easy to perform. Additional methods of evaluation that rely upon more sophisticated instrumentation were also discussed. This information, combined with the material presented in the Chapter 6, helps to provide a foundation on which interventions can be based. While it is not practical to incorporate all of the tests presented into a standard evaluation of a patient, it is hoped that the clinician will find many of the tests to be useful in a screening environment. When problems are detected, the patient can then be referred for more extensive evaluation.

▶ Case Study 7•1 Neuropathic Ulcer in a Patient with Type 2 Diabetes Mellitus

Case: A 73-year-old white female presents to the wound care center with a full-thickness (Shea stage III) ulceration over the lateral margin of her left great toe. (Fig. 7.7) She had experienced a similar ulcer in the same area several years previously, but it had healed with conservative care involving moist wound healing and off-weighting. The patient's history is significant in that she experienced a left cerebrovascular accident (CVA) 4 years earlier and has a residual right lower extremity hemiparesis.

Occupation/Employment: She is retired from work as a switchboard operator and spends the majority of her time playing cards with friends.

Social Information: She is single, widowed, and lives alone.

Past Medical History: History is significant for the CVA mentioned previously. In addition, the patient is noted to have type 2 diabetes, hypertension, vascular disease, hypercholesterolemia, congestive heart failure, and mild renal insufficiency.

Wound Assessment: Wound measures 1 cm² in surface area and 0.6 cm in depth. The wound base is pale in appearance. The wound does not appear to probe to bone and is classified by the University of Texas scale as a grade II-A. There is a 2-mm ring of undermining noted around the entire perimeter, and periwound callus is moderate.

Radiographic Findings: Radiographs of the left foot reveal swelling throughout the forefoot that is most pronounced in the area of the great toe. Bone quality appears normal, and joint spaces are well preserved. No periosteal elevation or acute fractures are noted. There is a mild hallux valgus present.

Laboratory Findings:

1. BUN (7–20 mg/dL) – 64 H

2. Creatinine (0.6–1.1 mg/dL) – 2.2 H

3. Glucose (80–115 mg/dL) – 126 H

4. Hemoglobin A$_{1c}$ (3.9%–6.1%) – 6.4 H

5. Hemoglobin (11.3–15.4 g/dL) – 11.0 L (improving from 8.4 four months earlier)

6. Hematocrit (34%–46%) – 32.5 L (improving from 25.0 four months earlier)

Vascular Status: Lower extremity pulses were nonpalpable but Doppler flow was detected in the dorsalis pedis and posterior tibial arteries. Ankle-brachial indices were greater than 1.3 and were deemed unusable due to vessel incompressibility. Capillary refill to the toes was delayed. Test for rubor of dependency was negative bilaterally. A 1+ pitting edema was present in both feet.

Sensory Status: Protective sensation was absent over the entire plantar foot bilaterally when tested with a 10-g Semmes-Weinstein monofilament. Sensation was intact to pinprick in the area of the wound.

Gait: Muscle weakness on the right side resulted in an unstable gait with pelvic drop to the left during stance phase on the right. Patient appears to use the left great toe a great deal for balance during stance phase on the left due to weakened swing phase on the right.

Conclusion: Patient appears to have developed a pressure ulcer of the left great toe secondary to neuropathic insensitivity and a valgus deformity of the digit. Wound healing is complicated by mild anemia, congestive heart failure with associated swelling, and renal insufficiency. In light of Doppler findings, a more definitive noninvasive vascular study is indicated. Current treatment should include neuromuscular rehabilitation of weakened muscles, evaluation for neurological splinting, and off-loading of the left great toe to promote healing. This will pose the greatest challenge due to patient's instability and inability to ambulate with many of the shoe and splint devices commercially available.

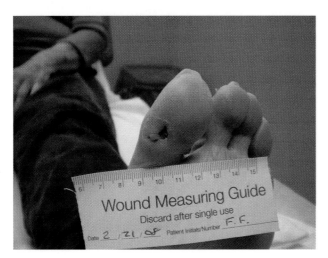

Figure 7•7 *Appearance of wound at the time of presentation to the wound care clinic.*

References

1. American Diabetes Association: Peripheral arterial disease in people with diabetes. Diabetes Care 2003; 26:3333–3341.
2. Hiatt, WR: Medical treatment of peripheral arterial disease and claudication. N Engl J Med 2001; 344:1068–1621.
3. Blume, PA, Key, JJ, Sumpio, BE: How to detect peripheral arterial disease. Podiatry Today 2004; 17:38–43.
4. White, C: Intermittent claudication. N Engl J Med 2007; 356:1241–1250.
5. Brandsma, JW, Robeer, BG, van den Heuvel, S, et al: The effect of exercise on walking distance of patients with intermittent claudication: A study of randomized clinical trials. Phys Ther 1998; 78:278–286.
6. Hiatt, WR, Regensteiner, JG, Hargarten, ME, et al: Superiority of treadmill walking exercise versus strength training for patients with peripheral arterial disease. Circulation 1994; 90:1866–1874.
7. American College of Sports Medicine: ACSM's Guidelines for Exercise Testing and Prescription, ed. 6. Baltimore, Lippincott Williams & Wilkins, 2005, p 58.
8. Wills, SJ: Calculating the ankle-brachial index. Adv Skin Wound Care 2000; 13:86.
9. Robson, MC, Cooper, DM, Aslam, R, et al: Guidelines for the treatment of venous ulcers. Wound Repair & Regen 2006; 14:649–662.
10. Patterson, GK: Vascular evaluation. In: Sussman, C, Bates-Jensen, BM (eds): Wound Care: A Collaborative Practice Manual for Health Professionals. Baltimore, Lippincott Williams & Wilkins, 2007, p 184.
11. Lawrence, JP: Physics and instrumentation of ultrasound. Crit Care Med 2007; 35:S314–S322.
12. Sheehan, P: Peripheral arterial disease in people with diabetes: Consensus statement recommends screening. Clin Diabetes 2004; 22:179–180.
13. Bonham, PA: Get the LEAD out: Noninvasive assessment for lower extremity arterial disease using ankle brachial index and toe brachial index measurements. J Wound Ostomy Continence Nurs 2006; 33:30–41.
14. Gerhard-Herman, M, Gardin, JM, Jaff, M, et al: Guidelines for noninvasive vascular laboratory testing: A report from the American Society of Echocardiography and the Society for Vascular Medicine and Biology. Vasc Med 2006; 11:183–200.
15. Zink, M, Rousseau, P, Holloway, GA: Lower extremity ulcers. In: Bryant, RA (ed): Acute and Chronic Wounds. St. Louis, Mosby, 1992, p 164.
16. Oubre, CM, et al: Retrospective study of factors affecting non-healing of wounds during hyperbaric oxygen therapy. J Wound Care 2007; 16:245–250.
17. Kalani, M, Brismar, K, Fagrell, B, et al: Transcutaneous oxygen tension and toe blood pressure as predictors for outcome of diabetic foot ulcers. Diabetes Care 1999; 22:147–151.
18. Shigematsu, K: Skin perfusion pressure. J Japanese Col Angiology 2005; 45:294–298.
19. Sample, R, Takkin, L, Anholm, J, et al: Predicting wound healing outcome: Skin perfusion pressure vs. transcutaneous pO$_2$. Wounds 2003; 15:A23–A34.
20. Eklof, B, Rutherford, RB, Bergan, JJ, et al: Revision of the CEAP classification for chronic venous disorders: Consensus statement. J Vasc Surg 2004; 40:1248–1252.
21. Kunimoto, B, Cooling, M, Gulliver, W, et al: Best practices for the prevention and treatment of venous leg ulcers. Ostomy Wound Manage 2001; 47:34–36.
22. van Bemmelen, P, Char, D, Giron, F, et al: Angiographic improvement alter rapid intermittent compression treat for small vessel obstruction. Ann Vasc Surg 2003; 17:224–228.
23. Montori, VM, Kavros, SJ, Walsh, EE, et al: Intermittent compression pump for nonhealing wounds in patients with limb ischemia. The Mayo Clinic experience (1998–2000). Int Angiol 2002; 21:360–366.
24. Marquez, RR: Wound evaluation. In: Gogia, PP (ed): Clinical Wound Management. Thorofare, NJ, Slack, 1995, p 15.
25. Akram, M, Riha, AZ, Cameron, JD, et al: Quantitative assessment of chronic venous insufficiency using duplex ultrasound and air plethysmography. J Vasc Ultrasound 2006; 30:23–30.
26. Corabian, P: An assessment of air plethysmography. Annu Meet Int Soc Technol Assess Health Care Int Soc Technol Assess Health Care Meet 1998; 14:71.
27. Patterson, GK: Vascular evaluation. In: Sussman, C, Bates-Jensen, BM (eds): Wound Care: A Collaborative Practice Manual for Health Professionals. Baltimore, Lippincott Williams & Wilkins, 2007, p 190.
28. Perkins, BA, Olaleye, D, Zinman, B, et al: Simple screening tests for peripheral neuropathy in the diabetes clinic. Diabetes Care 2001; 24:250–256.
29. Savic, G, Bergstrom, EMK, Frankel, HL, et al: Inter-rater reliability of motor and sensory examinations performed according to American Spinal Injury Association standards. Spinal Cord 2007; 45:444–451.
30. Bexter, C, Salter, M: Assessment. In: Salter, M, Cheshire, L (eds.): Hand Therapy: Principles and Practice. Oxford, Butterworth-Heinemann, 1997, p 47.
31. Dellon, AL, Mackinnon, SE, Crosby, PM, et al: Reliability of two-point discrimination measurements. J Hand Surg 1987; 12:693–696.
32. Dimitrakoudis, D, Bril, V: Comparison of sensory testing on different toe surfaces: Implications for neuropathy screening. Neurology 2002; 59:611–613.
33. Juma, A, Mandal, A: Vibration sensitivity testing with tuning fork–256 Hz or 512 Hz? Eur J Plast Surg 2007; 30:5–6.
34. Pestronk, A, Florence, J, Levine, T, et al: Sensory exam with a quantitative tuning fork: Rapid, sensitive, and predictive of SNAP amplitude. Neurology 2004; 62:461–464.
35. Mayfield, JA, Sugarman, JR: The use of the Semmes-Weinstein monofilament and other threshold tests for preventing foot ulceration and amputation in persons with diabetes. J Fam Pract 2000; 49(suppl):S17–S29.
36. Dyck, PT: Evaluation procedures to detect, characterize, and assess the severity of diabetic neuropathy. Diabetic Med 1991; 8:48–51.
37. Bell-Krotoski, JA: Light touch-deep pressure testing using Semmes-Weinstein monofilaments. In: Hunter JM, Schneider, LH, Mackin, EJ, et al (eds): Rehabilitation of the Hand, ed. 3. St. Louis, Mosby, 1984, pp 585–593.
38. Wood, WA, Wood, MA, Werter, SA, et al: Testing for loss of protective sensation in patients with foot ulceration: A cross-sectional study. J Am Podiatr Med Assoc 2005; 95:469–474.
39. Smieja, M, Hunt, DL, Edelman, D, et al: Clinical examination for the detection of protective sensation in the feet of diabetic patients. J Gen Intern Med 1999; 14:418–424.

chapter 8

Assessing and Controlling Bioburden

Dot Weir, RN, CWON, CWS

Acute wound healing has been described to occur in the overlapping cascade of events of inflammation, proliferation, and remodeling. These events are presumed to occur whether the wound is an acute surgical wound closed by primary intention or an open traumatic wound left to close by secondary intention through contraction, granulation, and epithelialization. The timing of these events will vary depending on a variety of factors including, but not limited to, the duration of wounding; the location, size, and depth of the wound; the causative factors; the presence of comorbid conditions that can delay healing; the patient's age; and certainly the presence of bacteria in numbers great enough to interfere with normal cellular events.[1]

Human skin can be considered the boundary between the human organism and the outside environment, providing an effective barrier to bacterial contamination and invasion into deeper tissues. By its very nature, the skin provides its own defense.

> **PEARL 8•1** Human skin can be considered the boundary between the human organism and the outside environment.

The dry, dead, keratinized cells on the surface prevent most microorganisms from infiltrating into deeper layers. In addition, cells from the stratum corneum are shed every day, and attached microorganisms slough off with them.[2] The normal pH range of the skin is 4 to 6.5.[3,4] The production of sebum from the sebaceous glands contributes to this low pH, making the skin a more hostile environment for microbial growth. Sebum is also high in lipids, which could serve as a nutrient to bacteria, but the fatty acid breakdown of the lipids produces toxic by-products that inhibit the growth of potentially pathogenic bacteria. Sweat, because of its low pH and high salt concentration, is also inhibitory to microorganisms.[2] Additionally, small populations of resident bacteria such as *Staphylococcus epidermidis* and skin diphtheroids help prevent colonization by more pathogenic bacteria such as *Staphylococcus aureus*[5] A breach of this boundary, or break in the skin, allows access for both pathogenic as well as normal residential skin flora to penetrate deeper tissues, which provide the warmth, moisture, decreased oxygen, and nutrients bacteria require to thrive and multiply.

The role of bacteria located in and on an open wound has been the subject of numerous citations in the literature over the past decades. Practitioners must understand the role that bacteria play in wound healing and nonhealing, appropriately assess and make clinical judgments based on the known or presumed level and host impact of any bacterial presence, and make treatment decisions based on the sum of all of this information.

Bioburden, according to the University of Rochester glossary, is the number of microorganisms with which an object is contaminated.[6] According to *Stedman's Medical Dictionary* the term *bioburden* is defined as the degree of microbial contamination or microbial load; the number of microorganisms contaminating an object.[7] By its truest definition, bioburden is a status that is assumed to be quantified relative to the object. In the often casual language of wound management and wound healing, the term bioburden is used often as a statement as to the presence of bacteria on a wound, as well as a qualitative descriptor of the bacterial status of a wound. As a result, it has also become a term used to document and consequently rationalize and support the use of various treatment alternatives, specifically dressings and devices known to impact surface wound bacteria, such as antiseptics, antimicrobial dressings, and biophysical agents such as ultrasound.

The mere presence of bacteria on the surface of an open wound is expected and frequently not an impediment for the eventual closure and ultimate healing of the wound.[1,8] The impact of these microorganisms, however, is directly related to their number and virulence, the presence of multiple types, and the host's resistance or ability to manage these organisms.

Defining and Describing Bacteria

Bacteria are microscopic, single-celled organisms that possess a prokaryotic type of cell structure, meaning their cells are noncompartmentalized, and their DNA (usually circular) can be found throughout the cytoplasm rather than within a membrane bound nucleus. They live practically everywhere.

Although some bacteria produce infectious diseases in humans (eg, cholera, syphilis, anthrax), some have been found to be beneficial. For example, bacteria in the gut aid in digestion. Other bacteria, often lactobacillus in combination with yeasts and molds, have been used for thousands of years in the preparation of fermented foods such as cheese, pickles, vinegar, wine, and yogurt.[9]

The identification and description of bacteria is a microbiological procedure using a language that is important to identify and define. On a microscopic level, there are numerous ways in which bacterial species are identified. On a practical level, there are commonalities in the language used in everyday practice that are important to understand.

Bacteria are identified and described based on their shape, the results of their Gram stain, their need or lack of need for oxygen, and the mode of growth.

Shape

While there is great variation in the shape, size, and arrangement of bacteria, they are most basically described by one of the three most common shapes: round or ball shaped, described as a coccus; cylindrical (longer than wide), described as a rod or bacillus; and a spiral-shaped cylinder, called a *spirillum* or *spirochete,* depending on the thickness and regularity of the spirals or coils. The description is broadened and further variation comes into play when there is a combination of two shapes, such as a rod that is short and plump, called a *coccobacillus,* when the bacteria are found in chains or clusters, paired together, and curved or twisted.

Gram Staining

Gram staining is a more than century-old laboratory method used in identifying and classifying bacteria as either gram-positive or gram-negative. One of the greatest advantages of this method is to provide rapid basic information for empirical management of an infection when a body fluid or biopsy is available.

This method is named for Hans Christian Gram, the Danish scientist who developed the technique in 1884 to make bacteria in specimens more visible. While it is not an infallible tool for diagnosis or identification, it is still widely used in hospital and community laboratories today and is based on a differentiation between two major cell wall types. A very basic description of the methodology is that a small sample of the bacterial culture is taken and smeared onto a slide that, when dry, is heated for a few seconds. Once cool, the smear is then flooded with the stain crystal or gentian violet, washed off, further stained with an iodine solution (Gram's iodine), and then again washed with a decolorizing agent such as alcohol or acetone. The slide is then again stained with a red dye (safranin or fuchsin) and rinsed a final time. After a final drying, the slide is examined under a microscope to see if the bacterial cell wall has retained the purple dye (gram-positive), lost the purple color (gram-negative), or retained a mix of the purple and red dyes (gram-variable). Common gram-positive bacteria include various species of the genera *Streptococcus, Staphylococcus, Enterococcus, Cornybacterium,* and *Listeria.* Common gram-negative bacteria include various species of the genera *Pseudomonas, Proteus, Escherichia, Klebsiella, Enterobacter, Serratia, Salmonella, Shigella,* and others.[10-12]

Oxygen Requirement

Bacteria are further differentiated by those that survive and grow in an oxygenated environment (aerobes), those that do not require oxygen to grow and may even die in the presence of oxygen (anaerobes), as well as those that can use oxygen but also have anaerobic methods of energy production (facultative anaerobes).

Mode of Growth

Clinicians speaking in general terms about bacterial growth in wounds, results of cultures, and bacterial targets for antibiotics and most of the topical dressings and agents are typically referring to free-floating or planktonic bacteria. Planktonic bacteria are free-living bacteria that are the populations that grow out in the laboratory flask or dish. They have been known for centuries, have surfaces that are relatively hydrophilic, and have a cell wall that is more susceptible to eradication by the host's immune system and targeted antimicrobials. Most of the knowledge of antibiotics is based on experiments done on planktonic bacteria.[13] The opposite mode of growth is the adherent, or sessile mode of growth, known as biofilm.

▶ **PEARL 8•2** Biofilms are complex communities of bacteria and other microorganisms that adhere to solid surfaces.

Biofilms are complex communities of bacteria and other microorganisms that adhere to solid surfaces. These communities are embedded in an extracellular polysaccharide matrix or glycocalyx, are associated with 65% of nosocomial infections, and are implicated in chronic infections in humans. Under the right conditions, all bacteria can grow a biofilm. They become a problem in wound healing due to several factors, including, but not limited to the following: (1) The biofilm bacteria are less susceptible to our immune defense system as well as antimicrobial agents due to the inability of phagocytic cells, antibiotics, and antimicrobial agents to penetrate the protective film. (2) Antibiotics are most effective in killing cells that are rapidly growing and dividing, so the slower growth of the bacteria within the biofilm contributes to reduced susceptibility. (3) The environment within the biofilm (pH, oxygen content) is altered, leading to the reduced activity of an antimicrobial agent. (4) The communication between the bacteria involves production of signaling molecules that can initiate a response to the environment when a critical density of bacteria (quorum) has been reached. This communication is known as *quorum sensing* and has been documented as playing a role in antibiotic resistance by promoting adaptive responses through coordination of bacterial behavior.[14-16]

In a study published by Garth et al, an analysis of the presence of biofilm found on acute and chronic wounds reported that 60% of the chronic wounds were found to contain biofilms versus only 6% of the acute wounds, providing evidence that biofilms are abundant in chronic wounds. Further research in this area is ongoing and warranted.[17]

▶ **PEARL 8•3** An analysis of the presence of biofilm found on acute and chronic wounds reported that 60% of the chronic wounds were found to contain biofilms versus only 6% of the acute wounds.

States of Bacterial Load in Chronic Wounds

There is wide agreement in the literature that all open wounds are considered to be contaminated regardless of the age of the wound. *Contamination* is defined as the presence of bacteria on wound surfaces with no replication or multiplication of the bacteria and no clinical host response.[18-20] The presence of some level of bacteria at the time of injury contributes to evoking the inflammatory response needed to begin the normal cascade of events resulting in wound repair. As time progresses, it is the presence of bacteria and the host's ability to balance the bacteria that seems to define the impact on wound healing.

▶ **PEARL 8•4** There is wide agreement in the literature that all open wounds are considered to be contaminated, regardless of the age of the wound.

The activity of replication on the wound surface begins the change in the dynamics between the host and the bacterial organisms. The environment on the wound surface offers an ideal milieu, providing warmth, moisture, oxygen, and nutrients for bacterial growth, promoting replication, *colonization*, and attachment of surface bacteria, while still not inciting a significant host response.

The point at which the bacteria multiplying on the surface begin to interfere with wound healing has been termed *critical colonization*, a term that was coined by Davis in 1996, yet to this day continues to be scrutinized.[21]

▶ **PEARL 8•5** The point at which the bacteria multiplying on the surface begin to interfere with wound healing has been termed *critical colonization*.

The principle that wounds are either infected or not, with quantitative laboratory confirmation to support the diagnosis, provides clinicians with a decade's worth of evidence with which to make clinical decisions.[22-24] The belief that the presence of pathogens could interfere with wound healing in the absence of a host response is viewed as a fundamental link to understanding the concept of critical colonization. So while the *clinical* definition of critical colonization is not universally accepted, clinicians and researchers generally agree that the term needs more definitive characterization in order to validate its consideration in infection management.[21]

Clinical signs of critical colonization have been described as a slowing or cessation of a wound's current healing trajectory demonstrated by a failure of wound margins to change. Additionally, the critically colonized wound often will exhibit increasing wound exudate with or without accompanying odor, the presence of friable, often exuberant bright red granulation tissue that bleeds easily, as well as areas of new necrosis. Suggested causative factors in the healing delay include the bacterial release of matrix metalloproteases (MMPs) and other proinflammatory mediators, the release of endotoxins during the lysis of the cell wall of gram-negative organisms, and exotoxins released by bacteria and fungi in general, as well as the competition between wound healing cells and bacteria for oxygen and nutrients. Additionally, bacteria can stimulate angiogenesis and lead to the production of a deficient or corrupt matrix. In clinical practice, assumed critical colonization is most often confirmed when intervention with an antimicrobial dressing or modality results in clinical improvement and resumption of wound healing.[21,25] (Fig. 8.1)

▶ **PEARL 8•6** Wound *infection* is described as the invasion of replicating bacteria into tissues and the deeper compartment of the wound, with subsequent host injury and disease.

Wound *infection* is described as the invasion of replicating bacteria into viable tissues and the deeper compartment of the wound, with subsequent host injury and disease. Depending on the location of the wound and the condition of the host, the presenting signs may be discrete or profound. A quantitative threshold of greater than 10^5 colony forming units per gram (CFU/g) of biopsy tissue has been used to define burn wound infection[8,26] and in the prediction of skin graft failure,[27] yet chronic wounds have been reported to go on to closure despite levels of microorganisms as great as 10^8 CFU/g of tissue.[8] Wound infection has also been defined in terms of the bacterial load and the virulence of the pathogens relative to the patient's level of resistance. The majority of chronic wounds are polymicrobial. Certain pathogens such as *S. aureus, Pseudomonas aeruginosa,* and β-hemolytic streptococci have been cited most often as the cause of delayed wound healing and infection.[1] Another study of chronic leg ulcers[28] reported that no single or group of microorganisms were more detrimental to wound healing; however, a significantly lower probability of healing

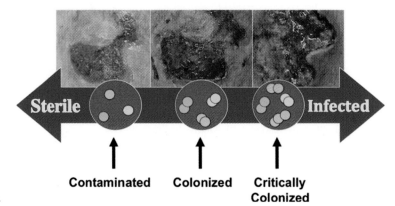

Figure 8•1 *Signs of critical colonization.*

was observed if four or more bacterial groups were present in any ulcer. This further indicates that microbial interactions may have an enhanced pathogenic effect, and that it is not just the presence of bacteria, but the type and pathogenicity of the organism and the interaction with the host that determines the resulting influence on chronic wound healing. The mere presence of bacteria may not increase the risk of infection, but the presence of one virulent β-hemolytic streptococcus should be considered significant and appropriate treatment initiated. Additionally, some combinations of bacterial species may develop synergy with each other resulting in previously nonvirulent organisms becoming virulent and causing damage to the host. For example, in diabetic foot ulcers, group B streptococci and *S. aureus* have been found to have synergistic hemolytic activity, and pathogens within the *Enterococcus* species may contribute to host injury when present with other pathogens.[29,30] Lastly, antimicrobial therapy targeting specific organisms may wipe out those pathogens, allowing the nontargeted bacteria to become more overwhelming.

Whereas bacterial quantity and virulence are important factors in wound infection, host resistance is also of notable and critical significance. Host resistance is defined as the ability of the host to mount an immune response in order to resist bacterial invasion and damage. This resistance can be impacted by a number of systemic and local factors. The ability to mitigate these factors has a direct influence on the impact that the bacteria will have on the wound and surrounding

tissues. See Table 8.1 for lists of local and systemic factors with the potential to impact host resistance. Clinical interventions to remove those factors that can be controlled may include but are not limited to wound debridement; interventions to control and improve comorbid conditions such as diabetes; vascular intervention; dietary management; counseling related to lifestyle changes; compression therapy; and advanced wound management choices to improve wound healing, such as topical biologics, negative pressure wound therapy, and hyperbaric oxygen.

Assessing the Wound

Determining the presence of a wound infection begins as a result of a clinical examination. The results of a microbiological test then validate the presence of the suspected offending organism(s) and confirm that the empirically prescribed antimicrobial agents appropriately target those organisms. Reliance on clinical evaluation alone, however, may lead to a false sense of security as to the infectious status of a wound. In a retrospective analysis by Serena et al,[31] the data from a phase IIB prospective, randomized, placebo-controlled clinical trial were examined to determine the accuracy of clinical examination in making the diagnosis of infection in venous leg ulcers. Of 614 screening biopsies obtained by impeccably strict standards, 122 were found to have a colony count greater than 10^6. Of the 352 patients eventually enrolled in

Table 8•1 Local and Systemic Factors Influencing Host Resistance	
Local	**Systemic**
Size, location, and age of the wound	Poorly controlled diabetes
Necrotic tissue or foreign bodies	Inadequate vascular perfusion
Presence of scar	Edema
Previous radiation	Immunosuppressive drugs
Inadequate or improper topical treatments	Malnutrition Alcohol and/or tobacco abuse Neutrophil disorders

the trial, 26% were found to have infected ulcers despite a lack of clinical signs, leading to the conclusion that the incidence of infection is grossly underestimated by clinical examination. Today, most hospitals perform surveillance-screening wound cultures on patients upon admission to the inpatient setting; but in the home care and outpatient setting, routine screening cultures are not done as a general rule, and reliance upon clinical evaluation remains the norm. The conventional fear is that routine culturing will lead to treatment of noninfecting bacteria with the end result of increasing resistance to available antibiotics.

> **PEARL 8•7** Determining the presence of a wound infection begins as a result of a clinical examination.

The guidelines published by the Wound Healing Society in 2006[32-35] recommend that if an infection is suspected in a débrided ulcer or if epithelialization from the margin in the venous, diabetic, and pressure ulcer (as well as contraction in the pressure ulcer) is not progressing within 2 weeks despite appropriate compression, pressure relief, and off-loading, the type and level of infection should be determined by a tissue biopsy or a validated quantitative swab technique.

Historically, the signs and symptoms of infection have been described as *rubor* (redness, erythema), *calor* (warmth), *dolor* (pain), and *tumor* (edema/swelling), as well as the presence of purulence. These classic heralding symptoms may be diminished or altered in the chronic wound environment and, conversely, may be also mistaken for inflammatory changes triggered by increased levels of inflammatory cytokines in the chronic wound environment. Other clinical signs and symptoms of chronic or secondary wounds validated by Gardner et al[36] include serous drainage with concurrent inflammation, delayed healing, discoloration of granulation tissue, friable granulation tissue, pocketing at the base of the wound, foul odor, and wound breakdown. The degree to which any of these 11 indicators may predict actual wound infection still seems to be related to the host response, but the patient presenting with increased wound pain, friable granulation tissue, foul odor, and wound breakdown warrants a thorough evaluation and attention to management as these signs and symptoms showed the greatest positive predictive value. See Figures 8.2 through 8.5 for clinical examples.

Wound Cultures

Beyond the assessment of the wound, the culture provides essential information to compare to the clinical picture, confirm the plan for treatment, or make appropriate changes. The patient presenting with the previously discussed clinical signs and symptoms of infection commands quick action based on the information available at the time, usually beginning treatment with antibiotics commonly sensitive to frequent pathogens in a particular wound type or, if available, based on antibiotic sensitivities to bacteria cultured previously from the wound. Collaboration with an infectious disease specialist is recommended in wounds

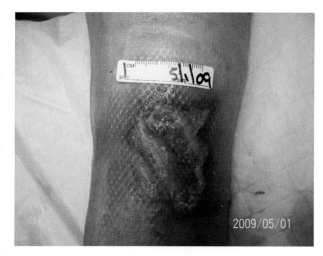

2009/05/01

Figure 8•2 *Example of colonized wound as evidenced by accumulation of debris and exudates on tissue surface, yet continued evidence of epithelialization from edges, indicating no interruption in the progression of healing.*

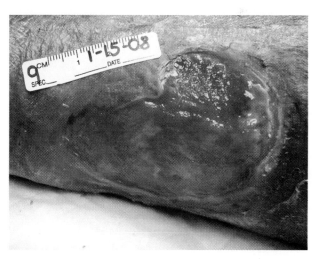

Figure 8•3 *Example of critically colonized venous ulcer that was previously granulating, but now presents with edematous, friable tissue, lack of continued progression of epithelial migration, and mild odor.*

culturing positive for multiple types of bacteria to assure treatment decisions are based upon current trends of known synergies and/or resistance in a particular hospital or community.

> **PEARL 8•8** Beyond the assessment of the wound, the culture provides essential information to compare to the clinical picture, confirm the plan for treatment, or make appropriate changes.

The appropriate method of obtaining a culture from a wound has been widely discussed and even debated over

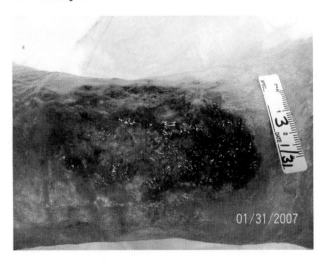

Figure 8•4 *Example of infected venous ulcer with increase in exudate, odor, and dark green discoloration to both exudate and tissue not present on previous evaluation. Tissue culture 4+ positive for* P. aeruginosa.

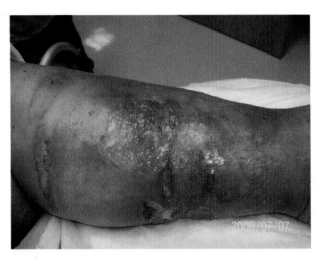

Figure 8•5 *Example of diffuse infection/cellulitis characterized by erythema, edema with bullous eruptions, noted to be warm, and reported to be painful by the patient.*

the years. The 72 hours required to obtain final results on standard laboratory cultures, regardless of the method, demands that the information provided be accurate in order to confirm treatment choices. Increasing growth of resistant strains of common pathogens further confirms this need.

The Terminology of Culturing Methods

Comparative information as to the accuracy and usability of results obtained from various techniques used to obtain a wound culture has been widely published.[8,36-39] The quantitative information that can be generated from a tissue biopsy remains the "gold standard"; and while it is the most common methodology used in research and clinical trials, it is likely the least often used in clinical practice.

▶ **PEARL 8•9** The quantitative information that can be generated from a tissue biopsy remains the "gold standard," and while it is the most common methodology used in research and clinical trials, it is likely the least often used method in clinical practice.

Regardless of the procedure used, there are two essential components to yielding the most accurate and valuable information. First, know the optimal time frame for transport of the specimen to the laboratory. Using culture specimen containers and tubes designed to stabilize and fix the bacteria, not promoting growth or death, allows a reasonable time frame for transport, especially for cultures taken in the home and freestanding clinics or institutions without a laboratory on the premises, such as outpatient wound care centers or skilled nursing facilities. Aerobic specimens contained in appropriate transport media will survive, and the media will not promote continued growth. Specimens obtained specifically for anaerobic culture should be placed into prereduced, anaerobically sterilized transport media.[18] Second, of equal or greater importance, carefully and accurately obtain the specimen.

A survey of the culturing practices by wound care professionals in the United States was undertaken in 2002.[8] Of the 345 respondents to the 34-item questionnaire, 79% were registered nurses, physical therapists, and physicians. The respondents had an average of 11 years of wound care experience, with 64% of their work time spent in direct wound care activities. When culturing wounds, 54% indicated that they routinely collect a swab only, while another 42% indicated that they routinely collected both swab and biopsy specimens, depending on the nature of the wound, confirming the frequency with which swab specimens were used. At the time of this nationwide survey, the results indicated that culturing of wounds may be a source of clinical information underutilized in health care, with the results showing that the majority of wounds (70%) were reported to be treated without cultures ever being performed, which compromises the use of results from posttreatment cultures. Furthermore, only 12% of the respondents reported routinely culturing wounds before beginning treatment regimens, and only 20% reported culturing when a treatment regimen had failed. Lastly, the respondents estimated that 79% of the wounds they did culture were found to be infected based on a positive laboratory report, thus reinforcing the need for more frequently culturing wounds.

Obtaining the Specimen

Regardless of the method, the practitioner's goal in obtaining a specimen for culture is to provide one as free of contaminants as possible. As a general rule, the ideal sample is one that is obtained

- after débridement and subsequent cleansing of the site with nonpreserved normal saline. Rationale: to obtain a specimen most representative of the actual bacterial status of the wound without contaminants.
- from an area of the wound most free of necrotic tissue if débridement is not possible. Rationale: necrotic tissue is

known to harbor bacteria that may not be invasive into wound tissue.

- away from intact skin and wound edges. Rationale: to avoid contamination of the specimen with normal skin flora or organisms that may be populating the periwound area and to avoid exposure to wound exudate or previous dressings.
- before instituting systemic antimicrobial therapy. Rationale: specimens collected after the initiation of antibiotic therapy may yield falsely low or nonexistent levels of sensitive bacteria, possibly leading the provider to alter or change an appropriate therapeutic agent.

Specimens are obtained by three methods: tissue removal, aspiration, and swab.

Tissue Removal

Methods of removal include obtaining biopsy tissue using a standard punch biopsy instrument and tissue obtained with other instruments such as a scalpel or curette. (See Fig. 8.6) When sending specimens for quantitative measurement, it is important to know the individual laboratory requirements for the size of the specimen. A 3-mm sample is typically required by most laboratories.

A consideration when obtaining a tissue specimen for bacterial culture is that the use of some topical and injectable anesthetic agents may influence bacterial survival through their antimicrobial properties.[40,41] In an in vitro study by Berg et al,[40] the effects of EMLA® (eutectic mixture of local anesthetic; AstraZeneca, Wilmington, DE), containing two anesthetic drugs (lidocaine 2.5% and prilocaine 2.5%), and lidocaine as a singular drug on common wound pathogenic bacteria was investigated. Five clinical isolates each of *S. aureas* (including one isolate of a methicillin-resistant strain), *E. coli, P. aeruginosoa,* and *Streptococcus pyogenes* were studied. EMLA was found to have a rapid-acting and powerful

antibacterial effect and should not be used before obtaining tissue samples for culture. Preservative-free lidocaine 1% solution as an injectable infiltrate was found to be safe for a wound biopsy performed within 2 hours. The use of a gel or solution of lidocaine applied topically was not addressed in this study. As a side note, the findings of the use of EMLA as a local anesthetic in other clinical procedures such as débridement are promising, as it may minimize the risk of iatrogenic bacterial spread and transient bacteremia.

> **PEARL 8•10** The use of some topical and injectable anesthetic agents may influence bacterial survival through their antimicrobial properties.

Using a tissue sample for culture is an advantage because it can enable identification of the organisms that have invaded beyond the wound surface in order to optimize antibacterial management. The disadvantage is that the technique is skill intensive and must be performed by a physician, podiatrist, or physician extender due to licensure restrictions. A safe assumption is that a majority of the bacterial cultures taken are done by nurses at the bedside, either in the home or institutional setting. This provides timeliness in obtaining the culture versus needing to transport the patient to a site of care where a tissue culture could be obtained, which would also add to the overall cost. Because it is an invasive procedure, it is also more painful, requiring local anesthetic in the sensate individual.

> **PEARL 8•11** The advantage of using a tissue sample for culture is to identify the organisms that have invaded beyond the wound surface to optimize antibacterial management.

Aspiration

The goal of aspirating a culture sample from a wound is to obtain fluid from below the wound bed, thereby avoiding surface contaminants. It is a method used more often to obtain a specimen from an abscess or loculated fluid collection. The skin over or adjacent to the area to be aspirated is prepared with povidone-iodine and allowed to dry for 60 seconds. A 10-mL syringe containing 0.5 mL of air, with a 22-gauge needle attached, is inserted through the skin toward the area to be aspirated. Suction is achieved by briskly withdrawing the plunger the length of the syringe to the 10-mL mark. The needle is then moved backward and forward through the tissue in the area. The plunger is then released back to the 0.5-mL mark, and the needle is withdrawn. The syringe is then capped and sent to the laboratory.[42] If the recapping of the syringe is against the policy of the site of care, the aspirated fluid may be gently injected into a sterile container and transported. The challenge of obtaining a culture using aspiration as a methodology is that, like a biopsy, it is an invasive procedure and technique is critically important; it is not likely to be performed by the bedside care provider. Overall, it is a technique rarely mentioned as used in general practice.

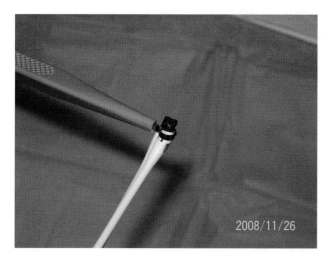

2008/11/26

Figure 8•6 *Tissue specimen that has been removed from the wound base tissues with a curette after débridement and cleansing of the wound.*

Swab

Swab cultures have historically been considered the least appropriate method by which to obtain a culture due to the potential for contamination by surface debris and skin contaminants; yet, as previously mentioned, obtaining specimens using swabs has been and continues to be the primary method used. Because of this fact, it is imperative for clinicians to use excellence in technique when obtaining the specimen. Modern wound dressings are designed to use moisture from the wound to maintain an ideal environment for healing and by design are left in place for several days. Unless the dressing is considered to be therapeutically antimicrobial, the accumulated exudate found upon removal of these dressings will often contain bacteria residing on the surface of the wound as well as the surrounding skin. Swabbing of this accumulated exudate will likely result in both higher numbers of microbes as well as lead to systemic treatment targeting organisms that are not negatively affecting the wound. Prior to obtaining the specimen, the wound surface should be cleansed with a nonpreserved, nonantimicrobial cleanser such as normal saline to remove surface debris, residual dressing material, and any coagulum easily removed from the surface. Additionally, wound débridement should be carried out if appropriate to remove necrotic and devitalized tissue, which will also harbor higher numbers of microorganisms.

The two swab techniques most often described in the literature are the Z-stroke and Levine's technique. The Z-stroke, as the name indicates, involves starting at the top of the wound, pressing the swab into the wound surface, and moving the swab from skin edge to skin edge in a "Z" pattern down to the bottom of the wound. The inherent challenge of this technique is the probability of contamination of the swab(s) with resident bacteria from the skin as well as from any devitalized tissue remaining on the wound surface. As mentioned, this may lead to overtreatment with antibiotics that may not be warranted, subject the patient to potential negative side effects of antibiotic use, and potentially kill off surface bacteria while allowing deeper contaminants to thrive and increase in numbers.

In 1976 Levine and colleagues[43] described a method for obtaining a viable sampling of aerobic bacteria on the surface of wounds. This method involves thoroughly cleansing the wound surface and identifying a 1-cm area of the wound that is free from necrotic tissue. The swab is rotated while applying pressure sufficient to express fluid from the wound tissue. This technique is thought to yield the most accurate results compared to the Z-stroke or, most certainly, swabbing residual exudate at the time of dressing removal.

Assessing the Culture Results

Final results of a wound culture generally take up to 72 hours to be reported. If Gram staining was ordered or is routinely carried out as the laboratory's standard procedure, these preliminary results can be available within hours and provide information helpful in establishing early treatment by identifying the organism(s) as gram-negative or gram-positive, as well as describing other components of the wound found within the specimen, such as the presence of white blood cells indicating that the patient is mounting an inflammatory response to the presence of the bacteria.

The reporting of culture results identifies the laboratory methodology used, and they are referenced in terms of qualitative, semiquantitative, and quantitative.

A *qualitative* culture is obtained by plating the specimen on solid media and identifying the organisms grown. *Semiquantitative* cultures are plated on solid media and then serially streaked into four quadrants. Results are reported as 1+ to 4+, identifying the number of quadrants in which growth of the bacteria occurred. *Quantitative* cultures are generally performed on tissue specimens, but swab specimens can also be used. Tissue specimens are homogenized and plated, whereas the swab specimens are serially diluted and plated. This technique allows for counting of colony forming units (CFUs) of the bacteria identified and is reported as CFUs per gram of tissue for wound biopsies and CFUs per square centimeter for swab cultures. As previously mentioned, soft tissue wound infections have been defined as cultures yielding greater than 10^5 CFU per gram or square centimeter of tissue; however, in chronic wounds this number needs to be considered within the context of the other clinical indicators previously described.

In addition to the specific bacteria being identified through one of these culturing techniques, antibiotic sensitivity tests based on the bacterial strain and antibiotics common to the setting, laboratory, or hospital are carried out. The final report will identify the organism(s) grown, the sensitivity (S) or resistance (R) to the antibiotics tested, and the minimum inhibitory concentration (MIC) relative to those antibiotics. The MIC identifies the lowest concentration of the antibiotic tested that resulted in inhibition or reduction of the inoculums, and as a general rule, the lower the MIC the more effective the antibiotic tested will be. This information, however, must be considered in relation to the species of the bacteria, other species identified, and possible synergies that may exist. Therefore, consultation with an infectious disease specialist may be warranted in the presence of multiple organisms, significant resistance, and in the patient experiencing persistent or recurring infections.

Osteomyelitis

Infection of the bone, or osteomyelitis, should be considered separately, as cultures taken of soft tissue may not accurately reflect bacterial penetration into bone. The absolute diagnosis of osteomyelitis is a difficult one, often resulting in expensive imaging or invasive bone biopsies. In 1995 Grayson et al[44] reported an 89% positive predictive value (PPV) and a 56% negative predictive value (NPV) in pedal ulcers of 75 patients with 76 ulcers known to be infected, in which bone could be probed using a stainless steel probe. The authors concluded that in patients with diabetes the ability to probe to bone (PTB) is strongly correlated with osteomyelitis and that specialized radiological and nuclear tests to diagnose osteomyelitis were unnecessary. Called the "poor man's bone scan," this seemingly conventional wisdom drove and continues to drive practice today.

In 2005 Shone et al[45] studied 81 patients with a total of 104 foot ulcers over a 5-week period. The ulcers were probed by one of two podiatrists following débridement. The diagnosis of osteomyelitis was determined by one of two expert diabetologists who were blinded to the PTB results. Diagnosis of osteomyelitis was based on the presence of clinical signs of infection in association with radiological evidence of bone destruction, supported when necessary by MRI and cultures of deep tissue samples. Osteomyelitis was diagnosed in 21 of the 104 ulcers. The PTB test was positive in 8 of the 21 ulcers and in 7 of 83 without associated bone infection, resulting in a 53% PPV and an 85% NPV.

In 2007 Lavery et al[46] also sought to assess the accuracy of the PTB test in diagnosing foot osteomyelitis. In this large 2-year study, the investigators enrolled 1666 consecutive diabetic individuals who underwent an initial standardized detailed foot assessment followed by examinations at regular intervals. The patients were instructed to come to the foot clinic if they developed a lower-extremity complication. Over a mean of 27.2 months, 247 patients developed a foot wound and 151 developed 199 foot infections. Osteomyelitis was found in 30 patients, 12% with a foot wound and 20% with a foot infection. The PTB test was highly sensitive (0.87%) and specific (0.91%). The PPV was only 0.57%, but the NPV was 0.98%. The authors concluded that the PTB test, when used in a population of diabetic patients with foot wounds, had a relatively low PPV, but a negative test may exclude the diagnosis.

In the final analysis, there is still debate as to whether the ability to probe to bone should be totally diagnostic in clinical practice. Unquestionably, if one is probing to bone in an obvious infected ulcer and soft or mushy bone is encountered, osteomyelitis is an obvious diagnosis. Care must also be taken to use caution in the degree of pressure used in probing a wound that is close to bone to avoid pushing through otherwise healthy tissue and creating a pathway to bone that was not previously present. In this era of increasing concerns related to medical liability, the total picture of the condition of the patient, the wound, and imaging studies will continue to drive the conclusion as to the presence or absence of bone infection.[47]

Additionally problematic is the diagnosis of osteomyelitis beneath pressure ulcers. In patients with deep nonhealing pressure ulcers, clinical evaluation poorly predicts the existence of underlying osteomyelitis. Neither clinical evaluation nor radiological examinations correlate well with the likelihood of finding histopathology diagnostic for bone infection. The bone scan often yields confusing results. While a bone scan is highly sensitive (almost 100%), it is poorly specific (less than 33%) due to the tendency of the nuclear molecules to concentrate in areas of bone that are affected by pressure-induced changes and in foci of heterotopic bone ossification. Therefore, bone scans should be used primarily for its NPV to rule out osteomyelitis rather than its low PPV for diagnosis. Diagnosis of osteomyelitis beneath pressure ulcers requires examination of bone tissue that is best obtained intraoperatively because osteomyelitis is likely to be a focal process; therefore, percutaneous biopsy may fail to sample truly infected bone.[48]

Controlling and Managing Bioburden

The foundation for controlling bioburden begins with rapt attention to detail in the care of the patient with a chronic wound. Support and correction of those factors that can impair resistance to infection are frequently overlooked as essential components in the plan to control infection. Detailed evaluation and management of nutrition, glycemic control, blood flow, edema management, and removal of trauma and pressure should be addressed as part of initial and then ongoing assessments of the patient.

> ▶ **PEARL 8•12** The foundation for controlling bioburden begins with rapt attention to detail in the care of the patient with a chronic wound.

The concept of wound bed preparation implies preliminary care to prepare a wound to heal. The foundation for wound bed preparation—cleansing, débridement of necrotic or nonviable tissue with attention to wound edges, and management and prevention of infection—must be part of every wound encounter and integrated into routine care. Wound cleansing and débridement as components of wound bed preparation will also be covered elsewhere in this book but cannot be overlooked as an essential component in the management of wound bioburden. The presence of necrotic tissue provides a nidus for bacterial growth and should be removed or débrided by the means appropriate to the locale of care. Those wounds in which débridement is not indicated (eg, an eschar on an ischemic heel) should be monitored frequently for signs of infection (separation and/or drainage at edges, erythema, induration, fluctuance).

Wound Cleansing

All wounds should be cleansed at the time of dressing change, before and after débridement, or in the event of contamination, using a neutral, nonirritating, nontoxic solution. Routine cleansing should be accomplished with a minimum of chemical and/or mechanical trauma.[22-24] An exception to this may be the recent application of a skin graft or bioengineered tissue, which should be left undisturbed; in this case, the surrounding skin should be cleansed.

The choice of solution or agent used, as well as the method of delivery, is driven by the condition of and local factors in the wound. There have been numerous citations in the literature spanning many years related to the toxicity of various solutions used for cleansing and disinfection in burn and wound care. Although definitive research is lacking, practice evidence suggests using a nontoxic cleaning solution in combination with a delivery device that will create sufficient mechanical force to remove the surface debris without injury to healthy tissue[3]

> ▶ **PEARL 8•13** The choice of solution or agent used, as well as the method of delivery, is driven by the condition of and local factors in the wound.

Decisions relative to wound cleansing must be made based on the condition of the wound surface. Years of argument against the use of antiseptics such as hydrogen peroxide, acetic acid, Dakin's solution, and povidone-iodine are based primarily on in vitro models demonstrating the ability of these agents to create an environment toxic to the viability of cells important in wound healing, such as fibroblasts, keratinocytes, and leukocytes. In 1919, Fleming[49] reported that antiseptics are not as effective against bacteria that reside in wounds as they are against bacteria in vitro. The presence of exudate, serum, or blood seems to decrease their activity. As a practical matter, the choice of solution used for wound cleansing should be made relative to the necrotic tissue, exudates, and general coagulum on the wound surface; the condition and hygiene of the patient; the area of the body on which the wound is located; and the potential for recent environmental or other contamination, such as due to incontinence.

Commercially available wound cleansers contain surface active agents that break the bond of contaminants and debris, allowing them to be rinsed away mechanically by the spraying, pouring, or wiping of the solution over the wound. The potential toxicity of these cleansers should be weighed against the need for more aggressive removal of surface debris and contaminants based on the assessment of the wound. Normal saline is an effective agent for wound cleansing when delivered with enough pressure to ensure adequate removal of surface debris. Pressures below 4 pounds per square inch (psi) are not sufficient to remove debris, and pressures exceeding 15 psi risk driving debris into rather than off of the tissues.[3]

Antimicrobial Agents and Dressings

In recent years there has been rapid growth in the options for managing and controlling bacterial activity on wound surfaces using targeted solutions and dressings that provide increased access as well as flexibility in meeting the environmental needs of the wound. Research relative to their use is typically aimed at providing FDA-required safety and efficacy testing, while other published information is primarily case- and usage-based studies and trials. The decision to use one of these agents or dressings should be driven by the wound assessment and the concern of critical colonization interfering with wound healing. The perceived efficacy of a chosen agent or product then becomes the reversal of the previously assessed colonization as evidenced by improvement in the wound appearance or progression toward healing.

Antiseptics and Wound Treatment Solutions

Decisions related to the solution choice to cleanse or treat a wound must be made with the goal of care in mind. The clean, granulating wound that needs only the residue from a previous dressing or treatment removed may be best served with isotonic saline or other nontoxic solution or cleanser. Conversely, the wound exhibiting odor, an abnormal color of the tissue or exudate, other signs of critical colonization, or necrotic tissue may benefit from a short course of an antimicrobial product to cleanse and/or counteract the negative effects of bacterial growth. A fitting question to be asked when making this decision should be "is the goal of care to clean or to disinfect?"

▸ **PEARL 8•14** The solution used to cleanse or treat a wound must be chosen with the goal of care in mind.

For disinfection or reduction of bioburden, common agents historically used have included, but are not limited to, hydrogen peroxide, Dakin's solution, acetic acid, and povidone-iodine. Their use was based on testing on bacteria in a fluid medium in the laboratory. In a chronic wound, these agents additionally bind to other forms of organic matter, resulting in reduced effectiveness against bacteria. The concentrations that would be effective in reducing bacteria are known to be toxic to cells important to wound healing, including leukocytes and fibroblasts, and their use in clean wounds should be avoided.[50]

Skin cleansers, those designed for use in care of the incontinent patient, should not be used as a wound cleanser. The surface active agents in these preparations are of a concentration sufficient to emulsify and lift adherent fecal matter from the skin and therefore are damaging to the cells of an open wound.

Therefore, if a wound surface is assessed to be colonized, as evidenced by the previously described exudates, odor, color change, and surface debris, the use of a commercial wound cleanser with or without an antimicrobial agent may be the product of choice. As previously mentioned, many cleansers that are effective at disinfecting the wound are biologically aggressive and result in the damage of essential cells within the wound site, inhibiting progression of the wound healing process. While it is essential to remove foreign debris, potential bioburden, and wound pathogens from the wound site, the wound cleanser of choice must also be noncytotoxic in order to promote the most favorable conditions for wound healing.

▸ **PEARL 8•15** While it is essential to remove foreign debris, potential bioburden, and wound pathogens from the wound site, the wound cleanser chosen must also be noncytotoxic in order to promote the most favorable conditions for wound healing.

A cleansing and moistening solution recently made available for clinical practice is hypochlorous acid (HOCl). It is available for single-patient use as a commercially available spray, and it is produced by electrolysis using a specific generator and specific electrolyte fluid for point-of-use care in the clinic setting. The resulting HOCl solution is stable for 72 hours in an opaque container at room temperature and for 14 days when refrigerated.

HOCl is a naturally occurring small molecule generated by white blood cells in the human body. An important attribute of the human body's immune system is its ability to instigate a rapid attack against invading pathogens by releasing highly potent oxidized molecules such as HOCl. After engulfing invading pathogens, neutrophils release an "oxidative burst" of HOCl that very quickly destroys the engulfed bacteria, virus, or fungi. The HOCl, produced by neutrophils, affects microbial cell permeability and kills microorganisms by binding to critical cell membrane components. This leads to the rupture of cell membranes and subsequent disintegration of microbial cells.[51]

Hypochlorous acid is indicated for use on diabetic ulcers, venous ulcers, stage I to IV pressure ulcers, and first- and second-degree burns. Efficacy in the treatment of chronic ulcers has been demonstrated. In a pilot evaluation, Selkorn et al observed that ulcer pain was significantly reduced and 45% of ulcers healed in patients treated with hypochlorous acid.[52] HOCl is nonsensitizing, nonirritating, and noncytotoxic. In vitro analysis of cell toxicity testing of keratinocytes and fibroblasts showed no negative effects. The pH of HOCl is approximately 5.4, close to the natural protective pH of human skin.[53] Clinically, HOCl has been found to reduce or eliminate odor on contact, soften dried exudate and callus, and break down surface debris and coagulum, making both easier to remove from the wound surface without trauma.

Topical Antibiotics

The use of topical antibiotics, as with systemic antibiotics, should be limited to agents targeting known or assumed bacteria and used for a defined period of time. Topical antibiotics can play an important role in the prevention and treatment of many primary cutaneous bacterial infections commonly seen. Possibly the greatest use for topical antibiotics is infection prophylaxis in superficial skin wounds, particularly when used with a dressing that occludes the wound.[54] Prophylactic topical antibiotic use makes particular sense for wounds in which the risk of infection is high, such as those that are likely to be contaminated (accidental wounds, lacerations, abrasions, and burns). Because all traumatic wounds should be considered contaminated, topical antibiotics are a logical measure to prevent wound infection.

> ▶ **PEARL 8•16** The use of topical antibiotics, as systemic antibiotics, should be limited to agents targeting known or assumed bacteria and used for a defined period of time.

The topical agents used most often in the treatment of superficial cutaneous bacterial infections are mupirocin, bacitracin, polymyxin B, and neomycin.

Mupirocin

Mupirocin, an inhibitor of bacterial protein synthesis, targets primarily gram-positive organisms, especially *S. aureus* and most streptococci. Many gram-negative pathogens, including enteric bacilli and other enterococci, are not affected. Activity is enhanced in an acid environment (pH 5.5), which is the normal pH of the skin, but mupirocin is temperature sensitive. Its most common use is for localized impetigo caused by *S. aureus* and *S. pyogenes* and for eradication of *S. aureus* from the anterior nares. It is available as a single-agent formulation for topical use or as an intranasal preparation. It is widely used for skin injuries in patients known to be colonized or at risk for colonization with methicillin-resistant *Staphylococcus aureus* (MRSA) and methicillin-sensitive *Staphylococcus aureus* (MSSA).

Bacitracin

Bacitracin interferes with bacterial cell wall synthesis and is primarily active against the gram-positive bacteria *S. aureus* and streptococci.[55] Most gram-negative organisms and yeasts are resistant. Topical bacitracin is effective for the treatment of superficial bacterial infections of the skin, such as impetigo, furunculosis, and pyoderma. Bacitracin is a component of many commercial products, both singly and as part of triple antibiotic ointment (TAO).

Polymyxin B

Polymyxin B acts to disrupt the integrity of the bacterial cell membrane and increase bacterial cell permeability. It is active against a wide range of gram-negative organisms, including *P. aeruginosa*, *Enterobacter*, and *E. coli*. Polymyxin B is available singly, combined with bacitracin, or as part of TAO.

Neomycin

A member of the aminoglycoside family of agents, neomycin interferes with bacterial protein synthesis. It is most commonly used to treat infections caused by aerobic gram-positive and gram-negative bacilli (*S. aureus* and *E. coli*) and to prevent infection in superficial abrasions, cuts, and burns. It is formulated alone, in combination with other antibiotics (bacitracin, polymyxin B, gramicidin), or with other agents, such as lidocaine, pramoxine, or hydrocortisone, and as part of TAO.

Triple Antibiotic Ointment

The development of combination antibiotic products has been driven by the principle that drugs with complementary or overlapping antimicrobial spectra may have additive or even synergistic interactions when combined. Choices of agents for combination products have therefore been influenced by the target mechanism of action of each, based on the hypothesis that combining agents having different mechanisms of action would enhance effectiveness while limiting the potential for antagonism.

The TAO components, bacitracin zinc, polymyxin B sulfate, and neomycin sulfate, provide a broad spectrum of activity. In vitro, the triple components of TAO have activity against both gram-positive (including the most common skin pathogens *S. aureus* and *S. pyogenes*) and gram-negative organisms (including *P. aeruginosa*).

Concerns of resistance, sensitivities, and potential for contact dermatitis should be considered. There are reports in the literature of increasing resistance to mupirocin, likely due to widespread use in community-acquired MRSA as well as in patients at high risk for MRSA.

Antimicrobial Wound Dressings

Management and treatment of the infected and critically colonized wound is a dilemma encountered by wound clinicians with increasing frequency and is of particular concern with the rising numbers of infections caused by drug-resistant organisms. As previously discussed, careful and frequent assessment to recognize changes in the wound indicating an impact by surface and invading bacteria is critical. Realizing that initial changes in the previously healing wound may indicate an initial host response to the presence of the bacteria enables clinicians to intervene and reduce the bacterial load topically, preventing continued replication and potential invasion into the deeper tissues.

In recent years there has been an appreciable increase in dressing options available to address local wound bioburden while simultaneously managing the local environmental needs of the wound, such as exudate and moisture balance, protection of the periwound skin, filling of wound space, coverage, protection, and insulation. Each dressing material brings unique yet familiar attributes commonly used to meet those needs. Additionally, Maillard and Denyer [56] itemized the features of an ideal antimicrobial dressing, including the following:

- Provides sustained antimicrobial activity
- Provides a moist wound healing environment
- Allows consistent delivery of the antimicrobial in the dressing over the entire surface of the wound
- Allows monitoring of the wound with minimum interference
- Manages exudate, if problematic
- Is comfortable
- Is conformable
- Provides an effective microbial barrier
- Absorbs and retains bacteria
- Avoids wound trauma on removal

The differentiating factor is the particular antimicrobial agent incorporated into the dressing. Antimicrobial agents are bound into or coated onto the dressing materials, acting as a barrier to outside contamination as well as interacting with wound exudate to further enhance the barrier effects and reduce bacterial load on the surface of the wound. Commonly used agents include silver, cadexomer iodine, honey, polyhexamethylene biguanide (PHMB), and the pigments crystal violet and methylene blue.

Cadexomer Iodine

The term *cadexomer iodine* actually describes a delivery system rather than an antimicrobial agent. Iodine has a broad spectrum of activity and works in many ways by disrupting cell walls and nuclei and facilitating oxidative killing of microorganisms and neutrophils.[57] It has been shown to be toxic at a cellular level in vitro.[58-60] In this novel delivery system, the iodine is contained within a cadexomer starch bead. As wound exudate is drawn up, it enters the cadexomer bead, causing its openings to swell and allowing a slow, sustained release of the iodine molecules; it maintains a steady-state 0.9% concentration at the wound bed, providing a nontoxic level for healing wounds. Iodine is brown, and iodide, which is the inactive form of iodine, is colorless. The dressing progresses from brown to colorless, indicating that the iodine has been used and as a signal to change the dressing. The dressing lasts for an average of 72 hours, depending on the amount of exudate, the size of the wound, and the amount of the dressing/gel used. Cadexomer iodine has also been shown to be effective against certain *S. aureus* in biofilm in vitro and in vivo.[60]

Honey

The use of honey has been documented as a treatment for open wounds for ages, having been mentioned in the Bible, the Koran, and the Torah. It was documented to be used in plasters by the Egyptians in 2000 BC, was found documented in medical writings from 1392, and has experienced a renaissance in recent years as a topic of clinical and scientific research in wound healing. It is primarily sourced from the *Leptospermum* species, and the medical-grade honey is gamma-irradiated to destroy commonly found *Clostridium* spores.

The antimicrobial activity of honey has been related to the high sugar content and low water activity, creating an osmotic effect that dehydrates the bacteria and, along with the acidic pH of 3.2 to 4.5, inhibits bacterial growth. The fluid shift resulting from this osmotic effect also contributes to creating a moist wound healing environment and reduced pain on dressing removal due to decreased potential for desiccation and adherence to the wound surface. The presence of the glucose oxidase enzyme added by bees to the nectar that they collect results in the production of hydrogen peroxide, which, although known to be toxic as a rinse, is 1000 times less toxic in honey. Honey dressings are available in an alginate, hydrocolloid, and paste form.[61-66]

Polyhexamethylene Biguanide

Polyhexamethylene biguanide (PHMB) is a biocide that has been used for many years with no known resistance. It is used in a variety of products, including wound care dressings, contact lens cleaning solutions, perioperative cleansing products, and swimming pool cleaners.[67,68] PHMB is a synthetic compound similar in structure to naturally occurring molecules produced by inflammatory cells to protect against infection. By attaching itself to the bacterial cell membrane, PHMB causes structural changes that kill the bacteria. Bacteria commonly protect themselves from resistance by pumping some antibiotics out of the cell using efflux pumps. The structural changes caused by the PHMB prevent the bacteria from using their efflux pumps to pump out the biocide.[68,69] The incorporation of PHMB into dressings, including gauze sponges, nonadherent dressings, foams, and a biosynthesized cellulose wound dressings, has been shown to be an effective barrier to protect a wound from outside contamination as well as to have bactericidal activity on relevant bacteria absorbed into the dressing material. The gauze sponges have also been used extensively as part of the dressing interface layer with numerous negative-pressure wound therapy devices.

Crystal Violet and Methylene Blue

The pigments crystal violet and methylene blue have been used in medicine for over 50 years as both laboratory stains[11] and as antiseptics that have bacteriostatic properties on multiple clinically relevant bacteria, including resistant strains such as methicillin-resistant *S. aureus* (MRSA). They are available commercially bound within a polyvinyl (PVA) alcohol foam, which when hydrated becomes a soft, conformable wound filler and contact dressing. The open cell structure of the foam allows the removal of wound exudate up and into the dressing where the active agents inhibit the growth of microorganisms. This unique uptake of exudate is visibly evident upon dressing removal, and the interaction of the exudate with the pigments will be noted to blanch out the color of the foam, providing visual evidence that the dressing should be changed. In clinical use, the foam also has been noted to reduce hypergranulation tissue, as well as flatten out slightly rolled wound edges, particularly in venous leg ulcers, allowing epidermal edge cellular migration. The dressing is changed every other day or more or less frequently, depending upon the level of exudate.[70]

Silver

Silver has been used for centuries, originally as vessels used to preserve water, and has had medicinal uses documented from AD 750. A renewed interest in the use of ionic silver in topical antimicrobial dressings has been widely documented and studied to assess its use to reduce bacterial growth and reduce the risk of wound infection, to manage active infections, and to reduce the risk of hospital-acquired wound infections. This renewed interest is largely attributed to its bactericidal efficacy at low concentrations and its relatively limited toxicity to human cells. Silver has proven antimicrobial activity, which includes antibiotic-resistant bacteria such as methicillin-resistant *S. aureus* (MRSA) and vancomycin-resistant enterococci (VRE). Renewed interest in clinical use also arises from advances in impregnation techniques and polymer technologies, resulting in numerous delivery systems in the form of dressing materials.[56]

There is an abundance of information published regarding the use of silver compared to other antimicrobial dressings and antimicrobial agents within dressings. This is in large part related to the number of years that silver has been used in wound management, with silver sulfadiazine having been available for over 40 years, particularly as a broad-spectrum antimicrobial used in managing burn wounds.[71] Silver sulfadiazine cream has a relatively short action, its penetration of the burn eschar is poor, and it forms a pseudo-eschar, requiring more frequent and often painful dressing changes.

Silver is biologically active when it is in soluble form, that is as Ag^+ or Ag^0 clusters. Ag^+ is the ionic form present in silver nitrate, silver sulfadiazine, or other ionic silver compounds. Ag^0 is the uncharged form of metallic silver present in nanocrystalline silver. Free silver cations have a potent antimicrobial effect that destroys microorganisms immediately by blocking the cellular respiration and disrupting the function of bacterial cell membranes. This occurs when silver cations bind to tissue proteins, causing structural changes in the bacterial cell membranes, which in turn cause cell death. Silver cations also bind and denature the bacterial DNA and RNA, thus inhibiting cell replication.[72]

Concerns related to the use of silver dressings revolve around the potential for development of resistance, the cellular toxicity, and the appropriate use of the right amount of silver at the right time. Percival et al[73] looked at the prevalence of silver resistance in bacteria from diabetic foot ulcers and found that the silver-resistance genes from these ulcers is low and appears to be confined to an enteric bacterium, *Enterobacter cloacae*, which is not known to be a primary wound pathogen. No evidence of resistance genes in wound pathogens such as *S. aureus* and *P. aeruginosa* was found in this study. This study also found that the low proportion of wound bacteria that possess silver-resistance genes are killed when challenged with silver-containing wound dressings.[73]

The toxicity of silver in cells and tissues has been assessed. Silver dressings that have been shown to be cytotoxic in vitro within 1 day showed no cytotoxicity in vivo after 1 week, suggesting that in vitro cytotoxicity is more sensitive than in vivo because there is no means of reducing toxicity via blood circulation, tissue reservoir, metabolism, or by dilution effects.[71]

Every dressing category (films, foams, alginates, hydrofibers, gels, gauze, contact layers, and composites) are available with a silver component in one form or another. No data exist to strongly support one type of dressing over another based on their silver "dosage." Assurance of intimate contact with the wound bed has been shown to increase the success of the dressing by avoiding the formation of voids (dead space) where bacteria may flourish. The clinical result is the definitive test of the dressing (ie, does it work in practice?).[71] Continued discretion in the judicious use of silver, as well as all antimicrobial dressings, is required to mitigate potential further resistance patterns in common wound pathogens in the future.

> ▶ **PEARL 8•17** Continued discretion in the judicious use of silver, as well as all antimicrobial dressings, is required to mitigate potential further resistance patterns in common wound pathogens in the future.

Summary

The management of known or perceived bioburden impacting chronic wounds requires a careful assessment of both the patient and the wound, and decisions as to the appropriate management of wounds will be made based upon this assessment. Careful attention to the actual or potential invasive bacterial infection should drive systemic treatment with antibiotics. Careful and appropriate culturing will confirm not only the presence of the bacteria and, if quantified, the potential impact on the host, it will also confirm that the chosen drug regimen is on target. The judicious use of topical antimicrobial agents and dressings must be based on the timely assessment of the wound surface, the recognition of changes that indicate increasing bioburden, and the supposition that this bacterial presence may interfere with the progression of healing.

> ▶ **PEARL 8•18** The judicious use of topical antimicrobial agents and dressings must be based on the timely assessment of the wound surface, the recognition of changes indicating increasing bioburden, and the supposition that this bacterial presence may be interfering with the progression of healing.

References

1. Martin, LK, Drosou, A, Kirsner, RS: Wound microbiology and the use of antibacterial agents. In: Falabella, AF, Kirsner, RS (eds): Wound Healing. Boca Raton, FL, Taylor & Francis Group, 2005, pp 83–101.
2. Cowan, MK, Talaro, KP: Infectious diseases affecting the skin and eyes. :In: Microbiology: A Systems Approach. New York, McGraw-Hill, 2006, pp 540–576.
3. Baranoski, S, Ayello, E, Tomic-Canic, M: Skin: an essential organ. In: Baranoski, S, Ayello, E (eds): Wound Care Essentials: Practice Principles. Ambler, PA, Lippincott Williams & Wilkins, 2008, pp 47–63.
4. Sussman, C: Assessment of the skin and wound. In: Sussman, C, Bates-Jensen, B (eds): Wound Care: A Collaborative Practice Manual for Health Professionals, ed. 3. Philadelphia, Lippincott Williams & Wilkins, 2007, pp 85–122.
5. Bowler, PG: The 10^5 bacterial growth guideline: Reassessing its clinical relevance in wound healing. Ostomy Wound Manage 49:44–53.
6. Wikipedia. Bioburden. Available at: http://en.wikipedia.org/wiki/Bioburden. Accessed 08/21/07.
7. Stedman, TL: Stedman's Medical Dictionary. Baltimore, Lippincott Williams & Wilkins, 2006.
8. Bamberg, R, Sullivan, PK, Conner-Kerr, T: Diagnosis of wound infections: Current culturing practices of US wound care professionals. Wounds 2002; 14:314–327.
9. Bacteria. Available at: http://www.biology-online.org/dictionary/Bacteria. Accessed 08/21/07.
10. Cowan, MK, Talaro, KP. Infectious diseases affecting the skin and eyesIn:Microbiology: A Systems Approach. New York, McGraw-Hill, 2006, pp 89–118.
11. Wikipedia. Gram staining. . Available at: http://en.wikipedia.org/wiki/Gram staining. Accessed 12/2/2007.
12. The Gram Stain. Available at: http://www.ncl.ac.uk/dental/oralbiol/oralenv/tutorials/gramstain.htm. Accessed 12/02/07.
13. Lee, EK, Lerner, BW: Plankton and planktonic bacteria. World of Microbiology and Immunology, 1: 2003. eNotes.com. Available at: http://www.enotes.com/microbiology-encyclopedia/plankton-planktonic-bacteria. Accessed 12/02/07.
14. Percival, SL, Bowler, PG: Biofilms and their potential role in wound healing. Wounds 2001; 16:234–240.
15. Bello, YM, Fallabella, AF, DeCaralho, H, et al: Infection and wound healing. Wounds 2001; 13:127–131.
16. Serralta, VW, Harrison-Balestra, C, Cazzaniga, AL, et al: Lifestyles of bacteria in wounds: Presence of biofilms? Wounds 2001; 13:29–34.
17. Garth, AJ, Swogger, E, Wolcott, R, et al: Biofilms in chronic wounds. Wound Rep Reg 2008; 16:37–44.
18. Landis, S, Ryan, S, Woo, K, et al: Infections in chronic wounds. In: Krasner, D.L., Rodeheaver, GT, Sibald, RG (eds): Chronic Wound Care: A Clinical Source Book for Healthcare Professionals, ed. 4. Malvern, PA, HMP Communications, 2007, pp 299–321.
19. Browne, A, Dow, G, Sibbald, RG: Infected wounds: Definitions and controversies. In: Falanga, V. (ed): Cutaneous Wound Healing. London, Martin Dunitz, 2001, pp 203–219.
20. Stotts, N: Wound infection: Diagnosis and management. In: Morison, MJ, Ovington, LG, Wilkie, K. (eds): Chronic Wound Care: A Problem-based Learning Approach. Mosby, 2004, pp 101–116.
21. White, RJ, Cutting, KF: Critical colonization—the concept under scrutiny. Ostomy Wound Manage 2006; 52:50–56.
22. Robson, MC, Cooper, DM, Aslam, R, et al: Guidelines for the treatment of venous ulcers. Wound Rep Reg 2007; 14:649–662.
23. Whitney, J, Phillips, L, Aslam, R, et al: Guidelines for the treatment of pressure ulcers. Wound Rep Reg 2007; 14:663–679.
24. Steed, DL, Attinger, C, Colaizzi, T, et al: Guidelines for the treatment of diabetic ulcers. Wound Rep Reg 2007; 14:680–692.
25. Schultz, GS, Sibbald, RG, Falanga, V, et al: Wound bed preparation: A systematic approach to wound management. Wound Rep Reg 2003; 11(suppl):S1–S28.
26. Robson, MC: Wound infection. A failure of wound healing caused by an imbalance of bacteria. Surg Clin North Am 1997; 77:637–680.
27. Robson, MC, Krizek, TJ: Predicting skin graft survival. J Trauma 1973; 13:213–217.
28. Trengove, NF, Stacey, MC, McGechie, DF, et al: Qualitative bacteriology and leg ulcer healing. J Wound Care 1996; 5:277–280.
29. Enoch, S, Harding, K: Wound bed preparation: The science behind the removal of barriers to healing. Wounds 2003; 15:213–229.
30. Dow, G, Browne, A, Sibbald, RG: Infection in chronic wounds: Controversies in diagnosis and treatment. Wounds 1999; 45:23–40.
31. Serena, T, Robson, MC, Cooper, DM, et al: Lack of reliability of clinic/visual assessment of chronic wound infection: The incidence of biopsy-proven infection in venous leg ulcers. Wounds 2006; 18:197–202.
32. Robson, MC, Cooper, DM, Aslam, R, et al: Guidelines for the treatment of venous ulcers. Wound Rep Reg 2006; 14:649–662.
33. Whitney, J, Phillips, L, Aslan, R, et al: Guidelines for the treatment of pressure ulcers. Wound Rep Reg 2006; 14:663–679.
34. Steed, DL, Attinger, C, Colaizzi, T, et al: Guidelines for the treatment of diabetic ulcers. Wound Rep Reg 2006; 14:680–692.
35. Hopf, HW, Ueno, C, Aslam, R, et al: Guidelines for the treatment of arterial insufficiency ulcers. Wound Rep Reg 2006; 14:693–710.
36. Gardner, SE, Frantz, RA, Doebbeling, BN: The validity of the clinical signs and symptoms used to identify localized chronic wound infection. Wound Rep Reg 2001; 9:178–186.
37. Bill, TJ, Ratliff, CR, Donovan, AM, et al: Quantitative swab culture versus tissue biopsy: A comparison in chronic wounds. Ostomy Wound Manage 2001; 47:34–37.
38. Ratliff, CR, Rodeheaver, GT: Correlation of semi-quantitative swab cultures to quantitative swab cultures from chronic wounds. Wounds 2002; 14:329–333.
39. Sullivan, PK, Conner-Kerr, TA, Hamilton, H, et al: Assessment of wound bioburden development in a rat acute wound model: Quantitative swab versus tissue biopsy. Wounds 2004; 16:115–123.
40. Berg, JO, Mössner, BK, Skov, MN, et al: Antibacterial properties of EMLA® and lidocaine in wound tissue biopsies for culturing. Wound Rep Reg 2006; 14:581–585.
41. Johnson, SM, Saint John, BE, Dine, AP: Local anesthetics as antimicrobial agents: A review. Sur Infect 2008; 9:205–213.
42. Lee, P, Turnidge, J, McKonald, PJ: Fine-needle aspiration biopsy in diagnosis of soft tissue infections. J Clin Microbiol 1985; 22:80–83.
43. Levine, N, Lindberg, R, Mason, A, et al: The quantitative swab culture and smear: A quick, simple method for determining the number of viable aerobic bacteria open wounds. J Trauma 1976; 16:89–94.
44. Grayson, ML, Gibbons, GW, Balogh, K, et al: Probing to bone in infected pedal ulcers. A clinical sign of underlying osteomyelitis in diabetic patients. JAMA 1995; 273:721–723.
45. Shone, A, Burnside, J, Chipchase, S, et al: Probing the validity of the probe-to-bone test in the diagnosis of osteomyelitis of the foot in diabetes. Diabetes Care 2006; 29:945; letter.
46. Lavery, LA, Armstrong, DG, Peters, EJG, et al: Probe-to-bone test for diagnosis diabetic foot osteomyelitis. Reliable or relic? Diabetes Care 2007; 30:270–274.
47. Steinberg, JS, Warren, JS: Point-counter point: Probe to bone: Is it the best test for osteomyelitis? Podiatry Today 2007; 20:5–54.
48. Gardner, SE, Frantz, RA: Wound bioburden. In: Baranoski, S., Ayello, E.A. (eds): Wound Care Essentials: Practice Principles, ed. 2. Ambler, PA, Lippincott Williams & Wilkins, 2008, p 107–109.
49. Fleming, A: The action of chemical and physiological antiseptics in a septic wound. Br J Surg 1919; 7:99–129.
50. Rolstad, BS, Ovington, LG: Principles of wound management. In: Bryant, RA, Nix, DP (eds): Acute & Chronic Wounds Current Management Concepts, ed. 3. Philadelphia, Mosby/Elsevier, 2007, p 420–421.
51. Drosou, A, Falabella, A, Kirsner, R.: Antiseptics on wounds: An area of controversy. Wounds 2003; 15:149–166.

52. Selkorn, FJ, Cherry, GW, Wilson, JM, et al: Evaluation of hypochlorous acid washes in the treatment of chronic venous ulcers. J Wound Care 2006; 15:33.

53. Wang, L, Bassiri, M, Najafi, R, et al: Hypochlorous acid as a potential wound care agent. Stabilized hypochlorous acid: A component of the inorganic armamentarium of innate immunity. J Burn Wounds 2007; 6:65–79.

54. Topical antibiotics. Available at: http://yenoh93.medceu.com/index/courses/dermanti.htm. Accessed 12/08.

55. Bonner, MW, Benson, PM, James, WD: Topical antibiotics in dermatology. In: In: Wolff K, Goldsmith LA Kats SI, et al, Fitzpatrick's Dermatology in General Medicine, ed. 5. New York, McGraw-Hill, 1999.

56. Maillard, JY, Denyer, SP: Focus on silver. EWMA Journal 2006; 6:5–7.

57. Cooper, ML, Laxer, JA, Hansbrough, JF: The cytotoxic effects of commonly used topical antimicrobial agents on human fibroblasts and keratinocytes. J Trauma 1991; 31:775–782.

58. Lineaweaver, W, Howard, R, Soucy, D, et al: Topical antimicrobial toxicity. Arch Surg 1985; 120:267–270.

59. Lineaweaver, W, McMorris, S, Soucy, D, et al: Cellular and bacterial toxicities of topical antimicrobials. Plast Reconstr Surg 1985; 75:394–396.

60. Akiyama, H, Oono, T, Saito M, et al: Assessment of cadexomer iodine against *Staphylococcus aureus* biofilm in vivo and in vitro using confocal laser scanning microscopy. J Dermatol 2004; 31: 529–534.

61. Ahmed, AKJ, Hoekstra, MJ, Hage, JJ, et al: Honey-medicated dressing: Transformation of an ancient remedy into modern therapy. Ann Plast Surg 2003; 50:143–148.

62. Eddy, JJ, Gideonsen, MD: Topical honey for diabetic foot ulcers (observations from practice). J Fam Pract 2005; 54:533–535.

63. Dunford, C, Cooper, R, Molan, P, et al: The use of honey in wound management. Nurs Stand 2000; 15:63–68.

64. Namias, N: Honey in the management of infections. Surg Infect 2003; 4:219–226.

65. Molan, PC: Potential of honey in the treatment of wounds and burns. Am J Clin Dermatol 2001; 2:13–19.

66. Lusby, PE, Coombs, A, Wilkinson, JM: *Honey*: A potent agent for wound healing? J Wound Ostomy Continence Nurs 2002; 29(6):295–300.

67. Mulder, GD, Cavorsi, JP, Lee, DK: Polyhexamethylene biguanide (PHMB): An addendum to current topical antimicrobials. Wounds 2007; 19:173–182.

68. Moore, K, Gray, D: Using PHMB antimicrobial to prevent wound infection. Wounds UK 2007; 3:96–102.

69. Cuttino, C, Mejza, B, Krause, S, et al. Balancing a dynamic wound environment: Multicenter experience with a novel antimicrobial foam dressing containing PHMB. Ostomy Wound Manage 2009; 55(3):4–22.

70. Hydrofera blue. Available at: http://www.hydrofera.com/hydro_blue.html. Accessed 10/08.

71. White, R, Cutting, K: Exploring the effects of silver in wound management—What is optimal? Wounds 2006; 18:307–314.

72. Fong, J, Wood, F: Nanocrystalline silver dressings in wound management: A review. Int J Nanomedicine 2006; 1(4):441–449.

73. Percival, SL, Woods, E, Nutekpor, M, et al: Prevalence of silver resistance in bacteria isolated from diabetic foot ulcers and efficacy of solver-containing wound dressings. Ostomy Wound Manage 2008; 54:30–40.

chapter 9

The Role of Imaging in Wound Care

Maureen Heldmann, MD

Abbie Kemper-Martin, MD, PhD, CWS, MLT, FACCWS

In general, radiologic imaging does not play a major role in therapy of the uncomplicated wound. However, wounds that fail to heal as expected can be further investigated with imaging to identify negative contributory factors that can then be ameliorated. Compromise of vascular inflow and efflux and deep infection may be factors in impaired wound healing, and occult foreign bodies present a nidus for continued inflammatory or infectious complication. Many radiologic examinations are available to augment clinical diagnosis and can be performed either alone or in combination. All imaging modalities have inherent advantages and disadvantages, and the optimal choice of examination is guided by patient attributes and clinical context.

This chapter is divided into technical and clinical sections, first providing a basis for understanding radiologic studies with a description of common contrast agents and precautions. Clinical examples of vascular and soft tissue imaging pertinent to wound care follow, depicting common pathologic conditions with normal comparisons. Varied anatomy is depicted with an emphasis on the lower extremity, and suggested imaging algorithms are presented.

Physics and Contrast
Physical Basis of Modalities

X-rays

The basic premise for conventional radiographs (x-rays) and computed tomography involves the passage of an x-ray beam through the patient and generation of an image from the radiation that reaches a receptor. The receptor may be as simple as a single sheet of film or as complicated as the data acquisition system of a multidetector computed tomography system, and the amount of radiation passing through the patient to make the image is determined by the density of the anatomic patient structures it traverses. The x-ray beam is a form of ionizing radiation, and as such is a potential carcinogen that should be used wisely for diagnostic imaging.

Arteriograms

Catheter arteriography is performed under direct visualization with fluoroscopy, a specialized type of radiographic machine that allows continuous, or "real-time", x-ray visualization. Patients lie recumbent on an x-ray table with a mobile x-ray tube and detector on either side. A needle puncture is made into an artery, usually in the groin, through which a catheter is placed for injection of contrast material. In complicated cases, the x-ray tube may be turned on many times in short bursts, and radiation exposure is on the order of minutes, rather than seconds.

Ultrasound

Ultrasound is similar to sonar, and employs a pulsed, focused, high-frequency sound beam delivered and received by an ultrasound transducer. The beam is variably absorbed, deflected, and transmitted by different tissue types, and the amplitude, or strength, of the reflected ultrasound energy returning to the transducer is processed to make a gray-scale ultrasound image. In the context of vascular ultrasound, the direction and speed of flowing blood can be determined by means of the Doppler effect. Sound energy returning from moving objects will experience a measurable change in frequency that can be correlated with elapsed time and other known mathematic parameters to calculate the velocity of flow. (Fig. 9.1) To assist visualization color coding can be assigned to flowing blood depending upon the speed and direction of flow.

Computed Tomography

Computed tomography (CT), formerly called computed axial tomography (CAT scan), is a density-based radiographic technique that utilizes an x-ray tube emitting an x-ray beam traveling rapidly around the patient, and a sophisticated detector and computer system to collect and construct the radiation reaching the detectors into an anatomic image. The patient lies supine on a CT table that moves rapidly through an aperture while the scan is being performed. The exam is generally complete in a few seconds, rather than minutes, but is diagnostic only, unlike catheter arteriography, which allows the operator to perform therapy. Since un-opacified blood is similar to many other tissues in density, sterile iodinated contrast material is injected intravenously to increase the density, and therefore the visualization, of the vessel lumen.

Magnetic Resonance Imaging

Magnetic resonance imaging (MRI) is based upon an entirely different principle than the other modalities described. The magnetic resonance scanner consists of a large superconducting magnet, radiofrequency transmitter, and receiver coils. When a patient is placed in the large magnet, the protons in their atoms align within the magnetic field. With variable radiofrequency pulses turned rapidly on and off, small changes in the atomic energy states can be detected and used to generate detailed images. MRI is very sensitive

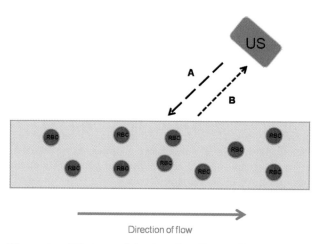

Figure 9•1 *Diagram of the Doppler effect in flowing blood. The frequency of a sound beam directed into (arrow A) and subsequently reflected from (arrow B) a blood vessel is changed in proportion to the speed and direction of blood flow. US, ultrasound transducer; RBC, red blood cell. Vessel lumen is depicted in blue.*

to physical differences between soft tissues and fluid, and image planes can be chosen to the anatomic plane of interest. Gadolinium contrast agents are often used, depending upon the clinical indication for the exam and body part examined, but flowing blood generates a signal of its own and may be detected without contrast agents in some cases. Examination times are considerably longer than computed tomography, often 10 to 20 minutes or more, depending upon the area being imaged. Because of the strong magnetic field, the MR environment is restricted to only those items that are not attracted to a magnet.

▶ **PEARL 9•1** The magnetic resonance (MR) environment is restricted to only those items that are not attracted to a magnet.

Wheelchairs, oxygen tanks, and cleaning equipment must be specially designed for use in the MR suite, and patients with implantable devices such as pacemakers or previous shrapnel injuries in proximity to vital structures are not suited to magnetic resonance imaging. Pre-scan questionnaires play a vital role in detecting such patients, preventing injury, and keeping everyone safe in the MR environment.

Nuclear Medicine

Nuclear medicine provides a unique tool in medical imaging and patient care. Although the detail, or resolution, obtained from nuclear medicine images is less than that from other modalities, these examinations offer functional information that is complementary to the anatomic data obtained by radiographs, ultrasound, CT, or MRI. A small amount of radioactivity in the form of a radionuclide is coupled to various stable compounds that localize to one or more organ systems to produce clinically useful radiopharmaceuticals. As the radionuclide decays, it emits a small amount of radioactivity that can be detected by a specialized camera. In the example of a nuclear medicine bone scan, the radiopharmaceutical would be a radionuclide-labeled phosphate injected intravenously, which is delivered to the skeletal structures through the vascular system and localizes to the bone over minutes to hours. The patient lies motionless on a table while a camera slowly moves around his or her body, capturing the small amount of radioactive decay emitted to make a picture. Nuclear medicine exams deliver a small amount of ionizing radiation to the patient, typically less than that from other exams that use x-rays.

Contrast Agents

Many formulations of contrast material are used in radiological imaging; the two groups most pertinent to this discussion are intravascular iodinated contrast for computed tomography and gadolinium-based intravascular agents used in magnetic resonance imaging.

Adverse reactions to intravascular contrast material are uncommon,[1] and vary from mild to life threatening. The reason some patients react negatively to radiographic contrast material is not well understood, but it is known that patients with pre-existing heart or kidney disease are at increased risk for reactions, as are those who have asthma, allergies, or a prior adverse event. Corticosteroid premedication regimens have been shown to decrease, but not eliminate, risk, and contrast agents should only be used when the benefit of information to be gained exceeds the potential risk and the same information cannot be obtained by another imaging modality without contrast material. In any radiological practice, care is given to pre-test identification of risk factors, hydration status, and immediate availability of emergency equipment and personnel.

Toxic renal effects of iodinated contrast administration are a significant contributor to in-hospital renal failure, and are of greatest concern in those patients with pre-existing renal insufficiency and diabetes mellitus. Patients with normal renal function are at very low risk for contrast-induced nephrotoxicity, and potential risk in those with cardiac or kidney disease may be reduced by careful patient selection, adequate hydration, choice of newer contrast agents, and possibly, premedication regimens aimed at decreasing renal risk.[2]

Specific mention is made of diabetic patients taking an oral antihyperglycemic medication containing the generic component metformin. Since metformin is excreted by the kidneys, any worsening of renal function may produce higher levels of drug in the blood than desired, placing the patient at risk for lactic acidosis. The accumulation of lactate in the blood has a high mortality, and although radiological contrast agents are not a direct cause of lactic acidosis, their potential to produce renal dysfunction in the diabetic population is a concern. For this reason, metformin should be temporarily discontinued in a patient undergoing imaging with an iodinated intravascular contrast agent and reinstituted only after renal function has been retested and documented as normal (generally 48 hours after the contrast injection).

> **PEARL 9•2** Metformin should be temporarily discontinued in a patient undergoing imaging with an iodinated intravascular contrast agent.

Gadolinium chelates are widely used as contrast agents for MRI and differ from iodine-based contrast in their chemical composition. In general, gadolinium contrast is much better tolerated than the contrast used for computed tomography, but patients with a history of allergies or previous contrast reactions are at increased risk for an adverse event with gadolinium. Another precaution has recently been described with gadolinium contrast agents with reference to their use in patients with renal impairment. In 2006 a rare disease consisting of skin swelling and tightening was first described in conjunction with the use of gadolinium MRI contrast in patients with impaired renal function.[3] Termed *nephrogenic systemic fibrosis*, the process has been found to involve other organs and

may be progressive or fatal. As more cases of possible causal affect accumulate, the Food and Drug Administration has issued a public health advisory and drug warning, which is available and updated on their website.[4]

Vascular Assessment—Arterial and Venous Systems

Multiple imaging options are available to determine normal arterial blood supply and to exclude venous disease. Vascular disease can be diagnosed and characterized, selecting patients for radiological or surgical intervention as appropriate.

Arterial Evaluation

Adequate delivery of oxygenated blood to the wound site may be limited by vascular disease when injury or atherosclerosis produces stenosis or occlusion of arterial inflow. The ankle-brachial index has long been used to estimate adequacy of arterial pressures in the lower extremities, and can be enhanced by plethysmography. (See Chapter 7 for additional information.) In this manner, the degree and level of arterial narrowing can be inferred, but the actual stenosis is not directly visualized.

The historical gold-standard for evaluation of the diseased artery has long been fluoroscopic or catheter angiography, a process in which a thin hollow tube is introduced directly into the vessel through a needle puncture. The catheter can then be advanced to the artery of interest and contrast material injected to produce a picture of the lumen. Advantages of this technique include the ability to intervene with balloon dilatation if a suitable stenosis is detected or to administer therapy such as drugs directly through the catheter when needed. However, catheter angiography is costly, time consuming, and invasive, and poses finite risks associated with the contrast agent and procedure. Bleeding from, or injury to, the blood vessel wall are well-known complications of vascular catheterization, with rates of 1.73% to 3.29%, depending upon the artery accessed.[5] Catheter angiogram findings of stenosis, occlusion, and balloon angioplasty are depicted in Figures 9.2 through 9.4.

Safer methods for diagnosing arterial disease have emerged with vascular applications of ultrasound (US), computed tomography, and magnetic resonance imaging. Rapid advancements in cross-sectional imaging such as CT and MRI now allow direct visualization of arterial and venous lumina in a noninvasive manner, using vascular contrast agents injected into peripheral veins without the need for large vessel catheterization.

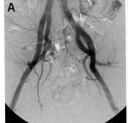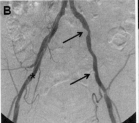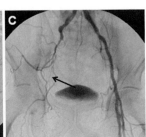

Figure 9•2 *Catheter pelvic arteriograms in three patients. A, normal iliac arteries; B, mild to moderate left iliac stenoses (arrows). The catheter can be faintly seen in the right iliac artery (*). C, right iliac artery occlusion (arrow).*

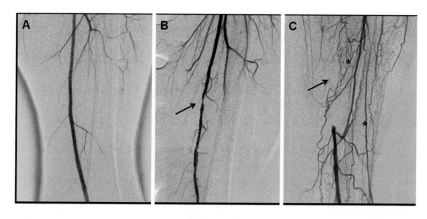

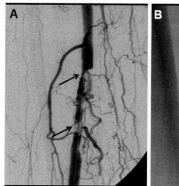

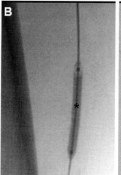

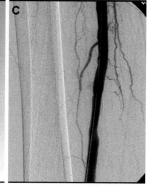

Figure 9•3 *Femoral artery catheter arteriograms in three patients. A, normal; B, moderate disease (arrow); C, a long segment occlusion (arrow). Many collateral vessels bypass the occlusion (*).*

Figure 9•4 *Femoral artery angioplasty. A severe femoral artery stenosis (arrows in A) is treated with balloon (*) dilatation angioplasty (B), with good result (C).*

Ultrasound of the aorta and peripheral arteries can be performed to assess the blood vessel wall for atherosclerotic plaque and lumen diameter for narrowing, and the addition of Doppler techniques allow determination of velocity, direction, and waveform analysis of flowing blood. Normal extremity arteries have uniform walls and taper smoothly as they branch into smaller blood vessels supplying the thigh, leg, and foot. The muscular compartments of the extremity at rest are supplied by arterioles that can dilate with activity to increase blood flow and oxygen delivery to the muscles but remain relatively constricted at rest. The arterial waveform in this high-resistance bed is therefore brisk and forward, or antegrade, in cardiac systole, with a short reversal of flow in early cardiac diastole due to elastic recoil of arterioles, followed by a smaller peak of forward flow before the next heartbeat. The characteristic waveform has three peaks and is therefore described as triphasic. (Fig. 9.5) Atherosclerosis is the result of plaques that form along the wall of the arteries and can be visualized protruding from the wall of the artery on ultrasound. (Fig. 9.6) As arterial disease progresses, collateral vessels may develop to maintain flow around the stenosis or occlusion; but these alternative pathways have lost their normal autoregulation, and the Doppler waveform appears low-velocity and antegrade throughout the cardiac cycle. The waveform from a collateral artery, or an artery distal to a stenosis, has a lower velocity and a slower peak, the so-called tardus-parvus waveform. Microbubble contrast agents injected intravenously increase the visibility of flowing blood but are not in widespread use. Advantages of ultrasound include a lack of ionizing radiation and the ability to perform portable examinations at the bedside of critically ill patients.

> ▶ **PEARL 9•3** The advantages of ultrasound include a lack of ionizing radiation and the ability to perform examinations bedside.

Multiple image planes can be obtained, anatomy can be viewed in real time during the examination, and very superficial structures can be evaluated. Difficulty visualizing deep structures, limited beam penetration in obese patients, in addition to dependence upon operator skill, are potential

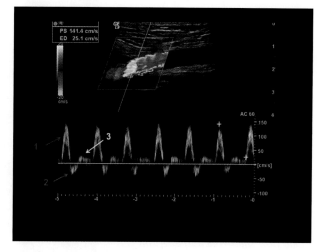

Figure 9•5 *Normal Doppler ultrasound waveform. Antegrade flow in systole (1) is followed by early diastolic flow reversal (2) and forward flow in late diastole (3).*

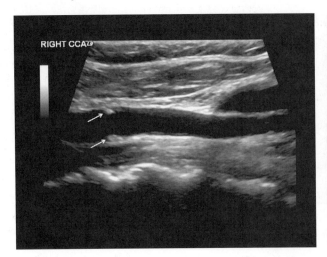

Figure 9•6 *Atherosclerotic carotid artery on US. The vessel wall is irregular, and two discrete plaques are denoted by arrows.*

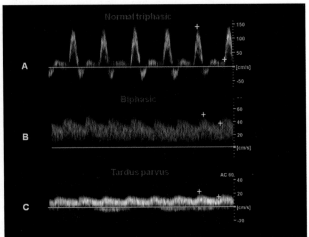

Figure 9•7 *Extremity arterial waveforms in health and disease. Normal triphasic (A). As arterial narrowing progresses, the peripheral muscle bed arterioles dilate. The waveform loses its high-resistance profile and reverse-flow phase and becomes biphasic (B) or monophasic with diminished velocity. When severe or occlusive, the artery distal to disease has a slow upstroke (tardus) and diminished peak (parvus) (C).*

disadvantages of this technique. Examples of normal and abnormal arterial walls, lumina, and waveforms are depicted in Figures 9.7 through 9.9.

CT angiography (CTA) is a term applied to the rapid acquisition of computed tomographic (CT) images through an arterial or venous region of interest after the intravenous injection of iodinated radiographic contrast. An upper extremity vein is the preferred injection site, and the contrast is administered by a power injector to achieve bright vascular enhancement. With state-of-the-art CT equipment and fast CT table movement, large anatomical regions such as the chest, abdomen, pelvis, and lower extremity arterial tree can be covered in a matter of seconds. The images can then be reprocessed to optimize the arterial information that can be gathered, displayed, and analyzed. Widely available software applications produce two- and

three-dimensional reconstructions for virtually limitless projections of the vessel lumen and wall, and semi-automated techniques allow bone to be "subtracted" to portray arteries alone. (Fig. 9.10) Calcified and noncalcified atherosclerotic plaque is well depicted, and quantitative software allows calculation of stenoses by diameter or area reduction. (Fig. 9.11) With greater than 90% sensitivity and specificity for hemodynamically significant lesions,[6] utilization of CT angiography has expanded rapidly and now includes investigation of extremely small vessels such as the coronary arteries. Although the advantages of computed tomography of the arterial and

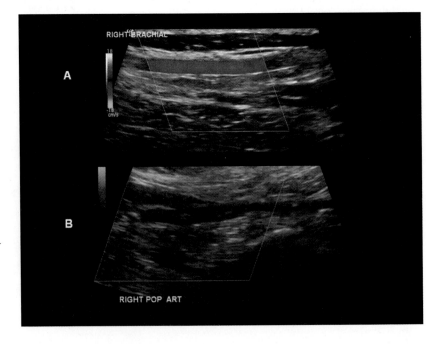

Figure 9•8 *Color Doppler flow. A normal upper extremity artery demonstrates complete luminal filling with blood flow color-coded to direction and velocity (A). (B) The artery contains very little color Doppler flow, compatible with severe disease.*

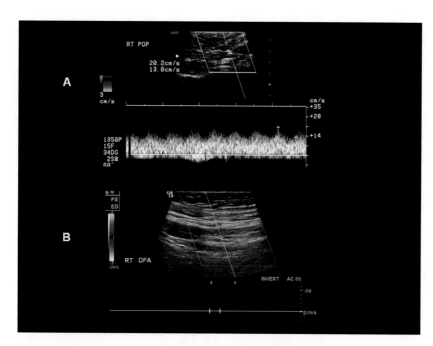

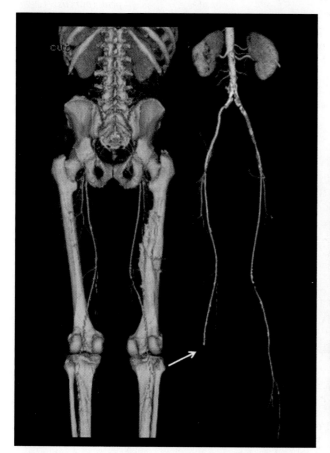

Figure **9•9** *Lower extremity arterial compromise in two patients. (A) Color flow is present, but the waveform is abnormally biphasic. The patient in (B) has no demonstrable flow in the deep femoral artery.*

venous systems include much shorter examination time and lower cost and risk than invasive catheter arteriograms, adverse drug effects of the contrast agent and the potential carcinogenic effects of ionizing radiation are still pertinent considerations in patient selection.

Magnetic resonance imaging is also applicable to interrogation of the vascular system, with multiple pulse sequences

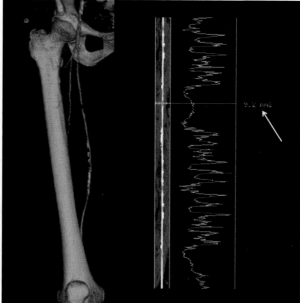

Figure **9•10** *Three-dimensional posterior view of CT arteriogram with bone subtraction. Interactive removal of bone allows better depiction of the left popliteal artery occlusion (arrow).*

Figure **9•11** *Three-dimensional right femoral artery CT arteriogram with quantitative analysis of lumen stenosis. The irregular arterial lumen diameter is depicted in green, and point-by-point measurements are available along the vessel (arrow).*

designed to evaluate the vessels, with or without contrast agents. Magnetic resonance angiography (MRA), unlike CTA, can be performed using only the inherent blood flow to obtain a picture, but most commonly gadolinium chelate intravenous agents are injected to produce vascular enhancement similar to the process described for CTA. Multiple anatomical regions, such as the arterial system of the abdomen, pelvis, and legs, can be imaged with a moving table technique, but magnetic resonance imaging takes somewhat longer than CT, cannot encompass the same amount of anatomy in a single exam, and does not have the resolution of nor depict calcifications as well as computed tomography. CT angiography may have some advantages over MR angiography,[7] but the major advantage of MRI over CT is that magnetic resonance imaging does not employ ionizing radiation, thus providing an alternative examination for those particularly sensitive to radiation, such as the pregnant or pediatric patient.

> **PEARL 9•4** The major advantage of magnetic resonance imaging (MRI) over computed tomography (CT) is that MRI does not employ ionizing radiation, making it useful for pregnant women and children.

Precautions regarding patient selection for magnetic resonance scans are described below, and both CT and MR tables have table weight limits that may decrease their availability to very obese patients. Examples of normal and abnormal MR angiograms are illustrated in Figures 9.12 and 9.13.

Venous Evaluation

Disease of the venous system is pertinent to wound care, such as venous valve incompetence, thrombosis, and stenosis. The primary modality for assessment of the deep venous system of the extremities is ultrasound, typically supplemented with

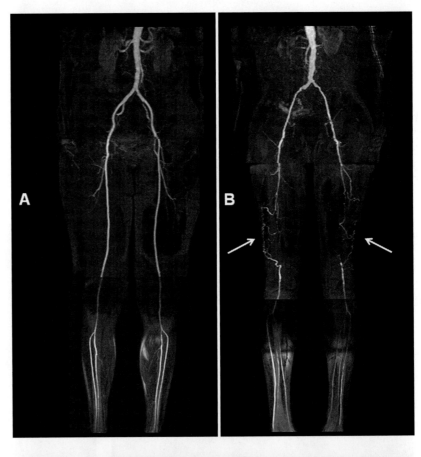

Figure 9•12 *Magnetic resonance arteriogram (MRA) of the aorta, iliac, and lower extremity arteries. Patient (A) has mild arterial wall irregularity, but no evidence of stenosis. Patient (B) has bilateral superficial femoral artery occlusion with reconstitution of popliteal arteries by collateral flow (arrow). Note that the exams are obtained as three separate images after sequential movement of the MR table and "pasted" together.*

Figure 9•13 *MRA of the superficial femoral arteries (SFA) in two patients. Patient (A) has smooth vessel walls and no evidence of stenosis. The arterial walls in patient (B) are more irregular, and there is a tight stenosis or short occlusion of the distal SFA (arrow).*

Doppler assessment of flow. As in the arterial system, the vein wall and lumen are both examined, with the addition of manual ultrasound transducer compression of the vein to temporarily obliterate the lumen and exclude thrombus.

> ▶ **PEARL 9•5** The primary modality for assessment of the deep venous system of the extremities is ultrasound.

The normal vein demonstrates a thin wall, complete compression, and forward (or antegrade) flow. (Fig. 9.14) Normal venous flow varies with respiration, increasing toward the heart with inspiration and slowing with expiration, and can be augmented with manual compression of the distal soft tissues, effectively "squeezing" more blood from the arm or leg into the vein. (Fig. 9.15) Extremity veins contain valves that limit backward flow during expiration, but varicose vein valves may become incompetent, with resultant retrograde blood flow that further potentiates vein enlargement. (Fig. 9.16) In patients with normal venous ultrasound examination results in whom valve incompetence is clinically suspected, the examination may be performed standing or with Valsalva maneuver to exaggerate the abnormality and increase sensitivity. All of these components are included in a comprehensive extremity venous ultrasound, which may be performed quickly, noninvasively, and portably at the bedside.

Thrombosis of the deep extremity veins (DVT) is a potentially life-threatening disorder with numerous medical and surgical risk factors including malignancy, immobilization, trauma, oral contraceptive use, and pregnancy. A venous clot may impair blood return to the heart, producing extremity swelling, and a thrombus can dislodge and travel through the heart to produce pulmonary thromboembolism (PTE). Venous thrombi are diagnosed by ultrasound when there is incomplete coaptation of vein walls with compression. Color Doppler flow in a clotted vein will be incomplete or absent,

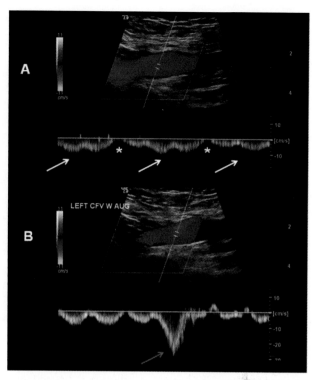

Figure 9•15 *Normal lower extremity venous waveform. The normal respiratory cycle is reflected in phasic changes (A). Cardiac blood return increases during inspiration (arrows) and decreases in expiration (*). Squeezing the distal leg increases, or augments, the blood return to the heart in a patent venous system (blue arrow in B).*

and the thrombus may be visualized as low-level echoes within the vein lumen. (Fig. 9.17) Poor or absent flow augmentation and loss of respiratory phasicity are indirect evidence of thrombosis and therefore potentially helpful but

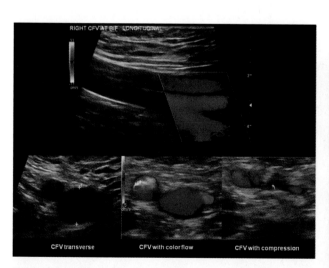

Figure 9•14 *Normal color Doppler ultrasound of the lower extremity venous system. The normal vein lumen contains no internal echogenic material, fills with color Doppler flow, and is completely compressible. Vein (blue) and artery (red) are color-coded by direction of flow. CFV, common femoral vein.*

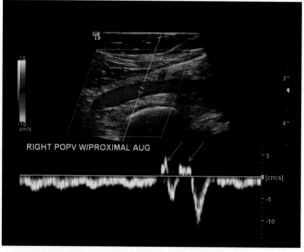

Figure 9•16 *Venous valve incompetence. Squeezing the leg above the vein being examined produces retrograde flow (blue arrows) in the lumen, indicating reflux of blood through an incompetent valve.*

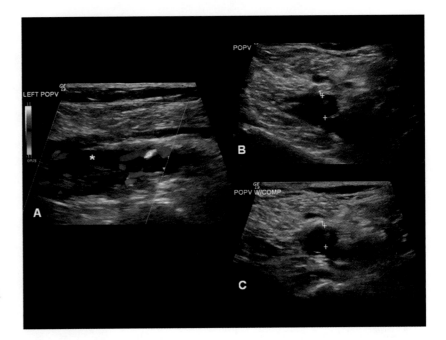

Figure 9•17 *(A–C) Lower extremity deep venous thrombosis. The vein lumen contains echogenic material (*), does not fill with color, and is not compressible (C).*

nonspecific signs. Ultrasound is excellent in the detection of proximal lower extremity deep venous thrombosis, but sensitivity drops off in the calf,[8] and the pelvic veins above the inguinal ligament are not well visualized with sonographic techniques.

CT venography (CTV) is a form of CT angiography in which intravenous contrast opacification and scanning are timed to the venous system. CTV can reveal an occlusive or nonocclusive thrombus (Fig. 9.18) and is used in some institutions in combination with CT angiography of the pulmonary arteries for comprehensive evaluation of suspected PTE and lower extremity DVT. CT venography is better able to confirm or exclude pelvic vein thrombosis than ultrasound, but is not portable and has the same disadvantages as CTA.

MRI can be utilized for venography (MRV) in much the same way as MR arteriography, but it is not as widely available as ultrasound and requires greater examination time and cost. Direct catheter-insertion venogram techniques are uncommonly performed for diagnosis in current radiological practice, but are appropriate when other studies are equivocal or when interventions such as thrombolysis, dilatation of stenosis, and stent placement are needed. (Fig. 9.19)

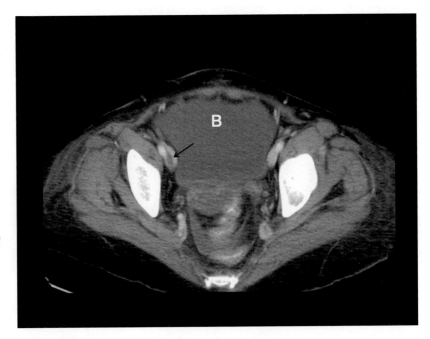

Figure 9•18 *CT venography. Computed tomography performed 2 to 3 minutes after contrast injection can detect iliac vein clot (arrow) in areas not amenable to ultrasound compression. B, urinary bladder.*

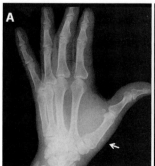

Figure **9•19** *Catheter venography for intervention. (A) A filling defect consistent with thrombus is present in an enlarged femoral venous lumen (white arrow), distal to a focal stenosis (black arrow). Balloon (*) dilatation (B) can improve the narrowing. (C) In some cases, stents may be placed.*

Soft Tissue Infection

Traumatized or poorly vascularized tissue is susceptible to breakdown, infection, and subsequent abscess development. Current imaging techniques facilitate the diagnosis of numerous causes of delayed wound healing, and are frequently used in therapeutic procedures such as abscess drainage and biopsy. This section will illustrate several causes of wound complication, from foreign bodies to deep soft tissue infection, including osteomyelitis.

Foreign Bodies

Retained foreign bodies may be a source of acute infection, or a contributory factor in chronic wounds, and are frequently located in the hands and feet. Wooden splinters, glass, and needles are commonly encountered foreign bodies, and the ability to recognize these objects on radiographs depends on their inherent density. (Fig. 9.20) Metal objects are easily recognizable (Fig. 9.20C) and glass fragments can be detected with radiography, but wooden foreign bodies are difficult to see with x-rays alone and require a high degree of suspicion for identification. Ultrasound is an excellent modality for the detection of superficially located foreign bodies, as nonanatomic material may reflect or block the ultrasound beam in a manner much different than the skin, subcutaneous fat, and muscle. Foreign bodies appear as bright reflectors on ultrasound (Fig. 9.21), and sensitivities and specificities of 90% and 96.7% have been reported for wooden foreign bodies as small as 2.5 mm.[9] However, the sound beam cannot penetrate very deep tissues, and the marrow cavity of bone is not amenable to ultrasound assessment. CT or MRI may detect clinically unsuspected foreign bodies during assessment of a chronic or draining wound, and both can be employed in select cases. However, they are more expensive than radiographs or ultrasound. The appearance of foreign bodies on CT and MRI is variable depending upon the density and composition of the material, and the surrounding inflammatory soft tissue reaction may predominate. A radiographically occult foreign body is illustrated in Figure 9.22.

Deep Soft Tissue Infection

Radiologic studies are not clinically necessary to diagnose soft tissue swelling and ulceration (Fig. 9.23) but provide a means to more precisely assess the extent of the inflammatory process and determine the tissues involved. Local symptoms such as pain and erythema are generally present, and deep soft tissue infections commonly manifest as focal collections of purulent material or abscesses. The tissue swelling produced by infection tends to be poorly defined, and subcutaneous air may be evident on radiographs from gas-forming organisms or abscesses. (Fig. 9.20B). Draining wounds or sinus tracts can be injected with contrast under direct x-ray visualization to confirm or exclude that an abscess communicates with underlying bone in an examination called a *fistulogram*. (Fig. 9.24) Ultrasound provides a rapid, inexpensive, readily available tool to detect superficial fluid collections, and real-time visualization affords guidance for diagnostic aspiration or therapeutic drainage. (Fig. 9.25). Sonographic features of soft tissue abscesses vary, with a classic appearance of a mixed echo collection with irregular borders (Fig. 9.26), often with internal debris, septation, and increased vascularity of the surrounding area.

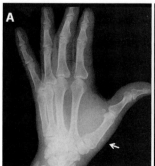
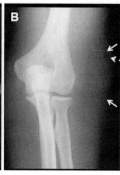
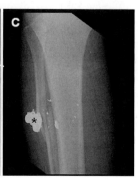

Figure **9•20** *Foreign bodies in three patients. (A) Small fangs are faintly seen on hand x-ray (arrow) after a snakebite. (B) Two needles are well depicted on radiographs, and a small gas collection (broken arrow) is consistent with recent soft tissue trauma or abscess. (C) Bullets and bullet fragments (*) are easily detected on radiographs due to the high density of metal.*

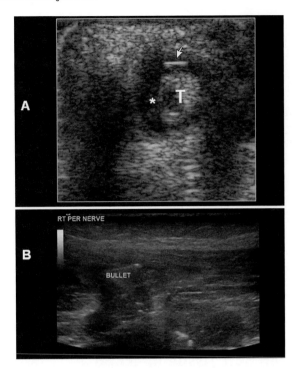

Figure 9•21 *US of foreign bodies. Two patients with superficial foreign bodies. (A) Transverse image of the finger. A small linear echo in close proximity to a long finger tendon (T) (arrow) represents a foreign body. A crescent of dark fluid within the tendon sheath is indicated (*). (B) Same patient as 9.20. (C) Longitudinal image of the leg. The bullet appears as a linear bright reflector of the ultrasound beam (annotated).*

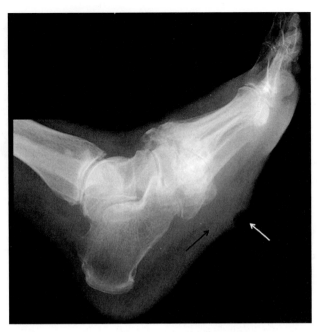

Figure 9•23 *Lateral radiograph of the foot. A soft tissue ulcer is evident on the midfoot plantar surface (white arrow). The underlying subcutaneous fat density is increased, consistent with edema or inflammation (black arrow; compare with the fat of the calcaneal heel pad).*

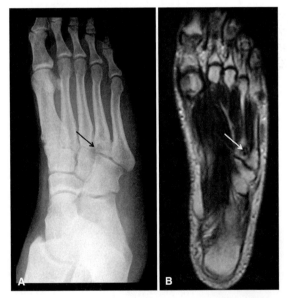

Figure 9•22 *Oblique radiograph (A) and axial MRI (B) of the right foot. Bone destruction is noted in the base of the fourth metatarsal and adjacent cuneiform and cuboid (black arrow). An unsuspected linear low-signal foreign body surrounded by a small amount of bright fluid is revealed on MR (arrow). Surgery recovered a football cleat embedded in the bone from an athletic incident months previously.*

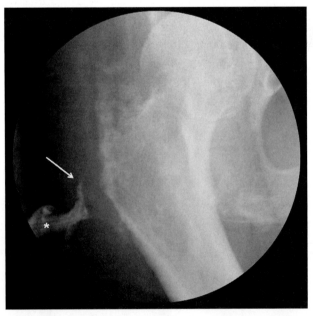

Figure 9•24 *Fistulogram. A catheter (*) is used to inject contrast material (arrow) into a sinus or draining wound tract. In this case, no communication with the underlying femur is demonstrated.*

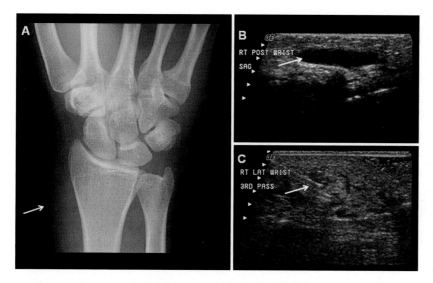

Figure 9•25 *US for diagnosis and therapy of soft tissue infection. This patient experienced persistent swelling, erythema, and pain after an animal bite despite antibiotic therapy. Radiograph of the region (A) revealed soft tissue swelling (arrow) with confirmation of an underlying fluid collection on US (arrow B). Aspiration recovered a small amount of purulent fluid, and total abscess evacuation was accomplished (C). Arrow indicates needle tip.*

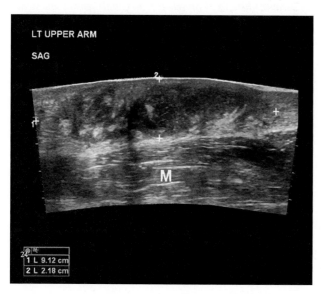

Figure 9•26 *Longitudinal US of soft tissue abscess. A large irregular collection with varying echogenicity lies deep to the skin and superficial to the muscle (M) in the lateral upper extremity. Surgical incision and drainage confirmed* S. aureus *abscess.*

(Fig. 9.27) For infections that are deeper and less amenable to ultrasound detection, CT with the addition of intravenous contrast may reveal an irregular or loculated fluid density collection with a rim of enhancement. (Fig. 9.28) Computed tomography can be used to guide drain placement in deep-set abscesses, allowing a minimally invasive alternative to open surgical procedures.

MRI is superior to CT in soft tissue assessment and can be used to identify even very small abscesses. Normal fat appears bright on the major pulse sequences used in clinical MRI, normal muscle is intermediate or gray, and cortical bone is perceived as a thin black line. When inflammation develops due to trauma or infection, the normal signal of fat in the subcutaneous tissues and bone marrow is changed, and the muscle signal may become altered in deep infections. As abscesses develop, collections of purulent material can be identified within the subcutaneous fat or muscle (Figs. 9.29 and 9.30), as a peripheral rim of enhancing vascular tissue surrounding a central necrotic or non-enhancing core. The depth of involvement, including components such as skin, subcutaneous tissue, fascia, muscle, periosteum, cortex, and bone marrow, can all be visualized. Examinations can be repeated to evaluate treatment efficacy without the cumulative radiation penalty of CT.

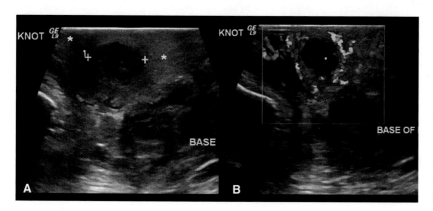

Figure 9•27 *Transverse US of scrotal soft tissue abscess. The scrotal wall is thickened (*), and a small mixed echo collection is measured on (A). With color Doppler, there is remarkable surrounding vascularity consistent with hyperemia (B). Drainage and culture return methicillin-resistant* S. aureus *(MRSA).*

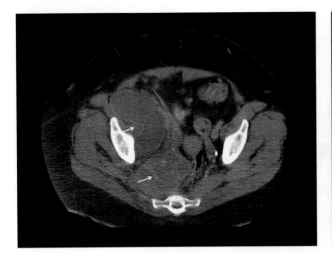

Figure 9•28 *CT of soft tissue abscess. In deep areas of the body not amenable to ultrasound, computed tomography can investigate for abscess. Loculated fluid density collections (arrows) with internal septation or surrounding inflammatory changes can be aspirated for diagnosis and treated percutaneously with catheter drainage.*

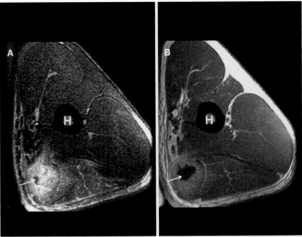

Figure 9•30 *MR of muscle infection. Axial/transverse images of the arm with T2 and T1 contrast-enhanced pulse sequences. (A) A poorly marginated bright signal abnormality involves the triceps muscle (arrow), with central low signal on T1 (arrow in B) and peripheral enhancement. S. aureus was diagnosed on needle aspiration. The normal marrow signal and dark cortex of the humerus (H) are maintained.*

Osteomyelitis

Osteomyelitis is the term used to describe infection of the bone and bone marrow and occurs through several pathways. Most commonly, organisms spread to the bone from an adjacent soft tissue infection, but they can also be directly inoculated into bone by penetrating injury or surgery or reach the bone marrow through the bloodstream. Trauma, ischemia, diabetes mellitus, and foreign bodies predispose to osteomyelitis, and clinical evidence of infection such as fever, pain, edema, erythema, and wound drainage are often present. The most common organism producing acute osteomyelitis is *Staphylococcus aureus*, although other bacteria or fungi

can occur with greater than general population frequency in intravenous drug abusers or patients with sickle cell disease or immunosuppression. Wound culture is virtually always performed to identify the causative pathogen and determine the most appropriate antibiotics to eradicate the infection. Diabetics and bedbound patients are two special groups at risk for osteomyelitis, the former typically in the foot as a consequence of impaired blood supply and sensation and the latter in the ischia and sacrum from pressure ulcers. In these instances, soft tissue breakdown exposes the osseous structures beneath, and infection can then extend contiguously to contaminate the bone.

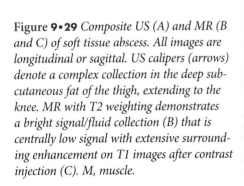
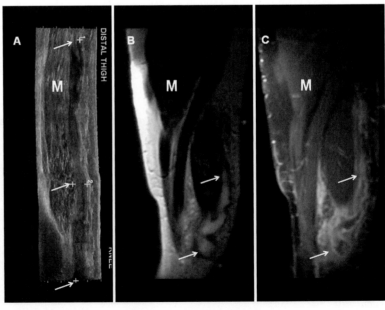

Figure 9•29 *Composite US (A) and MR (B and C) of soft tissue abscess. All images are longitudinal or sagittal. US calipers (arrows) denote a complex collection in the deep subcutaneous fat of the thigh, extending to the knee. MR with T2 weighting demonstrates a bright signal/fluid collection (B) that is centrally low signal with extensive surrounding enhancement on T1 images after contrast injection (C). M, muscle.*

Early in the course of the infection, x-rays of the affected area may demonstrate soft tissue ulceration or edema, but initial radiographs may be normal. Periosteal reaction and bone destruction generally require 10 to 14 days to develop (Fig. 9.31), and the sensitivity of radiographs for the detection of bone infection is limited.

> **PEARL 9•6** Periosteal reaction and bone destruction generally require 10 to 14 days to develop.

Since antibiotic treatment for bone infection must be more aggressive and continued for a longer period of time than therapy for soft tissue infection alone, the distinction is clinically important. CT is more sensitive than plain film radiography for findings such as bone erosion and periosteal reaction, and computed tomography can also identify adjacent soft tissue abscess or foreign bodies. Although osseous detail is better evaluated with CT, the initial findings of bone infection are marrow edema and inflammation, and the imaging modalities of greatest utility in the detection of early-stage osteomyelitis are magnetic resonance imaging and nuclear medicine bone scans.

> **PEARL 9•7** The imaging modalities of greatest utility in the detection of early-stage osteomyelitis are magnetic resonance imaging and nuclear medicine bone scans.

Magnetic resonance imaging signs of osteomyelitis include signal alteration compatible with increased marrow fluid and associated abnormal marrow enhancement. Evidence of marrow edema and inflammation is not specific for infection, but extensive marrow signal change and periosteal reaction support the diagnosis of osteomyelitis. Sinus tracts, abscesses, and cortical destruction may be present. (Fig. 9.32) The pattern and location of the signal intensity are important clues, as pedal osteomyelitis results almost exclusively from contiguous infections and is most frequent adjacent to the fifth and first metatarsophalangeal joints.[10] Imaging features of osteomyelitis may overlap with those of neuropathic arthropathy, complicating diagnosis, and the distinction between neuropathic diabetic foot disease and superimposed infection may be difficult.

Nuclear medicine scans using a radiopharmaceutical that is delivered to bone help to distinguish between bone and soft tissue inflammatory change when performed in three phases. Images acquired from the affected area immediately after the radiopharmaceutical is injected reflect the vascular supply or angiographic phase, and are followed by images in the blood pool (or soft tissue phase) minutes later and delayed (or bone phase) after several hours have elapsed. Hyperemia, or increased blood flow, is reflected as abnormally high delivery of the radiopharmaceutical to the inflamed region, and soft tissue inflammation is manifest as increased activity in the second, or blood pool, phase.

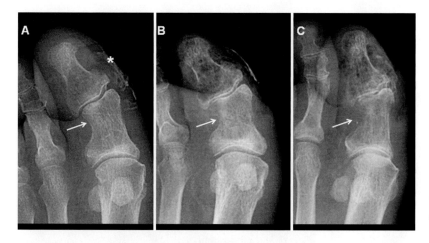

Figure 9•31 *Sequential radiographs of the foot in a diabetic with soft tissue ulceration. Early x-ray (A) demonstrates bandage material over the great toe (*), with intact lateral proximal phalangeal cortex (arrow). Over the course of 2 weeks (B and C), soft tissue gas is progressive and cortical destruction is evident (arrow).*

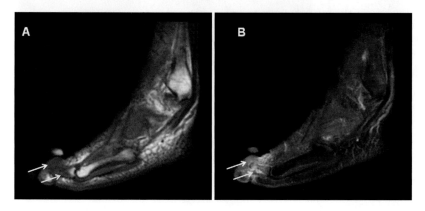

Figure 9•32 *(A and B) MR of the fifth toe in a diabetic patient with soft tissue infection. Signal changes are evident in both the soft tissue (white arrow) and bone marrow. There is abnormal enhancement of the phalangeal marrow (yellow arrow) and loss of cortical signal compatible with bone infection.*

Increased bone activity on the delayed phase is seen in a variety of conditions and is poorly specific. However, when increased uptake in the first two phases is coupled with abnormal accumulation of the radiopharmaceutical in the bone on delayed phase, osteomyelitis is likely. (Fig. 9.33) Nuclear medicine three-phase bone scans may be abnormal as early as 24 to 72 hours following infection onset, with the caveat that complicated cases such as those with neuropathic bone changes or recent fracture may be prone to false-positive bone scans. In this select population, the patient's white blood cells can be labeled with a radionuclide and reinjected intravenously. As leukocytes migrate to areas

▶ **PEARL 9•8** Nuclear medicine three-phase bone scans may be abnormal as early as 24 to 72 hours following onset of infection.

of inflammation, the radioactivity can be identified and localized to soft tissue or bone to raise specificity. (Fig. 9.34)

Infection lasting longer than 6 weeks is considered to be chronic and may be reflected by plain film findings of sclerosis, cortical thickening, sequestrum (a small island of dead bone within a cavity), or distorted local architecture. (Figs. 9.35 and 9.36).

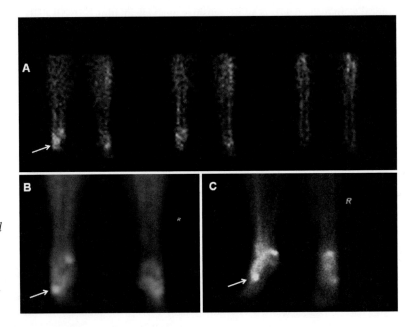

Figure 9•33 *Nuclear medicine three-phase bone scan. The radiopharmaceutical is asymmetrically delivered (flow phase A) to the left foot, and the soft tissue phase (blood pool B) depicts focal abnormality along the lateral fifth metatarsal. Hours later, the delayed phase (C) reveals increasing localization of the radiopharmaceutical to the bone (arrow) consistent with osteomyelitis.*

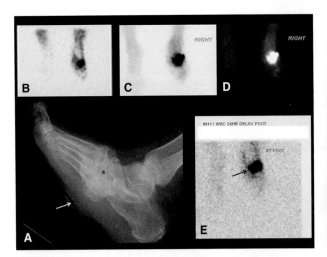

Figure 9•34 *(A) Composite foot radiograph, (B–D) nuclear medicine bone scan, and (E) tagged white blood cell scan. Plantar soft tissue swelling and gas (arrow) corresponded clinically to a chronic wound in a diabetic patient with midfoot distortion (*) compatible with neuropathic change. A three-phase bone scan (B–D) was positive. Tagged white cell scan pursued to increase specificity (E) is positive for focal increased uptake of the radiopharmaceutical in the midfoot consistent with active infection (arrow).*

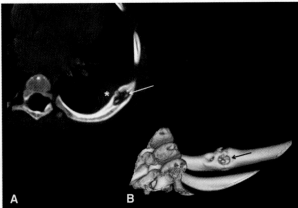

Figure 9•35 *Sequestrum on CT. Axial (A) and three-dimensional (B) reconstructed CT images of the left chest wall. A single left rib is expanded, and small bone fragments are contained within a cavity (arrow). The surrounding soft tissue is thickened (*). Incisional biopsy was positive for methicillin-resistant S. aureus.*

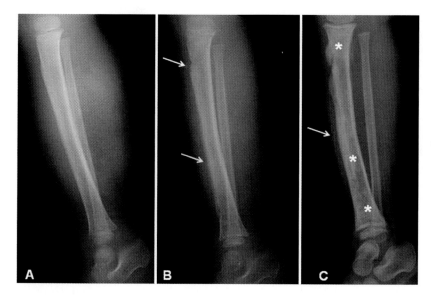

Figure 9•36 *Serial radiographs of the leg over a 4-week period. Initial film (A) is significant for diffuse soft tissue swelling. The tibia is intact. Over 12 days (B), the anterior tibia develops irregular ill-defined periosteal reaction (yellow arrow) and areas of bone destruction (white arrow). After 1 month (C), the anterior tibial cortex is cloaked in thick periosteal reaction (arrow), the tibial medullary canal is mottled (*), and the soft tissue has atrophied.*

Summary

Radiologic imaging is a powerful tool in the armamentarium of the clinician faced with the assessment of the non-healing wound. Venous, arterial, and soft tissue investigation can be pursued noninvasively to identify contributory factors such as stenosis, thrombosis, deep infection, or foreign bodies, and interventional techniques offer image-guided therapies in the vascular and musculoskeletal systems.

The choice of imaging modality depends upon the patient's overall condition, body habitus, and suspected pathology. The American College of Radiology (ACR) publishes evidence-based guidelines developed by expert panels to assist referring physicians and other health care providers in making the most appropriate imaging or treatment decision. Radiologic examinations are numerically ranked by appropriateness to the clinical context and the relative radiation level (RRL) each method delivers to the patient are included. ACR criteria for arterial disease/claudication, suspected venous thrombosis, and osteomyelitis in patients with diabetes mellitus are reproduced with permission in Tables 9.1, 9.2, and 9.3.[11] Many exams offer complementary information, and each modality has inherent advantages and limitations. The availability of equipment or personnel may influence the selection of imaging methods, and the ultimate decision regarding the appropriateness of any specific radiologic examination must be made by the referring physician and radiologist in light of the circumstances. A combination of studies may be needed to offer comprehensive patient care and direct treatment to achieve optimal outcome. Consultation with a local radiologist is suggested regarding precautions, contraindications, and contrast agents, especially in complex or particularly challenging cases.

Table 9•1	American College of Radiology: ACR Appropriateness Criteria®: Clinical Condition: Claudication-Suspected Vascular Etiology		
Radiologic Procedure	**Rating**	**Comments**	**RRL**
Ultrasound segmental Doppler pressures	9	Should be performed with exercise in this clinical scenario	None
aAngiography lower extremity	7	Indicated to guide intervention once vascular diagnosis is established by SDP-PVR, non-invasive imaging, and/or physical exam	Low
MRA lower extremity with contrast	8	See statement regarding contrast in text under "Anticipated Exceptions"	None
CTA lower extremity	8		Medium
US lower extremity with Doppler	6		None

Rating scale: 1, least appropriate; 9, most appropriate.
RRL, relative radiation level; SDP, segmental Doppler pressures; PVR, pulse volume recordings; MRA, magnetic resonance angiography; CTA, computed tomography angiography; US, ultrasound.
Reprinted with permission of the American College of Radiology. No other representation of this material is authorized without express, written permission from the American College of Radiology. You should access the ACR website at www.acr.org/ac for the most *current and complete* version of the ACR Appropriateness Criteria® topics.

Table 9•2 American College of Radiology: ACR Appropriateness Criteria®: Clinical Condition: Suspected Lower Extremity Deep Vein Thrombosis

Radiologic Procedure	Rating	Comments	RRL
US lower extremity duplex Doppler with compression	9		None
Venography pelvis	6	When other studies equivocal or an intervention is planned.	NS
MRI venography lower extremity	6	Demonstrated to be useful, but insufficient supporting data so far.	None
CT pelvis with contrast	6	As an adjunct to CTPA done for suspected PE.	Medium
Venography lower extremity	5	When other studies equivocal or an intervention is planned.	Medium
CT venography lower extremity (following arm injection)	5	As an adjunct to CTPA done for suspected PE.	Medium
Radionuclide venography lower extremity	3		Medium
X-ray lower extremity	2		Minimal
US continuous wave Doppler (nonimaging) lower extremity	1		None

CTPA, computed tomography pulmonary angiography; PE, pulmonary embolism; NS, not specified.
Reprinted with permission of the American College of Radiology. No other representation of this material is authorized without express, written permission from the American College of Radiology. You should access the ACR website at www.acr.org/ac for the most *current and complete* version of the ACR Appropriateness Criteria® topics.

Table 9•3 American College of Radiology: ACR Appropriateness Criteria®: Clinical Condition: Suspected Osteomyelitis in Patients with Diabetes Mellitus

Variant 1: Soft-tissue edema without ulcer or neuroarthropathy.

Radiologic Procedure	Rating	Comments	RRL
X-ray foot	9	Initial study. Radiographs and MRI are complementary. Both are indicated.	Minimal
MRI foot with contrast	9	Radiographs and MRI are complementary. Both are indicated. Useful for mapping devitalized areas preoperatively.	None
MRI foot without contrast	9	Radiographs and MRI are complementary. Both are indicated.	None
NUC Tc-99m 3-phase bone scan and In-111 WBC scan foot	4	If MRI contraindicated.	High
NUC Tc-99m 3-phase bone scan foot	1		Medium
NUC In-111 WBC scan and Tc-99m sulfur colloid marrow scan foot	1		High
NUC Tc-99m 3-phase bone scan and In-111 WBC scan and Tc-99m sulfur colloid marrow scan foot	1		High
US foot	1		None
CT foot without contrast	1		Minimal
FDG-PET foot	1		High

Rating scale: 1, least appropriate; 9, most appropriate.
RRL, relative radiation level; NUC, nuclear; WBC, white blood cell; FDG-PET, fluoro-deoxyglucose positron emission tomography; Tc, technetium; In, indium.
Reprinted with permission of the American College of Radiology. No other representation of this material is authorized without express, written permission from the American College of Radiology. You should access the ACR website at www.acr.org/ac for the most *current and complete* version of the ACR Appropriateness Criteria® topics.
Rating scale: 1, least appropriate; 9, most appropriate.
RRL, relative radiation level;
Reprinted with permission of the American College of Radiology. No other representation of this material is authorized without express, written permission from the American College of Radiology. You should access the ACR website at www.acr.org/ac for the most *current and complete* version of the ACR Appropriateness Criteria® topics.

Further Resources

Middleton, WD, Kurtz, AB, Hertzberg, BS (eds): Ultrasound: The Requisites. St. Louis, Mosby, 2004.

Mettler, FA, Guiberteau, MJ (eds): Essentials of Nuclear Medicine Imaging, ed. 3. Philadelphia, WB Saunders, 1991.

PA Kaplan, CA Helms, R Dussault, et al: Musculoskeletal Infection. In: Musculoskeletal MRI. Philadelphia, WB Saunders, 2001, pp 101–122, http://mrsafety.com

Resnick, D: Diagnosis of Bone and Joint Disorders, ed 4. Philadelphia, WB Saunders, 1995.

References

1. American College of Radiology. Manual on Contrast Media. Available at: www.acr.org/SecondaryMainMenuCategories/quality_safety/contrast_manual.aspx. Accessed 10/19/09.
2. Gleeson, TG, Bulugahapitiya, S: Contrast-induced nephropathy. Am J Roentgenol 2004; 183:1673–1689.
3. Grobner, T: Gadolinium—A specific trigger for the development of nephrogenic fibrosing dermopathy and nephrogenic systemic fibrosis? Nephrol Dial Transplant 2006; 21:1104–1108.
4. Available from: http://www.fda.gov/Drugs/DrugSafety/PostmarketDrugSafetyInformationforPatientsandProviders/ucm142911.htm accessed 11/8/09.
5. Hessel, SJ, Adams, DF, Abrams, HL: Complications of angiography. Radiology 1981; 138:273–281.
6. Heijenbrok-Kal, MH, Kock, MCJM, Hunink, MGM: Lower extremity arterial disease: Multidetector CT angiography—Meta-analysis. Radiology 2007; 245:433–439.
7. Ouwendijk, R, de Vries, M, Pattynama, PMT, van Sambeek, MRHM, et al: Imaging peripheral vascular disease: A randomized controlled trial comparing contrast-enhanced MR angiography and multi-detector row CT angiography. Radiology 2005; 236:1094–1103.
8. Kearon, C, Julian, JA, Math, M, et al. Noninvasive diagnosis of deep venous thrombosis. Ann Intern Med 1998; 128:663–677.
9. Jacobson, JA, Powell, A, Craig, JG, et al: Wooden foreign bodies in soft tissue: Detection at US. Radiology 1998; 206:45–48.
10. Ledermann, HP, Morrison, WB, Schweitzer, ME: MR image analysis of pedal osteomyelitis: Distribution, patterns of spread, and frequency of associated ulceration and septic arthritis. Radiology 2002; 223:747–755.
11. American College of Radiology. ACR appropriateness criteria. Available at: http://www.acr.org/SecondaryMainMenuCategories/quality_safety/app_criteria.aspx. Accessed 10/19/09.

chapter 10

Identification and Management of Atypical Wounds

Asha R. Patel, MD
Robert S. Kirsner, MD, PhD

Introduction

A variety of etiologies cause chronic wounds, which are frequently seen in medical practices around the world. These chronic wounds can be caused by long-standing diabetes mellitus (diabetic foot ulcers), poor arterial supply (arterial ulcers), venous insufficiency (venous leg ulcers), neurological deficit (neuropathic ulcers), and prolonged pressure (pressure ulcers or bed sores).[1] Wounds secondary to more unusual sources are called atypical wounds, and as a result, some are rare and intricate in nature. Atypical wounds have a spectrum of etiologies, including inflammatory processes, vasculopathies, infectious disease, metabolic disorder, genetic disease, neoplastic origination, and external trauma or injury.[2] It is estimated that out of 500,000 leg ulcers in the United States alone, an expected 10% are caused by atypical or unusual etiologies.[1] Therefore, it is essential for all health-care specialists to be familiar with this medical issue, including identification and treatment of unusual wound etiologies.

An atypical etiology for a wound must be considered within a differential diagnosis when (1) the location of the wound varies from that of a common or chronic wound, (2) the clinical presentation is unique and different from that of a common or chronic wound, or (3) the suspicious wound fails to respond to standard treatment regimens.[2,3] Since many atypical wounds tend to present similar to each other, a definitive diagnosis based on visualization alone is often difficult, and lesional biopsies are warranted and often crucial for diagnosis. Histopathological evaluation with adjunct studies such as special staining, tissue cultures, or immunofluorescence is essential to properly evaluate a wound once it is suspected to be of an atypical nature. It is also important that a comprehensive history and physical examination be undertaken to accurately diagnose the cause of the wound. Aspects of the patient's history to be taken into account during the workup are the following: epidemiological exposure, family history, personal or unusual habits, recreational and hobby activities, employment history, recent travel, sexual history, substance abuse history, known history of systemic illnesses, immunosuppression status, and laboratory blood testing.[3-5]

> ▶ **PEARL 10•1** An atypical etiology for a wound must be considered within a differential diagnosis when (1) the location of the wound varies from that of a common or chronic wound, (2) the clinical presentation is different from that of a common or chronic wound, or (3) the suspicious wound fails to respond to standard treatment regimens.

> ▶ **PEARL 10•2** Histopathological evaluation with adjunct studies such as special staining, tissue cultures, or immunofluorescence is essential to properly evaluate a wound once it is suspected to be of an atypical nature.

Inflammatory Etiologies

An inflammatory etiology of a wound is identified when the process resulting in ulcer formation primarily involves inflammation as the causative factor. Fundamentally, all skin ulcerations must have an inflammatory component; however, an inflammatory ulcer is defined as directly leading to cutaneous breakdown and ulcer formation.[6] There are a variety of interesting atypical wounds resulting strictly from an inherently inflammatory ulcer, namely vasculitis and pyoderma gangrenosum. In this chapter we will also discuss in detail other causes of inflammatory ulcers that are not as common.

Vasculitis

Cutaneous vasculitis is an umbrella term for a host of diseases distinguished by vascular inflammation of the arterioles, capillaries, and venules that may eventually lead to necrosis of the vasculature and end organ damage. With its all-encompassing pathogenesis, cutaneous vasculitis evidently displays a wide spectrum of clinical manifestations. The classic phenotype is leukocytoclastic vasculitis with palpable purpura; however, clinical presentation depends upon the organ involvement.[7,8] (Fig. 10.1) Clinically, the size of the underlying vessel affected determines the vasculitis appearance. Involvement of the superficial plexus of cutaneous vessels will most likely display a reticulated erythematous pattern (livedo reticularis), whereas inflamed larger and deeper vessels are more likely to reveal widespread ulcerative purpura and necrosis. The physician should also be alert to the fact that cutaneous involvement can reveal an underlying vasculitis in various end organs, such as the renal system, pulmonary system, central nervous system, and gastrointestinal tract.[9,10]

Tissue biopsies are crucial for diagnosing the specific type of vasculitis and should be sampled from lesions that are early in development, for example between 18 and 48 hours of the lesion's age.[10] Under a timely histopathological examination in lesions of leukocytoclastic vasculitis, pathology will show angiocentric segmental inflammation, fibrinoid necrosis, and a neutrophilic infiltrate around the blood vessel walls with erythrocyte extravasation.[7] Not only should the biopsy sample be taken early, but to attain a more accurate diagnosis it is recommended that the skin biopsy extend into the subcutis in order to identify the dominant inflammatory cell and the degree to which the vessels are affected.[11] Circulating immune antibody-antigen complexes are causative factors in many types of vasculitis.[12] These complexes deposit in blood vessel walls, and therefore special serological evaluations, histopathology special stains, and direct immunofluorescence can also be used if the clinical situation warrants further investigation.[10] If the biopsy is performed later in the course of wound development, pathology may not show immunoreactants as inflammatory cells present in the wound may lead to degrading of immunoglobulins present.[3]

If the diagnosis is confirmed by clinicopathological correlation, the causative agent must be addressed and treated. The etiology of cutaneous vasculitis is unknown in many cases, but the physician must look into the possibility of medications, postviral syndromes, malignancy, primary vasculitis, and connective tissue disorders causing the atypical wound. The ultimate diagnosis of a vasculitis-induced wound relies upon a complete history and physical examination, as well as relevant antibody testing, viral serologies, complement count, immunoglobulin studies, complete blood count, and skin biopsy.[7]

Disease that is limited to the skin will benefit from supportive care such as appropriate wound care dressings, warming, and elevation of the extremity. Medications with minimal side effects also typically instituted symptomatically including colchicine, dapsone, antihistamines, and NSAIDs.[10] Patients with evident widespread or refractory skin involvement with systemic vasculitis will have to undergo aggressive but carefully monitored treatment, which includes systemic steroids, anti-inflammatory agents, and immunosuppressants.[10,13]

> **PEARL 10•3** Cutaneous vasculitis is an umbrella term for a host of diseases distinguished by vascular inflammation of the arterioles, capillaries, and/or venules that may eventually lead to necrosis of the vasculature and end-organ damage.

Pyoderma Gangrenosum

Pyoderma gangrenosum (PG) is an inflammatory ulcerative disease that was originally described in 1930.[14] It was first suspected to be a bacterial infection that disseminated from either the gastrointestinal or pulmonary system to the skin. After many years of investigation, it was found that PG was actually a misnomer; it was neither an infection[15] nor was there a gangrenous component to the disease.[16] To date, the pathogenesis of PG is not completely understood, but it is recognized to be an independent autoinflammatory disease and not merely a cutaneous complication of other systemic diseases in most patients studied.[17] Currently, the gene associated with pyoderma gangrenosum has been identified,[18] and more studies of PG etiology are underway on a molecular level.

PG begins as either inflamed individual or groupings of folliculocentric pustules or fluctuant nodules, with or without bullae, typically on the lower extremities of middle-aged adults. These initial stages of PG may deteriorate into ulcers rapidly; therefore, it is crucial for the physician to inspect skin closely and institute appropriate evaluation. (Fig. 10.2) The pustular PG is typically seen in patients with inflammatory bowel disease (IBD), and the bullous PG may be a clue for an underlying myelodysplastic disease.[19] As these lesions

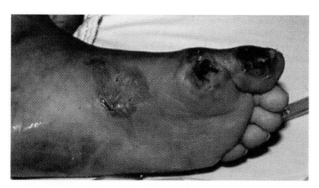

Figure 10•1 *Vasculitis. This patient has hemorrhagic and necrotic ulcers secondary to leukocytoclastic vasculitis.*

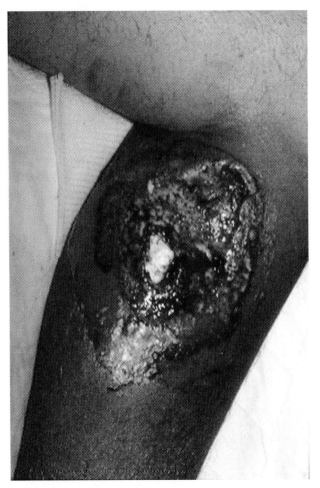

Figure 10•2 *Pyoderma gangrenosum. This is an upper leg ulcer with inflamed undermined borders due to pyoderma gangrenosum.*

described in 1997.[26] Although there is an association with a variety of diseases, PG is diagnosed as idiopathic in 25% to 50% of cases. Histopathology is generally supportive by demonstrating marked inflammation, but it is mainly used to help rule out other differential diagnoses.[20]

Treatment of PG can be an arduous task and is sometimes not completely curative; however, there is a growing body of literature that reports using local and systemic immunosuppressant therapy has significant response rates. For local and limited disease, topical or intralesional steroids are the standard of care. If disease is aggressive and extensive, systemic therapies should be instituted; however, their potent side effects will limit the medication course. Sulfonamides, sulfones, dapsone, or corticosteroids are commonly used; however, newer biological therapeutic agents are starting to gain recognition for PG treatment.[3,20] Success stories have been reported in the medical literature for a range of drugs, such as cyclosporine, mycophenolate mofetil,[27] infliximab,[28] and etanercept[29]; however, larger randomized controlled clinical trials (RCT) will have to evaluate the efficacy of these treatment modalities. The only treatment demonstrated to be effective in a RCT is an anti-tumor necrosis factor alpha (TNF-α) agent, infliximab.[30] Due to the breadth of PG clinical manifestations, treatment should be tailored to the individual and geared toward the extent of his or her disease.

Ulcerative Lichen Planus

Ulcerative lichen planus (ULP), also known as erosive lichen planus of the feet, is an unusual variant of lichen planus (LP). Primarily, middle-aged females are affected, and as diagnosis is often difficult, they often have this condition chronically for approximately 10 years before diagnosis.[31] ULP occurs largely on the palms and soles and presents as hyperkeratotic firm papules, nodules, and plaques with overlying scale and crusting. These lesions are generally positioned on a base of skin that is either atrophic or sclerotic in nature. ULP lesions are commonly found toward the peripheral margins of the palms and soles. Ulcers then spontaneously develop from these lesions, which can then be quite tender. Toenail dystrophy with or without complete nail loss and subsequent pterygium formation may concomitantly occur. Patients may also present with oral/genital mucosal erosions and cicatricial alopecia of the scalp, axillae, and/or pubic region.[19,31,32] Associations between ULP and autoimmune disorders such as rheumatoid arthritis,[33] sicca syndrome,[34] and Sjögren's syndrome[35] have also been reported in the literature.

Treatment of ULP can be problematic because of its chronic and recalcitrant nature. Management of ULP with topical therapeutic agents such as tacrolimus has been reported sparsely in the literature.[19,36] More success has been achieved with systemic therapeutics such as etretinate[37] and cyclosporine; however, surgical excision and grafting is thought to provide the best long-term results.[38] It is important to note that squamous cell carcinoma may develop within the ulcerations of ULP. Therefore, if a clinician finds a case of ULP refractory to standard treatments, skin biopsies are warranted to rule out cancer.[39]

Ulcerative Necrobiosis Lipoidica

Necrobiosis lipoidica diabeticorum was initially described in 1932[40] and is now considered an inflammatory ulcerative process. It was later discovered that there are a significant

deteriorate and evolve into more classic destructive ulcerations, PG becomes more distinguishable by its well-demarcated, undermined violaceous boggy borders and surrounding erythema. Early on, the center of the ulcer may display hemorrhagic crust, and later the center will demonstrate a yellow fibrinoid exudate. The ulcers undergo rapid growth and enlargement with associated fever, malaise, myalgias, and arthralgias, which make this disease devastating and lead to an increased morbidity. If the PG lesion does resolve, cribriform scarring is usually left behind.[14,19,20] Other clinical manifestations of PG include vegetative[21] and peristomal types.[22] Mechanistically in susceptible patients, pathergy plays a role in PG lesion development. Pathergy is described when lesions are induced to develop in areas of known trauma or injury.[20,23,24] It is estimated that approximately 25% of PG patients experience the pathergy phenomenon.[25]

PG is a diagnosis of exclusion, therefore it is important for the clinician to completely rule out any other local or systemic cause for the ulcer. PG can also be associated with other conditions such as IBD, arthritides, monoclonal gammopathies, hepatic disease, and hematological aberrations.[3,20] In addition, PG is a major component of PAPA syndrome (pyogenic arthritis, pyoderma gangrenosum, and acne), a genodermatosis first number of patients without an association with diabetes mellitus, therefore the "diabeticorum" was omitted from the name.[41] Now the disease process is called necrobiosis lipoidica (NL). Patients who do have an association with abnormal glucose metabolism, however, typically have diabetes mellitus type 1.[42] Generally, the bilateral pretibial region of young to middle-aged females is a classic location and presentation for NL lesions. These lesions are oval to round multiple plaques characterized by well-demarcated violaceous borders. The centers are brown to yellow, with a waxy atrophic texture.[19] (Fig. 10.3) Often blood vessels are seen coursing through the lesion.

NL is most likely to undergo ulceration in large lesions; in the literature, approximately 35% of patients undergo painful ulcerative NL.[43] Several case reports have appeared in the literature regarding malignant transformation within NL lesions.[44-51] Physicians must suspect an underlying squamous cell carcinoma in suspicious ulcers, and therefore biopsies in these situations are compulsory.

Treatment of NL is challenging. Topical and intralesional corticosteroids are considered first-line treatment modalities; however, long-term usage will instigate atrophy. An assortment of reports in the literature reflect the benefits of several various treatment options, such as systemic corticosteroids, topical mycophenolate mofetil, perilesional heparin, stanozolol, inositol niacinate, nicofuranose, ticlopidine, pentoxifylline, infliximab, niacinamide, systemic cyclosporine, clofazimine, pioglitazone, PUVA (psoralen plus ultraviolet light A), antiplatelet agents, excision and grafting, and the application of bioengineered skin.[19,42,52,53]

Ulcerative Sarcoidosis

Sarcoidosis is a chronic granulomatous systemic inflammatory condition that primarily affects the skin and pulmonary system.[54] The exact etiology of sarcoidosis is yet to be known; however, there is a strong T_H1-type cytokine presence that highly influences the growth of the characteristic granulomas.[55] It has also been hypothesized that this disease is a result of an autoimmune etiology or is a persistent inflammatory response to undegradable infectious antigens in vulnerable patient environments; however, no theories have been proven.[54] Sarcoidosis has been described in all ages, all races, and both genders. Generally, there is a bimodal age distribution between 25 and 35 years and later on between 45 and 65 years of age.[42]

It is estimated that 25% to 33% of sarcoidosis patients have cutaneous symptoms.[42,54] Cutaneous sarcoidosis is one of the dermatological diseases known as "the great imitators" because of the vast range of possible clinical presentations.[56] Cutaneous sarcoidosis can manifest as yellow, brown, red, or purple maculopapules, papules, nodules, or plaque-like lesions. These can appear on the face, extremities, buttocks, or trunk. Other variants include erythema nodosum, lupus pernio lesions, sarcoidosis infiltration of old scars or old injuries, and sarcoidosis causing scarring alopecia. Upon diascopy, applying pressure with a glass slide to induce blanching, the lesion will typically turn the color of "apply jelly."[42]

Ulcerative sarcoidosis is a variant of sarcoidosis, despite what was initially described by Boeck in 1899.[57] There were few case reports in the literature prior to the 1990s describing ulcers stemming from sarcoidosis lesions.[58,59] The ulcerative nature of sarcoidosis was first closely examined by Albertini and colleagues and was found to be most common in African-American women during young adulthood. Typically, the ulcers develop from cutaneous sarcoid lesions; however, they have been known to appear *de novo* or may be instigated by trauma. This disease is also predominantly on the lower extremities, and skin biopsies are the mainstay for a clear diagnosis. Corticosteroids were the most effective treatments, with methotrexate being used successfully only for refractory cases.[60] Another recent analysis mirrored Albertini's earlier results and found that 7 out of 147 patients presented with ulcerative-atrophic sarcoid lesions; all patients were of African-American descent, with five females and two males affected. All ulcers were on the pretibial location of the lower extremities, and biopsies were essential for diagnostic purposes. Most of the patients achieved complete reepithelialization of the ulcers with immunomodulatory therapy, such as antimalarials, low-dose prednisone, thalidomide, or mycophenolate mofetil.[61] Another recent report has supported the use of TNF-α inhibitors, such as adalimumab, which was proven to work effectively in a refractory sarcoidosis ulcer.[62]

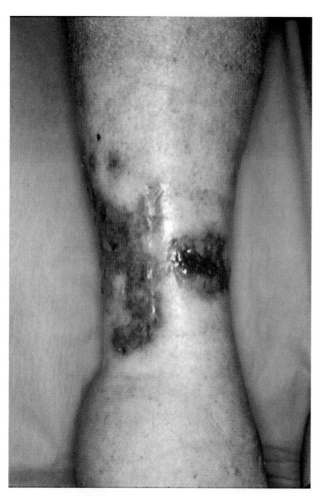

Figure 10•3 *Pictured is ulcerative necrobiosis lipoidica and a leg ulcer with atrophic waxy orange yellow center with ulceration present on the anterior aspect of the leg.*

▶ **PEARL 10•4** The ulcerative nature of sarcoidosis was found to be most common in African-American women during young adulthood.

Ulcerative Wegener's Granulomatosis

Wegener's granulomatosis (WG) is described as a triad of systemic vasculitis, necrotizing granulomatous inflammation of the upper and lower respiratory tracts, and glomerulonephritis. The pathogenesis is yet to be discovered; however, it is hypothesized that WG is an aggressive and exaggerated cell-mediated response to an unknown innate or environmental antigen. WG affects both genders equally and has an estimated prevalence in the United States of 3 in 100,000, with the mean age of diagnosis at approximately 40 years of age. Cutaneous WG manifests in only 20% of patients with early WG; however, 40% of WG patients will have cutaneous symptoms overall.[63] WG is classically diagnosed from clinical and laboratory findings and the presence of circulating antineutrophil cytoplasmic antibody (ANCA) directed against proteinase 3 (c-ANCA).[64]

Petechiae and palpable purpura are common presentations, with other skin lesions primarily presenting as painful subcutaneous nodules, papules, or vesicles.[65] Although ulcerative WG is not typical, it occurs in approximately 10% to 15% of cutaneous cases and occasionally mimics PG-like lesions. Ulcers can appear on the face and nose, elbows, upper and lower extremities, back, and perineum.[65-67] The standard of WG treatment is a combination of corticosteroids and cytotoxic drugs, such as cyclophosphamide. Once remission occurs, replacement of toxic drugs with less toxic medications such as methotrexate could be used to control and treat symptoms. Follow-up is extremely important in WG because relapse can be quite high, up to 50% of patients by 5 years of follow-up.[68]

Vasculopathic Etiologies

A vasculopathic lesion is the result of a small to medium vessel occlusion that typically occurs secondary to aberrant coagulation. Frequently, occlusion is caused by a thrombus or embolus and may be precipitated by antibodies directed against regulators of coagulation pathways. Depending upon the size of the occlusion and length of time it has been present, it will directly cause surrounding tissue to become hypoxic and eventually necrotic; usually, this may clinically present as livedo reticularis, petechiae, purpura, or ulcers.

Cryofibrinogenemia

Cryofibrinogenemia is an uncommon disorder characterized by cryoprecipitation of the patients' native fibrinogen, fibrin, fibronectin, albumin, and occasionally immunoglobulins and other plasma proteins. These precipitates cause a thromboembolic occlusion of the small to medium arteries, usually at distal extremities.[69,70] Essential, primary, or idiopathic cryofibrinogenemia develops spontaneously in previously healthy individuals, whereas secondary cryofibrinogenemia occurs in association with an underlying infectious process, inflammatory disease, malignancy, diabetes mellitus, autoimmune collagen vascular disease, or thromboembolic disease.[3,69] Individuals who have been diagnosed with cryofibrinogenemia are likely to be exposed to colder weather, and they also associate cold exposure with onset of symptoms[69]; this is logical as these fibrinogens tend to gel in the cold.[70] The cryofibrinogen clot precipitates in plasma at 39.2°F (4°C) and is soluble at 98.6°F (37°C).[69]

Cardinal signs of cryofibrinogenemia are purpuric to painful necrotic ulcerated lesions at distal sites of the body. Other clinical findings also may present as Raynaud's phenomenon, acral cyanosis, ecchymosis, livedo reticularis, and gangrene.[70] (Fig. 10.4) For diagnostic purposes, blood can be collected in anticoagulated tubes with sodium citrate and centrifuged at 37°C to prevent precipitation and consumption of all the fibrinogen. Biopsies can also be used, and fibrinogen precipitates should be visualized as occluding the small vessels. The actual precipitate, stained with hematoxylin and eosin (H&E), will be seen as eosinophilic intravascular deposits surrounded by inflammation.[71] The ulcerated lesions are very painful and typically present on the lower extremities. They are treatable, but frequent relapses may occur. Symptomatic treatment is standard as well as treatment of the underlying disorder if secondary cryofibrinogenemia is suspected. Fibrinolytic agents such as stanozolol have also been studied, which has been proven to reduce pain and improve clinical symptoms significantly.[3,72]

Cryoglobulinemia

Cryoglobulins are a complex of circulating immunoglobulins and proteins that precipitate in the cold and may also become soluble upon warming. Cryoglobulinemia occurs when these complexes form thrombi and eventually occlude vessels, thereby leading to clinical symptoms.[63] By classic definition, three types of cryoglobulinemia exist. Of these, one of the three typically causes cutaneous thrombosis. This type, type 1, is defined as noncomplexed monoclonal IgG or IgM; this type is usually seen in malignancies such as myeloma or in benign lymphoproliferative conditions such as Waldenström's macroglobulinemia. The other two types typically cause vasculitis. Type 2 is polyclonal IgG plus monoclonal IgM; this type is most commonly seen in infectious or inflammatory disease, however can be seen rarely in malignant conditions. Type 3 is polyclonal IgG plus polyclonal IgM; this type is strongly associated with hepatitis C (HCV) infection and HIV infection.[63,73] Mixed cryoglobulinemias

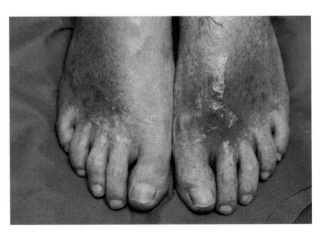

Figure 10•4 *This patient has ulcers due to Cryofibrinogenemia. Pictured are distal ulcers with atrophie blanche (porcelain white scars, telangiectasias, and dyspigmentation).*

are considered type 2 or type 3 because they are composed of both IgG and IgM,[63] and both can commonly cause a vasculitis-type picture that may lead to serious skin ulcers.[73]

The chief dermatological manifestation is a nonpruritic palpable purpura (in types 2 and 3), which may occur in up to 25% of patients with cryoglobulins. These lesions typically occur on distal extremities and dependent areas of the legs. Prolonged sitting or standing and exposure to cold may instigate a flare of the symptoms.[63] Other skin manifestations that are often seen are acral cyanosis, Raynaud's phenomenon, livedo reticularis, altered pigmentation of the skin, cold urticaria, and digital ulceration or gangrene. Extracutaneous manifestations of cryoglobulinemia include polyarthralgias, synovitis, neuropathy, and renal disease, such as glomerulonephritis.[63,74] In order for a diagnosis to be made, a skin biopsy is necessary not only to confirm but also to exclude other causes. Classically, the histopathological pattern in types 2 and 3 is leukocytoclastic vasculitis, while in type 1 noninflammatory vascular thrombi predominate. If additional studies are required, deposited immune complexes and complement identification by electrophoresis and special staining may allow further etiological differentiation.[74]

Treatment should be directed toward the histological finding as well as the underlying cause of the cryoglobulinemia. A quiescent malignancy, autoimmune disorder, or infectious disease must be tested for and ruled out, depending upon which type of cryoglobulinemia the patient has. Since HCV frequently plays an etiological role, treatment of the infection with interferon-α alone or in combination with ribavirin represents the standard protocol of treatment.[63,75] Plasmapheresis and immunosuppressants such as cyclophosphamide, in conjunction with steroids, have also been used as treatment for non-HCV–related, escalating cryoglobulinemia with success. In some additional cases, rituximab is being used as a treatment for recalcitrant cases with complete response, including ulcers. However, a large randomized controlled trial is yet to be performed to support these therapies efficacious.[75]

> **PEARL 10•5** Three types of cryoglobulinemia exist. Of these, one of the three typically causes cutaneous thrombosis. This type, type 1, is defined as noncomplexed monoclonal IgG, or IgM; this type is usually seen in malignancies such as myeloma or in benign lymphoproliferative conditions such as Waldenström's macroglobulinemia. The other two types typically cause vasculitis. Type 2 is polyclonal IgG plus monoclonal IgM; this type is most commonly seen in infectious or inflammatory disease, but rarely can be seen in malignant conditions. Type 3 is polyclonal IgG plus polyclonal IgM; this type is strongly associated with hepatitis C (HCV) infection and HIV infection.

Antiphospholipid Antibody Syndrome

Antiphospholipid antibody syndrome (APS) is defined by venous and/or arterial thrombosis, thrombocytopenia, and recurrent fetal loss. Antiphospholipid antibodies (aPLs) are immunoglobulins that are composed of IgG, IgM, or both. APS is associated with aPLs such as anticardiolipin antibodies, anti-β2

glycoprotein I antibodies, and a positive lupus anticoagulant test. APS can present as a primary disease or as a secondary illness associated with an autoimmune disorder such as systemic lupus erythematosus, an underlying malignancy, or an infectious disease process. This syndrome can manifest as a debilitating medical disease that affects nearly any organ system, including the pulmonary, central nervous, gastrointestinal and hepatic, renal, endocrine, and integumentary systems.[76,77]

The most common dermatological manifestation of APS is livedo reticularis. Thromboses in the vasculature may also result in ulcerations, gangrene of distal extremities, splinter hemorrhages, superficial venous thromboses, thrombocytopenic purpura, cutaneous infarcts, and anetoderma. (Fig. 10.5) Cutaneous ulcerations, frequently on the lower extremities, may clinically resemble pyoderma gangrenosum.[76,78] Treatment is focused on long-term anticoagulation and correcting any underlying medical condition. Women who are pregnant must be treated with a combination of aspirin and heparin. In cases that are severe and fulminant, treatment is complex and not always successful. Intravenous high-dose steroids and aggressive anticoagulation in conjunction with intravenous gamma globulin and repeated plasma exchanges with fresh-frozen plasma may limit progression of disease if used early.[76,77]

> **PEARL 10•6** Antiphospholipid antibody syndrome (APS) is defined by venous and/or arterial thrombosis, thrombocytopenia, and recurrent fetal loss.

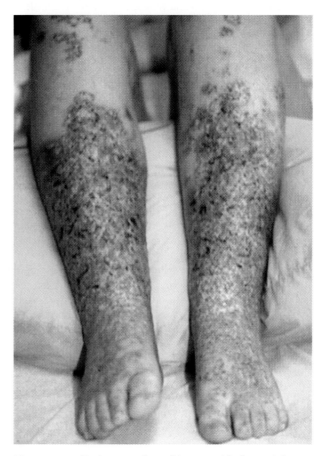

Figure 10•5 *Patients, such as this one, with the antiphospholipid antibody syndrome often have multiple necrotic ulcers secondary to small vessel thrombosis of both legs.*

Sickle Cell Disease Ulcers

Sickle cell disease (SCD) was first described in 1910 by Herrick, but it was unknown then whether this was a new disease or a manifestation of an existing medical condition.[79] Approximately 50 years later, it was discovered that the difference between normal and mutant hemoglobin is a single amino acid substitution.[80] SCD is caused by an amino acid substitution of valine for glutamic acid in the β hemoglobin chain, which leads to polymerization of the hemoglobin molecule in areas of low-oxygen tension, thereby leading to the sickle shape of red blood cells in deoxygenated environments.[81] SCD is notorious for the chronicity of the cutaneous ulcerations it produces, and the incidence is widely variable as well: SCD ulcers can manifest in 50% to 70% of Jamaican patients[82] and 5% to 10% of patients in other geographic locations.[83] Ulcerations on the lower extremities are most common and are usually characterized by a gradual yet aggressive course that can heal 3 to 16 times slower compared to ulcers of various other etiologies, including venous ulcers.[84] Patients with an active ulcer have a 146-fold increased risk of acquiring another ulcer in their lifetime.[85] Sickle cell ulcers are particularly recalcitrant and can lead not only to challenging medical issues but severe socioeconomic problems as well.

There are many theories regarding pathogenesis of SCD ulcers; however, the exact etiology has yet to be completely understood. Many theories focus upon the sickled red blood cell's rigid and inflexible shape causing frequent vascular obstructions in smaller blood vessels. These obstructions lead to tissue injury and upregulate the body's innate inflammatory response, promoting platelet aggregation and adhesion factors to further develop the blockage. This continued cycle of tissue injury and upregulation of inflammatory factors eventually cause tissue ulcerations and necrosis. Most patients with SCD also suffer from long-term underlying anemia, which contributes to hypoxic conditions, promoting necrosis.[83,85-87] A genetic component may also play a role, as there is also a known HLA correlation with SCD and ulcers. The relative risk for development of leg ulcers in patients with SCD who have both HLA-B35 and HLA-Cw4 is 17 times greater than that of SCD control patients without these antigens or those who had only one antigen.[88] SCD leg ulcer patients are likely to also have lower hemoglobin counts and higher levels of lactate dehydrogenase, bilirubin, aspartate aminotransferase, and reticulocytes when compared to age-matched, sex-matched SCD control patients without leg ulcers.[89]

SCD ulcers are typically found in the lower extremities in areas such as the pretibial region, dorsum of the feet, posterior heel, and medial/lateral malleolus. These areas are more prone to ulceration because they have decreased blood flow and are surrounded by less subcutaneous tissue. Ulcers are classically tender, round, and punched-out appearing, with or without peripheral brown hyperpigmentation and scaling. (Fig. 10.6A and B) The margins appear raised, and the base of the ulcer can be very deep. Necrotic slough in and around the ulcer is also typically present. These ulcers are sometimes reminiscent of venous ulcerations.[85]

For diagnostic purposes, patients should have peripheral smears and hemoglobin electrophoresis performed to establish levels of hemoglobin A, S, and F and severity of disease.[87]

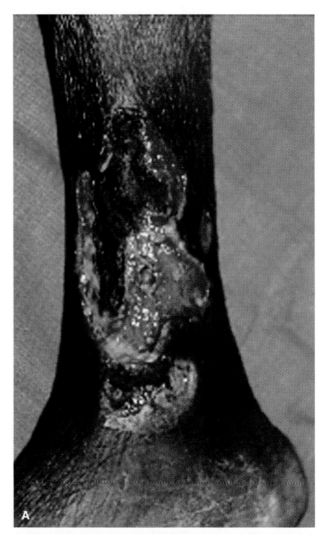

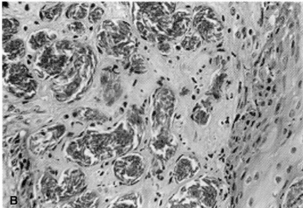

Figure 10•6 *(A and B) In this patient with sickle cell ulcer a diagnose is renderd by a combination of clinical and histologic picture in a patients with sickle cell disease. This patient has a lower extremity ulcer with overlying necrotic tissue, which a biopsy found sickled red blood cells within dermal blood vessels.*

Biopsies may not provide a diagnosis; however, one may be able to see sickled red blood cells within cutaneous blood vessels on histology.[90] Treatment of SCD ulcers revolves around prevention. Slight trauma and minor injuries can propagate formation of an ulcer; therefore, adequately fitting shoes and avoidance of bug bites and other small scrapes and bruises are critical. Edema of the lower extremities may also worsen ulcerations, therefore compression stockings, leg rest and elevation, and a sodium-free diet are recommended in patients at risk for venous or lymphatic disease. If patients have dry, cracking, or peeling skin, a thick emollient should be applied often to moisturize vulnerable fragile skin.[85,90]

Treatment modalities for active ulcers encompass topical dressings, surgery, and systemic interventions. Triple antibiotic ointments[91] and synthetic dressings have been proven to be efficacious in many chronic cases. The Unna boot, gauze impregnated with zinc oxide, in conjunction with compression wraps, leads to better control of edema and a faster healing time in SCD.[85] DuoDerm®, Solcoseryl®, Collistat®, and Apligraf® are all synthetic and bioderived dressings that have been effective in some reports; however, larger trials are needed to prove their efficacy, specifically in SCD ulcer patients.[84,85,92,93] Surgical interventions such as myocutaneous flaps are preferred over autologous split-thickness grafts because myocutaneous flaps have their own vascular supply and thus are able to thrive. Since areas of ulcerations are already inherently low on vascular supply, most other grafts fail. Therefore, a flap rich in its own blood supply will have a higher likelihood of survival.[94-96] In regard to systemic treatments, transfusions have been reported to aid healing in difficult cases. The goal for therapeutic blood levels is to keep the hemoglobin above 10 g/dL and reduce the hemoglobin S to less than 30%.[85,86] Standard SCD systemic agents such as pentoxifylline, hydroxyurea, and erythropoietin have also been suggested for refractory ulcers and have had some success.[85] Pain treatment should not be overlooked as it is a crucial part of a sickle cell patient's medication regimen. NSAIDs, prescription opioid medications, and antidepressants may need to be prescribed when warranted.[90]

Infectious Disease Etiologies

Infectious causes of atypical wounds may be due to a variety of bacterial, viral, fungal, or protozoal organisms. The etiological agent will primarily depend upon geographical location of the patient because certain organisms are native to specific regions of the world. The occupation or hobbies of the patient may also play a role in determining the cause of the infection as specific activities are directly related to exposure to various types of organisms. The patient's immunosuppression status is another factor to consider because the immunocompromised population is more vulnerable to both common and rare infectious disease, especially organisms that usually do not cause harm in a healthy patient.

Atypical Mycobacterial Infections

Atypical mycobacteria, also known as anonymous nontuberculous, nonlepromatous mycobacteria, began to be recognized and categorized in the 1950s as a human pathogen,

primarily causing disease in the lungs and skin.[97-99] The term *atypical* was first created by Pinner,[100] and currently there are 95 reported species in the genus *Mycobacterium*. Atypical mycobacteria are thin nonmotile, acid-fast bacilli that are ubiquitous worldwide.[101] Presently, these organisms have also emerged as a common and important cause of infectious disease because of the AIDS epidemic and increased usage of immunosuppressants for a variety of other illnesses.[102]

Atypical mycobacteria not only cause skin and soft tissue disease but also cause pulmonary infection, lymphadenitis, blood infection, catheter-related infections, and chronic granulomatous infections of the musculoskeletal system.[103] (Fig. 10.7A and B) Risk factors for cutaneous infection usually involve inoculation either by trauma, immunosuppression, or a chronic disease. Almost all atypical species have been reported as the causative agent in cutaneous disease. The most common species in the United States and Europe is *Mycobacterium marinum,* followed by *M. abscessus, M. fortuitum,* and *M. chelonae.*[102] *M. marinum* is particularly reported in patients who have had recent exposure to a home aquarium or who have a fish-related occupation.[101] Cutaneous lesions have a nonspecific and wide spectrum of presentation and can been visualized as verrucous papules, nodules, plaques, sinus tracts, diffuse cellulitis, and superficial or large ulcers, depending upon the specific atypical mycobacterial species.[97]

Because of the nonspecific nature of the clinical presentation, a skin biopsy specimen is required for tissue culture and histology. The polymerase chain reaction (PCR) technique can also be used to rush the diagnosis, but it does not give the antimicrobial susceptibility pattern of the bacteria; therefore, it should not be used to replace tissue culture but as an adjunct tool for diagnosis. Treatment regimens will differ depending on the causative organism because susceptibility to antibiotics will vary. Currently, clarithromycin is considered a superior drug in treating atypical mycobacterial infections; however, deeper and recalcitrant wounds will benefit from combination treatments. It is also recommended that medications be used continuously for at least 3 months to avoid relapse of infection.[101] In difficult ulcers, surgical excision, local heat therapy, and hyperbaric oxygen therapy have been successful.[97]

Deep Fungal Infections

Deep fungal infections are typically divided into two categories: subcutaneous and systemic mycoses. Subcutaneous mycoses usually arise when the infectious agent is introduced into the dermis or subcutis, usually through trauma or instrumentation. Once implanted beyond the epidermis, the fungus will most likely proliferate into a localized ulcerated infection and eventually may become systemic by dissemination through the lymphatic system and, more rarely, the bloodstream. Most cases of subcutaneous mycoses are found in Central and South America.[104] In systemic infections, the pulmonary system may be the first site of inoculation via inhalation, leading to a localized lung infection. This focus of infection may cause dissemination of fungal organisms, spread by the lymphatic and blood circulation, to other organs such as the skin.[105] Immunocompromised patients, such as AIDS patients, are more vulnerable and more likely to present with a systemic fungal infection.[104]

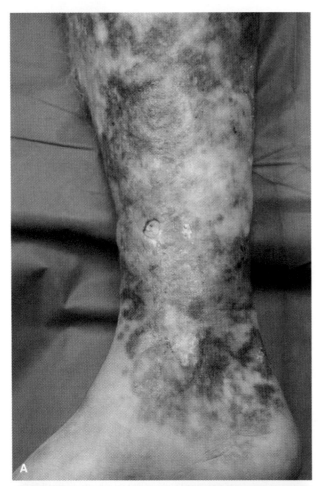

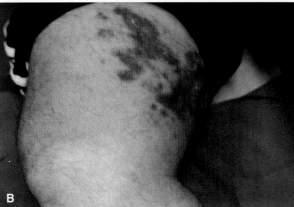

Figure 10•7 *(A and B) This patient has an ulcer due to an atypical mycobacterial infection with an indurated leg and thigh with cutaneous ulceration and deep-seated granulomatous inflammation.*

Chromomycosis, phaeohyphomycosis, sporotrichosis, entomophthoramycosis, lobomycosis, and rhinosporidiosis encompass the organisms that are typically involved in subcutaneous mycoses. Paracoccidioidomycosis, coccidioidomycosis, histoplasmosis, and cryptococcosis are the most common organisms involved in systemic mycoses.[105]

Certain deep fungal infections are native to limited regions of the world; therefore, a careful history of patient travel, recent geographical location, and unique exposures are helpful for diagnosis. Patients with unusual professions may also be at risk, thus a detailed occupational history is also warranted.

> ▶ **PEARL 10•7** Deep fungal infections are typically divided into two categories: subcutaneous and systemic mycoses. Subcutaneous mycoses usually arise when the infectious agent is introduced into the dermis or subcutis, usually via trauma or instrumentation. In systemic infections, the pulmonary system may be the first site of inoculation via inhalation, leading to a localized lung infection.

Chromoblastomycosis

Chromoblastomycosis is a subcutaneous mycosis also known as chromomycosis, cladosporiosis, verrucous dermatitis, phaeosporotrichosis, Pedroso's disease, and Fonseca's disease. This deep fungal infection is caused by the following pigmented fungi: *Cladosporium carrionii*, *Fonsecaea compacta*, *Fonsecaea pedrosoi*, *Phialophora verrucosa*, and *Rhinocladiella aquaspera*. Chromoblastomycosis is prevalent in tropical and temperate climates throughout the world, and the fungal organisms are commonly found in the soil, plants, or wood. Individuals with occupations in the rural farming and mining industries are particularly at risk. Trauma to the lower extremity is the typical scenario for contracting this infection.[104]

Initially, the inoculation site will present as a papule or nodule that evolves into a verrucous or granulomatous plaquelike lesion. Several of these lesions may coalesce to form a large mass, or they may remain separated. Excoriations, scaling, ulcerations, and crusting may also be evident on the lesions. Constitutional symptoms are not commonly associated with subcutaneous chromoblastomycosis. Skin scrapings with potassium hydroxide (KOH) 20% and a skin biopsy for tissue culture and histology are necessary for complete diagnosis.[104] Round pigmented bodies, also called "copper pennies," can be visualized in the dermis. These are pathognomonic for chromoblastomycosis and are referred to as "Medlar bodies" or "sclerotic bodies."[106]

Treatment for chromoblastomycosis is challenging, and success rates are very limited. In regard to oral antifungal medications, a combination of two drugs proves to be more efficacious than one; combinations that have been relatively successful include amphotericin B and 5-fluorocytosine, itraconazole and 5-fluorocytosine, and itraconazole and terbinafin.[107,108] Alternative treatment options reported in the literature include surgical excision, laser therapy, local heat treatments, and cryotherapy.[109] Radical surgery such as amputation may be required in cases that are intractable and disabling.[110]

Mycetoma

Mycetoma is a subcutaneous deep fungal infection also known as Madura foot or maduromycosis. There are three different subtypes of mycetoma depending upon the causative agent: actinomycotic mycetoma, eumycotic mycetoma, and botryomycosis. This infection is predominantly found in tropical and subtropical locations such as India, Africa, and Central and South America. Individuals typically contract mycetoma from exposure to contaminated soil, and risk factors include malnutrition, exposed cutaneous injuries, and lack of footwear. The foot, hand, thorax, and scalp are the most frequent inoculation sites on the body.[104,111]

The initial presentation of mycetoma frequently manifests as an asymptomatic papule that eventually progresses into edematous purulent draining sinuses, fistulae, and abscesses. The drainage is particularly unique as it is composed of pathognomonic grains, also known as sclerotia, which represent fungal colonies. The localized lesions of mycetoma may also invade the subcutaneous tissue into muscle and bone, causing cavitations. Diagnosis is based on patient history, clinical presentation, and results of a skin biopsy. A KOH scraping, Gram stain of the drainage, and bacterial and fungal tissue culture should also be performed to help with diagnostic evaluation. Special stains for histopathology should also be used to determine the subtype of mycetoma. The pathognomonic sclerotia should also be present during histopathology.[104,111] Treatment is challenging, and frequently surgical excision with wide margins in combination with long-term azole treatment offers the best result. In larger and deeper infections with bone involvement, amputation will most likely be the only viable treatment option.[112]

Sporotrichosis

Sporotrichosis, also known as rose gardener's disease, is a subcutaneous mycosis caused by the dimorphic fungal organism *Sporothrix schenckii*. The disease is a consequence of traumatic inoculation of the fungus deep into the skin, most commonly acquired via a prick by a contaminated rose thorn. However, in immunocompromised patients, inhalation is another mode of entry that leads to inoculation of the pulmonary system and subsequent dissemination to other organ systems. This fungal etiologic agent is prevalent globally and is most commonly found in soil, wood, and plants.[104]

The clinical presentation initially manifests as a solitary papule at the exact site of trauma. This primary lesion will ultimately ulcerate and drain. A characteristic cutaneous manifestation of sporotrichosis infection that appears weeks after the inoculation is lymphangitis and the appearance of subcutaneous nodules scattered along the lymphatic vasculature of the affected limb. The pattern along the lymphatic vessels is classic and is labeled as a "sporotrichoid pattern."[113]

The causative agent of sporotrichosis will rarely be visualized during pathological tests; however, if seen, they will be cigar-shaped. Periodic acid-Schiff (PAS) and silver stains may also aid visualization in histological studies. Treatment requires systemic medications; topical therapy is absolutely ineffective. Saturated solution of potassium iodide, itraconazole, and amphotericin B are effective, depending upon the severity of the infection.[104]

Paracoccidioidomycosis

Paracoccidioidomycosis, also known as South American blastomycosis or Brazilian blastomycosis, is a systemic mycosis caused by the dimorphic saprophyte *Paracoccidioides*

brasiliensis. It is native to Central and South American countries and is commonly found in soil and decaying vegetation. Individuals primarily contract this fungal disease through inhalation of the conidia. The pulmonary disease is typically mild; however, dissemination to other organ systems may follow. The infection progressively spreads, notably causing severe mucocutaneous disease. The face, oral mucosa, and nasal mucosa are primarily affected by painful, ulcerative, verrucous lesions. Lymphatic spread may also take place, subsequently leading to regional lymphadenopathy, typically in the cervical region. Besides inhalation, patients can also directly inoculate themselves through traumatic contact on the skin or in mucocutaneous areas of the body.[104,114]

Diagnosis is established by microscopic examination and identification of the organism in tissue culture. Narrow-based buds that resemble a "mariner's wheel" will most likely be seen.[104] Treatment involves chronic use of systemic agents such as amphotericin B, ketoconazole, itraconazole, or sulfonamides.[115]

Vibrio Vulnificus Infection

Vibrio vulnificus (*V. vulnificus*) is a gram-negative, halophilic bacillus that is found worldwide in marine and estuarial bodies of water. *V. vulnificus* also is found in many different types of fish and shellfish, such as sea bass, mullet, oysters, crabs, clams, and mussels. It is a rare cause of severe bacterial skin infections and overwhelming septicemia.[116] *V. vulnificus* infections occur most commonly in patients who are immunocompromised or suffering from an underlying hepatic disorder, diabetes, or renal disease.[116,117] The bacterial organism produces extracellular proteolytic and elastolytic enzymes and collagenases that invade and destroy human tissue, either the skin if inoculated externally or the small bowel mucosa if ingested.[117]

Clinically, infections will present as wound infections and sepsis. Septicemia is accompanied by a greater than 50% mortality rate.[116] Cutaneous infection occurs when *V. vulnificus* invades the body through a breach in the epidermal barrier, typically on the extremities during outdoor water activities such as fishing or sports.[117] Onset of symptoms begins hours to days after initial exposure to the bacteria.[116] Cutaneous manifestations of *V. vulnificus* can vary widely. These presentations are as follows: hemorrhagic bullae, erythema, pustules, generalized papules and macules, purpura, vasculitic lesions, necrotic ulcers, necrotizing fasciitis, gangrene, urticaria, erythema multiforme-like lesions, lymphangitis, lymphadenitis, cellulitis, and myositis.[116,117] Diagnosis is made by considering the clinical presentation and a careful patient history, taking into account any recent exposure to the ocean and/or raw seafood. Early treatment is essential, as mortality can be very high in some cases. Tetracycline or doxycycline is first-line therapy in conjunction with cefotaxime or ciprofloxacin as second-line agents. Local wound care should include antibiotic therapy and careful débridement of necrotic tissue.[116]

▶ **PEARL 10•8** *Vibrio vulnificus* infections occur most commonly in patients who are immunocompromised or suffering from an underlying hepatic disorder, diabetes, or renal disease.

Herpes Virus Infection

Herpes is a ubiquitous viral infection most commonly caused by herpes simplex virus type 1 (HSV-1) and herpes simplex virus type 2 (HSV-2). HSV-1 is a frequent etiologic agent in orofacial herpes, and HSV-2 is indicted as the cause of genital herpes; however, either strain can cause orofacial and genital herpes.[118]

Clinically, HSV typically presents on the lips, oral mucosa, and genitalia. (Fig. 10.8A and B) A burning or stinging sensation may herald development of the classic vesicular lesions. The neuropathic sensations will occur several days before classic dermatological manifestations. The early herpetic lesions largely present as macules or papules, progressing to the characteristic vesicles, which eventually lead to unsightly and painful erosions and ulcerations. HSV therapy has largely focused on antiviral management, seen in

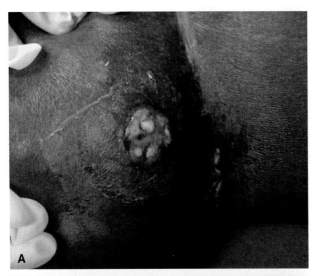

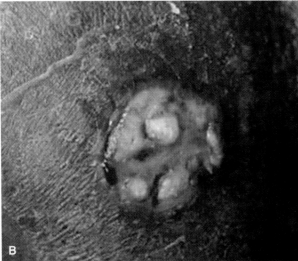

Figure 10•8 *(A and B) Patients with herpes simplex can develop partial thickness wounds as pictured here. This patient has a nonhealing ulcer on buttocks secondary to herpes simplex.*

the topical products available over the counter; however it has not focused on treatment of the resultant wounds. Recently it was proven that HSV causes partial-thickness wounds, wounds that extend beyond the basement membrane and into the dermis. With this valuable information and a review of previous literature, the conclusion was drawn that occlusion therapy would be the best method of wound care for recalcitrant HSV wounds. This hypothesis needs to be proven by implementing a novel occlusive wound dressing that will bind to mucosal surfaces.[119] In addition, standard local wound care, analgesics, and monitoring for further infection should be executed when caring for an HSV wound.

> **PEARL 10•9** Recently, it was shown that HSV causes partial-thickness wounds, wounds that extend beyond the basement membrane and into the dermis, suggesting occlusion therapy would be the best method of care for HSV wounds.

Necrotizing Fasciitis

Necrotizing fasciitis (NF) is a rare and deadly skin and soft tissue bacterial infection. It is described as a rapidly spreading inflammatory process that subsequently causes necrosis of the skin, subcutaneous tissue, and fascia. This disease has an exceptionally high morbidity and mortality rate, exceeding 70% if NF is left untreated.[120] Patients who are typically susceptible to developing NF are in immunocompromised states, such as cancer and AIDS patients.[121] Patients who have undergone serious or minor cutaneous trauma, such as burns and other injuries, are also vulnerable to NF.[120]

NF is classified as type 1 or type 2, depending upon the etiologic bacterial organism that is cultured from the wound. Type 1 NF is a polymicrobial infection from aerobic and anaerobic bacteria such as the following: *Bacteroides, Peptococcus, Fusobacterium, Clostridium, Corynebacterium, Streptococcus* (not group A), *Escherichia, Enterobacter, Proteus, Klebsiella, Serratia, Eikenella, Pseudomonas, Candida, Cryptococcus, Histoplasma, Vibrio, Staphylococcus, Shigella, Neisseria, Pasteurella,* and *Salmonella* species. Type 2 NF is caused by group A *Streptococcus* (*S. pyogenes*) with or without a *Staphylococcus* infection.[120]

NF can present as acute, subacute, or fulminant on any part of the body, but is commonly seen on the extremities. It initially presents as a lesion similar to cellulitis; there is surrounding poorly demarcated edema and erythema with overlying shiny, taut skin. Most characteristically at this early stage, the patient will present with pain out of proportion to the clinical findings. This is usually a warning sign for an invasive deep infection, and it is critical to start early management as soon as these symptoms arise to improve the patient's chance of survival. If left untreated, gangrene will set in and extend deep into the subcutis and between the fascial tissue planes. Suppuration and myonecrosis will subsequently take place, and lymphadenitis, lymphangitis, crepitation, and thromboses of the vasculature may also be seen in progressive cases. Metastases to other organ systems, constitutional symptoms, and multiorgan system failure will typically follow in fulminant NF cases.[120,122]

Management of NF is focused on surgical débridement, intravenous antimicrobial therapy, and supportive care. Tissue culture, gram staining, and sensitivity tests must be performed in order to diagnose the type of NF.[122] Polymicrobial NF management must include treatment that is against both aerobes and anaerobes, such as a combination of ampicillin-sulbactam plus clindamycin plus ciprofloxacin. Group A *Streptococcus* NF must be treated with clindamycin and penicillin.[123] For *Pseudomonas* coverage, an imipenem-cilastatin combination should be effective.[122] Intravenous immunoglobulin (IVIG) has been shown to reduce the mortality rate in patients with low serum levels of protective antibody counts; however, this treatment regimen has not yet been proven in a large randomized controlled trial.[123] In extensive cases that do not respond well to local wound care or IV antibiotics, further surgical débridement, fasciotomies, and skin and muscle grafts must be considered as the next treatment options. In extreme cases, amputation of the affected extremity may have to be performed in order to save the patient's life.[122]

Metabolic Disorder Etiologies

Metabolic diseases are unusual causes of severe cutaneous manifestations and chronic wounds. A metabolic disorder in particular, calciphylaxis, can be seen in end-stage renal disease (ESRD) patients on chronic hemodialysis. These patients subsequently develop secondary hyperparathyroidism, which eventually leads to deposition of calcium within soft tissue and the vasculature, causing tissue death and unique cutaneous findings.[124] Other metabolic derangements such as inadequate supply of nutrition to the body and metabolic disease such as diabetes mellitus may also manifest as unique cutaneous wounds.

Calciphylaxis

First reported in 1898, calciphylaxis is an uncommon disorder that clinically manifests as progressive cutaneous necrotic disease in ESRD patients.[125] Other names for this disease that have been used in the literature are calcific uremic arteriolopathy, calcifying panniculitis, metastatic calcinosis cutis, and necrotizing panniculitis.[124] Calciphylaxis affects approximately 1% to 4% of the dialysis population.[126]

The most common eliciting factor, secondary hyperparathyroidism, produces an elevated calcium-phosphate product and the subsequent development of cutaneous, subcutaneous, and vascular calcified bodies. Skin findings begin as erythematous to violaceous plaques in a vascular pattern, found nearly anywhere on the body and often in symmetric patterns. These plaques will consequently become necrotic and gangrenous, with eschar formations. (Fig. 10.9) Vesicles and hemorrhagic bullae may appear on the periphery of these plaques. If left untreated, these plaques will ulcerate and can eventually lead to autoamputation of the digit or extremity. Extreme pain is characteristic of this disease, along with an unusual debilitating skeletal myopathy.[124,127]

Diagnosis of calciphylaxis is usually based on clinical presentation by an ESRD patient. Serum laboratory testing for calcium and phosphate levels will also aid in diagnosis. An elevated parathyroid hormone reading, radiographic evidence of pipe-stem calcifications, and evidence found

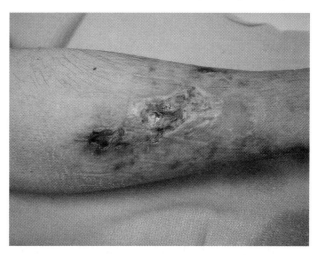

Figure 10•9 *Calciphylaxis may present with necrotic ulcer on the leg as seen here.*

during histopathology will also solidify the patient's diagnosis. Pathology findings of calciphylaxis include arterial medial calcification, intimal hyperplasia, intimal proliferation, adipocyte calcification, or infiltration of inflammatory cells.[124,127]

Management and treatment of calciphylaxis is focused on supportive care. Laboratory normalization of abnormal calcium and phosphorus levels may be accomplished by diet, binding agents, and parathyroidectomy. Tissue cultures must be performed to focus antibiotic treatment regimens, in case of infection. Local wound care and débridement of necrotic tissue is mandatory to prevent further wound infection. Hyperbaric oxygen therapy has also been proven to completely resolve cutaneous ulcers secondary to calciphylaxis.[124,127]

Neoplastic Etiologies

Chronic wounds and malignancies are intricately connected in many different ways. Chronic wounds have been known to gradually degenerate into a malignancy, most commonly squamous cell carcinoma. Malignancies may also degenerate into ulcerated chronic open wounds, occasionally seen in large basal cell carcinomas. In addition, certain wounds may be associated with malignancy such as chronic wounds secondary to vasculitis or PG.

Marjolin Ulcer

Dr. Jean-Nicholas Marjolin first reported his description of warty malignant-like changes of chronic ulcers in 1828.[128] The term *Marjolin ulcer,* which was initially published by DaCosta,[129] has presently been expanded to include malignant transformation of burns, chronic venous insufficiency ulcers, pressure ulcers, vaccination sites, fistulas, scars, frostbite, snakebites, osteomyelitis, pilonidal abscesses, hydradenitis suppurativa, herpes zoster, skin graft donor sites, dog bites, knife wounds, and gunshot wounds.[130] Malignant degeneration of a wound into a squamous cell carcinoma (SCC) chiefly affects middle-aged to elderly males who have had a preexisting condition for a chronic period of time, such as

20 to 50 years.[131] Etiology of malignant degeneration is unknown and controversial; however, most hypothesize it is an abnormality in the wound healing process caused by constant irritation, chronic environmental exposure, and repeated injury to the area of initial trauma.[130]

Management and treatment of Marjolin ulcer consists of surgical intervention with a local wide excision or Mohs micrographic surgery, depending upon location of the carcinoma. Amputation may also be indicated if the cancer is adherent to underlying tissue, if excision was too wide and unable to close, if bone necrosis has set in, or if excision causes decreased functionality of the affected body part.[132]

Traumatic Etiologies

Traumatic and external causes of atypical wounds include arthropod attacks, chemical agents, chronic radiation exposure, trauma, and factitial injuries. A detailed patient history, including recent and past exposures, travel history, and unusual activities or hobbies, along with the clinical examination, are the most valuable pieces of information in determining the cause of chronic wounds caused by external factors.

Spider Bites

There are a variety of spider species in the world that have been reported to cause significant local and systemic medical injury; however, the *Loxosceles* and the *Latrodectus* spider species are the most recognized in the United States to cause skin ulcers and necrosis.

The attack of *Loxosceles reclusa*, also known as the brown recluse spider, is initially a painless bite and is often disregarded.[133] In most cases, the bite will not progress, but in about 10% of patients there will be development to more significant wounds.[134] In these patients, the initial symptom is a sharp burning pain at the bite site in approximately 2 to 8 hours. The area will soon become erythematous, and vesicles may develop. Days later, the injured area will become a dusky blue violaceous color with a hardened center. Most bites will self-heal in 6 to 8 weeks, but on occasion, these injuries can invade into underlying subcutis and muscle tissue with associated necrosis and ulcerations. When ulcerations occur, healing will be quite slow, taking up to 6 months to heal completely. Constitutional symptoms such as malaise, fever, headaches, and arthralgias may coincide with these dermatological manifestations.[133]

For a loxoscelism diagnosis, tissue for a skin biopsy should be taken, and the biopsy may show dermal edema, thickening of blood vessel endothelium, leukocyte infiltration, intravascular coagulation, vasodilatation, destruction of blood vessel walls, and red blood cell exudate.[135] Preliminary treatment consists of routine first aid, such as limb elevation, immobilization, icing the wound, local wound care, tetanus prophylaxis, and analgesics. The use of systemic steroids may prevent the enlargement of progressing necrotic areas, and dapsone has been recommended for over 20 years as the standard treatment of care in adults.[133]

Latrodectus mutans, also known as the black widow spider, is found worldwide and is distinguished by the bright red hour-glass figure on its abdomen. The bite is painless and rarely noticed; however, it is followed by relentless pain, edema, and tenderness at the site of attack. Systemic symptoms such as headaches, nausea, hypertension, neuromuscular twitching, abdominal pain, and abdominal rigidity will usually follow and last for up to 3 days. Treatment includes supportive care such as icing, wound care, and calcium gluconate. There is currently no solid evidence of the effectiveness of different antivenins in humans or of the most appropriate route of administration. Randomized controlled trials are currently being held to determine the dosage and methods to effectively administer antivenin.[136]

Chemical Burns

A wide range of chemical products are capable of causing injury to the human skin, such as the following acids and alkalis: hydrofluoric acid, formic acid, anhydrous ammonia, cement, phenol, white phosphorus, elemental metals, nitrates, hydrocarbons, and tar.[137] These caustic chemicals will cause cutaneous damage by direct and indirect contact, and it may take only a single exposure to cause painful ulcers that are difficult to diagnose and treat. The lesions caused by alkalis are usually more severe when compared to acid injury, but most importantly, the degree of skin destruction is primarily based upon the chemical's concentration and the duration of initial and continual contact.[138] Copious irrigation with saline for at least 30 minutes to all areas exposed to the chemical agent is the initial standard of care for chemical burn victims. Certain chemicals require additional therapy because of their unique properties. If burned by hydrofluoric acid, one should apply 25% magnesium sulphate; if chromic acid is the culprit, it is best to excise the affected area, if possible; and if exposed to phenol, one should apply a 2:1 mixture of polyethylene glycol and ethanol.[139]

> ▶ **PEARL 10•10** Copious irrigation with saline for at least 30 minutes to all areas exposed to the chemical agent is the initial standard of care for chemical burn victims. Certain chemicals require additional therapy because of their unique properties. If burned by hydrofluoric acid, one should apply 25% magnesium sulphate; if chromic acid is the culprit, it is best to excise the affected area, if possible; and if exposed to phenol, one should apply a 2:1 mixture of polyethylene glycol and ethanol.

Radiation Dermatitis

Radiation therapy is a widely used treatment regimen, particularly in oncology patients. As with any medical procedure, there are side effects, and therefore an estimated 95% of patients who undergo radiation therapy develop a superficial reaction to the radiation in the immediate, acute, or delayed time frame. The intensity of a skin reaction is influenced by the total dose and type of radiation used, as well as the location, area, and volume treated.[140] After exposure to ionizing radiation exceeding 10 Gy, a local skin reaction is likely to develop. Localized erythema, edema, and pruritus are typically the initial mild symptoms.[141] Other manifestations include flaking or peeling, pigmentation changes, hair loss, decreased or absent perspiration, telangiectatic changes, edema, vesiculation, ulceration, and scarring. (Fig. 10.10) After discontinuation of radiation therapy, symptoms will most likely subside over time. The affected area must be kept clean, moist, and protected from further injury. The patient must also try to avoid skin breakdown by avoiding adhesive covers, harsh chemicals, or exposure to the sun. Minor injuries that are accompanied by burning and itching symptoms may benefit from a topical hydrogel or low-potency steroid cream. However, in particularly bothersome cases such as ulcerations, surgical excision, local wound care, and hyperbaric oxygen have been recommended.[140]

Dermatitis Artefacta/Factitial Dermatitis

The term *dermatitis artefacta* or *factitial dermatitis* is defined as a self-imposed injury that may masquerade as a component of another dermatological disease. Clinical presentation is widely varied and chronic ulcers are a possible manifestation. Clinically, these ulcers are unusually well-defined with sharp or linear edges in areas such as the extremities, abdomen, or anterior chest. These areas are usually affected because they are within reach for self-inflicted injury. Management

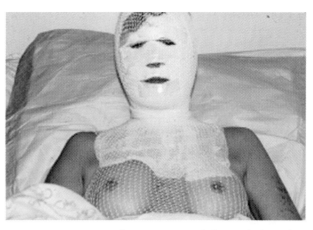

Figure 10•11 Pictured is a *patient with factitial ulcer of her face with dressing in place to limit access to afflicted area.*

includes a multidisciplinary collaboration with mental health professionals and a complete evaluation and treatment of any underlying psychological disease. It is also important to carefully monitor the patient and limit his or her access to the afflicted area (Fig. 10.11); for example, a heavy dressing or casting may have to be implemented to prevent further injuries.[142,143]

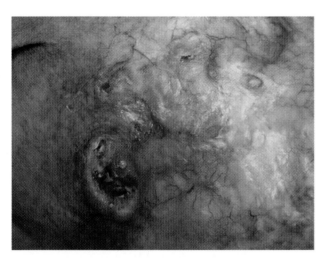

Figure 10•10 This is a *patient with breast cancer after surgery and radiation therapy with a nonhealing ulcer on chest wall.*

Summary

Atypical wounds are generally the result of an underlying condition, and therefore the initial step of management is to diagnose and treat the primary medical disease. Additional treatment targeted toward the wound is an essential component of successful healing, and anti-infectious medications, surgical intervention, and anti-inflammatory agents may have to be used. Local wound care is another critical factor in management, so a moist healing environment, compression dressings, and elevation of the wound are important. The body also has to be in top condition in order to heal well from the inside, thus correcting nutritional deficits and resolving any blood count discrepancies are necessary. In many cases, the complex nature of the diagnosis and treatment of atypical wounds requires a multidisciplinary approach between many medical specialties and health-care providers.

References

1. Phillips, TJ, Dover, JS: Leg ulcers. J Am Acad Dermatol 1991; 25:965–987.
2. Falabella, A, Falanga, V: Uncommon causes of ulcers. Clin Plast Surg 1998; 25:467–479.
3. Araujo, T, Kirsner, RS: Atypical wounds. In: Baranoski, S, Ayello, EA (eds.): Wound Care Essentials: Practice Principles. Philadelphia, Lippincott Williams & Wilkins, 2003, pp 381–398.
4. Anderson, J, Hanson, D, Langemo, D, et al: Atypical wounds: Recognizing and treating the uncommon. Adv Skin Wound Care 2005; 18:466, 468–470.
5. Panuncialman, J, Falanga, V: Basic approach to inflammatory ulcers. Dermatol Ther 2006; 19:365–376.
6. Kerdel, FA: Inflammatory ulcers. J Dermatol Surg Oncol 1993; 19:772–778.
7. Iglesias-Gamarra, A, Restrepo, JF, Matteson, EL: Small-vessel vasculitis. Curr Rheumatol Rep 2007; 9:304–311.
8. Lotti, T, Ghersetich, I, Comacchi, C, et al: Cutaneous small-vessel vasculitis. J Am Acad Dermatol 1998; 39:667–687.
9. Gibson, LE: Cutaneous vasculitis: Approach to diagnosis and systemic associations. Mayo Clin Proc 1990; 65:221–229.
10. Russell, JP, Gibson, LE: Primary cutaneous small vessel vasculitis: Approach to diagnosis and treatment. Int J Dermatol 2006; 45:3–13.

11. Carlson, JA, Chen, KR: Cutaneous vasculitis update: Neutrophilic muscular vessel and eosinophilic, granulomatous, and lymphocytic vasculitis syndromes. Am J Dermatopathol 2007; 29:32–43.

12. Jennette, JC, Falk, RJ: Small-vessel vasculitis. N Engl J Med 1997; 337:1512–1523.

13. Scott, DG, Watts, RA: Systemic vasculitis: Epidemiology, classification, and environmental factors. Ann Rheum Dis 2000; 59:161–163.

14. Brunsting, LA, Goeckerman, WH, O'Leary, PA: Pyoderma (echthyma) gangrenosum: Clinical and experimental observations in five cases occurring in adults. Arch Dermatol Syphilol 1930; 22:655–680.

15. Crowson, AN, Nuovo, GJ, Mihm, MC Jr., et al: Cutaneous manifestations of Crohn's disease, its spectrum, and its pathogenesis: Intracellular consensus bacterial 16S rRNA is associated with the gastrointestinal but not the cutaneous manifestations of Crohn's disease. Hum Pathol 2003; 34:1185–1192.

16. Greenbaum, SS: Phagedaena geometrica (Brocq). Inoculation studies with viable bacteria cultured from lesions of phagedaena geometrica (Brocq) (chronic burrowing ulcer and pyoderma gangrenosum). Arch Dermatol Syphilol 1941; 43:775–801.

17. von den Driesch, P: Pyoderma gangrenosum: A report of 44 cases with follow-up. Br J Dermatol 1997; 137:1000–1005.

18. Wise, CA, Gillum, JD, Seidman, CE, et al: Mutations in CD2BP1 disrupt binding to PTP PEST and are responsible for PAPA syndrome: An autoinflammatory disorder. Hum Mol Genet 2002; 11:961–969.

19. Hoffman, MD: Inflammatory ulcers. Clin Dermatol 2007; 25:131–138.

20. Callen, JP: Pyoderma gangrenosum. Lancet 1998; 351:581–585.

21. Langan, SM, Powell, FC: Vegetative pyoderma gangrenosum: A report of two new cases and a review of the literature. Int J Dermatol 2005; 44:623–629.

22. Sheldon, DG, Sawchuk, LL, Kozarek, RA, et al: Twenty cases of peristomal pyoderma gangrenosum: Diagnostic implications and management. Arch Surg 2000; 135:564–568.

23. Wolf, R, Lotti, T, Ruocco, V: Isomorphic versus isotopic response: Data and hypotheses. J Eur Acad Dermatol Venereol 2003; 17:123–125.

24. Papi, M, Didona, B, Chinni, LM, et al: Koebner phenomenon in an ANCA-positive patient with pyoderma gangrenosum. J Dermatol 1997; 24:583–586.

25. Powell, FC, Schroeter, AL, Su, WP, et al: Pyoderma gangrenosum: A review of 86 patients. Q J Med 1985; 55:173–186.

26. Lindor, NM, Arsenault, TM, Solomon, H, et al: A new autosomal dominant disorder of pyogenic sterile arthritis, pyoderma gangrenosum, and acne: PAPA syndrome. Mayo Clin Proc 1997; 72:611–615.

27. Hohenleutner, U, Mohr, VD, Michel, S, et al: Mycophenolate mofetil and cyclosporin treatment for recalcitrant pyoderma gangrenosum. Lancet 1997; 350:1748.

28. Tan, MH, Gordon, M, Lebwohl, O, et al: Improvement of pyoderma gangrenosum and psoriasis associated with Crohn's disease with anti-tumor necrosis factor alpha monoclonal antibody. Arch Dermatol 2001; 137:930–933.

29. Charles, CA, Leon, A, Banta, MR, et al: Etanercept for the treatment of refractory pyoderma gangrenosum: A brief series. Int J Dermatol 2007; 46:1095–1099.

30. Brooklyn, TN, Dunnill, MG, Shetty, A, et al: Infliximab for the treatment of pyoderma gangrenosum: A randomized, double blind, placebo-controlled trial. Gut 2006; 55:505–509.

31. Cram, DL, Kierland, RR, Winkelmann, RK: Ulcerative lichen planus of the feet. Bullous variant with hair and nail lesions. Arch Dermatol 1966; 93:692–701.

32. Sonnex, TS, Eady, RA, Sparrow, GP, et al: Ulcerative lichen planus associated with webbing of the toes. J R Soc Med 1986; 79:363–365.

33. Micalizzi, C, Tagliapietra, G, Farris, A: Ulcerative lichen planus of the sole with rheumatoid arthritis. Int J Dermatol 1998; 37:862–863.

34. Zijdenbos, LM, Starink, TM, Spronk, CA: Ulcerative lichen planus with associated sicca syndrome and good therapeutic result of skin grafting. J Am Acad Dermatol 1985; 13:667–668.

35. Tsuboi, H, Katsuoka, K: Ulcerative lichen planus associated with Sjögren's syndrome. J Dermatol 2007; 34:131–134.

36. Meyer, S, Burgdorff, T, Szeimies, RM, et al: Management of erosive lichen planus with topical tacrolimus and recurrence secondary to metoprolol. J Eur Acad Dermatol Venereol 2005; 19:236–239.

37. Joshi, RK, Abanmi, A, Jouhargy, E, et al: Etretinate in the treatment of ulcerative lichen planus. Dermatology 1993; 187:73–75.

38. Patrone, P, Stinco, G, La Pia, E, et al: Surgery and cyclosporine A in the treatment of erosive lichen planus of the feet. Eur J Dermatol 1998; 8:243–244.

39. Crotty, CP, Su, WP, Winkelmann, RK: Ulcerative lichen planus. Follow-up of surgical excision and grafting. Arch Dermatol 1980; 116:1252–1256.

40. Urbach, E: Beitrage zu einer physiologischen und pathologischin chemi der hant: Eine enue diabetische stoffwechsel dermatose, nekrobiosis lipoidica diabeticorum. Arch Dermatol Syph 1932; 166:273–285.

41. O'Toole, EA, Kennedy, U, Nolan, JJ, et al: Necrobiosis lipoidica: Only a minority of patients have diabetes mellitus. Br J Dermatol 1999; 140:283–286.

42. Howard, A, White, CR Jr.: Non-infectious granulomas. In: Bolognia, JL, Jorizzo, JL, Rapini, RP (eds.): Dermatology. New York, Mosby, 2003, pp 1455–1469.

43. Lowitt, MH, Dover, JS: Necrobiosis lipoidica. J Am Acad Dermatol 1991; 25:735–748.

44. Clement, M, Guy, R, Pembroke, AC: Squamous cell carcinoma arising in long-standing necrobiosis lipoidica. Arch Dermatol 1985; 121:24–25.

45. Kossard, S, Collins, E, Wargon, O, et al: Squamous carcinomas developing in bilateral lesions of necrobiosis lipoidica. Australas J Dermatol 1987; 28:14–17.

46. Beljaards, RC, Groen, J, Starink, TM: Bilateral squamous cell carcinomas arising in long-standing necrobiosis lipoidica. Dermatologica 1990; 180:96–98.

47. Gudi, VS, Campbell, S, Gould, DJ, et al: Squamous cell carcinoma in an area of necrobiosis lipoidica diabeticorum: A case report. Clin Exp Dermatol 2000; 25:597–599.

48. Imtiaz, KE, Khaleeli, AA: Squamous cell carcinoma developing in necrobiosis lipoidica. Diabet Med 2001; 18:325–328.

49. Santos-Juanes, J, Galache, C, Curto, JR, et al: Squamous cell carcinoma arising in long-standing necrobiosis lipoidica. J Eur Acad Dermatol Venereol 2004; 18:199–200.

50. McIntosh, BC, Lahinjani, S, Narayan, D: Necrobiosis lipoidica resulting in squamous cell carcinoma. Conn Med 2005; 69:401–403.

51. Lim, C, Tschuchnigg, M, Lim, J: Squamous cell carcinoma arising in an area of long-standing necrobiosis lipoidica. J Cutan Pathol 2006; 33:581–583.

52. Boyd, AS: Treatment of necrobiosis lipoidica with pioglitazone. J Am Acad Dermatol 2007; 57:S120–S121.

53. Stuart, L, Wiles, PG: Management of ulcerated necrobiosis lipoidica: An innovative approach. Br J Dermatol 2001; 144:901–922.

54. English, JC 3rd, Patel, PJ, Greer, KE: Sarcoidosis. J Am Acad Dermatol 2001; 44:725–743.

55. Kataria, YP, Holter, JF: Immunology of sarcoidosis. Clin Chest Med 1997; 18:719–739.

56. Fernandez-Faith, E, McDonnell, J: Cutaneous sarcoidosis: Differential diagnosis. Clin Dermatol 2007; 25:276–287.

57. Boeck, C: Multiple benign sarkoid of the skin. J Cutan Genitourin Dis 1899; 17:543–550.

58. Neill, SM, Smith, NP, Eady, RA: Ulcerative sarcoidosis: A rare manifestation of a common disease. Clin Exp Dermatol 1984; 9:277–279.

59. Verdegem, TD, Sharma, OP: Cutaneous ulcers in sarcoidosis. Arch Dermatol 1987; 123:1531–1534.

60. Albertini, JG, Tyler, W, Miller, OF 3rd: Ulcerative sarcoidosis. Case report and review of the literature. Arch Dermatol 1997; 133:215–219.

61. Yoo, SS, Mimouni, D, Nikolskaia, OV, et al: Clinicopathologic features of ulcerative-atrophic sarcoidosis. Int J Dermatol 2004; 43:108–112.

62. Philips, MA, Lynch, J, Azmi, FH: Ulcerative cutaneous sarcoidosis responding to adalimumab. J Am Acad Dermatol 2005; 53:917.

63. Hannon, CW, Swerlick, RA: Vasculitis. In: Bolognia, JL, Jorizzo, JL, Rapini, RP (eds.): Dermatology. New York, Mosby, 2003, pp 381–402.

64. Rao, JK, Weinberger, M, Oddone, EZ, et al: The role of antineutrophil cytoplasmic antibody (c-ANCA) testing in the diagnosis of Wegener's granulomatosis. Ann Intern Med 1995; 123:925–932.

65. Francès, C, Du, LT, Piette, JC, et al: Wegener's granulomatosis. Dermatological manifestations in 75 cases with clinicopathologic correlation. Arch Dermatol 1994; 130:861–867.

66. Fiorentino, DF: Cutaneous vasculitis. J Am Acad Dermatol 2003; 48:311–340.

67. Szõcs, HI, Torma, K, Petrovicz, E, et al: Wegener's granulomatosis presenting as pyoderma gangrenosum. Int J Dermatol 2003; 42:898–902.

68. Bacon, PA: The spectrum of Wegener's granulomatosis and disease relapse. N Engl J Med 2005; 352:330–332.

69. Amdo, TD, Welker, JA: An approach to the diagnosis and treatment of cryofibrinogenemia. Am J Med; 2004; 116:332–337.

70. Piette, W: Cutaneous manifestations of microvascular occlusion syndromes. In: Bolognia, JL, Jorizzo, JL, Rapini, RP (eds.): Dermatology. New York, Mosby, 2003, pp 365–380.

71. Lin, P, Phillips, T: Ulcers. In: Bolognia, JL, Jorizzo, JL, Rapini, RP (eds.): Dermatology. New York, Mosby, 2003, pp 1631–1649.

72. Kirsner, RS, Eaglstein, WH, Katz, MH, et al: Stanozolol causes rapid pain relief and healing of cutaneous ulcers caused by cryofibrinogenemia. J Am Acad Dermatol 1993; 28:71–74.

73. Rallis, TM, Kaduce, DP, Gerwels, JW: Leg ulcers and purple nail beds. Essential mixed cryoglobulinemia. Arch Dermatol 1995; 131:342–343, 345–346.

74. Braun, GS, Horster, S, Wagner, KS, et al: Cryoglobulinaemic vasculitis: Classification and clinical and therapeutic aspects. Postgrad Med J 2007; 83:87–94.

75. Tedeschi, A, Baratè, C, Minola, E, et al: Cryoglobulinemia. Blood Rev 2007; 21:183–200.

76. Asherson, RA, Francès, C, Iaccarino, L, et al: The antiphospholipid antibody syndrome: Diagnosis, skin manifestations, and current therapy. Clin Exp Rheumatol 2006; 24(suppl):S46–S51.

77. Gezer, S: Antiphospholipid syndrome. Dis Mon 2003; 49:696–741.

78. Schlesinger, IH, Farber, GA: Cutaneous ulceration resembling pyoderma gangrenosum in the primary antiphospholipid syndrome: A report of two additional cases and review of the literature. J La State Med Soc 1995; 147:357–361.

79. Herrick, JB: Peculiar elongated and sickle-shaped red blood corpuscles in a case of severe anemia. Arch Int Med 1910; 6:517–521.

80. Ingram, VM: Abnormal human haemoglobins. The comparison of normal human and sickle-cell haemoglobins by fingerprinting. Biochim Biophys Acta 1958; 28:539–545.

81. Ingram, VM: Abnormal human haemoglobins. The chemical difference between normal and sickle cell haemoglobins. Biochim Biophys Acta 1959; 36:402–411.

82. Serjeant, GR: Leg ulceration in sickle cell anemia. Arch of Intern Med 1974; 133:690–694.

83. Koshy, M, Entsuah, R, Koranda, A, et al: Leg ulcers in patients with sickle cell disease. Blood 1989; 74:1403–1408.

84. Gordon, S, Bui, A: Human skin equivalent in the treatment of chronic leg ulcers in sickle cell disease patients. J Am Podiatr Med Assoc 2003; 93:240–241.

85. Eckman, JR: Leg ulcers in sickle cell disease. Hematol Oncol Clin North Am 1996; 10:1333–1344.

86. Steinberg, MH: Predicting clinical severity in sickle cell anaemia. Br J Haematol 2005; 129:465–481.

87. Frenette, PS, Atweh, GF: Sickle cell disease: Old discoveries, new concepts, and future promise. J Clin Invest 2007; 117:850–858.

88. Ofosu, MD, Castro, O, Alarif, L.: Sickle cell leg ulcers are associated with HLA-B35 and Cw4. Arch Dermatol 1987; 123:482–484.

89. Nolan, VG, Adewoye, A, Baldwin, C, et al: Sickle cell leg ulcers: Associations with haemolysis and SNPs in Klotho, TEK and genes of the TGF-beta/BMP pathway. Br J Haematol 2006; 133:570–578.

90. Trent, JT, Kirsner, RS: Leg ulcers in sickle cell disease. Adv Skin Wound Care 2004; 17:410–416.

91. Baum, KF, MacFarlane, DE, Maude, GH, et al: Topical antibiotics in chronic sickle cell leg ulcers. Trans R Soc Trop Med Hyg 1987; 81:847–849.

92. La Grenade, L, Thomas, PW, Serjeant, GR: A randomized controlled trial of solcoseryl and duoderm in chronic sickle-cell ulcers. West Indian Med J 1993; 42:121–123.

93. Reindorf, CA, Walker-Jones, D, Adekile, AD, et al: Rapid healing of sickle cell leg ulcers treated with collagen dressing. J Natl Med Assoc 1989; 81:866–868.

94. Richards, RS, Bowen, CV, Glynn, MF: Microsurgical free flap transfer in sickle cell disease. Ann Plast Surg 1992; 29:278–281.

95. Khouri, RK, Upton, J: Bilateral lower limb salvage with free flaps in a patient with sickle cell ulcers. Ann Plast Surg 1991; 27:574–576.

96. Spence, RJ: The use of a free flap in homozygous sickle cell disease. Plast Reconstr Surg 1985; 76:616–619.

97. Groves, R: Unusual cutaneous mycobacterial diseases. Clin Dermatol 1995; 13:257–263.

98. Timpe, A, Runyon, EH: The relationship of atypical acid-fast bacteria to human disease: A preliminary report. J Lab Clin Med 1954; 44:202–209.

99. Runyon, EH: Anonymous mycobacteria in pulmonary disease. Med Clin North Am 1959; 43:273–290.

100. Pinner, M: Atypical acid-fast microorganisms. Am Rev Tuberc 1935; 32:424–445.

101. Dodiuk-Gad, R, Dyachenko, P, Ziv, M, et al: Nontuberculous mycobacterial infections of the skin: A retrospective study of 25 cases. J Am Acad Dermatol 2007; 57:413–420.

102. Wagner, D, Young, LS: Nontuberculous mycobacterial infections: A clinical review. Infection 2004; 32:257–270.

103. Petitjean, G, Fluckiger, U, Scharen, S, et al: Vertebral osteomyelitis caused by non-tuberculous mycobacteria. Clin Microbiol Infect 2004; 10:951–953.

104. Sobera, JO, Elewski, BE: Fungal diseases. In: Bolognia, JL, Jorizzo, JL, Rapini, RP (eds.): Dermatology. New York, Mosby, 2003, pp 1171–1198.

105. Rivitti, EA, Aoki, V: Deep fungal infections in tropical countries. Clin Dermatol 1999; 17:171–190.

106. Lokuhetty, MD, Alahakoon, VS, Kularatne, BD, et al: Zeil Neelson and Wade-Fite stains to demonstrate medlar bodies of chromoblastomycosis. J Cutan Pathol 2007; 34:71–72.

107. Bonifaz, A, Martinez-Soto, E, Carrasco-Gerard, E, et al: Treatment of chromoblastomycosis with itraconazole, cryosurgery, and combination of both. Int J Dermatol 1997; 36:542–547.

108. Gupta, AK, Taborda, PR, Sanzovo, AD: Alternate week and combination itraconazole and terbinafine therapy for chromoblastomycosis caused by Fonsecaea pedrosoi in Brazil. Med Mycol 2002; 40:529–534.

109. Santos, AL, Palmeira, VF, Rozental, S, et al: Biology and pathogenesis of Fonsecaea pedrosoi, the major etiologic agent of chromoblastomycosis. FEMS Microbiol Rev 2007; 31:570–591.

110. Elgart, GW: Chromoblastomycosis. Dermatol Clin 1996; 14:77–83.

111. Welsh, O, Vera-Cabrera, L, Salinas-Carmona, MC: Mycetoma. Clin Dermatol 2007; 25:195–202.

112. Ahmed, AA, van de Sande, WW, Fahal, A, et al: Management of mycetoma: Major challenge in tropical mycoses with limited international recognition. Curr Opin Infect Dis 2007; 20:146–151.

113. Ramos-e-Silva, M, Vasconcelos, C, Carneiro, S, et al: Sporotrichosis. Clin Dermatol 2007; 25:181–187.

114. Lupi, O, Tyring, SK, McGinnis, MR: Tropical dermatology: Fungal tropical diseases. J Am Acad Dermatol 2005; 53:931–951.

115. Menezes, VM, Soares, BG, Fontes, CJ: Drugs for treating paracoccidioidomycosis. Cochrane Database Syst Rev 2006; 19:CD004967.

116. Borenstein, M, Kerdel, F: Infections with Vibrio vulnificus. Dermatol Clin 2003; 21:245–248.

117. Serrano-Jaen, L, Vega-Lopez, F: Fulminating septicaemia caused by Vibrio vulnificus. Br J Dermatol 2000; 142:386–387.

118. Whitley, RJ, Roizman, B: Herpes simplex virus infections. Lancet 2001; 357:1513–1518.

119. Patel, AR, Romanelli, P, Roberts, B, et al: Treatment of herpes simplex virus infection: Rationale for occlusion. Adv Skin Wound Care 2007; 20:408–412.

120. Trent, JT, Kirsner, RS: Diagnosing necrotizing fasciitis. Adv Skin Wound Care 2002; 15:135–138.

121. Gannon, T: Dermatologic emergencies. When early recognition can be lifesaving. Postgrad Med 1994; 96:67–82.

122. Salcido, RS: Necrotizing fasciitis: Reviewing the causes and treatment strategies. Adv Skin Wound Care 2007; 20:288–293.

123. Gabillot-Carré, M, Roujeau, JC: Acute bacterial skin infections and cellulitis. Curr Opin Infect Dis 2007; 20:118–123.

124. Guldbakke, KK, Khachemoune, A: Calciphylaxis. Int J Dermatol 2007; 46:231–238.

125. Bryant, JH, White, WH: A case of calcification of the arteries and obliterate endarteritis, associated with hydronephrosis, in a child aged six months. Guys Hosp Rep 1898; 55:17–20.

126. Angelis, M, Wong, LL, Myers, SA, et al: Calciphylaxis in patients on hemodialysis: A prevalence study. Surgery 1997; 122:1083–1089.

127. Oh, DH, Eulau, D, Tokugawa, DA, et al: Five cases of calciphylaxis and a review of the literature. J Am Acad Dermatol 1999; 40:979–987.

128. Marjolin, JN: Ulcère: Dictionnaire de Medécine 1828; 21:31–50.

129. DaCosta, JC: Carcinomatous changes in an area of chronic ulceration, or Marjolin's ulcer. Ann Surg 1903; 37:496.

130. Hatzis, GP, Finn, R: Marjolin's ulcer: A review of the literature and report of a unique patient treated with a CO(2) laser. J Oral Maxillofac Surg 2007; 65:2099–2105.

131. Goldberg, DJ, Arbesfeld, D: Squamous cell carcinoma arising in a site of chronic osteomyelitis. J Dermatol Surg Oncol 1991; 17:788–790.

132. Kirsner, RS, Spencer, J, Falanga, V, et al: Squamous cell carcinoma arising in osteomyelitis and chronic wounds. Treatment with Mohs micrographic surgery vs amputation. Dermatol Surg 1996; 22:1015–1018.

133. Swanson, DL, Vetter, RS: Loxoscelism. Clin Dermatol 2006; 24:213–221.

134. Smith, DB, Ickstadt, J, Kucera, J: Brown recluse spider bite: A case study. J Wound Ostomy Continence Nurs 1997; 24:137–143.

135. Futrell, JM: Loxoscelism. Am J Med Sci 1992; 304:261–267.

136. Isbister, GK, White, J: Clinical consequences of spider bites: Recent advances in our understanding. Toxicon 2004; 43:477–492.

137. Edlich, RF, Farinholt, HM, Winters, KL, et al: Modern concepts of treatment and prevention of chemical injuries. J Long Term Eff Med Implants 2005; 15:303–318.

138. Bates, N: Acid and alkali injury. Emerg Nursing 1999; 7:21–26.

139. Newcomer, VD, Young, EM Jr.: Unique wounds and wound emergencies. Dermatol Clin 1993; 11:715–727.

140. Hunter, S, Langemo, D, Thompson, P, et al: Radiation wounds. Adv Skin Wound Care 2007; 20:438–440.

141. Caccialanza, M, Piccinno, R, Beretta, M, et al: Results and side effects of dermatologic radiotherapy: A retrospective study of irradiated cutaneous epithelial neoplasms. J Am Acad Dermatol 1999; 41:589–594.

142. Kwon, EJ, Dans M, Koblenzer, CS, et al: Dermatitis artefacta. J Cutan Med Surg 2006; 10:108–113.

143. Gupta, MA: Somatization disorders in dermatology. Int Rev Psychiatry 2006; 18:41–47.

chapter *11*

Wound Bed Preparation/ Débridement

Karen Albaugh, PT, DPT, MPH, CWS
Harriett Loehne, PT, DPT, CWS, FACCWS

Wound Bed Preparation

Over the years, the rationale for wound débridement has held the following unwavering goals: rid the wound of necrotic tissue, reduce the wound bacterial burden, and correct abnormal wound repair—all with the intention of facilitating the cascade of wound healing. With the introduction of "advanced" wound therapies, such as bioengineered skin and platelet-derived growth factors in the 1990s, it quickly became apparent that these therapies would not be effective unless a conducive environment for wound healing was established.[1] Since 2000, the concept of *wound bed preparation* has given a more focused approach to wound management and, consequently, to the value of débridement in the successful care of patients with chronic wounds. Falanga and Sibbald were among the first to coin the term *wound bed preparation.*[1,2] They have since defined the individual concepts within the model in numerous journal publications. At the crux of the model is the importance of débridement, bacterial control, and adequate moisture balance within the wound bed. These three points, at a minimum, are necessary to establish an environment conducive to healing.

The TIME framework was also inspired by Falanga's work and developed by the International Wound Bed Preparation Advisory Board. It was further refined by the European Wound Management Association (EWMA) as a means of capturing the essential components of wound examination and ensuring targeted interventions. TIME is an acronym for tissue management, infection or inflammation, moisture balance/imbalance, and epithelial or edge advancement.[3] Tissue management involves appropriate application of the various débridement strategies with an overall clinical outcome of a viable wound base. Infection necessitates appropriate assessment of the cellular processes hindering healing, such as the presence of excessive inflammatory cytokines and proteases and ultimately reduction of the bacterial burden and chronic inflammation. Moisture assessment requires the ongoing examination of the wound bed and the procurement of moisture-balancing dressings that prevent both dry environments and excessive fluid environments. And finally, the edge of the wound must be routinely examined to determine if any abnormalities exist or if advanced therapies are warranted to aid in wound contraction.

The overall concept of wound bed preparation continues to develop and take on a more holistic approach, emphasizing "the global management of the wound to accelerate endogenous healing or to facilitate the effectiveness of other therapeutic measures."[4] Use of the term has also led to the understanding that chronic wounds heal differently than do acute wounds and require a unique approach.[1] Experts now agree that the concept has come to involve several comprehensive elements necessary for wound bed preparation, not just examination of the wound bed itself. (Table 11.1) The foremost objective is to determine the "healability,"[2] or capacity to heal, of the patient. By taking a thorough assessment of the patient, not just his or her wound, factors such as comorbidities, blood supply, and nutrition are seen as instrumental considerations in a successful outcome. Wound bed preparation emphasizes a patient-centered approach, which does not resort to prescribed algorithms, but instead considers the individual factors affecting tissue healing in each patient. The patient is encouraged to take a more active role in the process. Examination of individual wound characteristics will tell the history of the wound as well as its ability to heal. The periwound, or surrounding skin, should be carefully observed to help predict potential to heal.

Among the recommendations put forth for wound bed preparation is to débride healable wounds, removing necrotic and infected tissue.[2] Necrotic tissue in the wound bed delays healing and prolongs the inflammatory response of the body's natural defense system. In addition, it serves as an ideal medium for bacterial colonization, leading to a cycle of continued tissue destruction. The body uses endogenous enzymes to help digest necrotic tissue; however, more rapid healing is possible with assistive modes of débridement. Often, pockets of space with necrotic or purulent fluid collection are unmasked during tissue débridement to reveal greater depths of tissue impairment. Once these areas have been rid of necrosis, wounds typically respond in a positive manner and convert from a chronic wound to an acute wound, thus resulting in more expeditious healing.

Removing necrosis is one of the first steps in restoring bacterial control and preventing infection. While it is not practical to think in terms of eradicating all bacteria, the risk for further wound impairment can be greatly lowered when measures are taken to reduce bioburden. Sustained bioburden tips the balance from contamination to critically colonized and then clinically infected. In these situations, the wound/host succumbs to the bacteria, and the wound bed is, in essence, ill-prepared for healing to take place. In the critically colonized wound, healing is at a standstill, with a net result of the wound status being no worse and no better. When infection occurs, the organisms or the virulence of those organisms reach numbers sufficient to overcome host resistance. This agent-host environment of poor bacterial

Table 11•1 Principles of Wound Bed Preparation[1-4]

Identify the cause	Complete a thorough assessment of blood supply and other host factors that may be influencing wound healing or nonhealing. Correct any issues and determine capacity to heal.
Patient-centered approach	Involve the patient in the healing process. Facilitate compliance through active participation, education, and support.
Assess the wound	Complete a thorough assessment of history and clinical characteristics (location, size, tissue composition, undermining, exudate, periwound, thickness of tissue involvement, and pain).
Débridement	Use surgical, sharp, mechanical, autolytic, enzymatic, or maggot débridement methods to remove necrotic or infected tissue from healable wounds. Nonhealable wounds should be managed conservatively, with only the removal of necrotic tissue.
Bacterial control	Assess and control for bacterial burden and infection. Treat the signs and symptoms of infection with appropriate anti-inflammatory, antibacterial, and antibiotic interventions.
Moisture balance	Choose cleansers that are noncytotoxic to healthy tissue. Select dressings that help to create moisture balance within the wound (not too wet, not too dry) and stimulate new tissue growth.
Monitor rate of healing	Continually monitor the rate of wound healing and modify the interventions when healing does not steadily progress. Consider adjunctive therapies and advanced wound agents to enhance healing when progress has slowed.

balance leads to a persistent inflammatory response and a myriad of cellular responses that further hinder the laying down of new granulation tissue and epithelial cells.

Moisture balance is seen as another key component of wound bed preparation. Since the 1960s, the concept of moist wound healing has been shown to be more effective than allowing wounds to dry out or be left open to air.[5] The selection and placement of moisture-retentive dressings will create an optimal environment for migration and proliferation of fibroblasts and epithelial cells. When choosing between the various dressings available to clinicians and patients, it is important to consider the dressing that best manages the physical characteristics observed in the wound bed. The overall goal to achieve moisture balance for proper wound bed preparation essentially involves choosing a dressing that absorbs excess exudate but does not allow the wound to dry out or *desiccate*. Proper control of the exudate will aid in preservation and protection of the surrounding periwound. It should be noted that this will typically involve several different dressing choices throughout the healing process. Clinicians should assess moisture balance with each dressing change and alter the therapeutic approach when wound characteristics change. Chapter 12 will present dressing selection and utilization in much greater detail.

Recent technology in skin equivalents has demonstrated a role for these products to enhance wound bed preparation when overall progress has slowed. Biological dressings should be considered once all other factors described above have been addressed and the wound is still not healing. Various biological dressings and agents aid in wound bed preparation by administering growth factors and providing collagen matrices or scaffolding for cell growth. However, the application of such expensive dressings will be futile if proper débridement, bacterial control, and moisture balance have not been achieved. For these reasons, wound débridement offers a vital step toward overall wound bed preparation.

▶ **PEARL 11•1** Wound bed management includes three key principles for optimizing wound healing: débridement of necrotic tissue, bacterial control, and moisture balance.

Débridement

Débridement is the removal of necrotic and infected tissues that interfere with wound healing. However, a review of the literature reveals a paucity of quality studies providing solid scientific evidence for the implementation of débridement.[6-8] For example, a Cochrane review of débridement in diabetic foot ulcers in 2002 disclosed only five randomized controlled trials eligible for review.[9] Due to the limited number of studies that met eligibility in measuring complete healing or rate of healing, there was no consensus regarding effectiveness between the multiple methods of débridement that exist. In theory, general clinical practice has included débridement for the purposes of identifying the true dimensions of the wounds, removing necrotic tissue, and converting a chronic wound to an acute wound.[2,10,11] Despite the gap between solid evidence involving randomized controlled trials and standard clinical practice, débridement is still a widely accepted component of wound management.

Débridement may be performed on partial or full-thickness wounds of any etiology. Several methods of débridement are available. When selecting a method to employ, clinicians should carefully consider efficiency, patient tolerance, patient medical status, cost, and skill level of the provider. Often, wounds will appear larger following débridement than before the procedure was started, especially in the case of surgical débridement. This possible outcome should be thoroughly explained to the patient prior to performing débridement to assist in patient-centered education and overall compliance.

This chapter will begin with a discussion of the importance of tissue identification. The evidence will be summarized for each of the different débridement methods: surgical, sharp, mechanical, autolytic, enzymatic/chemical, and maggot débridement therapy. Each method will discuss indications, contraindications, and precautions, as well as procedural considerations. The key components of débridement documentation and coding will be discussed, and a clinical case study will highlight several methods of débridement employed to help a patient reach full reepithelialization of a lower extremity wound.

Tissue Identification

Débridement of necrotic tissue poses several risks of harming viable or healthy tissue. The clinician must possess critical knowledge of the anatomy of tissue and the ability to distinguish between tissue types. Those qualified to perform tissue débridement must be able to identify nuances between viable and nonviable tissue to prevent iatrogenic trauma and unnecessary bleeding. The following is a review of the various tissue types and a description of the viable and nonviable presentations of each.

Skin

The integument is the largest organ in the body. It protects and insulates, regulates temperature, processes vitamin D, and facilitates sensory input. It is also the organ responsible for our general appearance, a function important to overall psychological and emotional well-being. Able to repair tissue, the layers of the skin and the essential cells within them routinely repair superficial and deep traumas experienced in everyday living. Each of the three layers—the epidermis, basement membrane, and dermis—provide a different function for protection or integument regeneration.

The *epidermis*, or stratum corneum, is the outermost layer and is composed of mostly dead keratinocytes. This avascular layer is present in varying thickness over the entire body. It generally sloughs off within 30 days as new keratinocytes, developing in the basement membrane, are moved to the surface. The epidermis is responsible for waterproofing the deeper tissues. It allows the skin to absorb some moisture, yet not lose all of the fluids from within the body.

The *basement membrane,* just below the epidermis, is the area in which keratinocyte cell turnover takes place. The basement membrane forms an undulating line between epidermis and dermis, thus connecting the two layers and preventing sliding of one layer over the other. Younger persons have greater redundancy of the undulation, thereby allowing more rapid cell proliferation and quicker healing. With aging, the basement membrane tends to flatten, producing less surface area at the junction, less cell turnover, and less adhesion between the layers of the skin. This is why more complications due to shearing and thinning of the epidermis occur in older individuals.

The *dermis* is the deeper, vascular layer of the skin, which provides nourishment and support for the basement membrane. The dermis is richly supplied with collagen, produced by fibroblasts. Fibroblasts are believed to be essential in wound repair and regeneration, as well as in the overall tensile strength of the integument. Blood vessels, hair follicles, sweat glands, and nerves are located within the dermis.

Subcutaneous Layer

The subcutaneous layer, located immediately below the dermis, provides insulation and cushioning. It is primarily composed of adipose tissue; however, it also contains superficial blood vessels, cutaneous nerves, and lymphatic vessels. The subcutaneous layer varies in thickness with each individual and throughout different parts of the body.[12] This layer can become easily damaged by infection or prolonged pressure. Adipose will normally appear as a pale yellowish-white, globular tissue. When damaged, adipose tissue will become dark yellow.

Fascia

Fascia is a shiny, white, dense connective tissue and is found beneath the subcutaneous layer, surrounding muscles and organs.[12] Caution should be taken when débriding near fascia as infection spreads easily along the smooth fascial planes of skeletal muscles. Incidental débridement of fascia may create a portal of entry for bacteria to the deeper structures of the body.[12]

Skeletal Muscle

Skeletal muscles provide support and function to the skeletal system. Healthy muscle will appear bright red due to its rich vascular supply. (Fig. 11.1) If visible in an open wound, one can observe the healthy contractile nature of the muscle. A dull, dusky appearance, as well as an avascular response, is observed when the muscle becomes necrotic.

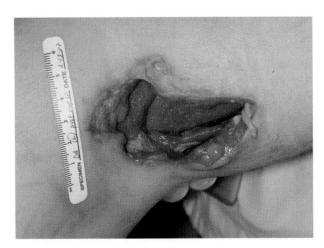

Figure 11•1 *Exposed healthy muscle.*

Tendon

Tendons and ligaments are dense bands of fibrous connective tissue composed mostly of water, with the remainder of the tissue consisting of collagen and glycosaminoglycans.[13] Although important in attaching muscles to bones and bones to bones, these structures have minimal sensory or vascular supply. Exposed tendon can be identified by moving the joint and watching the tendon glide within its sheath. Healthy tendon is shiny and white. If tendons are exposed or the sheath is damaged, they face serious risk of infection due to their limited vascular supply. The tendon will become necrotic if it dries out or desiccates. (Fig. 11.2) Therefore, stringent attempts should be made to keep exposed tendon moist. If kept adequately moist, the tendon may granulate over and receive collateral capillary support. (Fig. 11.3) Realignment of the collagen is possible after an

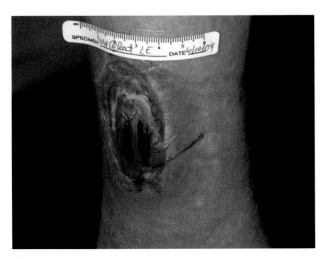

Figure 11•2 *Necrotic tendon.*

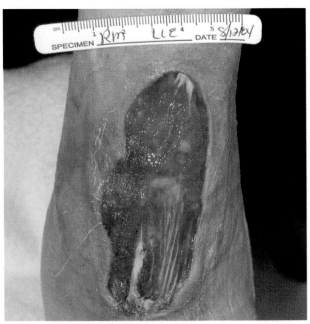

Figure 11•3 *Healthy tendon with granulation tissue surrounding it.*

initial period of immobilization followed by restoration of functional mobility.[13] Aggressive irrigation of the exposed tendon should be avoided as it may cause it to swell within the sheath and become impaired. Necrotic tendon should be débrided by a physician. Loss of the tendon will result in loss of function at that joint.

Bone

Bone is a hard, yet living form of connective tissue that provides structure and protection to the organs of the body. It is hard and white if healthy. (Fig. 11.4) The *periosteum,* or outer covering of the bone, provides nourishment to the bone tissue and is the site of new cartilage and bone formation.[12] With its rich vascular supply, granulation tissue can form over the periosteum as long as the periosteum is still intact and kept moist. However, should the periosteum become desiccated, the bone will become yellow and nonviable. *Compact* and *trabecular* (spongy) bone tissues are located on the inner aspect and will vary in thickness and amount, depending on the function needed by the bone. With exposure, these inner types of bone tissue easily desiccate and will not granulate over, predisposing it to the spread of infection. A bone from which the periosteum has been removed will die.[12]

A *joint* is a union between two or more bones. It is often surrounded by a ligamentous capsule containing lubricating synovial fluid. Incidental débridement or penetration into the capsule may create a portal of entry for bacteria and should be reported to the physician immediately.

Cartilage

The several forms of cartilage include *articular* cartilage (found at the end of bones), *fibrocartilage* (found in the menisci and at the insertions of tendons and ligaments onto the bone), and *elastic* cartilage (found in the ligamentum flavum, external ear, and epiglottis).[13] The primary purpose of cartilage is to cover and cushion the bones at the joints and tendons as they act as pulleys around the bones or other joint surfaces. Articular cartilage is composed of hyaline cartilage and collagen. It tends to be aneural and avascular; therefore, it does not regenerate well once damaged.[12]

Blood Vessels

Blood vessels include arteries, arterioles, capillaries, venules, and veins. These vessels are responsible for the delivery of blood to and from the tissues and organs. Knowledge of the circulatory system and the location of major arteries and veins

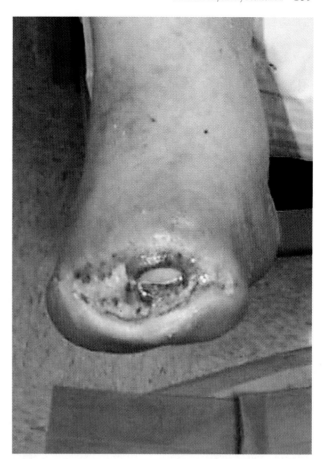

Figure 11•4 *Exposed metatarsal bone.*

is essential when employing débridement methods near these vessels.

Necrotic Tissues, Reparative Tissues, and Wound Drainage

Necrotic tissue is nonviable tissue. It is also described as necrotic fibrin, eschar, or scab. (Table 11.2) Necrotic fibrin ranges in color from yellow to tan, and its adherence may be loose *(slough)* to firmly adherent *(fibrin).* (Figs. 11.5 and 11.6) *Eschar* is composed of desiccated fibrin and is generally tightly adherent. Although often described as leathery, eschar may be soft or hard, depending on the moisture content. (Fig. 11.7) Removal of eschar is hastened by *cross-hatching,* or scoring

Table 11•2 Necrotic Tissue Types			
	Fibrin/Slough	Eschar	Scab
Nature	Moist	Moist to dry fibrin	Dehydrated body fluid
Adherence	Loosely to firmly	Firmly	Loosely to firmly
Appearance	Stringy	Concave	Convex
Texture	Soft and thick	Soft to hard, smooth and leathery	Rough
Color	Yellow, tan, gray	Yellow, brown, black	Yellow, brown, black

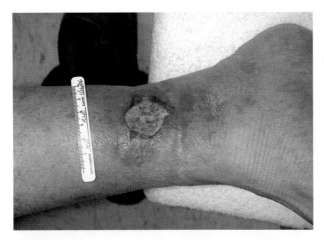

Figure 11•5 *Loosely adherent slough.*

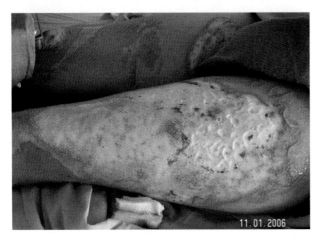

Figure 11•6 *Firmly adherent fibrin. (Courtesy of Luther Kloth)*

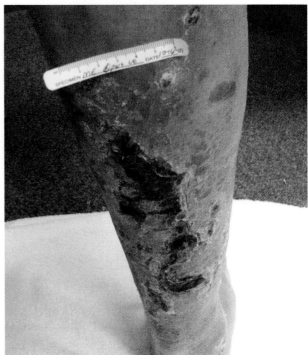

Figure 11•7 *Dry, desiccated eschar on a posterior lower extremity.*

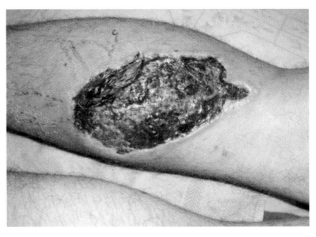

Figure 11•8 *A traumatic wound exhibiting a combination of granulation tissue, slough, necrotic fat, and eschar.*

the surface with a scalpel, which allows greater surface area permeation of enzymatic débriding agents and donated moisture. A *scab* develops when blood and body fluids are permitted to dry out on the surface of the open area. In contrast to the concavity of eschar, a scab usually appears convex and rough on the surface of the skin. A "biological bandaid," the scab serves to protect the superficial wound bed and to maintain a minimal level of sub-scab hydration, which provides moisture for slowly migrating epithelial cells. Thus, rehydration of a scab allows emulsification of the dried fluids and a more rapid healing time. Wounds often exhibit a combination of necrotic tissues at any given time. (Fig. 11.8)

Granulation tissue is the hallmark of wound repair in the fibroblastic phase. Healthy granulation tissue will appear bright or "beefy" red due to its vascular composition and rich collagen makeup. (Fig. 11.9) Granulation tissue will ultimately fill wound depths and defects. Unhealthy or friable granulation tissue appears dull, darker red, and bleeds easily. Friable granulation tissue is one of the clinical signs associated with localized infection. Occasionally, wounds will exhibit *hypergranulation*, a condition in which fibroblast and new capillary growth is excessive, resulting in a raised or "proud flesh" appearance of the granulation tissue as compared to the periwound. (Fig.11.10) Hypergranulation may be managed through chemical cauterization, the use of silver nitrate sticks, or the use of silicone or foam dressings.[14] The hypergranulated areas must be controlled before reepithelialization can occur.

Epithelial tissue resurfaces the wound by migrating over a granulated wound base. It is identified by its pale pink appearance. The epithelial cells will migrate in from the wound edges or appear as islands of new skin in the center of a granulated base. (Fig. 11.11) These islands will stimulate wound bed contraction and contact inhibition until, eventually, the entire wound base is resurfaced. Once resurfaced, the wound is said

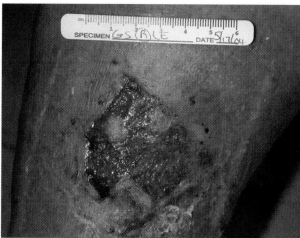

Figure 11•11 *Epithelial budding within granulation tissue.*

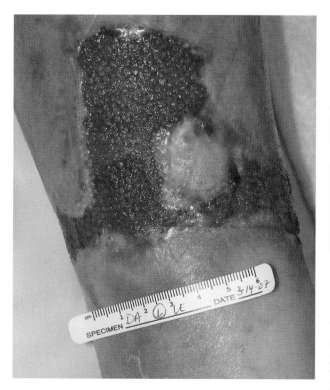

Figure 11•9 *Healthy granulation tissue.*

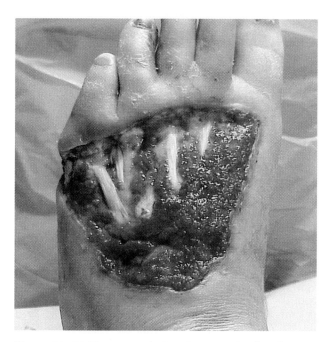

Figure 11•10 *Hypergranulation tissue proximal to the exposed tendons.*

to be reepithelialized, although the remodeling phase of wound healing occurring beneath the surface will continue for several months.

Healing tissues will exhibit drainage associated with keeping the underlying tissues and structures moist. *Transudate*, also called *serous* drainage, is clear or amber in color and is composed of water and 0.9% electrolytes. When tinged with blood, transudate is referred to as *serosanguineous*. *Exudate* describes a more viscous type of drainage, containing plasma proteins, neutrophils, and dead cells. As the number of neutrophils and dead cells increases, the drainage will become more viscous or thick. As a result, the drainage will also take on a yellow, tan, or brown appearance. The term *purulence* (pus) describes thick, yellow to brown, or even green drainage. It is often associated with an odor and localized infection.

Débridement Strategies

This section will discuss the various types of débridement. Table 11.3 summarizes each general strategy, the type of necrotic tissue removal, and examples of methods of débridement by that strategy.

Surgical Débridement

Surgical débridement is the removal of viable and nonviable tissue using sterile, sharp instruments. It has been recognized as the fastest, most effective way to remove debris and necrotic tissue.[11] A Cochrane collaboration review of débridement strategies for diabetic foot ulcers found only one randomized controlled trial that compared surgical débridement with conventional nonsurgical management.[9] The identified study demonstrated 95% of ulcers débrided by surgical means healed as compared to 79% of ulcers managed conservatively.[15] Although surgical débridement is still widely accepted in the treatment of diabetic neuropathic foot ulcers,[5,8] there was insufficient data from the Cochrane review to show whether there was statistical significance in the time it took to heal after surgical débridement.[8,9]

Indications, Contraindications, and Precautions

Wide excision involving the débridement of viable tissue beyond the visible borders of the wound is often deemed necessary to prepare the wound bed and ensure complete removal of necrotic and/or infected areas. It is used to convert a chronic wound into an acute wound.[2,11,16] It is also

Table 11•3 Débridement Strategies

Débridement Strategy	Selective or Nonselective Removal of Necrotic Tissue	Method
Surgical	Nonselective	Sharp instruments
Sharp	Selective	Sharp instruments
Mechanical	Nonselective	Soft abrasion
		Wet to dry
		Whirlpool
		Syringe and needle irrigation
		Jet lavage
		Pulsatile lavage with suction
		Negative-pressure wound therapy
Autolytic	Selective	Moist dressings
		Occlusive dressings
Enzymatic	Selective	Chemical
		Collagenases
		Fibrinolysins
		Proteolytic
Maggot	Selective	Sterile larvae

employed when areas of undermining could not otherwise be visualized. In addition, surgical débridement may be performed to remove hardware, necrotic bone, muscle, or tendon. This method of débridement is contraindicated for the patient who is medically unstable or who lacks vascular supply for adequate healing. Extreme caution must be used when considering surgical débridement with patients taking anticoagulants.[11]

> **PEARL 11•2** Surgical débridement is contraindicated in patients who are medically unstable or lack vascular supply. Extreme caution should be used when patients are taking anticoagulants or have clotting disorders.

Procedural Considerations

Surgical débridement may be performed only by a physician, podiatrist, or certified physician assistant. It is not within the scope of practice of other clinicians due to the excision of viable tissue. Surgical débridement is often associated with significant pain and a resultant bleeding base. A bleeding base is thought to be beneficial in stimulating the release of growth factors.[11] The patient usually requires medication with topical, oral, or intravenous analgesics or anesthesia prior to the procedure. Surgical débridement may be performed in an operating room or outpatient clinic rather than the bedside.

Sharp Débridement

Sharp débridement refers to the exclusive débridement of nonviable tissue using sterile scalpels, forceps, or scissors. Sharp débridement involves a more conservative débridement strategy, often leaving a thin margin of necrosis so viable tissue is not harmed in the process.[16] The removal

of necrosis and bacterial burden is still seen as a positive step toward preparing the wound bed and assisting in converting a chronic wound to an acute wound. Like surgical débridement, very little evidence exists related to sharp débridement. It is, however, widely accepted as standard practice in wound management.

Indications, Contraindications, and Precautions

Sharp débridement is effective in removing eschar, loose slough, or adherent fibrin. A secondary method of débridement is often employed to enhance effectiveness of the overall removal of necrotic tissue. For example, cross-hatching with a scalpel may be performed on desiccated eschar to allow more effective permeation of topical enzymes and donated moisture for further débridement.

Sharp débridement carries all of the previously mentioned concerns associated with surgical débridement in terms of knowledge of anatomy, assessment of adequate blood supply, and assurance of adequate clotting mechanisms. Sharp débridement is contraindicated in several situations. For example a noninfected pressure ulcer on the heel, covered with dry eschar, should be monitored and given adequate pressure relief rather than sharply débrided. The eschar itself may serve as a protective barrier for the wound in an otherwise compromised patient. Débridement would become indicated if the eschar softened or demonstrated clinical signs of infection. Sharp débridement is contraindicated in patients with dry gangrene, severely impaired arterial flow, or impaired clotting mechanisms. Ulcers due to pyoderma gangrenosum should not be sharply débrided as it has been shown to increase the wound size, propagate an inflammatory response, and further delay healing.[3,17] Caution should be used when débriding areas such as tunnels or undermining, where the edge between viable and nonviable tissue can not be easily determined. Caution should also be taken in sharply débriding wounds of individuals receiving anticoagulation therapies or those with low platelet counts.

▶ **PEARL 11•3** Ulcers due to pyoderma gangrenosum should not be sharply débrided as it has been shown to increase the wound size, propagate an inflammatory response, and further delay healing.[3,17]

Procedural Considerations

Clinicians performing sharp débridement must have knowledge of the relevant anatomy, ability to control bleeding if it should occur, and recognition of limitations of débridement.[15] Sharp débridement may be performed by those qualified to surgically débride, as well as other health-care providers, such as physical therapists and registered nurses, who demonstrate evidence of appropriate education and technical competence and who have written approval as defined in their state practice act.

The American Physical Therapy Association (APTA) clearly recognizes wound management as part of physical therapy practice. It is supported by core documents, including the *Normative Model to Physical Therapist Education*, the APTA Position on Model Definition of Physical Therapy, the Federation of State Boards of Physical Therapy's (FSBPT's) Model Practice Act, and the *Guide to Physical Therapy Practice*.[18] According to the Commission on Accreditation of Physical Therapy Education (CAPTE), an accredited physical therapist education program must include wound care in the curriculum. According to the APTA State Government Affairs Office, no state law or rule completely denies physical therapists from providing wound care or sharp débridement.[18] Several states have laws specifying the legal authority for physical therapists to perform wound débridement. These states are Arkansas, Arizona, California, Colorado, Hawaii, Kansas, Montana, New Hampshire, New Mexico, North Carolina, South Dakota, Tennessee, Texas, Utah, and Washington.[18] States that make no mention of wound care or sharp débridement in their physical therapist practice act allow physical therapists to perform wound débridement without restriction, provided the therapist has graduated from an accredited physical therapist education program.[18]

Sharp Débridement Instruments

Sterile forceps, scalpels, or scissors are the most frequently used instruments for sharp or surgical débridement. Débridement instruments may be disposable or reusable stainless steel, which can be cleaned using an autoclave or cold sterilizer. Suture removal kits are not designed for cutting tissue and should not be used for sharp or surgical débridement.

Tissue forceps, such as Adson forceps, may be serrated or nonserrated. Generally, the serrated forceps are more suitable for débridement since they have "teeth" to ensure accurate grasp of the tissue. Forceps can pick up and separate necrotic tissues from viable tissue in preparation for the coordinated removal of necrosis by scalpel or scissors. (Fig. 11.12)

Disposable scalpels come with the blade already attached. Nondisposable scalpel blade handles require the placement of a disposable blade onto a stainless steel handle. The most frequently used scalpel blades are #10, #11, and #15. (Fig. 11.13) A #10 blade is used for removal of a thick

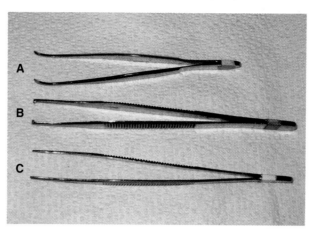

Figure 11•12 *Samples of curved, serrated, and standard forceps.*

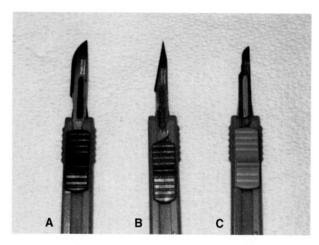

Figure 11•13 *Note the differences in shape between the #10 (A), #11 (B), and #15 (C) scalpel blades.*

callus or hyperkeratotic tissue. It is also helpful in large excisional, surgical débridement. A #11 blade is typically used for incision and drainage of superficial abscesses. A #15 blade is often the blade of choice for precise débridement or cross-hatching.

Several types of scissors are used in wound management. Bandage scissors have a blunt tip and are used to cut tape, sponges, or other dressing materials. They are not intended for tissue débridement. Tissue scissors may be straight or curved. The tips are generally very sharp. Dissection scissors are blunt and used for heavier tissue débridement. (Fig. 11.14)

Disposable use scalpels and instruments are designed for single use and must be disposed of in an appropriate sharps container. (Fig. 11.15) Reusable stainless steel instruments require sterilization in an autoclave or by cold sterilization. Practitioners should follow the autoclave manufacturer's instructions regarding sterilization. Cold sterilization requires that the instruments be cleaned with a brush and then placed in a container with a fixative added. The instruments are left in the cold sterilization solution for approximately 10 hours. The solution may be reused for 28 days.[19]

Stainless steel, surgical-grade instruments (except scalpel blades) should be sharpened on an as-needed basis. In most

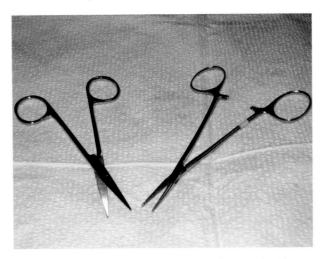

Figure 11•14 *Samples of iris scissors without and with teeth.*

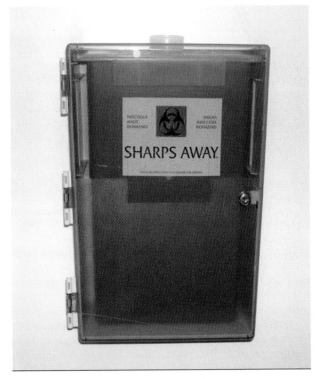

Figure 11•15 *Disposable sharp instruments must be placed in an approved sharps container.*

hospitals, the operating room supervisor will typically have the sharpening schedule dates. If used outside of a hospital setting, the instruments may need to be shipped out for service.

Reusable instruments should be placed in a stainless steel covered container with an enzymatic solution until they can be sterilized. A plastic puncture-resistant container with tight-fitting lid has also been approved by Occupational Safety and Health Administration (OSHA) for transport of contaminated instruments.[19]

Preparation and Technique for Sharp Débridement

Before beginning, make sure the room has adequate lighting and that all supplies are within easy reach. Basic setup should include properly fitting sterile gloves, a pair of sterile forceps, scissors, and a scalpel of the desired blade number. Adequate gauze or hemostatic agents should be accessible in the event of bleeding. Soiled dressings should be removed using clean gloves. Sterile gloves should be used for sharp débridement to prevent the introduction of additional bacteria into the wound bed.

Appropriate personal protective equipment (PPE) includes a face shield or goggles and mask, fluid-resistant gown, and hair cover. A standard waste container and an infectious waste container should be within reach. PPE should be changed or disinfected before it is used with another patient.

The patient should be placed in a comfortable position, providing adequate pressure relief as needed and optimal access to the wound. The treating clinician should be comfortable, relaxed, and able to perform the débridement with proper body mechanics.

Knowledge of anatomical structures and tissue types is of utmost importance before attempting sharp débridement. It is absolutely critical to know where and what to cut. Since sharp débridement involves the removal of only nonviable tissue, clinicians should look for areas where the necrotic tissue has demarcated from the viable tissue and presents an edge for picking it up. (Fig. 11.16) Débridement should progress in a slow fashion, carefully removing tissues in thin layers parallel to the wound base. Débridement should be stopped if pain or bleeding is encountered. When as much loose necrotic tissue has been removed as possible, the residual necrotic tissue can be rehydrated using a moisture-retentive dressing to facilitate sharp débridement on a subsequent visit. If hard eschar is present, it can be scored or cross-hatched using a scalpel and then covered with an enzymatic débriding agent or moisture-retentive dressing to facilitate softening of the eschar.

> **PEARL 11•4** Sharp débridement should progress in a slow fashion, carefully removing necrotic tissues in thin layers parallel to the wound base.

The proper technique for holding forceps is to place them between the thumb and forefinger. If another instrument is being used at the same time, the forceps may be used in either the dominant or nondominant hand. A scalpel should be held like a pencil (between tips of thumb, index, and middle finger) in the dominant hand. Except for scoring hard eschar, all cuts using a scalpel for excising nonviable tissue should be made parallel to the surface of the wound and in a single direction. "Sawing" of tissue is not recommended because the depth of penetration of the blade may reach deeper, healthy tissue. Tissue scissors should be held in the dominant hand using the thumb and ring finger. The index finger may be placed along the blades to steady them during cutting. Care should be taken not to probe with any of the instruments into areas that cannot be easily seen. Although the postdébridement measurements may be larger, the actual wound base and margins will be more evident following the procedure. (Figs. 11.17 and 11.18) The wound

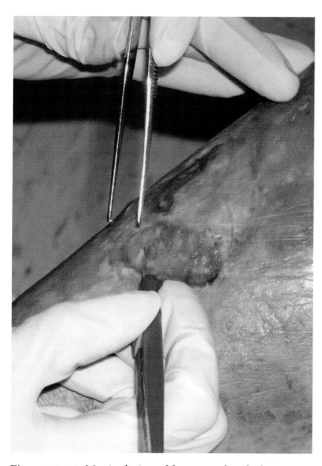

Figure 11•16 *Manipulation of forceps and scalpel to remove loose necrotic slough.*

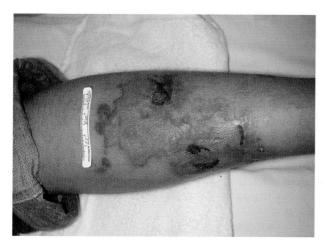

Figure 11•17 *Partial-thickness thermal burn before sharp débridement of blister.*

should be cleansed with normal saline solution. The sterile gloves and soiled débridement field should be removed and replaced with a clean field and gloves for wound redressing.

There are two major indications that sharp débridement has progressed into viable tissue: *pain* and *bleeding*. Débridement of viable tissue is beyond the scope of physical therapists

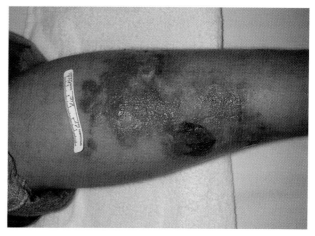

Figure 11•18 *Partial-thickness thermal burn after sharp débridement of blister.*

and nurses and should be avoided. Certain events may require the intervention of a physician if they should occur during sharp débridement.

Theoretically, there should be no pain associated with sharp débridement because it involves nonviable insensate tissue. However, occasionally with sharp débridement the necrotic tissue is tightly adhered to the surrounding healthy insensate tissue, which may be irritated during the procedure. A premedication order may be obtained from the physician to enhance patient comfort during débridement. Oral medication is typically administered 30 minutes prior to the procedure. Intramuscular injections, if warranted, should be given 10 minutes prior to the procedure. Intravenous (IV) medications are generally given right before the débridement is to be performed.[19] Topical analgesics, such as EMLA® (AstraZeneca Pharmaceuticals, Wayne, PA) or Xylocaine® 4% topical solution (AstraZeneca) may be placed on the wound in a thick layer, then covered with an occlusive dressing for 15 to 30 minutes before sharp débridement. The choice of pain control method is dependent on the patient's medical status and tolerance for the procedure.

Removal of nonviable tissue should not result in bleeding; however, because there is often close proximity of viable tissue to nonviable tissue, healthy tissue or vessels may become compromised during the procedure. Extreme caution must be used when débriding a patient on anticoagulant therapy. There are several important steps to follow if bleeding should occur.

For minor bleeding, firm pressure over the site of bleeding for a minimum of 10 minutes will generally be adequate for coagulation of blood. The pressure should be applied for the full 10 minutes, without lifting the dressing or your gloved finger to see if the bleeding has stopped. Once the bleeding has subsided, apply gauze dressings to the area. If the bleeding persists beyond 10 minutes, a silver nitrate stick or hemostatic agent, such as a Gelfoam® (Pfizer Inc., New York, NY) dressing, may be needed to assist with coagulation. These methods require a physician's order but can effectively stop bleeding from a superficial capillary that has been unresponsive to pressure.

▶ **PEARL 11•5** If bleeding should occur during sharp débridement, elevate the extremity and apply pressure for a full 10 minutes, without lifting the dressing or your gloved finger to see if the bleeding has stopped. Redress with gauze.

If the bleeding does not stop with any of the above-mentioned methods, the physician should be notified to determine if further treatments, such as sutures, are required. Regardless of the method chosen to achieve hemostasis, elevation and compression should be employed as soon as possible.

Dr. Wethe, a physician often quoted regarding débridement, once said, "all bleeding stops eventually." He is also quoted as having said, "bleeding you can hear is bleeding to fear." (Wethe, J: Unpublished material, 1997). If arterial bleeding is audible or the source of bleeding cannot be located, the physician should be called immediately.

The very nature of sharp débridement is not without risk of causing trauma or sepsis. Even the most careful clinician will, at some time, inadvertently débride viable tissue. Once again, knowledge of anatomy and the ability to differentiate structures make this a specialized skill that requires clinical competence before performing independently.

Sharp débridement should be terminated if wound edges become unclear, identifiable anatomical structures are visible, bleeding is not easily stopped, or the source of bleeding cannot be located.[20] These situations should be reported to a physician immediately. Additionally, if ever a clinician becomes nervous or uncertain while doing the procedure, sharp débridement should be terminated and a more conservative approach selected until the wound can be further assessed.

Mechanical Débridement

Mechanical débridement refers to removal of necrotic tissue using mechanical sources of energy applied directly to the nonviable tissue. Mechanical débridement includes soft abrasion débridement with gauze or swab, wet-to-dry dressings, hydrotherapy, and negative-pressure wound therapy. Other forms of mechanical débridement, such as the use of an antimicrobial solution, hypochlorous acid (HOCL), and the use of low-frequency ultrasound for débridement will be presented in Chapter 28. The advantages of mechanical débridement are that they help to soften or remove necrotic tissue. The main disadvantages of mechanical débridement, particularly with wet-to-dry and some of the hydrotherapy techniques, is that they are nonselective to necrotic tissue, often performed incorrectly, and many times result in trauma and pain to the wound bed. These will be discussed in further detail where applicable.

Soft Abrasion Débridement
Indications, Contraindications, and Precautions

Soft abrasion débridement is the removal of necrotic tissue using a gauze sponge or calcium alginate-tipped swab. Either technique is effective in the removal of nonadherent, moist necrotic tissue. The technique is generally ineffective with hard, dry eschar or adherent fibrinous necrotic tissue. Soft abrasion may be painful when applied over granulation tissue. Precautions should be maintained when attempting soft débridement with patients on anticoagulant therapy since aggressive friction with a gauze or swab may cause bleeding.

Procedural Considerations

This strategy may be employed daily as part of the cleansing process or on an as-needed basis. It should be discontinued when the wound no longer exhibits loose, moist necrotic tissue or if the necrotic tissue becomes dry and hard. Soft débridement by means of abrading the gauze along the wound edges and the immature, advancing epithelial cells can aid in preventing epibole (rolled wound edges) until the wound base adequately fills in. This may be painful for the patient and should generally be performed only once a day until the advancing epithelial cells are sufficiently held back.

Wet-to-Dry Dressings

Long thought to be a mainstay of wound care, *wet-to-dry dressings* are a nonselective method for débridement of necrotic tissue. If performed properly, the necrotic tissue adheres to the moist gauze dressing and, as the dressing dries, enmeshes in the woven fibers so that it is removed as the gauze is pulled from the wound base. This form of débridement has many disadvantages. If granulation tissue is present, this method will result in the removal of some granulation tissue, as well as necrotic tissue. Maceration, bleeding, and pain are often associated with this form of mechanical débridement. However, one small study suggests that larger-pore, 100% cotton, nonwoven sponges were more effective and less traumatic than smaller-pore sponges in removing necrotic tissue.[21] Another disadvantage is desiccation of the wound bed, which contradicts the principles of moist wound healing and wound bed preparation. There is also concern that this method of débridement is more time intensive and costly than other forms of débridement.

Indications, Contraindications, and Precautions

Wet-to-dry dressings would be indicated when the risk of harming healthy tissue does not exceed the benefit of removing necrotic tissue. It is most effective on loose, necrotic tissue that can adhere to the woven fibers of the gauze. It is not recommended for wounds exhibiting greater than 50% granulation tissue in the wound base. It should not be used on patients who are undergoing anticoagulant therapy. Due to the trauma to healthy granulation tissue, many experts recommend alternate forms of débridement and dressing selection.

Procedural Considerations

Premedication may be necessary to aid pain control and the patient's tolerance of the procedure. Wet-to-dry dressings are typically changed every 12 hours, or when the dressing has dried. An alternative to using this dressing type for mechanical débridement is to change the dressing every 8 hours so that it remains moist and is less painful to remove. Rehydration of the dressing before removal, or use of a wet-to-moist dressing, helps to minimize pain and damage to the epithelial cells and granulation tissue; however, mechanical débridement is less effective and the periwound could become macerated.

Hydrotherapy

There are several forms of hydrotherapy that fall under mechanical débridement category. These methods include whirlpool, syringe and needle irrigation, jet lavage, and pulsatile lavage with suction.

Whirlpool

Historically, submerging the wound in a *whirlpool* is one of the most commonly used methods of hydrotherapy for wound débridement. (Fig. 11.19) During the past 10 years, its use has declined due to lack of evidence and the emergence of newer, more efficient systems to irrigate and mechanically débride necrotic tissue. The whirlpool method involves immersion of the involved body part in a tank filled with water. A turbine mixes air and water to create agitation of the water. Although warm whirlpools are known to increase circulation, the intensity of the agitation may be detrimental to granulation tissue. When possible, care should be taken to avoid directly exposing the wound to the aeration from the turbine.

One of the major disadvantages of using the whirlpool is the inability to control the force coming from the turbine and the resultant pressure of water on the wound. In 1994 the Agency for Health Care Policy and Research (AHCPR) set a guideline for safe irrigation impact forces of 4 to 15 pounds per square inch (psi).[22] The exact force generated by turbines in a full-body or limb hydrotherapy tank is not known but is

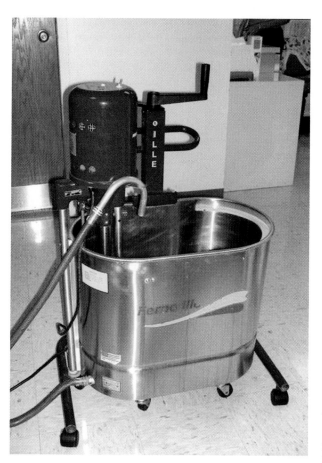

Figure 11•19 *An extremity whirlpool tank.*

assumed to exceed this, particularly if the extremity comes in close contact with the turbine. Animal studies have shown that forces greater than 15 psi may drive bacteria deeper into the tissue.[23] The whirlpool method is considered a nonselective form of débridement due to the potential to affect both nonviable and viable tissue.

Another disadvantage of hydrotherapy using a whirlpool is that it places the extremity in a gravity-dependent position. The positioning required is counterproductive for those patients who also exhibit distal extremity edema. Other techniques such as syringe and needle irrigation or pulsatile lavage with suction may be performed in a more discreet manner, with the patient's extremity in a nondependent position.

Whirlpools tend to overhydrate or macerate the wound and surrounding skin. Softening of toenail or fingernail beds, web spaces, and fissures may lead to areas of further bacterial contamination.[11] Callus around a neuropathic ulcer is softened by soaking in a whirlpool and may result in excess moisture accumulating beneath the callus, leading to further tissue destruction and possible infection.

Although whirlpool is intended to decrease bacterial load, cross-contamination has been a significant concern. There have been several studies identifying the risk of *Pseudomonas aeruginosa* contamination with whirlpool use.[24-26] Many of the risks for contamination were attributed to increased host susceptibility to the organism due to the age, disease, and increased hydration and temperature of the skin.[24-26]

Indications, Contraindications, and Precautions

The primary purpose of the whirlpool is for deodorizing, soaking, loosening, and softening adherent necrotic tissue. Whirlpool treatment is indicated for wounds predominately covered in loosely adherent necrotic tissue, exudate, or debris, or where the risk of harming healthy, granulating tissue is minimal. It is also used for removal of thick topical creams associated with burn care. It is not effective on adherent necrosis, eschar, or fibrinous tissue. Whirlpool, as a method for softening or loosening necrotic tissue, is often followed by another form of débridement, such as sharp, enzymatic, or autolytic débridement.

Whirlpool is contraindicated for patients with compromised cardiovascular or pulmonary function, acute phlebitis, or renal failure, as well as for patients with impaired cognitive status, unresponsiveness, or lethargy. It is contraindicated for dry gangrene because submersion would convert the wound to wet gangrene, placing it at greater risk for spread of infection. It is also contraindicated for soaking of a neuropathic foot, which has impaired sweat and sensory function. Soaking of a neuropathic foot wound has also been associated with maceration of the callus and increased risk for infection. Wounds due to severe arterial insufficiency or ischemia should not be placed in a whirlpool. Periwound skin exhibiting maceration or extremity edema is also contraindicated for whirlpool treatment. A full-body whirlpool should not be used for patients with bowel or bladder incontinence. (Table 11.4)

Precautions should be taken when using whirlpool for the following conditions: clean, granulating wounds or epithelialized tissue, new skin grafts, new flaps, and patients with venous insufficiency for which placing them in a dependent position

Table 11•4 Contraindications and Precautions to Whirlpool for Débridement	
Contraindications	**Precautions**
Compromised cardiovascular or pulmonary function	Clean, granulating wounds
Acute phlebitis	New skin grafts or flaps
Renal failure	Venous insufficient wounds
Impaired cognitive status, unresponsiveness, or lethargy	Distal extremity edema
Dry gangrene	Sensory impairment
Neuropathic feet	Diabetic ulcers/callus
Severe arterial insufficiency/ischemia	
Already macerated tissues	
Bowel or bladder incontinence (for full-body tanks)	

may contribute to further lower extremity edema. Patients with sensory impairments may be at risk for thermal burns.

> **PEARL 11•6** Contraindications to whirlpool therapy for wound healing include compromised cardiovascular or pulmonary function, dry gangrene, ischemic wounds, and neuropathic wounds.

Procedural Considerations

Whirlpools come in a variety of sizes and may accommodate individual limbs or be large enough to allow for immersion of the patient using a stretcher or lift. The whirlpool should be filled with tap water. Tanks must be thoroughly disinfected with an approved disinfectant between each use. Additives are not necessary but are often prescribed. Many whirlpool additives, such as povidone-iodine, chloramine-T (Chlorazine®) (Wisconsin Pharmacal Co., Jackson, WI), and sodium hypochlorite (Dakin's solution), have been shown to be cytotoxic to healthy tissue, and this practice has been discouraged.[22] The use of antiseptics will be discussed further in the section on enzymatic and chemical débridement.

Water temperatures should be kept between tepid (80° to 92°F) and neutral (92° to 96°F). Water temperatures in the tepid range have been associated with vasoconstriction in the limb and may chill the wound, slowing clotting and healing.[27] This may be a more appropriate temperature for patients who have compromised venous disease, for which warmer temperatures could cause excessive vasodilatation. Enhanced cellular function and optimal tissue repair has been seen when temperatures are maintained at the core temperature of the body (98°F).[28] Patients receiving whirlpool therapy should be carefully monitored for signs of systemic response to temperature. Thermal responses include an increase in heart and respiratory rates, sedation, analgesia, and muscle relaxation. Temperatures exceeding 98°F may place too much stress on patients with cardiovascular or pulmonary compromise and should also be avoided, especially when considering full-body immersion. Warming or thermal temperatures should also be avoided for patients with sensory loss or for those with compromised vascular systems that cannot effectively dissipate heat. Patients should be observed for changes in mental status or complaints of lightheadedness.

Setting up and disinfecting a whirlpool tank are labor-intensive duties for staff. An extremity tank can require up to 30 gallons of water for a treatment, and a full-body tank takes as much as 425 gallons of water.[19] Once the water is drained, a ring of exudate and loosened tissue is usually visible around the rim of the tank. The tank must be thoroughly cleaned with an approved disinfectant. The resilience of certain bacteria, such as *P. aeruginosa*, make it difficult to ensure the adequate cleansing of the hardware and components associated with the agitator, pipes, and drains. Aerosolization of vapors from the whirlpool during agitation may also contaminate surrounding surface areas such as chairs, floors, and sinks.

Due to safety concerns of water near electrical equipment, it is also recommended that staff remain in close proximity to the whirlpool treatment area. Caution should be taken as patients and clinicians enter and exit the whirlpool since the floor may be very slippery and hazardous.

Frequency and Duration

Whirlpool treatments range from 5 to 20 minutes, depending on the type of wound and medical condition of the patient. Whirlpool treatment once a day is generally sufficient for cleansing, deodorizing, and débriding a wound. More frequent cleansing and débridement by whirlpool is disruptive to endogenous enzymes and healing tissues. Treatment may continue for several days to weeks, but it should be discontinued when the wound bed is more than 50% granulated or when there is no measurable sign of healing.

Infection Control

Standard OSHA precautions and infection control policies should be followed by all personnel in the hydrotherapy area. Masks are appropriate to prevent inhalation of water droplets from the agitation of the whirlpool. Fluid-resistant gowns, hair covers, footwear covers, gloves, and face shields are recommended for personal protection during administration of treatment and cleaning of the whirlpool. All personal protective equipment (PPE) should be changed or disinfected when exiting the area and between each patient contact.

Syringe and Needle Irrigation

Hydrotherapy for mechanical débridement also includes the use of a 35-mL syringe with a 19-gauge needle or angio-catheter. The needle or catheter is held at a right angle to the wound to aid in flushing debris and reducing surface bacterial contamination. Saline or other topical irrigants are delivered from the syringe drain by gravity.

Indications, Contraindications, and Precautions

This method is indicated for clean wounds, small infected wounds, and wounds with loose slough. It is not appropriate for use on wounds with hard eschar or adherent fibrin because the impact pressure is too low to penetrate these types of tissues.

Procedural Considerations

With careful positioning, a basin can be placed to catch the irrigant runoff and prevent soaking the patient's bed. This mechanical débridement strategy is typically used once daily until the wound is free of loose debris or necrotic tissue. The main disadvantage of this strategy is that the irrigant pressure is approximately 8 psi, which is not recommended for irrigating in areas of tunneling or undermining. There is no suction associated with the treatment. As with the previously mentioned forms of hydrotherapy, the risk for splashing necessitates appropriate PPE use and infection control consideration.

Jet Lavage

Jet lavage provides wound irrigation using a pressurized stream of irrigation solution from a device such as a WaterPik® (Fort Collins, CO). Like the mechanical débridement methods previously mentioned, the purpose of this device is to cleanse, deodorize, and débride loose necrotic tissue. Among the disadvantages are the minimal control of pressure and the risk for setting impact pressures greater than 15 psi. Despite the decreased use of this device for mechanical débridement, it is recognized as one of the earliest irrigation tools in débridement and management of soft tissue wounds. It is also recognized as the basis for the development of the system currently known as pulsatile lavage with suction. These newer devices have eliminated many of the disadvantages associated with jet lavage by providing increased control of impact pressures, containment of splash, and a vacuum suction mechanism that stimulates granulation tissue formation.

Jet lavage also includes the use of oxygen and saline under pressure. The Jetox-ND® (DeRoyal, Powell, TN) device has a flexible cup-shaped tip that collects the saline in a mist form over the surface of the wound (Fig. 11.20) and is purported to gently cleanse and débride the wound bed.

High-velocity jet lavage systems, such as Versajet® (Smith & Nephew, London, UK), may be used in hydrosurgery for the débridement of adherent slough and fibrin. These systems use fluid pressures of 1500 to 12,000 psi for tissue excision and contaminant removal.

Indications, Contraindications, and Precautions

The WaterPik device is intended to be an oral cleanser; however, clinicians have used it to mechanically débride wounds that contain loose necrotic tissue. It is ineffective in the softening or removal of hard eschar or adherent fibrin.

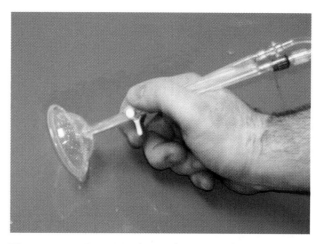

Figure 11•20 *Jetox-ND device. (Courtesy of DeRoyal, Powell, TN).*

Jetox-ND is indicated for the cleansing and débridement of diabetic, pressure, and venous ulcers, as well as burns.

Procedural Considerations

It is of utmost importance that the WaterPik device be used only on the lowest impact pressure setting of number 1, which correlates with 6 psi. Setting it at 3 produces 42 psi, and setting at 5 delivers more than 50 psi.[19] Studies have shown that at higher pressures granulation and epithelial tissues are damaged and bacteria can be driven deeper into the wound.[23] There is no suction available with this device. The risk for splash necessitates use of all of the required PPE discussed earlier. In addition, the device must be routinely disinfected between patients and treatments due to the risk for cross-contamination.

The impact pressure setting on the Jetox device can be adjusted by altering the flow from the oxygen source. (Fig. 11.21) For example, 9 L/min equals 4 psi, while a flow of 15 L/min equals 12 psi. DeRoyal also distributes Jetox-HDC®, which provides compressed oxygen and saline and a suction feature. Efficacy and aerosolization studies have not yet been published for these devices.

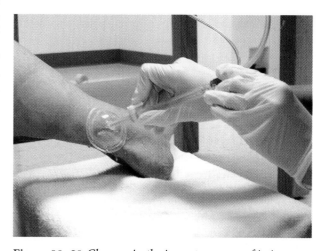

Figure 11•21 *Changes in the impact pressure of irrigant from a jet lavage device are made by adjusting the flow from the oxygen source.*

Pulsatile Lavage with Suction

Pulsatile lavage with suction (PLWS) utilizes mechanical energy as a débridement strategy that provides hydropressure cleansing and débridement of the wound bed with concurrent vacuum (suction) for removal of the irrigant solution, exudates, microorganisms, and debris. The devices were first used during the early 1980s by physicians in the operating room for irrigation during surgical procedures. Since the late 1990s, PLWS has been incorporated into physical therapy wound practice for pressurized irrigation and suction that together débride slough and cleanse the wound bed of bacteria and exudates.

One theory behind the benefit of PLWS in wound healing is that the positive pressure emitted from the irrigant source helps with cleansing and the negative pressure provided by the suction helps to stimulate granulation tissue. A pivotal study by Haynes et al indicated that granulation tissue formation increased as much as 12.2% per week in the subjects receiving PLWS compared to a 4.8% increase in granulation in subjects receiving whirlpool treatment.[29] Although the number of subjects was small ($n = 13$) and the researchers cited many variables that could additionally affect rate of closure, the researchers concluded that the group receiving PLWS had a faster mean closure rate than the group treated with a whirlpool.[29] Further research is needed to confirm this observation.

Another plausible theory for the benefits of PLWS in wound bed preparation is that mechanical irrigation lowers the bacterial count on the wound surface. Substantial literature exists on the use of lavage for bacterial reduction in soft tissue and bone.[30] Bhandari et al theorize that the pulsing of the irrigant produces recoil of the soft tissue, thereby dislodging particulate matter and bacteria.[31] Others believe the effectiveness of bacterial reduction is determined by the irrigation pressure.[32] Anglen et al concluded that the efficacy of bacterial removal was dependent on an interaction between the irrigation system, the wound environment, and the type of bacteria.[30] However, research indicates that an impact pressure that is too high, coupled with impaired host defense, may lead to higher infection potential.[23] Many of the studies in this area are orthopedically based and involve clinical trials with animals instead of human wounds. The literature defines pulsed lavage as delivery of an irrigation solution under pressure; however, many studies do not specify the impact pressure or if the lavage was coupled with suction. When impact pressure is stated, it is often greater than that of therapeutic PLWS. These discrepancies make it difficult to research the evidence specifically related to PLWS.

Hassinger et al explored the evidence for bacterial propagation with use of pulsatile lavage and compared the depth of bacterial penetration into soft tissue after high-pressure pulsatile lavage and low-pressure gravity flow lavage. They found each lavage group showed an increased depth of penetration ($P < 0.05$) compared to control.[23] High pressure lavage had increased depths of penetration when compared to the low-pressure gravity flow ($P < 0.05$).[23] In this study, low-pressure lavage was 3 psi, but high-pressure pulsatile lavage impact pressure was not stated.

Current guidelines for the use of lavage for wound management came from research showing 15 to 25 psi is the minimum effective level of pressure for adequate débridement.[33-34] Irrigation with 15 psi removed 84.8% of bacteria in a contaminated wound, as compared to 48.6% with 1 psi.[33-34] Much of the research for PLWS is in the form of case studies, and more controlled clinical research is needed. Until further research is published, the recommendation is for safe impact pressure to remain between 4 and 15 psi.[22]

Related to PLWS in mechanical effect, negative-pressure wound therapy has been shown to significantly reduce bacterial load in vivo.[35-36] Morykwas et al were able to demonstrate a significant reduction ($P < 0.05$) in porcine tissue bacterial counts after only 4 days of negative-pressure wound therapy.[36] Using vacuum pressures similar to those produced by PLWS (60–100 mm Hg), it appears likely that the suction effect of PLWS may be more effective than the irrigation forces in effectively decreasing wound bacterial burden.

Further investigation by Morykwas and colleagues suggest that the effect of the suction pressures seen with negative-pressure wound therapy systems, such as vacuum-assisted closure (V.A.C.) (KCI, San Antonio, TX), may contribute to faster granulation of the wound bed.[36] Theoretically, this work may explain why, in addition to cleansing and débriding, similar suction or vacuum pressures used in PLWS also produce clinical evidence of increased granulation tissue formation and depth fill in.[36-37]

Indications, Contraindications, and Precautions

PLWS is indicated for, but not limited to, cleansing and débridement of venous insufficient ulcers, neuropathic ulcers, pressure ulcers, postsurgical wounds, infected wounds, partial-take split-thickness skin grafts, and fasciotomies.[38] PLWS is appropriate to use on an infected, necrotic, or granulating wound. Specific treatment applicator tips for the PLWS device make it safe and effective when irrigating tracts, tunnels, and areas of undermining.[38] One of the major advantages of using PLWS over whirlpool treatment is that the limb can be properly elevated and the lavage can be site specific. This is particularly useful when a patient has an edematous limb or multiple venous insufficient ulcers. PLWS is also indicated when the location of the wound does not permit the use of a whirlpool, as in the case of treating a sacral ulcer, without access to a full-body whirlpool. It is also the hydrotherapy method of choice to irrigate a wound when a whirlpool would otherwise be contraindicated due to fever, incontinence, or decreased cognition. PLWS is a viable option when cleansing methods are challenged by such conditions as obesity, contractures, monitoring equipment, or isolation precautions. It can be performed at the bedside in a private room or in a designated treatment area.

There have been no known absolute contraindications to PLWS. However, only experienced clinicians should use PLWS to treat complex wounds, such those with fistulas, exposed cavity linings, or wounds with long tunnels into body cavities.

There are many precautions to consider when using PLWS. As with any débridement method, it is absolutely critical to know the anatomy of the area before beginning the procedure. General precautions should be taken for the use of PLWS over insensate areas, with patients taking anticoagulant medications, and those wounds with tunnels, tracts, or undermining that can not be fully seen. Use of PLWS in the following locations should be reserved for experienced clinicians due to the close proximity of vital structures: near major vessels; near cavity linings (such as the pericardium or peritoneum); at recent bypass or graft sites; at exposed bone, tendon or vessels; at recent grafts or flaps; and facial wounds.

Procedural Considerations

Possessing a strong educational background in anatomy and physiology, physical therapists are ideal practitioners to administer PLWS for débridement and wound bed preparation. Nevertheless, it is recommended to have a physician present when irrigating any of the above complex situations for the first time. Treatment should be stopped if the patient complains of increased pain during the procedure. Notify a physician if bleeding occurs during the treatment.

Three companies, Davol Inc. (Cranston, RI), Stryker Instruments (Kalamazoo, MI), and Zimmer Inc. (Warsaw, IN), currently manufacture and market pulsatile lavage with suction products. (Figs. 11.22, 11.23, 11.24) Each product is

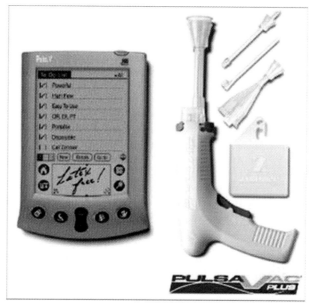

Figure **11•24** *Pulsavac Plus®. (Courtesy of Zimmer, Inc., Warsaw, IN).*

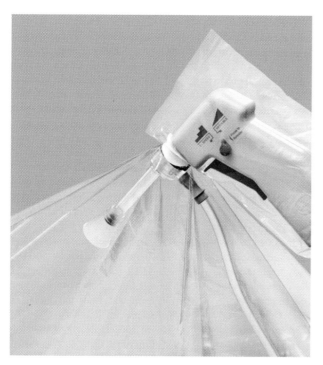

Figure **11•22** *Simpulse® Varicare® System with splash shield. (Courtesy of Davol Inc., Cranston, RI).*

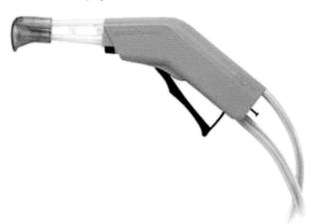

Figure **11•23** *SurgiLav®. (Courtesy of Stryker Instruments, Kalamazoo, MI).*

slightly different in its mechanics, setup, and outcomes. All three devices are distributed in kits containing the necessary handheld control unit, batteries, tubing, and spike for the saline bag. The facility in which the wound is treated will need to supply wall or portable suction, a regulator, one to two normal saline (0.9% sodium chloride) bags, and a collection canister for this therapeutic procedure.

Impact pressure in pounds per square inch (psi). An important consideration when choosing a PLWS system is whether the clinician can control the impact pressure of the irrigant during treatment. Ideally, impact pressure should be adjustable in increments of 1 psi. The Agency for Health Care Policy and Research (AHCPR) guidelines recommend the safe range for irrigation pressure to be between 4 and 15 psi.[22] Most wounds are adequately cleansed and débrided using 8 to 12 psi.[19] Tunnels should be treated more conservatively, with an impact pressure between 2 and 6 psi.[19] Reduction of bacterial levels in infected wounds can be best managed with a setting of 12 to 15 psi.[19] Impact pressures between 12 and 15 psi are also recommended in the presence of large amounts of exudate or necrosis. The clinician should obtain a signed order if the physician requests irrigation pressures greater than 15 psi. It is important to document the impact pressure setting in the treatment record.

▶ **PEARL 11•7** AHCPR guidelines recommend the safe range for irrigation pressure to be between 4 and 15 psi.[22] Most wounds can be adequately cleansed and débrided using 8 to 12 psi.[19] Tunnels should be treated more conservatively, with impact pressures between 2 and 6 psi.[19] Reduction of bacterial levels in infected wounds can be best managed with a setting of 12 to 15 psi.[19]

Irrigation delivery. The preferred irrigant solution is normal saline (0.9% sodium chloride) in bag form. Antibiotic or antiseptic solutions may be added at the physician's discretion. Saline bags should be warmed to 39° to 41°C. This can be accomplished using a fluid warmer or by resting the bag in hot tap water prior to treatment. The number of bags used will depend on the size of the wound and the amount of cleansing and débridement needed.

Each manufacturer makes a variety of exchangeable treatment tips to use with the PLWS device. Most of the tips are for use by physicians in the operating room. Physical therapists can effectively cleanse and débride the majority of patients' wounds using the soft splash shield tip for treating the surface of wounds and the long, flexible tip for tracts and undermining. When using the splash shield tip, it is important to maintain total contact with the wound bed to obtain the desired negative pressure and suction effect. During the treatment, the tip can be guided or molded with the therapist's fingers to adapt to the contours of the wound. (Fig. 11.25) The therapist should break the suction seal if it appears that the suction is too strong over a particular area. The long, flexible tip may be inserted into tunnels and cavities. It should be continuously inserted and retracted to aspirate exudate and loose necrotic tissue. The long, flexible tips have centimeter markings to indicate depth of insertion during the procedure. The same tip may be used on a single patient with multiple wounds during a single treatment session. If this is the case, it is recommended that the least-necrotic wounds be treated first.

Suction. The suction regulator should be set on a continuous mode between 60 and 100 mm Hg. Low-range suction is recommended when the wound is near a vessel, in a tunnel, an undermined area or near a cavity lining.[19] Suction should be decreased if bleeding is noted or if the patient complains of increased pain.

Single use only. The FDA and OSHA demand that the "single use only" directive be followed by any clinician performing PLWS. If the product is used more than once, PLWS is considered to be investigational and nonreimbursable. With the exception of the suction diverter attachments available from Davol and Stryker, all equipment is disposable and must be discarded in a white plastic bag with a biohazard label. Disposable suction canisters can be emptied in a commode before being discarded into a white biohazard bag.

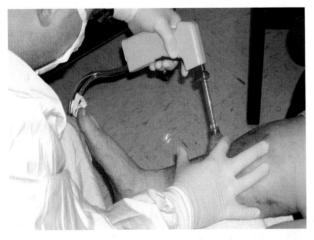

Figure 11•25 *Physical therapist's fingers mold PLWS shield to the wound surface to ensure full contact.*

The suction diverter attachments by Davol and Stryker allow the same handpiece to be used multiple times with the same patient, provided a new treatment tip is used each treatment session. This is only possible because the suction mechanism does not pass the wound effluent through the internal mechanism of the handpiece. Handpieces should be wiped clean, labeled with the patient's identification, and stored in a proper bag until the next treatment. The recommendation for re-use of the same device is up to five times, or 1 week, but this may vary by facility infection-control policies. Keep in mind that as battery life diminishes, so will the effectiveness of the impact[38] and vacuum pressures.

Although the disposable equipment adds to landfill accumulation, several parts of the product are recyclable.[19] The plastic kit containers and locking pins may be recycled. The batteries may be removed from the handpieces and used in other battery-operated devices.

Frequency and duration. Ideally, all wounds with less than 50% necrotic tissue should be treated with PLWS daily.[19] Wounds with more than 50% nonviable tissue or heavy exudate may be treated up to two times daily with PLWS.[19] When a fully granulated wound bed has been achieved, PLWS may be decreased to one to two times per week. Anecdotal reports by expert clinicians have suggested that PLWS, if used appropriately, does not destroy granulation tissue. Further research is needed in this regard. PLWS should be discontinued if there has been no decrease in necrotic tissue or if there has been no increase in granulation or epithelial tissue after 1 week.[19]

Infection control. All OSHA infection control guidelines and facility policies must be followed during administration of PLWS. Proper hand washing is to be emphasized before and after the procedure.

In 2002 Loehne et al described aerosolization of microorganisms during PLWS. Microorganisms were found as far as 8 feet away from the treatment area following a PLWS treatment.[39,40] As a result, specific procedural recommendations include that the patient be treated in a private room with walls and doors that close. Curtained or open gym areas are not acceptable.[40]

A study published in JAMA in 2003 highlighted the concerns with PLWS and aerosolization of bacteria.[41] An outbreak of multidrug-resistant *Acinetobacter baumannii* in a cohort of patients receiving PLWS occurred in a U.S. hospital.[41] The transmission of the bacteria was linked to improper PPE and probable aerosolization of the bacteria during the pulsatile lavage procedure. As a result, the Centers for Disease Control and Prevention (CDC) issued stricter infection control guidelines to prevent the nosocomial spread of infection when using this technology (Box 11-1). Under the new guidelines, no further outbreaks have been reported.

Only approved staff should be permitted in the area during treatment. Family or friends should be asked to leave for the duration of the procedure. Proper PPE for staff includes a face shield, mask, hair covering (with ears covered), fluid-proof (not fluid-resistant) gown with long sleeves, fluid-resistant shoe covers, and gloves that cover the cuffs of the gown. The new guidelines include the use of a surgical mask for the patient as well. All exposed items in the treatment field should be covered with a towel during the treatment procedure. Any linen in the room that was exposed to aerosolized blood or body fluid should be discarded in the soiled linen receptacles.

> ▸ **Box 11•1** | **Infection Control Guidelines for Use of Pulsatile Lavage with Suction**

- Treat the patient in a private room with walls and doors that close.
- Cover exposed supplies and patient belongings with a towel.
- Cover any exposed tubes, ports, etc, and any wounds not being treated.
- Consider having the patient wear a surgical mask.
- Do not permit family or visitors in the room during pulsatile lavage with suction (PLWS) treatment.

- Staff must wear appropriate personal protective equipment (PPE), including face shield, mask, hair covering, fluid-proof gown, fluid-resistant shoe covers, and gloves.
- Discard equipment and soiled linen in appropriate receptacles.
- Do not reuse "single use only" items.
- Thoroughly disinfect all horizontal surfaces, stretchers, wheelchairs, and carts after each treatment.

All horizontal surfaces, stretchers, wheelchairs, and carts used for treatment should be cleaned with an approved disinfectant after each treatment.

> ▸ **PEARL 11•8** PLWS treatments must occur in a private room with walls and doors that close. Curtained or open gym areas are not acceptable.[40]

Negative-Pressure Wound Therapy

Negative-pressure wound therapy (NPWT) is another form of mechanical débridement. It involves the application of negative pressure directly to the wound bed, through foam or gauze dressings, via a computerized vacuum pump. The negative-pressure dressing system assists with drainage removal and necrotic tissue débridement while maintaining a moist wound environment beneath an occlusive, protective seal. NPWT is believed to improve tissue perfusion,[36] enhance granulation tissue formation,[36,37] and reduce bacterial contamination.[35,36] Due to the recent increase in research on this modality and the surge in manufacturing of these devices, this form of débridement will be covered separately in Chapter 31.

Autolytic Débridement

Autolytic débridement, or autolysis, uses moisture-retentive dressings to facilitate the body's own endogenous enzymes in the breakdown of necrotic tissue. Autolysis is discreetly selective and requires minimal skill to perform. In a favorable environment, macrophages, neutrophils, and other phagocytic cells digest devitalized tissue by releasing proteolytic and collagenolytic enzymes that are normally present in wound fluid. Dressings that create this optimal environment include hydrogels, hydrocolloids, transparent films, and alginates. This form of débridement is typically painless. A Cochrane review of débridement strategies found the use of hydrogels was statistically more effective than the use of gauze when treating diabetic ulcers, resulting in a faster rate of healing.[8,9] Overall, autolytic débridement is the slowest of all methods of débridement, and the patient will need to be monitored closely for signs of infection.

Indications, Contraindications, and Precautions

Autolytic débridement is a conservative approach, indicated for dry or moist necrotic wounds and patients who cannot tolerate other, more aggressive forms of débridement. It is ideal for long-term care or home care settings in which visits may be infrequent or where caregivers can be easily instructed in the dressing application and signs or symptoms of infection.

The use of occlusive dressings for autolysis is contraindicated in the presence of clinical signs or symptoms of infection. In the event of serious infection, autolytic débridement should be discontinued at once.[42] Autolytic débridement using moist dressings is also contraindicated for wounds exhibiting dry gangrene. Converting a dry gangrene to a wet gangrene places the patient at greater risk for deeper infection. Dry gangrene should be kept dry. The same precautions would be in place for a patient with a dry, arterial insufficient ulcer.

Procedural Considerations

Rehydration of a scab or dried eschar is facilitated through the application of a moisture-retentive dressing such as a hydrocolloid or transparent film. Autolytic débridement is often used in conjunction with other débridement strategies such as cross-hatching to soften hard eschar in preparation for sharp débridement. Another example of autolytic débridement is the use of hydrogel to maintain a moist environment for a diabetic ulcer. The net result of autolysis is often a "soupy" exudate of liquefied slough and drainage, which may have a faint anaerobic odor upon dressing removal. (Fig. 11.26) The loose material is easily

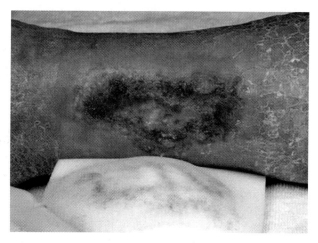

Figure 11•26 *Liquefied slough and exudate on a foam dressing after autolytic débridement.*

flushed out from the wound bed with gentle cleansing. Patients and caregivers using moisture-retentive dressings such as a transparent films or hydrocolloids should be instructed in recognizing the clinical signs and symptoms of infection and to notify their treating clinician immediately if they see such signs. Another form of débridement should be considered if a significant change in the necrotic tissue is not witnessed within 72 hours of applying a dressing for autolytic débridement purposes.[2,11]

Enzymatic/Chemical Débridement

Enzymatic débridement is a selective form of débridement involving the application of a topical enzymatic agent to promote emulsification of the devitalized tissue on the wound surface. Enzymatic agents include collagenases, fibrinolysins, and proteolytic enzymes, such as papain-urea. The type of enzyme selected is dependent on the clinical wound presentation. Collagenases selectively digest the collagen that binds nonviable tissue to the wound base.[11] Fibrinolysins inactivate fibrinogen and help to dilate blood vessels in the wound bed, thereby encouraging an inflammatory response.[11] Papain and urea work together to denature proteins, aiding in the digestion of fibrin in the wound bed.[11]

Several small studies have attempted to compare the effectiveness of each of the enzymatic agents available on the market; however, the literature is inconsistent regarding which agent is best. An animal model study comparing a fibrinolysin to a collagenase found the collagenase to be statistically more effective in both speed and reduction of necrosis.[43] The clinical effectiveness of collagenases and proteolytic enzymes was compared in a study by Alvarez et al involving 21 patients with pressure ulcers. The group receiving the papain-urea enzyme experienced significantly more effective reduction in the amount of black eschar and fibrin than the group receiving a collagenase (86.5% vs 37.3% at 3 weeks, 95.4% vs 35.8% at 4 weeks).[44] Both enzymes were found to be more effective on black eschar than on fibrin slough within the wound base.[44] Ayello and colleagues summarized the literature comparing collagenases and proteolytic enzymes by stating that collagenases appear to work slower because they work from the bottom of the wound up.[42] Papain-urea agents appear to initially work more rapidly because they débride from the top down.[42]

In general, enzymatic débridement is a slower method than sharp or surgical débridement, but a faster, more predictable method than autolytic débridement. It is usually less painful and traumatic than mechanical débridement.

Indications, Contraindications, and Precautions

Enzymatic débridement is most effective in softening large necrotic areas by denaturing the protein or necrotic collagen tissue in the wound base. Enzymatic agents can be used with infected wounds; however, close monitoring is advised since this method is significantly slower than surgical débridement.

Contraindications to enzymes include the concurrent use of chemicals or heavy metal ions, which may inactivate the enzymes. Hydrogen peroxide and heavy metals, such as silvers, should not be used with proteolytic enzymes, such as papain-urea. Silver- and zinc-containing dressings should not be used with collagenases since they alter the effective pH of the enzyme.[42] Enzymatic agents are less effective with heavily draining wounds because they tend to wash away. As a general precaution, some patients may experience transient irritation, pain, or periwound erythema with the use of enzymatic agents. Maceration of the periwound is possible if the ointment is applied too heavily or if there is significant drainage. Of all the enzymes, papain-urea does appear to produce more exudate in its emulsification of necrotic tissue and therefore may cause more maceration or periwound irritation.

Procedural Considerations

This method of débridement requires a physician's order and a prescription for the enzymatic agent. Collagenases typically come in a petroleum base. An example of a collagenase is Santyl® ointment (Healthpoint, Fort Worth, TX). Papain-urea products are typically prepared as hydrophilic ointments. Examples of these products include Ethezyme® (formerly manufactured by Ethex Corp., St. Louis, MO), and Accuzyme® (Healthpoint). Proteolytic enzymes may also contain chlorophyllin copper complex, which is reported to promote granulation and control odor.[45] The ointments containing chlorophyllin copper complex appear dark green in color. Examples of these products include Panafil® (Healthpoint) and Ziox 405® Ointment (Stratus Pharmaceuticals, Miami, FL). (Fig. 11.27) However, as of November 2008, papain-containing products have been recalled by the FDA due to safety concerns. They are no longer being manufactured or distributed. Collagenase is not part of the recall.

Before enzymatic débridement, the wound should be cleansed with normal saline. Permeation of the pharmacological agent is enhanced through cross-hatching the eschar to create greater surface area. Apply a thin layer of the enzymatic agent directly on the necrotic portions of the wound using a tongue depressor. A gauze dressing moistened with normal saline will help to activate the enzymes and provide moisture to the tissues.

> **PEARL 11•9** Permeation of the enzymatic agent is enhanced through cross-hatching the eschar to create greater surface area.

Collagenases are typically applied once a day. Proteolytic agents, such as those containing papain-urea, should be applied one to two times daily. Because they work slowly,

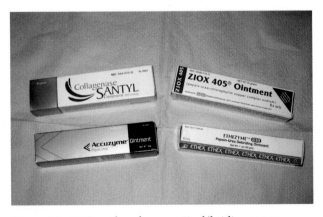

Figure 11•27 *Samples of enzymatic débriding agents.*

enzymatic débriders may be used for a few days to several weeks. They should be discontinued when necrotic tissue is no longer present. Although several manufacturers state that papain-urea with chlorophyllin copper complex products can be used until wound closure, no clinical studies have supported this recommendation. Ongoing use of a petroleum-based ointment may actually retard wound healing since a nonconductive oil-based medium will impede the physiological lateral voltage gradients that influence epithelial migration at the wound edge. Enzymes should be discontinued when there is no necrotic tissue present or when there has been a lack of progress in granulation tissue.

Chemical débridement involves the use of nonselective chemical substances, such as antiseptics or silver nitrate, for the removal of bacteria, foreign matter, and necrotic tissue. Chemical agents include the use of bleach and boric acid (Dakin's solution), hydrogen peroxide, acetic acid, povidone-iodine (Betadine®), chloramine-T (Chlorazene®), and chlorhexidine gluconate (Hibiclens®). The existing AHCPR guideline does not recommend the use of skin cleansers or disinfectants in wounds because of the cytotoxic effect they have on viable cells.[22] However, the AHCPR guidelines were established in 1994. Since then, in vitro research is emerging that suggests that some antiseptic agents are less toxic than once believed. In 2007 Kloth et al[46] found that chloramine-T was 100% effective against gram-positive bacteria tested in vitro, including *Staphylococcus aureus*, methicillin-resistant *S. aureus,* and vancomycin-resistant enterococcus, without fibroblast damage. Chloramine-T was also found to be highly effective in the reduction of *Escherichia coli* growth with minimal fibroblast damage.[46] There was little effectiveness noted in the reduction of *P. aeruginosa*.[46] The in vitro study did conclude that the negative effects of antiseptics, such as chloramine-T, are dependent on the concentration used and the time of exposure. Further in vivo research is needed to determine acceptable levels for sufficient organism kill rate without cytotoxic damage to fibroblasts. With additional research, the use of certain antiseptics in appropriate concentrations may again become acceptable in combination with mechanical débridement methods such as hydrotherapy and PLWS.

Indications, Contraindications, and Precautions

Antiseptic agents present an alternative to antibiotics in the reduction of bacterial contamination without posing a risk for bacterial resistance. Their effectiveness is typically viewed more in terms of bacterial reduction than in débridement capability.

In general, chemical agents are contraindicated for use in the presence of healthy granulation or macerated tissues. Tunnels and undermining can trap the solution, thus increasing the toxicity of the chemical. Previous research has not conclusively shown a reduction in superficial bacterial counts when using these chemicals on chronic wounds. The effervescence of hydrogen peroxide has not been shown to significantly remove necrotic tissue better than other methods of débridement. Many experts still feel that, even when diluted, the risks of these chemicals harming granulation tissue far outweigh any benefit as débriding agents.[3]

Cauterization as a method of chemical débridement would be indicated when hypergranulation is evident and the purpose is to even out the surface contours of the wound bed.

Procedural Considerations

Chemical cauterization with a silver nitrate stick entails twirling of the stick over the hypergranulated area until a gray or charred appearance is visible. The wound would then be cleansed and redressed. The clinician and patient should expect to see an increase in wound drainage since chemical cauterization does tend to precipitate an inflammatory response. The procedure is generally not painful, and results are usually seen after one to two treatments. A physician's order is needed for this form of débridement.

Maggot Débridement Therapy

Maggot débridement therapy (MDT) is also known as larval therapy, myiasis, biotherapy, or biosurgery. Its origin dates back as far as the 16th century, but it was William Baer[47] who first brought the use of sterile maggots for purposes of wound healing to the United States during the 1930s. The application of maggots decreased in the 1940s, but is now experiencing a resurgence in research and practice as clinical evidence has shown maggots to effectively ingest and reduce antibiotic-resistant strains of bacteria in the wound bed.

With this recurrent form of débridement, sterile larvae from the common green bottle fly, *Phaenicia (Lucilia) sericata* are applied to the wound surface. The larvae selectively ingest necrotic tissue and excrete proteolytic enzymes, which further denature the necrotic tissue.[47] Biological débridement is also thought to be antimicrobial, since the secretion of ammonia raises the wound pH.[48,49] Wound pH has been shown to increase from acid to neutral or slightly alkaline pH of 7 to 8.[49] The antibacterial effects of MDT have been attributed to the apparent ingestion of bacteria by the maggots. Studies have shown the gut of the larvae to be heavily contaminated with bacteria following débridement.[47] Other benefits noted with this type of débridement are reduction of odor and lack of pain with the procedure.

Research is now focusing on the effects of *P. sericata* on fibroblasts[50] and growth factor and cytokine release[51] as possible explanations for the increase in granulation tissue. Other evidence suggests that the maggots stimulate granulation tissue through a "micromassage" effect.[16,47] MDT has been successfully used in the treatment of pyoderma gangrenosum.[52] Sherman et al studied 21 outpatient subjects with nonhealing wounds.[53] Eight of the subjects were recommended for amputation. After MDT, only 3 subjects required surgical resection. Eleven subjects went on to heal without any further interventions.[53] Maggot therapy was also found to have a better healing outcome when compared to conventional treatment with patients who had pressure ulcers.[54]

This method of débridement has no reported toxicity or allergic reactions; however, some patients have reported a tingling, itching, or mild discomfort. Bleeding has been reported only in rare instances. Although the maggots have been shown to rapidly digest necrotic material, this method of débridement is slower than sharp or surgical débridement. Large, prospective, randomized trials have been hampered by lack of funding and aesthetic concerns.

Indications, Contraindications, and Precautions

MDT débridement is indicated for any nonhealing wound containing slough or other necrotic tissue. It is an alternative for débriding pyoderma gangrenosum for which surgical or sharp débridement is otherwise contraindicated.[52] MDT is contraindicated in the presence of severe infection, in wounds with inadequate blood supply, or with patients who have increased risk for bleeding.

Procedural Considerations

Sterile larvae from the green bottle fly is the only form of maggots used therapeutically for débridement. The number of larvae applied will vary depending on wound size. Although sources vary, the general recommendation is no more than 10 larvae per square centimeter, with fewer applied when necrosis is less prevalent. A fine, sterile mesh dressing is used to contain the larvae. The mesh is then covered with a hydrocolloid that sufficiently covers the treated area. The dressing is left in place for 1 to 3 days. Larvae will burrow down into crevices but not feed upon granulation tissue. Upon removal, the larvae will appear significantly larger in size. As they reach full-grown status, they will come to the surface of the wound and can be easily removed. (Fig. 11.28) The dressing and any remaining larvae should be double-bagged and sent for incineration. Several applications of sterile larvae may be needed, depending on the wound size and amount of necrosis.

Documentation of Débridement

Appropriate documentation of wound débridement is necessary from both a legal and clinical perspective. Documentation of débridement must include the type of débridement method selected, description of the tissues débrided, patient tolerance to procedure (whether any analgesia was necessary), and a description of any adverse events requiring physician notification. Additional information that may be necessary includes where the débridement procedure occurred, the type of wound bed irrigation, and the parameters of débridement strategy if applicable (ie, type of enzyme or impact and vacuum pressures of hydrotherapy procedure). Finally, a reassessment of the tissues postdébridement should describe the wound bed composition, periwound, drainage, follow-up

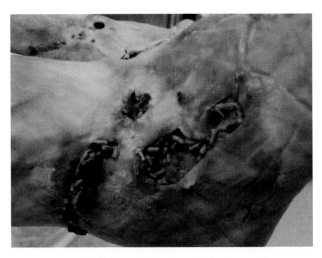

Figure 11•28 *Full grown larvae ready for removal. (Courtesy of Luther Kloth)*

dressing care, and any patient or caregiver education that may have taken place.

Coding for Débridement

Current Procedural Terminology (CPT®), published by the American Medical Association (AMA) describes the criteria for billing codes for various treatment interventions. As of January 1, 2006, the débridement codes for Active Wound Care Management by physician or nonphysician personnel are 97597, 97598, and 97602.[55] A description of these codes is provided in Table 11.5. The former code for selective débridement, 97601, has been deleted. The first two Active Wound Care Management codes are only to be used when sharp débridement with scissors, scalpel, and forceps or high-pressure water jet with or without suction is performed, without the use of anesthesia.[55] The codes are not timed but do require direct or one-on-one contact between the patient and provider. Clinicians should only submit for reimbursement when the skill level required meets the description of the procedural code. If multiple wounds are débrided during one visit, the total surface area should be calculated to determine if the total wound area is greater

Table 11•5	Débridement Codes
CPT code	**Description[55]**
97597	Removal of devitalized tissue from wound(s) by selective débridement without anesthesia (eg, high-pressure water jet with/without suction, sharp selective débridement with scissors, scalpel, and forceps), with or without topical application(s), wound assessment, and instruction(s) for ongoing care; may include use of a whirlpool, per session. Total wound(s) surface area less than or equal to 20 cm².
97598	Total wound(s) surface area greater than 20 cm².
97602	Removal of devitalized tissue from wound(s) by nonselective débridement without anesthesia (eg, wet-to-moist dressings, enzymatic, abrasion), including topical application(s), wound assessment, and instruction(s) for ongoing care, per session.

▶ **PEARL 11•10** To determine which CPT® code to use for sharp débridement or PLWS when multiple wounds are débrided during one visit, calculate the cumulative surface area to determine if the total wound area is greater than or less than 20 cm².

than or less than 20 cm². The codes include topical applications, wound assessment, and patient instruction.[55] Note that whirlpool may be included in this procedure and would not be billed separately.

Procedure code 97602 describes nonselective débridement, which may occur with autolytic, chemical, or enzymatic débridement. It is recommended that this code be used when there is evidence of change in the necrotic tissue as a result of the débridement method. The code includes topical applications, wound assessment, and any necessary patient instruction regarding dressings or care.[55]

Only physicians may use the débridement procedure codes in the 11040 to 11044 range. These codes reflect excisional débridement and are written to denote the surgical débridement of different levels of thickness in the skin and underlying structures. They may not be billed in conjunction with 97597, 97598, or 97602.[55]

Summary

This chapter has discussed the holistic concept of wound bed preparation, yet focused primarily on the débridement aspect of that framework. Knowledge of anatomy is paramount with any form of débridement. Therefore, a discussion of the different types of tissues and necroses was included to remind the clinician of that importance. Evidence was provided comparing the properties and effective outcomes of each débridement strategy. Guidelines for determining the most efficient and efficacious method of débridement have been presented. The type of débridement strategy chosen will depend on comfort level and training of the clinician, presentation of the wound and type of necrosis, presence or absence of infection, pain tolerance of the patient, and the débridement resources available.

▶ **Case Study 11•1**   **Débridement of a Crush Injury of the Foot**

History

Mr. McG is a 46-year-old male who presents with an ulcer on the plantar surface of his left foot. (Fig. 11.29) His medical history is unremarkable except for hypertension. Mr. McG is alert and oriented; he lives alone. He drives a truck for a living, but is currently on disability. He reports that 1 month ago, while assisting to disengage the trailer from the cab of the truck, the footer of the rig was inadvertently put down on his left foot. He was wearing steel-tipped boots at the time. The trailer was immediately jacked up, and Mr. McG was rushed to the emergency room. He was discharged from the hospital after

Figure 11•29 *Clinical presentation of Mr. McG's left foot upon initial examination at the wound center.*

radiographs were negative for fracture. Pulses were intact in the bilateral lower extremities. There were no open areas. Within a week, he developed progressive redness and darkening of the bottom of his left foot. His primary doctor treated the foot with bacitracin and gauze. He was seen by his doctor for 3 weeks before being referred to an outpatient wound care clinic.

Systems Review

Integument: The wound is located on the distal two thirds of the plantar surface of the left foot; the toes are not involved. It measures 13.6 cm × 8.8 cm × questionable depth; wound bed composition is 10% red, 20% necrotic yellow fat, and 70% dry black eschar. Periwound erythema extends approximately 2 cm surrounding the entire wound. There is a moderate amount of serosanguineous drainage with no odor detected.

Anthropometric Characteristics: Girth measurements of the left foot are approximately 2 cm larger than the right foot at the metatarsal aspect and arch; height is 5'11", and weight is 172 lb.

Joint Integrity, MMT, ROM, Posture: Lower extremity strength and range of motion (ROM) are within normal limits (WNL), except for the left ankle; ROM is decreased to neutral only; dorsiflexion is fair; unable to manual muscle test (MMT) plantarflexion due to tenderness with hand placement; standing and sitting posture appear to be normal.

Pain: Patient reports pain and occasional throbbing in the left foot. He rates his pain on a visual analog scale as 4 out of 10, especially at time of dressing changes and with prolonged ambulation. He uses over-the-counter pain relievers and reports that his pain deceases to 2 out of 10, but never really goes away.

Continued

▸ **Case Study 11•1** | **Débridement of a Crush Injury of the Foot—cont'd**

Ventilation, Respiration, Circulation: He has normal breath sounds at 16 breaths per minute, a resting heart rate of 72 beat per minute, and blood pressure of 138/82 with medication. He is negative for venous or arterial disease, with palpable 3+ dorsalis pedis and posterior tibialis pulses bilaterally.

Sensory and Reflex Integrity: Reflexes are intact. There is diminished sensation over areas of eschar and tenderness in wound perimeter and toes. He is intact to light touch on dorsum of foot and rest of lower extremities.

Motor Function, Gait, Balance: Independent with ADLs. He has an antalgic gait and tends to step on toes and not place the left heel fully down. His balance appears to be normal, yet guarded.

Orthotic, Prosthetic, Supportive, Assistive, and Adaptive Devices: He is wearing a cast shoe on the left foot and a regular sneaker on the right foot.

Aerobic Capacity and Endurance: Functional.

Self-Care and Home Management: Independent with current dressings and wound care. He lives independently in a two-story home.

Work and Community: He is employed as a truck driver, but is currently out on disability.

Tests and Measures

1. Girth measurements
2. Wound measurements
3. Wound culture

Recommended Interventions

Wound Management: A combination of strategies is recommended: sharp débridement (with scissors, scalpel, and forceps), enzymatic débridement (papain-urea enzyme), pulsed lavage with suction to remove nonviable tissue and decrease bacterial burden, antibiotics as needed to manage infection, support stocking of 15 to 20 mm Hg compression to decrease edema in the left foot and lower extremity, electrical stimulation combined with moist wound care to promote wound closure, complete off-loading of the left foot, and education regarding signs and symptoms of infection.

Exercise and Rehabilitation: He will be provided with crutches and crutch training to promote complete non-weight bearing on the left lower extremity while healing; general lower extremity exercise program to decrease left lower extremity edema and restore ankle muscle strength; and Achilles tendon stretching to increase ankle ROM.

Educational Considerations: Education includes the following: wound care, self-care issues, infection control, edema management.

Other Considerations: He is a possible candidate for skin grafting once necrotic tissue is removed and granulating base is established. He will need to moisturize newly healed tissue and be evaluated for appropriate footwear once the wound is reepithelialized.

References

1. Falanga, V: Classifications for wound bed preparation and stimulation of chronic wounds. Wound Repair Regen 2000; 8:347–352.
2. Sibbald, RG, Williamson, D, Orsted, HL, et al: Preparing the wound bed—Debridement, bacterial balance, and moisture balance. Ostomy Wound Manage 2000; 46:14–35.
3. Sibbald, RG, Schultz, GS, Falanga, V, et al: Preparing the wound bed: Focus on infection and inflammation. Ostomy Wound Manage 2003; 49:24–51.
4. Falanga, V: Wound bed preparation: Future approaches. Ostomy Wound Manage 2003; 49(suppl):30–33.
5. Winter, GD: Formation of the scab and the rate of epithelialization of superficial wounds in the skin of the young domestic pig. Nature 1962; 193:293–294.
6. Steed, DL, Donohoe, D, Webster MW, et al: Diabetic ulcer study group: Effect of extensive debridement and treatment on the healing of diabetic foot ulcers. J Am Coll Surg 1996; 183:61–64.
7. Bale, S: A guide to wound debridement. J Wound Care 1997; 6:179–182.
8. Smith, J, Thow, J: Update of systematic review on debridement—wound care. Diabetic Foot 2003; 6:12–16.
9. Smith, J.: Debridement of diabetic foot ulcers. Cochrane Database Syst Rev 2002; CD003556.
10. Edmonds, M, Foster, A: Stage 3: The ulcerated foot. In: Edmonds, M, Foster, A (eds): Managing the Diabetic Foot. London, Blackwell Science, 2000, pp 45–76.
11. Schultz, GS, Sibbald, R, Falanga, V, et al: Wound bed preparation: A systematic approach to wound management. Wound Repair Regen 2003; 11:1–28.
12. Moore, KL, Dalley, AF: Introduction to clinically oriented anatomy. In: Clinically Oriented Anatomy. Baltimore, Lippincott Williams & Wilkins, 2006, pp 2–73.
13. Tepper, SH, McKeough, DM: Injury, inflammation, and healing. In: Goodman, CC, Fuller, KS, Boissonnault, WG (eds): Pathology: Implications for the Physical Therapist. Philadelphia, Saunders, 2003, pp 120–152.
14. Sussman C: Assessment of the skin and wound. In: Sussman, C, Bates-Jensen, B (eds): Wound Care: A Collaborative Practice Manual for Health Professionals. Baltimore, Lippincott Williams & Wilkins, 2007, pp 85–122.
15. Piaggesi, A, Schipani, E, Campi, F, et al: Conservative surgical approach versus non-surgical management for diabetic neuropathic foot ulcers: A randomized trial. Diabetic Med 1998; 15:412–417.
16. Vowden, K, Vowden P: Wound bed preparation. World Wide Wounds. Available at: http://www.worldwidewounds.com/2002/april/Vowden/Wound-Bed-Preparation.html
17. Papageorgiou, KI, Matthew, RG, Kaniorou-Larai, MG, et al: Lessons of the week: Pyoderma gangrenosum in ulcerative colitis: Considerations for an early diagnosis. BMJ 2005; 331:1323–1324.

18. APTA State Government Affairs: APTA review of state PT practice acts: Wound care/debridement. Unpublished, 2002, amended 2006. www.apta.org, contact Director of State Government Affairs.

19. Loehne, HB: Wound debridement and irrigation. In: Kloth, LC, McCulloch, JM (eds): Wound Healing Alternatives in Management, ed. 3. Philadelphia, FA Davis, 2002, pp 203–231.

20. Leaper, D: Sharp debridement technique for wound debridement. World Wide Wounds. Available at: http://www.worldwidewounds. com/2002/december/Leaper/Sharp-Debridement.html. Accessed 10/23/09.

21. Mulder, GD: Evaluation of three non-woven sponges in the debridement of chronic wounds. Ostomy Wound Manage 1995; 41:62–67.

22. Bergstrom, N: Treatment of Pressure Ulcers. Clinical Practice Guideline. Quick Reference Guide for Clinicians. No. 15, Pub. No. 95–0652. Rockville, MD, U.S. Department of Health and Human Services, Public Health Service, Agency for Health Care Policy and Research, 1994.

23. Hassinger, SM: High-pressure pulsatile lavage propagates bacteria into soft tissue. Clin Ortho & Related Res 2005; 439:27–31.

24. Jacobson, JA: Pool-associated *Pseudomonas aeruginosa* dermatitis and other bathing-associated infections. Infect Control 1985; 6:398–401.

25. Solomon, SL: Host factors in whirlpool-associated *Pseudomonas aeruginosa* skin disease. Infect Control 1985; 6:402–406.

26. Shankowsky, HA, Heather A, Callioux, LS, et al: North American survey of hydrotherapy in modern burn care. J Burn Care Rehabil 1994; 15:143–146.

27. Sussman, C: Whirlpool. In: Sussman, C, Bates-Jensen, B (eds): Wound Care: A Collaborative Practice Manual for Health Professionals. Baltimore, Lippincott Williams & Wilkins, 2007, pp 644–664.

28. Kloth, LC, Berman, JE, Dumit-Minkel, S, et al: Effects of normothermic dressing on pressure ulcer healing. Adv Skin Wound Care 2000; 13:69–74.

29. Haynes, LJ, Brown, MH, Handley, BC, et al: Comparison of Pulsavac and sterile whirlpool regarding the promotion of tissue granulation (abstr). Phys Ther 1994; 74(suppl):S4.

30. Anglen, J, Apostoles, PS, Christensen, G, et al: Removal of surface bacteria by irrigation. J Orthop Res 1996; 14:251–254.

31. Bhandari, M, Adili, A, Schemitsch, EH, et al: The efficacy of low-pressure lavage with different irrigating solutions to remove adherent bacteria from bone. J Bone Joint Surg 2001; 83A:412–419.

32. Bahrs, C, Schnabel, M, Frank, T, et al: Lavage of contaminated surfaces: An in vitro evaluation of the effectiveness of different systems. J Surg Res 2003; 112:26–30.

33. Rodeheaver, GT, Pettry, D, Thacker, JG, et al: Wound cleansing by high pressure irrigation. Surg Gynecol Obstet 1975; 141:357–362.

34. Wheeler, CB, Rodeheaver, GT, Thacker, JG, et al: Side effects of high pressure irrigation. Surg Gynecol Obstet 1978; 143:775–778.

35. Morykwas, MJ, Argenta, LC: Use of negative pressure to decrease bacterial colonization in contaminated open wounds. Abstract presented at: the annual meeting of the Federation of American Societies for Experimental Biology Annual Meeting, New Orleans, LA, March, 1993.

36. Morykwas, MJ, Argenta, LC, Shelton-Brown EI, et al: Vacuum-assisted closure: A new method for wound control and treatment: Animal studies and basic foundation. Ann Plast Surg 1997; 38:553–562.

37. Morykwas, MJ, Argenta, LC: Use of negative pressure to increase the rate of granulation tissue formation in chronic open wounds. Abstract presented at: Federation of American Societies for Experimental Biology Annual Meeting, New Orleans, LA, March, 1993.

38. Loehne, HB: Pulsatile lavage with suction. In: Sussman, C, Bates-Jensen, B (eds): Wound Care: A Collaborative Practice Manual for Health Professionals. Baltimore, Lippincott Williams & Wilkins, 2007, pp 665–682.

39. Loehne, HB, Streed, SA, Gaither, B, et al: Aerosolization of microorganisms during pulsatile lavage with suction (abstr). Ostomy Wound Manage 2002; 48:75.

40. Streed, S: Aerosolization of microorganisms during pulsatile lavage. Presented at: The 1999 APIC Annual Educational Conference and International Meeting, Baltimore, MD, June, 1999.

41. Maragakis, LL, Cosgrove, SE, Song, X, et al: An outbreak of multidrug-resistant *Acinetobacter baumannii* associated with pulsatile lavage wound treatment. JAMA 2004; 292:3006–3011.

42. Ayello, EA, Cuddigan, JE: Debridement: Controlling the necrotic/cellular burden. Adv Skin Wound Care 2004; 17:66–75.

43. Mekkes, J, Zeegelaar, JE, Westerhof, W, et al: Quantitative and objective evaluation of wound debriding properties of collagenase and fibrinolysin/deoxyribonuclease in a necrotic ulcer animal model. Arch Dermatol Res 1998; 290:152–157.

44. Alvarez, OM, Fernandez-Obregon, A, Rogers, RS, et al: Chemical debridement of pressure ulcers: A prospective, randomized, comparative trial of collagenase and papain-urea for pressure ulcer debridement. Wounds 2000; 12:15–25.

45. Brett, DW: Chlorophyllin—A healer? A hypothesis for its activity. Wounds 2005; 17:190–195.

46. Kloth, LC, Berman, JE, Laatsch LJ, et al: Bactericidal and cytotoxic effects of chloramine-T on wound pathogens and human fibroblasts in vitro. Adv Skin Wound Care 2007; 20:3312–3345.

47. Nigam, Y, Bexfield, A, Thomas, S, et al: Maggot therapy: The science and implication for CAM—history and bacterial resistance. Evid Based Complement Alternat Med 2006; 3(Pt 1):223–227.

48. Thomas, S, Andrews, AM, Hay, NP, et al: The anti-microbial activity of maggot secretions: Results of a preliminary study. J Tissue Viability 1999; 9:127–132.

49. Nigam, Y, Bexfield, A, Thomas, S, et al: Maggot therapy: The science and implication for CAM—Maggots Combat Infection. Evid Based Complement Alternat Med 2006; 3(Pt 2):303–308.

50. Horobin, AJ, Shakesheff, KM, Pritchard, DI, et al: Maggots and wound healing: An investigation of the effects of secretions from *Lucilia sericata* larvae upon the migration of human dermal fibroblasts over a fibronectin-coated surface. *Wound Repair Regen* 2005; 13:422–433.

51. Mumcuoglu, K, Miller, J, Mumcuoglu, M, et al: Destruction of bacteria in the digestive tract of the maggot of *Lucilia sericata* (Diptera: Calliphoridae). *J Med Entomo* 2001; 38:161–166.

52. Rozin, A, Balbir-Gurman, A, Gilead, L, et al: Combined therapy for pyoderma gangrenosum. Ann Rheum Dis 2004; 63: 888–889.

53. Sherman, RA, Sherman, J, Gilead, L, et al: Maggot debridement therapy in outpatients. Arch Phys Med Rehabil 2001; 82:1226–1229.

54. Sherman, RA, Wyle, FA, Vule, M, et al: Maggot debridement therapy for treating pressure ulcers in spinal cord injury patients. J Spinal Cord Med 1995; 18:71–74.

55. American Medical Association: Current Procedural Terminology-CPT® 2007. American Medical Association 2006; pp 52, 416.

chapter 12

Dressings and Skin Substitutes

Liza G. Ovington, PhD, CWS, FACCWS

Introduction

This chapter provides an overview of wound dressings developed for the management of chronic wounds as well as a discussion of products commonly known as skin substitutes. At first glance, it may seem incongruous to cover wound dressings and skin substitutes in one chapter; however, if one seeks to generally define these two classes of products, the similarity becomes apparent. Wound dressings are a predominantly synthetic and heterogeneous group of medical devices that aid in the topical management of a wide variety of wound types and conditions and that vary greatly in their materials of composition as well as their purported mechanisms of action. Skin substitutes are a predominantly biological and heterogeneous group of substances that aid in the temporary or permanent closure of a wide variety of wound types and that may also vary greatly in their materials of composition and purported mechanisms of action. The differences between the two categories are specifically their materials of composition and proposed mechanisms of action. One might actually view skin substitutes as a natural progression of dressing technology. In clinical practice, these two categories of products are often used simultaneously and or sequentially in the course of wound management.

We begin this discussion with an examination of wound dressing categories and skin substitutes by looking at a description of the various materials of composition and their functions and mechanisms of action in the wound environment. This is followed by a discussion of the existing evidence for efficacy and utility in the health-care environment. It is not intended that this chapter be a discussion of individual wound

care products. A listing of several manufacturers and some of their more common products is presented in Chapter Appendix 1.

Dressings for Wound Care

Currently, there are over 400 different dressings commercially available for wound management in the United States.[1] (Table 12.1) Dressings for wound care are categorized by the Center for Medicare Services for reimbursement according to their composition, their dimensions, and whether they include a circumferential adhesive border. These reimbursement categories are shown in Table 12.2. More practically, dressings are categorized by health-care professionals based on their function in the wound environment, that is, what they do to facilitate the healing process. (Table 12.3).

The primary role of a dressing in the wound environment is to manage tissue moisture levels; however, this is a relatively new expectation in terms of wound dressing history. Up until the late 1970s, dressings for wound management allowed, or were even intended to promote, desiccation of the surface of the wound's exposed dermal tissues. Intact tissues are normally dry only at the level of the nonliving layer of the epidermis, the stratum corneum. Living tissues and cells function in an inherently moist environment that is normally maintained by the intact stratum corneum and skin lipids. Research has shown that open wounds are subject to high levels of evaporative moisture loss, which is primarily related to wound depth rather than etiology. Measurements made on the rate of moisture vapor loss from

Table 12•1 Commercially Available Wound Dressing Types

Dressing Material and Format	Number of Brands*
Alginate dressings	25
Collagen dressings	10
Composite dressings	28
Contact layers	13
Foam dressings	76
Gauze, nonimpregnated	44
Gauze, impregnated	23
Hydrocolloid dressings	46
Hydrogel dressing, gauze-impregnated form	18
Hydrogel dressings, sheet form	23
Hydrogel dressing, amorphous form	40
Specialty absorptive dressings	19
Transparent films	27
Wound fillers	10
Antimicrobial dressings	60

*According to Kestrel Health Information: WoundSource: The Kestral Wound Product Sourcebook. Hinesburg, VT, Kestral Health Information Inc., 2007.

venous ulcers averaged 188 mg/cm^2/day compared to that measured from nearby unwounded skin, which averaged 22 mg/cm^2/day, representing a ninefold increase in moisture loss when the epidermis is not present.[2]

The pivotal research of Winter and Maibach in the 1960s demonstrated in both animal and human models that wounds where this evaporative moisture loss was prevented by an occlusive film healed significantly more quickly than wounds in which unimpeded moisture loss resulted in tissue desiccation.[3,4] After this concept of *moist wound healing* became accepted, a variety of dressings designed to deliver it began to appear in the marketplace. Materials other than cellulose (gauze) began to be explored and exploited for their use as wound dressings. Ideally, a wound dressing should establish and maintain a balance of moisture in the wound tissues that is similar to their nonwounded or pre-wounded state. The concept of balance is important because excessive moisture levels created by an accumulation of wound exudates can promote tissue maceration and breakdown, which may interfere with the healing process just as deficient moisture levels can interfere with healing by causing tissue desiccation and cellular death. Topical wound dressings with the ability to balance tissue moisture levels are generally referred to as *moist wound healing dressings*, or more simply as *advanced dressings*.

> **PEARL 12•1** Central to the concept of "moist wound healing" is the fact that wounds heal faster when evaporative loss of fluid is minimized.

Table 12•2 Medicare Dressing Categories

HCPCS Code	Dressing Material and Format	Dressing Size
A6010	Collagen-based wound filler, dry form	Per gram
A6011	Collagen-based wound filler, gel/paste	Per gram
A6021	Collagen dressing	≤16 sq in
A6022	Collagen dressing	>16 ≤48 sq in
A6023	Collagen dressing	>48 sq in
A6024	Collagen dressing wound filler	Per 6 in
A6196	Alginate or other fiber gelling dressing	≤16 sq in
A6197	Alginate or other fiber gelling dressing	>16 ≤48 sq in
A6198	Alginate or other fiber gelling dressing	>48 sq in
A6199	Alginate or other fiber gelling dressing, wound filler	Per 6 in
A6200	Composite dressing, no adhesive border	≤16 sq in
A6201	Composite dressing, no adhesive border	>16 ≤48 sq in
A6202	Composite dressing, no adhesive border	>48 sq in

Continued

Table 12•2 Medicare Dressing Categories—cont'd

HCPCS Code	Dressing Material and Format	Dressing Size
A6203	Composite dressing, any adhesive border	≤16 sq in
A6204	Composite dressing, any adhesive border	>16 ≤48 sq in
A6205	Composite dressing, any adhesive border	>48 sq in
A6206	Contact layer	≤16 sq in
A6207	Contact layer	>16 ≤48 sq in
A6208	Contact layer	>48 sq in
A6209	Foam dressing, no adhesive border	≤16 sq in
A6210	Foam dressing, no adhesive border	>16 ≤48 sq in
A6211	Foam dressing, no adhesive border	>48 sq in
A6212	Foam dressing, any adhesive border	≤16 sq in
A6213	Foam dressing, any adhesive border	>16 ≤48 sq in
A6214	Foam dressing, any adhesive border	>48 sq in
A6215	Foam dressing, wound filler	Per gram
A6216	Gauze, nonimpregnated, nonsterile, no adhesive border	≤16 sq in
A6217	Gauze, nonimpregnated, nonsterile, no adhesive border	>16 ≤48 sq in
A6218	Gauze, nonimpregnated, nonsterile, no adhesive border	>48 sq in
A6402	Gauze, nonimpregnated, sterile, no adhesive border	≤16 sq in
A6403	Gauze, nonimpregnated, sterile, no adhesive border	>16 ≤48 sq in
A6404	Gauze, nonimpregnated, sterile, no adhesive border	>48 sq in
A6219	Gauze, nonimpregnated, any adhesive border	≤16 sq in
A6220	Gauze, nonimpregnated, any adhesive border	>16 ≤48 sq in
A6221	Gauze, nonimpregnated, any adhesive border	>48 sq in
A6222	Gauze, impregnated with other than water, normal saline, or hydrogel, no adhesive border	≤16 sq in
A6223	Gauze, impregnated with other than water, normal saline, or hydrogel, no adhesive border	>16 ≤48 sq in
A6224	Gauze, impregnated with other than water, normal saline, or hydrogel, no adhesive border	>48 sq in
A6228	Gauze, impregnated, water or normal saline, no adhesive border	≤16 sq in
A6229	Gauze, impregnated, water or normal saline, no adhesive border	>16 ≤48 sq in
A6230	Gauze, impregnated, water or normal saline, no adhesive border	>48 sq in
A6231	Gauze, impregnated, hydrogel	≤16 sq in
A6232	Gauze, impregnated, hydrogel	>16 ≤48 sq in
A6233	Gauze, impregnated, hydrogel	>48 sq in
A6234	Hydrocolloid dressing, no adhesive border	≤16 sq in
A6235	Hydrocolloid dressing, no adhesive border	>16 ≤48 sq in
A6236	Hydrocolloid dressing, no adhesive border	>48 sq in
A6237	Hydrocolloid dressing, any adhesive border	≤16 sq in
A6238	Hydrocolloid dressing, any adhesive border	>16 ≤48 sq in
A6239	Hydrocolloid dressing, any adhesive border	>48 sq in

Table 12•2 Medicare Dressing Categories—cont'd

HCPCS Code	Dressing Material and Format	Dressing Size
A6240	Hydrocolloid dressing, wound filler, paste	Per fluid ounce
A6241	Hydrocolloid dressing, wound filler, dry form	Per gram
A6242	Hydrogel dressing, no adhesive border	≤16 sq in
A6243	Hydrogel dressing, no adhesive border	>16 ≤48 sq in
A6244	Hydrogel dressing, no adhesive border	>48 sq in
A6245	Hydrogel dressing, any adhesive border	≤16 sq in
A6246	Hydrogel dressing, any adhesive border	>16 ≤48 sq in
A6247	Hydrogel dressing, any adhesive border	>48 sq in
A6248	Hydrogel dressing, wound filler, gel	Per fluid ounce
A6251	Specialty absorptive dressing, no adhesive border	≤16 sq in
A6252	Specialty absorptive dressing, no adhesive border	>16 ≤48 sq in
A6253	Specialty absorptive dressing, no adhesive border	>48 sq in
A6254	Specialty absorptive dressing, any adhesive border	≤16 sq in
A6255	Specialty absorptive dressing, any adhesive border	>16 ≤48 sq in
A6256	Specialty absorptive dressing, any adhesive border	>48 sq in
A6257	Transparent film	≤16 sq in
A6258	Transparent film	>16 ≤48 sq in
A6259	Transparent film	>48 sq in
A6261	Wound filler, gel/paste, not elsewhere classified	Per fluid ounce
A6262	Wound filler, dry form, not elsewhere classified	Per gram

Table 12•3 Wound Dressings Categorized by Functionality

Wound Dressing Function	Dressing Category
Moisture maintenance	Transparent films Hydrocolloids
Moisture absorption	Foams Alginates
Moisture addition	Hydrogels
Reduce bacterial levels (antimicrobial)	Silver-containing dressings Iodine-containing dressings
Reduce protease levels	Collagen dressings Collagen-ORC dressings
Reduce odor	Activated charcoal additive Cyclodextrin additive
Reduces pain	Ibuprofen-containing dressing Soft silicone dressings

Balancing Moisture in the Wound Environment

In terms of providing moisture balance, advanced dressings could theoretically fall into one of three general functional categories: maintaining adequate moisture, absorbing excess moisture (exudate), or adding needed moisture. Because wounds are dynamic entities that change over time, dressings from multiple functional categories may be appropriate for a single wound during its overall course of healing.

▶ **PEARL 12•2** Dressing should function to either absorb excessive moisture, add moisture in situations of desiccation, or maintain existing moisture balance.

In order for a topical dressing to maintain tissue moisture, it has to impede moisture vapor loss from the wound tissues, that is, not allow it to evaporate. The dressing also must neither remove nor add moisture but rather retain existing moisture levels in the tissues. Two types of advanced dressings that meet these criteria are transparent film dressings and hydrocolloid dressings. Transparent film dressings are thin, clear sheets of elastomeric polymers such as polyurethane, which are coated on one side with an adhesive. The films are impermeable to liquids and bacteria but permeable to gases. They have no ability to add or absorb moisture and can be helpful in maintaining adequate moisture in superficial wounds by themselves or in deeper wounds as a secondary dressing. Hydrocolloids are wafer-type dressings, which are complex formulations of elastomeric, adhesive, and gelling agents. Their basic formulation was derived from materials used in ostomy barrier products. Hydrocolloids are able to maintain tissue moisture but have a moderate absorptive capacity. Hydrocolloids do not absorb fluids rapidly, but they do possess a low rate of absorption that can be valuable when wound exudate levels are in transition from higher to lower quantities. Films and hydrocolloids represent some of the earliest types of advanced wound dressings to enter the commercial marketplace.

› **PEARL 12•3** Clear film and hydrocolloid dressings are two types of dressings noted for their ability to retain existing moisture levels in wounds.

Hydrocolloids are some of the most extensively evaluated dressings compared to other advanced dressing types. However, they have only rarely demonstrated significant improvement in wound healing outcomes. One small study in 31 venous leg ulcer patients did demonstrate a statistically significant improvement in wound closure for one type of hydrocolloid over another[5]; however, systematic reviews of many other comparative trials of hydrocolloids versus other types of advanced dressings have not demonstrated significant differences in wound closure.[6]

Examples of dressing categories that excel at absorption include calcium alginates and other types of gelling fibers, as well as polymer foams. Calcium alginates are biopolymers derived from seaweed and fashioned into dressings that are typically fiber-based, although powdered forms exist. The alginate fibers absorb wound exudate by swelling and then gelling to maintain a moist, humid environment at the wound surface while physically removing fluid from the tissue surface. The gelling results from an ion exchange between the calcium of the alginate fiber and sodium in the wound exudate.[7]

› **PEARL 12•4** Calcium alginate dressings help to absorb and maintain moisture through the gelling properties of the alginate fiber.

The alginate polymer is composed of a mixture of two monomer subunits, β-D-mannuronic acid (M type) and α-L-guluronic acid (G type). The ratio of M-type and G-type monomer units can vary; it may be an equal mixture, or it may have a higher ratio of one monomer to another. Based on their amount of M-type or G-type monomers, alginate dressings in general can be categorized as "wet integrity dressings" and "wet dispersible dressings." A wet integrity dressing has a high ratio of G-type monomer, swells only a little in wound fluid, and can be removed in one piece because the fiber does not gel to a great extent and retains its structural integrity. A wet dispersive dressing has a high ratio of M-type monomer, swells enormously in wound fluid, and is dispersed in the wound as the original fiber gels and loses structural integrity.[8] While these types of differences in handling characteristics may affect ease of use or clinician preference, different alginates do not appear to have different effects in wound healing when compared in controlled trials.[9]

Alginates in general have much of the flexibility of gauze dressings in that they may be layered, folded, or packed into wound cavities, sinuses, and undermined areas. Their gelling behavior makes them less likely to adhere to wound tissues than does gauze. A controlled comparison of an alginate versus saline-soaked gauze for packing cavity wounds demonstrated that patients found the alginate dressing significantly less painful upon removal, and clinicians also found it significantly easier to use.[10] One potential drawback of alginate dressings is that despite their gelling behavior, it is possible for them to dry out and adhere to the wound bed. A critical issue in the use of alginate dressings is the appropriate choice of secondary dressing to maintain that gelled state.

Foams are another option for management of excessive wound moisture and exudates and are typically composed of open-celled polymers such as polyurethane or polyvinyl alcohol. Foam dressings are highly variable from brand to brand and may contain one or more of the following components in addition to the foam core: a waterproof top coating or film, an adhesive border for attachment, and a full adhesive coating on the surface. While they are efficient exudate absorbers, they often do not have the flexibility of alginates in being able to address wounds with significant depth, undermining, or sinuses due to their quality of "memory." Memory refers to the inability to compress or fold foam and have it retain that altered shape. There are, however, certain foam products designed specifically for use in deep wounds that consist of porous pouches filled with chopped foam pieces or compressible foam layers capable of holding a wadded conformation.

› **PEARL 12•5** The "memory" quality of many foam dressings make them difficult to conform to certain wound cavity situations.

Like alginates, clinical comparisons of one foam dressing to another may identify differences in clinical or patient preference and ease of use, but do not demonstrate differences in healing outcomes.[11,12] In a large-scale postmarketing study of over 6000 patients, foam dressings have been shown to reduce frequency of dressing changes for exuding wounds in primary care compared to traditional dressings.[13]

Moisture donation is sometimes a desired property of a topical dressing when the tissues have begun to desiccate or when it is anticipated that they may desiccate over a particular time period. In order to donate moisture, a dressing must contain moisture or water. Hydrogel dressings exist in multiple formats containing varying amounts of water complexed in various polymer matrices. Hydrogels may be in the form of amorphous gels, three-dimensional sheets, or as amorphous gels impregnated into a carrier gauze or other mesh. Caution must be exercised so that these dressings do not create maceration in the wound. Different types of hydrogel dressings have not been proven to result in significant differences in wound healing when one was compared to the other.[14]

> ▶ **PEARL 12•6** The ability of a dressing to "donate" moisture to a wound is often desirable when desiccation is present or anticipated.

In general, when two types of advanced dressings have been compared to each other in randomized controlled trials, no significantly different effects on healing have been realized. Different types of foams have been compared to each other,[15] hydrocolloids have been compared to foams,[6-20] and hydrogels have been compared to hydrocolloids and saline-moistened gauze.[21] In none of these comparisons were statistically significant differences in healing outcomes demonstrated; however, there were often differences in parameters, such as ease of use, number of dressing changes, or cost of care. Each of these outcomes may present a real and differentiating value in different situations: Ease of use and frequency of dressing changes may be a critical issue for patients in home care settings or when performing self-care, and cost of care is an especially pertinent quality in a time of health-care prospective payment.

A variety of recent meta-analyses and systematic reviews of randomized comparisons of advanced dressings to traditional dressings or other advanced dressings in the treatment of venous leg ulcers, pressure ulcers, and surgical wounds healing by secondary intention have not shown any consistent or significant improvements in wound healing for one dressing versus another.

Chaby recently assessed the published evidence to support clinical efficacy of modern, advanced dressings in terms of multiple outcomes, including complete healing, avoidance of wound pain or complications, ease of use, exudate management, infection prevention, and costs.[22] Ninety-nine selected studies included both acute and chronic wound etiologies, but excluded burns. Studies were rated according to their level of evidence as A, B, or C. There were no A-level studies ("A" being large, powered, randomized controlled trials). Overall, it was found that study methodology was poor because it was not statistically powered; not containing heterogeneous patient populations; lacking objectivity, definition, and blinding of assessments; and not specifying important adjunctive treatments such as off-loading and compression. The study reported that there was some evidence in chronic wounds that hydrocolloid dressings were superior to saline and gauze in achieving complete healing and that alginates were superior to other advanced dressings in achieving wound area reduction. No meaningful data were found for acute wounds. The overall conclusion was that there was no convincing or strong evidence that one advanced dressing type was better than any other in acute or chronic wounds.

Other reviews have focused on evaluation of dressings efficacy in specific wound etiologies. A recent meta-analysis examined all randomized trials of dressings used under compression in the management of venous ulcers.[23] Forty-two trials met the inclusion criteria and involved 3001 patients and 3037 ulcers. Trials included comparisons of hydrocolloids, foams, and hydrogels to other advanced dressings and to nonadherent dressings. No trial showed a statistically significant benefit of any dressing over another in terms of ulcer healing. In most cases the specific dressing comparisons suffered from low statistical power; that is, they did not have a large enough sample size to be able to detect a difference, and even combining multiple trials did not improve power. However, one particular comparison, hydrocolloids versus nonadherent dressings, did have sufficient power—700 patients collectively—and no healing benefit was observed. This study echoes the findings of earlier systematic reviews of dressing effects in venous leg ulcers.[6,24] A similar systematic review was undertaken on the topic of dressing performance in pressure ulcers.[25] This review confirmed the efficacy of hydrocolloid dressings over conventional saline-moistened gauze dressings in the management of pressure ulcers. There were insufficient data to establish with any certainty that any other type of advanced dressing had greater healing efficacy than conventional dressings. Furthermore, there was insufficient evidence to consider that one type of advanced dressing was more effective than any other.

In a systematic review of dressings for the management of surgical wound healing by secondary intention, 13 evaluable trials were identified that included dressings such as foams, hydrocolloids, alginates, and gauze.[26] The analysis concluded that although the trials were weak in quality, there were no significant differences in wound healing for any of the dressing comparisons. They did note significant differences favoring the advanced dressings in terms of reduced pain and nursing time. A pivotal point in comparisons of advanced dressings to gauze appears to be outcomes in addition to healing.

> ▶ **PEARL 12•7** While few differences seem to exist in healing rates with various dressings, significant differences appear to exist with regard to reduced pain and provider time required.

Another recent review considered not only healing outcomes but also the cost-effectiveness outcomes (when available) of advanced dressings versus gauze.[27] When cost-effectiveness outcomes have been included, advanced dressings of many types tend to save money versus saline-moistened gauze despite their higher per unit price. The key to the cost savings is tied predominantly to reduction in overall materials cost to achieve a similar or better healing outcome, as well as reductions in labor costs (eg, longer dressing wear time, fewer dressing changes, less nursing time). This type of outcome is of particular interest in managed care and the current health-care environment of capitated payment in virtually all care settings.

Interestingly, the one wound etiology for which advanced dressings have consistently demonstrated a clinical benefit over gauze is in the management of an acute wound. A review of moist wound healing dressings in the management of split-thickness skin-graft donor sites included 58 randomized controlled trials and concluded that moist wound healing products were superior in terms of healing, pain/comfort, and infection rates.[28]

How to Make Dressing Choices

So, in the absence of a critical mass of data, how do clinicians select one dressing over another? A recent study tackled this question. Doctors, nurses, and patients in six surgery wards of a tertiary teaching hospital participated in a questionnaire designed to rate their preferences for particular dressing attributes as well as their willingness to pay for those attributes.[29] Six dressing attributes and two to three different performance levels of those attributes were identified. These included the following: time needed for complete wound healing (long or short), pain during dressing change (considerable or minimal), frequency of dressing changes (high or low), costs of wound care (high or low), required duration of hospitalization (long or short), and help needed for outpatient wound care (none, proxy, or visiting nurse). Compiling all the various combinations of the six dressing attributes by performance levels created 18 different product vignettes. Participants were asked to rate each product vignette as more or less ideal by choosing a number from 1 to 10 (with 10 being the most ideal combination of attributes and 1 being the least). Willingness to pay for each attribute was assessed separately.

All dressing attributes were found to significantly influence the judgment of the vignettes. The three attributes rated highest by all three groups were similar: lack of pain during dressing change, short duration of stay in the hospital, and faster healing time. However, the individual ranking by willingness to pay for each attribute varied significantly between the three participant groups. Physicians were willing to pay the most for a shortened hospital stay, while nurses were willing to pay the most for decreased pain at dressing change and patients chose rapid healing as their most valuable product attribute. These findings are of interest in that frequency of dressing change and independence in wound care were rated as the least-significant factors in the participants' preference, yet these are attributes on which dressing manufacturers tend to focus. Another finding of interest is that the nurses valued painless dressing change more than did the patient experiencing the dressing change. A potential limitation of this study may have been that the majority of the wounds were postsurgical or traumatic and therefore did not represent the patients and management challenges characteristic of chronic wounds.

An individual practitioner may make dressing selection decisions based on specific perceived healing characteristics of the dressing, but are these choices similar between practitioners? Vermeulen investigated this question by exploring the dressing selections by a group of physicians and nurses for agreement with each other as well as with an expert panel.[30] Seventy-nine physicians and 63 nurses from the department of surgery at a tertiary referral center viewed the same 18 photographs of open wounds (culled from a group of 90 to represent a variety of wound types and conditions) and selected what they thought were the most appropriate primary wound dressings from two groups of potential choices. The first group included three different types of gauze, and the second group included five different types of advanced dressings, all of which were available in the facility. An expert panel of one physician and three tissue viability nurses made the reference standard selections in both groups and were unanimous in their selections for the 18 wounds. The participants were also asked to select dressings for the wounds a second time in order to judge intraobserver agreement. Kappa values were computed to measure the levels of interobserver agreement, agreement with the expert panel and intraobserver agreement. Kappa values range from 0 to 1, with a value greater than 0.8 representing "very good" agreement, between 0.8 and 0.6 representing "good" agreement, between 0.6 and 0.4 representing "moderate" agreement, and than 0.4 "poor" agreement.

Agreement between either physicians as a group or nurses as a group on choices of either gauze dressings or advanced dressings was poor, with kappa values ranging from 0.07 to 0.23. Agreement between nurses was no better than agreement between physicians, contradicting the popular belief that nurses are more familiar with dressing characteristics. Agreement on dressing choices between the participants and the expert panel was similarly poor; however, the nurses' agreement with the expert panel was slightly higher than that of the physicians. For the physicians who made dressing selections twice, intraobserver agreement was moderate for gauze dressings and poor for advanced dressings. For nurses who made dressing selections twice, intraobserver agreement was also moderate for gauze and poor for advanced dressings. There was no correlation between agreement in wound dressing choice and level of clinical experience for either physicians or nurses.

An earlier similar study of wound dressing choices in a hospital setting found that appropriate selections were made in only 48% of cases.[31]

A more recent evaluation of the consistency of current wound care practices with evidence-based guidelines reported similar results in dressing selections for chronic wounds in four geographically diverse sites in the United States.[32] The sites examined wound patient medical records in a variety of care settings, including wound care centers, home health-care agencies, nursing homes, and inpatient units. The evidence-based guidelines identified for pressure ulcers, diabetic ulcers, and venous ulcers made only broad recommendations with regard to dressings, such as "use a moisture-retentive dressing" rather than recommending a specific category of dressings. However, there was little agreement in practice even with these broad recommendations. Upon reviewing the dressing choices in over 400 medical records, it was found that advanced dressings comprised only 42% of dressings ordered for diabetic ulcers, 44% of those for pressure ulcers and 59% of those for venous ulcers.

Such studies seem to indicate that there is a need for more evidence regarding the benefits and efficacy of advanced dressings, as well as for better clinician education on the selection and use of wound dressings. As we have seen earlier, comparative studies between advanced and conventional dressings, as well as within and between advanced dressing categories, have not yielded conclusive evidence of superior healing performance for one type of dressing versus another.

General Challenges in Generating Clinical Evidence for Wound Dressings

Chronic wounds are not the primary issue to be dealt with but rather are symptoms of underlying disease or multiple systemic and local conditions that have manifested in skin breakdown. Therefore, the topical dressing is but one aspect of care that will influence wound healing. For example, in clinical trials of dressings for diabetic foot ulcers, off-loading of the affected foot is a vital aspect of care. Patient nonadherence to off-loading regimens may negate any healing advantage provided by a topical dressing and affect the overall healing results of the study.

> ▶ **PEARL 12•8** The topical dressing is but one component in the management of a wound. The complex nature of the underlying disease must be of primary concern.

Patient populations may vary greatly in the wide variety of local and systemic factors that affect healing, especially during the temporal span of a wound healing trial. The healing of a chronic wound may be a protracted process, and wound healing trials typically run anywhere from 8 to 24 weeks in duration. It may be difficult to ensure patient homogeneity at the outset, much less throughout the trial. One particular educational tool developed by a team of clinicians and researchers identified 44 local, environmental, systemic, and biochemical factors that may significantly impact the wound healing process.[33,34]

Dressings are an important component of wound management; however, it may be difficult to isolate their specific effects from the plethora of other local, systemic, and social factors that impact wound healing.

At present, there is little comparative evidence to support a selection of a "best" dressing from a generic category such as foams, hydrocolloids, alginates, and hydrogels, or to support that any particular dressing in one material category is better than one in another category for a particular wound type. There has been no exhaustive comparison of the various dressing types, and indeed some types would not make any sense or even be used in the same type of wound. For example, one would not compare a transparent film to an alginate.

In clinical practice, multiple types of dressings are required to manage a single wound over its healing course. Achieving and maintaining tissue moisture balance with proper dressing selection is an art and depends on the dynamic equilibrium between a wound and its local and systemic environments. Consequently, it is exceedingly rare that anyone uses a single type of dressing for the duration of the wound healing process. The fact is that wounds are dynamic entities with changing characteristics (depth, exudate, bacterial levels), and it is precisely these characteristics that drive the choice of different dressings over time. However, the standard randomized controlled clinical trial demands static treatment of a wound with a single type of dressing for anywhere from 8 to 24 weeks and focuses on the outcome of complete wound closure. This is not reflective of real-life clinical practice, and this protocol

and the primary outcome of complete healing may not even be the best method to compare dressing performance and value in patient management. While it would certainly present logistical issues, a trial that compares systems of dressing types appropriate for the changing conditions of the wound may be an alternative.

> ▶ **PEARL 12•9** No one dressing is designed to carry a wound from conception to completion. Wound healing is dynamic and requires practitioners to alter care plans to meet changing wound needs.

For wound healing studies, it seems logical that we would want to know how many wounds healed or closed versus how many wounds did not. This is a quantitative outcome: We can count it. Wounds are either closed or not. But wound closure is not so black and white. A wound may decrease in size by a large amount and yet not completely close. This decrease in size is almost always a benefit to the patient, even though not technically a closure, so quantitative outcomes are often reported in terms of percentage of reduction of original wound volume or wound area. Healing data may also be reported in terms of the length of time it takes to reach wound closure or to reach a particular point of closure, for example 50% closure. If a wound becomes significantly smaller, it may mean that the patient can now self-manage the wound at home or be able to move from one care setting to another.

Increasingly, wound studies are including qualitative outcomes in their design and results—things that may not be discrete, but are important nevertheless. Examples of important qualitative outcomes of wound healing include parameters such as changes in patient perceived pain, changes in patient quality of life, changes in numbers of wound-related complications (such as infection or dehiscence) or in wound recurrence, and differences between products in terms of their ease of use by the clinician or the patient. These types of qualitative differences are usually measured by questionnaires using Likert scales.

There are also calls from the medical community to consider surrogate or other outcomes in wound healing trials to evaluate efficacy of new wound treatments, such as wound area reduction from baseline within a early time period (such as 2 to 4 weeks),[35] wound healing rates, or wound healing trajectories.[36,37]

The absence of better methodologies or more realistic protocols to evaluate the clinical performance of advanced dressings relative to other treatments may lead to their demise. Increasingly, health technology assessment groups, hospital formulary committees, and even insurance companies look for comparative evidence in order to make decisions regarding access to and reimbursement for new technologies, including advanced dressings. Standard evidence-based medicine hierarchies tout the randomized controlled trial as the epitome of comparative evidence, and there is little recognition of the aforementioned limitations of this methodology for assessing wound dressings. Patient access to advanced wound care dressings and even the development of new wound care dressings and other topical treatments may be restricted by this lack of evidence.

Beyond Moisture Balance: Balancing Bacteria in the Wound Environment

One of the more popular recent advances in dressing technology is the incorporation of additional ingredients targeted toward achieving a goal other than or in addition to moisture balance. A popular additional goal is topical antisepsis. Almost any of the dressing categories previously discussed are now available in an antimicrobial version. A more robust discussion of wound bacterial balance and antimicrobial dressings is provided in Chapter 8, so the topic will be only be briefly highlighted here.

Recently, new technologies have been applied to the incorporation and delivery of antimicrobial agents to the wound surface and may improve their use and acceptance. These technologies are most often aimed at creating a slow and sustained release of the antiseptic agent while maintaining adequate tissue moisture levels. Sustained release of an antiseptic agent enables lower concentrations to be used with greater antimicrobial efficacy and lower toxicity to host cells. The most prevalent antimicrobial agent incorporated into wound dressings by far is silver. Silver has been incorporated into a wide variety of dressing formats, including wound contact layers, foams, films, alginates, hydrocolloids, hydrogels, and fabrics. The silver may be incorporated in the form of a metallic coating on some aspect of the dressing, which interacts with oxygen in wound fluid to provide a sustained release of the antimicrobial silver ion. Alternatively, it may be incorporated as a silver compound, which dissociates in wound fluid to release the silver ion. The numerous wound dressings that contain and release silver may differ in the method of silver incorporation or in the amount of silver they contain or even the rate at which they release the silver ion; however, none of these differences have yet been shown to make a difference in terms of clinical performance.[38]

> ▶ **PEARL 12•10** Silver is one of the most common antimicrobial agents incorporated into wound dressings.

Other antimicrobial agents that have been incorporated into moisture-balancing dressings as delivery vehicles include iodine, polyhexamethylene biguanide, methylene blue, and gentian violet. To date, while there have been clinical trials comparing specific silver dressings to nonantimicrobial dressings or to silver-containing topical agents such as silver sulfadiazine or silver nitrate, there have been no head-to-head trials of one antimicrobial dressing versus another. Particular challenges with antimicrobial dressing studies are that their intended use is for wounds with a problematic level of bacteria, and it is impossible to ensure that wounds within or between the two treatment groups have the same number and types of bacteria. Additionally, one rarely measures the effect on bacteria as an outcome of the trial; rather, the effect on wound healing in terms of area reduction is measured. However, antimicrobial dressings are designed to address an impediment to healing (bacterial levels in excess of what the host can control), and early clinical signs of the benefit of an antimicrobial dressing may be more qualitative than quantitative, for example changes in exudate levels and tissue quality. Duration of use of the antimicrobial dressing is also challenging in that continued use of an antimicrobial dressing beyond the reduction in bacterial levels could actually delay healing through a negative impact on host cells.

In the absence of comparative clinical data, clinicians typically rely on data from standardized in vitro evaluations (log reduction studies and zone of inhibition studies) to establish the antimicrobial activity of the dressing and to select one antimicrobial dressing versus another based on other performance characteristics of the dressing such as conformability, absorbency, and ease of use.

Balancing Chemicals Other than Water in the Wound Environment

While moisture—or water—is a vital parameter to be balanced during the healing process of an open wound, there are other parameters—or chemicals—in the fluids and tissues of chronic wounds that may also require a balancing intervention. For example, oxygen is well known as one such chemical. Oxygen is delivered to the tissues through the vasculature, and we understand that without a sufficient blood supply, a wound is unlikely to heal. We assess oxygen levels with a variety of tools, such as transcutaneous oximetry and vascular testing. We currently address insufficient tissue oxygen levels with revascularization surgeries or hyperbaric oxygen treatment. Protein is another chemical target for balance to facilitate healing. We have multiple ways to assess a patient's systemic protein levels and a variety of nutritional supplements to increase it when deficient. Over the past decade, basic research has studied the biochemical milieu of healing wounds versus nonhealing wounds and has identified a variety of other chemicals that may be targets for balance in order to facilitate the healing process. In this new era of wound dressing, technologies are being developed with the purported abilities to address some of these newly recognized chemical imbalances.

Local levels of a variety of proteolytic enzymes, such a matrix metalloprotease (MMP) and elastase, have been found to be elevated in nonhealing wounds of many etiologies.[39,40] The metalloproteases are a family of structurally related enzymes that facilitate cellular migration through the extracellular matrix and also effect proteolysis by macrophages in the inflammatory phase of healing. Normal levels of MMPs rise from a low baseline, peak during the inflammatory phase of healing, and then decline as granulation and epithelialization proceed. In nonhealing wounds, MMPs appear to peak at a higher levels and remain persistently high, ultimately resulting in uncontrolled degradation of existing or newly deposited extracellular matrix components such as collagen, glycosaminoglycans, and proteoglycans, as well as degradation of the various growth factor proteins necessary to coordinate healing. The wound may appear clinically to arrest in the inflammatory phase of healing as a net result of this uncontrolled local proteolysis in the local wound environment. Elevated levels of MMPs are thought to develop due to a variety of causes, including high levels of bacteria in the wound, the presence of necrosis, and repetitive trauma in the wound environment.[41]

One dressing specifically targeted toward reducing local levels of MMPs in nonhealing wounds is a homogeneous mixture of 55% bovine collagen and 45% oxidized regenerated cellulose (ORC). When placed in a wound, the dressing binds any member of the MMP family of enzymes and renders them inactive, bringing their wound fluid levels back down into the ranges found in healing wounds, which is then thought to allow granulation tissue to accumulate and ultimately epithelialization to occur. The dressing's effects on key MMPs has been demonstrated in vitro using wound fluid collected from nonhealing chronic wounds. The mechanism of action has been postulated as the collagen moiety acting as a sacrificial substrate for the proteases, while the ORC moiety, with its multiple negative charges, dislodges the positively charged metal ions common to this family of enzymes. Loss of the metal ion destroys the three-dimensional shape of the proteases such that they can no longer bind any substrate.[42] More recently, it was shown in vivo that when the collagen-ORC dressing resulted in rapid healing progress, the measurable change was not simply reduction in proteases, but a reduction in the ratio of the proteases to their inhibitors.[43]

> **PEARL 12•11** Collagen-oxidized regenerated cellulose (ORC) dressings have been shown to be effective in reducing matrix metalloprotease levels in chronic wounds.

It has also been shown in vitro that the collagen-ORC material can protect growth factors from being degraded by MMPs. Therefore, a protease-modulating dressing may impact healing in complementary ways: by modulating elevated levels of proteases and by protecting local growth factor viability. Recently, a sulfonated polymer dressing with the ability to bind and inactivate proteases performed favorably when compared to the ORC-collagen material in vitro.[44]

Elastase is another protease that has been shown to be elevated in chronic wounds. The primary source of elastase in the wound is the neutrophil,[45] although it is also produced by bacteria.[46] Elastase has detrimental effects on the developing wound matrix similar to that of the MMPs, is one of the primary destructors of peptide growth factors,[47] and also has negative effects on cells such as fibroblasts.[46] While the ORC-collagen material has demonstrated activity against elastase,[43] chemically modified cotton wound dressings have also demonstrated in vitro activity against elastase levels.[48]

Nitric oxide (NO) is another biochemical target for modulation by topical dressings. NO is a very reactive, short-lived gas that is produced from suitable precursor molecules by the enzyme nitric oxide synthase (NOS). The amino acid L-arginine is a common precursor. The inducible NOS (iNOS) enzyme can be produced by a variety of cells, including neuronal cells, endothelial cells, platelets, neutrophils, macrophages, lymphocytes, wound fibroblasts, and proliferating keratinocytes.[49] Production of iNOS (and thereby NO)

is induced in these cells by inflammatory cytokines such as IL-1β, TNF-α, and interferon-γ. Once NO is produced, its lifetime in the body is extremely short because it is a free radical, a very reactive chemical species. NO is metabolized to nitrate (NO_3) and nitrite (NO_2) within seconds. Nitrate and nitrite levels can be measured in urine, plasma, or wound fluid as an indicator of NO synthesis.

NO has been found to be involved in some fashion in all of the phases of wound healing. Immunostaining for the inducible enzyme that produces NO from precursors revealed heavy staining in macrophages, in proliferating keratinocytes in the wound edges and hair follicles, and in dermal fibroblasts in wound tissue, but not in fibroblasts from normal nonwounded tissues.[50] A wound healing study using iNOS knockout mice revealed that these mice experienced a 31% delay in wound healing compared to control mice.[51] When the iNOS knockout mice were supplied with iNOS via an adenoviral vector, the delay was reversed. Another wound healing study in mice demonstrated that when the production of NO was inhibited, collagen deposition and wound-breaking strength decreased.[52] These data suggest that NO is involved in some stage of healing as well as the viability of a therapeutic approach to increasing local NO.

Early efforts to use dressing technology incorporating a NO precursor molecule to modulate local wound levels of NO resulted in local toxicity thought to be due to either the precursor itself or the carrier.[49] A later attempt to incorporate a different NO precursor into a hydrogel wound dressing for topical release of NO at the wound surface has shown promise both in vitro and in vivo.[53] Fibroblasts cultured with the NO-releasing hydrogel demonstrated higher production of extracellular matrix proteins than those cultured with the hydrogel vehicle. Additionally, wounds in diabetic mice treated with the NO hydrogel showed thicker granulation tissue and a greater reduction in wound area versus the treatment with the hydrogel vehicle.

Chronic wounds have often been described as being "stuck" in the inflammatory phase of wound healing. Biochemical research has validated this description by documenting elevated and persistent levels of inflammatory cytokines and reactive oxygen intermediates (chemical by-products of neutrophil and macrophage activity) in venous ulcers, and they may also be present in other etiologies.[54] These two classes of chemicals represent additional targets for modulation by dressings either through their composition or as a delivery system. There are currently available dressing materials with antioxidant properties (reduced production of oxygen species by cells and/or scavenging of existing free radicals) that may eventually prove valuable in reducing oxidative stress in the chronic wound.

> **PEARL 12•12** Biochemical research supports the concept of chronic wounds being "stuck" in the inflammatory phase of healing as evidenced by elevated levels of inflammatory cytokines.

Recently, an iodine-containing hydrogel has demonstrated in vitro free radical scavenging activity as well as inhibition of human neutrophil production of various reactive oxygen species.[55] Various honeys and a solution of metal ions and citric acid have also been shown to reduce human neutrophil production of reactive oxygen species such as hydroxyl radicals and hypochlorite anions.[56,57] Both of these materials have recently been incorporated into wound dressing materials.

There are also specialized dressings targeted to reduce wound pain (containing ibuprofen or tissue-friendly adhesives) and to adsorb wound odor (containing activated charcoal or cyclodextrin additives), parameters that deal less with the actual process of healing and more with the patient experience, which in itself may affect the process of wound healing. Early clinical trials with the ibuprofen-containing foam dressing have shown that it seems to reduce wound pain without adversely affecting healing.[58]

Evidence for the Value of Addressing Parameters Other than Water in the Wound Environment

While moisture content is relatively straightforward to evaluate by looking at the wound tissues, some of these other parameters being affected by newer advanced dressings are not easy to evaluate by simply looking; that is, we cannot see bacteria or other cell types, or enzymes or other chemicals. And while the parameter/cell/chemical of interest can be measured in a research laboratory, there are no available bedside diagnostics to rapidly measure that specific parameter either before or after we use the dressing that claims to target it. Therefore, as we see more and more dressings on the market that claim to address very specific issues in the wound environment, we are asked essentially to make an educated guess as to whether the condition that they address is present and to determine if the condition is being addressed, not by any specific measurement of that particular condition, but by an overall gestalt of whether the wound is getting better—for example, smaller, less odorous, better tissue quality, etc. This leads to new challenges in generating evidence for advanced dressings in addition to those previously discussed.

How do you measure the enzyme or reactive oxygen intermediate levels in a wound? How do you know what is normal for a particular patient or a particular point in the dynamic process of wound healing? At the very least, we should demand evidence that a dressing that claims to reduce bacteria or enzymes or another chemical can actually achieve that action in the best of conditions, for example, in vitro or ex vivo evidence of mechanism of action. But in many cases, there are no standard in vitro assays by which to measure these chemical parameters. Thus, different companies use different test methods and generate conflicting comparative results. To complicate things further, clinicians may use these highly specific dressings, but they are increasingly using them in sequence or in parallel with other dressings and technologies and for shorter periods of time than the course of a usual clinical trial in chronic wounds. It becomes more and more difficult to tease out a benefit of one product over another or to attribute that benefit to these new mechanisms of action.

Matrix Proteins as Dressings

Another general category of topical wound dressings includes those that employ materials of biological origin in an effort to generate a cellular response that may positively impact healing. Cells in native tissue live in a three-dimensional extracellular matrix composed of a variety of proteins and glycosaminoglycans. The extracellular matrix of tissue is thought to play important roles in the wound healing process by acting as a depot for chemicals, regulating intercellular communication, and providing a scaffold for cellular migration. Dressings that comprise matrix components are thought to play a role in accelerating healing by mimicking these roles.

Collagen dressings originally entered the market as absorption dressings, but they are unique and can do more than simply manage moisture. Collagen derived from animal sources, including cowhide, cow or chicken tendon, and pig intestine, is now available in different forms for use as wound dressings. Once the collagen protein is extracted from the original animal source, it can be processed into a wide variety of final physical formats such as gels or pastes, powders or granules, and sheets or sponges. Depending on the physical format, the collagen dressing may be capable of absorbing wound exudate; however, absorption is not the primary function of a collagen-based wound dressing. Collagen is bioresorbable, can act as a matrix in the wound environment, and has been shown to be chemotactic for key cells in the healing process. In addition, collagen can act as a sacrificial substrate for metalloproteases in the wound environment. These functions of collagen are independent of wound exudate levels, and management of wound exudate should be addressed with an appropriate secondary dressing. Collagen dressing products have been evaluated versus conventional dressings in a variety of clinical trials involving chronic and acute wounds with positive results.[59-62] Secondary dressings used over collagen depend on the wound exudate levels.

> **PEARL 12•13** Collagen from a variety of animal sources, including cowhide, cow or chicken tendon, and pig intestine, have been extracted and processed into a variety of physical formats for dressings such as gels, pastes, powders, granules, sheets, and sponges.

Another recently introduced matrix-based dressing is a viscous solution of amelogenin proteins (extracellular matrix proteins from porcine tooth enamel) in a propylene-glycol alginate carrier. This dressing is thought to provide a temporary extracellular matrix for cellular attachment and migration. The amelogenin dressing with compression therapy was compared to compression therapy alone in a 12-week trial of 83 patients with venous leg ulcers and achieved a statistically significant difference in wound area reduction as well as wound-related pain.[63] These differences in wound healing and pain were maintained in a follow-up evaluation 12 weeks after the end of the original study.[64]

Other matrix materials have been investigated as topical wound dressings in addition to collagen. Hyaluronan is one of the predominant glycosaminoglycans found in extracellular matrix and is thought to play a role in cellular proliferation and migration. Hyaluronan-based dressings have been evaluated in venous leg ulcers and diabetic foot ulcers and have demonstrated positive results in terms of complete wound healing and wound area reduction.[65-67] Dressings comprising hyaluronan esters have also demonstrated inherent antioxidant properties in vitro.[68]

Skin Substitutes and Topical Wound Management

Skin substitutes were originally designed to replace autografts, harvesting of a patient's own skin to apply to a burn or wound somewhere else on his or her body. Because in many cases the patient may not have enough undamaged skin to harvest and because harvesting the autograft creates its own wound to be treated, scientists have for some time been exploring ways to create nonautologous skin grafts—or substitutes for the patient's own skin—that can provide the same benefits as an autograft without creating a donor site wound.

Normal skin consists of multiple layers and cell types, extracellular matrix proteins, and other chemicals, as well as adnexal structures such as hair follicles, sweat glands, sebaceous glands, blood vessels, and nerves. To date, there are no skin substitute products that completely replicate normal, uninjured skin. Rather, most of the products are matrix components and/or cells in various combinations. As we have seen earlier in this chapter, wound dressings have moved toward incorporating matrix materials (collagen, hyaluronan), so skin substitutes can be viewed in some ways as a natural progression of dressing technology.

▸ **PEARL 12•14** To date, there are no skin substitutes that are capable of completely replicating normal, uninjured skin.

Currently available skin substitutes may consist of dermal cells, epidermal cells, or both, supported by a biodegradable matrix (Table 12.4). Depending on the source of the cells or matrix, the skin substitute may be referred to as autologous (source is the patient), allogeneic (source is a human other than the patient), or xenogeneic (source is another species).

Our discussion here will focus on the allogeneic skin substitutes. These types of skin substitutes are often referred to as bioengineered tissue products and can consist of matrix materials alone, matrix materials with epidermal cells, matrix materials with dermal cells, or a matrix populated with both types of cells. The basic recipe for a living skin substitute is as follows: A three-dimensional matrix or scaffold is created from a substance that is bioabsorbable, such as collagen or suture material (polyglycolic acid, polylactic acid). Dermal tissue cells, epidermal cells, or both are added to the matrix. The cells typically come from neonatal circumcision tissues. The right nutrients and environment are then supplied for the cells to grow within or on top of the matrix (eg, in vitro tissue culture). Products containing both dermal and epidermal cells are referred to as *bilayered*, and typically their manufacture incorporates a step in which the epidermal layer is allowed to stratify and even develop a stratum corneum by allowing a duration of exposure to an air-liquid interface. The final, cell-populated products are then either cryopreserved for shipping and thawed immediately before use or shipped at a controlled temperature with adequate nutrients to keep the cells viable for a limited period of time between shipping and application to a patient. Noncellular products may have less stringent temperature requirements and a longer shelf life.

In clinical use, the skin substitute products are cut to the exact size of the wound and applied to a clean wound bed. Depending on the specific product and application, the skin substitutes can be meshed prior to use in order to increase surface area coverage and allow drainage of exudate. They may be attached to the wound in a variety of ways, including the use of sutures, staples, or a simple compression dressing. They do require a moist environment for cell survival and function, which can be provided and maintained by the advanced dressings previously discussed.

Skin substitutes containing living human cells have been a topic of research and development for more than a decade, and there are currently several commercial offerings on the market. The commercial names of many of these products incorporate the word *graft*; however, this may be misleading in that skin substitutes are not grafts in the sense of an autograft, which "takes" or becomes an integrated part of the wound over which it is placed.

Initially it was believed that the skin substitute "took," meaning that the allogeneic cells became integrated into the patient's healed tissue. However, studies in both acute and chronic wounds treated with skin substitutes have revealed that skin substitutes do not take. One such study examined acute, deep dermal wounds created and treated with either an

Table 12•4	**Skin Substitute Types**		
Type	**Components**		**Examples**
Epidermal	Autologous or allogeneic keratinocytes grown in tissue culture or on a carrier film or matrix		Epicel®
Dermal	Allogeneic dermal cells (usually fibroblasts) grown on a support structure such as a film or biodegradable matrix		Dermagraft®
	Extracellular matrix proteins or chemicals only		Integra® Alloderm®
Bilayer	Allogeneic epidermal and dermal cells on a film or matrix		Apligraf®

autologous skin graft or a bilayered skin substitute.[69] Healing took 4 to 9 weeks, and biopsies of the wounds were performed over the healing period and tissue was analyzed by immunohistochemical and polymerase chain reaction techniques to detect the Y chromosome of the allogenic cells (derived from neonatal foreskins). Allogenic DNA was detected in the skin substitute–treated wounds for the first 4 weeks. All later time points were negative, except for the results of one biopsy at week 6. A study in venous leg ulcers used similar techniques to detect allogeneic DNA in 10 patients treated with a bilayered skin substitute at multiple time points up to 3 weeks.[70] Allogeneic DNA was detected in two patients at 4 weeks and in no patients at 8 weeks postgrafting.

Results such as these led to the theory that rather than "taking," the living cells in these skin substitutes stimulated healing from the wound edge by producing growth factors and other chemicals that activated the native wound cells to migrate and proliferate. The skin substitute could therefore be viewed as acting as a "smart" dressing that could actually interact with the wound environment at the cellular level or as having a pharmacological effect on the wound. This theory is supported by studies that have documented the production of over 15 different growth factors and cytokines by bilayered skin substitutes in vitro.[71,72] The absolute mechanism of action by which skin substitutes promote healing is not completely understood, however.

▶ **PEARL 12•15** Skin substitutes have been demonstrated not to "take," but rather they serve as a stimulant for the patient's own healing.

Several studies have raised the issue of the importance of the fibroblast cell in bilayered products. One particular cell culture study examined the effect of fibroblasts on epithelialization.[73] The study seeded keratinocytes on collagen matrices that had previously been seeded overnight with increasing numbers of fibroblasts and then raised the matrix to the air-liquid interface to examine epithelial structure over a 2-week culture period. In the absence of fibroblasts, the epithelial cells stratified into only three or four layers, but when fibroblasts were present, there was an increase in both keratinocytes proliferation and stratification. The improvements in epidermal morphology were more pronounced, and a basement membrane began to develop when fibroblasts were allowed to grow in the matrices for a week versus overnight. Another study examined the source of the fibroblast as a critical factor in the healing effects of skin substitutes.[74] This study prepared dermal substitutes by seeding matrices with fibroblasts derived from the papillary dermis or with fibroblasts derived from adipose tissue and culturing them for 2 weeks. Analysis of the matrices after the 2 weeks revealed that the matrix populated with the adipose fibroblasts had deposited more collagen and less glycosaminoglycans and were more contracted than those populated with the papillary dermis fibroblasts. These matrices were then applied to full-thickness wounds in mice. After 3 weeks, only the wounds treated with the adipose fibroblast matrix were completely epithelialized and were better vascularized than the wound treated with the papillary fibroblast matrix. Adipose-derived fibroblasts were shown to be morphologically different from the papillary dermal fibroblasts and also to express actin fibers, which is a marker for the myofibroblast phenotype important in wound contraction.

Thus, it appears that the effects of skin substitutes on the wound healing process may depend on not only the expression of soluble mediators and matrix materials from the living cells but also on the source and particular activities of those living cells for the finite period of time that they are viable in the wound. Skin substitutes have been used successfully in the treatment of burn wounds as well as diabetic and venous ulcers. Conclusive meta-analyses and systematic reviews of their relative efficacy in these wounds are hampered by the diversity of skin substitutes.[75]

An area in which skin substitutes have shown promise is that of "smart" dressings, which can deliver specific growth factors to the wound. Preliminary studies have shown that the cells of skin substitutes can be genetically modified to overexpress target molecules such as growth factors, which would then be temporarily delivered to the wound environment. This approach to gene therapy is attractive since the skin substitute cells are known to eventually die out in the wound, removing the fear of uncontrolled cell growth (a theoretical risk if native cells are modified). An early study used retroviral transduction techniques to modify keratinocytes and fibroblasts to express platelet-derived growth factor (PDGF) and then used these cells to create three types of bilayered skin substitutes by populating a collagen matrix with transduced cells of both types, or normal keratinocytes with transduced fibroblasts, or transduced keratinocytes with normal fibroblasts.[76] The skin substitutes were cultured for 2 weeks and shown to express PDGF throughout the culture period. They were then applied to wounds in athymic mice where PDGF production continued for up to 2 weeks after surgery.

More recently, skin substitutes have shown early promise as delivery systems for potentially more than just wound healing, but for disease state management as well. Human epidermal cells have been genetically modified to produce insulin.[77] The modified cells were used to create stratified epidermal substitutes that secreted insulin at the basal layer and may have promise as an alternative means of insulin delivery for treatment of diabetes by using a patient's autologous epidermal cells to create an insulin-producing skin graft.

Summary

The nature and variety of topical "coverings" for wounds is moving on a steady trajectory in both their materials of manufacture and their roles in and effects on wound healing. This trajectory aims for a "perfect" replacement for lost tissues, a product that results in tissue regeneration as opposed to tissue repair. Wound dressings are one such topical covering for wounds that have moved from simply covering the wound and absorbing exudate to the more robust concept of managing tissue hydration and managing other chemicals that may become imbalanced over time in the environment of a chronic, nonhealing wound. Specific dressing technologies have evolved to assist in bacterial control, enzyme control, free radical quenching, and even pain management, with concomitant benefits of reductions in clinician time spent in topical management. There has also been a logical merging of the dressings trajectory with that of skin substitutes, with the two having complementary and often common clinical goals, and in some cases common materials of composition. Skin substitutes aim to more closely mimic the role and contribution of the tissue cells and extracellular matrix components in healing and focus on the deconstruction and packaging of those tissue elements into more sophisticated topical coverings for wounds. However, skin substitutes can benefit from the effects of wound dressings, and wound dressings could become carriers for various cellular components of skin substitutes: The two are on a collision course that could end in overall benefit.

No wound covering, regardless of its sophistication, can simultaneously address the multitude of factors involved in wound healing; therefore, the variety of wound dressings and skin substitutes are valuable tools to be selected as appropriate and used in sequential fashion over the course of managing a particular patient with a nonhealing wound. A foundation in understanding the broad functional categories and mechanisms of action of both dressings and skin substitutes will facilitate their efficient and best use in wound management.

▶ Case Study 12•1 | Clinical Decision Making: Dressings

A rural nursing home is faced with decreasing budgets and staff. They embark on a project to consolidate their formulary of wound coverings while maintaining the flexibility to effectively manage their wound patient population, which tends to be primarily stage II and III pressure ulcers. What minimum combination of dressing types would offer that flexibility?

In order to select the appropriate dressing to meet the demands of this population, decision makers must first be aware of the unique properties of the individual dressing types outlined in this chapter. How each dressing functions to control exudate, facilitate debridement, and protect the wound from further deterioration must be considered, in addition to cost effectiveness that can be accomplished by using dressings that can remain in place on the patient's wound for longer periods of time.

Hydrocolloid dressings are effective in managing more shallow stage II ulcers, and they allow 2- to 3-day dressing changes, depending on exudate levels. Hydrocolloids could also be used on healing stage III ulcers as they begin to granulate and become shallower. In addition to providing a proper moisture balance in the wound, hydrocolloid dressings are highly occlusive and provide an excellent barrier to outside contamination.

An alginate dressing, for absorption capacity and its ability to address cavity wounds, would be another useful type of dressing for their formulary. Alginates do not have the same reactive properties that are seen with saline-moistened gauze and can easily be removed from the wound with minimal trauma. Because of the absorptive power, these dressing can often be left in place for longer periods than gauze dressing and prove more cost effective.

In addition to standard alginate dressings, silver alginate may be a valuable option to have on their formulary. Silver alginates not only provide the same type of absorptive property as traditional alginates but also serve to help control wound bioburden.

References

1. 2007 Buyer's Guide. Ostomy Wound Manage 2007; 53:85–140.
2. Wu, P, Nelson, EA, Reid, WH, et al: Water vapour transmission rates in burns and chronic leg ulcers: Influence of wound dressings and comparison with in vitro evaluation. Biomaterials 1996; 17(14):1373–1377.
3. Winter, GD: Formation of scab and the rate of epithelialization of superficial wounds in the skin of the young domestic pig. Nature 1962; 193:293–294.
4. Hinnman, CD, Maibach, HI: Effect of air exposure and occlusion on experimental human skin wounds. Nature 1963; 200:377–378.
5. Límová, M, Troyer-Caudle, J: Controlled, randomized clinical trial of 2 hydrocolloid dressings in the management of venous insufficiency ulcers. J Vasc Nurs 2002; 20(1):22–32.
6. Palfreyman, SJ, Nelson, EA, Lochiel, R, et al: Dressings for healing venous leg ulcers. Cochrane Database Syst Rev 2006; 3:CD001103.
7. Thomas, S: Alginate dressings in surgery and wound management. J Wound Care 2000; 9(Pt 1):56–60.
8. Simpson, NE, Stabler, CL, Simpson, CP, et al: The role of the CaCl2-guluronic acid interaction on alginate encapsulated betaTC3 cells. Biomaterials 2004; 25(13):2603–2610.
9. Limová, M: Evaluation of two calcium alginate dressings in the management of venous ulcers. Ostomy Wound Manage 2003; 49(9):26–33.
10. Dawson, C, Armstrong, MW, Fulford, SC, et al: Use of calcium alginate to pack abscess cavities: A controlled clinical trial. J R Coll Surg Edinb 1992; 37:177–179.
11. Vanscheidt, W, Sibbald, RG, Eager, CA: Comparing a foam composite to a hydrocellular foam dressing in the management of venous leg ulcers: A controlled clinical study. Ostomy Wound Manage 2004; 50:42–55.
12. Franks, PJ, Moody, M, Moffatt, CJ, et al: Randomized trial of two foam dressings in the management of chronic venous ulceration. Wound Repair Regen 2007; 15(2):197–202.
13. Diehm, C, Lawall, H: Evaluation of Tielle hydropolymer dressings in the management of chronic exuding wounds in primary care. Int Wound J 2005; 2(1):26–35.
14. Eisenbud, D, Hunter, H, Kessler, L, et al: Hydrogel wound dressings: Where do we stand in 2003? Ostomy Wound Manage 2003; 49(10):52–57.
15. Banks, V, Harding, EF, Harding, K, et al: Evaluation of a new polyurethane foam dressing. J Wound Care 1997; 6(6):266–269.
16. Seeley, J, Jensen, JL, Hutcherson, J: A randomized clinical study comparing a hydrocellular dressing to a hydrocolloid in the management of pressure ulcers. Ostomy Wound Manage 1999; 45(6): 39–44, 46–47.

17. Banks, V, Bale, S, Harding, K: The use of two dressings for moderately exuding pressure sores. J Wound Care 1994; 3(3):132–134.

18. Banks, V, Harding, K: Comparing two dressings for exuding pressure sores in community patients. J Wound Care 1994; 3(4):175–178.

19. Thomas, S, Banks, V, Bale, S, et al: A comparison of two dressings in the management of chronic wounds. J Wound Care 1997; 6(8):383–386.

20. Bale, S, Squires, D, Varnon, T, et al: A comparison of two dressings in pressure sore management. J Wound Care 1997; 6(10):463–466.

21. Mulder, G, Altman, M, Seeley, J, et al: Prospective randomized study of the efficacy of hydrogel, hydrocolloid, and saline-moistened dressings on the management of pressure ulcers. Wound Rep Reg 1993; 1:213–218.

22. Chaby, R, Senet, P, Vaneau, M, et al: Dressings for acute and chronic wounds. Arch Dermatol 2007; 143(10):1297–1304.

23. Palfreyman, S, Nelson, EA, Michaels, JA: Dressings for venous leg ulcers: Systematic review and meta-analysis. BMJ 2007; 335:244.

24. Bouza, C, Muñoz, A, Amate, JM: Efficacy of modern dressings in the treatment of leg ulcers: A systematic review. Wound Repair Regen 2005; 13(3):218–229.

25. Bouza, C, Saz, Z, Muñoz, A, et al: Efficacy of advanced dressings in the treatment of pressure ulcers: A systematic review. J Wound Care 2005; 14(5):193–199.

26. Vermeulen, H, Ubbink, DT, Goossens, A, et al: Systematic review of dressings and topical agents for surgical wounds healing by secondary intention. Br J Surg 2005; 92(6):665–672.

27. Jones, AM, San Miguel, L: Are modern wound dressings a clinical and cost-effective alternative to the use of gauze? J Wound Care 2006; 15(2):65–69.

28. Wiechula, R: The use of moist wound-healing dressings in the management of split-thickness skin graft donor sites: A systematic review. Int J Nurs Pract 2003; 9:2, S9–S17.

29. Vermeulen, H, Ubbink, D, de Zwert, F, et al: Preferences of patients, doctors and nurses regarding wound dressing characteristics: A conjoint analysis. Wound Rep Reg 2007; 15:302–307.

30. Vermeulen, H, Ubbink, D, Schreuder, S, et al: Inter- and intra-observer (dis)agreement among physicians and nurses as to the choice of dressings in surgical patients with open wounds. Wounds 2006; 18:286–293.

31. Bux, M, Malhi, JS: Assessing the use of dressings in practice. J Wound Care 1996; 5:305–308.

32. Jones, KR, Fennie, K, Lenihan, A: Evidence-based management of chronic wounds. Adv Skin Wound Care 2007; 20(11):591–600.

33. Johnson & Johnson: Core Healing Principles: A Systemic Approach to Wound Care. Pocket guide. Available at: http://www.regranex.com/content/backgrounders/www.regranex.com/www.regranex.com/CHP_Pocket_Guide.pdf. Accessed 10/26/09.

34. Available at: http://www.vnaa.org/vnaa/g/?h=html/Wound_Healing_principles.html. Accessed 03/03/08.

35. Sheehan, P, Jones, P, Giurini, JM, et al: Percent change in wound area of diabetic foot ulcers over a 4-week period is a robust predictor of complete healing in a 12-week prospective trial. Plast Reconstr Surg 2006; 117(suppl):239S–244S.

36. Steed, DL, Hill, DP, Woodske, ME, et al: Wound-healing trajectories as outcome measures of venous stasis ulcer treatment. Int Wound J 2006; 3(1):40–47.

37. Robson, MC, Hill, DP, Woodske, ME, et al: Wound healing trajectories as predictors of effectiveness of therapeutic agents. Arch Surg 2000; 135(7):773–777.

38. Ovington, LG: The truth about silver. Ostomy Wound Manage 2004; 50(suppl):1S–10S.

39. Trengove, NJ, Stacey, MC, MacAuley, S, et al: Analysis of the acute and chronic wound environments: The role of proteases and their inhibitors. Wound Repair Regen 1999; 7:442–452.

40. Wysocki, AB, Staiano-Coico, L, Grinnell, F: Wound fluid from chronic leg ulcers contains elevated levels of metalloproteinases MMP-2 and MMP-9. J Invest Dermatol 1993; 101(1):64–68.

41. Ovington, LG: Overview of matrix metalloprotease modulation and growth factor protection in wound healing. Ostomy Wound Manage 2002; 48(Pt 1, suppl):3–7.

42. Cullen, B, Watt, PW, Lundqvist, C, et al: The role of oxidised regenerated cellulose/collagen in chronic wound repair and its potential mechanism of action. Int J Biochem Cell Biol 2002; 34(12):1544–1556.

43. Schönfelder, U, Abel, M, Wiegand, C, et al: Influence of selected wound dressings on PMN elastase in chronic wound fluid and their antioxidative potential in vitro. Biomaterials 2005; 26(33):6664–6673.

44. Vachon, DJ, Yager, DR: Novel sulfonated hydrogel composite with the ability to inhibit proteases and bacterial growth. J Biomed Mater Res A 2006; 76(1):35–43.

45. Barrick, B, Campbell, EJ, Owen, CA: Leukocyte proteinases in wound healing: Roles in physiologic and pathologic processes. Wound Repair Regen 1999; 7:410–422.

46. Schmidtchen, A, Holst, E, Tapper, H, et al: Elastase-producing *Pseudomonas aeruginosa* degrade plasma proteins and extracellular products of human skin and fibroblasts, and inhibit fibroblast growth. Microb Pathog 2003; 34(1):47–55.

47. Yager, DR, Chen, SM, Ward, SI, et al: Ability of chronic wound fluids to degrade peptide growth factors is associated with increased levels of elastase activity and diminished levels of proteinase inhibitors. Wound Repair Regen 1997; 5:23–32.

48. Edwards, JV, Howley, PS: Human neutrophil elastase and collagenase sequestration with phosphorylated cotton wound dressings. J Biomed Mater Res A 2007; 83(2):446–454.

49. Bauer, JA, Rao, W, Smith, DJ: Evaluation of linear polyethyleneimine-nitric oxide adduct on wound repair: Therapy versus toxicity. Wound Repair Regen 1998; 6:569–577.

50. Paulsen, SM, Wurster, SH, Nanney, LB: Expression of inducible nitric oxide synthase in human burn wounds. Wound Repair Regen 1998; 6(2):142–148.

51. Yamasaki, K, Edington, HD, McClosky, C, et al: Reversal of impaired wound repair in iNOS deficient mice by topical adenoviral mediated iNOS gene transfer. J Clin Invest 1998; 101(5):967–971.

52. Schaffer, MR, Tantry, U, Gross, SS, et al: Nitric oxide regulates wounds healing. J Surg Res 1996; 63(1):237–240.

53. Masters, KS, Leibovich, SJ, Belem, P, et al: Effects of nitric oxide releasing poly(vinyl alcohol) hydrogel dressings on dermal wound healing in diabetic mice. Wound Repair Regen 2002; 10(5):286–294.

54. Wlaschek, M, Scharffetter-Kochanek, K: Oxidative stress in chronic venous leg ulcers. Wound Repair Regen 2005; 13(5):452–461.

55. Beukelman, CJ, van den Berg, AJ, Hoekstra, MJ, et al: Anti-inflammatory properties of a liposomal hydrogel with povidone-iodine (Repithel) for wound healing in vitro. Burns 2008; 34(6):845–855; Epub ahead of print.

56. van den Berg, AJ, van den Worm, E, van Ufford, HC, et al: An in vitro examination of the antioxidant and anti-inflammatory properties of buckwheat honey. J Wound Care 2008; 17(4):172–174, 176–178.

57. Van den Berg, AJ, Halkes, SB, van Ufford, HC, Hoekstra, MJ, Beukelman, CJ: A novel formulation of metal ions and citric acid reduces reactive oxygen species in vitro. J Wound Care 2003; (10):413–418.

58. Gottrup, F, Jørgensen, B, Karlsmark, T, et al: Less pain with Biatain-Ibu: Initial findings from a randomised, controlled, double-blind clinical investigation on painful venous leg ulcers. Int Wound J 2007; 4(suppl):24–34.

59. Gao, ZR, Hao, ZQ, Li, Y, et al: Porcine dermal collagen as a wound dressing for skin donor sites and deep partial skin thickness burns. Burns 1992; 18(6):492–496.

60. Di Mauro, C, Ossino, AM, Trefiletti, M, et al: Lyophilized collagen in the treatment of diabetic ulcers. Drugs Exp Clin Res 1991; 17(7):371–373.

61. Donaghue, VM, Chrzan, JS, Rosenblum, BI, et al: Evaluation of a collagen-alginate wound dressing in the management of diabetic foot ulcers. Adv Wound Care 1998; 11(3):114–119.

62. Van Gils, CC, Roeder, B, Chesler, SM, et al: Improved healing with a collagen-alginate dressing in the chemical matricectomy. J Am Podiatr Med Assoc 1998; 88:452–456.

63. Vowden, P, Romanelli, M, Price, P: Effect of amelogenin extracellular matrix protein and compression on hard-to-heal venous leg ulcers. J Wound Care 2007; 16(5):189–195.

64. Romanelli, M, Kaha, E, Stege, H, et al: Effect of amelogenin extracellular matrix protein and compression on hard-to-heal venous leg ulcers: Follow-up data. J Wound Care 2008; 17(1):17–18, 20–23.

65. Taddeucci, P, Pianigiani, E, Colletta, V, et al: An evaluation of Hyalofill-F plus compression bandaging in the treatment of chronic venous ulcers. J Wound Care 2004; 13(5):202–204.

66. Colletta, V, Dioguardi, D, Di Lonardo, A, et al: A trial to assess the efficacy and tolerability of Hyalofill-F in non-healing venous leg ulcers. J Wound Care 2003; 12(9):357–360.

67. Vazquez, JR, Short, B, Findlow, AH, et al: Outcomes of hyaluronan therapy in diabetic foot wounds. Diabetes Res Clin Pract 2003; 59(2):123–127.

68. Moseley, R, Walker, M, Waddington, RJ, et al: Comparison of the antioxidant properties of wound dressing materials— carboxymethylcellulose, hyaluronan benzyl ester and hyaluronan, towards polymorphonuclear leukocyte-derived reactive oxygen species. Biomaterials 2003; 24(9):1549–1557.

69. Griffiths, M, Ojeh, N, Livingstone, R, et al: Survival of Apligraf in acute human wounds. Tissue Eng 2004; 10:1180–1195.

70. Phillips, TJ, Manzoor, J, Rojas, A, et al: The longevity of a bilayered skin substitute after application to venous ulcers. Arch Dermatol 2002; 138(8):1079–1081.

71. Brem, H, Young, J, Tomic-Canic, M, et al: Clinical efficacy and mechanism of bilayered living human skin equivalent (HSE) in treatment of diabetic foot ulcers. Surg Technol Int 2003; 11:23–31.

72. Spiekstra, SW, Breetveld, M, Rustemeyer, T, et al: Wound-healing factors secreted by epidermal keratinocytes and dermal fibroblasts in skin substitutes. Wound Repair Regen 2007; 15(5):708–717.

73. el-Ghalbzouri, A, Gibas, S, Lamme, E, et al: Effect of fibroblasts on epidermal regeneration. Br J Dermatol 2002; 147(2):230–243.

74. Wang, HJ, Pieper, J, Schotel, R, et al: Stimulation of skin repair is dependent on fibroblast source and presence of extracellular matrix. Tissue Eng 2004; 10(7-8):1054–1064.

75. Pham, C, Greenwood, J, Cleland, H, et al: Bioengineered skin substitutes for the management of burns: A systematic review. Burns 2007; 33(8):946–957.

76. Supp, DM, Bell, SM, Morgan, JR, et al: Genetic modification of cultured skin substitutes by transduction of human keratinocytes and fibroblasts with platelet-derived growth factor-A. Wound Repair Regen 2000; 8(1):26–35.

77. Lei, P, Ogunade, A, Kirkwood, KL, et al: Efficient production of bioactive insulin from human epidermal keratinocytes and tissue-engineered skin substitutes: Implications for treatment of diabetes. Tissue Eng 2007; 13(8):2119–2131.

Manufacturers and Wound Products

AcryMed Inc.

12232 SW Garden Place
Portland, Oregon 97223
(503) 624-9830 or (888) ACRYMED
Fax: (503) 639-0846
Website: www.acrymed.com

SilvaSorb™
FlexiGel™

C.R. Bard Inc., Bard Medical Division

8195 Industrial Blvd.
Covington, Georgia 30014-2655
(770) 784-6100 or (800) 526-4455
Fax: (770) 784-6218
Website: www.bardmedical.com

Biolex™ Wound Gel
Vigilon® Wound Dressing

Bertek Pharmaceuticals Inc. (UDL Laboratories)

1718 Northrock Court
Rockford, Illinois 61103
(800) 848-0462
Fax: (815) 282-9391
Website: www.udllabs.com

BIOBRANE®
FLEXZAN™
Hydrocol®
SORBSAN™

BioCore Medical Technologies Inc.

1605 SW 41st St.
Topeka, Kansas 66609
(800) 577-4801
Fax: (785) 267-1900
Website: www.biocore.com

Medifil™ Pads
Medifil™ Particles
Medifil™ Gel

Carrington Laboratories Inc.

2001 Walnut Hill Lane
Irving, Texas 75038
(800) 527-5216
Fax: (972) 518-1020

CarraFilm™ Transparent Film Dressing
CarraDres™ Clear Hydrogel Sheet
CarraGauze® Hydrogel Wound Dressing Pads
CarraGauze® Packing Strips
CarraSmart™ Film Dressing
CarraSmart™ Foam Dressing
CarraSmart™ Hydrocolloid
CarraGinnateSorb™ H Calcium Alginate Wound Dressing
CarraSorb™ M Freeze-Dried Gel Wound Dressing
Carrington Bordered Gauze

Coloplast Corp.

1955 West Oak Circle
Marietta, Georgia 30062
(770) 281-8400 or (800) 533-0464
Fax: (770) 281-8501
Website: www.coloplast.com

Biatain™ Foam Dressing
Comfeel® Plus Clear Dressing
Comfeel® Plus Contour Dressing
Comfeel® Plus Pressure Relief Dressing
Comfeel® Plus Triangle Dressing
Comfeel® Plus Ulcer Dressing
Comfeel® Powder
Contreet®
Purilon Gel
Comfeel® Ulcer Care Dressing
Seasorb™ Alginate Dressing
Woun'Dres® Natural Collagen Hydrogel Wound Dressing

ConvaTec

100 Headquarters Park Dr.
Skillman, New Jersey 08558
(800) 422-8811 (clinic) or (800) 582-6514 (customer
  service)
Fax: (800) 523-2965
Website: www.convatec.com

AQUACEL™ Hydrofiber Wound Dressing
AQUACEL™ Hydrofiber Wound Packing (rope), Sterile
CombiDERM™ ACD Absorbent Dressing, Sterile
CombiDERM™ Non-Adhesive Absorbent Dressing, Sterile
DuoDERM® CGF® Control Gel Formula Border Dressing,
  Sterile (squares)
DuoDERM® CGF® Control Gel Formula Border Dressing,
  Sterile (triangles)
DuoDERM® CGF® Control Gel Formula Dressing, Sterile
DuoDERM® Extra Thin CGF® Dressing, Sterile
DuoDERM® Hydroactive®, Sterile
DuoDERM® Sterile Hydroactive Paste
SignaDRESS™ Sterile Dressing
Versiva®

Derma Sciences Inc.

214 Carnegie Center, Ste. 100
Princeton, NJ 08540
(609) 514-4744
Fax: (609) 514-0502
Website: www.dermasciences.com

Algicell™Ag
MediHoney™

DeRoyal Industries Inc., DeRoyal Wound Care

200 DeBusk Lane
Powell, Tennessee 37849
(423) 938-7828 or (800) 251-9864
Fax: (423) 362-1230
Website: www.deroyal.com

Algidex AG®
Covaderm® Adhesive Wound Dressing
Covaderm Plus® Adhesive Barrier Wound Dressing
Covaderm Plus® Tube Site Dressing
Covaderm Plus® V.A.D.
Multidex® Maltodextrin Wound Dressing
Multipad™ Non-Adherent Wound Dressing
Polyderm™ Border with COVADERM® Tape Hydrophilic
  Polyurethane Foam Dressing
Sofsorb®
Stretch Net™ Tubular Elastic Dressing
Transeal® Transparent Wound Dressing

Ferris Mfg. Corp.

16W300 83rd Street
Burr Ridge, Illinois 60521-5848
(630) 887-9797 or (800) POLYMEM
Fax: (630) 887-1008
Website: www.polymem.com

PolyMem® Adhesive Dressings
PolyMem® Alginate Dressings
PolyMem® Non-Adherent Dressings
PolyWic™ Wound Filler
PolyMem® Wound Measuring Grid

HEALTHPOINT

2600 Airport Fwy
Fort Worth, Texas 76111
(817) 900-4000 or (800) 441-8227
Fax: (817) 900-4100
Website: www.Healthpoint.com

CURASOL™ Gel Wound Dressing
CURASOL™ Hydrogel Saturated 4×4
HYROFERA BLUE™
IODOFLEX™ Pad Wound Cleaning Dressing
IODOSORB® Gel Wound Cleaning Dressing
OASIS® Wound Matrix

Hollister Inc.

2000 Hollister Drive
Libertyville, Illinois 60048
(847) 680-1000 or (800) 323-4060
Fax: (847) 918-3994
Website: www.hollister.com

Restore™ Calcium Alginate Dressing
Restore™ Calcium Alginate Dressing with Silver
Restore™ Contact Layer Dressing
Restore™™ Contact Layer Dressing with Silver
Restore™ Hydrocolloid Dressing
Restore™ Extra Thin Hydrocolloid Dressing

Johnson & Johnson Medical, Inc.

2500 Arbrook Blvd.
Arlington, Texas 76014
(800) 255-2500
Fax: (817) 262-4129
Website: www.jnjgateway.com

ACTISORB™ Dressing
BIOCLUSIVE™ MVP Select Transparent Dressing
BIOCLUSIVE™ Select Transparent Dressing

BIOCLUSIVE™ Transparent Dressing
FIBRACOL™ Collagen Alginate Wound Dressing
FIBRACOL™ PLUS Collagen Wound Dressing with
 Alginate
PROMOGRAN™ PRISMA Matrix Dressing

Kendall Healthcare Products Co.

15 Hampshire Street
Mansfield, Massachusetts 02048
(508) 261-8000 or (800) 962-9888
Fax: (508) 261-8271
Website: www.kendallhq.com

Aquaflo® Hydrogel Dressing
Conform® Stretch Bandages
Curafil® Gel Wound Dressing
Curafil® Hydrogel Impregnated Gauze
CURAFOAM® Hydrophilic Foam Wound Dressing
CURAFOAM PLUS® Foam Dressing
CURAGEL® Hydrogel Island Wound Dressing
CURAGEL® Hydrogel Wound Dressing
Curasorb® Calcium Alginate Dressing
Curasorb® Zinc
CURITY® Packing Strips, Iodoform
CURITY® Packing Strips, Plain
KERLIX® Bandage Rolls
KERLIX® AMD Roll
Polyskin® II Transparent Dressing
TELFA® Dressings
TELFA® Island Dressing
ULTEC® Hydrocolloid Dressings
ULTEC® PRO Alginate Hydrocolloid Dressing
Vaseline® Petroleum Gauze
Xeroform Petroleum Gauze
XEROFLO® Gauze Dressings

Medline Industries Inc.

One Medline Place
Mundelein, Illinois 60060
(800) 633-5463
Fax: (847) 949-3012
Website: www.medline.com

Arglaes Antimicrobial Barrier Film
Avant Gauze™ Non-Woven Gauze
Bulkee II™ Gauze Bandage
Bulkee™ Super Fluff Sponge
Derma-Gel Hydrogel Wafer
Exuderm™ Hydrocolloid
Exuderm LP™ Hydrocolloid
Exuderm RCD™ Hydrocolloid
Exuderm Ultra Hydrocolloid
Exuderm Sacrum Hydrocolloid

Maxorb™ Hydrofiber Alginate
Medfix Dressing Retention Roll
Medline ABD Pad
Medline Bordered Gauze
Medline Oil Emulsion Dressings
Medline Packing Strips
Medline Petroleum Dressings
Medline Xero-Form Dressing
SilvaSorb® Gel
SkinTegrity™ Hydrogel
SkinTegrity™ Hydrogel Impregnated Gauze
StrataSorb™ Composite Island
SureSite™ Transparent Film
TenderWet™ Active

Molnlycke Health Care

5550 Peachtree Parkway, Ste. 500
Norcross, Georgia 30092
(678) 250-7900 or (800) 882-4582
Fax: (678) 250-7984
Website: www.molnlycke.com

Alldress® Absorbent Film Dressing
Hypergel®
Mefix®
Mefilm™
Melgisorb™
Mepiform™
Mepitel®
Mepilex™
Mepore™
Mesalt®
MitraflexR Plus
Normlgel®

MPM Medical Inc.

801 Stadium Drive, Ste. 109
Arlington, Texas 76011
(817) 861-8570 or (800) 232-5512
Fax: (817) 861-8531
Website: www.mpmmedicalinc.com

MPM Conductive Gel Pad™
MPM DermaSeal™
MPM Excel Gel™
MPM Excel™ Hydrocolloid
MPM Flex-Gel™
MPM GelPad™
MPM Hydrogel Dressing™
MPM Multi-Layered Dressing
MPM Regenecare™
MPM Sof-Foam
MPM Wet Dressing (Sterile Saline)
MPM WoundGard
Repel Wound Dressing

Smith & Nephew Inc., Wound Management Division

11775 Starkey Road
P.O. Box 1970
Largo, Florida 33779-1970
(727) 392-1261 or (800) 876-1261
Fax: (727) 392-6914 or (727) 392-0797
Website: www.snwmd.com

Acticoat™
Algisite™ M
Allevyn™
Allevyn™ Adhesive
Allevyn™ Cavity Wound Dressings
Allevyn™ Island Dressing
CICACARE™
Conformant 2® Wound Veils
CovRSite™
DRYNET® Wound Veils
EXU-DRY®
EXU-DRY® Wound Dressing
Flexigel Hydrogel Sheet
Flexigel Strands Absorbent Wound Dressing
IntraSite™ Gel
Iodoflex® Pad
OpSite™ Flexigrid
OpSite™ Flexifix
OpSite™ Plus
OpSite™ Post-Op
OpSite™ Transparent Dressing
PRIMAPORE™
RepliCare™
RepliCare™ Absorbent Paste
RepliCare™ Thin
SoloSite™ Gel Conformable Wound Dressing

Southwest Technologies Inc.

1746 Levee Road
North Kansas City, Missouri 64116
(816) 221-2442 or (800) 247-9951
Fax: (816) 221-3995
Website: www.swtechinc.com

Elasto-Gel™
Elasto-Gel™ Cushions/Pressure Pads
Elasto-Gel™ Island
Elasto-Gel™ Plus
HyCure™ Collagen Wound Filler

3M Health Care

3M Center, Building 275-4E-01
St. Paul, Minnesota 55144-1000
(612) 736-1723 or (800) 228-3957
Fax: (612) 737-7678
Website: www.3m.com/healthcare

3M™ Microdon™ Soft Cloth Adhesive Wound Dressing
3M™ Reston™ Self-Adhering Foam Pad & Roll
3M™ Tegaderm™ Ag Mesh
3M™ Tegaderm™ Alginate Dressing
3M™ Tegaderm™ Transparent Dressing
3M™ Tegaderm™ +Pad Transparent Dressing with Absorbent Pad
3M™ Tegaderm™ Hydrocolloid
3M™ Tegagel™ Hydrogel Wound Filler
3M™ Tegagel™ Hydrogel Wound Filler with Gauze
3M™ Tegagen™ HG (High Gelling) Alginate Dressing
3M™ Tegagen™ HI (High Integrity) Alginate Dressing
3M™ Tegapore™ Wound Contact Material
3M Tegasorb™ Hydrocolloid Dressing
3M Tegasorb™ Thin Hydrocolloid Dressing

chapter 13

Topical Agents

Kevin Y. Woo, MSc, PhD, RN, ACNP, GNC(C), FAPWCA

R. Gary Sibbald, BS, MD, FRCPC (MED), FRCPC (DERM), Med

Topical agents can be selected to optimize local chronic wound care, but they will be completely ineffective without a holistic approach to patient care. Chronic wounds are often complex, recalcitrant to healing, and may persist for months or years due to underlying disease processes or complications. According to findings from control populations in randomized controlled trials (RCTs), a wound that is not 30% smaller by week 4 will usually not heal by week 12.[1,2] The exact mechanisms that contribute to poor wound healing remain elusive but likely involve an interplay of systemic and local factors. The wound bed preparation (WBP) model was proposed by Sibbald et al.[3-5] to systematically manage chronic wounds and optimize achievable patient outcomes. (Fig. 13.1)

Topical therapy choices are different for healable versus nonhealable wounds. Although complete healing may seem to be the logical goal for most patients, some wounds do not have the ability to heal due to inadequate vasculature, a cause that is not treatable, or coexisting medical conditions/medications that prohibit the healing process. Healable wounds have adequate tissue perfusion and the cause has been corrected or compensated with treatment. In addition, patients with these wounds do not have any other factors that would inhibit healing, including coexisting medical conditions (e.g., advanced cancer), negative protein balance, advanced anemia or prescribed medication (e.g., immunosuppressive drugs) that would prevent normal healing.

A maintenance wound is different from a healable wound or a nonhealable wound. A maintenance wound has the ability to heal but either the patient does not consistently adhere to treatment or the health-care system may restrict access to appropriate resources. To put this in a meaningful context, this type of wound classification system helps clinicians and patients identify a common realistic outcome goal. (Table 13.1)

Moist interactive healing is contraindicated in nonhealable wounds. Instead, local wound care involves conservative débridement without causing bleeding, bacterial reduction, and moisture reduction. (Fig. 13.2) These wounds are best treated with antiseptics when healing is not immediately achievable (uncontrolled deep infection) or when bacterial burden is more of a concern than tissue toxicity (maintenance or nonhealable wounds).

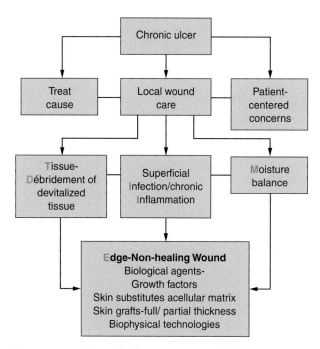

Figure 13•1 *Wound bed preparation model.*[3-5]

Table 13•1 Wound Classification According to Healing Ability			
Wound Prognosis	**Treat the Cause**	**Blood Supply**	**Coexisting Medical Condition/Drugs**
Healable	Yes	Adequate	Does not prevent healing
Maintenance	No*	Adequate	Possibly prevents healing
Nonhealable or palliative	No	Usually inadequate	May prevent healing

*Cause not treated due to lack of patient adherence or health system factors preventing access to resources

Non-healable and maintenance wounds

Figure **13•2** *Nonhealable and maintenance wounds.*

> ▶ **PEARL 13•1** Topical antiseptics for nonhealable and maintenance wounds may decrease superficial bacterial counts and therefore the likelihood of subsequent organism invasion into deeper viable tissue. (Table 13.2)

Topical Antiseptic Agents

In the past Betadine (Purdue Frederick, Norwalk, CT), which consists of 10% povidone-iodine (PVP-I) in an aqueous solution, was one of the most extensively used broad-spectrum topical antiseptics. Free iodine that is released from the PVP-I molecules exerts it antimicrobial property by combining irreversibly with tyrosine residues of proteins, disrupting the formation of hydrogen bonding by amino acids and nucleotides, oxidizing sulfhydryl (—SH) groups, and reacting with sites of unsaturated fatty acids.[6] These oxidative reactions produce a deleterious effect on mitosis and normal cellular metabolism and will ultimately lead to cell death. In vitro, PVP-I is toxic to human fibroblasts, even when diluted to a low concentration.[7] In a study of chronic leg ulcers,[8] PVP-I was compared with silver sulfadiazine and chlorhexidine digluconate. Healing rates improved by 4% to 18% and time to healing was reduced by 2 to 9 weeks using PVP-I (all *P* values <0.01). In a retrospective 42-patient chart review by Woo et al,[9] the majority of patients with nonhealable and maintenance wounds treated with topical povidone-iodine (10%; not cadexomer iodine) improved: 28% achieved complete closure and an additional 45% had reduced wound size despite their low probably for sustained healing. The final surface areas of these wounds were significantly smaller than the initial measurements in this chronic wound cohort of patients (Wilcoxon signed ranks test, *P* = 0.011).

Polyhexamethylene biguanide (PHMB) is another commonly used antiseptic related to chlorhexidine. It is a cationic molecule also known as polyhexanide and polyaminopropyl biguanide. It disrupts the integrity of the bacterial cytoplasmic membrane, causing the precipitation of cell contents and death. The evidence suggests that PHMB is not only effective against individual bacteria in their planktonic state but also sessile bacteria in biofilms.[10] Motta and associates demonstrated that PHMB impregnated in gauze resulted in a decrease in the number of organisms present in the wound. [11] In vitro, PHMB killed *Pseudomonas* in the presence of human wound fluid.[12] Mulder et al reported a study of PHMB-impregnated dressings in 26 chronic wounds.[13] The bacteria count obtained by semiquantitative methodology was reduced over the 7-week study period. The average wound size was reduced by 25% from 6.79 cm² to 4.57 cm². Unlike silver-coated dressings, PHMB was not able to produce a zone of inhibition in vitro, suggesting that limited antimicrobial activity would be released

Table 13•2 Antiseptics Most Commonly Used in Wound Care

Class and Agent	Action	Effect in Healing	Effect on Bacteria	Comments
Alcohols Ethyl alcohol Isopropyl alcohol	Dehydrates proteins and dissolves lipids.	Cytotoxic. May cause dryness and irritation on intact skin.	Bactericidal and virucidal.	Used as a disinfectant on intact skin. Stings and burns if used on open skin.
Biguanides 0.02%–0.05% chlorhexidine	Acts by damaging the cell membranes.	Relatively safe. Little effect on wound healing. Toxicity—small effect on tissue.	Highly bactericidal against gram-positive and gram-negative organisms.	Highly effective as hand washing agent and for surgical scrub. Binds to stratum corneum and has residual effect.
Halogen compounds Sodium hypochlorite (eg, Hygeol, Eusol, Dakin's solution)	Lyses cell walls.	Acts as a chemical débrider and should be discontinued with healing tissue.	Dakin's solution and Eusol (buffered preparation) can select out gram-negative microorganisms.	High pH causes irritation to skin.
1% Iodine (povidone) (eg, Betadine)	Oxidizes cell constituents, especially proteins at –SH groups; iodinates proteins and inactivates them.	Povidone-iodine Cytotoxicity depends on dilution. Potential toxicity in vivo related to concentration and exposure.	Prevents and controls bacterial growth in wounds. Resistance has not been reported. Broad spectrum of activity, although decreased in the presence of pus or exudate.	Toxicity is of concern with prolonged use or application over large areas Potential for thyroid toxicity

Class and Agent	Action	Effect in Healing	Effect on Bacteria	Comments
Organic acid Acetic (0.25%–1%)	Lowers surface pH.	Cytotoxicity in vitro; in vivo toxicity is concentration dependent.	Effective against *Pseudomonas*. May be useful for other gram-negative rods and *S. aureus*.	Often burns and stings on application.
Peroxides 3% Hydrogen peroxide	May induce cell death by oxidative damage.	Can harm healthy granulation tissue and may form air emboli if packed in deep sinuses.	Very little to absent antimicrobial activity.	Acts more like a chemical débriding agent by dissolving blood clots and softening slough. Safety concerns for deep wounds due to reports of air embolisms.
Tinctures Gentian violet	Very weak antiseptic.	Potential carcinogen and cytotoxic. May cause erosions, ulcers, or areas of necrosis, especially on mucous membranes.	Kills gram-positive organisms and some yeasts such as *Candida*; more effective at higher pH, but can select out overgrowth of gram-negative organisms.	High irritancy potential and occasional allergies.
Mercurochrome	A very weak antiseptic with action inhibited in the presence of organic debris.	Epidermal cell toxicity.	Not enough data available.	Contact allergen and irritant; systemic toxicity and rare death through topical application; possible aplastic anemia.
Cetrimide (quaternary ammonium)	Disrupts membranes, may inactivate some proteins.	High toxicity to tissues.	Gram-positive and gram-negative organisms.	Good detergent, but very irritating to open wounds.

© Modified by Sibbald and Woo 2008

to the surrounding areas.[14] When PHMB dressings were applied on contaminated wounds in a porcine model, only 20% achieved complete reepithelialization over 21 days compared to 95% with silver-coated dressings.[14]

Acetic acid lowers the wound surface pH, and this discourages the proliferation of *Pseudomonas*. White vinegar is 5% acetic acid, and this can be diluted 1:5 or 1:10 with water to achieve lower concentrations (1.0% or 0.5%) that are less likely to cause burning and stinging. Other antiseptic agents and associated effects and concerns are summarized in Table 13.2.

Topical Pain Agents

Pain is a common occurrence in patients with chronic wounds. Although mounting evidence suggests that pain is often exacerbated by treatment and dressing change or other procedures, a substantial proportion of patients also experience wound-related pain at rest, often associated with the wound etiology. The complexity of wound-associated pain (WAP) is illustrated in Figure 13.3.

Dressing removal may be painful due to dried-out materials, aggressive adhesives, adherent granulation tissue/capillary loops growing into the product matrix, and the gluelike nature of dehydrated or crusted exudate.

> **PEARL 13•2** Removal of gauze dressing is traumatic and more painful than any other advanced moisture-balance dressings, including foam,[16] alginates,[17,18] and hydrocolloid dressings.[19]

The use of "atraumatic" dressings is considered the most important strategy to avoid wound surface trauma and patient distress. Nonadherent layers can also be used effectively for reducing dressing adhesion to the wound and preventing local damage and pain on removal.[20-23] For more in-depth coverage of wound-related pain see Chapter 22.

To minimize systemic side effects, topical agents provide a useful alternative, with NSAIDs and capsaicin demonstrating promising results. Several randomized controlled trials were conducted to evaluate the effectiveness of ibuprofen-releasing foam (licensed in Europe and Canada, but not in the United States as of 2009) for the treatment of persistent and temporary wound pain.[24,25] Patients experienced a significant reduction of

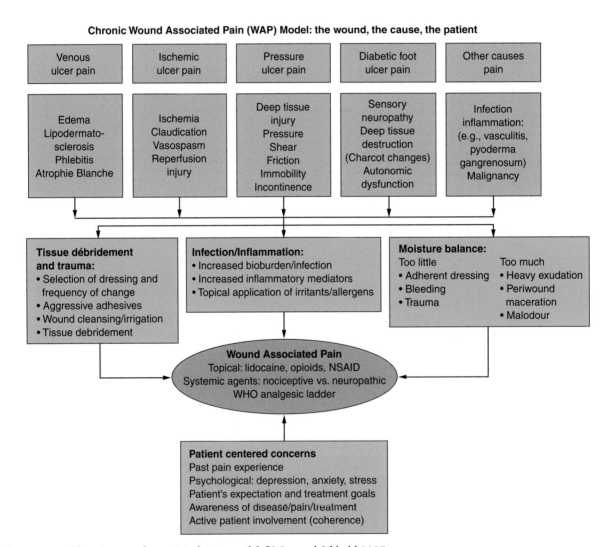

Figure 13•3 *Chronic wound-associated pain model.* ©*Woo and Sibbald 2007*

local wound-associated pain as early as the first evening after the application of the dressing. This dressing is only effective for local pain in the presence of wound exudate and an absence of infection.

The investigational use of topical morphine has demonstrated positive results in several studies; however, this formulation is not commercially available and the lack of pharmacokinetic data has precluded the routine clinical use of these compounds at this time. To reduce pain, topical anesthetics may be suitable for use prior to painful intermittent procedures. The use of an eutectic mixture of lidocaine and prilocaine, EMLA® Cream (AstraZeneca Pharmaceuticals, Wilmington, DE) has produced effective pain relief during débridement of venous leg ulcers.[26] This product is not licensed for direct ulcer application in the United States, but has approval for this indication in Canada and Europe.

Topical Débridement Agents

Débridement is a crucial step to prepare the wound bed by removing devitalized tissue that acts as a proinflammatory nidus and growth media for bacteria.[27] Bacterial metalloproteases and other proinflammatory mediators can cause further tissue damage and the formation of devitalized tissue. It is common for a chronic wound to have an increase in senescent cells less responsive to cellular signaling, with a coexistent decrease in growth factors and diminished cellular-signaling responses.[28,29] Débridement can remove senescent cells and biofilms, which may therefore promote healing in a stalled wound.[30] Although several research findings corroborate the value of sharp débridement in promoting wound healing, this method of débridement may not always be feasible due to pain, bleeding potential, cost, and the lack of clinician expertise.

Alternatively, autolytic débridement removes nonviable tissue through promoting the activities of phagocytic cells and endogenous enzymes. Enzymatic débridement provides addition of exogenous agents such as proteolytic enzymes, including collagenase, streptokinase, streptodornase, trypsin-chymotrypsin, papain-urea,[31] and plant enzymes (fig, pineapple), to accelerate the débridement process.[32-34] While comparative and descriptive studies have documented the selective benefits of enzymatic débridement, well-designed randomized controlled trials are lacking.

Papain was first described and used as a débriding agent in 1940 by Glasser.[35] Since then, a combination of papain-urea-chlorophyllin has been made commercially available for clinical use. Papain is an enzyme derived from the fruit of the papaya tree (*Carica papaya*). It facilitates débridement by breaking down proteins that contain cysteine residues over a wide pH range (pH 3 to 12). In moderate concentrations (10% to 25%), urea has been used as a humectant and moisturizer. At a higher concentration, urea's role in this enzymatic combination is to enhance the proteolytic action of papain through exposing the cysteine structure by altering the hydrogen bonds and disulfide bridges of the targeted tissue.[36] This makes the combination of products twice as effective. As mentioned in Chapter 11, in 2008 the FDA recalled papain-containing products due to safety concerns. Thus they are no longer being manufactured or distributed.

▶ **PEARL 13•3** Collagenase, papain-urea, and polyacrylate wet dressings promote enzymatic or autolytic débridement.

Collagen is a fundamental component of skin, composing over 75% of the dry weight of skin tissue. Collagenase is a water-soluble proteinase derived from bacteria that specifically breaks down collagen into gelatin.[38] Previous work demonstrated that both collagenase and papain-urea were more effective against denatured (devitalized) proteins than against nondenatured (native) proteins.[39] In one study of patients with pressure ulcers, papain-urea débriding ointment was significantly more effective ($P<0.0167$) than the collagenase ointment in reducing the amount of necrotic tissue at weekly evaluations.[40] Papain-urea preparations may be associated with local pain or an increase in existing pain, and when this happens clinicians should observe the wound carefully for infection.

Bromelain is a crude pineapple extract that contains various proteolytic enzymes capable of antithrombotic and fibrinolytic activities. In a murine model, topical bromelain (35% in a lipid base) facilitated complete débridement of necrotic tissue in burn wounds in 2 days as opposed to 10 days required with collagenase.[41] Fibrinolysin cleaves fibrin-containing blood clots and dissolves fibrinous material to facilitate wound débridement by macrophages. The enzyme DNAase depolymerizes deoxyribonucleoproteins and deoxyribonucleic acids in the necrotic tissue to produce a clean wound surface. These agents do not interact with living tissue and are not likely to delay healing. Peter et al demonstrated that fibrinolysin-DNAase may also promote healing by improving wound blood supply at the arteriolar and capillary levels.[42] Previous studies fail to demonstrate the superiority of any one agent over the other in wound débridement.[43,44] In a randomized controlled trial, Falabella et al found no significant difference in the removal of purulent exudate or necrotic tissue between the fibrinolysin-DNAase combination and a placebo ointment in patients with chronic leg ulcers over a 3-week study period.[45] Healing outcomes were similar between the two groups.

A randomized controlled trial ($n = 42$) compared the use of collagenase with a fabric dressing infused with Ringer's solution–soaked polyacrylate particles for 21 days in patients with chronic leg ulcers. Polyacrylates bind to MMPs and bacterial cell walls, assisting the removal of both of these harmful factors in healing. Wounds were evaluated weekly for the amount of eschar and slough, the area of healthy granulation, and the reepithelialized area.[46] Slough on the wound surface was reduced by 19% with polyacrylate wet dressing and by 9% with collagenase during the first 14 days. These results were not statistically significant.

Desloughing may be hastened by lowering wound pH, but the use of organic and inorganic acids and other chemical agents are discouraged in light of the potential for pain. Biological débridement by inoculating larva that feed on the necrotic wound tissue and exudate is gaining popularity. Despite the potential benefits of maggot therapy, this therapy is not innocuous, and local painful reactions are not uncommon.[47,48] Emerging evidence suggests that novel débridement methods including some kilohertz ultrasonic technologies and Versajet™ Hydrosurgery System (Smith & Nephew, Largo, FL) may be relatively pain free, but acceptance of these devices into some wound care practices is hindered by cost and in a few cases the need for an operating room instead of the ambulatory clinical setting.[49]

Topical Antimicrobial Agents

Chronic wounds are invariably colonized by microorganisms representing a complex ecology. In fact, more than 90% of chronic wounds host polymicrobial flora containing a range of 1.6 to 4.4 bacterial species per ulcer.[50] Increased surface bacterial burden or critical colonization can be deleterious to wound healing. Bacteria produce endotoxins and exotoxins that are toxic to the cellular wound microenvironment. Although gram-positive organisms predominate in wounds initially, other microorganisms are usually detected in chronic wounds (gram-negative organisms and then anaerobes in devitalized tissue). Poor wound healing has been associated with the presence of four or more bacterial species. Together these microorganisms aggregate to produce biofilms and exchange virulence factors, rendering them more difficult to be eliminated over time.

When considering the therapeutics and strategies for the management of wound infection, the chronic wound environment can be divided into four levels or compartments: surface, superficial, surrounding and deep, and systemic. This conceptualization allows clinicians to evaluate the extent of bacterial damage and select the most appropriate treatment modality to address the bioburden. (Table 13.3)

All chronic wounds are colonized with bacteria at the first level, the surface, but meticulous infection control must be exercised to avoid cross-contamination. A secondary dressing provides temporary coverage and may function as a barrier to block contaminants from entering the wound. Remember that bacteria have the ability to penetrate through multiple layers of gauze dressings. The second level, the superficial compartment, extends approximately 1 to 3 mm below the wound surface. Some bacteria will critically colonize the superficial, relatively hypoxic wound environment, but not all species have the virulence to invade the deep compartment. Many active ingredients in dressings are released into the wound surface compartment, but they require wound fluid or exudate to diffuse into the tissue. Alternatively, bacteria can be entrapped and sequestered in the microarchitecture of a dressing where they may be inactivated.

The third compartment is also considered as the surrounding and deep compartment in a chronic wound. Systemic agents usually recommended as topical agents are not able to penetrate into the deep compartment. An effective topical antimicrobial may still be considered to eliminate the bacteria that percolate to the superficial compartment where the circulation may be less than optimal. Last, if the infection is promulgated systemically, systemic parenteral agents must be considered.

By focusing on salient clinical signs to separate superficial and deep compartment involvement (Table 13.4),[51] clinicians can identify and differentiate wounds with increased bacterial burden that may respond to topical antimicrobials as well as deep infection that usually requires the systemic antimicrobial agents (Table 13.3).

Cutting and Harding proposed that evidence of red friable, exuberant granulation, increased discharge and new devitalized tissue along with other criteria are related to infection.[52] In Gardiner's study, a checklist was formulated based on validated symptoms and signs of infection, such as increased pain, wound enlargement, new areas of breakdown, and odor.[53] In patients with diabetes, wounds that probe to bone are considered associated with osteomyelitis until proven otherwise.[54] However, there is no evidence that any individual sign or symptom can independently and reliably identify wound infection.[55]

Based on literature review, Sibbald, Woo, and Ayello created the mnemonic NERDS and STONEES to categorize the two levels of bacterial damage or infection.[51] A validation study of these signs was conducted in a cohort of 111 patients with leg and foot ulcers.[56] The sensitivity and specificity for each sign is listed in Table 13.5. It is recommended that two or three of these signs be identified for the diagnosis in each level. If increased exudate and odor are present, additional signs are needed to determine if the damage is superficial, deep, or both.

Table 13•3 Compartment Model of Chronic Wound Bacterial Burden and Infection		
4 S's of Bacteria and Skin		
Level	**Bacterial Status**	**Treatment**
Surface	• Contamination	Infection control: Alcohol rinse and hand washing
Superficial	• Colonization • Critical colonization (increased bacterial burden, localized infection, covert infection)	Topical antimicrobial
Surrounding and deep	• Infection	Systemic agents
Systemic	• Sepsis	Parenteral therapy

© Modified by Woo and Sibbald 2008

Table 13•4 NERDS and STONEES

Superficial and Deep: Critical Colonization and Infection

Superficial: Treat topically	**N.E.R.D.S.** • **N**on-healing • **E**xudate increases • **R**ed and bleeding • **D**ebris • **S**mell	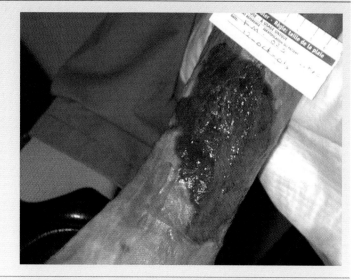
Deep: Treat systemically	**S.T.O.N.E.E.S.** • **S**ize is bigger • **T**emperature increases • **O**s (probes, exposed) • **N**ew breakdown • **E**xudate increases • **E**rythema, edema • **S**mell	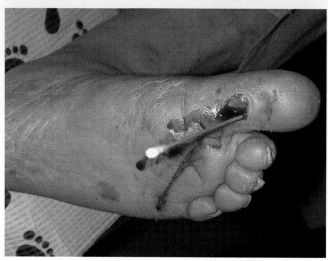

© Sibbald, Ayello, and Woo 2007.

With the emergence of bacteria that are resistant to commonly used antibiotics, the increased use of topical antimicrobial agents may become a sensible option for selected local wound care.

▶ **PEARL 13•4** Silver (in its aqueous ionized state) is a broad-spectrum antimicrobial agent that has been demonstrated to be effective against yeast, mold, and a large number of gram-positive and gram-negative microorganisms, aerobes, and several antibiotic-resistant strains such as methicillin-resistant *Staphylococcus aureus* (MRSA) and vancomycin-resistant enterococci (VRE).

The widely used 1% silver sulfadiazine (SSD) cream is an effective antimicrobial agent, but it does not promote autolytic débridement or moisture balance properties that are central to the WBP paradigm. This topical cream has a relatively meager amount of active ionized silver and larger amounts of the silver metal in the nonionized form that may be systemically absorbed.[58] The combinations of silver and sulfa ingredients are responsible for the antimicrobial property and should be avoided in people with sulfa allergies. Furthermore, repeated applications tend to leave heavy deposits of pseudoeschar-like debris on the wound surface. Over the years, a plethora of silver-based dressings in various concentrations, forms, vehicles, and functionalities have been introduced. Differences in

Table 13•5 Sensitivity and Specificity Summary of the Signs and Symptoms Associated with Superficial and Deep Bacterial Burden

	Signs and Symptoms	Sensitivity, % (Woo)[57]	Sensitivity, % (Grayson)[54]	Specificity, % (Woo)[57]	Specificity, % (Grayson)[54]
	Superficial				
N	Nonhealing	32	81	47	64
E	Exudate	70	18–55	64	64–72
R	Red friable tissue	45	82	86	76
D	Debris (discoloration)	62	64	78	56
S	Smell	37	36	86	88
	Deep and surrounding				
S	Size increasing	50	Not evaluated	83	Not evaluated
T	Temperature (>4°F) (heat)	76	18	71	84
O	Os (probe to bone)	40	Not evaluated	81	Not evaluated
N	New breakdown	37	46	89	100
E	Edema/erythema	87	55–64	44	68–72
E	Exudate	70	18–55	64	64–72
S	Smell	37	36	86	88
	Pain	Not evaluated	36	Not evaluated	100

› **Box 13•1   Key Considerations for the Selection of Silver Dressings**

When and How to Use SILVER

S—Signs of increased bacterial burden
I—Ionized silver concentration
L—Log reduction over time (kill time)
V—Vehicle for moisture balance
E—Effects on viable cells
R—Resistance

© Woo and Sibbald 2007

dressings have generated many unsettled disputes concerning the ideal properties of silver for the management of chronic wounds. (Box 13.1)

In an in vitro study, Castellano et al evaluated and compared the antimicrobial properties of eight silver-impregnated dressings against *Staphylococcus aureus, Staphylococcus faecalis, Pseudomonas aeruginosa,* and *Escherichia coli.*[59] All dressings demonstrated their abilities to inhibit bacterial growth. Quantitative analysis after 72 hours of incubation indicated that the four bacteria were less susceptible to the dressings with the lowest silver concentration. We must use caution interpreting in vitro data for clinic practice.

Randomized controlled trials with silver dressings in chronic wounds have been performed with moderate-release silver foam dressing (Contreet™, Coloplast Corp., Minneapolis, MN). In an efficacy study,[60] patients with venous disease and mixed (arterial and venous) disease were randomized to receive either compression with the silver-releasing foam (Contreet) or a foam dressing alone. All patients had stalled wounds and one of the following additional complaints: an increased exudate, increased pain, odor, or abnormal granulation tissue on the surface. At week 4, there was a 45% reduction in the silver foam group wound size compared to a 25% reduction in the ulcer size for the foam comparator ($P = 0.05$). In addition, there was noticeable improvement in odor and exudate management with less leakage. Results are also available from a larger efficiency RCT that enrolled 619 patients from 80 wound clinics around the world and compared best local practices with the same silver foam dressing.[61] In this study of chronic wounds (eg, leg, foot and pressure ulcers), the silver foam was compared to the local best clinical practice. The 4-week relative reduction in ulcer size was 50% for the silver foam dressing compared to 34% for the local best practices (*P*<0.01). There was also a significant and accelerated reduction in odor and wound fluid leakage. These results were consistent with the conclusions of a topical silver dressing systematic review for "infected" (surface critical colonization in our definition) chronic wounds.[62] Silver-containing foam dressings promoted a greater reduction of ulcer size but did not significantly increase complete wound closure.

Bergin and Wraight failed to locate any study pertaining to the use of silver dressings for the treatment of foot ulcers that would qualify for the Cochrane systematic review criteria.[63] Chambers et al reviewed silver treatments for leg ulcers.[64] The three studies included in the review compared silver sulfadiazine (SSD) cream with other inert dressings. No significant difference in healing was found.

In addition to silver dressings, topical antibiotics and antibacterial agents are available to combat superficial bacterial burden. (Table 13.6) In one study, polymyxin B sulfate was compared with 3% hydrogen peroxide, 1% povidone-iodine, 0.25% acetic acid, and 0.5% sodium hydrochloride in experimentally induced blister wounds that were inoculated with *S. aureus*.[65] Bacteria was eliminated by the neomycin-polymyxin B–bacitracin combination after two applications. Contaminated blister wounds treated with the triple antibiotic ointment healed significantly faster (mean = 9 days) than wounds

Table 13•6 Commonly Used Topical Antibacterial Agents

Agent	Vehicle	Staphylococcus aureus	Streptococcus	Pseudomonas	Anaerobe	Comments
Gentamicin sulphate* Cream/ointment	Alcohol cream base or petrolatum ointment	√	√	√		*Good broad-spectrum versus gram-negative bacteria. *Topical use may increase resistance.
Metronidazole gel/cream/ solution	Wax-glycerin cream and carbogel 940/propylene glycol gel				√	Good anaerobe coverage and wound deodorizer.
Mupirocin 2% Cream Ointment Nasal ointment	Polyethylene glycol (ointment) Paraffin/glycerine (nasal ointment)	√	√			*Good for MRSA. *Excellent topical penetration. *Used predominantly for perirectal, nasal colonization.
Polymyxin B sulphate Bacitracin zinc	White petrolatum ointment	√	√	√		Broad-spectrum. Low cost.
Polymyxin B sulphate Bacitracin zinc, neomycin**	White petrolatum ointment	√	√	√		Neomycin is a potent sensitizer and may cross-react with other aminoglycosides in 40% of cases.
Polymyxin/ gramicidin	Cream	√	√	√		Broad-spectrum coverage.
Silver sulfadiazine (SSD)	Water-miscible cream	√	√	√		*Do not use in sulfa-sensitive individuals. *Short half-life. Neutropenia is possible. *May leave pseudoeschar on wounds.

*Used systemically; **contains common sensitizer.
© Sibbald and Woo 2007.

treated with any antiseptic and those receiving no treatment. Another randomized trial compared mupirocin cream to oral cephalexin in the treatment of infected superficial wounds from laceration or abrasion. The intention-to-treat success rate was similar (83%) in both groups. Topical mupirocin cream was as effective as oral cephalexin for the treatment of secondarily infected wounds.

Increasing attention is paid to honey as an antimicrobial agent due to its osmotic activity, low pH, production of hydrogen peroxide, specific plant-derived factors and other unknown properties.[66] Molan reviewed clinical evidence for the use of honey as a wound dressing.[68] Seventeen randomized controlled trials were identified, with only two trials involving chronic wound patients. Most studies demonstrated favorable results, but there are several methodological flaws in these studies.

> **PEARL 13•5** Diagnosis of wound infection is based on clinical signs. Consider NERDS and STONEES.

Topical Anti-Inflammatory Agents

Many of the stalled chronic wounds demonstrate markedly increased activity of inflammatory cells and associated mediators perpetuated by recurring tissue trauma (e.g., pressure, bacterial growth, leukocyte trapping, or ischemic reperfusion injury.) The inflammatory cells are needed to remove nonvitalized tissue and to allow regeneration of granulation tissue, but this prolonged and superfluous inflammatory response can be deleterious.

> **PEARL 13•6** Inflammatory cells secrete cytokines that increase vascular permeability and promote cellular migration, resulting in the production of excess exudation. Under these conditions, wound healing is often stalled because degradation of extracellular matrix and growth factors occur more rapidly than their synthesis, hindering the wound from progressing toward the proliferative phase and ultimately reepithelialization.

Matrix metalloproteases (MMPs) are a family of metal-dependent enzymes. There are 23 MMPs or matrices identified, including a number of proteases that are involved in the degradation of extracellular matrix. Based on substrate preference, MMPs are grouped into collagenases, gelatinases, stromelysins, and matrilysins, as the most predominant classes. In chronic wounds, the overexpression of proteolytic enzymes can perturb the exquisite balance favoring degradation over remodeling processes.[69]

Trengove et al compared the protease activity in a number of wound types.[70] They sampled wound fluids from patients after surgery (mastectomy) with those who have chronic wounds, including mixed vessel disease, diabetic ulcers, and pressure ulcers. The mean protease level in chronic wound fluid was almost 60 times higher than those in acute wounds (59.9 µg MMP Eq/mL versus 0.75 µg MMP Eq/mL; $P < 0.001$). The levels of protease observed in chronic wound fluid may account for a relatively high degradation (mean 28.1%) of epidermal growth factor compared to acute samples (mean 0.6%, $P < 0.001$). More importantly, of all the subjects who were diagnosed with venous leg ulcers, the protease levels were rectified and drastically reduced by 49% ($P < 0.01$) following 2 weeks of hospital treatment. Overall, the analyses of chronic wound fluid revealed that nonhealing wounds have a low level of mitogenic activity, a high concentration of cytokines (e.g., TNF-α, IL-1),[21] high levels of proteases, and low levels of protease inhibitors.[71]

Silver has been shown to have anti-inflammatory properties. In a randomized controlled trial,[61] 619 chronic wound patients received either a silver foam dressing or the dressing considered to be the local best practice. The amount of wound fluid is an indirect measure of underlying tissue inflammation. All patients exhibited moderate exudate level at inclusion. After 4 weeks of treatment, patients with the silver dressing demonstrated significant reduction of wound fluid ($P = 0.0055$).

Serial biopsies were performed in a study of stalled venous ulcers (12 evaluable patients over 12 weeks).[72] The biopsy samples were analyzed for quantitative microbiology and histology. The results demonstrated a selective anti-inflammatory action of a high-releasing silver dressing with a decrease in neutrophils related to a decrease in *S. aureus* counts. The silver demonstrated a selective anti-inflammatory effect with increased lymphocytes related to faster healing. The venous ulcers in this study were 94% smaller over the 12 weeks, and 4 ulcers completely healed in about 9 weeks.

Summary

The wound bed preparation paradigm is an organized approach to the diagnosis and treatment of a person with a chronic wound. It is always important to treat the cause and address patient-centered concerns, including incorporating new topical approaches to wound-related pain.

This paradigm is altered when a chronic wound is not healable or is considered to be a maintenance wound. In this situation conservative débridement is combined with moisture and bacterial reduction that can be facilitated with the use of antiseptic agents, especially povidone-iodine and chlorhexidine derivatives (PHMB).

For healable wounds, topical treatments are available for débridement, surface increased bacterial burden, persistent inflammation, moisture balance, and stalled chronic wounds (the last two are discussed in other chapters). Topical débridement options include enzymatic agents and the autolytic débriding properties of calcium alginates, hydrogels, hydrocolloids, and adhesive films. Increased bacterial burden in the surface compartment of a chronic wound needs to be distinguished from the deep and surrounding skin infection that requires systemic antimicrobial agents. We have introduced the NERDS and STONEES mnemonic to help health-care providers make this clinical decision. For surface increased bacterial burden, there are a number of silver dressings available with differing concentrations of released ionized silver combined with different moisture-balance components; these need to be matched to wound characteristics. Topical antibiotics are less desirable in many clinical situations because they do not provide moisture balance, may induce allergies, and commonly induce bacterial resistance. We also realize that chronic wounds may be stalled in the inflammatory stage, and there are a number of anti-inflammatory agents, including silver, that can be used topically. The clinician has a toolkit of several topical agents, as seen in the tables in this chapter, which are designed to facilitate informed clinical decision making to optimize patient outcomes.

References

1. Tallman, P, Muscarc, E, Carson, WH, et al: Initial rate of healing predicts complete healing of venous ulcers. Arch Dermatol 1997; 133:1231–1234.
2. Margolis, DJ, Allen-Taylor, L, Hoffstad, O, et al: The accuracy of venous leg ulcer prognostic models in wound care systems. Wound Repair Regen 2004; 12:163–168.
3. Sibbald, RG, Williamson, D, Orsted, HL, et al: Preparing the wound bed: Debridement, bacterial balance, and moisture balance. Ostomy Wound Manage 2000; 46:14–35.
4. Sibbald, RG, Orsted, H, Schultz, GS, et al: International Wound Bed Preparation Advisory Board. Canadian Chronic Wound Advisory Board. Preparing the wound bed 2003: Focus on infection and inflammation. Ostomy Wound Manage 2003; 49:23–51.
5. Sibbald, RG, Orsted, HL, Coutts, PM, et al: Best practice recommendations for preparing the wound bed: Update 2006. Adv Skin Wound Care 2007; 20:390–405.
6. Banwell, H: What is the evidence for tissue regeneration impairment when using a formulation of PVP-I antiseptic on open wounds? Dermatology 2006; 212(Suppl):66–76.
7. Balin, AK, Pratt, L: Dilute povidone-iodine solutions inhibit human skin fibroblast growth. Dermatol Surg 2002; 28:210–214.
8. Fumal, I, Braham, C, Paquet, P, et al: The beneficial toxicity paradox of antimicrobials in leg ulcer healing impaired by a polymicrobial flora: A proof-of-concept study. Dermatology 2002; 204(suppl):70–74.
9. Woo, K, Etemadi, P, Coelho, S, et al: The use of Betadine in nonhealing wounds. Poster presentation at: European Wound Management Association, Glasgow, UK, 2007.
10. Gilbert, P, Das, JR, Jones, MV, et al: Assessment of resistance towards biocides following the attachment of micro-organisms to, and growth on, surfaces. J Appl Microbiol 2001; 91:248–254.
11. Motta, GJ, Milne, CT, Corbett, LQ: Impact of antimicrobial gauze on bacterial colonies in wounds that require packing. Ostomy Wound Manage 2004; 50:48–62
12. Werthen, M, Davoudi, M, Sonesson A, et al: *Pseudomonas aeruginosa*-induced infection and degradation of human wound fluid and skin proteins ex vivo are eradicated by a synthetic cationic polymer. J Antimicrob Chemother 2004; 54:772–779.
13. Mulder, GD: Polyhexamethylene biguanide (PHMB): An addendum to current topical antimicrobials. Wounds 2007; 19:173–182.
14. Wright, JB, Lam, K, Olson, ME, et al: Is antimicrobial efficacy sufficient? A question concerning the benefits of new dressings. Wounds 2003; 15:133–142.
15. Vermeulen, H, Ubbink, DT, Goossens, A, et al: Systematic review of dressings and topical agents for surgical wounds healing by secondary intention. Br J Surg 2005; 92:665–672.
16. Meyer, LJM: Randomized comparative study of Cutinova cavity dressing for the treatment of secondary healing wounds after abdominal surgery and abscess cavities in comparison with traditional therapy. The Cochrane Central Register of Controlled Trials. In: The Cochrane Library, Issue 1. Chichester, UK, John Wiley, 2003.
17. Guillotreau, J, Andre, J, Flandrin, P, et al: Calcium alginate and povidone iodine packs in the management of infected post operative wounds: Results of a randomized study. Br J Surg 1996; 83:861.
18. Cannavo, M, Fairbrother, G, Owen, D, et al: A comparison of dressings in the management of surgical abdominal wounds. J Wound Care 1998; 7:57–62

19. Viciano, V, Castera, JF, Medrano, J, et al: Effect of hydrocolloid dressings on healing by second intention after excision of pilonidal sinus. Eur J. Surg 2000; 166;229–232.
20. Meaume, S, Van de Looverbosch, D, Heyman, H, et al: A study to compare a new self adherent soft silicone dressing with a self adherent polymer dressing in stage II pressure ulcers. Ostomy Wound Manage 2003; 49(9):44–51.
21. Viamontes, L, Temple, D, Wytall, D, et al: An evaluation of an adhesive hydrocellular foam dressing and a self-adherent soft silicone foam dressing in a nursing home setting. Ostomy Wound Manage 2003; 49:48–52.
22. Gleaves, JR, Eldridge, K: Silicone sheeting as an alternative to elastic bandages in dressing lower extremity amputations. Ostomy Wound Manage 2004; 50:8, 10.
23. White, R: The benefits of honey in wound management. Nurs Stand 2005; 20:57–64.
24. Sibbald, RG, Coutts, P, Fierheller, M, et al: A pilot (real-life) randomised clinical evaluation of a pain-relieving foam dressing: (ibuprofen-foam versus local best practice). Int Wound J 2007; 4(suppl):16–23
25. Gottrup, F, Jorgensen, B, Karlsmark, T, et al: Less pain with Biatain-Ibu: Initial findings from a randomised, controlled, double-blind clinical investigation on painful venous leg ulcers. Int Wound J 2007; 4(suppl):24–34.
26. Briggs, M, Nelson, EA: Topical agents or dressings for pain in venous leg ulcers. Cochrane Database Syst Rev 2003; 1:CD001177.
27. Landis, S, Ryan, S, Woo, K, et al: Infections in chronic wounds. In: D Krasner, G Rodeheaver, RG Sibbald (Ed.), Chronic Wound Care: A Clinical Source Book for Healthcare Professionals, ed 4. Malvern, PA, HMP Communications, 2007, pp 299– 321.
28. Bergan, JJ, Schmid-Schonbein, GW, Smith, PD, et al: Chronic venous disease. N Engl J Med 2006; 355:488–498.
29. Medina, A, Scott, PG, Gahary, A, et al: Pathophysiology of chronic nonhealing wounds. J Burn Care Rehab 2005; 26:306–319.
30. Brem, H, Sheehan, P, Rosenberg, H, et al: Evidence-based protocol for diabetic foot ulcers. J Plast Reconstr Surg 2006; 117:193S–209S.
31. Weir, D, Farley, KL: Relative delivery efficiency and convenience of spray and ointment formulations of papain/urea/chlorophyllin enzymatic wound therapies. J Wound Ostomy Continence Nurs 2006; 33:482–490.
32. Klasen, HJ: A review on the nonoperative removal of necrotic tissue from burn wounds. Burns 2006; 26:207–222.
33. Bott, R, Crissman J, Kollar, C, et al: A silicone-based controlled-release device for accelerated proteolytic débridement of wounds. Wound Repair Regen 2007; 15:227–235.
34. Falabella, AF: Débridement and wound bed preparation. Dermatol Ther 2006; 19:317–325.
35. Glasser, ST: A new treatment for sloughing wounds: A preliminary report. Am J Surg 1940; 50:320.
36. McCallon, S: Enzymes for wound healing and débridement. Extended Care Product News 2007; 120:30–35.
37. Brett, DW: Chlorophyllin-A healer? A hypothesis for its activity. Wounds 2005; 17:190–195.
38. Zacur, H, Kirsner, RS: Débridement: Rationale and therapeutic options. Wounds 2002; 14:2s–6s.
39. Hebda, PA, Lo, CY: The effects of active ingredients of standard debriding agents—papain and collagenase—on digestion of native and denatured collagenous substrates, fibrin, and elastin. Wounds 2001; 13:190–194.

40. Alvarez, OM, Fernandez-Obregon, A, Rogers, RS, et al: A prospective randomized comparative study of collagenase and papain-urea for pressure ulcer debridement. Wounds 2002; 14:293–301.

41. Klaue, P, Dilbert, G, Hinke, G: Tierexperimentelle Untersuchungen zur enzymatischen Lokalbehandlung subdermaler Verbrennungen mit Bromelain. Therapiewoche 1979; 29:796–799.

42. Peter, FW, Li-Peuser, H, Vogt, PM: The effect of wound ointments on tissue microcirculation and leucocyte behaviour. Clin Exp Dermatol 2002; 27:51–55.

43. Fischer, H, Gilliet, F, Hornemann, M, et al: Enzymatic debridement in venous ulcus cruris. Report of a multicenter clinical comparative study with various enzyme preparations. Fortischr Med. 1984; 102:293–293.

44. Pullen, R, Popp, R, Volkers, P, et al: Prospective randomized, double-blind study of the wound-debriding effects of collagenase and fibrinolysin/deoxyribonuclease in pressure ulcers. Age Ageing 2002; 31:126–130.

45. Falabella, AF, Carson, P, Eaglstein, WH, et al: The safety and efficacy of a proteolytic ointment in the treatment of chronic ulcers of the lower extremity. J Am Acad Dermatol 1998; 39(Pt1):737–740.

46. Konig, M, Vanscheidt, W, Augustin, M, et al: Enzymatic versus autolytic debridement of chronic leg ulcers: A prospective randomised trial. J Wound Care 2005; 14:320–323.

47. Steenvoorde, P, Budding, T, Oskam, J: Determining pain levels in patients treated with maggot debridement therapy [erratum J Wound Care 2006; 15(2):71]. J Wound Care 2005; 14:485–488.

48. Kitching, M: Patients' perceptions and experiences of larval therapy. J Wound Care 2004; 13:25–29.

49. Attinger, CE, Janis, JE, Steinberg, J, et al: Clinical approach to wounds: Debridement and wound bed preparation including the use of dressings and wound-healing adjuvants. Plast Reconstr Surg 2006; 117(suppl):72S–109S.

50. Gibbins, B: The antimicrobial benefits of silver and the relevance of microlattice technology. Ostomy Wound Manage 2003; 49:4–7.

51. Sibbald, RG, Woo, K, Ayello, EA: Increased bacterial burden and infection: The story of NERDS and STONES. Adv Skin Wound Care 2006; 19:447–461.

52. Cutting, KF, Harding, KG: Criteria for identifying wound infection. J Wound Care 1994; 3:198–201.

53. Gardner, SE, Frantz, RA, Doebbeling, BN: The validity of the clinical signs and symptoms used to identify localized chronic wound infection. Wound Repair Regen 2001; 9:178–186.

54. Grayson, ML, Gibbons, GW, Balogh, K, et al: Probing to bone in infected pedal ulcers. A clinical sign of underlying osteomyelitis in diabetic patients. JAMA 1995; 273:721–723.

55. Nelson, EA, O'Meara, S, Craig, D, et al: A series of systematic reviews to inform a decision analysis for sampling and treating infected diabetic foot ulcers. Health Tech Assess 2006; 10:iii–iv, ix–x, 1–221.

56. Woo, K, Alavi, A, Botros, M, et al: A transprofessional comprehensive assessment model for persons with lower extremity leg and foot ulcers. Wound Care Canada 2007; 5(suppl):s34–s47

57. Woo, KY, Sibbald, RG: A Cross-sectional validation study of using NERDS and STONEES to assess bacterial burden. Ostomy Wound Manage 2009; 55(8):40–48.

58. Woo, KY, Ayello, EA, Sibbald, RG: SILVER(c) versus other antimicrobial dressings: best practices! Surg Technol Int 2008; 17:50–71.

59. Castellano, JJ, Shafii, SM, Ko, F, et al: Comparative evaluation of silver-containing antimicrobial dressings and drugs. Int Wound J 2007; 4(2):114–122.

60. Jorgensen, B, Price, P, Andersen, KE, et al: The silver-releasing foam dressing, Contreet foam, promotes faster healing of critically colonised venous leg ulcers: A randomised, controlled trial. Int Wound J 2005; 2:64–73.

61. Munter, KC, Beele, H, Russell, L, et al: Effect of a sustained silver-releasing dressing on ulcers with delayed healing: The CONTOP study. J Wound Care 2006; 15:199–206.

62. Vermeulen, H, van Hattem, JM, Storm-Versloot, MN, et al: Topical silver for treating infected wounds. Cochrane Database of Sys Rev 2007; 1:CD005486.

63. Bergin, SM, Wraight, P: Silver based wound dressings and topical agents for treating diabetic foot ulcers. Cochrane Database of Syst Rev 2006; 1:CD005082.

64. Chambers, H, Dumville, JC, Cullum, N: Silver treatments for leg ulcers: A systematic review. Wound Repair Regen. 2007; 15:165–173.

65. Leyden, JJ, Bartelt, NM: Comparison of topical antibiotic ointments, a wound protectant, and antiseptics for the treatment of human blister wounds contaminated with Staphylococcus aureus. J Fam Pract 1987; 24:601–604.

66. Lusby, PE, Coombes, A, Wilkinson, JM: Honey: A potent agent for wound healing? J Wound Ostomy Continence Nurs 2002; 29:295–300.

67. George, NM, Cutting, KF: Antibacterial honey (medihoney): In vitro activity against clinical isolates of MRSA, VRE, and other multiresistant gram-negative organisms including *Pseudomonas aeruginosa*. Wounds 2007; 19:231–236.

68. Molan, PC: The evidence supporting the use of honey as a wound dressing. Lower Ext Wounds 2006; 5:40–44.

69. Hanson, D, Langemo, D, Thompson, P, et al: Understanding wound fluid and the phases of healing. Adv Skin Wound Care 2005; 18:360–362.

70. Trengove, NJ, Stacey, MC, MacAuley, S, et al: Analysis of the acute and chronic wound environments: The role of proteases and their inhibitors. Wound Repair Regen 1999; 7:442–452.

71. Menke, NB, Ward, KR, Witten, TM, et al: Impaired wound healing. Clin Dermatol 2007; 25:19–25.

72. Sibbald, RG, Contreras-Ruiz, J, Coutts, P, et al: Bacteriology, inflammation, and healing: A study of nanocrystalline silver dressings in chronic venous leg ulcers. Adv Skin Wound Care 2007; 20:549–558.

chapter *14*

Diabetic Foot Ulcerations

Edward Mahoney, MSPT, DPT, CWS

Introduction

There are an estimated 23.6 million people in the United States with diabetes, which is roughly 7.8% of the population.[1] Although comprising less than 8% of the total population, people with diabetes account for more than 60% of nontraumatic lower limb amputations. In the year 2004, approximately 71,000 nontraumatic lower-limb amputations were performed in people with diabetes.[2] The total annual economic cost of diabetes in 2004 was estimated to be $174 billion dollars.[1] One of the major complications of diabetes is lower extremity amputation, which is often preceded by ulcer formation. It can be difficult to identify the cause of complications because there are so many factors that play a role in the development of foot problems. As the number of people diagnosed with diabetes and the number of foot complications associated with it continues to rise, it is becoming even more important to develop an understanding of the factors leading to ulceration and, ultimately, strategies to correct them.

This chapter reviews the management of diabetic foot ulceration. The etiology of diabetic foot complications and the evaluation and management of the diabetic foot are discussed. Treatment focuses on prevention of complications and managing complications that do occur.

Sensory Neuropathy

In order to understand the development of diabetic foot ulceration, there must be a general understanding of the relationship between diabetes and neuropathy. Neuropathy associated with diabetes is referred to as polyneuropathy because it affects sensory, motor, and autonomic nerves. The nerve damage is typically symmetrical and starts with the feet, but it can also affect the hands. Neuropathy progresses from distal to proximal in what is referred to as a stocking and glove distribution. Sensory neuropathy is considered to be the leading cause of the development of diabetic foot ulcers.[3] A prospective study by Boyko and colleagues showed loss of protective sensation (LOPS) to be independently related to foot ulcer risk.[4] A person without sensation is at a much greater risk of developing an ulceration of the foot than a person with intact sensation. In some studies, LOPS was present in over 80% of diabetic patients with foot wounds.[5] The cause of neuropathy in diabetics appears to be multifactorial. The basis for these changes appears to be related to hyperglycemia. Increased blood sugars are thought to damage the nerve directly and cause indirect damage by decreasing blood flow to the nerves.[6] Evidence for nerve damage has been substantiated by nerve conduction studies that showed that diabetics had significantly more abnormalities than nondiabetics.[7]

Sensory Examination

There are several quick and easy ways to assess for protective sensation in the diabetic foot, including monofilament testing, tuning forks, and bioesthesiometers. These are discussed in detail in Chapter 7.

Motor Neuropathy

The second component of the peripheral nervous system that is affected by diabetes is the motor system. Atrophy of the intrinsic muscles of the foot is common in diabetes and is apparent on MRI during the subclinical phase of diabetic neuropathy.[8,9] The atrophy in the muscles has a strong correlation to measurements of peripheral nerve function, indicating that there is a link between muscle atrophy and diabetic neuropathy.[9] Problems associated with motor neuropathy include loss of strength, range of motion, and balance. These are evident in foot deformities such as pes cavus, claw toes, hammer toes, plantar-flexed rays, and hallux valgus, all of which are commonly encountered with diabetes. Denervation of the muscles of the foot has been linked to a loss in muscle mass and increased plantar pressures during walking.[10] Several studies have investigated the link between muscle atrophy and neuropathy. Anderson and associates examined the volume of foot intrinsic muscles using cross-sectional MRI images in diabetic patients with and without neuropathy and in nondiabetics. The group with neuropathy was found to have approximately half the muscle volume of the other two groups. Results showed no significant difference between the diabetics without neuropathy and the nondiabetics.[8] Evidence for intrinsic muscle atrophy is supported by Bus and colleagues, who also found neuropathic subjects to have less cross-sectional area of intrinsic muscles compared to a control group of nondiabetics.[11] This loss of muscle mass may affect strength of the intrinsic musculature of the foot, which can lead to muscle imbalances between antagonistic pairs of muscle groups.[12] One of the most common examples is the imbalance between the toe flexors and extensors, leading to claw toe deformity. Claw toe deformity involves flexion of

the proximal interphalangeal (PIP) joint and flexion of the distal interphalangeal joint (DIP). (Fig. 14.1)

The imbalance between the flexors and extensors contributes to the pes cavus (high arch) deformity. In the normal foot, the metatarsal fat pad cushions the metatarsal heads from excess pressure. When the toe flexors are overpowered by toe extensors, this fat pad is pulled distally into the sulcus of the toes. In this position, the metatarsal heads are unprotected and have more pressure on them during weight-bearing because the force is no longer dissipated through the fat pad.[13] Ultimately, ulceration may result due to high pressure in spots that are not anatomically suited to bear weight. Common areas of breakdown include the dorsum of the PIP joint and the distal aspect of the distal phalanx beneath the toenail.[13] Similar problems with weight-bearing on intolerant areas develop with hammer toes—PIP flexion and DIP extension—and with mallet toes—PIP extension and DIP flexion. These areas can quickly develop a callus, which can lead to ulceration if not addressed.

> ▷ **PEARL 14•1** The displacement of the fat pad distally can often be reduced by applying pressure just proximal to the metatarsal heads. This causes the fat pads to realign over the metatarsal heads and reduces claw toe deformities. If the fat pads can be moved, a metatarsal bar may be beneficial in the patient's footwear.

The majority of diabetic lower extremity ulcers occur in the forefoot.[14] During the normal biomechanics of gait, approximately 50% of the body weight is transferred through the first ray during late stance phase, and 50% is dispersed through the other four rays. Any alteration in the normal biomechanics of gait will change the force distribution in the foot. As either higher amounts of force or similar amounts of force for longer durations are imposed on the tissues, the risk of tissue damage increases. A loss of muscle mass will have similar effects to the displacement of the fat pad previously mentioned. It will result in less cushioning between the metatarsal heads and the ground. Although the total area for weight bearing decreases, the same amount of

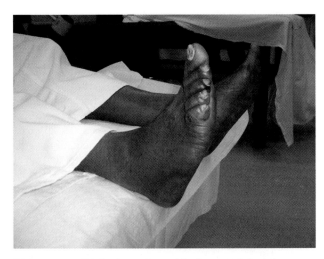

Figure 14•1 *Diabetic patient with claw toe deformity.*

force is still present and results in a higher pressure on any given area. This increased pressure is a major causative factor in the development of any neuropathic wound. In addition to changes in the amount of muscle mass, there are structural changes associated with diabetes that serve to increase the risk for ulceration. Among these changes are an increase in forefoot-to-rear foot pressure ratios and a decrease in dorsiflexion range of motion.[10,15] A loss of dorsiflexion has been associated with increased forefoot pressures and a weight shift toward the first metatarsal and the hallux.[16,17] Other impairments in joint mobility such as hallux limitus, hallux valgus, and Charcot arthropathy (discussed later in this chapter) also increase the risk of ulceration in the neuropathic foot.

Motor Examination

The clinical examination of the motor changes associated with neuropathy can be divided into three basic sections: muscle-strength testing, range-of-motion testing, and identification of deformities. As previously discussed, muscle weakness places the foot at a higher risk for foot ulceration by altering the normal stresses placed on the foot. It is important to palpate the metatarsal heads to assess for elevated skin temperatures, callus buildup, or displacement of the fat pad distally because all are risk factors for future ulceration. Strength of both the extrinsic and intrinsic musculature of the foot and ankle should be assessed during the examination.

Limitations in range of motion for the foot and ankle are often apparent with diabetes. Assuming the hip and knee are able to move through the full range, the ankle needs to range from at least 25 degrees of plantarflexion to 7 degrees of dorsiflexion for a normal gait pattern.[18] If the foot is unable to dorsiflex, it becomes a rigid lever during the push-off phase of the gait cycle. This will cause an increase in pressure and thus an increased likelihood of ulceration at the forefoot. Pressure can be exacerbated with ankle deformities such as overpronation, which has been linked to hallux ulceration.[19] In the foot itself, a limitation in first metatarsophalangeal extension, known as hallux limitus, also serves to increase the pressure and risk of ulceration on the first toe during gait. Hallux range of motion has been shown to be significantly reduced in diabetic patients with a history of a hallux ulcer.[19]

The physical exam must take note of any deformities or prominent areas, including bunions, hallux valgus, prominent metatarsal heads, or Charcot deformity. Combining any one of these deformities with insensate skin puts the patient at a much greater risk for ulceration. (Table 14.1)

Autonomic Neuropathy

The autonomic nervous system is a division of the peripheral nervous system consisting of sympathetic and parasympathetic subdivisions. In the foot, the autonomic system helps to regulate moisture balance, blood flow, skin integrity, and hair and nail growth. Impairments in the autonomic system are manifested in the diabetic foot as changes in the skin and nails, with dry, cracked, and fissured skin common in diabetes. (Fig. 14.2) One proposed reason for these abnormalities is a reduction in the skin lubrication performed by sebaceous and sweat glands. Sweat glands are known to atrophy in autonomic neuropathy.[20] The second mechanism for the development of dry skin relates

Table 14•1 High Risk Areas Associated with Selected Deformities	
Deformity	**Area at Risk for Ulceration**
Claw toes	Dorsum of toes, distal tip of toes, MTH
Hammer toes	Dorsum of toes, MTH
Mallet toes	Distal tip of toes
Excess pronation	Medial forefoot
Excess supination	Lateral forefoot
Hallux limitus	First MTH, great toe
Hallux valgus	Dorsal/medial first MTH
Charcot foot	Midfoot
Equinas foot	MTH and heels
Previous amputation	Adjacent weight-bearing areas

MTH, metatarsal head.

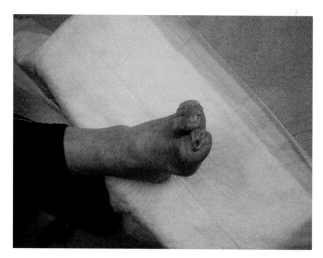

Figure 14•2 *Autonomic changes associated with diabetes.*

to the autonomic system's role in regulating blood flow. The sole of the foot contains arteriovenous shunts that are controlled by the autonomic system. With neuropathy, the blood is circulated away from the sole because the shunts remain dilated, drying out the skin on the plantar aspect of the foot.[20]

▶ **PEARL 14•2** Instruct patients with diabetes to lubricate their feet at least once a day. They should use creams that do not have an alcohol base and avoid applying lotion between the toes. Patients with diabetes should not soak their feet because this will only lead to further drying and cracking of skin.

Examination of the Skin

According to Aye and Masson, approximately 30% of patients with diabetes will have some form of dermatological problems related to diabetes.[20] Skin should be inspected for signs of cracking, redness, cuts or abrasions, maceration, callus buildup, and infection. In the nondiabetic foot, cracks and fissures are most common at the heel, but may be located anywhere on the diabetic foot. These are precursors to infection.[5,20] Special attention needs to be paid to the areas between the toes due to the risk of fungal infections. Thick callus buildup should be débrided to reduce pressure in that area and to assess for the presence of an ulcer underneath.[21]

Vascular Complications

Although neuropathy remains the primary causative factor leading to ulceration in the diabetic foot patient, whether that wound goes on to heal in a timely manner is greatly influenced by vascular status.[22] Diabetic patients with peripheral vascular disease have a significantly higher 5-year amputation rate following ulceration than do diabetics without peripheral vascular disease,[23] and they are at an increased risk of developing foot infections.[24] Ebskov and Josephsen reported that 18.8% of amputations due to diabetic gangrene required further amputation of the ipsilateral side within 4 years. Even more astounding, the risk of contralateral amputation within the first 4 years following a lower limb amputation due to diabetic gangrene was 44.3%.[25] Recent studies corroborate this data, finding peripheral vascular disease to be an independent risk factor for amputation.[23,24] Vascular involvement in diabetic patients with foot ulcerations is common and is usually diffuse in the lower limb. It is most severe in the arteries below the knee.[26]

An examination of the vascular system should be a routine part of every diabetic foot examination, whether or not the patient has an ulcer. This process is discussed in detail in Chapter 7.

Footwear Evaluation

A thorough diabetic foot examination must include an evaluation of footwear. Proper-fitting shoes are crucial due to the LOPS, foot deformities, and vascular compromise that are often associated with diabetes. It is best to check for proper shoe fit (Box 14.1) in weight-bearing and to check in the afternoon because of swelling that occurs throughout the day with prolonged upright positioning. The clinician must pay close attention to fit, especially if neuropathy is present, as that will

> **Box 14•1** **Proper Shoe Fit**

- The shape of the shoe conforms to the shape of the foot.
- There is a ⅜- to ½-inch space between the end of the shoe and the longest toe.
- The first metatarsophalangeal joint is at the widest part of the shoe.
- The toe box is deep and wide enough for toe spread and toe clearance.
- Laces or straps adjust for a snug fit over the instep.
- There is a snug fit around the heel.

limit the patient's ability to provide feedback as to comfort. A well-fitting shoe should provide support during the gait cycle and provide protection to the foot. If either of these conditions is not met, the potential for the shoe to cause ulceration will be present.

Local Factors Leading to Ulceration

Most diabetic foot ulcers are caused by some combination of sensory, motor, autonomic, or vascular problem. With the possible exception of vascular wounds, such as dry gangrene, most of these factors require an external stimulus to develop ulceration. For example, those with sensory loss do not automatically develop an ulcer; they develop an ulcer due to an excess amount of pressure that they are unable to feel. Local factors such as increased pressure are often precursors to the development of ulceration. Among the local factors commonly encountered are infection, improper foot care, improper footwear, the presence of previous injury sites, and the development of neuropathic fractures.

Infection

Diabetic patients are at a much higher risk of developing foot infections than are the general population.[24] Lavery and colleagues performed a longitudinal study on over 1600 diabetic patients enrolled in an outpatient clinic during a 2-year span. In that time span, people who developed a foot infection were over 55 times more likely to be hospitalized and more than 150 times more likely to have an amputation.[24] Hyperglycemia has proven to be a causative factor as seen by an increased number of infections in diabetics.[27,28] Hyperglycemia in diabetics may impair the body's ability to fight infection by reducing the effectiveness of the leukocytes.[27] With a normal immune response, there should be an elevated white blood cell count in addition to clinical signs of fever and chills. As Armstrong and coworkers reported, leukocyte values often remain within the normal range in diabetics because of their weakened immune response.[29] The lessened immune response limits the body's ability to fight the infecting pathogen and can quickly turn into a limb-threatening problem. This impaired response may also affect the clinician's ability to diagnose the presence of infection in the diabetic foot. Characteristic signs of infection including pain, fever, chills, and elevated white blood cell counts all may be blunted in diabetics.[30] Due to the subtlety of the signs of infection, a very thorough clinical examination must be performed to ensure that infection is not missed. Attention should be paid to the areas between the toes and any areas of dry, cracked skin, as they are ways for bacteria or fungi to enter the body. Of particular concern during the evaluation of a diabetic foot wound is the depth of the ulcer. As the ulcer gets progressively deeper and involves underlying structures, the risk of amputation increases. When infection is also present, the rate of amputation is higher than in deep noninfected ulcers and in superficial infections.[31]

Infecting pathogens in superficial diabetic foot ulcers tend to be primarily gram-positive aerobic bacteria. Deeper infections tend to be polymicrobial, may involve aerobic and anaerobic bacteria, and frequently have resistant strains of pathogens.[27,32]

One aspect of infection that is often overlooked is the role of fungus. The presence of fungal infections appears to be low compared to bacterial infections, but they do occur, especially in chronic ulcers.[33,34] The presence of fungal infections should be considered when a diabetic foot ulceration is in an unusual location, such as below the nail or between the toes. They should also be considered in wounds that are not healing despite proper antibiotic treatment and local wound care.[34]

Based on these studies that examined the relationship between depth and infection, and ultimately amputation, one of the most important aspects of the wound assessment is examining the depth of the wound. Treatment choices may be altered depending on wound depth regardless of the presence of other signs of infection. For example, a total contact cast would not be applied to a wound probing to bone due to the higher likelihood of infection. Ultimately, wounds may penetrate deep enough to cause an infection in the bone, or osteomyelitis.

Diagnosis of Osteomyelitis

Osteomyelitis, an inflammation of the bone caused by an infectious agent, usually bacteria, is present in up to two thirds of patients with severe limb-threatening infections and is a frequent cause of hospitalization for diabetics.[35] Most infections are confined to the soft tissue; however, many can progress to osteomyelitis. The gold standard for diagnosing osteomyelitis is a bone biopsy, which is expensive and may be impractical in some settings.[36] Aside from removing the bone to determine if osteomyelitis is present, diagnosing osteomyelitis can be difficult, as the infection may not be initially apparent radiographically during the first 2 weeks. Other imaging modalities have been used to diagnose osteomyelitis, including MRI, three-phase bone scans, and In-labeled leukocyte scanning, but these, too, are expensive and require a skilled professional to interpret the results.[36] Often, a simple probe-to-bone test is used clinically to diagnose osteomyelitis. The basis for this test is that if bone is open to the environment and can be probed with a sterile instrument, then bacteria can also reach the bone. A test is considered to be positive if the bone or periosteum is able to be palpated with a sterile probe.[37] This test is simple and time efficient to perform in the clinic. Several authors have studied the usefulness of the probe-to-bone test as a diagnostic tool for osteomyelitis. Lavery and associates performed a longitudinal cohort study comparing the accuracy of the probe-to-bone test to diagnose osteomyelitis in diabetic patients with bone cultures. The positive predictive value of the probe-to-bone test was found to be low and the negative predictive value to be high.[37] The results from Shone et al support these conclusions of a high negative-predictive value and a low positive-predictive value.[38]

These results suggest that a negative test—one in which the bone is not contacted—may be effective at excluding the diagnosis of osteomyelitis. A positive test—one in which the bone is able to be probed—does not necessarily mean that osteomyelitis is present. The positive predictive values for the two studies previously mentioned ranged from 53% to 62%, meaning a positive test only correlated with a diagnosis of osteomyelitis just over half the time. As a result, the diagnosis must be correlated with clinical examination and radiographic tests as indicated. Upon initial presentation, pain may not be evident due to the lack of pain fibers in cancellous bone and possible sensory neuropathy. Physical examination may be difficult because those with diabetes often have a blunted immune response and thus do not readily exhibit the clinical signs of infection. Examination should still test for signs of local infection and include a sensory and vascular examination, in addition to any blood work or tissue cultures being performed.

Once the diagnosis of osteomyelitis has been made, treatment should begin immediately. The course of treatment will depend upon the extent and duration of the infection. Treatment may include antibiotics, either intravenously or orally. In general, the course of antibiotic treatment will be longer than that of a soft tissue infection: a minimum of 6 weeks and usually up to 12 weeks.[39] When antibiotic therapy is ineffective and amputation is a better option, the goal should be to maintain as much of the foot as possible without compromising healing in order to maximize function.

Charcot Arthropathy

Charcot arthropathy is a relatively uncommon complication that can affect people with a variety of peripheral nerve diseases, including Hansen's disease, syphilis, alcohol abuse, and diabetes mellitus.[40-42] The combination of the dramatic rise in diabetes and the decrease in both Hansen's disease (formerly leprosy) and syphilis has resulted in the majority of Charcot neuroarthropathies occurring in diabetics. Rajbhandari and colleagues reported a prevalence of Charcot neuropathy in diabetics ranging between 0.1% and 0.4%, which is similar to that reported in other studies.[40,43] Although rare compared to complications such as peripheral neuropathy and vascular disease, Charcot deformities are important to understand as they have been identified as independent risk factors for the development of diabetic foot ulcers.[4]

The Charcot foot was first described by Jean-Martin Charcot in 1868. His initial theory was that the cause of the destructive process originated centrally. In this theory, damage to the autonomic nerves leads to an increased blood supply because the blood vessels remain dilated. This, in turn, leads to resorption of the bone by osteoclasts and leads to weakness and fractures.[40,44] Shapiro and colleagues investigated the effect of Charcot neuroarthropathy on vasomotion, which is a normal rhythmic contraction of the arteries of the dorsum of the foot. They found vasomotion to be impaired in diabetic neuropathy, but intact in healthy controls and in diabetics with Charcot arthropathy.[45] In addition, blood flow increased in response to increased temperatures in the control and Charcot group, but not in the neuropathy group. These findings, albeit in a small sample of individuals, indicate that a decrease in blood flow accompanying neuropathy may protect the foot from Charcot changes by preventing bone resorption.[45]

A second theory states that the development of the Charcot foot is caused by repeated traumatic events to the joint.[44] These traumatic events may have gone completely unnoticed by the patient at the time of injury due to the lack of sensation. As a result, the patient may not seek immediate attention and may continue to walk on the affected limb without relieving pressure. This constant pressure on an injured joint prolongs the inflammatory process. Gough and colleagues have previously established that the acute inflammatory phase stimulates bone resorption, which in turn can lead to fractures.[46] Most likely, it seems that the true cause of Charcot arthropathy is a combination of these two theories. One thing that both theories have in common is that they both start with a neuropathic joint.[41,44] People who are able to sense pain will alter their movement mechanics to reduce strain on the joint and thus allow the inflammatory phase to subside, whereas people with sensory loss will not. (Fig. 14.3)

A major factor in the healing potential of the acute Charcot foot is the duration between injury and the beginning of treatment, with better outcomes for those who are treated early.[40] This time is often prolonged because patients frequently do not seek immediate medical attention due to their lack of sensation. Even when patients do seek medical attention, the diagnosis of Charcot arthropathy is often missed, and the patient is begun on an ineffective treatment plan. In these cases, the patient may have already progressed to the point of deformity prior to initiating proper treatment. Refer to the case study as an example of how delayed diagnosis can impact the outcome of a Charcot foot.

Diagnosis of Charcot Arthropathy

As demonstrated in the case study, Charcot arthropathy may be misdiagnosed as cellulitis, osteomyelitis, or a variety of inflammatory diseases.[42] It would be prudent for the clinician to treat a swollen, warm, neuropathic foot that does not have an open wound as if it were a Charcot foot until it is diagnosed otherwise. If a wound is present, the diagnosis is complicated even further because of the increased likelihood of soft tissue infection or, in the case of exposed bone, osteomyelitis.[24]

> **PEARL 14•3** Any time there is pain in an insensate foot it should be a red flag for the practitioner. Pain in the insensate foot can be considered pathological until proven otherwise because it is often apparent with Charcot arthropathy or infection.

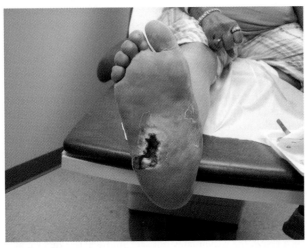

Figure 14•3 *Midfoot ulceration resulting from Charcot arthropathy.*

▶ **Case Study 14•1** Charcot Arthropathy Complicated by a Delayed Diagnosis

Mrs. W. is a 58-year-old Caucasian female who presented to the clinic with pain and swelling in the right foot and ankle for the past 2 weeks. Her past medical history was significant for type 2 diabetes mellitus for 13 years, hypertension, hypercholesterolemia, and osteoporosis. She also reported smoking "about a half pack" of cigarettes per day. Mrs. W. reported there was no known cause to her injury, as she didn't remember dropping anything on her foot or twisting it in any way. She stated she went to the local emergency room 10 days ago, where she had x-rays taken, and was diagnosed with a mild case of cellulitis. She has completed a course of antibiotic therapy, but reported that pain, redness, and swelling had not improved.

Upon physical examination, Mrs. W. was observed to be ambulating with an antalgic gait pattern, without an assistive device. The right foot was warm to the touch and had diffuse redness around the ankle and dorsum of the foot. She was unable to feel the 10-g monofilament during sensory testing in any of the testing locations on her feet. Both dorsalis pedis pulses could be palpated, but the right was much stronger than the left. Ankle joint mobility was impaired; it measured 2 degrees of passive dorsiflexion. Infrared temperature readings showed the right foot to be 6° to 8°F warmer than the left, with the largest difference being on the dorsum on the tarsal region.

In the case study, even if cellulitis was suspected, off-loading and immobilizing the joint could have been performed. If it had, there would have been less inflammation and, more importantly, the patient would not have been doing more damage walking on the unprotected joint over the past 10 days. Based on information presented by Chanteleu and Seabold and their respective colleagues, this cautious approach to management of the neuropathic foot may be justified due to the poor ability of radiographs to detect Charcot fractures in the early stage.[47,48] A diagnosis made solely on the basis of plain film radiography may not identify a Charcot fracture until it is more severe and harder to treat. MRI is much more sensitive in detecting early-stage Charcot changes.[40,47] It is also much more expensive and not as likely to be used to detect the presence of a subtle fracture, especially in a clinical setting. As a result, an early diagnosis, which leads to better functional outcomes, must incorporate a thorough history and physical examination in addition to radiographs.[40]

The clinical evaluation should begin with a thorough history focusing on past medical history, including duration of diabetes, presence of peripheral neuropathy, osteoporosis, and trauma to the foot, as all have been indicated as causative factors in the development of a Charcot fracture.[40,42,49] It is important to note that the subjective history of trauma may not be reliable due to the lack of sensation. Physical findings leading to the diagnosis of Charcot arthropathy may include loss of protective sensation, edema, erythema, increased local temperature, vascular abnormalities, and pain in the foot.[44,47] For information on sensory testing, refer to the Assessing the Sensory System section in Chapter 7. During an acute Charcot process, the local temperature will be elevated compared to the contralateral side. Qualitative assessment can be performed through palpation with the back of the hand, but a more accurate assessment can be obtained using an infrared thermometer.[50,51] (Fig. 14.4)

Medical infrared thermometers can display temperatures to the nearest 0.1°F or °C. They do not require contact with the skin and are an excellent option for producing quantitative data to assist in determining the appropriate intervention. Theoretically, assessing the local temperature will provide information regarding whether the tissue is being stressed. This idea was confirmed in studies conducted at the National Hansen's Disease Center.[52] To limit the variability in the temperature readings, patients should rest with both shoes off for 10 minutes prior to taking temperature readings. Readings are then recorded at the plantar aspects of the heel, midfoot, forefoot, and on the dorsum of the foot bilaterally. At present, there are no definitive guidelines to determine what constitutes a significant temperature difference between feet. This author considers an abnormal reading to be over 3°F difference. This value is consistent with the values reported by Armstrong and colleagues and others.[43,53] Temperature readings can also be used to monitor treatment progression and identify areas of concern before they are visually apparent.[53] Patients with Charcot fractures should remain partial weight-bearing in total contact casts (TCC) until the temperature readings have stabilized to within 3°F of the same area on the contralateral foot. It is important to note that a high temperature is not diagnostic for Charcot arthropathy; it indicates only that there is an inflammatory process occurring in that area.

The next clinical sign that is often apparent is a bounding pulse. This occurs as a result of blood vessels remaining dilated after a traumatic event due to autonomic neuropathy.[44] The implications for excessive blood flow, namely increased osteoclast activity, in the acute Charcot foot have been discussed previously in this chapter. Over time the bounding pulse will return to normal as the inflammatory process

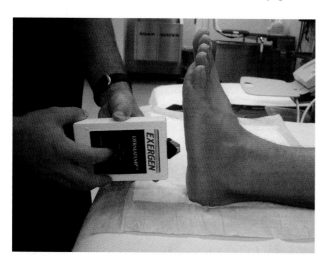

Figure 14•4 *Infrared thermometer for temperature assessment.*

subsides in the foot. Although the pulses should be assessed at each visit, it is more accurate to use infrared temperature readings to monitor the effectiveness of interventions because they offer quantitative data.[51]

Risk Reduction for Diabetic Foot Ulcerations

Ben Franklin said it best: "an ounce of prevention is worth a pound of cure." It is doubtful that he was referring to diabetic foot care, but it applies nonetheless. Key components of risk reduction include education, routine foot care, and fitting with proper footwear. For more information on education for prevention of diabetic foot ulceration, refer to Chapter 15.

Routine foot care and inspection require a multidisciplinary approach to address all the needs of the patient with diabetes. Many of the complications associated with diabetes, including retinopathy, nephropathy, and diabetic foot complications, have been linked to elevated blood glucose levels.[54] The American Diabetes Association recommends all diabetics have their hemoglobin A_{1c} tested a minimum of twice a year, with the target level of 7% or less, as increased glycosylated hemoglobin levels have been associated with diabetic complications.[54] In addition to proper medical management, every diabetic should have a foot exam at least once a year to help identify feet that are at risk for ulceration before problems arise.[54] Patients should be educated to remove their shoes and have their feet inspected at every doctor visit, whether they are there specifically for a foot examination or not. Each examination should consist of a visual and palpable examination for signs of sensory, motor, and autonomic neuropathy, along with a vascular assessment and footwear evaluation. Special attention should be given to areas between the toes to assess for maceration and signs of fungal infections as well as any cracks or fissures present, as they are routes of entry for pathogens.

Routine foot care should also be performed during these office visits. Callus and nail care should be performed because both can lead to ulceration if problems are left unchecked. Young and associates found a significant reduction in peak pressure reductions following callus removal in diabetic patients.[21] It is thought that the callus acts as a foreign body and thus increases the pressure in the affected area. Removing the callus would have the same effect on pressure relief as would removing a rock from the shoe. It is important to stress the risks of performing at-home surgery on calluses. Callus removal should be done by a trained professional with sterile equipment. Patients with sensory neuropathy, poor eyesight, reduced blood flow, or hypertrophic nails should not perform their own nail care either. Nail care can be done with nail clippers and rotary tools when nails are too hypertrophic to cut with standard nail clippers.

> ▸ **PEARL 14•4** The nails should be trimmed straight across and not rounded on the edge to prevent nails from growing into the skin. Nail and callus care should be performed frequently enough to prevent buildup that increases the risk for ulceration, either directly or by altering shoe fit.

In addition to proper foot care, a vital component to risk reduction is recommending and fitting protective footwear as indicated. Patients with mild deformities such as claw toes or previous toe amputations can be fitted with custom-molded orthotics and extra-depth shoes with a built-in rocker sole. Brodsky and colleagues compared the effectiveness of five common materials used for orthotics. They analyzed compression, combined shear-compression, and force distribution on soft-grade Plastazote® (Zotefoams, Croydon, UK), medium-grade Pelite® (Inoac Corp, Gifu, Japan), Spenco® (Spenco Medical Corp., Waco, TX), PPT® (Langer Inc., Deer Park, NY), and Sorbothane® (Sorbothane Inc., Kent, OH). All materials were compressed 10,000 times, and results showed the highest amount of compression in the Plastazote. Some rebound in the thickness of the material was noted in Plastazote and Pelite, but not in the other materials. Once the material had been stressed, it compressed faster in subsequent trials. During the shear-compression test, the Plastazote still had the greatest amount of compression out of the five materials tested, but it did not compress as much as it did in the compression test. The authors also pointed out that the shear-compression may be a more important variable to assess because it simulates walking, whereas compression in a perpendicular direction only simulates standing. On the other end of the spectrum, PPT did not compress at all under either condition. The third variable analyzed was force distribution. At low levels, there were not significant differences between the materials, but as the force was increased, Pelite was found to be most effective, followed by Plastazote, Spenco, PPT, and Sorbothane.[55] A benefit of the soft materials for the management of neuropathic feet is the moldability, which is not possible in a rigid orthosis. A soft material for the orthotic, such as Plastazote, may be effective in reducing pressure initially, but the trade-off for these softer materials is that they need to be inspected and replaced more frequently than do rigid orthotics. The perfect insert material would be durable and provide stability to the foot while reducing pressure. To achieve this, more than one type of material may be used to fabricate a multilayer orthotic. Many of the orthotics can be made relatively quickly in the clinic, which can be very important when trying to avoid problems transitioning from a more aggressive off-loading device to a diabetic shoe after ulcerations have closed. When orthotics are being fabricated to off-load healed ulceration sites, additional material may be used on the undersides of the orthotics to increase pressure relief. Placing the material on the underside of the orthotic reduces the risk of blisters and abnormal pressure gradients around the area being off-loaded by maintaining a smooth surface against the skin.

> **PEARL 14•5** Use lipstick to ensure that the materials are in the correct spot to off-load the area of concern. Place the orthotic in the shoe and use the lipstick to mark the closed ulcer site. Have the patient stand in the shoes and then remove them to ensure the imprint left on the orthotic is properly protected.

Once an orthotic has been fabricated, it must be fitted in an appropriate shoe to provide maximal benefit. Diabetic footwear has been shown to reduce pressure in the forefoot and rear of the foot and increase pressure in the middle part of the foot, which is beneficial since the majority of diabetic foot ulcers occur in the forefoot.[56] A therapeutic shoe should be made of materials that are firm enough to allow pressure distribution, but soft enough to prevent injury. The depth of the toe box must be sufficient to accommodate the insert and any deformity that may increase pressure on the dorsum of the foot, such as clawing of the toes. (Fig. 14.5)

Similarly, the material that comprises the top of the shoe is important. Traditionally, leather has been the material of choice because of its ability to adapt to the shape of the foot, but newer materials, such as Zennon™ (Dr. Zen Inc., Heathrow, FL), which is a spandex-like material, have become more common. Improperly fitted footwear has been implicated as the cause of 21% to 76% of ulcers or amputations.[57] Even if shoes are properly fitted, they are worthless unless the patient is compliant with wearing them at all times. In patients lacking protective sensation, compliance is often harder to enforce because they lack proprioceptive feedback and thus may not realize the benefit of proper-fitting shoes. Conflicting data exists concerning the effectiveness of diabetic footwear to prevent ulceration.[57] Chantelau and Uccioli, among others, have published evidence supporting the use of therapeutic footwear for ulcer prevention, showing a reduction in ulcer formation in those wearing therapeutic footwear compared to those without.[58,59] Hsi and associates reported decreased pressure on the forefoot and rear foot with a rocker bottom outsole and a molded foot orthosis during walking compared to the subject's normal footwear.[56] A review article by Cavanaugh points out that many of the studies showing no benefit to diabetic footwear are not standardized to ensure that all patients are wearing the same type of shoe, and some of the materials used to fabricate the shoes have also been questioned.[57]

The general consensus in the literature appears to be that therapeutic footwear with a rocker bottom is most effective in reducing forefoot pressure.[57,60,61] The rocker bottom shoe is designed to slow down the forefoot loading response during the gait cycle as the heel comes off the ground and the weight shifts forward. It has been shown to significantly reduce both pressure and shear forces over the metatarsals during gait.[62]

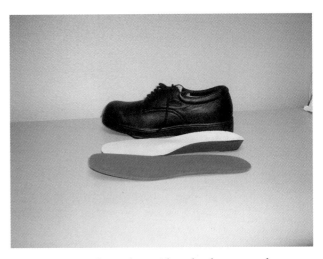

Figure 14•5 *Diabetic shoe with rocker bottom and removable insoles.*

The exact placement of the axis of the rocker bottom should be determined based on the area of the foot at highest risk for ulceration. Van Schie and colleagues found the most effective placement of the axis of the rocker bottom to be at 55% to 60% of the shoe length to reduce metatarsal head pressure. For the toes, the optimal position was found to be at 65% of the shoe length.[60] Nawoczenski and colleagues reported an axis at 50% of the shoe length to be most effective for off-loading the forefoot as a whole.[62] The traditional rocker bottom shoe has a built-up heel and midfoot, with a 30-degree upward angle of the forefoot of the shoe. This design was intended to prevent push-off from the forefoot during the terminal stance phase of gait. The point at which the forefoot of the shoe angles upward becomes the axis that the shoe rotates around during gait. The farther posterior this axis is placed the thicker the sole will be in order to prevent the forefoot from contacting the ground. In order for the rocker bottom to be effective, the sole of the shoe needs to be rigid. If it is not, the shoe will bend as the patient progresses through the gait cycle and will not effectively off-load the forefoot. The awkward appearance of the traditional rocker bottom shoe may be problematic because it may reduce patient compliance. Instead, lower-profile rocker shoes may provide a balance between function and style that will increase compliance and, ultimately, reduce the risk of ulceration. Diabetic shoes are now typically fabricated with a curved sole that is much less noticeable than the traditional rocker bottom shoe. As the patient walks, the shoe rolls forward on the rounded sole, slowly transferring the weight from the heel anteriorly, which gives the appearance of a more normal gait pattern.[62] Once the appropriate shoe and orthotic is fitted, the patient must be educated to check feet regularly for signs of pressure, and a wearing schedule should be set up to allow the foot to adjust to the orthotic.

Management of Diabetic Foot Ulcerations

To this point we have identified a multitude of factors that put the diabetic foot at risk for ulceration. These factors include sensory, motor, and autonomic neuropathy; vascular changes; infection; and repeated stress on at-risk tissue. Despite improved educational programs and the American Diabetes Association's recommendation that all diabetics receive an annual foot examination to identify high-risk feet, diabetic foot ulcers continue to be a major health-care problem.[1] A review by Crawford and associates reported an incidence of foot ulcers in diabetics ranging from 8% to 17%.[63] One of the most invaluable aspects of the management of diabetic foot ulcerations is proper education to reduce the chance of ulcer formation in the first place.

In the event that ulceration does occur, it must be determined whether it can be managed conservatively or if it will require a surgical intervention. Several wound care assessment tools exist to aid the clinician in making this determination. Among these are the Wagner grading system (Table 14.2) and the University of Texas Classification System for diabetic foot wounds.[31,64] The University of Texas Classification System stages diabetic foot wounds based on depth of the ulcer and

Table 14•2 Wagner Scale	
Grade	Description
0	Intact skin
1	Superficial ulcer
2	Deep ulcer
3	Deep, infected ulcer
4	Partial-foot gangrene
5	Full-foot gangrene

whether the wound is infected, ischemic, or both. This classification system is outlined in Chapter 6, (Table 6.14).

Wound assessment should consist of a vascular and sensory assessment of the foot, accurate measurements of the wound, including depth, and evaluation for the presence of signs of infection. If the wound is determined to be noninfected and nonischemic, treatment should initially focus on the removal of nonviable tissue through débridement.[65] Refer to Chapter 11 for further information on appropriate debridement strategies. In the diabetic foot, callus buildup has been shown to cause excess pressure and should be débrided from the wound.[21] Following appropriate débridement and cleansing of the wound, wounds should be dressed with sterile dressings that promote moist wound healing and do not reduce the effectiveness of off-loading devices. (Fig. 14.6)

Off-Loading Devices

The key component to addressing ulcers in weight-bearing areas is the removal of the stress that caused the ulcer. Just as a specialty bed may be used to alter the weight-bearing stress that caused a sacral ulcer, a variety of devices are used to minimize stress on the foot caused by walking. Off-loading methods range from cutouts that fit inside the patient's shoe to the total contact cast.

Total Contact Cast

The total contact cast was first used in the United States by Dr. Paul Brand to treat neuropathic foot wounds caused by leprosy (now Hansen's disease) and has become the gold standard for off-loading diabetic forefoot ulcers. The total contact cast differs from a cast fabricated for immobilization in that it is designed to conform to the shape of the leg to transmit weight through the cast. The toes are enclosed to prevent injury and to prevent any foreign objects from entering. The goal of the cast is pressure reduction, which can be accomplished by reducing the force being applied or by increasing the area over which the force is applied. The total contact cast has the advantage of doing both. The larger surface area of the cast during contact with the ground reduces pressure on any one location. Also, since the cast is designed to closely fit the contours of the leg, a percentage of the total body weight will be transferred to the cast and off the foot, thus reducing force on the wound.[66] The combined effects of these two mechanisms serve to make the cast an effective method of pressure

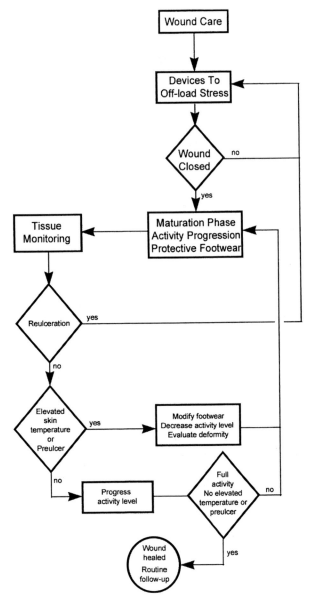

Figure 14•6 *Management of foot ulcerations.*

reduction for the foot. The initial total contact cast had minimal padding and did not have a relief area for the wound itself. Over time, the total contact cast has changed and is now typically applied with foam padding over the toes and the wound. Birke and colleagues reported similar pressure results in a true total contact cast and a padded cast.[67] In addition, areas that are susceptible to injury in the cast, including the malleoli, navicular, and tibial crest are padded with felt. The rest of the foot and leg should be padded with cotton cast padding to reduce the risk of ulceration.[68] Although some concern remains that creating a relief area in the cast by padding directly over the wound will lead to excessive pressures in the periwound, Petre and colleagues have found improved pressure relief by isolating the wound.[69] Clinically, the risk of breakdown can be reduced by beveling the edges of the padding to avoid large pressure gradients at the wound margin.

Total contact casts are effective in reducing pressure on forefoot ulcerations, but can also be dangerous if not used appropriately. Total contact casting should only be used on Wagner grade 1 or 2 ulcers. It should not be used in the presence of infection, arterial disease, deep wounds, or fluctuating edema.[68,70] Care must also be taken to avoid impingement of the peroneal nerve at the fibular head. The cast should be applied by a trained clinician due to the potential for ulceration if improperly applied. Prior to cast application, the wound must be evaluated to rule out any of the contraindications listed above. Cleanse and débride the wound as needed, and dress the wound with an appropriate dressing. It is important to consider the length of time the cast will be in place when choosing a dressing. Once the wound is dressed, separate the toes with lamb's wool to prevent maceration and apply a stockinet layer to the entire foot and leg, up to the knee, that fits snugly but does not compress the leg. Pad the leg and foot as previously described. When applying padding to the toes, end the padding at the toe sulcus rather than covering the metatarsal heads to increase the area of the foot that will be bearing weight. (Fig 14.7A) Next, apply a plaster layer to the foot and leg, usually two to three rolls, depending on the size of the leg, and cover with three rolls of fiberglass. (Fig 14.7B) Note that there is some evidence that using a fiberglass-only cast may reduce plantar pressure similarly to a traditional plaster total contact cast when compared in healthy subjects.[71] The benefit of an all-fiberglass cast is the faster drying time, which eliminates the need to maintain a non-weight-bearing status for the first day after the cast is applied. A drawback to the fiberglass method is that it is harder to achieve intimate contact with the foot than it is with the plaster cast. In either method, it is imperative to maintain the ankle at 90 degrees or even at slight dorsiflexion during the application of the cast. If the patient is casted in plantarflexion, initial contact during gait will occur at the forefoot and will lead to hyperextension at the knee. This can result in anterior tibial ulcers and damage to the knee joint. The easiest method to keep the ankle in neutral is to position the patient prone, with the knee flexed to 90 degrees while casting. This helps to ensure that tightness in the gastrocnemius does not prevent dorsiflexion. After the cast is applied, a rocker bottom or a cast shoe can be applied to the plantar surface of the cast to aid in gait (Fig 14.7C).

Patients should be instructed to avoid getting the cast wet and to notify the clinician at the first sign of increased odor, heavy drainage, discomfort, change in the fit of the cast, or excessive swelling above the cast. Strongly caution the patient to avoid cutting the cast off at home or sticking objects inside the cast if it is causing problems. The patient should be fitted with an assistive device such as crutches or a walker because the cast is intended to be partial weight-bearing.

Piaggesi and associates examined the histology of neuropathic foot wounds following casting. They found reduced inflammatory cells and higher amounts of fibroblasts present in neuropathic foot ulcers treated with a total contact cast for 20 days compared to a group that had not been casted.[72] The histological improvement helps to explain the link between pressure reduction caused by the cast, which

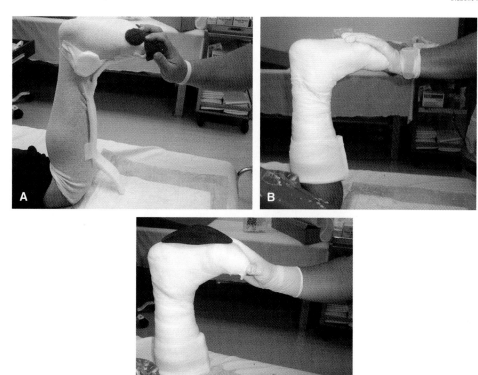

Figure 14•7 *Total contact cast. (A) Padding. (B) Plaster application. (C) Completed cast with rocker bottom.*

has been documented in numerous studies, and the promotion of wound healing.[66,67,72,73]

Walking Splints

Despite a general acceptance and a healthy amount of evidence to support the total contact cast as the gold standard for off-loading, it is not widely used. In cases for which the cast is contraindicated, a custom walking splint may be a viable alternative. The custom splint is fabricated in a manner similar to that of the total contact cast. As is true of the cast, an ulcer on the plantar aspect of the foot is off-loaded well with a splint due to the custom fit of the plaster and minimal padding. Both use stockinet as the contact layer and selectively pad high-risk areas to prevent skin breakdown. The splint is padded with foam at the wound site, toes, and the posterior heel. It is padded with felt at the malleoli, but does not require padding on the dorsum of the foot and the tibial crest, as they will not be covered by the splint. The leg is then lightly padded with a thin layer of cast padding. Once all padding is in place, the patient must be positioned in prone position, as during cast fabrication, to aid in dorsiflexion. Plaster strips are applied on the plantar aspect of the foot and posterior aspect of the leg. A compression wrap is then used to hold the splint on the leg. The splint may be preferred instead of a cast because it can be removed for wound inspection, cleansing, and dressing changes. The splint also has the advantage of being a viable option when infection or ischemia is present, as the wound is able to be seen and treated with antimicrobial dressings if needed. Pressure relief may not be quite as effective as it is in the cast because the walking splint does not fit as tightly to the leg and may allow shifting in the splint. This snug fit is thought to be useful in reducing pressure at the wound site.[74] In order for the splint to be effective, the patient must wear it at all times and use the appropriate assistive device. The fact that the splint can be removed by the patient at home may be detrimental to healing if it is removed and the patient bears weight without it in place. The idea of "forced compliance" in which the patient is off-loaded 100% of the time in the cast is not available with the splint. Another drawback to both the splint and total contact cast is that they require a skilled clinician and are somewhat time consuming to apply properly.

Prefabricated Cast Walkers

In response to the needs of clinicians for a time-saving, easy-to-use off-loading mechanism, several different types of prefabricated devices have been developed. These devices are more commonly used than casting or custom splinting because they do not require advanced skills and are faster to apply. Prefabricated removable cast walkers have proven to be effective in pressure reduction in numerous studies.[75-77] The walking boot with a rigid rocker bottom sole helps to promote a more natural gait pattern without shifting weight to the forefoot.[14] The fixed ankle also helps to reduce the amount of weight that is transferred to the forefoot during gait. Some of the walking boots, such as the Royce Active Walker® (Ossur North America, Aliso Viejo, CA), as shown in Figure 14.8, have modifiable inserts that can be adjusted to further reduce pressure on the wound.

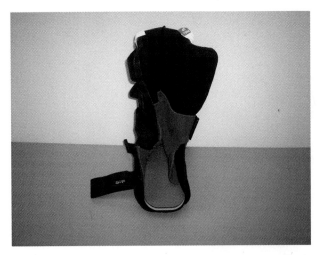

Figure 14•8 *Removable cast walker (Royce Active Walker).*

Lavery and coworkers found this boot to be the most effective of the cast walker boots and to be comparable to the total contact cast in off-loading.[76] The Royce Active Walker has a three-layer insole made of Poron® (Rogers Corporation, Rogers, CT), ethylene vinyl acetate, and another layer of Poron.[70] These layers are cut into removable hexagons that can be pulled out of the boot to create a relief area at any point on the foot. When the hexagons are removed to off-load a particular area, the edges should be beveled down to reduce the pressure gradient from the relief site and adjacent areas. It may also be helpful to fill in the hole created by removing the hexagon pegs with soft foam, such as Sifoam® (Knit-Rite Inc., Kansas City, KS). This helps to prolong the life of the boot by keeping the remaining pegs in place, and it also prevents the foot from bottoming out. Several studies have shown different brands of walking boots to be at least as effective as the cast for pressure relief.[70,76-79] There is also a large amount of evidence in the literature that identifies the cast as a superior method of healing wounds compared to removable walkers.[66,67,72,73,80,81]

Since the cast and removable walkers both have the ability to reduce pressure at the wound site and immobilize the foot, it has been suggested that the improved outcomes often seen with total contact casting may be related to the fact that it cannot be removed by the patient. A study by Katz and colleagues compared the effectiveness of a total contact cast to a removable cast walker that was made irremovable by wrapping fiberglass around it. In this study, 80% of the patients treated with the irremovable cast walker healed within 12 weeks, compared to 74% of the patients treated with a total contact cast, which was not a statistically significant difference between groups.[77] They also reported comparable rates of complications in both groups. A similar study by Armstrong and associates compared healing times for diabetic foot ulcers treated in a traditional removable cast walker and in a cast walker with a plaster bandage to prevent removal. Converting the cast walker to make it irremovable significantly reduced healing times compared to the removable walker group.[82] If an irremovable device is used to off-load the foot, the same contraindications for total contact casting should be considered because the foot cannot be examined between clinic visits. The cast walker, irremovable or not, may be a viable alternative to casting for neuropathic foot ulcers as long as a major deformity is not present. Casting may be preferred when a deformity is present, because accommodation of the deformity is limited in the rigid shell of the removable walker.

Other Off-Loading Devices

Many devices that are less cumbersome than a cast or walker that covers the entire lower leg have been developed for the treatment of foot ulcers. Regardless of the type of device used, the general principle of reducing pressure to promote wound healing remains the same. When choosing an appropriate device, the wound location, wound severity, patient compliance, and patient's ability to use the device safely must all be considered. A common device for off-loading the forefoot is the OrthoWedge® shoe by Darco (Darco International, Huntington, WV). (Fig. 14.9) It is designed with an elevated toe area, compared to the rear of the shoe, to shift weight posteriorly to the heel and midfoot.

Proper fitting of this shoe is critical for it to be effective. The OrthoWedge shoe is designed to off-load only from the metatarsals distally. With a proper fit, the area to be off-loaded should be distal to the portion of the sole that is in contact with the ground, and the toes should still be protected by the front of the shoe. An analysis of patients' gaits should be performed to ensure they are safe with balance and that they are taking small enough steps that the distal end of the shoe is not contacting the ground during the push-off phase of gait. Although there is a 10-mm thick, removable insole, the OrthoWedge shoe provides a relatively firm weight-bearing surface for the foot. The benefit of this rigid surface is that it limits the transfer of weight from the rear foot and midfoot to the forefoot during normal walking. A disadvantage is that there is very little pressure difference from the wound to other areas on the forefoot. Birke and colleagues addressed this issue and assessed the effectiveness of pressure relief at the great toe using a wedge shoe that was modified with a soft insert and relief area, a wedge shoe with a soft insert but no relief, and

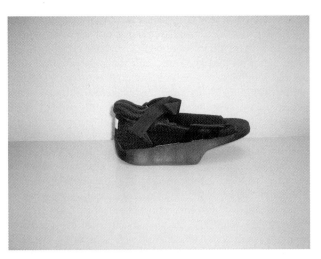

Figure 14•9 *OrthoWedge shoe (Darco).*

an unmodified wedge shoe. They found the OrthoWedge shoe with the soft insert and toe relief to be significantly more effective at reducing pressure on the toe than the wedge shoe with a soft insert, which in turn was more effective than the OrthoWedge alone.[83] The OrthoWedge shoe with the soft insert and toe relief is frequently used for forefoot ulcers that are on a prominent area resulting in excess weight-bearing compared to the surrounding tissue. It is a simple adjustment that provides an extra degree of off-loading at the intended site without sacrificing the rigidity of the OrthoWedge. Combining a wedge shoe with an adhesive felt foam dressing applied directly to the foot has also been shown to increase off-loading over a wedge shoe alone.[84]

Wedge shoes may be difficult to wear for patients with balance issues or for patients who have wounds bilaterally. Many patients wearing a wedge shoe for an extended period of time often report they have back discomfort due to the height difference between the affected and unaffected sides. In these cases, a shoe that is lower to the ground may be beneficial. One such shoe is the DH® shoe by Royce Medical Co. (Ossur North America, Aliso Viejo, CA). The sole of this shoe is the same as the removable cast walker discussed previously, with Velcro® (Velcro USA, Manchester, NH) pegs that can be removed to accommodate an ulcer. Unlike the cast walker, the shoe does not have a rigid shell to immobilize the ankle, nor does it have a rocker sole to reduce forefoot loading pressure. This shoe is generally tolerated well by people with balance issues or for those with bilateral ulcers. Additionally, the device can be used in conjunction with bulky dressings because the toe box is deep. Since the insole of the shoe has pegs along the entire surface, the DH shoe is not limited to treatment of forefoot problems as are the wedge shoes. Unlike the wedge shoe, the DH shoe has a flexible outer sole that permits weight transfer distally during gait. Although this facilitates a more normal gait pattern, it can put more pressure on a forefoot ulcer during the late stance phase of the gait cycle. As with the removable cast walkers, any of the shoe devices can be removed by the patients, which raises the concern of patient compliance. (Fig. 14.10)

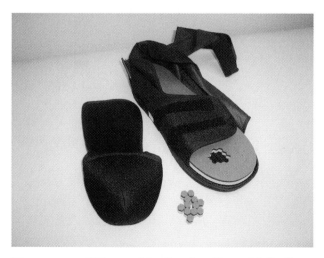

Figure 14•10 *DH wound-healing shoe (Royce Medical).*

A technique used to off-load an ulcer that is less cumbersome than a cast but not as easy to remove as a shoe is accommodative felt padding. Adhesive padding is applied directly to the periwound skin, with a cutout for the wound, and the patient is placed in a surgical shoe. Accommodative felt dressings have been shown to reduce peak pressure on ulcerated areas compared to walking barefoot. When the dressing is combined with a wedge shoe, the amount of pressure reduction was found to be superior to the wedge shoe alone.[84] Healing rates of accommodative felt padding were found to be comparable to total contact casting when ulcer width and location were accounted for.[85] The accommodative felt padding may be favorable in some instances due to the low cost compared to a prefabricated device and the ability of the practitioner to customize the padding based on ulcer location and size. The fact that the dressing is applied directly to the foot and always remains in place may be useful for a patient nonadherent to therapy for whom total contact casting is not appropriate.

Walking Strategies

Since it is not possible to cast someone forever, and the patient will inevitably walk barefoot at some point while being treated with removable devices, teaching effective walking strategies to reduce pressure on the forefoot may be helpful. A review article by Kwon and colleagues examined several different alterations to the normal gait pattern that have been attempted for pressure reduction.[86] One of the strategies used was a shuffling gait pattern designed to limit the transfer of forces to the forefoot by walking with the foot flat throughout the gait cycle. This pattern showed a drastic reduction in peak plantar pressures under the first and second metatarsals and the hallux compared to normal walking in patients without pathology.[87] Part of the reduction in force may be attributed to the shuffling pattern of gait, and part of the reduction may be due to the slower gait speed. Several authors have studied the relationship between gait speed and force on the forefoot. In patients with and without impairments, slower walking speeds were associated with smaller ground reaction forces when walking.[88-90] Another walking pattern that has been proposed involves training patients to decrease push-off from the ankle and increase hip flexion to pull the leg forward during gait. Mueller and colleagues based this idea on findings that this was a normal accommodation to diminished plantar flexor torque in diabetic patients. This pattern was tested on seven male patients with diabetes mellitus and peripheral neuropathy and showed a 27% reduction in forefoot peak plantar pressures.[91]

In most cases, an assistive device such as a cane, crutches, or walker should be used in addition to the off-loading device. When walking with crutches or a walker, it is possible to completely off-load the foot by walking without bearing weight. With a cane, pressure reduction has been shown to be greatest when it is used in the contralateral hand. Using a cane in the contralateral hand appears to reduce lateral forefoot pressure more than medial pressures.[92] The same study also reported increased pressures on the unaffected foot at the great toe and first metatarsal when using a cane. The potential for causing ulceration on the unaffected foot must be taken into account when determining the appropriate method for off-loading.

Permanent Footwear

The combination of appropriate off-loading, proper wound care, and a compliant patient results in closure for the majority of diabetic foot ulcers. Maintaining a closed wound often presents a major challenge as the patient transitions to higher activity levels and back to less restrictive footwear. There cannot be an interim period between use of the treatment device and fitting with permanent footwear during which the patient is walking on an unprotected foot. When shoes and orthotics are fabricated, the wearing schedule and the importance of checking feet regularly need to be discussed with the patient to reduce the risk of recurrent ulceration. The previous ulceration site is a major risk factor for a future ulcer, and the patient should therefore be fitted with permanent footwear as discussed previously.[54] In cases in which a severe deformity is present, custom-molded shoes, rather than custom inserts, may be required to accommodate the foot and reduce risk of future problems.

> **PEARL 14•6** Footwear that can be slipped on quickly may increase compliance when people awaken in the night to use the bathroom. Custom sandals can be fabricated in the clinic and can be a useful alternative to shoes for short walks in the house.

Management of Charcot Arthropathy

Managing Charcot arthropathy presents a unique set of challenges to the clinician. During an acute episode, foot instability and inflammation are both problematic. Initial treatment should focus on immobilizing the joint and reducing weight-bearing to halt the inflammatory process. The most common method for management involves total contact casting to immobilize and off-load the foot. Some controversy remains over whether bearing weight should be permitted on the cast during this stage.[93,94] Strictly prohibiting weight-bearing will obviously put less strain on the affected foot, but concern remains over putting excess stress on the unaffected limb as well as bone density changes associated with not bearing weight. Often, bedrest and no weight-bearing is extremely difficult, if not impossible, for patients to maintain for the extended amount of time required to heal a Charcot foot. As a result, total contact casting is the treatment of choice for an acute Charcot arthropathy because it reduces the load on the foot as well as immobilizes the joint. An additional benefit to the cast is the reduction of edema in the foot. When a patient presents with an acute Charcot foot, the edema is often drastic and may necessitate cast changes on a frequent basis until the edema has stabilized. The patient should be instructed to contact the clinician if the cast becomes too loose or is pistoning up and down. In addition to the risk of iatrogenic

ulcers from cast movement, a loose cast on a Charcot foot is problematic because it is not effectively immobilizing the joint and will not arrest the progression of deformity. If casting is used, casts are typically changed every 1 to 2 weeks until skin temperature has normalized compared to the contralateral side, edema is reduced, and radiographic evidence of healing is present. The literature reports duration of casting that is necessary before patients return to less restrictive footwear ranges from 8 to 12 weeks if nonweight-bearing, 18 weeks with partial weight-bearing, and up to 12 months for certain locations of Charcot fractures.[40,93,95-97] A successful course of therapy involving casting should result in a healed fracture with minimal deformity that will not prevent the patient from walking with protective footwear. At times, either due to severity of the fracture or a delay in treatment, deformity will result and may lead to ulceration, which may complicate healing.

An off-loading device used in the treatment of Charcot arthropathy is the Charcot restraint orthotic walker (CROW). (Fig. 14.11) This device is a bivalved device that fully

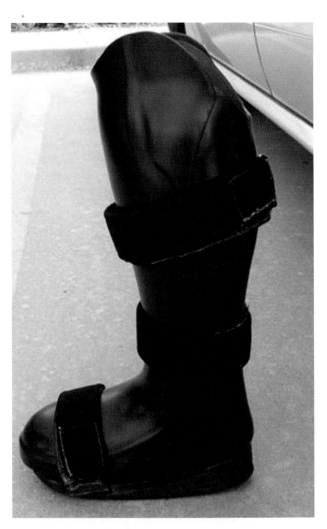

Figure 14•11 *Charcot restraint orthotic walker (CROW).*

encloses the foot and functions as a custom-fit ankle-foot orthosis. The outer shell is constructed of polypropylene and is rigid to lock the foot in neutral. The inner lining is constructed of molded foam plastic, and the plantar surface is a Plastazote insert layer. The CROW is held in place with several Velcro straps and provides a snug fit to the leg. The close fit helps to keep the edema in the foot and ankle under control. The outer sole of the boot is a rocker bottom to facilitate a more normal gait pattern with the immobile ankle. The CROW is often used after casting, which is used initially during the acute phase. Transition from a cast to a CROW or other removable cast walker should not take place until the temperature of the affected area and the corresponding area on the contralateral side are within 1°C for 2 consecutive weeks.[95] This transition is generally well accepted by patients, and they report increased satisfaction with the CROW compared to casting.[96] Benefits include the ability to take the boot off for bathing and sleeping and the ease of application and removal. The CROW can be used for extended periods of time before the patient returns to permanent footwear, with location of Charcot injury and patient compliance being major factors in determining the duration. Morgan and colleagues reported CROW usage in excess of 3 years after initial casting in several patients.[96] When temperatures have stabilized to within 1°C for 1 month with the use of the CROW, the patient can be transitioned to prescription footwear.[95] In cases of severe deformity that cannot be protected by prescription footwear, and when surgery is not a viable option, the CROW boot may be used as a permanent device. Generally, reconstructive surgery should be performed if a deformity places the foot at risk for ulceration or if it cannot be accommodated with conservative management. Refer to Chapter 24 for further information on surgical management of Charcot arthropathy.

Other conservative management strategies include pulsed electromagnetic fields, electrical stimulation, and pulsed, low-intensity ultrasound. The goal of these treatments is to stimulate bone formation at the fracture site. A review by Strauss and Gonya discussed several studies on both animals and humans supporting the use of ultrasound on nonhealing fractures. Ultrasound is thought to strain the fracture site and promote bone growth similar to the method proposed by Wolff's law, which states that bone will be generated in response to stress.[44] An abundance of studies examining the effect of modalities on bone healing exist, but few deal specifically with healing Charcot fractures. One study that did examine the effects of low-intensity ultrasound reported successful treatment in 28 out of 29 patients with Charcot arthropathy after previous treatments had failed.[98] Hanft and colleagues found shorter healing times in Charcot joints treated with combined magnetic field electrical bone stimulation and casting compared to casting alone.[99] A benefit of these bone-stimulating devices is that they can often be used concurrently with casting to immobilize the joint. It is important to keep in mind that these are adjuncts to therapy, and immobilization is of primary importance in healing a Charcot foot.

An additional aspect of treatment that is useful in the management of Charcot arthropathy is medical management of osteoporotic changes associated with both the Charcot process and the prolonged duration of limited weight-bearing during treatment. Bone, like any other tissue, will respond to stress placed upon it. When the stress is at an adequate level, it will cause bone to adapt by increasing its density. When bones are not being loaded, as in a cast, they begin to lose that density. Diabetics, as a group, are thought to be at an increased risk of low bone density due to impaired renal function.[50] During an acute Charcot process, dysfunction of the autonomic nerves leads to dilation of blood vessels and ultimately excessive bone resorption.[40] All of these factors combine to put a patient with a Charcot fracture at a high risk for complications related to bone mineral density. Potential complications include recurrent fractures when the patient attempts to transition back to walking and potential complications with internal fixation due to weak bone. Bisphosphonates inhibit osteoclastic bone resorption and are often used in the treatment of osteoporosis and Paget's disease. Two different studies examined the effectiveness of the bisphosphonate medication pamidronate (Novartis Pharmaceutical Corp., East Hanover, NJ) in the management of Charcot arthropathy. Both studies involved a single infusion of pamidronate and determined that it resulted in a significant decrease in bone resorption.[100,101] Both authors reported promising results with bisphosphonates related to reducing bone loss associated with Charcot fractures, but they pointed out that further studies were still needed to determine the true efficacy of the drug for this group of patients.

Summary

The effective management of patients with diabetic foot complications must begin with an understanding of the normal mechanics of the foot and any alterations that may be caused by diabetes. Effective treatment and prevention strategies depend upon thorough foot inspection by both the patient and the clinician to limit the severity of any complications that may develop. The combination of abnormal pressures and sensory loss predispose the diabetic foot to ulceration. Once ulceration is present, healing may be complicated by factors such as infection, continued ambulation on an insensate foot, or diminished blood flow, which is also related to diabetes. As a result, the most effective treatment may be proper education and preventative measures to ensure that ulceration does not occur. This chapter outlines the assessment of the diabetic foot, as well as strategies for prevention and treatment of ulcers that do occur.

Evaluation of the diabetic foot, including sensory, motor, and autonomic neuropathy, as well as evaluation of the vascular status and footwear, are discussed in this chapter. Prevention and treatment strategies, including off-loading techniques for active ulcers and appropriate footwear to prevent ulceration, are also discussed. Special consideration is also paid to Charcot arthropathy evaluation and management.

References

1. American Diabetes Association. American Diabetes Association home page. Available at: www.diabetes.org/diabetes-basics/diabetes-statistics. Accessed 11/11/09.
2. National Center for Chronic Disease Prevention and and Health Promotion. Diabetes Public Health Resource. National diabetes fact sheet 2005: General information and national estimates on diabetes in the United States. Available at: www.cdc.gov/diabetes/pubs/pdf/ndfs_2007.pdf. Accessed 11/11/09.
3. Steeper, RA: Critical review of the aetiology of diabetic neuropathic ulcers. J Wound Care 2005; 41:101–103.
4. Boyko, E, Ahroni, J, Stensel, V, et al: A prospective study of risk factors for diabetic foot ulcer: The Seattle diabetic foot study. Diabetes Care 1999; 22:1036–1042.
5. Armstrong, D, Lavery, L: Diabetic foot ulcers: Prevention, diagnosis, and classification. Am Fam Physician 1998; 57:1325–1332.
6. Park, T, Park, J, Baek, H: Can diabetic neuropathy be prevented? Diabetes Res Clin Pract 2004; 66:53–56.
7. Vinik, A, Kong, X, Megerian, J, et al: Diabetic nerve conduction abnormalities in the primary care setting. Diabetes Technol Ther 2006; 8:654–662.
8. Anderson, H, Gjerstad, M, Jakobsen, J: Atrophy of foot muscles: A measure of diabetic neuropathy. Diabetes Care 2004; 27:2382–2385.
9. Greenman, R, Khaodhiar, L, Lima, C, et al: Foot small muscle atrophy is present before the detection of clinical neuropathy. Diabetes Care 2005; 28:1425.
10. Mueller, M, Hastings, M, Commean, P, et al: Forefoot structural predictors of plantar pressures during walking in people with diabetes and peripheral neuropathy. J Biomech 2003; 36:1009–1017.
11. Bus, S, Yang, Q, Wang, J, et al: Intrinsic muscle atrophy and toe deformity in the diabetic neuropathic foot: A magnetic resonance imaging study. Diabetes Care 2002; 25:1444–1450.
12. van Schie, C, Vermigli, C, Carrington, A, et al: Muscle weakness and foot deformities in diabetes: Relationship to neuropathy and foot ulceration in Caucasian diabetic men. Diabetes Care 2004; 27:1668–1673.
13. Laing, P: The development and complications of diabetic foot ulcers. Am J Surg 1998; 176:11S–19S.
14. Reiber, G, Vileikyte, L, Boyko, E, et al: Causal pathways for incident lower-extremity ulcers in patients with diabetes from two settings. Diabetes Care 1999; 22:157–162.
15. Caselli, A, Pham, H, Giurini, J, et al: The forefoot-to-rearfoot plantar pressure ratio is increased in severe diabetic neuropathy and can predict foot ulcerations. Diabetes Care 2002; 25:1066–1071.
16. Mandato, M, Nester, G: The effect of increasing heel height on forefoot peak pressures. J Am Podiatr Med Assoc 1999; 89:75–80.
17. Zimny, S, Schatz, H, Pfohl, M: The role of limited joint mobility in diabetic patients with an at-risk foot. Diabetes Care 2004; 27:942–946.
18. Olney, S: Gait. In: Levangie, P, Norkin, C (eds): Joint Structure and Function: A Comprehensive Analysis, ed. 4. Philadelphia, FA Davis, 2005, p 527.
19. Nube, V, Molyneaux, L, Yue, D: Biomechanical risk factors associated with neuropathic ulceration of the hallux in people with diabetes mellitus. J Am Podiatr Med Assoc 2006; 96:189–197.
20. Aye, M, Masson, E: Dermatological care of the diabetic foot. Am J Clin Dermatol 2002; 3:463–474.
21. Young, M, Cavanagh, P, Thomas, G, et al: The effect of callus removal on dynamic plantar foot pressures in diabetic patients. Diabet Med 1992; 9:55–57.
22. Zimny, S, Schatz, H, Pfohl, M: Determinants and estimation of healing times in diabetic foot ulcers. J Diabetes Complications 2002; 16:327–332.
23. Moulik, P, Mtonga, R, Gill, G: Amputation and mortality in new-onset diabetic foot ulcers stratified by etiology. Diabetes Care 2003; 26:491–494.
24. Lavery, L, Armstrong, D, Wunderlich, R, et al: Risk factors for foot infections in individuals with diabetes. Diabetes Care 2006; 29:1288–1293.
25. Ebskov, B, Josephsen, P: Incidence of reamputation and death after gangrene of the lower extremity. Prosthet Orthot Int 1980; 4:77–80.
26. Graziani, L, Silvestro, A, Bertone, V, et al: Vascular involvement in diabetic subjects with ischemic foot ulcer: A new morphologic categorization of disease severity. Eur J Vasc Endovasc Surg 2007; 33:453–460.
27. Gallacher, S, Thomson, G, Fraser, W, et al: Neutrophil bactericidal function in diabetes mellitus: Evidence for association with blood glucose control. Diabet Med 1995; 12:916–920.
28. Joshi, N, Caputo, G, Weitekamp, M, et al: Infections in patients with diabetes mellitus. N Engl J Med 1999; 341:1906–1912.
29. Armstrong, D, Perales, T, Murff, R, et al: Value of white blood cell count with differential in the acute diabetic foot infection. J Am Podiatr Med Assoc 1996; 86:224–227.
30. Gleckman, R, Shakeri, M: Infection in the diabetic foot: What to look for and how to treat. Consultant 1997; 37:2396–2398.
31. Armstrong, D, Lavery, L, Harkless, L: Validation of a diabetic wound classification system: The contribution of depth, infection, and ischemia to risk of amputation. Diabetes Care 1998; 21:855–859.
32. Fung, H, Chang, J, Kuczynski, S: A practical guide to the treatment of complicated skin and soft tissue infections. Drugs 2003; 63:1459–1480.
33. Mlinaric Missoni, E, Vukelic, M, de Soy, D, et al: Fungal infections in diabetic foot ulcers [letter to the editor]. Diabetic Med 2005; 22:1124–1125.
34. Heald, A, O'Halloran, D, Richards, K, et al: Fungal infections of the diabetic foot: Two distinct syndromes. Diabetic Med 2001; 18:567–572.
35. Grayson, M: Diabetic foot infections—Antimicrobial therapy. Infect Dis Clin North Am 1995; 9:143–161.
36. Bonham, P: A critical review of the literature: Diagnosing osteomyelitis in patients with diabetes and foot ulcers. J Wound Ostomy Continence Nurs 2001; 28(Pt 1):73–88.
37. Lavery, L, Armstrong, D, Peters, E, et al: Probe-to-bone test for diagnosing diabetic foot osteomyelitis—reliable or relic? Diabetes Care 2007; 30:270–274.
38. Shone, A, Burnside, J, Chipchase, S, et al: Probing the validity of the probe-to bone test in the diagnosis of osteomyelitis of the foot in diabetes. Diabetes Care 2006; 29:945.
39. Bonham, P: A critical review of the literature: Antibiotic treatment of osteomyelitis in patients with diabetes and foot ulcers. J Wound Ostomy Continence Nurs 2001; 28(Pt 2):141–149.
40. Rajbhandari, S, Jenkins, R, Davies, C, et al: Charcot neuroarthropathy in diabetes mellitus. Diabetologia 2002; 45:1085–1096.
41. Chantelau, E, Onylee, G: Charcot foot in diabetes: Farewell to the neurotrophic theory. Horm Metab Res 2006; 38:361–367.
42. Slowman-Kovacs, S, Braunstein, E, Brandt, K: Rapidly progressive Charcot arthropathy following minor joint trauma in patients with diabetic neuropathy. Arthritis Rheum 1990; 33:412–417.
43. Fabrin, J, Larsen, K, Holstein, P: Long-term follow-up in diabetic Charcot feet with spontaneous onset. Diabetes Care 2000; 23:796–800.
44. Strauss, E, Gonya, G: Adjunct low intensity ultrasound in Charcot neuroarthropathy. Clin Orthop Relat Res 1998; 349:132–138.
45. Shapiro, S, Stansberry, K, Hill, M, et al: Normal blood flow response and vasomotion in the diabetic Charcot foot. J Diabetes Complications 1998; 12:147–153.
46. Gough, A, Abraha, H, Li, F, et al: Measurement of markers of osteoclast and osteoblast activity in patients with acute and chronic Charcot neuroarthropathy. Diabet Med 1997; 14:527–531.
47. Chantelau, E, Richter, A, Schmidt-Grigordiadis, P, et al: The diabetic Charcot foot: MRI discloses bone stress injury as trigger mechanism of neuroarthropathy. Exp Clin Endocrinol Diabetes 2006; 114:118–123.

48. Seabold, J, Flickinger, F, Kao, S: Indium-111-leukocyte/technetium-99m-MDP bone and magnetic resonance imaging: Difficulty of diagnosing osteomyelitis in patients with neuropathic osteoarthropathy. J Nucl Med 1990; 31:549–556.

49. Young, M, Marshall, A, Adams, J, et al: Osteopenia, neurological dsyfunction, and the development of Charcot neuroarthropathy. Diabetes Care 1995; 18:34–38.

50. Hastings, M, Sinacore, D, Fielder, F, et al: Bone mineral density during total contact cast immobilization for a patient with neuropathic (Charcot) arthropathy. Phys Ther 2005; 85:249–256.

51. Armstrong, D: Monitoring healing of acute Charcot's arthropathy with infrared dermal thermometry. J Rehabil Res Dev 1997; 34:317–321.

52. Beach, R, Thompson, D: Selected soft tissue research: An overview from Carville. Phys Ther 1979; 59:30–35.

53. Armstrong, D, Lavery, L, Liswood, P, et al: Infrared dermal thermometry for the high-risk diabetic foot. Phys Ther 1997; 77:169–177.

54. American Diabetes Association. Position statement: Standards of medical care in diabetes—2007. Diabetes Care 2007; 30:S4–S41.

55. Brodsky, J, Kourosh, S, Stills, M, et al: Objective evaluation of insert material for diabetic and athletic footwear. Foot Ankle 1988; 9:111–116.

56. Hsi, W, Chai, H, Lai, J: Comparison of pressure and time parameters in evaluating diabetic footwear. Am J Phys Med Rehabil 2002; 81:822–829.

57. Cavanaugh, P: Therapeutic footwear for people with diabetes. Diabetes Metab Res Rev 2004; 20:S51–S55.

58. Uccioli, L, Faglia, E, Monticone, G, et al: Manufactured shoes in the prevention of diabetic foot ulcers. Diabetes Care 1995; 18:1376–1377.

59. Chantelau, E, Haage, P: An audit of cushioned diabetic footwear: Relation to patient compliance. Diabet Med 1994; 11:114–116.

60. van Schie, C, Ulbrecht, J, Becker, M, et al: Design criteria for rigid rocker shoes. Foot Ankle Int 2000; 21:833–844.

61. Busch, K, Chantelau, E: Effectiveness of a new brand of stock 'diabetic' shoes to protect against diabetic foot ulcer relapse. A prospective cohort study. Diabet Med 2003; 20:665–669.

62. Nawoczenski, D, Birke, J, Coleman, J: Effect of rocker sole design on plantar forefoot pressures. J Am Podiatr Med Assoc 1988; 78:455–460.

63. Crawford, F, Inkster, M, Kleijnen, J, et al: Predicting foot ulcers in patients with diabetes: A systematic review and meta-analysis. QLM 2007; 100:65–86.

64. Lavery, L, Armstrong, D, Harkless, B: Classification of diabetic foot wounds. Foot Ankle Surg 1996; 35:528–531.

65. Steed, D, Attinger, C, Colaizzi, T, et al: Guidelines for the treatment of diabetic ulcers. Wound Repair Regen 2006; 14:680–692.

66. Leibner, E, Brodsky, J, Pollo, F, et al: Unloading mechanism in the total contact cast. Foot Ankle Int 2006; 27:281–285.

67. Birke, J, Sims, D, Buford, W: Walking casts: Effect on plantar foot pressures. J Rehabil Res Dev 1985; 22:18–22.

68. Birke, J, Patout, C: The contact cast: An update and case study report. Wounds: A Compendium of Clinical Research and Practice 2000; 12:26–31.

69. Petre, M, Tokar, P, Kostar, D, et al: Revisiting the total contact cast: Maximizing off-loading by wound isolation. Diabetes Care 2005; 28:929–930.

70. McGuire, J: Pressure redistribution strategies for the diabetic or at-risk foot. Adv Skin Wound Care 2006; 19(Pt 2):270–277.

71. Hartsell, H, Brand, R, Frantz, R, et al: The effects of total contact casting materials of plantar pressures. Foot Ankle Int 2004; 25:73–78.

72. Piaggesi, A, Viacava, P, Rizzo, L, et al: Semiquantitative analysis of the histopathological features of the neuropathic foot ulcer. Diabetes Care 2003; 26:3123–3128.

73. Myerson, M, Papa, J, Eaton, K, et al: The total contact cast for management of neuropathic plantar ulceration of the foot. J Bone Joint Surg Am 1992; 74:261–269.

74. Coleman, W, Brand, P, Birke, J: The total contact cast: A therapy for plantar ulceration on insensitive feet. J Am Podiatr Med Assoc 1984; 74:548–552.

75. Beuker, B, Van Deursen, R, Price, P, et al: Plantar pressure in off-loading devices used in diabetic ulcer treatment. Wound Repair Regen 2005; 13:537–542.

76. Lavery, L, Vela, S, Lavery, D, et al: Reducing dynamic foot pressures in high-risk diabetic subjects with foot ulcerations: A comparison of treatments. Diabetes Care 1996; 19:818–821.

77. Katz, I, Harlan, A, Miranda-Palma, B, et al: A randomized trial of two irremovable off-loading devices in the management of plantar neuropathic diabetic foot ulcerations. Diabetes Care 2005; 28:555–559.

78. Hartsell, H, Fellner, C, Saltzman, C: Pneumatic bracing and total contact casting have equivocal effects on plantar pressure relief. Foot Ankle Int 2001; 22:502–506.

79. Lawless, M, Reveal, G, Laughlin, R: Foot pressures during gait: A comparison of techniques for reducing pressure points. Foot Ankle Int 2001; 22:594–597.

80. Armstrong, D, Lavery, L, Kimbriel, H, et al: Activity patterns of patients with diabetic foot ulceration: Patients with active ulceration may not adhere to a standard pressure off-loading regimen. Diabetes Care 2003; 26:2595–2597.

81. Armstrong, D, Nguyen, H, Lavery, L, et al: Offloading the diabetic foot wound: A randomized clinical trial. Diabetes Care 2001; 24:1019–1022.

82. Armstrong, D, Lavery, L, Wu, S, et al: Evaluation of removable and irremovable cast walkers in the healing of diabetic foot wounds: A randomized controlled trial. Diabetes Care 2005; 28:551–554.

83. Birke, J, Lewis, K, Penton, A, et al: The effectiveness of a modified wedge shoe in reducing pressure at the area of previous great toe ulceration in individuals with diabetes mellitus. Wounds: A Compendium of Clinical Research and Practice 2004; 16:109–114.

84. Birke, J, Fred, B, Krieger, L, et al: The effectiveness of an accommodative dressing in offloading pressure over areas of previous metatarsal head ulceration. Wounds: A Compendium of Clinical Research and Practice, 2003; 15:33–39.

85. Birke, J, Pavich, M, Patout, C, et al: Comparison of forefoot ulcer healing using alternative off-loading methods in patients with diabetes mellitus. Adv Skin Wound Care 2002; 15:212–215.

86. Kwon, O, Mueller, M: Walking patterns used to reduce forefoot plantar pressures in people with diabetic neuropathies. Phys Ther 2001; 81:828–835.

87. Zhu, H, Wertsch, J, Harris, G, et al: Foot pressure distribution during walking and shuffling. Arch Phys Med Rehabil 1991; 72:390–397.

88. Cook, T, Farrell, K, Carey, I, et al: Effects of restricted knee flexion and walking speed on the vertical ground reaction force during walking. J Orthop Sports Phys Ther 1997; 25:236–244.

89. Andriacchi, T, Ogle, J, Galante, J: Walking speed as a basis for normal and abnormal gait measurements. J Biomech 1977; 10:261–268.

90. Zhu, H, Harris, G, Wertsch, J: Walking cadence effect on plantar pressures. Arch Phys Med Rehabil 1995; 76:1000–1005.

91. Mueller, M, Sinacore, D, Hoogstrate, S, et al: Hip and ankle walking strategies: Effect on peak plantar pressures and implications for neuropathic ulceration. Arch Phys Med Rehabil 1994; 75:1196–1200.

92. Wertsch, J, Loftsgaarden, J, Harris, G, et al: Plantar pressure with contralateral versus ipsilateral cane use. Arch Phys Med Rehabil 1990; 71:772.

93. Frykberg, R, Mendeszoon, E: Management of the diabetic Charcot foot. Diabetes Metab Res Rev 2000; 16:S59–S65.

94. Armstrong, D, Lavery, L: Acute Charcot's arthropathy of the foot and ankle. Phys Ther 1998; 78:74–80.

95. Armstrong, D, Todd, W, Lavery, L, et al: The natural history of acute Charcot's arthropathy in a diabetic foot specialty clinic. Diabet Med 1997; 17:357–363.

96. Morgan, J, Biehl, W, Wagner, W: Management of neuropathic arthropathy with the Charcot Restraint Orthotic Walker. Clin Orthop Relat Res 1993; 296:58–63.

97. McCrory, J, Morag, E, Norkitis, A, et al: Healing of Charcot fractures: Skin temperature and radiographic correlates. The Foot 1998; 8:158–165.

98. Kristiansen, T: The effect of low power specifically programmed ultrasound on the healing time of fresh fractures using a Colles' model. J Orthop Trauma 1990; 4:227–228.

99. Hanft, J, Goggin, J, Landsman, A, et al: The role of combined magnetic field bond growth stimulation as an adjunct in the treatment of neuroarthropathy/Charcot joint: An expanded pilot study. J Foot Ankle Surg 1998; 37:510–515.

100. Jude, E, Selby, P, Burgess, J, et al: Bisphosphonates in the treatment of Charcot neuroarthropathy: A double-blind randomised controlled trial. Diabetologia 2001; 44:2032–3037.

101. Anderson, J, Woelffer, K, Holtzman, J, et al: Bisphosphonates for the treatment of Charcot neuroarthropathy. J Foot Ankle Surg 2004; 43:285–289.

chapter 15

Diabetes and Wound Care

Pamela Scarborough, PT, MS, CDE, CWS, FACCWS

Both the World Health Organization (WHO) and the International Diabetes Federation (IDF) consider worldwide diabetes prevalence to be at epidemic proportions. The IDF estimates that in 2010 more than 285 million people globally had diabetes and that this number is likely to increase to over 438 million by 2030.[1] In the United States, type 2 diabetes (T2DM) is increasing faster than our health system can effectively support. Current national statistics estimate there are approximately 23.6 million individuals with diabetes and about 5.7 million people with T2DM who are undiagnosed.[2,3]

The impact of diabetes on overall health is far-reaching. Diabetes is a leading cause of adult blindness, lower-limb amputation, kidney disease, and nerve damage. Moreover, two thirds of people with diabetes die from heart disease or stroke. Beyond the existing diabetes epidemic, an estimated 57 million people are considered to have either the metabolic syndrome or what is now called "at risk for diabetes" (formerly prediabetes) and are not only at risk for developing type 2 diabetes,[3] but their at risk for diabetes condition creates an environment that accelerates macrovascular disease. This in turn increases risk for stroke, coronary artery disease, and peripheral vascular disease at an earlier age and with more severe manifestations. Clearly, diabetes has a staggering negative impact on overall health. This chapter will examine its deleterious effects on the wound healing process specifically.

Definition and Description of Diabetes Mellitus

Diabetes mellitus (DM) is a group of metabolic diseases characterized by hyperglycemia resulting from defects in insulin secretion, insulin action, or both. The chronic hyperglycemia of diabetes is associated with long-term damage, dysfunction, and failure of various organs, especially the eyes, kidneys, nerves, heart, and blood vessels.[4] The etiology of diabetes has a variety of pathophysiologies. However, it is important to keep in mind that the etiology and pathophysiology of diabetes are complex and to date are incompletely understood. The three most frequently encountered forms of diabetes include type 1 diabetes mellitus (T1DM), type 2 diabetes mellitus (T2DM), and gestational diabetes (GDM).

Type 1 diabetes mellitus (T1DM), which accounts for 5% to 10% of those affected with the disease, was previously called insulin-dependent diabetes mellitus (IDDM), or juvenile-onset diabetes. T1DM results from cellular-mediated autoimmune destruction of the pancreatic beta cells resulting in an absolute deficiency in insulin secretion.[4] To survive, people with T1DM must administer insulin daily. T1DM usually occurs in children and young adults, although disease onset can occur at any age. Risk factors include autoimmune abnormalities, genetics, or environmental triggers.

Type 2 diabetes (T2DM), accounting for 90% to 95% of those affected, was previously called non-insulin-dependent diabetes mellitus (NIDDM), adult-onset diabetes, or secondary onset diabetes. T2DM is a progressive disease caused by a combination of complex metabolic disorders that result from coexisting defects of multiple organ sites, such as insulin resistance in muscle and adipose tissue, a progressive decline in pancreatic insulin secretion, unrestrained hepatic glucose production, inappropriate glucagon secretion, diminished production of gastrointestinal incretins, as well as other hormonal deficiencies and impairments.[5]

Gestational diabetes mellitus (GDM) is defined as any degree of glucose intolerance during pregnancy. The definition applies regardless of whether insulin or lifestyle modification is used for treatment or whether the condition persists after pregnancy.[4] During pregnancy, treatment to normalize maternal blood glucose levels is required to avoid complications for both mother and infant. GDM imparts a lifetime risk for type 2 diabetes, although the risk is highest 5 to 10 years after delivery. In women with a history of GDM, even 10 years postpartum, the risk of developing diabetes is 70% higher than in a comparable group of women without GDM. The children of women with a history of GDM also are at increased risk for obesity and diabetes compared to other children.[6]

Other types of diabetes result from causes such as genetic defects in beta-cell function, genetic defects in insulin action, diseases of the exocrine pancreas (eg, cystic fibrosis), and drug- or chemical-induced impairments (such as in the treatment of AIDS or after organ transplantation).[4]

Regardless of the pathophysiology, the devastating effects of diabetes that result from chronic hyperglycemia are readily apparent to all who work in the health-care arena. Chronic complications of diabetes include macrovascular disease (atherosclerosis), such as coronary, cerebral, and peripheral vascular disease; microvascular disease, including retinopathy, nephropathy, and neuropathies; infections; difficulty with wound healing; and orthopedic abnormalities. In addition, studies have shown a decrease in cognitive function in patients with diabetes compared to age-equivalent peers. The cognitive impairment can be a major issue when viewed in relation to the complex tasks necessary for diabetes self-management. Consider the complicated pharmaceutical and nutritional regimes many of these individuals face on an ongoing daily basis.[7,8]

To mitigate the impairments and complications from diabetes it is important that blood glucose levels remain as close to "normal" ranges as possible. Blood glucose levels are regulated by a balance between the aforementioned hormones, types and amounts of foods consumed, and amount and types of physical activity engaged in by the individual. Extensive education and behavior modifications are required for people to acquire the knowledge and skills necessary to successfully control their blood glucose. Daily diabetes management rests primarily with the patient or a caregiver if the patient is unable to administer his or her medications and prepare food. Currently, there are well-established optimal blood glucose levels and diagnostic criteria for normal blood glucose, at risk for diabetes, and a diagnosis of diabetes mellitus. (Table 15.1) Impaired fasting glucose (IFG) and impaired glucose tolerance (IGT) are risk factors for future diabetes and for cardiovascular disease (CVD).[4,9]

Impact of Diabetes Mellitus on Wound Healing

Impaired wound healing is a well-recognized complication of diabetes. However, the pathophysiological relationship between diabetes and faulty healing is complex and multifaceted. Normal wound healing involves coordinated intricate interactions between cellular activities, growth factor activation, and connective tissue formation, all of which are negatively impacted in people with diabetes. In addition, microvascular and macrovascular, neuropathic, immune function, biochemical, and hormonal abnormalities each contribute to the altered tissue repair processes in patients with diabetes and hyperglycemia. A consensus on the exact pathogenesis of defective healing related to diabetes has yet to be conclusively determined. However, research has identified several mechanisms of dysfunction that shed light on the wound healing conundrum in this patient population. What is known is that patients with diabetes present a unique challenge as the impact of diabetes extends beyond glycemic control, affecting protein synthesis, white cell function, oxygen transportation and utilization, and growth factor availability.[10]

For purposes of organizing this discussion, the accepted and postulated dysfunctions associated with diabetes and hyperglycemia, in particular, are organized according to effects on overall physiological health, followed by effects specific to the commonly accepted wound healing phases of hemostasis (coagulation), inflammation, proliferation, and remodeling (maturation). (Table 15.2) Please refer to Chapter 2 for the discussion of normal wound healing.

General Physiological Effects

Microcirculatory damage exists in the skin and subcutaneous tissue of patients with diabetes and impairs the wound healing

Table 15•1 Criteria For the Diagnosis of Increased Risk and Diabetes in Adults[4]			
Stage	Fasting Plasma Glucose Test*	Casual Plasma Glucose Test† or A1c Test	Oral Glucose Tolerance Test‡
Normal	<100 mg/dL		2-hr PPG <140 mg/dL
At Risk for Diabetes (impaired glucose tolerance)	≥100 to 125 mg/dL	A1c 5.7–6.4%	2-h PPG ≥140–199 mg/dL
Diabetes	≥126 mg/dL	≥200 mg/dL (plus symptoms)	2-h PPG ≥200 mg/dL
Diabetes		A1C > 6.5%**	

PPG, postprandial glucose.
†Casual means testing any time of day without regard to time since last meal; symptoms are the classic ones of polyuria, polydipsia, and unexplained weight loss.
‡Fasting means no calorie intake for 8 hours.
**The A1C should be performed in a laboratory using a method that is NGSP certified and standardized to the DCCT assay.

Table 15•2	Impact of Diabetes Mellitus and Hyperglycemia on the Phases of Wound Healing				
Phase	**Cell**	**Normal Function**	**Normal Outcome**	**Impairment with Hyperglycemia**	**Outcome with Hyperglycemia**
Coagulation/ hemostasis	Platelets	Platelets aggregate and release clotting factors, growth factors, and cytokines (PDGF) and TGF-ß	Clotting; bleeding controlled Formation of fibrin plug Initiation of inflammatory responses	Delay in fibrin plug formation Delay/decrease in release of growth factors and cytokines Microvascular hemodynamics impaired Abnormal vascular autoregulatory capacity	Platelet irregularity Delayed fibrin plug formation leaves wound open longer Decreased local growth factors and cytokine production Leads to delayed recruitment of inflammatory cells
Inflammation	Neutrophils and macrophages	Early: • Neutrophils remove foreign materials, bacteria, and damaged tissue Late: • Macrophages continue the process of phagocytosis • Release of more PDGF and TGF-ß	Chemotaxis, adherence Phagocytosis by neutrophil and macrophages Intracellular killing Débridement Signaling to begin proliferation phase	Decreased release of growth factors and cytokines from neutrophils and macrophages Impaired migration, adherence, and phagocytosis by neutrophils and macrophages Thickened arterial basement membrane	Delayed inflammatory response Poor endogenous débridement Chronic inflammatory state Increased bioburden Patient at higher risk for infections
Proliferation	Fibroblasts Endothelial proliferation Myofibroblasts transformation Keratinocyte proliferation and migration	Fibroblasts migrate and proliferate Release of growth factors and matrix proteins Collagen synthesis Angiogenesis Growth factor-induced contraction via myofibroblasts Keratinocyte proliferation and migration	Granulation tissue formation Extracellular matrix replaces provisional fibrin matrix Reepithelialization Wound closure	Poor cellular response to growth factors and chemokines Impaired fibroblast proliferation, migration, and function Excessive activation of proteases Impaired contraction by myofibroblast	Reduced angiogenesis Impaired granulation tissue formation Impaired Diminished contraction of wound Friable and poorly functioning granulation tissue Wound stuck in cycle of chronic inflammatory state
Maturation	Fibroblasts Keratinocytes	Collagen production, transformation Matrix, remodeling Type III to type I collagen deposition	Wound returns to ~80% of former tensile strength	Ineffective matrix turnover	Collagen matrix cross-linked Ineffective matrix turnover Reduced ultimate strength of repair tissue

PDGF, platelet-derived growth factor; TGF-ß, transforming growth factor-ß.

processes. A functional microcirculation is needed for tissue nutrition, removal of waste products, initiation of inflammatory responses, and temperature regulation; therefore, disruption of the microvascular system adversely impacts wound healing.[11] Macrovascular changes resulting from diabetes also adversely affect healing. In fact, the macrovascular changes begin with blood glucose levels below that for diagnosis of diabetes (at risk for diabetes). These vascular changes impede wound healing by contributing to hypoxia.

Chronic hyperglycemia contributes to thickening of the basement membrane through a cascade of events at both the cellular and tissue levels. (For a review, see Konstantinos et al.[11]) Thickening of the basement membrane, in turn, presents several complications for wound healing due, in part, to impaired vascular reactivity and limited hyperemia. A thickened and rigid basement membrane restricts the normal hyperemic response to tissue damage, resulting in hypoxia. In addition, there is a corresponding alteration of membrane charge affecting capillary permeability. Persistent hyperglycemia encourages the conversion within the endothelial cells of glucose to sorbitol, which cannot diffuse across the cell membrane thus causing cellular edema. This edema results in metabolic alterations, membrane function alteration, and additional basement membrane thickening.[11]

Studies and scholarly thought have suggested that the adverse effects of intracellular hyperglycemia on cellular functions contribute to the underlying mechanism of early diabetic cataracts and peripheral neuropathy.[12] Furthermore, hyperglycemia impairs glucose diffusion through pores of cell membranes, creating a dehydrating effect. The increased osmotic pressure in the extracellular fluids causes water to transfer out of the cells; loss of glucose via the urine causes osmotic diuresis. This results in urinary losses of electrolytes and water, leading to both extracellular and intracellular dehydration.[13] Dehydration contributes to wound healing impairments from several perspectives, including decreasing the body's blood volume, which in turn decreases oxygen and nutrient delivery to the wound bed. Water is required to transport nutrients to and from the cells; therefore, dehydration impedes this transport system and interrupts cellular function.[14]

Research showing an increase in apoptosis of bone cells in hyperglycemic environments suggests a potential connection to Charcot foot syndrome. Increased apoptosis of bone cells results in a net loss of bone as bone resorption outpaces bone formation.[15,16] In addition, impairment of cellular mediators such as platelet-derived growth factor, basic fibroblast growth factor, and vascular endothelial growth factor, during the wound healing processes in diabetes is implicated as a contributing cause of faulty wound healing.[17]

Advanced Glycation End Products

In the presence of hyperglycemia, a process of nonenzymatic glycation occurs in which proteins or lipids become nonenzymatically glycated and oxidized after contact with aldose sugars. In nonenzymatic glycation, glucose chemically attaches to the amino group of proteins, creating a stable molecule that then accumulates over the surface of cell membranes and structural and circulating proteins. At this stage, these molecules are called Amadori products, and they are stable, yet reversible. However, in long-term hyperglycemic environments, further glycation of proteins and lipids occurs, causing molecular rearrangements in Amadori products that lead to the generation of advanced glycated end products (AGEs), which are nonreversible.[12,18]

The development of AGEs occurs during the normal aging process but is accelerated in hyperglycemic environments. The AGEs process is one of the mechanisms that contributes to the pathophysiology of vascular disease in both diabetes and the aging process.[19,20]

The cellular damage caused by formation of AGEs may include modifications of extracellular structural proteins such as collagen and intracellular proteins.[20] Another mechanism by which AGE-modified proteins may alter cellular function is by binding to receptors, such as the receptor for

AGEs (RAGE), to produce a cascade of cellular signaling events, such as activation of mitogen-activated protein kinase (MAPK), which can lead to cellular dysfunction.[18] AGEs may fluoresce, produce reactive oxygen species (ROS), bind to specific cell surface receptors, and form cross-links in the tissues.

The impact of AGEs on wound repair is multifaceted, with effects evident in the inflammatory, proliferative, and remodeling phases. In the inflammatory phase, the presence of AGEs results in altered tissue oxygen delivery,[21] diminished or altered growth factor activity,[22-24] and altered vascular structure and dysfunction.[25]

Effects of Diabetes on the Hemostatic/Coagulation Phase

As discussed in Chapter 2, under normal conditions during the coagulation phase there is an immediate fibrin plug formation as platelets aggregate at the wound site. The platelets release various growth factors and cytokines that cause recruitment of inflammatory cells. However, when there is a hyperglycemic environment, there is a delay in the fibrin plug formation, which leaves the wound open to contaminants, in addition to a delayed or decreased release in the growth factors and cytokines, causing an impaired recruitment of the inflammatory cells.[26] When the arrival of inflammatory cells is delayed, the wound is at greater risk for infection. Because of the delayed inflammatory response, patients with diabetes and hyperglycemia are at higher risk for more frequent and severe infections.[27]

Effects of Diabetes on the Inflammatory Phase

The inflammatory phase of wound repair is thought to last 3 to 7 days with the introduction of polymorphonuclear cell functions, including chemotaxis, adherence, phagocytosis, and the intracellular killing neutrophils to the wounded area. These important cells lyse and clear away nonviable cellular components in addition to secreting cytokines and a variety of growth factors that initiate the next phase (proliferative) of wound repair.[27,28]

In patients with hyperglycemia and poorly controlled diabetes, neutrophils are deficient in nearly all inflammatory functions, including chemotaxis (migration to inflammatory sites), adherence, phagocytosis (ingestion of bacteria), release of lytic proteases, production of reactive oxygen species, and apoptosis (programmed cell death). Similarly, monocytes in patients with diabetes suffer impairment of both chemotaxis and phagocytosis.[29-32]

The delayed influx of inflammatory cells into wounded tissue leads to a sustained state of chronic inflammation once the inflammatory cells do establish residence. Potent inflammatory forces unique to the diabetic environment arise that sustain the generation of proinflammatory cytokines, including tumor necrosis factor (TNF) and tissue-destructive matrix metalloproteinases (MMPs). There is also an inhibitor to the MMPs called tissue inhibitors of metalloproteinases (TIMPs). The MMPs and TIMPs work together in normal circumstances to facilitate the production of the extracellular matrix (ECM). Disruption of the normal MMP and TIMP balance has been discovered in chronic diabetic wounds and wound fluid as well as in excisional wounds of genetically diabetic mice. These proteases contribute to increased proteolytic activity, causing a disruption of the formation of new ECM. In addition, these circumstances have the potential for diminishing stimulation of cell proliferation due to lack of proper scaffolding upon which cells can become attached.[26] Also, aberrant matrix cross-links due to AGEs prevent the efflux of inflammatory cells from the wound environment, exacerbating the chronic, local inflammatory cytokine production. This stall in the inflammatory phase prevents the wound from progressing to matrix deposition (the proliferative phase) and ultimately to the remodeling phase in which collagen matrix matures.[20,22]

Furthermore, research has verified that the defects in the microbicidal function of neutrophils and monocytes are a major contributing factor to the development of bacterial infection, which in turn contributes to the increased morbidity and mortality observed in patients with diabetes.[29,33,34]

Effects of Diabetes on the Proliferative Phase

The absence or deficiency of insulin in diabetes mellitus, which impairs metabolism of carbohydrates, fat, and proteins, is well-established. With regard to wound healing, such metabolic activity is necessary for cellular activities and tissue synthesis. Insulin is required for glucose to enter cells. Glucose supplies energy for fibroblastic and polymorphonuclear (PMN) activities during wound healing. Altered glucose metabolism, as seen in diabetes mellitus, impairs wound healing through defective metabolism of these nutrients, which reduces the fibroblastic/PMN activity necessary for normal wound healing.[11]

As the connective tissue cell responsible for collagen deposition, the fibroblast function is essential for healing tissue injury. There is mounting evidence demonstrating selective impairments in aspects of fibroblast behavior important for tissue repair, including proliferation and collagen synthesis, deficiency of proangiogenic growth factors, prolonged inflammatory state, significantly enhanced rate of programmed cell death (apoptosis),[35] and impaired cell migration and wound contraction.

In a study of fibroblasts harvested from diabetic *db/db* mice, cell migration was impaired, MMP-9 was overexpressed, and diabetic fibroblasts were unable to produce normal levels of vascular endothelial growth factor (VEGF) at baseline or in response to hypoxia. Additional research is ongoing to better understand how glucose and hypoxia interact to diminish angiogenic growth factor expression in fibroblasts.[36] In another *db/db* mouse study, fibroblast-specific apoptosis was observed in diabetic mice in the peak healing period after bacteria-induced connective tissue damage. The reduced numbers of fibroblasts resulted in diminished collagen I and III expression and significantly reduced formation of new connective tissue matrix.[37] Such impairments in collagen deposition and connective tissue matrix would result in impaired angiogenesis and granulation tissue formation.

As described by Boykin and Baylis,[38] the research literature has established the critical importance of nitric oxide (NO) in wound healing through its mediation of angiogenesis, the formation of granulation tissue and collagen deposition, epidermal migration, and ongoing microvascular homeostasis. The NO-mediated enhancement of vascular (endothelial) modulation has also been implicated as a factor in functional recovery of cutaneous vascular beds after ischemia-reperfusion injury and local tissue flap survival. Optimal NO activity is necessary for full expression and receptor upregulation of VEGF and platelet-derived growth factor (PDGF). In conditions that reduce NO production, such as diabetes, impaired wound healing has been reported. In addition, evidence suggests a reduction in NO has been associated with decreased collagen accumulation, wound tensile strength, type I and III collagen gene expression, VEGF expression, granulation tissue formation, and wound microvascular perfusion. Also, successful recombinant topical PDGF-BB (becaplermin; Regranex®) therapy for chronic lower-extremity ulcers in patients with diabetes may depend on optimal NO production. In the not too distant future it may be clinically feasible to assess deficient wound NO bioactivity using wound fluid NO measurements, which may also function as a diagnostic tool for the prediction of impaired wound healing and a functional way of monitoring treatments designed to promote the healing of chronic wounds.[38]

Based on a preliminary clinical study, elevated homocysteine levels appear to be a risk factor for impaired wound healing by significantly reducing wound NO bioactivity. Additionally, elevated fasting homocysteine levels appear to be more common among patients with diabetes and neuropathic ulcers (63% incidence) than among lower-extremity ulcer patients without diabetes (47% incidence). Further research is needed to evaluate how elevated homocysteine levels antagonize NO production, wound NO bioactivity, and potentially the integrity of provisional wound matrix formation.[38]

Effects of Diabetes on the Remodeling Phase

The remodeling phase is the last stage of wound repair and can last up to, and perhaps longer than, 2 years. As mentioned in the Chapter 2, scar tissue never regains its original tensile strength. In diabetes, collagen synthesis is markedly decreased, resulting in chronic connective tissue complications. The defect in collagen metabolism in diabetes affects the collagen peptide production level as well as the posttranslational modification of collagen degradation.[17] As mentioned earlier, low levels of insulin or impaired insulin hormone functions contribute to defective collagen synthesis in the proliferative and maturation phases of wound healing. In addition, the process of enhanced AGEs production, nitric oxide impairments, and proinflammatory cytokines all contribute to grossly altered collagen remodeling during the maturation phase.[22-26]

Glycemic Control in Persons with Diabetes

Improved glucose levels will enhance outcomes for patients with chronic wounds and diabetes. Blood glucose levels closer to normal augment immune defenses, decrease the risk for developing both microvascular and macrovascular disease, improves wound healing outcomes, and contributes to an overall sense of "health" for the patient.

Screening and Diagnosis for Individuals at Risk for Diabetes

Considering the large number of Americans with undiagnosed diabetes and who are at risk for this disease, early detection and treatment is imperative for addressing the diabetes epidemic in the United States. At this point, those at risk for diabetes do not attract the same amount of medical attention as diabetes, but this will probably change as the medical community becomes more aware of the impairments and complications caused by this stage in the sequelae leading to overt T2DM. The National Institutes of Health reports that people at risk for diabetes, a glucose level higher than normal (100–125 mg/dl and an A1c of 5.7–6.4% fasting), will develop the disease within 10 years without aggressive intervention. The at risk category describes those metabolic states that occur when blood glucose levels are elevated but remain below levels used for diagnosing diabetes. Some risk factors that put an individual in the category for being at risk for diabetes cross over to diabetes as well.[4,5] (Box 15.1)

As mentioned earlier in this chapter, T2DM is a progressive disease. Individuals transition from normal glucose levels, to at risk for diabetes, and finally into the full-blown disease state of diabetes. Early intervention for preventing complications from diabetes, regardless of the pathophysiology, whether it is due to T2DM, T1DM, GDM, or other causes, is the key to prevention of microvascular and macrovascular complications. The American Association of Clinical Endocrinologists (AACE) recommends all individuals 30 years or older who are at risk for having or developing type 2 diabetes be screened annually. See Table 15.1 for a review of the clinical interpretation of plasma glucose concentrations. The ADA has not previously recommended the use of A1C for diagnosing diabetes, in part due to lack of standardization of the assay. However, A1C assays are now highly standardized. In an updated report an international expert committee recommended the use of the A1C test to diagnose diabetes with a threshold of ≥6.5%. The ADA affirmed recommending the diagnostic test should be performed using a method certified by the National Glycohemoglobin Standardization Program (NGSP) and standardized or traceable to the Diabetes Control and Complications Trial (DCCT) reference assay. Point-of-care A1C assays are not sufficiently accurate at this time to use for diagnostic purposes.[4]

Diabetes Care
Assessment of Diabetes Control

As wound care specialists or clinicians who care for patients with chronic wounds and the comorbidity of diabetes, it is of paramount importance that the degree of control for the disease be ascertained. The most readily recognized and recommended method for determining the success of a diabetes management program is the glycosylated hemoglobin test (A_{1C}). The A_{1C} test provides a measure of overall glycemic control. It is the average glycemia over the previous 2 to 3 months. The ADA, AACE, and IDF glycemic targets are shown in Table 15.3.[5,39-41] A newer method of reporting glycosylated hemoglobin has been developed and correlates more closely

---

⏵ **Box 15•1** **Risk Factors for Diabetes Mellitus**

- Family history of diabetes
- Cardiovascular disease
- Overweight or obese state
- Sedentary lifestyle
- Latino/Hispanic, Non-Hispanic black, Asian American, Native American, or Pacific Islander ethnicity
- Previously identified impaired glucose tolerance or impaired fasting glucose

- Hypertension
- Increased levels of triglycerides, low concentrations of high-density lipoprotein cholesterol, or both
- History of gestational diabetes
- History of delivery of an infant with a birth weight greater than 9 pounds
- Polycystic ovary syndrome
- Psychiatric illness

From: AACE Diabetes Mellitus Clinical Practice Guidelines Task Force. American Association of Clinical Endocrinologists medical guidelines for clinical practice for the management of diabetes mellitus. Endocr Pract 2007; 13(suppl 1):1–68. Used with permission.

Table 15•3 **Targets for Glycemic Control**

	ADA[4]	IDF[56]	AACE[5]
A_{1C}	<6.5%	<6.5% (T2DM) 7%–7.5% (T1DM)	<6.5%
Fasting	70–130 mg/dL	<110 mg/dL	<110 mg/dL
Postprandial (1–2 hr after beginning of meal)	<180 mg/dL	<145 mg/dL	<140 mg/dL

ADA, American Diabetes Association; IDF, International Diabetes Foundation; AACE, American Association of Clinical Endocrinologists.

with the patient's blood glucose monitor results. This test is called the estimated average glucose (eAG) mg/dL. (Table 15.4) Patients with diabetes use self-monitoring of blood glucose (SMBG) to assist in managing their daily lives when they have diabetes. They use this monitoring technique to help identify where they are from a blood glucose perspective on a day by day basis. When patients consistently monitor their blood glucose they can determine how different foods, activity, illness, and stress affect their glucose excursions giving them some objective information to assist in making decision about modifying aspects of their lives as best they can to keep them on track to optimal health. In addition, in recent years technologies for continuous monitoring of interstitial glucose have entered the market.[39]

Diabetes care is complex and multifaceted, requiring a team approach to patient-centered care, with the patient being an integral member of the team. While the medical team leader is the physician or advanced-practice nurse, who uses input, education services, and treatments from other healthcare providers, the management that occurs on a daily basis is provided by patients themselves (or caregivers when patients are too impaired to do self-care). All members of the team ultimately contribute to the patient's self-management. The team may include, but is not limited to, physicians, nurse practitioners, physician assistants, nurses, dietitians, pharmacists, mental health professionals, and rehabilitation and exercise specialists. (Fig. 15.1) Two important concepts inherent in the patient-centered approach to care are that (1) the person with diabetes assumes an active role in his or her care and that (2) care is individualized. To these ends, multiple strategies and techniques should be used to provide the necessary education and development of problem-solving skills in the various aspects of diabetes management. The care should include diabetes self-management education (DSME).[39,42]

Table 15•4 Estimated Average Glucose (eAG)[57]		
%	**Average Blood Glucose (mg/dL)**	**eAG mg/dL**
12	298	380
11	269	310
10	275	240
9	240	212
8	205	183
7	170	154
6	135	126
5	100	97

eAG, estimated average glucose.

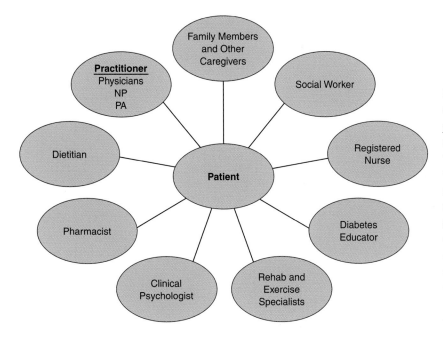

Figure **15•1** *An interdisciplinary model of patient-centered care for patients with diabetes. Examples of types of physicians who may be involved in the treatment of patients with diabetes include, but are not limited to, family practice physicians, internists, endocrinologists, cardiologists, podiatrists, and physical medicine and rehabilitation physicians. Not all patients will use the services of professionals represented here, and other types of health-care providers not represented here may be involved, depending on the patient's needs.*

Diabetes Self-Management Education

DSME, also known as diabetes self-management training, is defined as an ongoing, collaborative process involving the person with diabetes (or the caregiver or family) and the diabetes educator. It is through this collaborative process that the learner gains the knowledge and skills needed to modify his or her behavior and successfully self-manage the disease and its related conditions. The overall aims of DSME are to help the patient achieve optimal health status, improve their quality of life, and reduce the need for costly health care. According to the American Association of Diabetes Educators (AADE), there are seven key self-care behaviors for DSME.[43] (See Box 15.6.)[43] Additionally, the diabetes educator provides psychosocial support to the person with diabetes, including behavior strategies for establishing and maintaining a healthy lifestyle.

The four steps of DSME are as follows:

1. Assessment of the individual's specific education needs
2. Identification of the individual's specific diabetes self-management goals
3. Education intervention directed toward helping the individual achieve identified self-management goals
4. Evaluation of the individual's attainment of identified self-management goals.[43]

According to the American Association of Clinical Endocrinologists (AACE), DSME should be continued as an ongoing intervention to accommodate changes in the treatment plan and patient status.[5] This ongoing education and review of key self-management skills is of vital importance when dealing with patients who have complications from the diabetes disease process, including those with wounds. Often patients become so discouraged that their self-management care suffers, which exacerbates diabetes complications, especially wound healing.

> ▶ **PEARL 15•1** Patients with chronic nonhealing wounds often need a refresher course and extra support regarding their diabetes self-management skills. Consider a referral to a DSME program or diabetes educator to help support these patients during this difficult time. Many of these people need help managing their diabetes while the wound healing process is taking place, especially in the presence of infection.

Diabetes and Aging

Diabetes impairments actually shadow the symptoms of aging at the micro- and macrolevels we associate with "old age." By adding diabetes to the aging process, older patients end up with more severe compromises at an earlier age that manifest globally.

Glycemic Management

Goals of Management

The ADA and AACE have specific recommendations for glycemic control.[4,5,44] (Table 15.5) The diabetes management plan should be directed to help patients achieve glycemic levels as near normal as possible without inducing clinically significant hypoglycemia. Hypoglycemia occurs when blood glucose (BG) levels drop below 50 to 70 mg/dL or any time the patient has hypoglycemic symptoms. This drop can cause confusion, headache, fatigue, incoordination, and weakness. BG can plummet due to missed or poorly timed meals, intense exercise, insulin overdose, and/or accidentally taking oral medications more than once in a prescribed time period. (Table 15.6) Hypoglycemic symptoms can also occur in a patient who has been running chronically high BG levels that drop rapidly and dramatically in a short period of time (eg, from 350 mg/dL to 180 mg/dL).[3] This often happens when the patient's body has become accustomed to the chronic hyperglycemia. When the

Table 15•5 Diabetes Management Goals of Therapy (Nonpregnant Patients)	
Blood glucose before meals	90–130 mg/dL (normal <100 mg/dL)* <100 mg/dL** 100–125 mg/dL***
Blood glucose 2 hr after meals	<180 mg/dL* (peak) <140 mg/dL**
Blood glucose at bedtime	110–150 mg/dL* (normal <110 mg/dL)
Blood glucose at 3:30 a.m.	Goal = 100 mg/dL*
Blood glucose before exercising	100 mg/dL* If <100 mg/dL, snack before exercising (one carbohydrate (15 g) for every 30 minutes) If type 1 diabetes with blood glucose >250 mg/dL, caution against exercise, check ketones, drink water, and notify doctor (may need to increase insulin)
A_{1c}	<6.5%*,**,***
Ketones	Negative
Blood pressure	≤130/80 mmHg*,**,*** if ≥1 g proteinuria, ≤125/75 mm Hg

Table 15•5 Diabetes Management Goals of Therapy (Nonpregnant Patients)—cont'd

Triglycerides	<150 mg/dL
LDL cholesterol	<100 mg/dL
HDL cholesterol	≥40 mg/dL
Microalbuminuria	<30 mg/24 hr
eGFR	≥60***
Body mass index (BMI)	<25 (Overweight 25–29.9; Obesity ≥30)

*American Diabetes Association. Clinical practice recommendations. Diabetes Care 2008; 31(suppl 1):
**AACE Diabetes Mellitus Clinical Practice Guidelines Task Force. American Association of Clinical Endocrinologists medical guidelines for clinical practice for the management of diabetes mellitus. Endocr Pract Vol 13 (Suppl 1), May/June 2007:1–68.
***Diabetes Tool Kit, Fifth Edition (2009). Available at: http://www.dshs.state.tx.us/diabetes/hctoolkt.shtm. Accessed 1/17/10.

Table 15•6 Common Medications Affecting Blood Glucose Levels

Interacting Drug	↑ Blood Glucose	↓ Blood Glucose	Notes
Allopurinol		X	Decreased renal tubular secretion of chlorpropamide.
Androgens/anabolic steroids		X	Mechanism unknown.
Anticoagulants, oral		X	Interfere with metabolism of tolbutamide, chlorpropamide.
Asparaginase I	X*	X**	*Hyperglycemia associated with inhibition of insulin synthesis. **Hypoglycemia reported occasionally.
Aspirin		X	
Beta-adrenergic antagonists	X	X	Both hypo- and hyperglycemic response have been reported. May alter physiological response to, and subjective symptoms of, hypoglycemia, May reduce hyperglycemia-induced insulin release or decrease tissue sensitivity to insulin.
Calcium channel blockers	X	X	Hypoglycemia reported with verapamil. Hyperglycemia reported with diltiazem, nifedipine.
Cholestyramine	X*	X**	*Cholestyramine reduces absorption of coadministered drugs. **Cholestyramine may enhance effects of acarbose. Interactions may be avoided by administering cholestyramine 2 hr apart from other medications.
Chloramphenicol		X	Decreased hepatic metabolism and/or protein-binding displacement of tolbutamide, chlorpropamide.
Chloroquine		X	Mechanism unknown.
Cimetidine/possible other H₂ antagonists		X	
Clofibrate		X	
Corticosteroids	X		Increased gluconeogenesis; transient insulin resistance.
Cyclosporine	X		
Diazoxide	X		Inhibition of insulin secretion.
Dicumarol		X	Inhibits hepatic metabolism of tolbutamide, chlorpropamide.

Continued

Table 15•6 Common Medications Affecting Blood Glucose Levels—cont'd

Interacting Drug	↑ Blood Glucose	↓ Blood Glucose	Notes
Disopyramide		X	Most susceptible: elderly or patients with renal or liver impairment.
Diuretics	X		
Estrogen products	X		Mechanism not known.
Ethanol (alcohol)	X*	X**	*Chronic alcohol ingestion my increase metabolism of sulfonylurea. Alcohol ingestion, especially with carbohydrate-based drinks (beer, mixed drinks) has caloric effect. **Intrinsic hypoglycemic effect; impairs gluconeogenesis and increases insulin secretion. Effect is potentiated if alcohol consumed without food or in fasting state.
Fluoxetine	X	X	Hypoglycemia and hyperglycemia have been reported.
Gemfibrozil		X	
Guanethidine		X	Intrinsic glycemic effect. Protein-binding displacement of certain sulfonylureas.
NSAIDs	X		Possible intrinsic hypoglycemic effect.
			Protein-binding displacement (tolbutamide, tolazamide).
Monoamine oxidase inhibitors		X	
Isoniazid	X		Increase glycogenolysis.
Nicotinic acid (niacin)	X		Dose dependent when lipid-lowering doses are used. Insignificant effect as vitamin-supplement dose.
Octreotide	X	X	Hypoglycemia and hyperglycemia have been reported.
Oral contraceptives	X		Mechanism not known for hyperglycemic effect.
Pancrelipase/pancreatic enzymes	X		Do not administer these agents concurrently with acarbose.
Pentamidine	X	X	Initially hypoglycemia; hyperglycemia may occur days/months after initiation of therapy.
Phenothiazines	X	X	Hypoglycemia observed with some phenothiazines, hyperglycemia with others.
Phenytoin	X		Decreased insulin secretion.
Probenecid		X	
Protease inhibitors	X		
Rifampin	X*	X**	*Increased metabolism of chlorpropamide, glyburide, tolbutamide. **Possible intrinsic hypoglycemic effect.
Salicylates		X	Various effects upon chlorpropamide, tolbutamide kinetics: displacement from protein binding, decreased urinary excretion, and/or altered metabolism.
Sympathomimetics	X		Increases glycogenolysis and gluconeogenesis.
Tacrolimus	X		
Thyroid products	X		Once euthyroid status is achieved, diabetes medications may need to be adjusted to compensate for glycemic effect of thyroid product.
Urinary acidifiers		X	Interferes with chlorpropamide excretion.

BG drops to the more normal range, the patient's body experiences relative hypoglycemic symptoms. Although the BG levels are in a more optimal range, the patient experiences the symptoms of hypoglycemia. Thus, it is important to gradually bring BG levels down over a period of days or weeks in people who have been experiencing significantly elevated BG levels over extended periods of time.

People often think having glycemic control is the only goal for diabetes. However, there are additional considerations and targets that are as important as glucose control.[4,5,44] (See Table 15.5.)

Medical Nutrition Therapy

The cornerstone of diabetes management is medical nutrition therapy (MNT). According to the American Diabetes Association, the goals of MNT that apply to individuals with diabetes are as follows:

1. Achieve and maintain
   - blood glucose levels in the normal range or as close to normal as is safely possible.
   - a lipid and lipoprotein profile that reduces the risk for vascular disease.
   - blood pressure levels in the normal range or as close to normal as is safely possible.
2. Prevent, or at least slow, the rate of development of the chronic complications of diabetes by modifying nutrient intake and lifestyle.
3. Address individual nutrition needs, taking into account personal and cultural preferences and willingness to change.
4. Maintain the pleasure of eating by limiting food choices only when indicated by scientific evidence.[45]

For many people this is commonly a difficult lifestyle change to make. Slight changes impact glucose control. Encouraging the patient to change nutrition patterns gradually is acceptable. Incremental changes create habits that contribute to more permanent lifestyle changes.

The American Diabetes Association (ADA) has made this process easier. In September 2006, ADA released new food guidelines to help people with diabetes devise personalized food plans. The ADA gives guidelines for dealing with excess weight, preventing diabetes, managing T1DM and T2DM, eating well during pregnancy, preventing complications, and treating low blood glucose levels. The guidelines regarding carbohydrates, fats, and protein have recently been updated with a friendlier view toward the low-carbohydrate approach to nutrition. There is now respectable evidence showing low-carbohydrate (CHO) diets are effective for addressing the metabolic syndrome, minimizing postprandial blood glucose excursions, and contributing to weight loss. In addition to closely monitoring carbohydrates, which have the highest impact on blood glucose levels, foods with a lower glycemic index may also help improve blood glucose control.[45] Overall, there is a growing body of evidence that low-CHO diet interventions are more effective, at least in the short term, in reducing weight and improving insulin sensitivity without significant adverse cardiovascular effects. However, more clinical trials need to be conducted to assess the effectiveness of varying degrees of low-CHO diet on weight, glycemic control, hypertension, and lipid profiles in patients with T2DM to resolve current controversies.[46]

MNT is complicated and needs to be individualized. The input of a dietitian will be of great help to this patient population. When wounds are included in the mix with diabetes, special considerations will need to be given to proteins, vitamin and minerals—all of which should be viewed from the patient's perspective.[45,47,48]

Physical Activity

Exercise has many well-described health benefits for people with diabetes, including improved glycemic control and insulin action, blood pressure and lipid control, and increased cardiovascular fitness, mental health, and generalized stamina. As mentioned earlier, T2DM is a progressive disease. It is therefore important to note that the American Diabetes Association has concluded that lifestyle interventions, including physical activity and exercise alone, reduce the risk of progression from impaired glucose tolerance (IGT) to T2DM, stating that there is compelling evidence that increased physical activity and modest weight loss reduce the incidence of T2DM in individuals with IGT.[49] Reviews of the health benefits of physical activity demonstrate that both aerobic and resistance exercise are associated with decreased risk of T2DM.[50]

A recent Cochrane review found that exercise significantly improves glycemic control, improves the body's response to insulin, and reduces visceral adipose tissue and plasma triglycerides—but not plasma cholesterol—in people with T2DM, even without weight loss, as participants may build muscle.[51] In people with both T1DM and T2DM, physical activity is considered one of the three pillars of management, along with meal planning and medication; however, a sedentary lifestyle is a problem in the general population, with attendant issues of adherence. Physical activity for people with T2DM is recommended. Based on the individual's willingness and ability, exercise should be introduced gradually, with individualized, specific, and attainable goals. A suggested regimen is increased frequency and duration of physical activity, 3 to 5 days per week for up to 30 to 45 minutes. T1DM and T2DM patients who take medication, including insulin, should be given specific instructions for how to either adjust their medication accordingly or ingest carbohydrate for the planned periods of physical activity.[52] Despite its importance, as with nutrition, increasing physical activity is often a difficult change to make for people with diabetes; however, eliminating one of the three pillars of diabetes management effectively weakens the treatment plan by one third.

The American Association of Diabetes Educators (AADE) recently recommended a broad, unstructured approach to promoting physical activity by encouraging patients to incorporate more physical tasks (eg, household chores, walking, gardening, yard work) into their daily lives, recognizing that people who are willing to engage in structured exercise will benefit even more and citing the importance of helping patients problem solve to overcome barriers to participation. However, the AADE does not make specific recommendations for the exercise prescription.[53] Recommendations for frequency, duration, and types of exercise exist, although a discussion of these factors is beyond the scope of this chapter. It is of interest to note, however, that the effects of a single bout of exercise on insulin sensitivity lasts for 24 to 72 hours, depending on the structure of the activity.[54] An excellent exercise algorithm has been published by the Texas Diabetes Council (www.texasdiabetescouncil.org), and the

American College of Sports Medicine and American Heart Association have published recommendations for physical activity in older adults, including those with T2DM.[55] The ADA recommends a combination of aerobic, resistance, and stretching exercise. To minimize risk, a thorough pre-participation medical evaluation should be performed to help determine the most appropriate physical activity and exercise interventions. Exercise is a powerful modality and should be treated with the same respect as medications to reduce the risk of exercise-induced complications and side effects.

The ADA recommends that before beginning a program of physical activity more vigorous than brisk walking, people with diabetes be assessed for conditions that might be associated with increased likelihood of cardiovascular disease, that might contraindicate certain types of exercise, or that might predispose participants to injury (eg, severe autonomic neuropathy, severe peripheral neuropathy, preproliferative or proliferative retinopathy). The patient's age and baseline level of physical activity should also be considered.[54] Since diabetes is a chronic progressive disease, physical activity, like medication, needs to be an ongoing, permanent component of the management plan. The overarching goal is to encourage incorporation of physical activity into the participant's lifestyle to produce lasting change. In summary, physical activity interventions including exercise for patients with prediabetes, overt diabetes, and diabetes-induced complications are beneficial in improving homeostasis, lipid control, and an overall sense of well-being.

Medication Management

The drug armamentarium for glycemic control for patients with diabetes is fairly large and growing as the impairments related to diabetes are better understood. The different drugs and combination therapies address different pathophysiological mechanisms. For those with T1DM, the medication regime is somewhat simplified as this group of people must take insulin to survive. They incorporate their insulin therapy into their lifestyle, basing daily insulin administration on the number of CHOs they eat, their physical activities, and the results of self-monitoring of blood glucose (SMBG). The exogenous insulin in essence takes the place of the defunct beta cells in the pancreas. Insulin is administered multiple times during the day to effect what is known as "tight control" in an effort to mimic normal blood glucose excursions as closely as possible.[5] (See Table 15.7.)

Table 15•7 Pharmacokinetics of Available Insulin Preparations

Insulin, Generic Name (Brand)	Onset	Peak	Effective Duration
Rapid-acting			
Insulin aspart injection (NovoLog®)	5–15 min	30–90 min	<5 hr
Insulin lispro injection (Humalog®)	5–15 min	30–90 min	<5 hr
Insulin glulisine injection (Apidra®)	5–15 min	30–90 min	<5 hr
Insulin human (rDNA origin) inhalation powder (Exubera®)[2]	5–15 min	30–90 min	5–8 hr
Short-acting			
Regular	30–60 min	2–3 hr	5–8 hr
Intermediate, basal			
NPH	2–4 hr	4–10 hr	10–16 hr
Long-acting, basal			
Insulin glargine injection (Lantus®)*,†	2–4 hr‡	No peak	20–24 hr
Insulin detemir injection (Levemir®)*,†,3	3–8 hr	No peak	5.7–23.2 hr
Premixed			
75% Insulin lispro protamine suspension/25% insulin lispro injection (Humalog Mix 75/25)	5–15 min	Dual	10–16 hr
50% Insulin lispro protamine suspension/50% insulin lispro injection (Humalog Mix 50/50)[4]	5–15 min	Dual	10–16 h
70% Insulin aspart protamine suspension/30% insulin aspart injection (NovoLog Mix 70/30)	5–15 min	Dual	10–16 hr
70% NPH/30% regular	30–60 min	Dual	10–16 hr

NPH, neutral protamine Hagedorn
*May require two daily injections in patients with type 1 diabetes mellitus.
†Assumes 0.1–0.2 U/kg per injection. Onset and duration may vary significantly greatly by injection site.
‡Time to steady state.
From: AACE Diabetes Mellitus Clinical Practice Guidelines Task Force. American Association of Clinical Endocrinologists medical guidelines for clinical practice for the management of diabetes mellitus. Endocr Pract 2007; 13(suppl 1):1–68. Used with permission.

T2DM is more complicated due to the fact that the disease is multifactorial, with impairments of several organs and tissues. Different drug classifications target different impairments. In addition, because T2DM is a progressive disease, it requires medication changes in doses, classes, and combinations to keep blood glucose levels as normal as possible. As type 2 diabetes progresses, it becomes more difficult to control with a single drug. When monotherapy fails to manage blood glucose levels, the logical next step is combination therapy.[5] (Box 15.2) Because the major classes of medications available to treat T2DM have complementary mechanisms of action, they are often used in combination therapy in individual patients. Sulfonylureas and glinides both work primarily by increasing insulin secretion from the beta cells; however, the main difference in these classes of drugs is that while the sulfonylureas primarily impact fasting blood glucose levels, the glinides work only on postprandial glucose excursions and have a relatively low potential for drug-induced hypoglycemia. Thiazolidinediones (TZD) are insulin sensitizers that increase glucose uptake into muscle. The biguanides have a favorable effect on fasting blood glucose by suppressing glucose production in the liver. The alpha-glucosidase inhibitors are not as efficacious for reducing overall glycemia as sulfonylureas, thiazolidine thiazolidinedione diones, or biguanides; however, they are useful for reducing postprandial blood glucose spikes, as they delay glucose uptake in the intestine and thereby inhibit glucose absorption.[56-59] (Table 15.8)

The goal of combination therapy is to combine the effects of two or more drugs to reach the desired A_{1c} level. Ideally, the two drugs combined would have two different mechanisms of action, such as a drug that stimulates insulin secretion and a drug that improves insulin sensitivity. Some of the most popular combinations are (see Box 15.2)[5]

1. sulfonylurea with biguanide (metformin)
2. metformin and thiazolidinedione
3. sulfonylurea and thiazolidinedione[5]

If glycemic control is not accomplished with oral medications alone, adding insulin to the drug regimen or using insulin alone can be an effective next step. Often, insulin must be introduced to the medication regime as the beta cells gradually fail and the patient becomes move insulin resistant. (See practice considerations in Box 15.3.)

▸ **Box 15•2** **Examples of Pharmacological Regimens for Treating Type 2 Diabetes Mellitus**

Patients with Type 2 Diabetes Mellitus Naïve to Pharmacologic Therapy

Initiate monotherapy when HbA_{1c} levels are 6% to 7%.
  Options include:
  • Metformin
  • Thiazolidinediones
  • Secretagogues
  • Dipeptidyl-peptidase 4 inhibitors
  • Alpha-glucosidase inhibitors
Monitor and titrate medication for 2 to 3 months.
Consider combination therapy if glycemic goals are not met at the end of 2 to 3 months.
Initiate combination therapy when HbA_{1c} levels are 7% to 8%. Options include:
  • Secretagogue + metformin
  • Secretagogue + thiazolidinedione
  • Secretagogue + alpha-glucosidase inhibitor
  • Thiazolidinedione + metformin
  • Dipeptidyl-peptidase 4 inhibitor + metformin
  • Dipeptidyl-peptidase 4 inhibitor + thiazolidinedione
  • Secretagogue + metformin + thiazolidinedione
  • Fixed-dose (single pill) therapy
  • Thiazolidinedione (pioglitazone) + metformin
  • Thiazolidinedione (rosiglitazone) + metformin
  • Thiazolidinedione (rosiglitazone) + secretagogue (glimepiride)
  • Thiazolidinedione (pioglitazone) + secretagogue (glimepiride)
  • Secretagogue (glyburide) + metformin
Rapid-acting insulin analogs or premixed insulin analogs may be used in special situations.

Inhaled insulin may be used as monotherapy or in combination with oral agents and long-acting insulin analogs.
Insulin-oral medications: All oral medications may be used in combination with insulin. Therapy combinations should be selected based on the patient's self-monitoring of blood glucose profiles.
Initiate/intensify combination therapy using options listed above when HbA_{1c} levels are 8% to 10% to address fasting and postprandial glucose levels.
Initiate/intensify insulin therapy when HbA_{1c} levels are >10%.
  Options include: Rapid-acting insulin analog or inhaled insulin with long-acting insulin analog or NPH premixed insulin analogs.

Patients with Type 2 Diabetes Mellitus Currently Treated Pharmacologically

The therapeutic options for combination therapy listed for patients naïve to therapy are appropriate for patients being treated pharmacologically.
Exenatide may be combined with oral therapy in patients who have not achieved glycemic goals. Approved exenatide + oral combinations:
  • Exenatide + secretagogue (sulfonylurea)
  • Exenatide + metformin
  • Exenatide + secretagogue (sulfonylurea) + metformin
  • Exenatide + thiazolidinedione
Pramlintide may be used in combination with prandial insulin.
Add insulin therapy in patients on maximum combination therapy (oral-oral, oral-exenatide) whose HbA_{1c} levels are 6.5% to 8.5% .
Consider initiating basal-bolus insulin therapy for patients with HbA_{1c} levels >8.5%.

From: AACE Diabetes Mellitus Clinical Practice Guidelines Task Force. American Association of Clinical Endocrinologists medical guidelines for clinical practice for the management of diabetes mellitus. Endocr Pract 2007; 13(suppl 1):1–68. Used with permission.

Table 15•8 Current Medications for Type 2 Diabetes

Generic/Class	Brand Names	Target Organs	Mode of Action	% ↓ in A$_{1c}$*	Side Effects	Limitations/Contraindications
Metformin/biguanides	Glucophage®, Glucophage XR®, Fortamel®, Riomet®	Liver, adipose tissue, skeletal muscle	↓ Hepatic glucose production; ↓ insulin resistance in periphery	0.8–3.0	Nausea/GI upset, diarrhea (5%–10% intolerant)	Contraindicated in renal impairment; caution in heart failure, liver impairment
Glyburide Glipizide Glimepiride/sulfonylureas/secretagogues (second generation)	Diabeta® Glucotrol® Amaryl®	Pancreas	Stimulate insulin secretion via Na/K channel activation	0.9–2.5/0.6–1.9	Hypoglycemia, weight gain	
Acarbose Miglitol/alpha-glucosidase inhibitor	Precose® Glyset®	Small intestine, pancreas	Alpha-glucosidase inhibitor	0.4–1.3	GI disturbance	Poorly tolerated, limited efficacy
Pioglitazone Rosiglitazone/thiazolidinediones	Actos® Avandia®	Peripheral tissues, liver	PPARgamma activation	1.1–1.6	Weight gain, fluid retention	Contraindicated in heart failure; rosiglitazone not recommended in IHD
DPP-IV inhibitors	Januvia®	Liver	↓ Hepatic glucose production postprandial	0.6–0.8	Hypoglycemia in combination with SU Skin rashes	
Exenatide	Byetta®	Stomach, liver, pancreas, brain	Enhancement of incretin action, by inhibiting breakdown of GLP-1 and GIP GLP-1 mimetic, simulates insulin secretion	~1.0	Nausea, vomiting Hypoglycemia in combination with SU Pancreatitis	Injectable
Insulin	See insulin chart	Insulin receptors	Direct activation of insulin receptor	Variable	Hypoglycemia, weight gain	Injectable

Data from: Sodium-Glucose Transporter 2 Inhibitors: New Therapeutic Targets, New Therapeutic Options in the Treatment of Type 2 Diabetes Mellitus CME Release Date: March 31, 2008; Available at: http://www.medscape.com/viewprogram/9072_pnt. Accessed 4/8/08.
*Data from: Inzucchi SE. Oral antihyperglycemic therapy for type 2 diabetes: Scientific review. JAMA. 2002;287:360–372; Inzucchi SE, McGuire DK. New drugs for the treatment of diabetes: Incretin-based therapy and beyond. Circulation 2008;117(Pt 2):574–584.

> **Box 15•3** **Responsibility of the Wound Care Team**

It is the responsibility of the wound care team to ensure the patient's diabetes management plan is adequate to allow the best wound healing opportunities possible. This entails, at minimum, evaluating blood glucose patterns and reviewing medications, in addition to reviewing any pertinent laboratory values. One of the best ways to evaluate the overall management is to obtain a recent A_{1c}. If the patient's blood glucose levels are out of range for optimal wound healing, the wound care physician or practitioner is required to intervene. Be especially aware of elevated blood glucose levels in the face of infections, including wound-related infections or from other sources. This is a common occurrence in patients with diabetes and may necessitate initiation of insulin until the infection resolves and blood glucose levels stabilize. Referrals to the endocrinologist or practitioner supervising the diabetes management plan or to a diabetes educator for updates on diabetes self-management strategies may be appropriate.

> **Box 15•4** **Treatment Consideration for Patients with Wounds and Diabetes**

- Tight glycemic control—foundation for care
- Débridement of necrotic tissue and dysfunctional cells
- Vascular management of ischemia
- Infection control
- Moist wound healing principles
- Adjunctive modalities to facilitate wound closure
- Nutrition that supports wound healing
- Off-loading of bony prominences and wounded soft tissue

Remember: Diabetes with associated hyperglycemia impairs healing regardless of the wound etiology.

> **Box 15•5** **Angiogenic Therapies for Patients with Diabetes and Wounds Compromised by Hyperglycemia**

- Growth factors
- Sharp débridement
- Bioengineered tissue
- Electrical stimulation
- Ultrasound energy
- Hyperbaric Oxygen
- Negative-pressure wound therapy
- Photo therapy

> **Box 15•6** **The AADE™ 7-Self-Care Behaviors for DSME**

1. Healthy eating
2. Being active
3. Monitoring
4. Taking medication
5. Problem solving
6. Healthy coping
7. Reducing risks

With permission from American Association of Diabetes Educators. Diabetes education. Available at: http://www.diabeteseducator.org/export/sites/aade/_resources/pdf/Diabetes_Education_Definition.pdf. Accessed May 28, 2008.

Challenges for the Clinician and Patient with Diabetes and Chronic Wounds

There are challenges in caring for this patient population. The person with diabetes and wounds needs adequate knowledge in order to manage their DM in addition to wound self-care. Many of our patients with chronic wounds and diabetes do not have all the information they need to adequately manage the DM, especially in the face of a chronic wound and the further stress the wound places on their systems. Many of these people live with varying levels of depression. With depression, diabetes self-management care can become severely compromised, which in turn will create more challenges for wound healing. There are financial considerations and challenges that impact every aspect of medical care, from managing their DM to wound care. And last there is burnout. The patient becomes "burned out" from living with DM continuously, with no respite. The wound care team can become burned out when trying to help this patient population and may become frustrated when they perceive the patient is not providing optimal DM self-care and thereby "sabotaging" the wound care plan. The psychosocial impact of DM alone is life altering. Add chronic complications that frequently accompany the disease, including unsightly, odoriferous, and difficult-to-manage wounds, and one is able to comprehend why these patients and the clinicians that serve them have such a difficult road. There are no easy answers or pat formulas for these challenges. Care providers must all do the best they can and give the most comprehensive support within their means to these patients and their families.

Summary

Current evidence demonstrates that diabetes inhibits all phases of wound healing via impaired functions of the primary cells responsible for wound repair in addition to decreased efficacy of cytokines and growth factors. The accumulation of AGEs, nitric oxide dysfunction, decreased insulin availably or insulin resistance, and altered homocysteine levels all contribute to this complex host of impairments affecting wound healing. Research in human and animal models has identified many of these changes at the molecular levels that contribute to delayed wound healing; however, more research is needed to completely understand how the disease state of diabetes contributes to faulty tissue repair. What we see clinically is that the linear progression of wound repair with which we are familiar becomes disjointed when diabetes and hyperglycemia become part of the mix. Intrinsic pathobiological abnormalities and extrinsic factors combine to create an even more complex microenvironment that contributes to an altered or delayed path to healing.[60]

Resources

Following are some important websites related to diabetes.

American Diabetes Association: http://www.diabetes.org

American Association of Clinical Endocrinologist: http://www.aace.com

American Association of Diabetes Educators: http://www.aadenet.org

International Diabetes Federation: http://www.idf.org

Diabetes: http://www.noah-health.org/en/endocrine/diabetes/. This is a part of New York Online Access to Health (NOAH).

Diabetes Directory: http://www.mendosa.com/diabetes.htm

Diabetes Monitor: http://www.diabetesmonitor.com. This is one of the most valuable websites for people with diabetes.

Juvenile Diabetes Research Foundation International: http://www.jdf.org/

The National Diabetes Information Clearinghouse: http://diabetes.niddk.nih.gov/

National Institute of Diabetes and Digestive and Kidney Disease: http://www.niddk.nih.gov

Texas Diabetes Council: http://www.dshs.state.tx.us/diabetes/

References

1. 2009 International Diabetes Federation: atlas@idf.org; 166 Chaussée de la Hulpe, B-1170 Brussels, Belgium.
2. National Institute of Diabetes and Digestive and Kidney Diseases (NIDDK), National Institutes of Health, U.S. Department of Health and Human Services: National Diabetes Statistics, 2007. NIH Publication No. 08–3892. Available at: http://diabetes.niddk.nih.gov/dm/pubs/statistics/#estimation. Accessed 11/18/09.
3. U.S. Department of Health and Human Services, Centers for Disease Control and Prevention. National diabetes fact sheet: General information and national estimates on diabetes in the United States, 2005. Available at: http://apps.nccd.cdc.gov/DDTSTRS/template/ndfs_2005.pdf. Accessed 11/30/08.
4. Diagnosis and classification of diabetes. . Diabetes Care 2010; 33:S11–S61. Available at: http://care.diabetesjournals.org/content/33/Supplement_1/S11.full#sec-1
5. Rodbard, HW: American Association of Clinical Endocrinologists medical guidelines for clinical practice for the management of diabetes mellitus. Endocr Pract 2007; 13(suppl):1–68.
6. Overview of diabetes in children and adolescents. National Diabetes Education Program (NDEP). U.S. Department of Health and Human Services. Available at: http://ndep.nih.gov/diabetes/youth/youth_FS.htm#Gestational. Accessed 01/17/10.
7. Arvanitakis, Z, Wilson, RS, Li, Y, et al: Diabetes and function in different cognitive systems in older individuals without dementia. Diabetes Care 2006; 29:560–565.
8. Sinclair, AJ, Girling, AJ, Bayer, AJ: Cognitive dysfunction in older subjects with diabetes mellitus: Impact on diabetes self-management and use of care services: All Wales Research into Elderly (AWARE) Study. Diabetes Res Clin Pract 2000; 50:203–212.
9. Nathan, DM, Davidson, MB, DeFronzo, RA, et al: Impaired fasting glucose and impaired glucose tolerance: Implications for care. Diabetes Care 2007; 30:753–759.
10. Vowden, P, Vowden, K: The management of diabetic foot ulceration. In: Falanga, V (ed): Cutaneous Wound Healing. London, Martin Dunitz, 2001, pp 319–341.
11. Ekmektzoglou, KA, Zografos, GC, Kourkoulis, SK, et al: A concomitant review of the effects of diabetes mellitus and hypothyroidism in wound healing. World J Gastroenterol 2006; 12:2721–2729.
12. Khan, MN: The influence of diabetes on wound healing. The Diabetic Foot 2005; 8:144,146,148,150,152–153.
13. Ferguson, M, Cook, A, Rimmasch, H, et al: Pressure ulcer management: The importance of nutrition. Medsurg Nurs 2000; 9:163–175.
14. Posthauer, M: Hydration: Does it play a role in wound repair? Adv Skin Wound Care 2006; 19:97–102.
15. He, H, Liu, R, Desta, T, et al: Diabetes causes decreased osteoclastogenesis, reduced bone formation, and enhanced apoptosis of osteoblastic cells in bacteria stimulated bone loss. Endocrinology 2004; 145:447–452.
16. Chau, D, Edelman, S: Osteoporosis and diabetes. Clin Diabetes 2008; 20:153–157.
17. Dinh, T, Pham, H, Veves, A: Emerging treatments in diabetic wound care. Wounds 2002; 14:2–10.
18. Sheetz, M, King, G: Molecular understanding of hyperglycemia's adverse effects for diabetic complications. JAMA 2002; 288:2579–2588.
19. Kislinger, T, Fu, C, Huber, B, et al: N(epsilon)-(carboxymethyl)lysine adducts of proteins are ligands for receptor for advanced glycation end products that activate cell signaling pathways and modulate gene expression. J Biol Chem 1999; 274:31740–31749.
20. Goldin, A, Beckman, JA, Schmidt, AM, et al: Advanced glycation end products; sparking the development of diabetic vascular injury. Circulation 2006; 114:597–605.
21. Watala, C, Golanski, J, Witas, H, et al: The effects of in vivo and in vitro non-enzymatic glycosylation and glycoxidation on physicochemical properties of haemoglobin in control and diabetic patients. Int J Biochem Cell Biol 1996; 28:1393–1403.
22. Goova, MT, Li, J, Kislinger, T, et al: Blockade of receptor for advanced glycation end-products restores effective wound healing in diabetic mice. Am J Pathol 2001; 159:513–525.
23. Duraisamy, Y, Slevin, M, Smith, N, et al: Effects of glycation on basic fibroblast growth factor induced angiogenesis and activation of associated signal transduction pathways in vascular endothelial cells: Possible relevance to wound healing in diabetes. Angiogenesis 2001; 4:277–288.
24. Twigg, SM, Joly, AH, Chen, MM, et al: Connective tissue growth factor/IGF-binding protein-related protein-2 is a mediator in the

induction of fibronectin by advanced glycosylation end-products in human dermal fibroblasts. Endocrinology 2002; 143:1260–1269.

25. Ido, Y, Chang, KC, Lejeune, WS, et al: Vascular dysfunction induced by AGE is mediated by VEGF via mechanisms involving reactive oxygen species, guanylate cyclase, and protein kinase C. Microcirculation 2001; 8:251–263.

26. Blakytny, R, Jude, E: The molecular biology of chronic wounds and delayed healing in diabetes. Diabet Med 2006; 23:594–608.

27. Baum, CL, Arpey, CJ: Normal cutaneous wound healing: Clinical correlation with cellular and molecular events. Dermatol Surg 2005; 31:674–686.

28. Werner, S, Grose, R: Regulation of wound healing by growth factors and cytokines. Physiol Rev 2003; 83:835–870.

29. Hatanaka, E, Monteagudo, PT, Marrocos, MS, et al: Neutrophils and monocytes as potentially important sources of proinflammatory cytokines in diabetes. Clin Exp Immunol 2006; 146:443–447.

30. Gupta, S, Koirala, J, Khardori, R, et al: Infections in diabetes mellitus and hyperglycemia. Infect Dis Clin N Am 2007; 21:617–638.

31. Waltenberger, J, Lange, J, Kranz, A: Vascular endothelial growth factor-A-induced chemotaxis of monocytes is attenuated in patients with diabetes mellitus: A potential predictor for the individual capacity to develop collaterals. Circulation 2000; 102:185–190.

32. Katz, S, Klein, B, Elian, I, et al: Phagocytotic activity of monocytes from diabetic patients. Diabetes Care 1983; 6:479–482.

33. Joshi, N, Caputo, G, Weitekamp, M, et al: Infections in patients with diabetes mellitus. N Engl J Med 1999; 341:1906–1912.

34. McManus, L, Bloodworth, R, Prihoda, T, et al: Agonist-dependent failure of neutrophil function in diabetes correlates with extent of hyperglycemia. J Leuko Biol 2001; 70:395–404.

35. Al-Mashat, HA, Kandru, S, Liu, R, et al: Diabetes enhances mRNA levels of proapoptotic genes and caspase activity, which contribute to impaired healing. Diabetes 2006; 55:487–495.

36. Lerman, OZ, Galiano, RD, Armour, M, et al: Cellular dysfunction in the diabetic fibroblast. Impairment in migration, vascular endothelial growth factor production, and response to hypoxia. Am J Pathol 2003; 162:303–312.

37. Liu, R, Desta, T, He, H, et al: Diabetes alters the response to bacteria by enhancing fibroblast apoptosis. Endocrinology 2004; 145:2997–3003.

38. Boykin, JV, Baylis, C: Homocysteine—A stealth mediator of impaired wound healing: A preliminary study. Wounds 2006; 18:101–116.

39. American Diabetes Association Position Statement: Standards of Medical Care in Diabetes, 2008. Diabetes Care 2008; 31(suppl):S12–S54.

40. Silink, M, Mbanya, J: Global standardization of the HbA$_{1c}$ assay—The consensus committee recommendations. Diabetes Voice 2007; 52:33–34.

41. IDF Clinical Guidelines Task Force: Glucose control levels. In: Global Guidelines for Type 2 Diabetes. Brussels International Diabetes Federation, 2005. Available at: http://www.idf.org/ Global_guideline. Accessed 10/31/09.

42. American Diabetes Association: Report of the task force on the delivery of diabetes self-management education and medical nutrition therapy. Diabetes Spectrum 1999; 12:44–47.

43. American Association of Diabetes Educators. Diabetes education. Available at: http://www.diabeteseducator.org/export/sites/aade/ _resources/pdf/Diabetes_Education_Definition.pdf. Accessed 05/28/08.

44. Texas Diabetes Council: Diabetes Tool Kit, Fifth Edition (2009). Available at: http://www.dshs.state.tx.us/diabetes/hctoolkt.shtm. Accessed 1/17/10.

45. ADA. Nutrition recommendations and interventions for diabetes: A position statement of the American Diabetes Association. Diabetes Care 2008; 31(suppl):S61–S78.

46. Worth, J, Soran, H: Is there a role for low carbohydrate diets in the management of type 2 diabetes? QJ Med 2007; 100:659–663.

47. Nielsen, JV, Joensson, EA: Low-carbohydrate diet in type 2 diabetes: Stable improvement of bodyweight and glycemic control during 44 months follow-up. Nutr Metab Lond 2008; 5:14.

48. Stern, L, Iqbal, N, Seshadri, P, et al: The effects of low-carbohydrate versus conventional weight loss diets in severely obese adults: One year follow-up of a randomized trial. Ann Intern Med 2004; 140:778–785.

49. Sigal, RJ, Kenny, GP, Wasserman, DH, et al: Physical activity/exercise and type 2 diabetes. A consensus statement from the American Diabetes Association. Diabetes Care 2006; 29:1433–1438.

50. Warburton, DER, Nicol, CW, Bredin, SSD: Health benefits of physical activity: The evidence. CMAJ 2006; 174:801–809.

51. Thomas, DE, Elliott, EJ, Naughton, GA: Exercise for type 2 diabetes mellitus. Cochrane Database Syst Rev 2006; 3:CD002968.

52. Clinical Guidelines Task Force, International Diabetes Federation: The IDF 'Global guideline for type 2 diabetes': background and methods. Diabetes Voice, 2006; 51:S2–S4.

53. American Diabetes Association position statement. Diabetes and exercise. Diabetes Educ 2008; 34:37–40.

54. American Diabetes Association consensus statement. Physical activity/exercise and type 2 diabetes. Diabetes Care 2006; 29:1433–1438.

55. Nelson, ME, Rejeski, WJ, Blair, SN, et al: Physical activity and public health in older adults. Recommendation from the American College of Sports Medicine and the American Heart Association. Circulation 2007; 116:1094–1105.

56. American Diabetes Association: ADA-SAP™ Module 1: Basic principles of management of type 2 diabetes 2007. Available at: http://www.proevalinc.com/medical/diabetes/ADASAP1.php. Accessed 1/17/10.

57. Sodium-glucose transporter 2 inhibitors: New therapeutic targets. New therapeutic options in the treatment of type 2 diabetes mellitus. Available at: http://www.medscape.com/viewprogram/9072_pnt. Accessed 1/17/10.

58. Inzucchi, SE: Oral antihyperglycemic therapy for type 2 diabetes: Scientific review. JAMA 2002; 287:360–372.

59. Inzucchi, SE, McGuire, DK: New drugs for the treatment of diabetes: Incretin-based therapy and beyond. Circulation 2008; 117(Pt 2):574–584.

60. Falanga, V: Wound healing and its impairment in the diabetic foot. Lancet 2005; 366:1736–1743.

Venous Insufficiency and Ulceration

Joseph M. McCulloch, PhD, PT, CWS, FACCWS, FAPTA

It has been suggested that approximately 90% of the estimated 600,000 leg ulcers seen annually in the United States are due to chronic venous disease or mixed arteriovenous insufficiency.[1] In addition, 5% to 8% of the world's population is affected by venous disease, making this a costly problem from both an economic and quality-of-life perspective.[2-4] As individuals age, ulcer prevalence appears to increase exponentially.[5] Anderson and associates noted that leg ulcers develop in 1% of the population over 70 years old; this incidence rises to 5% by age 90.[6] In patients over age 65, 82% of the leg ulcers seen were secondary to venous insufficiency. These findings correlate well with earlier reports that indicated an 80% to 90% predominance of venous ulceration.[7]

This chapter presents information about the pathogenesis and management of wounds resulting from venous insufficiency. Because of the complimentary role the lymphatic system plays in venous system function, some aspects of lymphatic system physiology will be included. For a more detailed discussion of lymphatic disease and treatment, however, the reader is referred to Chapter 18.

Overview of Anatomy and Physiology of the Phlebolymphatic System

Blood vessels are composed of five major elements: endothelial cells, basement membranes, elastic tissue, smooth muscle, and collagen. Endothelial cells line all blood vessels and lymphatics.[8] Because of their location between the fluid components of blood or lymph and the tissue, endothelial cells are responsible for maintaining vascular homeostasis.[9] Integrity of the endothelial lining is essential for normal blood flow. Damage to the lining results in blood cells sticking at the point of injury, subsequently forming a clot.

While veins, like arteries, have intimal, medial, and adventitial layers, the proportions of tissue in each layer vary. Overall, venous walls are much thinner. The smooth muscle and elastic proportions of venous walls are less developed in comparison to arterial walls. The venous adventitia is proportionally thicker.[10] Venous walls are much more distensible than arterial walls, however, allowing veins to better accommodate variations in blood volume and serve as a reservoir. In fact, more than 60% of the body's blood volume is contained in veins and venules.[11] Unlike arteries, veins contain valves that allow regulating the direction of blood flow toward the heart.

In the leg, perforating veins penetrate the fascia, providing the connection between the deep and superficial veins. Valves direct the flow of blood from superficial to deep veins in the legs. Venous sinusoids within the calf musculature connect to form intramusuclar plexi, which join the peroneal veins. In contrast, the valves in veins of the foot direct blood from deep to superficial veins, thus explaining how the saphenous veins are filled without direct contact with the capillary beds.[12]

In the legs, because of the valves, blood flow is assisted by contractions of skeletal muscle. This function is known as the skeletal muscle pump. In contrast, blood flow in the abdomen and chest is assisted by movement of the diaphragm. This tunction is known as the respiratory pump.[13]

The lymphatics are thin-walled, permeable vessels that are not part of the blood circulatory system. Lymphatics have blind ends through which interstitial fluid and components such as plasma proteins diffuse. The fluid is carried to the point where the largest lymph vessels empty into the veins in the lower back. Thus, lymphatics carry fluid from interstitial spaces back into the bloodstream, thus assisting the venous system.

Larger lymphatics are formed by the anastomosis of smaller lymphatics. Although they closely resemble the structure of veins, the media are poorly developed. Like veins, lymphatics are supplied with valves to assist flow toward the venous system.[14] Many lymphatics empty into lymph nodes, collections of lymphocytes joined by connective tissue and penetrated by lymphatic channels. The lymph nodes filter all lymph that passes through them.

Lymphatic vessels act in concert with veins to remove interstitial fluid. Any obstruction in the veins or lymph vessels can therefore result in the accumulation of tissue fluid (edema). The management of this problem is addressed in detail in Chapters 18 and 30.

Venous Insufficiency
Pathogenesis

Venous pressure, measured in the foot vein of a person in the upright position, is proportional to the height of the column of blood between the foot and the right side of the heart. Typically, this pressure ranges from 60 to 90 mm Hg.[15] As the individual ambulates, muscle pumps in the feet and legs push venous blood from the lower extremities, thereby reducing ambulatory venous pressure. As the calf pump fails, pressure begins to rise in the veins and ulcerations may result. Ambulatory venous hypertension is widely accepted as the primary cause of venous ulcerations.[16,17]

> **PEARL 16•1** The calf muscle pump is critical to blood flow in the lower extremities. Failure of the calf pump can result in significant venous hypertension.

It was demonstrated over a decade ago by Nicholaides and associates that patients with ulcers all had pressures greater than 90 mm Hg.[18] There appeared to be a linear correlation with the increase in pressures and the risk of developing ulcers. Why this elevated pressure resulted in microcirculatory injury to the skin was less well understood. Various theories have been proposed: for example, the development of a pericapillary fibrin cuff and plugging of capillaries by activated leukocytes (white blood cells, or WBCs).

High ambulatory venous pressure can result from a variety of causes. Four major disruptive mechanisms are venous thrombosis, obstruction, dilatation, and hemorrhage. In addition, impaired lymphatic drainage, although not necessarily a cause of venous insufficiency, can substantially perpetuate chronic microcirculatory changes that may occur.[19]

Venous Thrombosis

Venous thrombosis begins as platelets adhere to the endothelial wall. Continued aggregation results in the deposition of a fibrin mesh, encouraging further platelet adherence. As the lumen becomes completely occluded, several events ensue. Clinically, the patient begins to exhibit swelling, warmth, and lower extremity pain. Within days of occlusion, fibrinolysin begins to act upon the thrombus, putting the individual at risk of embolization. Although embolization may or may not occur, inflammation of the adjacent vessel wall results. Unfortunately, during the entire sequence of events, valve damage typically occurs and places the patient at risk for future venous problems.[20,21]

Venous Obstruction

Venous obstruction from any source can result in ambulatory venous hypertension. The extent to which this obstruction leads to significant dysfunction and ulceration depends on the duration and anatomical location of the obstruction.

> **PEARL 16•2** Whether venous obstruction leads to significant dysfunction is determined by duration and location of the obstruction.

Obviously, the longer an obstruction persists, the longer the high pressure is sustained and the greater the damage that is inflicted. Obstruction of superficial veins, or even their surgical excision, seldom results in ulceration because numerous collateral vessels can compensate for the loss. Obstruction of a deep vein, however, can cause major peripheral problems. Edema is one clinical manifestation that can indicate that degree of obstruction.

Venous Dilatation

Venous dilatation, or varicosity, is a manifestation of venous hypertension rather than a cause. Varicose veins are permanently dilated, suprafascial, tortuous veins. Although generally a result of sustained high venous pressure, varicosities may also be genetic, appearing just after adolescence. Whether the defect lies in the valve, the vein wall, or both is not fully understood.[22] Varicosities are frequently subdivided into primary and secondary, depending on whether they are due to heredity or obstruction, respectively.

Hemorrhage

A final factor contributing to venous insufficiency and ulceration is hemorrhage. Hemorrhage can actually be considered a possible concurrent problem with any of the previously identified conditions. A hematoma can develop following any hemorrhage, or there can be a significant blood loss.

Venous Ulcer Pathogenesis

Although it is accepted that venous insufficiency ulcerations result from inadequate circulation to the skin and subcutaneous tissues, the exact pathophysiology leading to ulceration remains a source of some confusion. As stated by Ennis and Meneses,[23] much greater attention has been directed toward the diagnosis and treatment of arterial disorders than to venous disorders. Reasons for this are many, but they include vascular surgeon interest and general awareness of atherosclerosis and heart disease in the general population. Another major factor addressed by Dalsing et al is the lack of an adequate animal model to study venous disease.[24]

While venous ulcer pathogenesis may not be fully understood, there is consensus that a properly functioning calf pump is critical to the healthy venous system.[25] The calf pump refers to emptying of the deep veins of the calf by contraction of the gastrocnemius and soleus muscles. This process is obviously facilitated by ambulation and can be compromised by muscular weakness, valvular incompetence, or outflow obstruction. Generally, ambulation results in a decrease in resting venous pressure. When any of the previously mentioned problems is present, however, ambulatory venous hypertension results and the likelihood of ulceration increases.

> **PEARL 16•3** When valves are functioning properly, ambulation generally helps to lower resting venous pressure. However, with valvular obstruction, outflow obstruction, or muscle weakness, venous hypertension and ulceration risks increase.

Homans' Theory

John Homans is a name closely associated with venous disease. One of the first tests taught to students when evaluating for deep vein thrombosis bears his name, Homans' sign.[26] Homans was noted for being the first individual to document the role played by incompetent valves of the communicating veins as a cause of venous ulceration.[23,27] He went on to discuss the concept of "stasis" and stated that ulceration actually developed because the stagnant blood was poorly oxygenated. Later work by Dormandy demonstrated that venous blood has a normal, if not increased, level of oxygenation.[28] Despite this new understanding, the term "venous stasis" remains in common use today.

> **PEARL 16•4** Although the concept of stasis as the cause of venous ulceration is unsubstantiated, the term "venous stasis" continues to be used.

Fibrin Cuff

Great interest surfaced in 1982 when two British researchers, Browse and Burnand, discovered the presence of a pericapillary fibrin cuff around the venous capillaries in persons with venous disease.[29] They proposed that venous hypertension secondary to a dysfunctional calf muscle pump resulted in increased loss of plasma proteins (particularly fibrinogen) through endothelial pores, and the polymerization of the fibrinogen resulted in fibrin deposition. The fibrin cuff that resulted was postulated to restrict the diffusion of oxygen into subcutaneous tissues and skin. This process is represented graphically in Figure 16.1.

Subsequent work by Michiels and Falanga et al have challenged this theory.[9,30] Michiels suggested that if the fibrin layer contained 5% fibrin, similar to that seen in a blood clot, there would be no significant impairment in oxygen delivery. Additionally, Falanga and his group showed that while fibrin cuffs did exist, they were discontinuous around the capillaries, and the venous ulcers healed even when cuffs were present.

> **PEARL 16•5** While pericapillary cuffs do exist, the degree to which they contribute to venous ulcer pathogenesis is questionable since the cuffs tend to be discontinuous and do not completely block oxygen transport.

Leukocyte Trapping

In 1988 Coleridge-Smith and colleagues postulated another theory of venous ulcer pathogenesis.[31] The theory, known as leukocyte trapping, was first suggested by Moyses et al.[32] The theory proposed that increased venous pressure altered the differential between the arteriolar and venular sides of the capillary bed, which lead to trapping of leukocytes in the postcapillary venules.[23,33,34] Evidence supports a central role for the abnormal interaction between WBCs and endothelial cells in venous ulcer pathogenesis.[35-37] Elevated

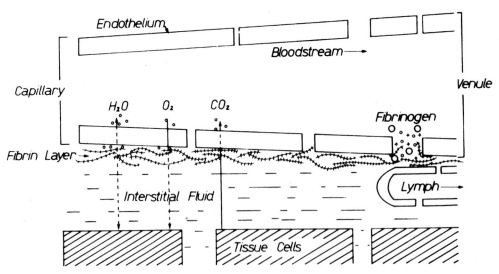

Figure 16•1 *Diagram of a capillary, showing an enlarged pore at the venous end leaking fibrinogen into the interstitial fluid, where it polymerizes to form a layer of fibrin. (From Browse and Burnand: The cause of venous ulceration. Lancet 1982; 2:244. Used with permission.)*

WBC counts have long been associated with coronary, cerebral, and peripheral vascular diseases.[38-40] In chronic venous disease, the cells become sequestrated in legs and become activated. (Fig. 16.2) During activation, they may release proteolytic enzymes that subsequently cause the formation of free radicals. The free radicals damage the capillaries, making them more permeable to large molecules and allowing additional leukocyte trapping.[31] In addition, trapped cells can act as a barrier to the diffusion of oxygen and nutrients.[41]

WBCs tend to become trapped when legs are held motionless in a dependent position.[32] Approximately 5% of the circulatory WBCs become trapped in normal individuals when the leg is held dependently. This is in contrast to 30% trapping in individuals with venous insufficiency.[42,43] Trapped cells are poorly deformable and adhere to the endothelium.

Leukocyte trapping does appear to be a controllable phenomenon. For example, when the leg is elevated, most of the WBCs return to circulation. Likewise, leukocyte trapping is decreased in individuals whose extremities are compressed.[38]

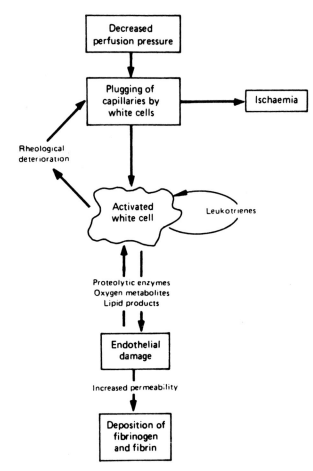

Figure **16•2** *Proposed mechanism by which trapping of white blood cells in peripheral circulation results in formation of venous ulcers. (From Coleridge Smith, P., et al: Causes of venous ulceration: A new hypothesis. Br Med J 1988; 295:172. Used with permission.)*

> ▶ **PEARL 16•6** Allowing legs to hang dependently can lead to 5% of circulating leukocytes becoming trapped in normal subjects. Fortunately, most of the cells return to circulation with leg elevation.

Ischemia-Reperfusion Theory

Following the initial work of Coleridge-Smith et al previously mentioned,[31,34] Greenwood and coworkers suggested the idea of ischemia-reperfusion as the main cause of venous ulceration.[35] They postulated that patients with chronic venous insufficiency (CVI) may have a low-level, long-term injury secondary to ischemia-reperfusion. This situation was felt to have lasted for months to years before skin ulcerated. They investigated this hypothesis through two studies. The first examined free radicals and the other ischemia-reperfusion. It was demonstrated that leg dependency caused ischemia in the venous-insufficient limb. With limb elevation, tissues were again perfused, but with perfusion came a larger release of free radicals.

It appears almost counterintuitive to suggest that reperfusion of a tissue would lead to cellular injury when perfusion is obviously necessary for tissue survival. The adverse effects, however, have been reported with organ transplantation,[44,45] cerebral vascular accidents,[46] myocardial infarction,[46,47] and other conditions.[48-50]

The mechanisms by which ischemia-reperfusion injury works is similar in all organ systems.[50] Reactive oxygen metabolites and inflammation are key components of the process. When dealing with chronic venous insufficiency, however, the situation is a bit more complicated. Individuals with CVI go through repetitive phases of ischemia-reperfusion. As the limb is held dependent, edema results, leading to tissue ischemia. Reperfusion is accomplished as the extremity is elevated or compressed. In patients who are ambulatory, this repetitive sequence of events becomes unavoidable.

Work by Vanscheidt and associates suggests that individuals with chronic venous insufficiency have circulatory WBCs that appear primed and more susceptible to activation and trapping.[51] Furthermore, the process of leukocyte trapping and ischemia-reperfusion have been found to evoke not just a local inflammatory response, but also a systemic one.[49,50,52] Better understanding of the pathophysiology of ischemia-reperfusion injury have lead to development of various management strategies, including anti-inflammatory medication, antioxidants, and compliment therapy.[49,50]

Clinical Features of Venous Disease

Venous ulceration should not be thought of as a distinct state, but rather a process that, if detected and addressed early, may prevent actual ulceration. Chen and Rogers present a progression of disease involving three overlapping stages[53]: preulceration, ulceration, and healing.

The preulceration stage is that period in which there is no visible sign of an open skin wound, but in which conditions exist that, without intervention, may result in ulceration. At this stage, there is evidence of an increased proliferation of fibrous tissue and signs of oxidative stress. As fibrosclerosis worsens, the skin takes on an indurated quality termed *lipodermatosclerosis*.

In acute inflammatory states, this may be mistaken for bacterial cellulitis.[16] Skin pigment changes such as hemosiderosis may be evident with or without associated edema.

> ▶ **PEARL 16•7** In acute inflammatory states, lipodermatosclerosis can be mistaken for bacterial cellulitis.

Hemosiderosis occurs when red blood cells leak from the capillaries, become trapped in the pericapillary tissue, and undergo lysis, causing the release of the pigment hemosiderin from the hemoglobin.

Treatment approaches during this stage typically involve elevation, compression, exercise, and possibly vein surgery. Some success has been reported with pharmaceutical management with such agents as aspirin, escin, hydroxyethylrutoside, Daflon®, and pentoxifylline.[53-56]

The ulcerative stage of venous disease occurs when inflammation increases to the point that the balance between fibrous tissue proliferation and tissue damage tips toward damage. It is suggested by Chen and Rogers that the ulcers actually may become chronic due to this imbalance persisting and tissue destruction surpassing tissue deposition.[53] The classic presentation of a venous ulcer is one involving the medial leg (gaiter region) and is irregular in shape, with well-defined borders.[57] The ulcer depth tends to be partial thickness, and the borders are erythematous. Hyperpigmented periwound skin, noted during the preulcer stage, persists. The wound base takes on a very convoluted appearance, and granulation tissue begins to proliferate. Depending on the stage of ulcer development and the exudate levels, fibrin deposits may be evident in the wound base. (Fig. 16.3)

Venous ulcers are typically more shallow and less painful than ischemic ulcers of comparable size. Size varies greatly, although the fascia and deep structures are not usually exposed. The borders are flat, slopping into a shallow crater, with epithelium visible at the borders as healing occurs. During highly exudative stages, the periwound skin may be wet and eczematous. (Fig. 16.4)

Venous ulcers tend to develop slowly and can exist for years, even decades. Repeated episodes of infection and cellulitis often

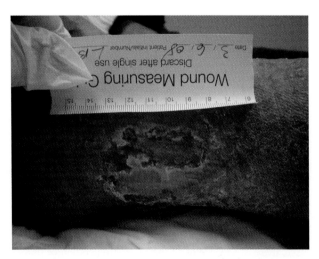

Figure 16•3 *Venous ulceration with fibrin deposition.*

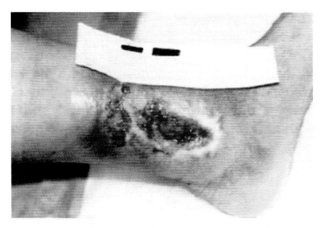

Figure 16•4 *Appearance of venous insufficiency ulcer at admission.*

result in damage to the lymphatic system and subsequent lymphedema. Additionally, substantial loss of ankle function can occur because of fibrosis and bony anklylosis.[7]

Not all medial malleolar ulcers are caused by this disease. Sindrup and associates demonstrated that up to 50% of patients with medial leg ulceration had an active arterial component to the disease.[58] Other conditions such as vasculitis, cryofibrinogenemia, basal cell and squamous cell carcinoma, and antiphospholipid syndrome can result in similar ulcerations.[59,60] Any ulcer that does not respond to appropriate conservative therapy should have a biopsy performed to obtain a definitive diagnosis.

The third stage of CVI to ulceration discussed by Chen and Rogers is the healing stage. This stage requires that the deposition-destruction imbalance swings back toward deposition. Current evidence suggests that in order for this to occur, the hostile chronic wound environment must be improved. In order to accomplish this, a multidisciplinary approach is encouraged.[61] This involves fluid management in the wound bed, edema management in the extremity, and possible surgical management of the venous system.

Venous Ulcer Management

The mainstay of management for CVI and ulceration is compression therapy. The importance of the topic warrants its independent discussion in Chapter 29. In addition to compression therapy, attention must be directed to management of the ulcer and other means besides compression that can affect calf pump function.

Dressings

Selecting the proper dressing for a venous ulcer is no different from selecting dressings for any other type of wound. The principle is always to select the dressing that can maintain the proper wound moisture balance. The dressing selected will vary depending on wound size and level of exudation. Venous ulcers traditionally tend to be very moist. This is especially true in the more chronic stages of the disease process when ulcers can be quite large. In such instances, a highly absorbent dressing such as thick foam, calcium alginate, or hydrofiber are often indicated. In situations in which significant fibrin deposition is present, hydrocolloid dressings may be useful in facilitating autolytic débridement. In all cases, the dressing selected should be able to be used in concert with compression therapy. Other dressing options are presented in detail in Chapter 12.

Exercise

As noted previously, calf muscle pump dysfunction is a central causative factor in development of venous ulcerations. Any condition leading to diminished calf pump function is thereby contributing to the problem.

From a rehabilitation perspective, several things must be considered. The first is ankle range of motion. As noted by Belczak et al, patients with C6 disease (active ulceration) had significantly decreased motion at the talocrural joint compared to other groups.[62] Whether the loss of motion led to the calf pump dysfunction or was a result of it remains to be determined. It should be obvious, however, that restricted ankle mobility leads to changes in both stride length and effective contraction of the calf musculature. Placing patients on walking and stretching program should be beneficial.

Several researchers have also examined the effects of exercise on improved calf muscle function. Yang et al noted that calf ejection fractions increased and residual fractions decreased when patients were placed into an intensive 6-week exercise program that involved a series of heel rises with the ball of the feet elevated 5 cm on a step.[63] Although calf function was improved, there was no change in venous reflux.

Padberg et al also studied the effects of calf muscle pump functioning with exercise.[64] Thirty-one patients were randomized into a control ($n = 13$) or exercise ($n = 18$) group. All patients were supplied with compression hosiery (30–40 mm Hg). The exercise group received physical therapy consisting of isokinetic exercise. Improved calf muscle pump function, similar to that reported by Yang et al, was noted. In addition, improved dynamic calf strength after a 6-month program was demonstrated.

▶ Case Study 16•1 — Ulceration Secondary to Venous Insufficiency

A 42-year-old white female presents with an ulcer on the medial aspect of the left ankle as demonstrated in Figure 16.4. The ulcer has been present for several months, and the patient has been trying to manage the drainage and swelling with gauze bandages and elastic wraps. The patient stated that she had experienced ulcers previously in the same location and that they had healed and recurred on several occasions. Ulcer pain was reported at 3/10. This worsens slightly with prolonged standing and improves with leg elevation and bedrest. Most recently, the condition began to worsen because the patient began a new job as a department store greeter. This requires her to spend long hours standing.

Drainage from the wound has been moderate to heavy, and the periwound tissue has begun to macerate. No infection is evident at the present time, and there are no signs of deep vein thrombosis or arterial compromise. Swelling is noted in the left lower extremity, and calf girth is 2 cm greater on the left than the right. Range of motion of the left ankle is limited by a 5-degree plantarflexion contracture.

Initial efforts in treatment were aimed at reducing lower extremity swelling. This was handled by using intermittent pneumatic compression (50 mm Hg for 30 minutes) followed by application of a hydrofiber dressing and an Unna boot, which was changed weekly. At clinic visits, the wound was cleansed with pulsatile lavage with suction and a new dressing and compression wrap applied. Within 2 weeks, drainage reduced considerably, and periwound maceration began to resolve. Loss of ankle motion was addressed by stretching and a treadmill walking program.

Figure 16.5 is a photograph of the lower extremity after 4 weeks of compression therapy, then again after the ulcer had completely resolved. At this point, the patient was fitted for custom gradient support stockings with instructions to have the stockings refitted every 6 to 12 months to prevent ulcer recurrence.

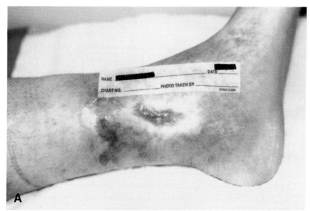

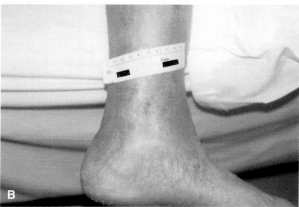

Figure 16•5 *Appearance of limb (A) after several weeks of compression therapy. (B) When healed.*

Summary

In discussing venous ulcer etiology, it is best to think of the wound not as a disease, but rather as a manifestation of disease. The disease actually progresses "silently" until signs of preulceration develop. If appropriate interventions don't occur, the patient goes on to skin ulceration.

In this chapter, an overview of the most common theories of venous insufficiency have been presented. The stages of ulcer development have been discussed and interventions outlined that, when combined with effective compression therapy, frequently lead to ulcer resolution.

The chronic nature of venous ulcers means that quite often many health-care professionals may be involved in caring for a particular patient. Interdisciplinary communication is essential to the team approach and is the key to coordinated wound management education. When wound closure is successful, the patient must not be led to think that the disease is cured. This becomes instead a life-long disease process that can be managed with compliant care.

References

1. Trent, JT, Falabella, A, Eaglstein, WH, et al: Venous ulcers: Pathophysiology and treatment options. Ostomy Wound Manage 2005; 51:38-53.
2. Samson, H, Showalter, D: Stockings and the prevention of recurrent venous ulcers. Dermatol Surg 1996; 22:373–376.
3. Vanhoutte, P, Corcaud, S, DeMontrion, C: The demographics of venous disease of the lower limbs. Angiology 1997; 48:557–558.
4. Ruckley, C: Socioeconomic impact of chronic venous insufficiency and leg ulcers. Angiology 1997; 48:67–69.
5. Margolis, DJ, Bilker, W, Santanna, J, et al: Venous leg ulcer: Incidence and prevalence in the elderly. J Am Acad Dermatol 2002; 46:381–386.
6. Anderson, E, Hansson C and Swanbeck G: Leg and foot ulcer prevalence and investigation of the peripheral arterial and venous circulation in a randomized elderly population: An epidemiological survey and clinical investigation. Acta Derm Venereol Suppl (Stockh) 1993; 73:57–61.
7. Phillips, T, Dover, J: Leg ulcers. J Am Acad Dermatol 1991; 25:965–987.
8. Van De Graaff, K: Human Anatomy, ed. 3. Dubuque, IA, William C. Brown, 2002, p 805.
9. Michiels, C, Arnould, T, Janssens, D: Interactions between endothelial cells and smooth muscle cells after their activation by hypoxia: A possible etiology for venous disease. Int Angiol 1996; 15:124–130.
10. Grollman, S (ed): The Human Body: Its Structure and Physiology, ed. 2. New York, Macmillan, 1969, p 191.
11. Starr, C (ed): Basic Concepts in Biology, ed. 4. Pacific Grove, CA, Brooks/Cole, 2000, p 565.
12. Lofgren, E: Chronic venous insufficiency. In: Spittel, J (ed): Clinical Vascular Disease. Philadelphia, FA Davis, 1983, p 135.
13. Oates, C: Cardiovascular Haemodynamics and Dopple Waveforms Explained. New York, Cambridge University Press, 2001, p 192.
14. Moore, K, Dalley, A: Clinically Oriented Anatomy. Philadelphia, Lippincott Williams & Wilkins, 2006, p 1248.
15. Hannson, C: Optimal treatment of venous (stasis) ulcers in elderly patients. Drugs Aging 1994; 5:323–334.
16. Coleridge-Smith, P: Pathogenesis of chronic venous insufficiency and possible effects of compression and pentoxifylline. Yale J Biol Med 1993; 66:47–59.
17. Niren, A, Bergan, J: Chronic venous ulcer. BMJ 1997; 314:1019–1022.
18. Nicolaides, AN, Hussein, MK, Szendro, G, et al: The relation of venous ulceration with ambulatory venous pressure measurements. J Vasc Surg 1993; 17:414–419.
19. Whiston, R, Hallett, MB, Davies, EV, et al: Inappropriate neutrophil activation in venous disease. Br J Surg 1994; 81:695–698.
20. Johnson, B, Manzo, R, Bergelin, R, et al: Relationship between changes in the deep venous system and the development of the postthrombotic syndrome after an acute episode of lower limb deep vein thrombosis: A one-to-six-year follow-up. J Vasc Surg 1995; 21:307–313.
21. Kahn, S, Ginsberg, J: Relationship between deep venous thrombosis and the postthrombotic syndrome. Arch Intern Med 2004; 164:17–26.
22. Regan, B, Folse, R: Lower limb venous dynamics in normal persons and children with varicose veins. Surg Gynecol Obstet 1971; 132:15–18.
23. Ennis, W, Meneses, P: Standard, appropriate, and advanced care and medical-legal considerations: Venous ulcerations. Wounds 2003; 15(Pt 2):107–122.
24. Dalsing, M, Ricotta, J, Wakefield, T, et al: Animal models for the study of lower-extremity chronic venous disease: Lessons learned and future needs. Ann Vasc Surg 1998; 12:487–498.
25. Browse, NL, Burnand, KG, Irvine, AT, et al (eds.): Physiology and functional anatomy. In: Diseases of the Veins. London, Arnold Publisher, 1999, pp 49–65.
26. Baker, W: Diagnosis of deep venous thrombosis and pulmonary embolism. Med Clin NA 1998; 82:459–476.
27. Homans, J: The etiology and treatment of varicose ulcers of the leg. Surg Gynecol Obstet 1917; 24:300–311.
28. Dormandy, J: Pathophysiology of venous leg ulceration-an update. Angiology 1997; 48:71–75.
29. Browse, N, Burnand, K: The cause of venous ulceration. Lancet 1982; 2:243–245.
30. Falanga, V, Kirsner, R, Katz, MH, et al.: Pericapillary fibrin cuffs in venous ulceration: Persistence with treatment and during ulcer healing. J Dermatol Surg 1992; 18:409–414.
31. Coleridge-Smith, P, Thomas, P, Scurr, JH, et al: Causes of venous ulceration: A new hypothesis. BMJ 1988; 296:1726–1727.
32. Moyses, C, Cederholm-Williams, S, Michel, C: Haemoconcentration and the accumulation of white cells in the feet during venous stasis. Int J Microcirc Clin Exp 1987; 5:311–320.
33. Cheatle, TR, Scott, HJ, Scurr, JH, et al: White cells, skin blood flow, and venous ulcers. Br J Dermatol 1991; 125:288–290.
34. Coleridge-Smith, P: The causes of skin damage and leg ulceration in chronic venous disease. Int J Low Extrem Wounds 2006; 5:160–168.
35. Greenwood, J, Edwards, A, McCollum, C: The possible role of ischemia-reperfusion in the pathogenesis of chronic venous ulceration. Wounds 1995; 7:211–219.
36. Nash, G, Shearman, C: Neutrophils and peripheral arterial disease. Crit Ischemia 1992; 2:15–20.
37. Nicolaides, A: Chronic venous disease and the leukocyte endothelium interaction: From symptoms to ulceration. Angiology 2005; 56(suppl):s11–s19.
38. Bradbury, A, Murie, J, Ruckley, C: Role of the leukocyte in the pathogenesis of vascular disease. Br J Surg 1993; 80:1503–1512.
39. Jackson, M, Collier, A, Nicoll, JJ, et al: Neutrophil count and activation in vascular disease. Scott Med J 1992; 37:41–43.
40. Greenberg, D, Simon, R, Aminoff, M: Clinical Neurology, ed. 7. New York, McGraw Hill, 2005, p 297.
41. Franzeck, U, Bollinger, A, Huch, R, et al: Transcutaneous oxygen tension and capillary morphologic characteristics and density in patients with chronic venous incompetence. Circulation 1984; 70:806–811.
42. Thomas, P, Nash, G, Dormandy, J: White cell accumulation in the dependent legs of patients with venous hypertension: A possible

mechanism for trophic changes in the skin. BMJ 1992; 296:1693–1695.

43. Loosemore, T, Dormand, J: Etiology and Pathophysiology of Leukocyte Adhesion. Oxford, Oxford University Press, 1995, p 447.

44. Ng, C, Wan, S, Yim, A: Pulmonary ischaemia-reperfusion injury: Role of apoptosis. Eur Respir J 2005; 25:356–363.

45. Kupiec-Weglinski, J, Busuttil, R: Ischemia and reperfusion injury in liver transplantation. Transplant Proc 2005; 37:1653–1656.

46. Schaller, B, Graf, R: Cerebral ischemia and reperfusion: The pathophysiologic concept as a basis for clinical therapy. J Cereb Blood Flow Metab 2004; 24:351–371.

47. Moens, A, Claeys, M, Timmermans, J, et al: Myocardial ischemia/reperfusion-injury, a clinical view on a complex pathophysiological process. Int J Cardiol 2005; 100:179–190.

48. Kong, S, Biennerhassett, L, Heel, K: Ischaemia-reperfusion injury to the intestine. Aust N Z J Surg 1998; 68:554–561.

49. Eltzschig, H, Collard, C: Vascular ischaemia and reperfusion injury. Br Med Bull 2004; 70:71–86.

50. Mustoe, T, O'Shaughnessy, K, Kloeters, O: Chronic wound pathogenesis and current treatment strategies: A unifying hypothesis. Plast Reconstr Surg 2006; 117:35S–41S.

51. Vanscheidt, W: Leg ulcer patients: No decreased fibrinolytic response but white cell trapping after venous occlusion of the upper limb. Phlebology 1992; 7:92–96.

52. Calam, M: Arterial disease in chronic leg ulceration: An underestimated hazard. Lothian and Forth Valley leg ulcer study. BMJ 1987; 294:929–931.

53. Chen, W, Rogers, A: Recent insights into the causes of chronic leg ulceration in venous diseases and implications on other types of chronic wounds. Wound Rep Regen 2007; 15:434–449.

54. Layton, A, Ibbotson, SH, Davies, JA, et al: Randomised trial of oral aspirin for chronic venous leg ulcers. Lancet 1994; 344:164–165.

55. Flick, R: Three treatments for chronic venous insufficiency; escin, hydrosyethylrutoside, and Daflon. Angiology 2000; 51:197–205.

56. Jull, A, Waters, J, Arroll, B: Pentoxifylline for treatment of venous leg ulcers: A systematic review. Lancet 2002; 359:1550–1554.

57. Zimmet, S: Venous leg ulcers: Modern evaluation and management. Dermatol Surg 1999; 3(suppl):S1–S12.

58. Sindrup, J, Groth, S, Antrop C, et al: Coexistence of obstructive arterial disease and chronic venous stasis in leg ulcer patients. Exp Dermatol 1987; 12:410–412.

59. Falanga, V: Venous ulceration. J Dermatol Surg Oncol 1993; 19:764–771.

60. Phillips, T, Salman, S, Rogers, G: Nonhealing leg ulcers: A manifestation of basal cell carcinoma. J Am Acad Dermatol 1991; 25:47–49.

61. Schultz, G, Sibbald, R, Falanga V, et al: Wound bed preparation: A systematic approach. Wound Rep Regen 2003; 11(suppl):S1–S28.

62. Belczak, C, Cavalheri, G, Jr, de Godoy, JMP, et al: Relationship between talocrural joint mobility and venous ulcer. Jornal Vascular Brasileiro 2007; 6:2.

63. Yang, D, Vandongen, Y, Stacey, M: Effect of exercise on calf muscle pump function in patients with chronic venous disease. Br J. Surg 1999; 86:338–344.

64. Padberg, F, Johnston, M, Sisto, S: Structured exercise improves calf muscle pump function in chronic venous insufficiency: A randomized trial. J Vasc Surg 2004; 39:79–87.

chapter 17

Conservative Management of Arterial Ulceration

Amy M. Brogle, MSPT, CWS

In order to be effective in the challenging environment of chronic extremity ulcer management, clinicians must have a thorough understanding of arterial disease in its presentation and management. Venous wounds account for a majority of lower-extremity ulcerations in industrialized countries (approximately 80%–90%). Within that population, mixed disease presentation, or the presence of both venous and arterial insufficiency is estimated to occur in about 25% of those cases.[1,2] This chapter provides a framework for evaluation and treatment of arterial ulceration.

Pathophysiology, Etiology of Arterial Insufficiency

Oxygen is essential in the air we breathe and in the most basic cellular processes: It sustains life on innumerable physiological levels. Ischemia, or the lack of oxygen via blood supply to the body's tissues, is the fundamental problem underlying arterial insufficiency (AI). Common nomenclature exists, and the terms arterial insufficiency, arterial disease, peripheral vascular disease (PVD), and peripheral arterial disease (PAD) may be used interchangeably. Clearly, "PVD" is a less specific term, as the reference may be venous or arterial, and "AI" or "PAD" is preferred in medical communication.

Ischemia may affect any tissue of the body; it may be classified as cerebral, visceral, or, as in the focus of this chapter, peripheral. Cerebral ischemia is seen most commonly with a cerebrovascular accident (CVA), or thrombolytic stroke, whereas visceral ischemia may affect any organ system from

gastrointestinal, as seen with ischemic bowel, to cardiac, with myocardial infarction. Peripheral ischemia, or PAD, manifests as claudication and extremity ulceration.

PAD is a broad term used to describe a number of disorders that ultimately lead to reduction of blood flow to the extremities. Symptoms occur when the arterial lumen is narrowed by greater than 50%.[3] Patients may be asymptomatic, even with greater than 50% blockage. A thorough examination is key to detection. This narrowing may occur as a result of atherosclerotic plaque formation, primary or secondary inflammatory states, thrombus, or a combination of these. Severity of PAD may be quantified using grading systems such as the older Fontaine system,[4,5] which reports severity in terms of patient symptoms, or the more recent Rutherford categories.[4,6,7] The Rutherford categories offer traditional grades that are advised for clinical use and categories that are intended for use in clinical research.[7] With each of these tools, the most severe classifications are tissue loss, ulceration, and gangrene. (Tables 17.1 and 17.2)

> **PEARL 17•1** Individuals with PAD may be asymptomatic, even with greater than 50% blockage.

Tissue ischemia may be viewed in categories according to acuity and cause. First, ischemic states may be reached acutely through thrombosis, embolism, or constriction secondary to excessive pressures (ie, compartment syndrome). Cases of acute ischemia are medical emergencies. In contrast, chronic causes such as arteriosclerosis obliterans

Table 17•1 Fontaine System for Grading Peripheral Arterial Disease[4]

Stage	Description
I	Asymptomatic
IIa	Mild claudication
IIb	Moderate-severe claudication
III	Ischemic rest pain
IV	Ulceration or gangrene

Table 17•2 Rutherford System for Grading Peripheral Arterial Disease[4,6,8]

Grade	Category	Description
0	0	Asymptomatic
I	1	Mild claudication
I	2	Moderate claudication
I	3	Severe claudication
II	4	Ischemic rest pain
III	5	Minor tissue loss—nonhealing ulcer
III	6	Major tissue loss—gangrene above metatarsals

will characteristically develop over a number of years.[9] Estimates suggest a 20% prevalence of PAD in those older than 70 years of age.[10,11] Surprisingly, approximately 70% to 80% of these individuals will be asymptomatic.[12,13] In these individuals collateralization, or development of supplementary flow around a blocked site, is the likely explanation for the lack of symptomatology. It is also a differentiating factor between chronic and acute arterial disease.[3]

Classes of PAD

In addition to classification as acute or chronic, a number of underlying causes may contribute to arterial disease. The most common classes are occlusive, inflammatory, and vasomotor.[14] Often, these will overlap, but will be described distinctly for understanding. Another classification used is organic versus functional. Organic causes of arterial disease are structural alterations that lead to occlusion, such as blockage due to tissue damage or chronic inflammation. Functional causes, on the other hand, refer to short-term, nonstructural changes such as vasospasm that is seen temporarily in Raynaud's disease.[15]

Occlusive disease results primarily from atherosclerosis; examples include arteriosclerosis obliterans, arterial thrombosis, and arterial embolism. These are classified as *organic PAD*. *Inflammatory* disorders, often referred to as vasculitides, include polyarteritis nodosa, arteritis, hypersensitivity arteritis, Takayasu's arteritis, and thromboangiitis obliterans. Systemic inflammatory states, such as systemic lupus erythematosus (SLE) and dermatomyositis, may also have extremity manifestations and relative arterial insufficiency.

The most common among the *vasomotor* disorders to be recognized clinically are Raynaud's phenomenon, reflex sympathetic dystrophy (RSD), acrocyanosis, and erythromelalgia. This group of disorders may also be described as *functional* PAD, referring to the altered sympathetic control of vasomotor responses to the environment.[14] Arterial aneurysm may also be classified among the vasomotor disorders for the purpose of this chapter, but is defined as a dilative disorder that will be unlikely to cause tissue necrosis as compared to the aforementioned diseases. Table 17.3 summarizes the classifications to be discussed in greater detail.

Arteriosclerosis Obliterans

The most common occlusive disease, accounting for about 95% of cases of PAD, is arteriosclerosis obliterans.[3,14] It is also the most significant disease in terms of ulcer development.[16] The underlying cause of obstruction is atherosclerosis.

Table 17•3 Classification of Arterial Insufficiency

Obstructive (Organic)	Inflammatory (Organic)	Vasomotor (Functional)
Arteriosclerosis obliterans	Thromboangiitis obliterans	Raynaud's disease
Thromboangiitis obliterans*	Vasculitis	Acrocyanosis
Sickle cell disease	• Polyarteritis nodosa	Erythromelalgia
Acute obstruction	• Systemic lupus erythematosus	
• Emboli	• Takayasu's arteritis	
• Thrombus		
• Compartment syndrome		

* Thromboangiitis Obliterans may be classified as both inflammatory and obstructive.

▶ **PEARL 17•2** *Arteriosclerosis* and *atherosclerosis* will often be used interchangeably; while this is often acceptable, there are distinctions. Arteriosclerosis is simply hardening of the arteries, or loss of arterial wall elasticity. Atherosclerosis, the most common form of arteriosclerosis, refers to plaques of fatty deposits, or "atheromas," forming in the intima of the arteries.

Atherosclerosis gradually develops as fatty streaks build up on the normally smooth endothelial vessel lining. A number of factors may contribute to this phenomenon. First, arterial wall damage occurs secondary to noxious substances in blood or by the physical stress of hypertension. Next, larger molecules from the blood, such as cholesterol, may enter and collect in the area as the lining is now more jagged. At the same time, a platelet aggregation response will attempt to plug up this "injured" site. While this physical obstruction forms, biochemical changes further increase risk of occlusion. Among these changes is the attraction of white blood ells (WBCs) via the inflammatory response. The resultant plaque that forms may be stable or unstable. A stable clot will statically contribute to occluding the arterial lumen and reduce perfusion to distal tissues. An unstable clot may ultimately dislodge into a thrombotic occlusion in a smaller distal vessel or an embolization.[17] Defined simply by the American Heart Association, a thrombus is a blood clot that forms inside a blood vessel or cavity of the heart, and an embolus is a blood clot that moves through the bloodstream until it lodges in a narrowed vessel and blocks circulation.[18]

This pathophysiology of plaque development seen in PAD is the same as in development of coronary artery disease (CAD). This means there is substantial risk of coronary artery or cardiac compromise in patients who are diagnosed with peripheral vascular disease. In addition, PAD has been shown to be an independent predictor of cardiovascular complications and death.[19,20] This correlation is crucial for the health professional to understand. When treating those who have undiagnosed PAD, but have significant coronary history, suspicion and caution is warranted. The reverse also holds true; those patients who are undergoing treatment for PAD and report "no heart trouble" are in need of education about the close relationship between PAD and coronary disease, as well as their modifiable risk factors.[3,4] The most influential of the modifiable risk factors for PAD are smoking, diabetes, hypertension, and hyperlipidemia.[21-25] Additional risk factors identified for PAD are summarized in Table 17.4.[4]

Many would suspect limb amputation to be the major threat to this group, but the true threats to life expectancy are cerebrovascular and cardiovascular events such as heart attack and stroke.[13] Large-scale studies such as the ATTEST study, which took place in France in 2003, confirm this misconception. In a population of patients with known atherosclerotic disease (PAD and CAD), cardiovascular risk was consistently underestimated and undertreated, and amputation risk was overestimated in the group with diagnosed PAD.[26]

Studies have shown that 84% to 90% of patients with PAD are current or past smokers.[27,28] Smoking is closely linked with arterial risk due to its chemical effects on smooth muscle, resultant systemic vasoconstriction, and inflammation.

Table 17•4 Risk Factors for Peripheral Arterial Disease

Nonmodifiable	Modifiable
Age >70	Smoking
Male gender	Diabetes
Diabetes*	Hypertension
Hypercoagulable states	Hypercholesterolemia
Hyperhomocysteinemia	Obesity

*There is a "non-modifiable" risk of diabetes due to family history, yet the onset of type 2 diabetes is impacted by factors such as diet and exercise.

▶ **PEARL 17•3** Circulation may improve in just 4 weeks after smoking cessation. In 1 year, the risk of coronary heart disease and heart attack is cut in half.

Diabetes is also prevalent in this population. According to the Framingham Heart Study, glucose intolerance with diabetes has been shown to be more strongly related to development of claudication than CAD or CVA. These patients may have three to four times more risk of PAD than their nondiabetic age matches.[22] As in atherosclerotic plaque development, hypertension can increase risk of PAD if not controlled, with risk increasing as hypertension increases.[19,23,24]

Vascular surgery is often indicated to preserve distal flow in this group; options discussed further in this chapter include open and endovascular techniques such as bypass grafting, stenting, angioplasty, and thrombolytic procedures.

Intermittent Claudication

Intermittent claudication is a hallmark symptom of arterial insufficiency. It is defined as cramping of the calf, thigh, or buttock brought on by a specific amount of activity, usually walking, which relents within 5 to 10 minutes if the patient rests.[29] Symptoms are often correlated with the patient's ankle-brachial index (ABI) value, or the comparison of systolic flow to the ankle compared to the upper arm. These findings may give indications of prognosis or disease severity. Intermittent claudication may begin to manifest when patients have an ABI value of less than 0.8.[30]

So what is claudication pain exactly? Imagine the calf pump pushing blood back to the heart during ambulation, assuming an intact venous system. Blood is drained out of working muscles with each contraction. In the healthy state, arteries pump new blood in with equal efficiency to fuel the working muscles with oxygen and nutrients. As activity progresses in an insufficient arterial state, the refill phase cannot match the venous return. The total blood and oxygen available to the muscles diminishes because the inflow is less than the outflow. An ischemic state results; muscles feel strangulated, and this is significantly painful. Local sensory receptors may be activated due to accumulation of lactate and other metabolites.[3] Rest allows the arterial system to catch up and refill the thirsty muscle, thereby providing relief. Since metabolic needs of the muscle help drive claudication onset, increasing intensity of activity on stairs or an incline will induce pain faster in these patients.

▸ **PEARL 17•4** Exercise can actually help to decrease the "supply versus demand" imbalance in ischemic conditions.

Cramping pain that is not triggered by activity, but rather brought on by rest, known as "rest pain," is typical of an ABI value of less than 0.5.[30] This pain may be constant and is often worse at night. Patients will report sleeping with their legs over the side of the bed or have a very difficult time maintaining antigravity positions. Now picture the system under no exertional stress; the arteries are *still* unable to keep up with the oxygen needs of the muscle. This state may be indicative of the patient with "critical limb ischemia."[8,31] At this point, surgical consultation is essential as patients with rest pain are among the group more likely to progress to surgery or amputation.[32]

The location of claudication pain may also clue the clinician as to the anatomical site of occlusion. Pain in the buttocks or thigh is likely due to aortoiliac disease, or Leriche's syndrome. This is a syndrome seen mostly in men. It is a narrowing or blockage of the lower aorta where it divides into the common iliac arteries.[30] Calf pain is associated with femoral-popliteal obstruction.[32] Foot and arch pain is associated with distal obstruction of the plantar and tibial arteries.

When claudication is suspected, musculoskeletal evaluation should rule out other causes, such as spinal stenosis. With stenosis, pain in the legs will not be as predictable, will take longer to recover or require seated rest position, and will not be triggered in flexed walking postures when the foramen is allowed space.[33] The patient with venous insufficiency will have distinct patterns of activity tolerance as well. Table 17.5 summarizes differential diagnosis of claudication.

Treatment of claudication by pharmacological means and with supervised exercise has been shown to improve patient's quality of life.[34-36] Such pain is known to be significantly disabling to everyday life. Standardized scales that reflect the HRQOL (health-related quality of life) and are validated for functional evaluation of patients with claudication include the SF-36 (Medical Outcomes Study) and the WIQ (Walking Impairment Questionnaire).[35,37,38]

Supervised exercise is well supported in the literature as a primary treatment for claudication; this is shown in over 20 randomized controlled trials (RCTs).[5,34,36] It has been shown to be superior to pharmacological means. Even with this evidence, programs are infrequently used due to lack of third-party reimbursement, patient convenience, and motivation for hospital-based programs.[5] Successful supervised exercise programs are advised to be at least three times weekly, with short bouts of treadmill walking over a 50- to 60-minute period, with monitoring of maximum walking time and distance. The structured exercise provides benefits due to improved oxygen metabolism, angiogenesis for collateral circulation, improved blood viscosity, or simply improvement of walking economy.[35] In comparison to casual recommendations to increase activity and walk daily, supervised programs have repeatedly proved superior. One study did report favorable calf muscle characteristics among patients with PAD who reported higher general activity levels, and therefore advice regarding daily walking or activity is not necessarily insignificant.[39]

Thromboangiitis Obliterans

Thromboangiitis obliterans (TOA), or Buerger's disease, is the next most prevalent of the arterial occlusive diseases. It has been estimated that 12 to 20 cases per 100,000 are diagnosed annually.[40] The major risk group includes male smokers between 20 and 45 years of age.[41,42] The disease differs from arteriosclerosis obliterans (AO) in that atheromas are not the primary cause of obstruction. Distal ischemia of the upper and lower extremities is linked with vasoconstriction and inflammation of the small- and medium-sized arteries and veins, which causes obstruction and may be accompanied by thrombus formation.[14]

Table 17•5 **Differential Diagnosis of Leg Pain and Claudication**			
	Intermittent Claudication	**Spinal Stenosis**	**Venous Insufficiency**
Type of pain	Cramping/throbbing	Burning or shooting pain with weakness	Heavy, achy pain
Pain location	Calf, thigh, or buttock	Along dermatome distribution down leg	Thigh or groin most commonly, sometimes calf
Onset	Predictable walking distance Onset sooner with incline/stairs	After walking; may or may not be predictable distance Able to walk farther on incline[34]	With prolonged dependency and walking
Relieving factors	Rest, legs dependent	Sitting Flexed spine posture, longer rest periods	Elevation of extremity
Other	Reproducible with walking distance or sooner with high intensities Presence of other arterial signs	May be unpredictable; rest alone may not improve unless spine angle changes	Likely have other signs of venous insufficiency, edema, varicosities

▶ **PEARL 17•5** It is rare for a non-nicotine user to have thromboangiitis obliterans.

Classically, these patients will present with involvement of two or more extremities. Clinical presentation may begin with claudication pain that occurs in the arch of the foot due to plantar and tibial artery involvement.[33] It is important to differentiate these reports from plantar fasciitis, which will have characteristic pain that is worse in the morning and is local to the plantar fascia insertion on the calcaneus.[43] They may initially present with multiple distal lesions or gangrene. When TOA is suspected, arteriography of bilateral upper and lower extremities is useful. Arteriography in this group will demonstrate presence of "corkscrew collaterals," or small winding collateral circulation around sites of occlusion. This collateralization typically is not as effective in prevention of symptoms and necrosis as it is with arteriosclerosis. Arteriography will also reveal characteristic proximal flow preservation and marked distal occlusion.[41]

Many patients diagnosed with TOA experience multiple digit amputations. Absolute smoking cessation is the only known method of risk reduction, prevention of disease progression, and prevention of amputation. The major long-term risk for patients with TOA is amputation if they continue to smoke; there is not a direct threat to life expectancy as seen in arteriosclerosis obliterans.[41] Vascular surgery is not generally indicated, as there is little chance of locating a distal vessel with sufficient integrity to receive a bypass graft or stent.

Sickle Cell Disease

Sickle cell disease may be classified as an occlusive vascular disorder that affects both the arterial and venous systems. Extremity wounds are highly prevalent in this population. Red blood cells become rigid when bound to sickled hemoglobin and deoxygenated at the capillary level.[16] These sickled red blood cells become trapped and cause physical obstruction of capillary beds in addition to biochemical changes that cause local tissue ischemia.[44] These obstructions may occur in the skin or in organ systems. Patients may present with chronic hypoxemia of the skin due to the above microvascular changes in the skin, compounded by systemic hypoxemia from the pulmonary system. The pulmonary system influences wound healing since fibrosis and organ ischemia are sequelae of the disease process.[44,45] Although an ischemic state is a factor in these wounds, they more often present clinically with signs of venous insufficiency. Management of these wounds therefore relies on edema control and should follow guidelines for management of venous insufficiency (VI) in correlation with clinical examination findings. Bedrest and elevation during a sickle cell pain crisis with ulceration is suggested.[46]

Acute Occlusion

Acute interruption of blood flow to an extremity is a medical emergency. Vessel blockage may be precipitated by embolus from a proximal source or a local thrombus. In either case, prognosis of limb salvage will depend greatly on length of time from injury to reperfusion. An embolism will classically present with the five P's: pistol shot (acute pain onset), pale, painful, pulseless, paresthetic leg. A sixth P is added often:

poikilothermia, meaning cooling of the limb to the ambient temperature.[47] Embolus maybe diagnosed in patients without prior PAD but with significant coronary history in which a clot dislodges from the aorta or heart and gets trapped at a distal bifurcation, causing sudden interruption of flow without collateral backup. Thrombosis, on the other hand, is the more common cause of acute ischemia and is seen in patients with preexisting claudication, which rapidly declines as a thrombus is added on top of an already narrowed arterial lumen. This may be referred to as "acute on chronic ischemia." Thrombosis, unfortunately, is also linked with acute graft occlusion following peripheral bypass grafting.[48]

▶ **PEARL 17•6** If circulation is not restored 6 to 8 hours following onset of paresthesia with vessel blockage, the risk of amputation is high.

Medical management involves embolectomy or open surgical revascularization if neurological deficits are present.[47] Other options include catheter-directed thrombolytic therapy (CDT) and percutaneous isolated limb perfusion (PILP), which is delivery of high-dose antithrombolytics to a localized vascular bed.[49]

Trauma may also threaten distal perfusion and limb viability, as seen in compartment syndromes. Compartment syndromes have been documented following trauma of lower extremity fractures, as well as ankle sprains, or as a result of exertional stress in athletes.[50-52] They differ from acute arterial occlusive etiologies in that the arteries, veins, and nerves are compressed by edema and high tissue pressures. When suspected, assessment of pulses, sensation, and motor function will predict limb salvage. Surgical management involves fasciotomy and subsequent wound care as indicated. (Fig. 17.1)

Vasculitides

Inflammatory causes of peripheral ischemia are recognized widely. Each of the necrotizing vasculitides, or vasculitis, vary greatly in presentation and often have characteristic systemic organ manifestations. In general, the term *vasculitis* broadly defines disorders of inflammation and necrosis of blood vessel walls that may occur in arteries or veins in any region of the body.[53]

While specific diagnostic criteria and management is considered beyond the scope of this chapter, the commonly seen disorders will be briefly discussed. All forms of vasculitis may present with extremity necrosis and impaired wound healing; therefore, collaboration with the primary physician to treat the underlying pathology is paramount to effective management of wounds due to the vasculitides conditions.

Polyarteritis nodosa is characterized by inflammation of the small and medium vessels of most organ systems. Primary complaints will center around one or more organ systems; for instance, musculoskeletal complaints are myalgias and arthralgias. Systemic lupus erythematosus (SLE) is a chronic autoimmune disorder that affects multiple organ systems. It is characterized by periods of exacerbation and remission. Skin lesions are associated with inflammation of the small and medium vessels of the skin. When skin lesions are present, it often indicates there is a significant inflammatory process

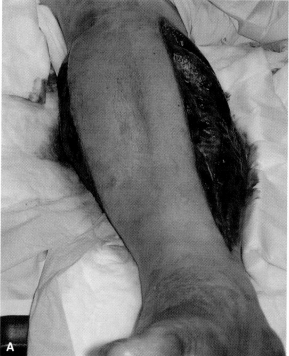

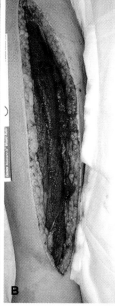

Figure **17•1** *Classic lower-extremity wounds following two-compartment fasciotomy. Note the edema and convexity of muscle bellies in the right leg (A). Decompression of edema will be paramount to healing. The left leg (B) demonstrates normalization of edema; this wound will likely achieve closure sooner than the right.*

occurring in the organ systems as well.[16,54] These patients may present with chronic circular lesions and recurrent mucous membrane lesions.[32] (See Fig 17.2.) In addition, inflammatory ulcers may present with characteristic purple margins or the presence of livedo reticularis, which will provide clues to underlying vasculitis.[54,55]

A challenge of clinical management of these inflammatory disorders is that the necessary pharmacological interventions often include corticosteroids, which may delay healing due to anti-inflammatory effects in most patients. Steroids have been linked to delayed healing in all phases of repair.[56,57] Although counterintuitive, often the risk associated with steroid use and nonhealing in this population is outweighed by the needed anti-inflammatory effects of the drugs on the underlying pathology. It is the author's experience, as has been documented by others,[58] that some patients heal *faster* while inflammation is managed aggressively since it is the underlying cause of necrosis. This may not be the case with many patients, as steroids have been shown to inhibit phagocytosis, collagen synthesis, and angiogenesis. Proper steroid selection may help to regulate a flow through all healing phases while preventing a chronic inflammatory state.[58] Topical and systemic vitamin A have also been recommended and used with success to counteract these effects in the wound bed.[56]

> ▶ **PEARL 17•7** Some debate remains as to the most effective dosage and delivery mode of vitamin A. Always confirm the most current research and clinical practice.

Takayasu's arteritis (TA) is another less common form of vasculitis. TA affects large and medium vessels, often the aorta. Inflammation in these cases may cause occlusion or dilation (aortic aneurysm). The disorder most commonly affects young women and is not a common cause of extremity ulceration. Rather, TA may have a host of symptoms centrally or peripherally, including claudication.[59,60]

Vasomotor Disorders

Vasomotor disorders or functional PAD include Raynaud's disease, acrocyanosis, and erythromelalgia. The common feature among them is the altered sympathetic nervous system control over arterial dilation and constriction.

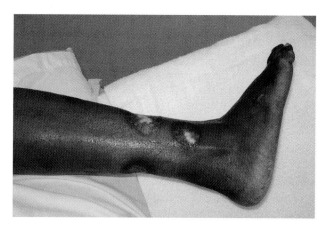

Figure **17•2** *Multiple wounds in a patient with systemic lupus erythematosus. Observe multiple scarred areas of healing along with active wounds on the posterior leg and toes. This patient presented with significant pain and mixed arteriovenous signs and symptoms. She responded well to moist semiocclusive dressings and light compression.*

Raynaud's disease is a rare disease of unknown etiology in which distal sites such as the fingertips, toes, and nose undergo rapid, brief periods of vasospasm. In the nonpathological state, cold temperatures for a prolonged period of time will provoke shunting of blood to internal organs for survival, which sacrifices distal perfusion. This is the natural reaction in extreme temperature that leads to frostbite. With Raynaud's, the reaction occurs prematurely with brief exposure to low temperatures or may be induced by emotional stress.[61]

Acrocyanosis refers to the bluish discoloration of the hands and sometimes the feet due to spasm of superficial vessels. Erythromelalgia is the periodic sensation of burning heat, pain, and redness in the skin due to dilation of the superficial arterioles of the skin. While these disorders do not commonly cause extremity wounds, prolonged or repeated episodes may eventually result in distal tissue necrosis.[9]

Clinical Features of Arterial Ulcerations

Arterial ulceration and gangrene are the most advanced integumentary result of any of the aforementioned diseases. As stated, the majority of clinical cases of ulceration will be attributable to arteriosclerosis obliterans. A broad understanding of differential diagnosis within the described causes of AI and among other causes of ulceration is essential in the wound management arena. Clinicians need to have the ability to discern signs of arterial involvement using a thorough history, exam, and evaluative process. The following section will present the most common findings in the patient exam when AI is one component of the patient's diagnosis.

History

Differential diagnosis of extremity wounds begins with thorough history. Referrals to wound centers and clinics may not be more specific than "70 year old with lower extremity wound," therefore effective and safe management relies on an accurate working diagnosis. Etiology should always be hypothesized to establish indications and contraindications for possible interventions. Thorough vascular examination will guide the clinician to safe treatment choices. The most crucial interventions for which the clinician needs to establish circulatory status are the implementation of sharp débridement and the use of compression devices. Compression, the cornerstone to management of venous insufficiency, may have significant implications for healing and limb preservation in those with compromised arterial flow. Débridement, a crucial component of wound bed preparation, may also be limb or life threatening in the presence of arterial compromise.

▸ **PEARL 17•8** Rule of thumb: "Know before you go." Screen circulatory status regardless of diagnosis.

As outlined in discussion of patient examination (Chapter 6), in addition to past medical history, past surgeries, and documentation of medications, a clear picture of the current wound progression and behavior is paramount to rule out arterial insufficiency. Questions should explore the duration of wound presence to establish trends of slow or poor healing in the past and currently. Mode of onset of the current wound will also be important, as well as pain behaviors and the influence of positioning.

Medical History

Patient factors should be considered, such as age, gender, diabetes mellitus (DM), hypercholesterolemia, hypertension, and CAD, as these are all associated with increase risk of PAD.[13,30,41] Other less powerful risk factors include hypercoagulable states and hyperhomocysteinemia. Presence of these comorbidities should alert the clinician to possible arterial insufficiency. In the presence of uncontrolled diabetes, it is also notable that a patient's clinical presentation may not be typical in regard to claudication and pain reports when neuropathy and impaired mobility may be present. Patients with neuropathic ulcerations should therefore always be screened for circulatory status. According to Sumpio and colleagues' research review, outcomes in a high-risk diabetic group are optimal with aggressive revascularization along with débridement and diligent wound management strategies.[62]

Social History

As discussed throughout the pathophysiology section of this chapter, smoking has highly detrimental effects on wound healing and is a major risk factor for the development of PAD.[63] Smoking has been shown to increase systemic vasoconstriction, slow fibroblast migration, and decrease epithelial integrity.[64] Moderate alcohol intake and regular physical activity have been shown to be protective factors in the development of arterial insufficiency.[21,65,66]

▸ **PEARL 17•9** The key word in alcohol's protective role is *moderation*. The slight blood-thinning effect is beneficial in occlusive disorders, but in excess may depress immunity and slow healing.

Wound Age

Patients with AI will often report stubborn presence of seemingly insignificant scrapes and cuts. They may have a history of "slow healing" on their feet or legs. When wounds or small cuts fail to heal within expected time frames, AI should be ruled out. Ulcers that do not heal along anticipated healing pathways described in Chapter 2 may be defined as chronic.

Onset

Wounds due to AI will often have traumatic onset. These "traumas" are typically not severe; it may be bumping a shin on a picnic table or stubbing a toe that leads to nonhealing ulceration in this group. In contrast to venous wounds, which may have slow onset of edema and apparent stress to the tissues that ultimately ulcerates, arterial ulcers have a more acute onset. In addition, given the prevalence of AI in the diabetic population, neuropathic wounds with concomitant AI are common.

Pain Patterns

Patients will often complain of significant pain associated with arterial wounds: They are generally more painful than a venous wound. Pain reports may be specific to the wound site or the extremity in general. Relief will be reported with legs in a dependent position whereas elevation or resting with legs in a neutral position will be painful. Patients may use strategies known as "dangling" to use gravity assistance to relieve pain while sitting: This may lead many to sleep while seated to avoid the pain of antigravity postures. Edema may become a complicating factor in these individuals as they will have reduced activity and excessive time spent in dependent positions. Patients may also report the feeling of cold feet or numbness of the lower legs and feet. This should prompt the clinician to rule out both neuropathy and ischemia. As described earlier, intermittent claudication will be reported as severe cramping or burning pain that is brought on by a predictable walking distance in ambulatory patients. Rest pain is a sign of more advanced disease. Along with claudication, patients may describe the feeling of numbness, coldness, or tingling on exertion. This is due to ischemia of the peripheral nerves as the maximally dilated arterioles of the muscles "steal" blood from cutaneous and peripheral nerves to try to meet the demands of working muscles.[67]

Examination Findings
Ulcer Appearance

Arterial wounds will be located on surfaces that are susceptible to minor traumas, such as the anterior tibia, lateral leg, or distal toes. In addition, wounds are often in more distal sites, such as the toes or ankle, by nature of the distance from the heart and the effect of atherosclerotic changes on smaller distal vessels. Distal vessels and capillary beds behave like crowded city streets, easily congested with a few vehicles. It takes many more vehicles to congest a major central highway (aorta, proximal vessels); therefore, distal ischemia and wounds are more common than in proximal locations in the presence of atherosclerosis. Wounds may also be present on pressure areas, especially in the neuropathic patient or in immobile, bed-bound individuals. The heels and lateral malleolus will be the most susceptible.

Gangrene may be present and is described as "dry" or "wet." Dry gangrene is complete ischemia along with neuropathy of tissues, which leads essentially to mummification of the body part, often a toe. (Fig. 17.3) Its margins clearly delineate between viable and nonviable tissues. In many cases, these digits may autoamputate. If there are no signs of infection, sites should be protected, kept dry, and should not be treated with topical products or local débridement. Wet gangrene, on the other hand, is neuroischemia coupled with deep infection, or septic vasculitis. It is malodorous, boggy, and has potential to cause significant systemic sepsis. Urgent vascular consultation is indicated when wet gangrene is suspected.[68] Clinically, the line between living and necrotic tissue (line of demarcation) becomes vague, pus or foul drainage may exude, and periwound tissues may become edematous and erythematous.

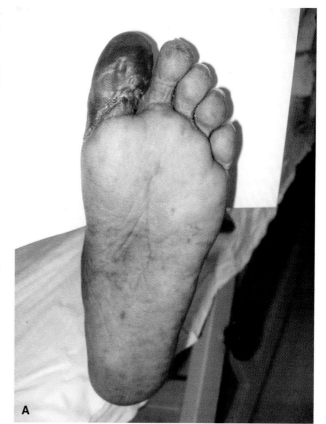

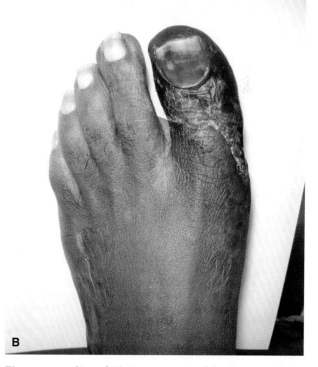

Figure 17•3 *(A and B) Dry gangrene of the first toe. This site is stable, as there is no edema, drainage, or associated cellulitis. The line of demarcation is easily seen as the point where living tissue meets "mummified" necrotic tissue.*

Often, a characteristic sweet and pungent odor will accompany these changes.

> ▶ **PEARL 17•10** Wound odors can be difficult to convey in words. Once you have smelled gangrene or *pseudomonas* colonization, you will know it!

Arterial ulcers are deprived of oxygen; therefore, they will appear pale, generally dry, with little drainage or eschar, and will have clearly demarcated or "punched out" margins. (Fig. 17.4) Arterial ulcers will have variable size and depth, but in general will be deeper than a venous wound because there is often necrosis through skin and superficial tissues into exposure of tendons, ligaments, and even bone.[1,16] Nonviable tissue is very common, and colors of anatomical structures will turn dusky when they become ischemic. (Table 17.6) Granulation, if present, will be pale, and epithelial growth is not likely. There may be erythema or cellulitis of intact surrounding skin. Differentiation of these periwound skin changes should be made to diagnose infection as opposed to dermatitis or allergic reaction to topical dressings or products.

Examination

Observation of the Involved Limb

Those with arterial compromise will present often with thin and pale lower extremities. *Trophic changes* of the skin will be observed, which include atrophy of skin and muscle; shiny, dry, scaly appearance of skin due to poor maintenance of hydration and nutrition; poor turgor; loss of hair; and poor nail growth. (Fig.17.5)

Skin temperature and color will be influenced by arterial insufficiency as well. Skin may be cool to palpation, with a gradient from distal to proximal. The sole of the foot may appear pale with elevation of the extremity as blood returns to the heart and the arterial system cannot overcome gravity to refill.

> ▶ **PEARL 17•11** Be sure to observe the sole of the foot since color changes in darkly pigmented skin tones is difficult to detect.

Muscle strength and girth should be assessed. It is common to find muscle weakness and atrophy in the hands and feet when arterial obstruction advances. Weakness and muscle wasting may be observed distally first. As pain of claudication or ulceration limits functionality, this may compound declines in functional strength.

Tests and Measures

In addition to a thorough history and observational examination, a vascular assessment may be performed noninvasively in the clinical setting. Additional testing modalities are performed in the vascular laboratory or are done surgically, as outlined in Box 17.1. Tests that require no tools other than the clinician's hands and observational skills are pulse palpation, rubor of dependency, capillary refill, and venous refilling time

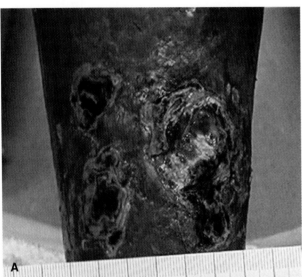

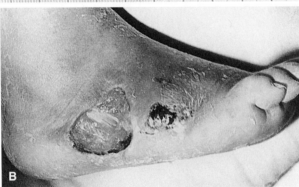

Figure 17•4 *(A) Arterial ulceration of the anterior tibia with well-defined margins, dry eschar, full-thickness necrosis to muscle tissue, and surrounding erythema. Mild accompanying edema suggests mixed arteriovenous presentation. (B) Typical arterial ulceration of the lateral foot with dry wound bed and exposed tendon.*

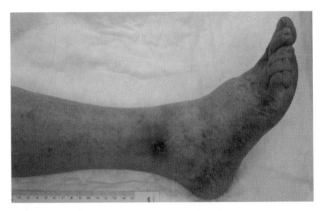

Figure 17•5 *Trophic changes of the extremity associated with arterial insufficiency and advanced age (>90). The skin is shiny and pale, and there is no hair growth on the lower leg. Atrophy of intrinsic foot muscles is evident with the clawing position of the toes.*

Table 17•6 Qualitative Markers of Viable Versus Necrotic Tissues

	Healthy/Viable	Necrotic	Significance
Skin Epidermis/ dermis	Pink/blanches with pressure (+ capillary refill)	Purple/deep maroon (deep necrosis) Nonblanchable (superficial or deep necrosis) May develop bullae	Watch for periwound skin changes, especially in traumatic wound sites. *Bullae and severe ecchymosis following trauma to †LE.
Subcutaneous fat	Pale yellow Spongy Intact individual cells	Bright yellow, brown, or green Slimy Notice oily drainage in area	Assess for undermining. *Failing partial forefoot amputation in neuroischemic foot.
Fascia	White Tough, thin fibrous	Gray/yellow Loosely adhered/mobile	"Stop and think" layer Separates superficial from deep structures. *Fascial necrosis following extensive débridement of Fournier's gangrene.
Muscle	Red Springy with palpation Bleeds with dressing removal Contracts on command	Dusky, dark red/maroon, brown, or black Soft/mushy with palpation Poor bleeding	Full-thickness tissue loss. If extensive necrosis, advise surgical débridement to effectively salvage viable tissue. *Transtibial amputation with ischemia.
Tendon	White Tiny vascular network visible on surface when peritenon intact Strong adherence of fibers in bundle	Yellow/gray Stringy/loose fibers with palpation/ débridement	Full-thickness tissue loss. *Note poorly defined edges in necrotic anterior tibial tendon.
Bone	Ivory/pale pink when periosteum intact 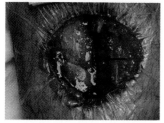	Dry/dusky gray 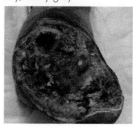	*High suspicion of osteomyelitis when bone exposed.[68] *Transmetatarsal amputation in patient with ‡DM2; green residue is enzymatic débriding ointment.

*As seen in corresponding image; †LE = lower extremity; ‡DM2 = type 2 diabetes

> **Box 17•1** **Tests and Measures Used in Diagnosis of Peripheral Arterial Disease**

Clinical Testing: Clinician Only

- Pulse palpation
- Capillary refill
- Venous refill
- Rubor of dependency

Vascular Laboratory Tests: Noninvasive

- Ankle-brachial index (ABI)*
- Toe brachial index (TBI)*
- Transcutaneous partial pressure of oxygen (TcPo$_2$)*
- Segmental Doppler ultrasonography
- Duplex Doppler imaging
- Pulse volume recordings

Invasive Testing

- Angiography
  MRA
  CTA

*May be performed by qualified clinician outside a vascular laboratory

Table 17•7 **Clinical Features of Arterial Ulcerations**

Location	Distal sites Toes, lateral malleolus Dorsal surfaces/exposed to small traumas
Appearance	Pale Dry with little drainage "Punched out"; clearly defined margins Necrosis, eschar, or gangrene common Poor epithelial migration
Limb characteristics	Thin with muscle atrophy Pale skin appearance Decrease distal hair growth Dystrophic nail growth Poor skin turgor Cool to palpation Edema in advanced stages
Basic clinical test results	Pulse: Diminished or absent Rubor of dependency: + Capillary refill: >3 seconds Venous filling time: >15 seconds ABI: ≤0.8

ABI, ankle-brachial index

tests. Edema should be assessed for possible mixed vascular etiology; this is discussed in detail in Chapter 16. The other more involved but noninvasive tests include ankle-brachial index (ABI), toe brachial index (TBI), and transcutaneous partial pressure of oxygen (TcPo$_2$) tests. The procedure for performing these is outlined in detail in Chapter 7.

Patients will have positive findings on the rubor of dependency test: bright red/deep purple appearance of the sole of the foot in dependent position following pallor with elevation. There will also be delayed venous refilling of greater than 15 seconds and capillary refill delay of greater than 3 seconds in the presence of arterial compromise.

Diminished peripheral pulses should be expected in these patients. For pulse palpation, it is advised to assess femoral, popliteal, posterior tibial (PT), and dorsalis pedis (DP) pulses. Distally, PT assessment is advised over DP alone because some patients may have congenitally absent dorsalis pedis pulses.[69,70] Pulse palpation alone is often not sufficient diagnostically since the presence of pulses has not been shown in multiple studies to rule out AI.[71,72] These basic clinical exam findings are summarized in Table 17.7.

When pulses are nonpalpable, Doppler and ABI testing are indicated. Several authors report the ABI as being both a specific and sensitive reference for the diagnosis of PAD.[4,30,73] A 2007 report of a retrospective review of high-risk patients assessed with ABI found independent predictive validity of the ABI on mortality rates.[19] One limitation of the ABI is false elevation of the value in the presence of incompressible arteries seen with diabetes.[4,24,61] The toe index is advised in these situations.[69] In addition, it may not be uniformly specified in many cases which artery in the foot was used for testing or if the test was performed at rest versus after exercise.[24]

Further information can be obtained as to local skin perfusion by transcutaneous oxygen tension measurements, or TcPo$_2$. This test has been shown to be a strong linear predictor of healing probability and extent of ischemia.[74] Prognosis for healing can generally be established with these diagnostic tests, which are summarized in Table 17.8. When patients present with these values upon examination, healing may not be likely without revascularization.

More involved but noninvasive tests performed in a vascular laboratory are indicated when any of the tests discussed above reveal abnormal findings. These tests include segmental Doppler systolic pressures and pulse volume waveform recordings (PVR).[30,80] These will provide more detailed information as to disease severity and location of obstruction anatomically.

Invasive image testing such as angiography is indicated only for patients who have an established diagnosis and for whom surgical intervention is planned. Angiography may be

Table 17•8 **Indicators of Poor Healing Prognosis with Diagnostic Tests**

Test	Finding
ABI	<0.4[41]
Toe pressure	<30 mm Hg[1,69]
TcPo$_2$	<40 mm Hg[75,76] <20–30 mm Hg[73,77–79]
Ankle systolic pressure	<50 mm Hg[12]

visualized with magnetic resonance (MR) or computed tomography (CT). These tests are discussed in detail in Chapter 9 on diagnostic imaging.

Treatment of Arterial Ulcers

Conservative management of arterial ulcers is a challenge to the health-care professional in any setting. Effective management will follow from a comprehensive examination and evaluation of findings as described earlier. The key components to achieving healing include *local care* (wound bed preparation, dressing selection, modalities, and management/prevention of infection), *limb protection* (bedrest, pressure reduction), and *risk factor reduction*. In addition to these management factors, medical, surgical, nutritional, and social service collaboration must occur where appropriate to address these complex cases with an effective interdisciplinary approach. The treating clinician, whether a physician, nurse, physical therapist, or occupational therapist, must recognize when conservative measures are not sufficient and revascularization, more aggressive medical management, or amputation should be considered.

> **PEARL 17•12** Limb protection is a group effort, especially in an inpatient setting. Clear communication and monitoring are a must.

Since these wounds are often extremely challenging to manage, patience on the part of the clinician and the patient is crucial. How do we know when our efforts are hopeless? A 2005 study by Marston and colleagues attempted to answer this question. In a retrospective view of prospectively collected cases at the University of North Carolina Wound Management Center, they looked at the outcomes of conservative treatment of 169 limbs in 142 patients with arterial insufficiency (defined as ABI of less than 0.7 or toe pressure of less than 50 mm HG). The patients included in the review had "uncomplicated, stable limb ulcers" and were in an outpatient clinic; therefore, their findings should not be applied to acute, infected, and hospitalized patients. Their data revealed that at 12 months, 23% of patients required amputation, and wound healing was eventually achieved in 52% of patients.[81] In stable, efficiently managed cases, healing is possible, and clinicians and patients may anticipate slow progress when revascularization is not feasible.

Clinicians must remember that even the best advanced wound care practices, dressings, and modalities may not be enough if the wound is fundamentally not "healable," defined by Sibbald and colleagues as "a wound that has adequate blood supply and favorable host factors that will promote healing if the wound bed is adequately prepared."[78] This balance feels contradictory at times since healing may be achieved in many seemingly grim prognoses by advanced modalities and good care. Constant reevaluation of patient and wound factors collaboratively will provide the best outcomes. Advanced treatment strategies, which are indicated in cases of recalcitrant healing, will be discussed in the following section. They are part of an aggressive nonsurgical approach to wound management, especially when surgery is not an option.

Local Care

Wound Bed Preparation

Wound bed preparation for arterial wounds will follow good wound care practices as outlined for any chronic or acute wound. This includes removal of necrotic tissue, proper cleansing and irrigation, and selection of the appropriate dressings and adjunctive therapies to promote healing.

To débride or not to débride . . . that is the question. Accurate identification and safe removal of necrotic tissue can be complex in the presence of arterial compromise. Wound care referrals requesting débridement may range from closed stable eschars to open draining wounds, and this range must be appreciated in the decision-making process. Open wounds that are uninfected and draining should be débrided of necrotic tissue as often as necessary to promote healing and prevent infection. Complete necrosis of wound tissues, especially in conjunction with diminished arterial flow, is an indication for surgical débridement if healing is the goal of therapy. Surgical procedures will often occur in series, as seen in Figure 17.6. The patient shown presented with poorly controlled type 2 diabetes and a ABI of 0.25. Conservative management was attempted on the partial forefoot amputation. An initial surgical débridement was then performed, with further resection of the metatarsals. Necrosis continued to advance despite optimum wound care, and the patient ultimately underwent femoral-popliteal bypass grafting and wound débridement, which resulted in an ABI greater than 0.6 and observable improved health of the wound tissues. The patient went on to complete healing with split-thickness skin grafting and accommodative footwear.

A stable eschar should never be débrided until healing potential and local perfusion are confirmed. "Stable" means the site has dry adhered margins, no surrounding cellulitis, and no undiagnosed sources of systemic infection. In the presence of

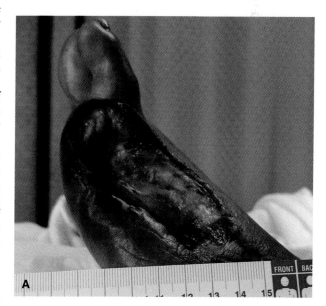

Figure 17•6 *Partial forefoot amputation before (A and B) and after (C) femoral-popliteal bypass grafting in a patient with type 2 diabetes and arterial insufficiency.*

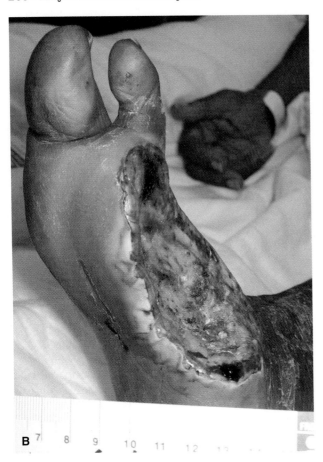

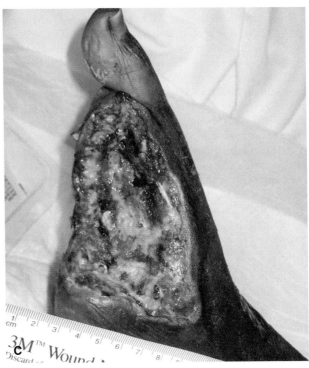

Figure 17•6 *Cont'd*

an ABI of 0.8 or less, the goal of treatment will be maintenance of the stable eschar, with protection from pressure, friction, and infection, and close daily monitoring to ensure no decline.[1] It is important to educate both the patient and other staff involved in care regarding this goal and your rationale. Essentially, these stable eschars act as a barrier for the patient as would intact skin. Especially in the presence of poor functional mobility and confounding medical comorbidities, removal of this stable cover often creates significant risk of nonhealing complications. See Figure 17.7 for a guide to the decision-making process for these eschars.

▶ **PEARL 17•13** Listen to mom! Don't pick! Fingernails carry large amounts of hidden bacteria and pose infection risk to compromised patients.

An unstable eschar will present with separation of the roof from the wound edges; it may have drainage, purulence, foul odor, or surrounding cellulitis. Unstable or "soft" eschars, along with clinical indicators of arterial compromise, should prompt surgical consultation. In these situations, nonsurgical débridement may be appropriate if the site is uninfected and healable,[78] but it is advisable to make a collaborative decision to that effect since the risk associated with nonhealing is great and amputation or vascular correction may be appropriate.

Dressing Selection

Dressing selection for arterial wounds will follow the same decision-making process as for any complex wound. While anecdotal evidence exists in patient-by-patient scenarios, little evidence exists to say one dressing is superior over another in treating this group. A 2006 Cochrane review sought to determine superiority of dressing selection as evidenced by randomized controlled trials or clinical controlled trials for arterial wounds. They located 37 potential studies, 2 of which met inclusion criteria. The review concluded that no clear evidence exists to advise any particular dressing for wounds due to arterial insufficiency.[2] Good care will include dressing selection appropriate to address particular needs of the local and systemic wound factors. Since arterial ulcers are generally dry, primary dressings with the ability to donate and maintain moisture, such as hydrogels, hydrocolloids, or impregnated gels, tend to do best. While alginate and hydrofiber dressings are indicated for highly exuding wounds, in the author's experience these may be premoistened with saline or sterile H_2O to provide a moist environment to a low-exuding wound if gels are not available.

When selecting secondary dressings, it is important to note the fragility or general state of the surrounding tissues. Avoidance of harsh adhesives or irritants may save the patient from developing new traumas surrounding the wound in question.

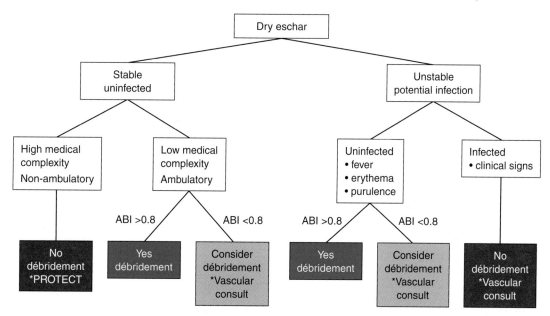

Figure 17•7 *Decision tree in the presence of a closed eschar. "Débridement" implies necrotic tissue removal–sharp, enzymatic, or autolytic as appropriate. Surgical débridement is considered within surgical referral scope. Green means "go," red means "stop," yellow means "proceed with caution as outlined."*

In the author's experience, when an occlusive environment is needed, yet adhesives are contraindicated, secondary dressing selection can be tricky. Petroleum-impregnated gauze has been useful in these situations to maintain a semiocclusive environment. Frequent dressing change in this population is advised. Especially in severe cases of ischemia or postoperative revascularization, changes may occur quickly and need to be monitored. Signs of infection and progressive ischemia should be assessed. Since infection poses considerable risk to the patient with arterial insufficiency, dressings with antimicrobial properties such as silver, iodine, or polyhexamethylene biguanide (PHMB) are frequently used.

> ▶ **PEARL 17•14** If an adhesive dressing is the best option for the treatment of someone with fragile skin, a spot test away from the wound margins is useful to establish basic tolerance for the adhesive product.

Given the growing need for wound management in health care as the population ages, infinite dressing options are available to the clinician. It is important to consider relative cost effectiveness, ease of application, reports of associated pain, and healing outcomes when selecting dressings for these complex wounds.

Patients may present with mixed arteriovenous etiology. It is advised to treat the underlying arterial insufficiency first,[82] and proceed with caution when considering the use of compression according to the patient's ABI values. This decision should take into account patient factors such as ambulatory status and the ability to place legs horizontally, rather than never leaving the dangling position. Clinicians may decide that it is beneficial to use inelastic compression devices that retard advancing edema in these cases without adding static elastic compression. For patients with an ABI of 0.8 or more, it is generally advised to use compression devices. Some authors report cautious use of light compression levels in the group of patients with ABI of 0.6 to 0.8 and report ABI of 0.5 or less as the absolute contraindication for compression.[1,74,83]

Management and Prevention of Infection

The biggest risk for those with ischemic ulcers is infection. It is often the deciding factor that leads ultimately to amputation in this group. The predisposition for necrotic tissue is one risk factor that makes ischemic wounds susceptible to infection, which is why skilled, aggressive débridement of necrotic tissue in draining arterial ulcers is paramount. Reduced tissue oxygenation also provides an inviting environment for aerobic and anaerobic bacteria.[84] The first intuitive solution is antibiotic therapy, but there may be questionable effectiveness of intravenous administration when arterial disease is present. How much of a selected drug reaches the target (infected wound site) in an individual who has the ability to transport only a fraction of the needed blood to the lower extremities? Poor perfusion is the underlying factor limiting healing potential to begin with! A possible solution lies in the use of local antimicrobial agents administered through approved modalities or dressings. Topical antimicrobials will not be effective against deep compartment infections. If infection appears to be advancing beyond the wound margins or probes to the bone, systemic therapy is indicated.[85]

Advances are being made in balancing the promotion of a healing environment with safe bacterial reduction using antimicrobial dressings. Antimicrobial dressings must have low cytotoxicity, that is, low risk of harm to viable tissues. Many topical substances demonstrate this effect: They promote closure while reducing local colonization. Examples of topical antimicrobials with acceptable cytotoxic levels include ionic and nanocrystalline silver, silver sulfadiazine, polyhexamethylene biguanide (PHMB), and cadexomer iodine.[78] If a wound is determined to be nonhealable and the need for antiseptic effect is greater than concerns for cytotoxicity, a number of agents are suggested. For example, while waiting for a patient to be stable for a revascularization or in an end-of-life situation in which no drastic surgical measures are indicated, topical agents that may be used include sodium hypochlorite, hydrogen peroxide, crystal violet, quaternary ammonium, chlorhexidine, acetic acid (0.5%–5%), or povidone iodine.[78]

To appreciate the relative infection risk in ischemic versus venous and diabetic ulcers, a 2000 observational study by Schmidt et al is referenced. The authors used swab cultures and tracking of healing progress to compare 63 patients over a 4-month period with "severe, nonhealing leg ulcers." The patients were divided into classifications of "ischemic, venous, and diabetic (further divided into diabetic-neuropathic and diabetic-ischemic)." Among the proposed study questions, they set out to determine the following: "What consequences do positive wound smears carry for the healing process of different types of ulcers?"[84] Their results were very telling. Multiple conclusions were drawn, and the most relevant to this discussion are summarized in Table 17.9.

While this is a single small-scale study, the outcomes are important because they expose the impact of infection on not only the ischemic limb, but especially in the groups with concomitant diabetes and arterial disease. The patients with ischemia and diabetes had significantly higher presence of clinical infections and relative amputation risk as compared to venous and nondiabetic ischemic patients.

Modalities

When standard care, combined with revascularization (as appropriate), diligent wound bed preparation, dressing selection, and risk factor reduction do not achieve healing, a number of adjunctive treatment modalities may be considered. It has been reported that clinicians may expect increasing wound size in ischemic ulcers due to advancing necrosis from hypoxic conditions.[77, 78] This may be the case, but one must also recognize when such observations do not reverse with aggressive conservative management in reasonable time frames. The following section will briefly address the usefulness of emerging and accepted modalities, including electrical stimulation, negative pressure wound therapy, ultrasound, hyperbaric oxygen therapy, circulator devices, and pneumatic compression devices, as they relate to ischemic ulcers. Each of these modalities is described in further detail throughout the text. They are all suggested augmentations to care and should not replace vascular surgery consultation. In addition, other adjunctive treatments, such as pulsed lavage with suction (PLWS) and UV-C light, may be beneficial.

Electrical Stimulation

Electrotherapy has been used for wound healing with positive outcomes in many studies. In fact, electrical stimulation, or E-stim, has the largest number of clinical trials of any adjunct modality to support its use in wound care.[86] In particular, the use of HVPC (high-voltage pulsed current) has been shown to promote microcirculation and healing of ischemic wounds and increase perfusion of periwound tissues.[76,87,88] Electrical currents and polarity placement is designed to attract or repel ionized cells such as neutrophils, macrophages, fibroblasts, or epidermal cells at the appropriate healing phase.[89] In their 2004 study of infrapopliteal ischemic wounds, Goldman and colleagues suggest HVPC to facilitate arterial vasodilation and dermal angiogenesis.[87] They also demonstrate statistically significant improvements in periwound $TcPo_2$. Use of HVPC was hypothesized to be necessary until restoration of $TcPo_2$ values to within normal limits (>30–40 mm Hg).[77]

The risk of infection of arterial ulcers was emphasized earlier. Low-voltage pulsed current (LVPC) was recently assessed as to its effects on gram-positive and gram-negative bacteria in vitro. Positive polarity was favorable in the degree of log reduction of bacteria in this model.[90]

Table 17•9 Relationship of Clinical Infection with Swab Findings, Wound Healing, and Amputation				
Total All Types	**Ischemic**	**Venous**	**Diabetic-Neuropathic**	**Diabetic-Ischemic**
Probability (%) of clinical infection with (+) swab				
55%	69%*	22%*	67%	75%*
Percentage that went on toward healing† with (+) clinical infection confirmed				
Not reported	20%‡	100%‡	50%‡	Not reported
Relative amputation risk correlated with (+) clinical infection				
58%	67%	0%	50%	80%

*Statistically significant difference between venous and ischemic or diabetic-ischemic wounds (P = 0.015).
†Progress toward healing defined as wounds that reduced in size >15% within the study period of 3 months.
‡Statistically significant difference between venous and ischemic or diabetic-ischemic wounds (P = 0.007).
Adapted from Schmidt, K, et al: Bacterial population of chronic crural ulcers: Is there a difference between the diabetic, the venous, and the arterial ulcer? VASA 2000; 29:62–70.

Negative Pressure Wound Therapy

The use of subatmospheric pressure to treat wounds has been in U.S. practice for over two decades. Introduced in 1995 by Kinetic Concepts Inc. (San Antonio, TX), the V.A.C.® device has been used to promote vacuum-assisted closure in acute, chronic, postsurgical, and diabetic wounds.[91,92] Since then, other devices have been marketed that also provide negative pressure wound therapy (NPWT). It has been proposed that NPWT provides active decompression of local wound fluid, which restores microcirculation and promotes oxygen delivery to the tissues for angiogenesis.[93] This effect is promising for relatively ischemic wounds. In the author's experience, NPWT should be used with caution in patients with an ABI of less than 0.6. NPWT will promote perfusion to wounds in the presence of adequate flow; that is, it will not replace revascularization, but is an excellent adjunct following vascular surgery to reduce healing time. In addition, in marginal cases or in cases of unacceptable surgical risk and a low-exuding wound, anecdotal evidence suggests using NPWT with the following factors in mind: lower pressures (75–100 mm Hg), increased frequency of dressing change, and the addition of hydrogel to ensure moisture balance. NPWT should be discontinued if necrosis advances or desiccation of the wound bed occurs, and it should not be applied to already dry tissues that have no drainage. In addition, it is important to protect the patient from pressure necrosis resulting from the rigid tubing by using padding or strategic placement of the tubing, as well as staff education.

▶ **PEARL 17•15** When using negative-pressure wound therapy, extra foam from the dressing kit may provide a simple cushion under the tubing path to protect bony prominences.

Ultrasound

Noncontact, low-frequency (40 kHz) ultrasound is emerging as a promising therapy indicated for cleansing and débridement of chronic wounds. MIST® therapy (Celleration Inc., Eden Prairie, MN) uses a fine saline mist to deliver ultrasound waves. Positive healing outcomes have been demonstrated in multiple small-scale clinical studies.[94-97] One proposed method of efficacy is promotion of microcirculatory blood flow to the wound bed. Kavros et al reported a prospective, parallel-group, randomized controlled trial of 70 patients with nonhealing ulcers and critical limb ischemia. The study compared use of MIST plus standard of care three times per week for 12 weeks to standard care alone. Sixty-three percent of patients in the MIST therapy group, compared to 29% of those in the standard care group, reached greater than 50% reduction in wound size at 12 weeks ($P < 0.001$). The authors found $TcPo_2$ baseline values to correlate with healing potential.[98]

Hyperbaric Oxygen Therapy

Hyperbaric oxygen therapy (HBOT) aims to increase local tissue oxygen delivery via the inhalation of 100% oxygen in a pressurized environment of two to three times the atmospheric pressure at sea level.[98] The therapy is advised for patients with recalcitrant and ischemic wounds. Since HBOT is known to be costly, time consuming, and to pose possible risks of O_2 toxicity or barotraumas, identification of patients who may benefit is important. Use of HBOT is advised if patients show a greater than10 mm Hg increase in $TcPo_2$ from baseline, first breathing room air and then breathing 100% O_2.[88,99] The proposed mechanism of hyperoxygenation to ischemic wounds is rational. The mechanism of action is proposed to be more than simply reversal of hypoxic conditions. It is suggested that hyperoxic states facilitate gene function and signal transduction, as well as complement growth factor production.[100] The utility of hyperbaric O_2 is very promising, although randomized controlled trials proving its efficacy are lacking.[101] Small groups of patients with ischemic wounds have been identified to respond favorably to the therapy when appropriately screened for treatment.[99,102]

Pneumatic Compression Devices

Compression devices are typically advised for the management of venous insufficiency and proposed with caution in patients with mixed arteriovenous pathology. Intermittent pneumatic foot compression (IPC) has been studied as a therapy to augment arterial lower-extremity flow as well.[103,104] Foot and/or calf compression in patients with stable intermittent claudication has resulted in significant increases in walking distance and collateral circulation. It is theorized to mimic the calf muscle pump when levels of external pressure do not exceed diastolic pressure and are timed appropriately with systole so that pressures do not impede already impaired arterial inflow.[78] Models include the ArtAssist® device (ACI Medical, San Marcos, CA), often prescribed for in-home usage.[34] Konstantinos et al found a 110% median increase in absolute claudication distance in subjects who completed a 4.5-month daily intermittent pneumatic compression (IPC) treatment compared to controls. They also noted improvements in resting and postexercise ABI values.[103] A limitation to these findings is the fact that patients who participated in the study used the IPC device at home 4 hours a day throughout the 4.5-month period. The cost effectiveness and practicality of such use have not been established. For some patients with disabling claudication, this time sacrifice may be worthwhile. The other modality, which surpasses these results consistently, is *supervised* walking interventions; no clinical value has been proven with unsupervised advice to "walk more."[35,36,105]

▶ **PEARL 17•16** Although not proven, advising general activity may promote fitness to act as a buffer to obesity, hypertension, and diabetes risk, all of which are linked with claudication.

Protection

Protection of limbs with active arterial ulceration and prevention strategies in those with intact skin is crucial. First, when patients show signs of advancing arterial disease, they should be educated on skin and foot care to prevent ulceration. Good skin care includes conservative care of minor cuts and scrapes and avoiding peeling of scabs. Patients should be taught to moisturize dry skin, which will help maintain pliability to prevent minor skin tears due to dryness. In addition, soaking the feet should be avoided, as this promotes dehydration of the skin as well. Skin and nail care in this group should also be handled conservatively. Especially in the face of concomitant diabetic neuropathy with nail hypertrophy, patients are advised to seek professional care from a podiatrist or physical therapist for nail trimming and callus care. Footwear selection should be attended to as well. Patients should avoid narrow shoes and seek supportive shoes with adequate depth and width that will not cause blistering due to friction. Finally, dress stockings and restrictive clothing that provide compression should not be worn.

▶ **PEARL 17•17** In treating dryness, patients should avoid lotions containing alcohol, which can promote dryness.

Aggressive medical management of ulceration involves bedrest in severe cases. Positioning schedules should be used, along with active range of motion, to preserve joint mobility and prevent contracture due to immobility. Mattress selection should take into consideration each patient's functional mobility status to protect and off-load active ulceration as well as prevent necrosis of other pressure sensitive areas. Even the dorsal surface of the foot and toes should be protected from friction due to heavy blankets. Devices that tent or raise the sheets at the end of the bed are useful for this purpose. Elevation of the head of the bed to place the heart higher than the legs is suggested to improve perfusion to the distal extremity.[33]

Protective devices for the foot are plentiful. Among the optimal strategies available to clinicians, heel protection is vital. Heel-lift boots should be selected with regard for the needs of the patient and with attention to proper fit. Caution is advised with prefabricated rigid splint or ankle-foot orthoses (AFOs). These devices may have plastic or metal parts that can easily cause pressure necrosis if the fit and functionality are not monitored closely. The safest devices are made of soft material that suspends the heels and have lateral support to protect the malleoli. There are many options available. A promising support device on the market that provides safe heel protection, warmth with lamb's wool lining, and permits ambulation is the Rooke Boot® (Osborn Medical, Utica, MN). Its design follows from studies reporting positive effects of warmth on TcPo$_2$ via attenuation of sympathetic tone in the extremity.[106]

Risk Factor Reduction

Patient education as to the variables of arterial disease that are in their control is very important to disease management. Along with medical and pharmacological management of confounding conditions, patients should be advised on smoking cessation, weight control, and the value of exercise. Nicotine from smoking is a powerful vasoconstrictor and inhibits fibroblast migration for healing.[63,107] The many chemicals in cigarettes promote endothelial injury and atherogenesis and may promote increases in LDL levels,[108] which are related to atherosclerosis. Weight management and exercise have been shown to reduce cardiovascular and circulatory risk in many studies, and both are known to influence cholesterol profiles, blood glucose levels, blood pressure, and circulation. Patients should be educated that medical and surgical management from the health-care team will not be as effective as they could be in the presence of poor lifestyle choices: Patients are a crucial component of the "team."

▶ **PEARL 17•18** Clinicians should familiarize themselves with local support groups and smoking cessation resources to help guide their patients to stop smoking.

Medical and Pharmacological Management

Primary medical and pharmacological treatment goals are to decrease cardiovascular risk, increase walking distance, and prevent critical limb ischemia.[109] Optimal limb and ulcer care, as already highlighted, is also crucial.[110] In the case of the inflammatory conditions or other underlying comorbidities, these should be managed with the primary physician to allow the patient's body to achieve a healing-friendly environment. Collaboration with primary physicians in the management of existing comorbidities such as hypertension (HTN), DM, and hyperlipidemia should be addressed in the treatment of PAD. Blood glucose levels should be managed pharmacologically and with lifestyle modification such as diet and exercise.

Pharmacological approaches to PAD are much more commonly seen in both medical literature and in the marketing world. Every other television commercial is for a new drug for cardiac and vascular health; this is a sign of our times, and we need to readily answer questions for our patients on the drugs' underlying actions and benefits. The commonly discussed PAD drugs are designed and tested in patients with claudication as a main outcome variable. Studies demonstrating effects on wound healing with use of these drugs is scarce. The most widely recognized drugs in the literature to improve walking time include statins, angiotensin-converting enzyme (ACE) inhibitors, antiplatelet drugs, and vasodilators. Brief explanations of the actions of these drugs follow, with examples of trade names in parenthesis. The examples are not exclusive.

Hypertension and hypercholesterolemia have been closely linked with severity of arterial disease. Statins, such as atorvastatin (Lipitor®; Pfizer, NY, NY), simvastatin (Zocor®; Merck, Whitehorse Station, NJ), and rosuvastatin (Crestor®; Astra Zeneca, Wilmington, DE) are among the most commonly prescribed drugs for hypercholesterolemia. They are effective in reducing LDL levels through the action of 3-hydroxy-3-methyl-glutaryl-CoA HMG-CoA) inhibitors, controlling cholesterol production in the body. ACE inhibitors, such as lisinopril (Prinivil®; Merck, and Zestril®; Astra Zeneca) will help manage HTN with peripheral vasodilation to decrease peripheral resistance. They act by blocking the action of angiotensin-converting enzyme, which is a strong vasoconstrictor.[111] The following drugs aim to improve extremity flow and are prescribed for claudication. Clopidogrel (Plavix®; Bristol Myers Squibb, New York, NY), which reduces platelet reactivity, acts by blocking the ADP receptor of platelets via the glycoprotein IIb/IIIa pathway.[28] Clopidogrel has been compared to aspirin in the CAPRIE study, which found a reduction of cardiovascular risk (ischemic stroke, myocardial infarction, or vascular death) that favored the use of clopidogrel.[28] Pentoxifylline (Trental®; Sanofi-Aventis, Bridgewater, NJ) is a phosphodiesterase (PDE4) inhibitor that improves red blood cell mobility, thereby reducing blood viscosity and improving efficiency of flow.[36] Cilostazol (Pletal®; Otsieka America Pharmaceutical Inc., Rockville, MD) is a phosphodiesterase III inhibitor that promotes vasodilation and decreases platelet aggregation.[35,36] Growth factors such as vascular endothelial growth factor (VEGF) and supplements such as L-arginine, a nitric oxide precursor, are also being studied.[5,36]

Surgical Options

Revascularization procedures are considered for patients with obstructive PAD, but not inflammatory or vasculitides conditions. Candidates must be ambulatory, with acceptable surgical risk factors and correctable anatomic lesions shown through arteriography. They must also have at least one of the following: rest pain, disabling claudication, or a nonhealing ulcer.[32] Norman and colleagues add that "diagnostic uncertainty" and presence of significant carotid stenosis or aneurismal disease may also warrant referral.[13] Note that surgical correction only relieves the most obstructive blockage for limb salvage; it does not reverse the process of new development of obstruction. Surgical candidates need to be educated about this fact and the risk of graft failure if modifiable risk factors are not addressed.[41]

Options for revascularization include open surgical procedures such as bypass grafting and endovascular procedures, including angioplasty, atherectomy, or stenting procedures. A bypass grafting procedure is essentially a detour around diseased vessels with redirection to patent distal vessels. Angiography preoperatively will provide a road map for the vascular surgeon as to location of obstruction and available distal connections. Common anatomical courses include femoral to popliteal arteries (fem-pop), femoral to distal tibial or peroneal arteries (fem-distal), axillary to femoral (axillo-fem), or aorta to one or both femoral arteries (aorto-bifem). Bypass grafting has been shown to be most successful when the patient's own saphenous vein is used as the graft material (SVG). In cases where this is not optimal, synthetic material such as polytetrafluoroethylene (PTFE or Gore-Tex®; W.L. Gore & Associates, Flagstaff, AZ) is used.[66] Percutaneous transluminal angioplasty (PTA) is a procedure that involves passage of a wire, followed by a balloon catheter, from the femoral artery down beyond the identified site of occlusion. Once the catheter is in location, the balloon is inflated to press and flatten atheromas on the arterial wall and ultimately widen the arterial lumen. Stenting is the permanent placement of a tubular mesh prosthetic (usually wire) that supports the arterial lumen, widening the passageway for blood. It is inserted at an area of narrowing using the balloon technique, which expands the mesh to desired width.[112] Atherectomy may be thought of as the "Roto-Rooter" procedure because it consists of catheter-guided shaving and removal of plaques. A 2007 study assessed whether open versus endovascular options for revascularization were superior in terms of outcome for diabetic patients. The authors concluded these options were equivocal as a first option, and the more important conclusion was the recommendation for early revascularization in this population.[113]

The discussion of surgical interventions for PAD is not complete without mentioning amputation. We refer here to amputation in the presence of chronic vascular disease, specifically, and not traumatic amputation, although the psychological processes will have similarities. Recall that amputation is not currently the major threat to life expectancy, but rather cardiovascular events threaten patients with PAD. In those with diabetes as an additional factor, amputation continues to pose a significant risk, especially in the face of neuropathy.[114] The decision for amputation will be made primarily by the vascular surgeon in conjunction with the patient and supporting disciplines when healing is not likely or infection poses risk to the patient's life. Elective amputations will flow from what is often a grueling struggle to heal a very "sick" limb. Often the pain and stress of trying to achieve healing in these difficult cases becomes more physically and mentally demanding than is manageable. Patients benefit from knowing that the unrelenting wound and extremity pain associated with critical ischemia are relieved following major amputation. It is a positive step when the patient is healthy enough to support a prosthesis or function at wheelchair level. They have a better chance to resume a life not driven by pain.[114] Psychological factors clearly play a role for the patient dealing with a chronic wound who may be facing amputation, no matter the underlying pathology. Open communication and professional counseling is very important for the emotional state of each individual. Referral to a clinical psychologist is appropriate before and after major amputation.

Summary

Arterial insufficiency is a significant challenge to the wound care professional. One of the keystones to management is the recognition that these cases require multidisciplinary care and communication. Healing successes will occur when a combination of clinician decision-making skills, and social, medical, pharmacological, preventative, and educational factors work together. A tremendous number of conservative measures may promote healing in cases with a very grim prognoses. It is therefore important to be optimistic and realistic at the same time, recognizing the available aggressive nonsurgical approaches available, as well as the cases that do not respond favorably. Clinicians should feel confident asking for team input in these complex cases for the best outcomes. It is additionally important to recognize at-risk groups for education regarding prevention and management of modifiable risk factors, especially smoking cessation and diabetes. (Fig. 17.8)

▶ **PEARL 17•19** Don't go it alone! Interdisciplinary care is key to successful outcomes.

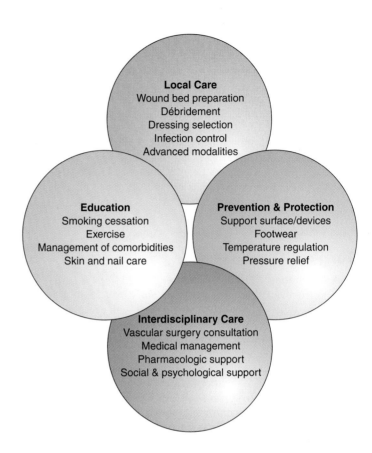

Figure 17•8 *Considerations for conservative management of arterial ulceration.*

▶ **Case Study 17•1** | **Arterial Insufficiency**

Joseph P. is an 80-year-old male with a 7-week history of a nonhealing sore on his left anterior shin that developed after he walked inadvertently into a concrete slab in his poorly lit work shed. His medical history is remarkable for a 3-year history of renal insufficiency and HTN, controlled with low-sodium diet and ACE inhibitors. He recently describes feeling nervous and "jumpy" quite often. He was a moderate drinker until this past year and has a 20 pack-year smoking history (20 cigarettes [1 pack] per day for 60 years). He has a past surgical history of carotid endarterectomy 4 years ago and cataract surgery 5 years ago; otherwise, his medical history is unremarkable. He presents with increasing concern over the cut on his left leg, which he says has begun to hurt more and is looking larger. He has not sought treatment until now because "it seemed like a little scrape." He has been covering it with triple antibiotic ointment and a large adhesive bandage.

Systems Review

Integument: Bilateral lower extremities are pale with little hair growth. His toenails are thickened and yellow, and skin appears fragile. The left anterior tibia presents with 3 × 1.4-cm partial-thickness wound extending to the anterior tibial tendon. The wound base has adhered fibrin, pale granulation at margins, and scant cloudy serosanguineous drainage. There is a foul odor, along with a 2-cm ring of erythema, and the site is exquisitely tender to palpation.

Anthropometric characteristics: Bilateral lower extremities appear thin, with high arches and clawing of the toes. He is 5'7", and his weight is 140 lb.

Joint Integrity, Manual Muscle Testing (MMT), Range of Motion (ROM), Posture: Joint mobility is within functional limits throughout bilateral lower extremities. Strength is 5–/5 in quadriceps and hamstrings and 4+/5 in bilateral gastrocnemius/soleus. Patient reports he used to walk down to the corner store (approximately 10 blocks), but now his legs hurt so badly after four blocks that he does not go anymore. Posture is slightly flexed through the trunk and lower extremities.

Pain: He reports pain at 10/10 when he tries to walk too far. Pain goes away when he rests, but occasionally has begun to wake him up at night. He sleeps in his recliner, and this helps sometimes.

Ventilation, Respiration, Circulation: Breath sounds with mild crackles in lower lobes are audible, and the rate is 16 breaths per minute. Heart rate is 82 bpm, and blood pressure is 155/85 on medications. Posterior tibialis and dorsal pedal pulses are nonpalpable. Posterior tibial artery Doppler signal is faint, and the signal is not audible in the dorsalis pedis artery. An ABI has been scheduled for next week in the vascular laboratory, scheduled following his last nephrologist's appointment when the walking pain was reported.

▶ Case Study 17•1 | Arterial Insufficiency—cont'd

Sensory and Reflex Integrity: Protective sensation is intact in bilateral feet; Achilles and patellar reflexes are brisk.

Motor Function, Gait, Balance: He is mostly independent in activities of daily living. His wife handles the cooking, and he assists with household cleaning and handy-work. He was walking the dog until the leg pain became so bad, now he only goes out occasionally, walks less than three to four blocks, and experiences severe pain. There are no balance or proprioceptive deficits.

Orthotic, Prosthetic, and Supportive Devices: He uses no assistive device. He has tried to use his wife's cane, but it doesn't help the leg pain.

Aerobic Capacity and Endurance: He has functional aerobic capacity. He reports "panic attacks" and "losing his breath, and chest tightening" when walking. This seems to pass if he rests, but sometimes it becomes frightening and he takes longer to catch his breath.

Work and Community: He works as a shuttle bus driver in his town 20 hours per week.

Tests and Measures:

1. Pulse assessment
2. ABI
3. Rubor of dependency
4. Cardiac workup to rule out cardiac chest pain and shortness of breath versus anxiety
5. Absolute claudication distance
6. Blood chemistry including WBC count

Recommended Interventions

Wound Management:

- Vascular consultation and laboratory findings to establish arterial status and presence of infection should be initiated.

- Systemic antibiotics should be prescribed if WBC count is elevated.
- Silver impregnated hydrogel or foam dressing should be used with daily dressing change.
- Irrigation and sharp débridement of ulcer to tolerance is indicated since it is open and is likely colonized or infected. Once circulatory status is determined, an idea of healing prognosis will be established.
- Care should remain conservative as long as patient factors show the lesion to be healable and good wound care is begun including:
  - Treatment three to five times a week with noncontact ultrasound or electrical stimulation is advised as adjunctive modalities.
  - In the presence of exposed tendon, relative immobilization with a walking boot will promote healing.
  - If infection or necrosis appear to be advancing, or if distal perfusion is not found to be adequate to support healing, surgical revascularization should be considered.

Exercise and Rehabilitation: There will be a referral to physical therapy for initiation of a supervised walking program for claudication.

Education: Smoking cessation, wound care, nutritional support services will be topics for patient education.

Other Considerations: Smoking cessation support, psychological support for possible anxiety, and recent changes in health status will be provided. Cardiovascular workup should be completed given the high correlation with cardiac risk in the presence of peripheral arterial disease.

References

1. Bonham, PA: Assessment and management of patients with venous, arterial, and diabetic neuropathic lower extremity wounds. AACN 2003; 4:442–456.
2. Bradley, NEA: Dressings and topical agents for arterial leg ulcers (review). The Cochrane Collaboration, London, John Wiley, 2002, pp 1–16.
3. Cassady, SL: Peripheral arterial disease: A review of epidemiology, clinical presentation, and effectiveness of exercise training. Cardiopulm PT 2004; 15:6–12.
4. Omran, AK: Diagnosis and risk assessment of lower extremity peripheral arterial disease. J Endovasc Ther 2006; 13(suppl II): II-10–II-18.
5. Nehler, MR, Wolford, HW: Natural history and non-operative treatment of chronic lower extremity ischemia. In: Rutherford, RB (ed): Vascular Surgery, ed. 6. Philadelphia, Elsevier Saunders, 2005, pp 1083–1094.
6. Suggested Standards for Reports Dealing with Lower Extremity Ischemia. Prepared by the Ad Hoc Committee on Reporting Standards, Society for Vascular Surgery/North American Chapter, International Society for Cardiovascular Surgery. J Vasc Surg 1986; 4:80–94.
7. Dayal, R, Kent, KC: Standardized reporting practices. In: Rutherford, RB (ed): Vascular Surgery, ed. 6. Philadelphia, Elsevier Saunders, 2005, pp 41–52.
8. Rutherford, RB, Baker, DJ, Ernst, C, et al: Recommended standards for reports dealing with LE ischemia: Revised version. J Vasc Surg 1997; 26:517–538.
9. The Merck Manual of Medical Information, Home Ed. 2. Whitehouse Station, NJ, Merck & Co., 2003, Chapters 31–34.
10. Newman, AB, Shemanski, L, Manolio, TA, et al: Ankle-arm index as predictor of cardiovascular disease and mortality in the cardiovascular health study. Arteriosclero Thromb Vasc Biol 1999; 19:538–545.

11. Diehm, C, Schuster, A, Allenberg, JR, et al: High prevalence of PAD and comorbidity in 6880 primary care patients: A cross-sectional study. Atherosclerosis 2004; 172:195–205.

12. Baumgartner, I, Redha, F, Baumgartner, RW, et al: Management of PVD. Annu Rev Med 2005; 56:249–272.

13. Norman PE, Eikelboom, JW, Hankey, GJ, et al: Peripheral arterial disease: Prognostic significance and prevention of atherosclerotic complications. Med J Aust 2004; 181:150–154.

14. Goodman, CC: The cardiovascular system. In: Goodman, CC, Boissonnault, WG (eds): Pathology: Implications for the Physical Therapist. Philadelphia, WB Saunders, 1998, pp 318–326.

15. Hirsch, A, Haskal, Z, Hertzer, N: ACC/AHA Guidelines for the management of peripheral arterial disease. Circulation 2006; pp 1487–1488.

16. McCulloch, JM: Management of wounds secondary to vascular disease. In: McCulloch, JM, Kloth, LC (eds): Wound Healing Alternatives in Management, ed. 3. Philadelphia, FA Davis, 2002, pp 418–424.

17. Garcia, LA: Epidemiology and pathophysiology of lower extremity peripheral arterial disease. J Endovasc Ther 2006; 13(suppl II): 11–3–9.113–119.

18. Heart and Stroke Encyclopedia. American Heart Association. Available at: www.americanheart.org. Accessed 08/18/07.

19. Thatipelli, MR, Pellikka, P, McBane, R, et al: Prognostic value of ankle-brachial index and dobutamine stress echocardiography for cardiovascular morbidity and all-cause mortality in patients with peripheral arterial disease. J Vasc Surg 2007; 46:62–70.

20. Criqui, MH, Langer, RD, Fronek A, et al: Mortality over a period of 10 years in patients with peripheral arterial disease. N Engl J Med 1992; 326:381–386.

21. Dormandy, J, Rutherford, RB: Management of peripheral arterial disease. TASC Working Group. Trans-Atlantic Intersociety Concensus (TASC). J Vasc Surg 2000; 31:S1–S296.

22. Gordon, T, Kannel, WB: Predisposition to atherosclerosis in the head, hearts, and legs. The Framingham Study. JAMA 1972; 221:661–666.

23. Fowkes, FGR, Housley, E, Cawood, EHH, et al: Edinburgh artery study: Prevalence of asymptomatic and symptomatic peripheral arterial disease in the general population. Int J Epidemiol 1991; 20:384–392.

24. Hiatt, WR, Hoag, S, Hamman, RF, et al: Effect of diagnostic criteria on prevalence of peripheral artery disease. The San Luis Valley Diabetes Study. Circulation 1995; 91:1178–1479.

25. Murabita, JM, D'Agostino, RB, Silbershatz, H, et al: Intermittent claudication. A risk profile from the Framingham Heart Study. Circulation 1997; 96:44–49.

26. Blacher, J, Cacoub, P, Luizyet, F, et al: Peripheral arterial disease versus other localizations of vascular disease: The ATTEST Study. J Vasc Surg 2006; 44:315–318.

27. Smith, GD, Shipley, MJ, Rose, G: Intermittent claudication, heart disease risk factors, and mortality. The Whitehall Study. Circulation 1990; 82:1925–1931.

28. CAPRIE Steering Committee. A randomized blinded trial of clopidogrel versus aspirin in patients at risk of ischemic events (CAPRIE). Lancet 1996; 348:1329–1339.

29. Berkow, R, Beers, MH (eds): The Merck Manual of Medical Information Home Edition. Whitehouse Station, NJ, Merck & Co, 1997, pp 130–136.

30. Federman, DG, Bravata, DM, Kirsner, RS: Peripheral arterial disease: A systemic disease extending beyond the affected extremity. Geriatrics 2004; 59:26–36.

31. Dormandy, J, Heeck, L, Vig, S, et al: The fate of patients with critical leg ischemia. Semin Vasc Surg 1999; 12:142–147.

32. Rubano, JJ, Kerstein, MD: Arterial insufficiency and vasculitides. J Wound Ostomy Continence Nurs 1998; 25:147–157.

33. Kisner, C, Colby, LA (eds): Therapeutic Exercise: Foundations and Techniques Philadelphia, FA Davis, 2002, pp 622–624, 708–715.

34. McCulloch, J: Physical modalities in wound management: Ultrasound, vasopneumatic devices, and hydrotherapy. Ostomy Wound Manage 1995; 41:30–37.

35. Lumsden, AB, Rice, TW: Medical management of peripheral arterial disease: A therapeutic algorithm. J Endovasc Ther 2006; 13(suppl II): 19–29.

36. Regensteiner, JG, Stewart, KJ: Established and evolving medical therapies for claudication in patients with peripheral arterial disease (Review). Nat Clin Prac 2006; 3:604–610.

37. Regenister JG, Steiner, JF, and Hiatt, WR, et al: Exercise training improves functional status in patients with peripheral arterial disease. J Vasc Surg 1996; 23:104–115.

38. Regenister JG, Ware, JE, McCarthy, WJ, et al: Effect of Cilostasol on community-based walking ability and health related quality of life in patients with peripheral arterial disease: Results of six randomized controlled trials. J Am Geriatr Soc 2002; 50:1939–1946.

39. McDermott, MM, Greenland, K, Liu, JM, et al: Physical activity, walking exercise, and skeletal muscle characteristics in patients with peripheral arterial disease. J Vasc Surg 2007; 46:87–93.

40. Lie, JT: The rise and fall and resurgence of thromboangiitis obliterans (Buerger's disease). Acta Pathol Jpn 1998; 39:153–158.

41. deWolfe, VG: Chronic occlusive arterial disease of the lower extremities. Cardiovasc Clin 1983; 13:15–35.

42. Lazarides, MK, Georgiadis, GS, Papas, TT, et al: Diagnostic criteria and treatment of Buerger's disease: A review. Int J Low Extrem Wounds 2006; 2:89–95.

43. Al Shami, AM, Souvlis, T, Coppieters, MW, et al: Biomechanical evaluation of two clinical tests for plantar heel pain: The dorsiflexion-eversion test for tarsal tunnel syndrome and the windlass test for plantar fasciitis. Foot Ankle Int 2007; 28:499–505.

44. Hamm, R, Rodrigues, J, Weitz, IC: Pathophysiology and multidisciplinary management of leg wounds in sickle cell disease: A case discussion and literature review. Wounds 2006; 18:277–285.

45. Eckman, JR: Leg ulcers in sickle cell disease. Hematol Oncol Clin North Am 1996; 10:1333–1344.

46. Sickle cell anemia. Department of Health and Human Services, National Institute of Health. Available at: http://www.nhlbi.nih.gov/health/dci/Diseases/Sca/SCA_WhatIs.html. Accessed 09/30/07.

47. Whitman, B, and Foy, C: Management of acute leg ischaemia. In: Beard, JD, Murray, S. (eds): Pathways of Care in Vascular Surgery. Shrewsbury, UK, tfm Publishing, 2002, pp 99–105.

48. Rajagopalan, S, Mckay I, Ford, I, et al: Platelet activation increases with the severity of peripheral arterial disease: Implications for clinical management. J Vasc Surg 46:2007; 485–484.

49. Ali, AT, Kalapatapu, VR, Bledsoe, S, et al: Percutaneous isolated limb perfusion with thrombolytics for severe limb ischemia. Vasc Endovascular Surg 2005; 39:491–497.

50. Ashworth, MJ, Patel, N: Compartment syndrome following ankle fracture-dislocation: A case report. Orthop Trauma 1998; 12:67–68.

51. Zachariah, S, Taylor, L, Kealey, D, et al: Isolated lateral compartment syndrome after Weber C fracture dislocation of the ankle: A case report and literature review. Injury 2005; 36:345–346.

52. Freidericson, M, Wun, C: Differential diagnosis of leg pain in the athlete. J Am Podiatr Med Assoc 2003; 93:321–324.

53. Fries, JF, Hunder, GG, Bloch, DA, et al: The American College of Rheumatology 1990 Criteria for the Classification of Vasculitis. Arthritis Rheum 1990; 33:1065–1067.

54. Panuncialman, J, Falanga, V: Basic approach to inflammatory ulcers. Dermatologic Therapy 2006; 19;365–376.

55. Pullen, RL: Managing cutaneous vasculitis in a patient with lupus erythematosus. Dermatol Nurse 2007; 19:21–26.

56. Sussman, C, Bates-Jensen, BM: Wound healing physiology: Acute and chronic. In: Sussman, C, Bates-Jensen, BM (eds): Wound Care: A Collaborative Practice Manual for Health Professionals, ed. 3. Philadelphia, Lippincott Williams & Wilkins, 2007, pp 21–51.

57. Stotts, N, Wipke-Tevis, D: Co-factors in impaired wound healing. In: Krasner, D (ed): Chronic Wound Care: A Clinical Sourcebook for Health Professionals, ed. 2. Wayne, PA, Health Management Publications, 1997, pp 64–71.

58. Fellows, J: Pyoderma gangrenosum and leg ulcers associated with vasculitis: Importance of addressing the underlying disease process when treating inflammatory wounds. J Wound Ostomy Continence Nurs 2006; 33:81–82.

59. Teravaert, JW, Kallenburg, C: Neurologic manifestations of systemic vasculitides. Rheum Dis Clin North Am 1993; 19:913–940.

60. What you need to know about Takayasu's arteritis: The Vasculitis Clinical Research Consortium. Cleveland Clinic, July 7, 2006; Available at: http://my.clevelandclinic.org/disorders/Takayasu_Arteritis/hic_Takayasus_Arteritis.aspx Accessed 08/10/07.

61. Hillegass, EA: Cardiovascular diagnostic tests & procedures. In: Hillegass, EA, Sadowsky, HS (eds): Essentials of Cardiopulmonary Physical Therapy, ed. 2. Philadelphia, WB Saunders, 2001, pp 370–373.

62. Sumpio, BE, Lee, T, Blume, P, et al: Vascular evaluation and arterial reconstruction of the diabetic foot. Clin Podiatr Med Surg 2003; 20:689–708.

63. Fowler, B, Jamrozki, K, Norman, P, et al: Prevalence of peripheral arterial disease: Persistence of excess risk in former smokers. Aust NJZ Pub Health 2002; 26:219–224.

64. Wong, LS, Martins-Green, M: First hand cigarette smoke alters fibroblast migration and survival: Implications for impaired healing. Wound Repair Regen 2004; 12:471–484.

65. Camargo, CA, Stampfer, MJ, Glynn, RJ, et al: Prospective study of moderate alcohol consumption and risk of peripheral arterial disease in US male physicians. Circulation 1997; 95:577–580.

66. Housley, E, Leng, GC, Donnan, PT, et al: Physical activity and risk of PAD in the general population. Edinburgh Artery Study. J Epidemiol Commun Health 1993; 47:475–480.

67. Black, JM: Management of clients with vascular disorders. In: Black, JM, Hawks, JH (eds): Medical Surgical Nursing Clinical Management for Positive Outcomes, ed. 7, vol 2. Philadelphia, Elsevier Saunders, 2005, pp 1509–1545.

68. Gough, S, Bradbury, A: The diabetic foot. In: Beard, JD, Murray, S (eds): Pathways of Care in Vascular Surgery. Shrewsbery, UK, tfm Publishing, 2002; pp 39–46.

69. Bonham, P: A critical review of the literature: Diagnosing osteomyelitis in patients with diabetes and foot ulcers. J Wound Ostomy Continence Nurs 2001; CN28(Pt 1):73–78.

70. Criqui, M, Fronek, A, Klauber, MK, et al: The sensitivity, specificity, and predictive value of traditional clinical evaluation of PAD: Results from non-invasive testing in a defined population. Circulation 1985; 71:516–522.

71. Lundkin, M, Wikson, J, Perakyla, T, et al: Distal pulse palpation: Is it reliable? World J Surg 1999; 23:252–255.

72. Moffiatt, C, O'Hare, B: Ankle pulses are not sufficient to detect impaired arterial circulation in patients with leg ulcers. J Wound Care 1995; 4:134–138.

73. Khan, NA, Rahim, SA, Anand SS, et al: Does the clinical examination predict lower extremity peripheral arterial disease? JAMA 2006; 295:536–546.

74. Padberg, FT, Back, TL, Jr., Thompson, PN, et al: Transcutaneous oxygen (TcPo$_2$) estimates probability of healing in the ischemic extremity. J Surg Res 1996; 60:365–369.

75. Bonham, P, Flemster, B: Guidelines for management in patients with lower extremity arterial disease. J Wound Ostomy Continence Nurs, 2002; WOCN clinical practice guideline series; no. 1.

76. Ballard, J, Eke, CC, Bunt, TJ, et al: A prospective evaluation of transcutaneous oxygen measurements in the management of diabetic foot problems. J Vasc Surg 1995; 22:485–492.

77. Goldman, R, Brewley, B, Zhou, L, et al: Electrotherapy reverses inframaleolar ischemia: A retrospective, observational study. Adv Skin Wound Care 2003; 16:79–89.

78. Sibbald, RG, Orsted, H, Schultz, GS, et al: Preparing the wound bed: Focus on infection and inflammation. Ostomy Wound Manage 2003; 49:24–51.

79. Vella, A, Carlson, LA, Blier, B, et al: Circulator boot therapy alters the natural history of ischemic leg ulceration. Vasc Med 2000; 5:21–25.

80. Kohler, TR, Andros, G, Porter, JM: Can duplex scanning replace arteriography for lower extremity disease? Ann Vasc Surg 1990; 4:146–161.

81. Marston, WA, et al: Natural history of limbs with arterial insufficiency and chronic ulceration treated without revascularization. J Vasc Surg 2006; 44:108–114.

82. Vijayaraghavan, KS, et al: Chronic non-healing ulcer of the lower limb with mixed arteriovenous pathology. Int J Low Extrem Wounds 2004; 3:47–48.

83. Ghauri, AS, Nyamekye, I, Grabs, AJ, et al: The diagnosis & management of mixed arterial/venous leg ulcers in community-based clinics. Eur J Vasc Endovasc Surg 1998; 16:350–355.

84. Schmidt, K, Debus, ES, Jeberger, S, et al: Bacterial population of chronic crural ulcers: Is there a difference between the diabetic, the venous, and the arterial ulcer? VASA 2000; 29:62–70.

85. Wheat, LJ, Allen, SD, Henry, M, et al: Diabetic foot infections: Bacteriologic analysis. Arch Intern Med 1986; 146:935–940.

86. Kloth, LC: Physical modalities in wound management: UVC, therapeutic heating and electrical stimulation. Ostomy Wound Manage 1995; 41:18–27.

87. Goldman, R, Rosen, M, Brewley, B, et al: Electrotherapy promotes healing and microcirculation of infra-popliteal ischemic wounds: A prospective pilot study. Adv Skin Wound Care 2004; 17:284–290, 292–294.

88. Petrofsky, J, Schwab, E, Lo, T, et al: Effects of electrical stimulation on skin blood flow in controls and in and around stage III and IV wounds in hairy and non-hairy skin. Med Sci Monit 2005; 11:CR309–316.

89. Hess, CL, Howard, MA, Attinger, CE: A review of mechanical adjuncts in wound healing: Hydrotherapy, ultrasound, negative pressure wound therapy, hyperbaric oxygen, and electrostimulation. Ann Plast Surg 2003; 51:210–218.

90. Daeschlein, G, Assadian, O, Kloth, LC, et al: Antibacterial activity of positive and negative polarity low-voltage pulsed current (LVPC) on six typical gram-positive and gram-negative bacterial pathogens of chronic wounds. Wound Repair Regen 2007; 15:399–403.

91. Argenta, LC, Morykwas, MJ: Vacuum assisted closure: A new method for wound control and treatment: Clinical experience. Ann Plast Surg 1997; 38:562–576.

92. Vuerstack, JDD, Vainas, T, Wuite, J, et al: State-of-the-art treatment of chronic leg ulcers: A randomized controlled trial comparing vacuum-assisted closure (VAC) with modern wound dressings. J Vasc Surg 2006; 44:1029–1038.

93. Clare, MP, Fitzgibbons, TC, McMullen, ST, et al: Experience with vacuum assisted closure negative pressure technique in the treatment of non-healing diabetic and dysvascular wounds. Foot Ankle Int 2002; 23:896–901.

94. Leidl, DA, Kavros, SJ: The effect of mist ultrasound transport technology on cutaneous microcirculatory blood flow. Presented at Symposium on Advanced Wound Care, 2001.

95. Schenck, EC, Kavros, SJ: The use of mist ultrasound transport technology for the promotion of chronic wound healing. Presented at Symposium on Advanced Wound Care, 2001.

96. Kavros, SJ: The use of low-frequency ultrasound in the treatment of chronic foot and leg ulcerations: A 51 patient retrospective analysis. Presented at Symposium on Advanced Wound Care, 2005.

97. Ennis, WJ, Valdes, W, Gainer, M, Meneses, P: Evaluation of clinical effectiveness of mist ultrasound therapy for the healing of chronic wounds. Adv Skin Wound Care 2006; 19:437–446.

98. Kavros, SJ, Miller, JL, Hanna, SW: Treatment of ischemic wounds with non-contact low-frequency ultrasound: The Mayo Clinic experience: 2004–2006. Adv Skin Wound Care 2007; 20:221–226.

99. Grolman, RE, Wilkerson, DK, Taylor, J, et al: Transcutaneous oxygen measurements predict a beneficial response to hyperbaric oxygen therapy in patients with non-healing wounds and critical limb ischemia. Am Surg 2001; 67:1072–1080.

100. Davidson, JD, Mustoe, TA: Oxygen in wound healing: More than a nutrient [editorial]. Wound Repair Regen 2001; 9:175–177.

101. Roeckl-Wiedmann, I, Bennett, M, Kranke, P: Systematic review of hyperbaric oxygen in the management of chronic wounds. Brit J Surg 2005; 92:24–32.

102. Markus, YM, Bell, MJ, Evans, AW: Iscemic scleroderma wounds successfully treated with hyperbaric oxygen therapy. J Rheumatol 2006; 33:1694–1696.

103. Delis, KT, Nicolaides, AN, Wolfe, JH, et al: Improved walking ability and ankle brachial pressure indices in symptomatic peripheral

vascular disease with intermittent pneumatic foot compression: A prospective controlled study with one-year follow-up. J Vasc Surg 2000; 31:650–661.

104. Ramaswami, G, D'Ayala, M, Hollier, LH, et al: Rapid foot and calf compression increases walking distance in patients with intermittent claudication: Results of a randomized study. J Vasc Surg 2005; 41:749–801.

105. Kakkos, SK, Geroulakos, G, Nicolaides, AN, et al: Improvement of the walking ability in intermittent claudication due to superficial femoral artery occlusion with supervised exercise and pneumatic foot and calf compression: A randomized controlled trial. Eur J Vasc Endovasc Surg 2005; 30:164–175.

106. Rooke, TW, Hollier, LH, Osmundson, PJ: The influence of sympathetic nerves on transcutaneous oxygen tension in normal and ischemic lower extremities. Angiology 1987; 38:400–410.

107. Wong, LS, Martins-Green, M: Effects of second hand smoke that can lead to impaired healing and fibrosis. Mol Biol Cell 2003; 14:355.

108. Kelly, SP, Gough, MJ: Risk factor modification. In: Beard, JD, Murray, S (eds): Pathways of care in vascular surgery, ed. 1. Shrewsbury, UK, tfm Publishing, 2002, 9–18.

109. Duprez, DA: Pharmacological interventions for peripheral arterial disease. Expert Opin Pharmacother 2007; 8:1465–1477.

110. Mohler, ER: Therapy insight: Peripheral arterial disease and diabetes—From pathogenesis to treatment guidelines. Nat Clin Pract Cardiovasc Med 2007; 4:151–162.

111. Peripheral Vascular Disease Index. Available at: http://www.medicinenet.com/peripheral_vascular_disease/page6.htm#toci. Accessed: 08/24/07.

112. Derubertis, BG, Faries, PL, McKinsey, JF, et al: Shifting paradigms in the treatment of lower extremity vascular disease: A report of 1000 percutaneous interventions. Ann Surg 2007; 246:415–422.

113. Dick, F, Diehm N, Galimanis A, et al: Surgical or endovascular revascularization in patients with critical limb ischemia: Influence of diabetes mellitus on clinical outcome. J Vasc Surg 2007; 45:751–761.

114. Neilsen, CC: Etiology of amputation. In: Lusardi, MM, Neilsen, CC (eds): Orthotics and Prosthetics in Rehabilitation. Woburn, MA, Butterworth-Heinemann, 2000, 327–336.

chapter 18

Lymphedema Complicating Healing

Heather Hettrick, PT, PhD, CWS, MLT, FACCWS

Introduction

Lymphedema is a chronic, incurable condition that is characterized by an abnormal collection of fluid owing to an anatomical alteration of the lymphatic system.[1] Throughout the world, it is estimated that one person in 30 is afflicted with lymphedema.[2] Lymphedema can lead to significant impairments in function, integumentary disorders, pain, and psychological issues. Appropriate identification of this disease can allow intervention and improve functional and aesthetic outcomes and patient quality of life. This chapter will describe the function of the lymphatic system and the etiologies of lymphedema. Examination, intervention, and preventive measures will be discussed, as well as impairments associated with lymphedema, including loss and restoration of function and other complications involving the integument.

Etiology

The lymphatic system has two main functions. The first is to provide significant immune function by protecting the body from disease and infection via production, maintenance, and distribution of lymphocytes. The second function is the facilitation of fluid transport from the interstitial tissues back into the bloodstream. This fluid transport maintains normal blood volume and eliminates chemical imbalances in the interstitial fluid.[3] The substances transported by the lymphatic system are called *lymphatic loads* and consist of protein, water, cellular debris, and fat (from the digestive system). These lymphatic loads are filtered by regional and central lymph nodes prior to reentry into the venous blood system.

The *lymphatic capillaries*, the beginning of the lymphatic system, abound in the dermis at the dermal-epidermal junction, forming a continuous network over the entire body, with the exception of the central nervous system (CNS) and cornea.[3] (Fig. 18.1) Unlike blood capillaries that consist of continuous tubules of endothelial cells, lymphatic capillaries consist of overlapping endothelial cells. A surrounding fiber net of *anchoring filaments*, arranged around the lymph capillaries, enables these vessels to stay open even under high tissue pressure.[4] (Fig. 18.2) The lymphatic loads are collected by the lymph capillaries and flow into bigger lymph vessels called *precollectors*, which then drain into *collectors*. Lymph collectors have segments called *lymph angions,* which are the sections between two valves in a lymph collector. Valves are spaced every 6 to 20 mm, and the frequency of contraction of lymph angions at rest is 6 to 10 contractions per minute.[5] The contraction of smooth muscle in each angion (called *lymphangiomotoricity*) generates the propulsive force of lymph flow along the lymph vessel. This is aided by a large number of valves inside the collectors, which enable the one-way flow of lymph. The propulsion directs the lymph fluid into regional and central lymph nodes to be filtered. (Fig. 18.3) Ultimately, the lymph fluid empties into the venous system through the left and right venous angles. The left and right venous angles are junctions between the subclavian and jugular veins at the level of the clavicles.

The amount of lymphatic load transported by the lymphatic system is dependent upon the same forces that propel blood in

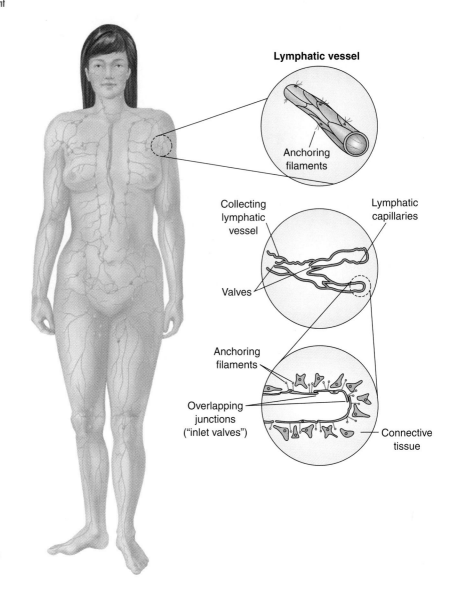

Lymphatic vessel

Anchoring filaments

Collecting lymphatic vessel

Lymphatic capillaries

Valves

Anchoring filaments

Overlapping junctions ("inlet valves")

Connective tissue

Figure 18•1 *Schematic of lymphatic system.*

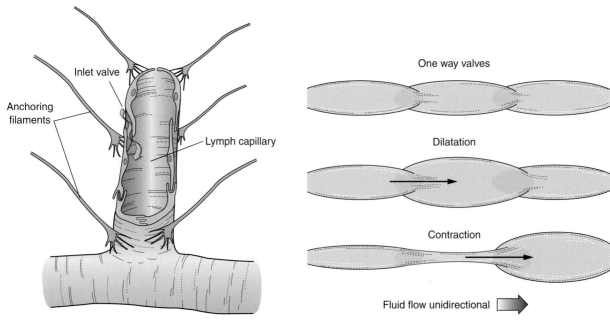

Inlet valve

Anchoring filaments

Lymph capillary

Figure 18•2 *Schematic of anchoring filaments.*

One way valves

Dilatation

Contraction

Fluid flow unidirectional ▶

Figure 18•3 *Schematic of lymphangiomotoricity.*

the blood capillaries. The *Starling equilibrium equation* (see Table 18.1) describes the balance of capillary filtration and reabsorption.[4,6] The transport of fluid through the membrane of blood capillaries depends on four variables: blood capillary pressure, colloid osmotic pressure of the plasma proteins, colloid osmotic pressure of the proteins located in the interstitial tissue, and tissue pressure. (Table 18.1) *Ultrafiltration* is defined as blood capillary pressure greater than the colloid osmotic pressure of plasma proteins. *Reabsorption* is defined by blood capillary pressure being less than the colloid osmotic pressure of plasma proteins.[4]

A shift in Starling equilibrium toward an increase in ultrafiltration (such as occurs in cases of inflammation or venous hypertension) or decreased colloid osmotic pressure (associated with hypoproteinemia) can cause an increased amount of lymphatic load placing a higher burden on the lymphatic system. A healthy lymphatic system is generally able to prevent or decrease the amount of acute edema. Under normal conditions the transport capacity of the lymphatic system is approximately 10 times greater than the physiological amount of the lymphatic loads. This is known as the *functional reserve of the lymphatic system*.[4] (Fig. 18.4) As long as the lymphatic load remains lower than the transport capacity of the lymphatic system, the lymphatic compensation is successful. If the lymphatic load exceeds the transport capacity, edema will occur. This is called *dynamic insufficiency* of the lymphatic system; the lymph vessels are intact but overwhelmed. (Fig. 18.5) The result is edema, which can usually be successfully treated with elevation, compression, and decongestive exercises (any basic exercise to facilitate the muscle pump).[4]

Lymphedema is caused by *mechanical insufficiency* or *low-volume insufficiency* of the lymphatic system. The transport capacity drops below the physiological level of the lymphatic loads. (Fig. 18.6) This means the lymphatic system is not able to clear the interstitial tissues, and an accumulation of high protein fluid is the result. This is recognized as *lymphedema or lymphostatic edema*.[4] The decisive difference between lymphedema and virtually all other types of edema is the high content of plasma proteins in the interstitial fluid. Over time (several months to years), this can lead to fibrosis of all affected tissue structures and is readily evident in the texture and consistency of the involved integument.[7] (Fig. 18.7)

Sometimes the etiology of edema is uncertain, and there is no clear clinical distinction between lymphedema and other types of edema. Some swelling may be a mixture of both edema and lymphedema as the functional reserve of the lymphatic system is exceeded or the lymph transport capacity

Table 18•1	Starling Equation
$$J_v = K_f\,[P_c - P_{if} - \sigma\,(\pi_p - \pi_{if})]$$	
Symbol	**Definition**
$P_c - P_{if}$	Hydrostatic pressure gradient
$\pi_p - \pi_{if}$	Colloid osmotic pressure gradient
K_f	Permeability of water and small solutes
σ	Permeability of plasma proteins
J_v	Capillary filtrate
J_l	Lymphatic return
$J_v > J_l$	Edema

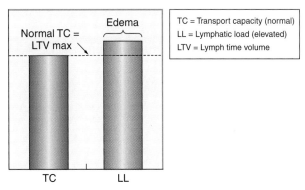

Figure **18•5** *Dynamic insufficiency. TC, transport capacity; LL, lymphatic load; LTV, lymph time volume.*

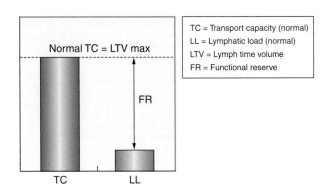

Figure **18•4** *Functional reserve of the lymphatic system.*

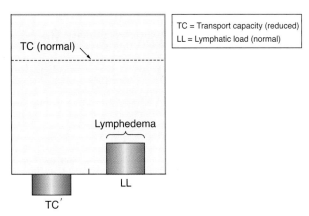

Figure **18•6** *Mechanical insufficiency.*

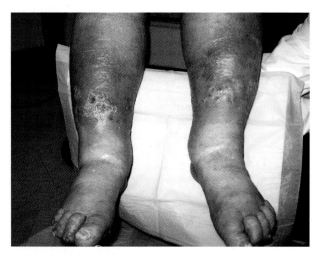

Figure 18•7 *Bilateral lymphedema with fibrosis.*

is compromised.[8] The progression of lymphedema from the patient's first perception of "heaviness" and nonresolving edema to irreversible fibrotic changes takes time. In an effort to standardize the associated integumentary changes, staging and classification systems have been developed. The staging system is used clinically to describe the subjective and objective integument changes. The classification system is used for unilateral limb involvement and is based on circumferential limb measurements. Tables 18.2 and 18.3 depict the stages and

classification systems for lymphedema. Early accurate diagnosis, patient education, and appropriate treatment will decrease the amount of time needed to achieve limb reduction, skin changes, and overall improvement or restoration of function.[3]

> ▶ **PEARL 18•1** A healthy lymphatic system is generally able to prevent or decrease the amount of acute edema. Under normal conditions the transport capacity of the lymphatic system is approximately 10 times greater than the physiological amount of the lymphatic loads.

> ▶ **PEARL 18•2** The decisive difference between lymphedema and virtually all other types of edema is the high content of plasma proteins in the interstitial fluid.

The etiology of lymphedema is currently classified into two major categories: *primary* and *secondary lymphedema.* Primary lymphedema is caused by a condition that is either hereditary or congenital. In the United States it is estimated that approximately 2 million people have primary lymphedema.[9] Eighty-three percent of primary lymphedema cases manifest before the age of 35 (*lymphedema precox*) and 17% manifest after the age of 35 (*lymphedema tardum*).[10] Onset of primary lymphedema can occur at birth (Milroy's disease or Meige's disease), yet most often the onset is during puberty or around the age of 17. Eighty-seven percent of all cases of primary lymphedema occur in females, and the lower extremities are more often involved than other body parts.[11]

Table 18•2 Stages of Lymphedema

Stages of Lymphedema	Description
Subclinical	Patient begins to feel "heaviness" in limb; fibrotic changes and fluid accumulation can occur before visible swelling or pitting. Approximately 50% of patients with minimal edema report a feeling of heaviness or fullness of the extremity.
Stage 1	Reversible lymphedema: accumulation of protein-rich fluid, elevation reduces swelling. Tissue pits on pressure.
Stage 2	Spontaneously irreversible lymphedema: proteins stimulate fibroblast formation, connective and scar tissue proliferate. Minimal pitting, even with moderate swelling.
Stage 3	Lymphostatic elephantiasis: hardening of dermal tissues, papillomas of the skin, tissue appearance elephant-like. (Not everyone progresses to this stage).

Adapted from Casley-Smith, JR, Casley-Smith, JR: *Modern Treatment for Lymphoedema*, 5th edition. Malvern, South Australia, Australia, The Lymphedema Association of Australia, Inc., 1997; Kelly, DG: *A Primer on Lymphedema*. Upper Saddle River, NJ, Prentice Hall, 2000.

Table 18•3 Classification for Lymphedema

Classification for Lymphedema	Description
Mild	Less than 3 cm differential between affected limb and unaffected limb.
Moderate	3–5 cm differential between affected limb and unaffected limb.
Severe	5+ cm differential between affected limb and unaffected limb.

Adapted from Casley-Smith, JR, Casley-Smith, JR: *Modern Treatment for Lymphoedema*, 5th edition. Malvern, South Australia, Australia, The Lymphedema Association of Australia, Inc., 1997; Kelly, DG: *A Primer on Lymphedema*. Upper Saddle River, NJ, Prentice Hall, 2000.

Secondary lymphedema is caused by some identifiable insult to the lymphatic system.[11] Secondary lymphedema etiologies include inflammation, infection, radiation therapy, surgery, filariasis (parasitic infection), trauma, iatrogenic alterations, artificial self-induced lymphedema, benign or malignant tumor growth, or chronic venous insufficiency.[11] About 2.5 to 3 million people in the United States have been diagnosed with secondary lymphedema.[9] One third of patients who undergo mastectomy (with lymph node resection) secondary to breast cancer develop secondary lymphedema of the upper extremity.[12] Radical lymph node dissection with prostate cancer causes lymphedema of one or both legs and often the genitals in more than 70% of the cases.[13] Secondary lymphedema is usually unilateral; however, it may present in both limbs. It is important to note, however, that involvement of the limbs and presentation of the edema is generally not symmetrical. One limb will appear larger, and it is this limb that should first be addressed with intervention strategies.

Lymphedema can lead to numerous health-related and emotional problems. Of concern is the high risk of infection and skin changes associated with chronic lymphedema, particularly for patients who do not receive intervention. Fluid accumulation in the tissues is an ideal medium for pathogen growth, and cellulitis and venous-type ulceration (particularly of the lower extremities) can be a common occurrence for patients with lymphedema. Patients also experience embarrassment and social barriers due to increased limb size, discomfort, diminished movement and function of the affected limb or limbs, and difficulty donning and doffing clothing and shoes, any of which may compromise a person's quality of life.[8]

Examination

A thorough physical examination is critical in correctly diagnosing lymphedema.[14] The diagnosis of lymphedema is made in most cases by patient history, systems review, inspection, palpation, and a few select noninvasive tests such as volume or girth measurement. At present, the only clinical test that has been shown to be a reliable and valid method to diagnose lymphedema is *Stemmer's sign*.[15,16] This is a thickening of the skin over the proximal phalanges of the toes or fingers of the involved limb and the inability to "tent" or pick up the skin. (Fig. 18.8) If positive, it is a definite indication of lymphedema; if negative, its absence is not certain (ie, a secondary lymphedema may have started in the thigh but not have progressed to the foot).[17] When the Stemmer's sign is negative, it is appropriate to treat the edema with conventional interventions of elevation, rest, and compression. If the edema does not respond to conventional interventions, it should be monitored, and regular reassessment should be conducted as the underlying pathology may be an early lymphedema.

A thorough history is essential to correctly identify lymphedema. The history should include the following:

- *Symptoms.* Onset of the symptoms (swelling, heaviness of limb), length of time since initial onset, and the triggering event (ie, a bee sting, sprained ankle, recent surgery or trauma), should be included if known.

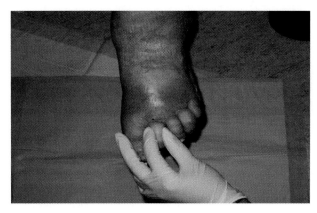

Figure 18•8 *Stemmer sign.*

- *Current and past medical history, including traumatic events and surgery.* This should also include all current medications, health-risk factors, coexisting problems (ie, cancer diagnosis, obesity, cardiac problems, venous insufficiency), and family history.
- *Pain and/or associated discomfort.* Significant pain may suggest additional tests and measures to determine if a secondary problem exists, such as venous or arterial compromise or an underlying orthopedic condition. Most patients with lymphedema report heaviness and associated discomfort in lieu of pain due to the large amounts of fluid in the tissues.
- *Functional status and activity level.* Does the patient report a loss in function or difficulty doing activities of daily living due to the swelling? How active or inactive is the patient, and in what type of activities does the person participate and enjoy?
- *Review of social habits such as smoking, diet and nutritional habits, and physical fitness and weight management strategies.* A diet does not exist for lymphedema, but a low-sodium diet in combination with good hydration and nutritional habits is recommended.
- *Past treatment and intervention history.* Some interventions may have led to an exacerbation of the symptoms, such as improper compression, sole use of a pneumatic compression pump, thermal modalities, and/or deep massage.[18]

Following the history, a brief systems review should be performed. Specifically, a review of the cardiopulmonary, integumentary, musculoskeletal, and neuromuscular system will help the clinician identify health problems that may require referral to another health professional, and it may help identify specific tests and measures to use to complete a thorough patient assessment. In addition, it is important to review the patient's affect, cognition, language, and learning style to optimize the examination and intervention strategies.

Tests and measures that should be included for patients with lymphedema or those at risk for developing lymphedema follow.[19] Characteristic findings common with lymphedema are presented.

1. *Integumentary integrity:* Assessment consists of extensive palpation and inspection, including texture (rough, orange peel-like); color (red, brown, darker than the

person's natural color); pitting status (slow or hard to pit); fibrosis (hardening of the skin and tissues); temperature (involved limb may feel warmer upon palpation); deepening of skin folds (skin may fold over ankle or wrist joint similar to a rubber band effect); nail quality (thickened and/or discolored); Stemmer's sign test; and presence of cysts/fistulas, papillomas, or ulcers (defects in the integument such as lesions and/or benign growths). (Fig. 18.9)

2. *Anthropometric characteristics:* Volume measurements using water displacement and girth measurements comparing circumferential limb segments of the involved and noninvolved limb are the most common noninvasive assessments of the lymphedematous limb.[20] If the involvement is bilateral, baseline measurements should be taken on both limbs for future comparison. Tonometry (measurement of fluid mobility by recording tissue deformation) and bioelectrical impedance analysis (amount of extracellular water and total water content) are newer methods that can assist with detecting subclinical lymphedema.[21,22]

3. *Joint integrity and mobility, muscle performance, range of motion and posture:* Patients with lymphedema will present with significant limitations in manual muscle strength tests and goniometry (range of motion) due to the heaviness of the limb from the excessive fluid burden. Biomechanical compensations such as gait deviations and overuse of the noninvolved limb can negatively affect joints and posture.

4. *Pain:* Pain should be differentiated from discomfort or heaviness. The location is important to determine if the pain is related to the lymphedema or another problem. The use of a visual analog scale can objectify the patients' pain response and help to differentiate pain from discomfort. Pain may be related to other patient comorbidities (ie, peripheral vascular disease, orthopedic or neuromuscular pathologies), or it could be an indicator of infection (ie, cellulitis). Further evaluation should explore the true nature of the pain so the appropriate intervention can be implemented.

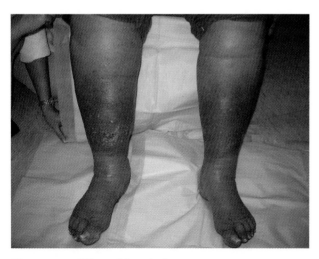

Figure 18•9 *Bilateral lymphedema.*

5. *Arousal, mentation, and cognition:* The results of these evaluations are important as patient education and compliance are paramount for successful management. Patients require extensive education and support to learn how to manage lymphedema and how to prevent exacerbations and/or associated complications. Verbal instruction, demonstration, and patient-appropriate literature will help to empower patients with lymphedema.

6. *Ventilation, respiration, and circulation:* When the lower extremities are involved, a vascular exam consisting of an ankle-brachial index and the use of a handheld ultrasound Doppler to assess pulses is important to determine venous and arterial integrity. A pulmonary review (part of the systems review) will determine the patient's tolerance to deep breathing and resisted breathing, which are components of lymphedema intervention.

7. *Sensory and reflex integrity:* These characteristics are particularly important with associated complications such as diabetes and circulatory disorders so as to recognize and prevent further injury. Loss of protective sensation in the feet, measured by a 5.07- or 10-g Semmes-Weinstein monofilament, should be identified so education and appropriate shoes and inserts can be provided.

8. *Motor function, gait, locomotion, and balance:* Establishing the patient's functional baseline will promote the individualized exercise prescription, aiding compliance and positive outcomes. In clinical practice, it appears that the larger the lymphedematous limb, the more common and advanced the compensations and impairments present in motor function, gait, locomotion, and balance.

9. *Orthotic, prosthetic, supportive devices, assistive and adaptive devices:* Identification of need will assist with the rehabilitation and prevention components of treatment by improving safety and facilitating independence.

10. *Aerobic capacity and endurance:* Establishing baseline will promote individualized exercise prescription, assisting with compliance and improved outcomes.

11. *Self-care and home management:* It is imperative to determine the needs of the patient to effectively implement treatment interventions. The patient's ability or lack of ability to participate will directly impact the course of care, particularly self-management of lymphedema.

12. *Community and work/school integration or reintegration and environmental, home, and work/school barriers:* Patient and family education, modification of lifestyle, and maintenance and prevention strategies should consider the patient's home, work, and school life for optimal results.[18]

▶ **PEARL 18•3** The diagnosis of lymphedema is made in most cases by patient history, systems review, inspection, palpation, and a few select noninvasive tests, such as volume or girth measurement.

Wound Care Interventions

Meticulous skin and nail care is a significant part of lymphedema intervention and prevention. The goal is to prevent skin breakdown and infection. However, many patients present with skin lesions due to the destructive nature of chronic lymphedema and the excessive fluid burden on the tissues. (Fig. 18.10) The excess fluid commonly associated with chronic lymphedema increases the diffusion distance, the distance oxygen, nutrients, and blood are required to travel from the capillaries to the cells and tissues of the skin. A high fluid burden on the tissues could also result in systemic infection, as stagnant fluid is present for pathogen growth. Tissue lesions common with lymphedema, due to the impaired lymph vascular system and/or to other comorbid conditions, may present from simple superficial excoriations to multifarious ulcers with complex etiologies. Vascular and inflammatory ulcers, fungating wounds, radiation burns, minor traumas, and failed surgical sites are all potential skin lesions that may present in patients with lymphedema. To appreciate the relationship of lymphedema to wound healing, clinicians should review their understanding of venous ulceration and chronic venous insufficiency (Chapter 16), because the pathophysiology and clinical presentation are related.[1]

In chronic venous insufficiency (CVI), edema does not develop as long as the lymphatic system can compensate for the increased venous pressure. When the lymphatic system becomes overwhelmed, a condition called *phlebolymphatic*

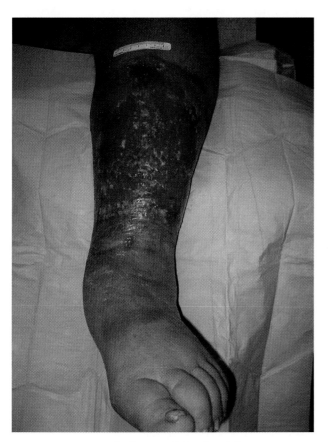

Figure 18•10 *Lymphedema and skin breakdown.*

insufficiency is created, meaning the combined carrying capacity of the local veins and lymphatics can no longer handle the buildup of fluid in the tissues.[5] Altered physiology of lymphatic drainage plays a major role in the etiology of edema, chronic leg ulcers, and chronic venous hypertension. At first, *lymphodynamic insufficiency* develops, followed by the physical destruction of the lymphatic vessels, causing lymphostatic edema and safety valve insufficiency, a form of secondary lymphedema.[5] Wounds are common with this clinical presentation, and lymph drainage and compression can help decrease the severity of the ulceration.[1] Appropriate wound management, combined with specific lymph drainage around the ulcer helps to rid the wound of cellular debris and toxins.[5] Care should be taken to drain the fluid away from the ulcer to prevent wound congestion, and additional drainage techniques should be used on the proximal extremity to promote the lymphatic flow toward regional lymph nodes. (Specific drainage techniques are discussed in the section on lymphedema intervention.)

Cellulitis (erysipelas) is the most common complication of primary and secondary lymphedema. Cellulitis is a painful inflammation of the soft tissue that is characterized by expanding local erythema, palpable local lymph nodes in 50% of the cases, and associated fever and chills.[13] Caused by an acute streptococcus infection, the smallest injuries can be the portal of entry for the bacteria, leading to a local or systemic infection. Seventy percent of cellulitis cases are caused by simple injuries such as cuts, abrasions, insect bites, local burns, and interdigital mycosis.[13] Treatment requires local antibiotics and/or persistent systemic antibiotic therapy in addition to patient education about preventative measures, as recurrence is frequent, thereby further limiting lymph transport capacity.[13] (Fig. 18.11)

Local wound infection is common as the moist or wet environment is conducive to pathogen growth. Treatment involves addressing the underlying infection, if present, with appropriate systemic and topical antibiotics. Local wound care should involve managing the often copious exudate while maintaining adequate compression. Hydrofibers, alginates, and other absorptive dressings should be considered in the presence of exuding wounds. Four-layer bandage systems (ie, Profore™, Smith & Nephew, Largo, FL; Dyna-Flex™, Johnson & Johnson, New Brunswick, NJ) are effective for absorbing excess drainage and provide the necessary and vital compression. With compression and control of lymphedema, the associated wounds will heal in the majority of cases.[1] Once the systemic and/or local infection has resolved, specific lymphedema interventions (manual lymph drainage, compression, exercise, and skin and nail care) should begin or resume.

Compression is the cornerstone of lymphedema therapy. The degree of swelling, presence of skin breakdown, diabetes, arterial insufficiency, and chronic congestive heart failure must be considered.[1] The Unna boot, short-stretch bandage, long-stretch bandage, cotton padding, self-adherent crepe dressing, and combination wraps are among the variety of compression bandages used in the treatment of lymphedema. In applying compression, frequently reassessing the condition of the limb (ie, limb size reduction) and matching the dressing to the patient's diagnosis and wound status is critical.[1]

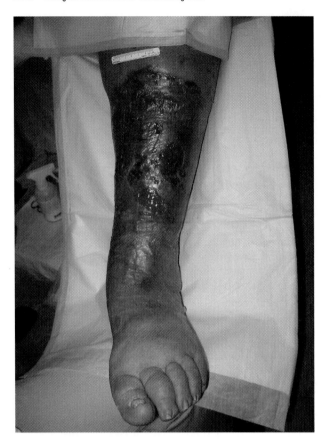

Figure 18•11 *Lymphedema and infection.*

Bandages used in compression differ in elasticity and extensibility. Bandages also have varying amounts of resting and working pressure. Resting pressure is that which is exerted on the skin by the elastic whether or not the patient is moving or activating a muscle pump. Working pressure is pressure exerted on the skin when contracting muscles push against a compression bandage. (Fig. 18.12) Short-stretch bandages have a high working pressure and low resting pressure. Short-stretch bandages (ie, Comprilan®, BSN-Jobst Inc., Charlotte,

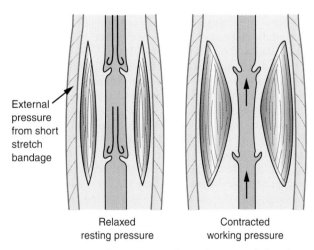

Figure 18•12 *Working pressure from short stretch bandage.*

NC) stretch 20% of their original length compared to long-stretch bandages (ie, elastic wraps) that stretch up to 190% of their original length. When the limb is at rest, short-stretch bandages supply a comfortable degree of support (without a tourniquet effect), but the total pressure increases significantly when the muscles contract against fixed resistance. This creates an effective, intermittent massage that forces interstitial fluid into functioning lymph collectors. Therefore, the compression wrap becomes a dynamic part of the wound dressing or treatment for patients with lymphedema.[1]

> **PEARL 18•4** Tissue lesions common with lymphedema, due to the impaired lymph vascular system and/or to other comorbid conditions, may present from simple superficial excoriations to multifarious ulcers with complex etiologies.

> **PEARL 18•5** Compression is the cornerstone of lymphedema therapy.

Lymphedema Interventions

Once the diagnosis of lymphedema has been made, it is essential that the appropriate interventions be used to address the patient's impairments. Treatment should involve specific interventions for lymphedema, integument and wound management strategies, and rehabilitation for functional impairments. Long-term management requires prevention and maintenance strategies to decrease the risk of exacerbations, infections, and other associated impairments.

Lymphedema is a manageable disease with the right treatment and intervention. The goal of lymphedema therapy is to get the patient back to a subclinical or latency stage, regardless of their diagnosed stage or classification. In most cases, this can be readily achieved with *complete decongestive therapy* (CDT). CDT, a two-phase intervention for lymphedema, is noninvasive, highly effective, cost-effective, and can reduce and maintain limb size.[23-25] The proposed benefits of CDT include opening collateral lymphatic drainage pathways, increasing pumping by the deep lymphatic pathways, and reducing and breaking down fibrotic tissue.[14,24]

Phase 1, or the intensive phase, involves meticulous skin and nail care, manual lymphatic drainage (MLD), bandaging, exercise (in bandaging), and the use of a compression garment (at the end of phase 1). Phase 2, or the self-management phase, involves the patient wearing a compression garment during the day and bandaging at night, exercise (in the garment or bandage), meticulous skin and nail care, and self-MLD as needed.[25]

Manual lymph drainage is a specialized manual technique based on physiological principles of lymph flow and lymph vessel emptying. MLD affects the lymph system by moving lymph fluid opposite natural flow patterns and around blocked areas toward collateral vessels, anastomoses, and uninvolved lymph node regions; increasing lymph angiomotoricity; increasing the volume of transported lymph fluid; increasing pressure in the lymph collector vessels; improving lymph transport capacity; and potentially increasing arterial blood flow.[24,26-32]

External pressure from short stretch bandage

Relaxed resting pressure

Contracted working pressure

In Europe, phase 1 of CDT includes twice-daily visits for an average of 4 to 6 weeks. In the United States (due to health-care constraints) CDT is limited to daily visits for 3 to 4 weeks for the upper extremity and 4 to 6 weeks for the lower extremity.[25] Phase 2 begins when phase 1 ends (plateau in limb reduction as indicated by weekly girth measurements) and may continue for up to 18 months after CDT initiation. The duration and intensity of treatment are dependent upon the clinical stage of lymphedema. Stage 1 and 2, mild and moderate lymphedema, are more easily managed than stage 3 or severe lymphedema. Patient compliance is paramount, and management is a life-long process. The stages and classifications help health-care professionals determine the intensity of the therapy as well as plan the potential duration of the interventions.

Functional limitations should be addressed according to patient needs. Often, as a limb reduces in size, function is improved. However, patients often require a basic exercise prescription to improve strength, flexibility, and cardiovascular health.

Several other interventions are worthy of discussion as they are often implemented for the management of edematous and lymphedematous limbs. These include the following: intermittent compression pumps, diuretics, and biophysical technologies.

> **PEARL 18•6** CDT (complete decongestive therapy) is a two-phase intervention for lymphedema that is noninvasive, highly effective, and cost-effective that can reduce and maintain limb size.

Intermittent Pneumatic Compression

Intermittent pneumatic compression pumps can be harmful to patients with lymphedema when they are used inappropriately. These pumps successfully mobilize fluid; however, proteins may remain in the affected tissues. This can promote more fluid to accumulate, as proteins are hydrophilic and cause the area to become even more fibrotic. If a pump is used without manual lymphatic drainage (MLD), the mobilized fluid may collect in the torso from the upper extremity or in the groin area from the lower extremities. The pumps do not reroute lymph fluid, as does MLD. It is highly recommended to use a pump only at the end of phase 2 of complete decongestive therapy (CDT) in combination with manual lymph drainage. The pump should not be used to decongest, but rather to maintain the benefits of CDT. For further information on pneumatic compression, please refer to Chapter 30 on compression.

Diuretics

A second treatment consideration is the use of diuretics. Diuretics also mobilize fluid out of the affected areas and increase the blood volume. The proteins, however, remain in the affected tissues, drawing in more water, which ultimately leads to more fibrosis. Some patients may have comorbidities that require the use of diuretics, such as congestive heart failure, certain kidney disorders, or high blood pressure. As long as the physician is managing the patient for the specific condition that requires a diuretic, then the diuretic should be continued. If the diuretic is solely being used to manage lymphedema, it is important to discuss other treatment options such as CDT with the physician and suggest that the diuretic be discontinued.

Biophysical Technologies

Electrical stimulation is not recommended with patients who have lymphedema. Electrical stimulation can increase local blood flow, leading to active hyperemia. Active hyperemia can trigger or exacerbate lymphedema. In relation to active hyperemia, heat modalities, cold modalities, and basic therapeutic massage should not be used on lymphedematous limbs. Although widely used for pain management, there is not sufficient evidence to support the use of transcutaneous electrical nerve stimulation (TENS) for the management of lymphedema-related discomfort. Anecdotally, the conventional setting with TENS has been utilized for lymphedema-related discomfort. Conventional TENS that utilizes a biphasic, charge balanced wave form does not induce a local hyperemia as do other forms of electrical stimulation, and it is believed to reduce pain by nociceptive inhibition. Gentle stretching exercises and manual traction may also diminish pain symptoms.

Approaches for Prevention

Patients must be educated about the preventative measures and risk factors as currently understood. Patients must also avoid activities that can trigger a further decrease of the transport capacity of the lymph vessels or unnecessarily increase the lymphatic fluid and protein load of the lymphatic system in an affected region.[18]

Lymphedema may be triggered or exacerbated by the following factors (these factors are based on clinical expert opinion and anecdotal evidence):

- Infection, integument insult, and threats to skin integrity, such as pet scratches, gardening-related injuries, insect bites, contusions, injections, intravenous cannulation, application of artificial nails, poor foot care, vigorous and repetitive housework, and blood pressure measurements on the involved extremity should all be avoided.
- Obesity and body fluid volume fluctuations are beginning to be associated with the development of lymphedema. Other predisposing factors include pregnancy, weight gain, chronic venous insufficiency, certain medications, and related complications from other health problems that lead to fluid retention or weight gain. These factors can stretch and permanently damage the lymphatic vessels, resulting in lymphedema.
- Age can influence the progression of lymphedema after onset, and fatigue and structural changes of the body systems related to aging can impact and weaken the lymphatic system, making it less efficient. Specifically, a weakened or diseased integumentary, cardiopulmonary, or musculoskeletal system can compromise the lymphatic system either from direct damage or from its inability to assist in lymphatic propulsion by ineffective circulatory, respiratory, or muscle pump action.
- Systemic or local events that cause hyperemia of the involved limb tissues can all trigger or exacerbate lymphedema. These include but are not limited to hot packs, hot tubs, summer weather, sun bathing, handling hot foods, aggressive massage, overuse of involved limb, infection, and soft tissue sprains and strains.

• Pressure changes resulting from airplane travel, scuba diving, prolonged wearing of tight clothing over areas at risk, and sleeping for long periods of time on the limb at risk are all activities that should be avoided. Subtle pressure changes can affect Starling equilibrium and trigger or exacerbate lymphedema. If air travel is necessary, the use of compression bandages or garments during flight is imperative.[11]

Certain activities may be of high risk, medium risk, or beneficial for patients with upper and lower extremity lymphedema. The Academy of Lymphatic Studies has issued exercise-risk guidelines for patients with lymphedema. (Table 18.4)

Patients should be properly educated regarding exercise and activities of daily living that are safe and beneficial for them to perform. The goal of exercise is to improve lymphatic flow without adding undue stress to the impaired lymphatic system. Exercise programs should be prescribed and progressed at a pace to ensure compliance and enable the effects of the exercise to be monitored and altered if required. Individual exercise programs should be equivalent to the patient's fitness level and directed by a therapist or clinician with knowledge of exercise progression, lymphedema contraindications, and risk factors.

Prevention strategies and adherence to maintenance programs are essential to decrease the risk of exacerbation and/or injuries that can lead to infection and subsequent lymphedema.

Table 18•4 High-Risk, Medium-Risk, and Beneficial Upper- and Lower-Extremity Exercises for Lymphedematous Limbs		
Upper-Extremity High Risk	**Upper-Extremity Medium Risk**	**Upper-Extremity Beneficial**
Gardening	Jogging/running	Swimming
Racquet sports	Biking (minimize grip)	Lymphedema exercise (gentle exercises to induce a muscle pump)
Golf	StairMaster®,* (minimize grip)	Walking
Shoveling snow	NordicTrack™,† (minimize grip)	Self MLD
Moving furniture	General weight lifting	Yoga
Carrying heavy luggage		Water aerobics
Carrying grocery bags		
Scrubbing		
Weight lifting with arm		
Gripping activities		
Lower-Extremity High Risk	**Lower-Extremity Medium Risk**	**Lower-Extremity Beneficial**
Running	Light jogging	Walking
Intense biking	Biking longer than 30 min	Easy biking 10–20 min
Moving furniture	Skating longer than 20 min	Lymphedema exercise
Soccer	Golfing	Easy skating 10–15 minutes
Hockey	Volleyball/tennis (easy)	Swimming
Long periods of sitting or standing	Upper-extremity weight lifting	Calf pumps
Weight lifting with legs	NordicTrack longer than 15 min	NordicTrack 5–10 min
StairMaster longer than 15 min	StairMaster longer than 5 min	Deep breathing exercises
Wrestling	Easy horseback riding	Yoga
Intense sport activities		Water aerobics

MLD, manual lymphatic drainage.
Adapted from the *Academy of Lymphatic Studies Course Manual*, 2001. Academy of Lymphatic Studies, Sebastian, FL.
*Nautilus Inc., Vancouver, WA.
†ICON Health & Fitness, Logan UT.

▶ **PEARL 18•7** The goal of exercise is to improve lymphatic flow without adding undue stress to the impaired lymphatic system.

Common Functional Impairments and Recommendations for Restoration of these Impairments

Lymphedema can significantly impact a patient's functional status and quality of life. Because lymphedema is a progressive disease, early intervention and identification of the disease is important to improve patient outcomes. Once limb reduction has been achieved with CDT, associated functional limitations should be addressed.

Due to the significant size of some lymphedematous lower limbs, patients often have difficulty with ambulation, basic mobility tasks, and balance. Community ambulation and negotiation of stairs and curbs can be challenging for patients with lower-extremity lymphedema. To compensate for the accumulated fluid burden with increased limb size and weight, the patient may alter their gait pattern and biomechanics related to ambulation. Patients may present with a wide base of support and externally rotated feet to accommodate for the lymphedematous limb and to compensate for balance discrepancies. Overuse and strain of the noninvolved extremity can further impair a person's mobility status. If the patient has bilateral lower-extremity lymphedema, these compensations may be further exacerbated. Additionally, patients often are deconditioned and have limited cardiovascular endurance. Initiating CDT to reduce limb size will facilitate improvements in gait and ambulation activities. Providing patients with appropriate assistive devices will enhance safety and reduce complications related to biomechanical compensations. Basic exercise prescription for cardiovascular endurance and strengthening will provide overall improvement in mobility tasks and enhance home and community ambulation skills.

Other impairments associated with lymphedema include limitations in range of motion (due to large fluid volumes), decreased strength (related to diminished use), and difficulty with upper-extremity function and activities of daily living when the lymphedema is present in the hand and/or arm. Range of motion should improve as limb volume decreases. Individualized exercise prescription including range of motion and therapeutic exercise will improve function by restoring range and strength for both fine motor and gross motor activities. Compliance with exercise prescription is improved if activities are broken down into frequent, short sessions throughout the day. In addition, lifestyle modifications and adherence to compression therapy will augment functional outcomes.

Lymphedema is often referred to as a hidden epidemic; however, it is a manageable disease. Identification and intervention at any stage can improve functional and cosmetic outcomes. Recognizing and addressing the associated impairments related to lymphedema will enhance outcomes and patient satisfaction. Additionally, patient education and compliance with treatment is paramount for the successful management of this disease.

▶ **Case Study 18•1** ▏ **Evaluation and Management of Lymphedema Following Prostate Cancer Surgery**

History

Mr. H is a 52-year-old male with a 2-year history of bilateral lower-extremity secondary lymphedema. His medical history is remarkable for prostate cancer with nodal resection, type 2 diabetes mellitus for 8 years, and hypertension. Mr. H is alert and oriented, and he cares for his wife who has advanced multiple sclerosis. Mr. H reports he developed lymphedema 3 months after the interventions for prostate cancer. He does not recall the triggering event other than gradual swelling that did not resolve. Past and current treatment includes elevation, elastic wraps, and the use of a pneumatic compression pump twice a week for the last 4 months.

Systems Review

Integument: Mr. H has positive Stemmer's sign bilateral lower extremities; fibrosclerotic skin changes; hard pitting edema; nail changes; 12 cm × 12 cm partial-thickness ulcer on anterior left lower extremity that drains copious serous fluid, which appears clinically infected; and deepening of skin folds at ankle mortise, on the left more than the right.

Anthropometric Characteristics: The left lower extremity is approximately 2 cm larger than right lower extremity. His height is 5'11" and weight 240 lb.

Joint Integrity, Manual Muscle Test (MMT), Range of Motion, Posture: The patient has diminished proprioception in bilateral ankles, fair strength in lower extremity flexors and extensors, and limited range of motion due to excessive edema at bilateral ankles and knees. Patient reports difficulty negotiating stairs and ambulating greater than 200 feet. His stance is significant for externally rotated feet with broad base of support, weak abdominal musculature, and exaggerated lumbar lordosis.

Pain: Patient reports discomfort and heaviness in his legs. Pain at the wound site is rated 3 out of 10 on a visual analog scale.

Ventilation, Respiration, Circulation: Patient has normal breath sounds, with 14 breaths per minute. His resting heart rate is 78 beats per minute, and blood pressure is 140/80 with medication. He is negative for venous and arterial disease. Doppler pulses are present and bounding in posterior tibialis, dorsalis pedis, and popliteal arteries, bilaterally.

Continued

▶ **Case Study 18•1** | **Evaluation and Management of Lymphedema Following Prostate Cancer Surgery—cont'd**

Sensory and Reflex Integrity: The patient has loss of protective sensation in bilateral feet, but reflexes are intact.

Motor Function, Gait, Balance: He is independent in ADLs. He demonstrates a wide base of support with gait and has difficulty walking longer than 20 minutes or 200 feet due to limb fatigue. Safety and righting reflexes are present with stance and mobility.

Orthotic, Prosthetic, Supportive, Assistive, and Adaptive Devices: None.

Aerobic Capacity and Endurance: These are functional, yet diminished.

Self Care and Home Management: He is independent with self-care. He maintains the home and cares for his debilitated wife. His daughter assists with dressing changes and elastic wrap bandaging.

Work and Community: He is employed as computer analyst.

Tests and Measures

1. Girth measurements
2. Semmes-Weinstein monofilament
3. Handheld Doppler
4. Stemmer's sign
5. Blood chemistry, including HbA1c

Recommended Interventions

Wound Management: Topical and systemic antibiotics should be used to manage infection. Primary dressings may include silver-impregnated dressings, hydrofibers, or alginates, followed by absorbent secondary dressings and a four-layer bandage system for compression.

Lymphedema Management: After infection has been addressed, treat left lower extremity before right lower extremity with CDT (performed by trained therapist); sequence may be phase 1 left, phase 2 left while beginning phase 1 right, and complete phase 2 right. During phase 1 (intensive or decongestive phase), daily treatment combining skin and wound care (as needed), manual lymph drainage, bandaging, and education are essential until the limb is decongested. Once limb girth measurements reach a plateau, the patient seamlessly enters phase 2 (self-management phase) in which the patient assumes responsibility for maintaining, managing, and improving the results achieved in phase 1.

Exercise and Rehabilitation: General individualized program of cardiovascular conditioning and strengthening should be prescribed. He should consult with nutritionist and certified diabetic educator for weight management and diabetes education.

Educational Considerations: Education should take place for lymphedema management, wound care, self-care issues, diabetic foot care, and diabetes management.

Other Considerations: He should receive custom shoes with accommodative inserts, single-prong cane for community ambulation, social services consultation for home health assistant regarding basic family needs, and referral to lymphedema support group through Lymphedema Association of North America® (LANA, Wilmette, IL).

References

1. Macdonald, JM: Wound healing and lymphedema: A new look at an old problem. Ostomy Wound Manage 2002; 47:52–57.
2. Casely-Smith, JR, Casley-Smith, JR: Frequency of lymphedema. In: Casely-Smith, JR, Casley-Smith, JR (eds.): Modern Treatment for Lymphoedema. Malvern, Australia, The Lymphedema Association of Australia, 1997, pp 81–84.
3. Kelly, D: Anatomy and Physiology of the Lymphatic System with Clinical Implications. A Primer on Lymphedema. Upper Saddle River, NJ, Prentice Hall, 2002, pp 3–27.
4. Zuther, J: Understanding lymphedema. PT & OT Today 1997; 18–22.
5. Weissleder, H, Schuchhardt, C: Physiology. In: Weissleder, H, Schuchhardt, C (eds.): Lymphedema Diagnosis and Therapy. Koln, Viavital Verlag, 2001, pp 25–34.
6. Kramer, GC, Lund, T, Herndon, D: Pathophysiology of burn shock and burn edema. In: Herndon, D (ed.): Total Burn Care. New York, WB Saunders, 2002, pp 78–87.
7. Weissleder, H, Schuchhardt, C: Pathophysiology. In: Weissleder, H, Schuchhardt, C (eds.): Lymphedema Diagnosis and Therapy. Koln, Viavital Verlag, 2001, pp 35–48.
8. Weiss, J, Spray, B: The effect of complete decongestive therapy on the quality of life of patients with peripheral lymphedema. Lymphology 2002; 35:46–58.
9. Chikly, B: Lymphedema: An Overview. Silent Waves: Theory and Practice of Lymph Drainage Therapy. Scottsdale, AZ, International Health & Healing, 2001, pp 168–170.
10. Casely-Smith, JR: Alterations of untreated lymphedema and its grades over time. Lymphology 1995; 28:174–185.
11. Kelly, D: Lymphedema. A Primer on Lymphedema. Upper Saddle River, NJ, Prentice Hall, 2002, pp 29–41.
12. Weissleder, H, Schuchhardt, C: Primary lymphedema. In: Weissleder, H, Schuchhardt, C (eds.): Lymphedema Diagnosis and Therapy. Koln, Viavital Verlag, 2001, pp 98–117.
13. Weissleder, H, Schuchhardt, C: Secondary lymphedema. In: Weissleder, H, Schuchhardt, C (eds.): Lymphedema Diagnosis and Therapy. Klon, Viavital Verlag, 2001, pp 118–246.
14. Rockson, SG: Workgroup III: Diagnosis and management of lymphedema. Cancer 1998; 83:2882–2885.
15. Stemmer, R: Ein Klinisches Zeichen Zur Fruhund Differential Diagnose Des Lymphoedemas. VASA 1976; 5:261–262.
16. Foldi, E: Uber Das Stemmersche Zeichen. Vasomed 1997; 9:189.
17. Casely-Smith, JR, Casley-Smith, JR: Diagnosis of lymphedema and implications for treatment. In: Casely-Smith, JR, Casley-Smith, JR (eds.): Modern Treatment for Lymphedema. Malvern, Australia, The Lymphedema Association of Australia, 1997, pp 94–97.

18. Kelly, D: Patient Management. A Primer on Lymphedema. Upper Saddle River, NJ, Prentice Hall, 2002, pp 45–62.

19. APTA.: Guide to physical therapist practice. Model definition of physical therapy for state practice acts. Phys Ther 1997; 77:1178.

20. Stanton, AB, Badger, C, Sitzia, J: Non-invasive assessment of the lymphedematous limb. Lymphology 2000; 33:122–135.

21. Chen, HC, O'Brien, B, Pribaz, JJ, et al: The use of tonometry in the assessment of upper extremity lymphoedema. Br J Plast Surg 1988; 41:399–402.

22. Cornish, BH, Chapman, M, Hirst, C, et al: Early diagnosis of lymphedema using multiple frequency bioimpedance. Lymphology 2001; 34:2–11.

23. Boris, M, Weindorf, S, Lasinski, G: Lymphedema reduction by non-invasive complex lymphedema therapy. Oncology 1994; 8:95–106.

24. Hwang, JH, Kwon, J, Lee, KW, et al: Changes in lymphatic function after complex physical therapy for lymphedema. Lymphology 1999; 32:21.

25. Kelly, D: Complete Decongestive Therapy. A Primer on Lymphedema. Upper Saddle River, NJ, Prentice Hall, 2002, pp 65–99.

26. Franzeck, UK, Spiegel, I, Fischer, M, et al: Combined physical therapy for lymphedema evaluated by fluorescence microlymphography and lymph capillary pressure measurements. Vasc Res 1997; 34:306–311.

27. Foldi, E, Foldi, M, Clodius, L: The lymphoedema chaos: A lancet. Ann Plast Surg 1989; 22:505–515.

28. Casley-Smith, JR: Varying total tissue pressures and the concentration of initial lymphatic lymph. Microvasc Res 1983; 25:369–379.

29. Mortimer, PS: The measurement of skin lymph flow by isotope clearance reliability, reproducibility, injection dynamics, and the effect of massage. J Invest Dermatol 1990; 95:677–682.

30. Olszewski, WL, Engeset, A: Intrinsic contractility of prenodal lymph vessels and lymph flow in human leg. Am J Physiol 1980; 239: H775–H783.

31. Smith, A: Lymphatic drainage in patients after replantation of extremities. Plast Reconstr Surg 1987; 79:163–168.

32. Eliska, O, Eliskova, M: Are peripheral lymphatics damaged by high pressure manual massage? Lymphology 1995; 28:21–30.

chapter 19

Prevention and Treatment of Pressure Ulcers

Laurie M. Rappl, PT, CWS
Stephen H. Sprigle, PT, PhD
Renee Trahan Lane (case study contributor), PT, ATP

A *pressure ulcer* is localized injury to the skin and/or underlying tissue, usually over a bony prominence, as a result of pressure or pressure in combination with shear and friction.[1] Because most pressure ulcers are preventable, they can be one of the most unnecessary, and often tragic, manifestations of wounds on the human body. Knowledge of the body sites at risk and prevention methods—such as the appropriate choice and use of support surfaces for both the bed and the chair, as well as correct positioning on both the bed and the chair—are of utmost importance for individuals with mobility deficits. In addition, fitted protective devices, including shoes or orthotics, frequent repositioning, positioning to off-load the risk sites, and proper nutrition and hygiene can dramatically reduce the occurrence and recurrence of these ulcers.

As with all dermal ulcers, treating the underlying cause of pressure ulcers is the most important principle. Treating the ulcer site with topical agents, dressings, and biophysical energies is not enough: Pressure must be removed from the ulcer site.[2] Unfortunately, applying this principle is challenging because pressure ulcers are commonly found on all weight-bearing areas of the body, such as the sitting surface or the recumbent surface in the person's acquired or preferred positions. Prevention and treatment require knowledge of the physiological responses to the physical changes in tissues that lead to pressure ulcers, such as pressure, shear, heat, moisture, and friction. This knowledge provides a foundation for the clinician to address the causative physical factors and the person's overall risk level and to determine safe positions that

remove pressure on those body areas at highest risk. This information is used to determine the proper body positions in sitting and recumbent postures and the equipment required to achieve those optimal positions.

This chapter presents information concerning factors the caregiver must consider when treating persons at risk for, or who have, pressure ulcers due to mobility deficits. The chapter focuses on prevention and treatment of pressure ulcers through appropriate body positioning and selection of bed surfaces and seat cushions. In addition, the detrimental effects of improper positioning on the integument and on other body systems are described.

The Pressure Ulcer Problem
Incidence and Prevalence

The reported incidence and prevalence rates related to pressure ulcer formation show the devastating toll this diagnosis has on health, quality of life, and health-care costs. The Centers for Medicare and Medicaid Services (CMS) reported that in fiscal year 2006, 323,000 Medicare recipients had a diagnosis of pressure ulcers as a secondary condition and that these persons incurred, on average, $40,381 in hospital costs.[3] Pressure ulcers have been cited as the cause of 115,000 deaths and cost $55 billion annually.[4] Of course, the costs of pressure ulcers extend far beyond the medical costs incurred for treatment. Personal and societal costs from inactivity and missed educational, vocational, and recreational pursuits almost certainly outpace any medical costs.

In 2001 the National Pressure Ulcer Advisory Panel performed an extensive literature review in an attempt to define changes in the incidence and prevalence of pressure ulcers in the United States over the preceding decade.[5] This effort resulted in a compilation of studies covering different care settings and diagnoses. Incidence and prevalence studies and cost assessment studies use a variety of approaches and methods, thereby hindering a clear comparison of data over time and across studies. Nonetheless, reported data paint a clear picture of the widespread problem and the associated costs.

Studies in long-term care (LTC) settings include analyses of existing databases, retrospective analyses of medical charts, and prospective studies. Studies using large data sets such as the MDS (minimum data set), found the prevalence rates in LTC facilities ranging from 2.3% to 12%.[6-8] Using the Braden scale, Horn et al retrospectively studied over 2400 residents who were deemed "at risk" for pressure ulcer development at 109 LTC facilities.[9] Over 50% of the subjects did not develop an ulcer during the study, 19% developed a new ulcer, 22% had an existing pressure ulcer, and 6% had an existing ulcer and developed a new pressure ulcer. In 1996, Xakellis and Frantz estimated the cost to heal a stage III or IV pressure ulcer in the long-term care facility, including hospitalization, to be at $10,185, with a standard deviation of $27,635.[10] When they calculated the cost of treatment for all stage I to IV pressure ulcers from their initial occurrence in long-term care through their natural history, including hospital treatment of complications, the mean cost to close one ulcer was found to be $2,731, with a standard deviation of $12,184.

Whittington and Briones conducted a 6-year study of incidence and prevalence in acute care settings.[11] Prevalence ranged from 14% (2001–2002) to 17% (1999), and incidence ranged from 7% (2001, 2003, 2004) to 9% (2000). A separate economic analysis concluded that 2.5 million pressure ulcers are treated annually in acute care settings, with an estimated cost of $2.2 to $3.6 billion.[12] Allman et al studied the costs associated with pressure ulcers that developed in acute care settings.[13] Mean unadjusted hospital costs increased 2.7 times, from $13,924 to $37,288 ($P = 0.0001$), and mean lengths of stay increased 2.4 times, from 12.8 days to 30.4 days ($P = 0.0001$). Allman's $37,288 figure is very close to the $40,381 figure reported by CMS as stated earlier.

Pressure ulcers are an international problem. Woodbury and Houghton reported the following pressure ulcer prevalence rates in Canada in 2004: 25.1% for acute care settings, 29.9% in non-acute care settings, 22.1% in mixed health settings, and 15.1% in community care. The overall estimate of the prevalence of pressure ulcers in all health-care institutions across Canada was 26.0%.[14]

Spinal cord injury (SCI) represents the diagnosis with the best pressure ulcer data, which is compiled by the multicenter Model Spinal Cord Injury System. According to the most recent data from the National Spinal Cord Injury Database, 24% of people with SCI experience a pressure ulcer during their rehabilitation hospital stay and 15% experience an ulcer within the first postinjury year.[15,16] Researchers have estimated that 5% to 85% of individuals with SCI will develop a pressure

ulcer during their lifetime.[17-19] A 2005 multicenter cohort study by Chen et al involving nine Model Spinal Cord Injury Systems showed a significant trend toward increasing pressure ulcer prevalence in recent years (1994–2004 vs 1984–1993).[15] Pressure ulcer risk appeared to remain steady during the first 10 years after injury, but increased 15 years after injury. Annual U.S. treatment costs for pressure ulcers in this population are approximately $1.3 billion, accounting for 25% of the total cost of medical care for those with SCI.[20]

▶ **PEARL 19•1** The Model Spinal Cord Injury System collects extensive data on pressure ulcers within this population. According to the most recent data, 24% of people with SCI experience a pressure ulcer during their rehabilitation hospital stay, 15% experience an ulcer within the first year postinjury, and between 50% and 85% will develop a pressure ulcer in their lifetimes.

Of individuals with conditions such as spinal cord injury and spina bifida whose conditions cause them to be in sitting-dependent positions for extended periods, approximately 75% are estimated to experience skin breakdown at some time. Of that group, 75% will have a recurrence of breakdown.[2,21-24] Chronic, nonhealing ulcers often necessitate closure by myocutaneous flap, but several reports have indicated that failure rates for flap surgeries fall between 76% and 91%.[21-23] As a result, surgeons are becoming more discerning when considering candidates for flap surgeries.

Causative Factors

The formation of pressure ulcers is influenced by many factors. By definition, tissue loading or external pressure is the primary factor in the development of pressure ulcers. However, other factors have been identified that impact the ability of tissues to withstand loading. An understanding of these factors can help clinicians focus pressure ulcer prevention strategies and address the myriad tradeoffs associated with implementing these strategies. Risk factors are often categorized as either extrinsic (ie, normal pressure, friction, shear, moisture) or intrinsic (ie, nutritional status, medical condition, age-related skin changes, tissue temperature, and vascular competency). Several of these factors will be discussed.

▶ **PEARL 19•2** Pressure is the defining causative factor in the development of pressure ulcers, but factors such as shear, friction, heat, and moisture also contribute to make the tissues vulnerable to breakdown.

Magnitude and Duration of Pressure

Research shows that the damaging effects of pressure are related to both its magnitude and duration. Over short periods of time, tissues can withstand higher loads than they can over longer periods of time. Kosiak first demonstrated this characteristic by applying loads to the trochanters and ischial tuberosities of dogs.[25] High loads for short durations and low loads for long durations induced ulcers, with the time-at-pressure curve following an inverse parabola. Reswick and Rogers,[26] who followed human subjects with spinal cord injury, determined this same pressure-time relationship and created a now-familiar figure to illustrate this important concept.

The pressure-time relationship offers useful, albeit general, guidance to clinicians about external loading on tissues. A natural extension of the work by Kosiak targeted the definition of a "safe" pressure threshold, below which no tissue damage would occur.

To date, research has corroborated the relationship between tissue damage and pressure magnitude and duration, but it has not defined a critical loading threshold above which ischemia occurs. Several studies have used controlled experimental approaches to determine the pressure at which blood flow to tissue ceases, with significantly varying results. Lassen and Holstein found that the pressure required for vascular occlusion approximated diastolic pressures when the measured region approached the heart level.[27] Holloway et al found that blood flow decreased as external pressure approached mean arterial pressure and occlusion was reached around 120 mm Hg.[28] Ek and associates found a "weak positive correlation" between blood flow during loading and systolic blood pressure.[29] Sangeorzan and associates determined that 71 mm Hg was needed to occlude flow over "soft" sites, but only 42 mm Hg occluded flow over "hard" sites.[30] Bennett and colleagues measured occlusion pressure in nondisabled subjects and found 100 to 120 mm Hg necessary to occlude vessels in "low-shear" conditions and 60 to 80 mm Hg needed in the presence of "high shear."[31] In reviewing the results of these studies, the single prudent conclusion that can be made is that the tolerance of tissue to external loading varies across people and the anatomical sites of loading. If one accepts this conclusion, then pressure ulcer prevention strategies must be based on individual needs and reflect the current understanding of clinical and physiological situations that influence the load-bearing integrity of tissues.

> **PEARL 19•3** Many research studies have applied pressure to the skin and measured the resulting changes in blood flow. The conclusion based upon these studies is that the tolerance of tissue to external loading varies widely across people and the anatomical sites of loading. This conclusion indicates that pressure ulcer prevention strategies must be based upon individual evaluation.

Friction and Shear

Friction and shear are both noted as risk factors for pressure ulcers and are erroneously used synonymously. *Friction* is the resistance to motion in a parallel direction relative to the common boundary of two surfaces.[32] When the body slides upon a surface, frictional forces can abrade tissue at the boundary. As a result, the dermal papillae are exposed, creating an inflammatory reaction that results in leakage of watery transudate (serous fluid) from the damaged area. Friction that results in damage to the epidermis makes the underlying tissues very vulnerable to further damage from pressure, shear, and maceration, thus providing an opening for pathogens to enter the body and increasing the risk of infection. Friction is a force that applies tangential or shear forces to the skin under many conditions.

Despite increasing risk of tissue damage, friction is needed to maintain postural stability. Without friction, people would slide out of beds and wheelchairs. Thus, clinicians must acknowledge that friction is ever present while attempting to minimize the damaging effects of friction and shear.

Cushions and support surfaces manage friction in different manners. Certain construction and cover materials are designed to minimize friction effects at the body-support surface interface. Segmented nylon air bladders offer a lower frictional surface than a polyvinyl chloride-covered (PVC-covered) air mattress. A contoured foam cushion will hold a client in the seat better than a flat cushion with a viscous fluid top layer. However, this increased stability comes, in part, from increased friction at the body-support surface interface, and this may not be desirable for an individual.

Shear can refer to either shear stress, the force acting tangentially on an area of an object, or shear strain, the deformation of an object in response to shear stresses.[32] When sitting or lying in bed, shear strain results from all the forces that cause the deformation of buttock tissues, including normal forces from gravity, shear stress, and frictional forces at the body-support surface interface. Research has shown that the presence of shear stresses on tissues reduces the tissues' ability to withstand normal loads.[33-35] In other words, tissues are at higher risk for damage in the presence of shear.

> **PEARL 19•4** Shearing forces cause distortion in tissues along fascial planes. This may cause damage to tissue below the surface of the skin that surrounds the wound opening, resulting in undermining and tunneling; therefore, tissue damage can extend well beyond the surface opening of the ulcer.

Clinicians can help reduce shear strain resulting from a user sliding on a support surface by addressing posture and stability. Preventing sliding in bed is the reason behind limitations in head-of-bed elevation. As one inclines the bed, the body tends to slide downward, exposing the sacrum to shear and friction. Combining head elevation with knee elevation can help counteract this sliding tendency so that a person can assume a more functional posture. Reducing the sliding tendency in a seated posture is also important for skin integrity and function. When a seated person slides forward on a wheelchair, the pelvis rotates posteriorly, thereby exposing the sacrum and coccyx to damaging loads. Moreover, sliding forward or the resistance to sliding also induces shear strain throughout the buttocks. Reducing the sliding tendency may be done via attention to the seat-to-back angle of the wheelchair and to the proper sizing of the wheelchair seat. A backrest that is too vertical and seats that are too long or short are contributors to postural instability that result in sliding.

> **PEARL 19•5** Seat and backrest dimensions and angles affect postural stability. A vertical backrest and horizontal seat encourages the person to slide forward in the seat into a kyphotic posture. Similarly, a seat that is too long or short can promote a kyphotic posture. A kyphotic seated posture exposes the sacrum and coccyx to pressure and friction.

Temperature and Moisture

Skin temperature and moisture are often linked when describing the microclimate of the tissues when assessing support surfaces. These two variables are linked because, as skin temperature rises, perspiration occurs, thereby increasing skin moisture. Of course, skin temperature can increase without a concomitant increase in moisture (low-humidity or high-ventilation situations) and moisture can occur without high temperature. Nonetheless, both factors should be considered in pressure ulcer prevention.

Over 100 years ago, van't Hoff postulated that for every 10° rise in tissue temperature, local tissue metabolism increases two to three times.[36-38] Subsequent testing found that a rise of 1°C in skin temperature causes a 10% increase in tissue metabolism.[38] When cutaneous heat buildup occurs with external loading, tissue loading impedes the delivery of blood and nutrients at a time when the need for both is heightened. Recent research into tissue temperature and tissue loading has produced very interesting results. Patel et al studied the influences that both pressure and temperature have on blood flow.[39] Kokate found that pressure ulcer formation was prevented in pigs when tissue temperature was decreased to 25°C.[40] Lachenbruch published an interesting review and secondary analysis of temperature and loading.[41] He performed a simple analysis using published data and proposed the following relationship: an 8°C decrease in skin temperature is equivalent to a 29% reduction in interface pressure. While the specifics of this relationship must be confirmed, Lachenbruch rightly advocates attention to skin temperature

Research related to tissue moisture has also produced information applicable to pressure ulcer prevention. Several studies have shown that the friction coefficient of skin increases with moisture.[42-44] Excessive moisture can also macerate tissue, resulting in a reduced ability to withstand external forces. While these results do not mean that clinicians should seek dry skin, it does identify the need to understand and monitor skin moisture when addressing tissue integrity.

The clinician, caregiver, and client must take appropriate steps to curb excessive heat and moisture buildup in the tissues that are predisposed to pressure ulceration or that are ulcerated. Such steps may include adjusting medications, repositioning to ventilate all tissues periodically, and using barrier creams to keep excessive moisture off of the skin. Durable medical equipment, such as support surfaces, seat cushions, and positioners (eg, heel protectors and wedges) must be evaluated for their heat-dissipation properties.[41,45,46]

Supports and their covers also have a huge impact on how moisture is managed. Support surfaces and cushions that permit airflow via a breathable cover and cushioning material are better able to dissipate moisture than those that do not. Some "incontinence" covers are breathable, being made from fabric that prevents water passage but allows air flow. These have advantages over covers that block both air and water flow, but at a higher cost.

Proper positioning in bed and chair can alleviate temperature and moisture buildup. Moreover, proper positioning of a person in bed and wheelchair allows for enhanced functional movement and activity. A regular unweighting, via a lifting pressure relief or leaning activity, helps dissipate heat from the cushion's surface. Ensuring that a person can achieve a functional posture in bed or wheelchair promotes more movement and, therefore, better dissipation of heat and moisture. Alternatively, very active users will have a higher workload, which can lead to sweating. A judicious clinical guideline is that if a person regularly sweats on a particular support bed surface or wheelchair cushion, other options should be investigated.

> ▸ **PEARL 19•6** Temperature and moisture can contribute to tissue damage. Proper selection of support surfaces, cushions, and positioning devices, along with proper positioning in bed and wheelchair, can alleviate temperature and moisture buildup. Regular unweighting, by lifting pressure reliefs, leaning, or changing position, can dissipate heat and moisture.

Other Physical Factors

External factors related to equipment may also contribute to pressure ulcer formation. Inappropriate equipment such as bed surfaces (often called support surfaces), seats and seat cushions on chairs and wheelchairs, back supports, and orthotic devices that do not fit correctly may cause excessive pressures against the skin and underlying tissues. Ill- or tight-fitting clothing and shoes, lifting devices, belts or restraints, wheelchair parts, and foreign objects such as catheters are all potential contributors to the formation of pressure ulcers.

Intrinsic Factors

In addition to extrinsic physical factors, several intrinsic factors can magnify the effects of pressure applied to the skin, making it more susceptible to pressure ulcer development. Intrinsic factors include muscle atrophy, medications, and comorbid medical conditions as described below.

Muscle Atrophy

Muscle atrophy resulting from aging, physical deconditioning, or neuromuscular damage decreases the natural padding of well-vascularized muscle and soft tissue mass between vulnerable bony prominences and the skin. Little tissue other than skin and adipose tissue is left to absorb and disperse pressure forces. Thus, pressure is concentrated over a smaller area, increasing the vulnerability to pressure ulcer development.

Medications

Medications such as steroids, antiprostaglandins, antineoplastics, and anti-inflammatory drugs are known to have a negative effect on wound healing. Chemotherapy and radiation therapy can also affect wound healing by interfering with tissue repair processes. Anticoagulants suppress the early inflammatory response and increase cellular apoptosis, adversely affecting wound healing.[47]

Malnutrition

Protein calorie malnutrition is associated with many severe health problems, including an increased incidence of pressure ulcers, poor wound healing, and poor tensile strength of scar tissue. Certain substances play a key role in wound healing. Albumin is the major plasma protein and serves many functions. It maintains plasma oncotic pressure; functions as a carrier for metabolites, enzymes, drugs, and hormones in the bloodstream; and is an amino acid donor for extrahepatic tissue synthesis. Many nutrients are involved in collagen synthesis during wound healing, including copper, calcium, vitamin C, and vitamin A. Proliferation of fibroblasts and increased epithelialization are associated with normal dietary levels of protein, zinc, and vitamin A.

A serum albumin level less than 2.5 g/dL is commonly used as a benchmark for malnutrition.[48] In a study of 232 nursing home residents, Pinchcofsky-Devin and Kaminski found a direct correlation between incidence of pressure ulcers and malnutrition.[49] All subjects in the severely malnourished group—those with serum albumin levels less than 2.3g/dL (normal range, 3.5–5.0 g/dL) and total lymphocyte counts less than 1080—had pressure ulcers. In a prospective descriptive study of 150 tube-fed patients with and without wounds, Pompeo found that those with wounds require higher levels of protein than those without wounds and that protein requirement is affected by wound size and severity.[50] Furthermore, he found that in order to improve low prealbumin levels in those with wounds, higher levels of protein than are commonly recommended were required.

> **PEARL 19•7** Research has demonstrated a relationship between incidence of pressure ulcers and poor nutrition. A serum albumin level less than 2.5 g/dL is commonly used as a benchmark for malnutrition. In people with wounds, a higher level of protein than is commonly recommended is needed to improve low prealbumin levels.

Medical Conditions

Medical conditions such as AIDS, diabetes, rheumatoid arthritis, cancer, and certain dermatological conditions may create immunological compromise that impairs tissue healing. Edema, often associated with numerous medical conditions, causes high internal tissue pressures by stretching interstices, resulting in increased tension on the skin. Edema secondary to inflammation impairs pressure ulcer healing by compressing small vessels, thus creating tissue hypoxia. Edema also contributes to vascular ulcers by allowing leakage of fibrinogen and red blood cells into interstitial fluid, which causes tissue hypoxia.

Damage to the central nervous system such as spinal cord injury causes significant changes in the tissues below the site of cord damage. Loss of protective sensation leads to unrelieved pressure on bony prominences for longer periods of time, both in sitting and in recumbency. Atrophy of muscle tissue below the level of the lesion gradually reduces the soft tissue padding naturally found around bony prominences and concentrates the pressures borne on those prominences. The sitting-dependent position and decreased ease of mobility often leads to a sedentary lifestyle and a general state of deconditioning, placing the body at risk for multiple complications. Lack of movement in the extremities slows circulation and contributes to changes in the structure of blood vessels and tissue perfusion. Vasomotor tone is compromised, leading to unopposed vessel distension and a decrease in blood pressure and blood perfusion through tissues. As a result of compromised perfusion, oxygen and nutrient delivery to the tissues is diminished.[51] Damage to the autonomic nervous system leads to dryness of the skin and loss of thermoregulatory control. Microscopically, dermal collagen becomes thickened and less elastic. The epidermis also atrophies.[52]

All persons at risk for pressure ulcers must be educated in pressure ulcer prevention techniques. The major educational points are listed in Box 19.1.

> **Box 19•1 Skin Care Education Program for Patients At-Risk for Pressure Ulcers**

Hygiene

- Keep the skin clean and dry. Dampness from sweat, urine, or excess water can cause maceration, making the skin more vulnerable to pressure ulcers.

Skin Checks

- Check the skin on insensate areas twice daily, morning and evening, for skin blemishes, breaks, or irritation. Do this independently, using a handheld mirror to see posterior areas, or ask a trained caregiver for assistance.
- Look for areas of unusual redness that do not blanch when pressed with a finger or that do not resolve overnight.

Seat Cushions

- Have a seating expert at a rehabilitation center who specializes in spinal cord injury (SCI) help you choose a cushion that will help control posture and pressure.
- Use a seat cushion that will distribute body weight evenly or that will eliminate weight from bony prominences that are most at risk.

- Compare the ability of several seat cushions to reduce pressure by having a pressure mapping study to give a more objective indication of the pressures created by body weight.

Weight Shifts

- Try to completely relieve pressure on the skin of the buttocks every 15 to 30 minutes for at least 1 full minute.

Sleeping Positions and Surfaces

- Change sleeping position frequently throughout the night. Try to sleep on sides or stomach to give the skin on the posterior surface of the body a long length of time with complete pressure relief.
- Find a mattress overlay, or a mattress, that allows you to wake up in the morning with no reddened areas. Persons with SCI who are at low risk for ulcers, who move frequently, and who eat well and maintain good hygiene, may need only a mattress overlay. Those at high risk for ulcers, who have difficulty achieving changes of

▶ **Box 19•1** | **Skin Care Education Program for Patients At-Risk for Pressure Ulcers—cont'd**

position during the night or who have frequent redness on weight-bearing areas, may need to use a therapeutic replacement mattress.

Nutrition

• Eat well-balanced meals.
• Drink noncaffeinated and nonalcoholic beverages to keep skin hydrated.

Safety Measures

• Avoid touching hot surfaces to insensate areas, for example, sitting on hot car upholstery or in hot bathwater that has not been tested with a sensate part of the body.

• Do not place insensate areas near or on hot water or furnace/heater pipes.
• Avoid placing pots, pans, or cups of hot liquid on the lap.

Clothing

• Avoid constrictive clothing: Get clothing with flat seams if possible.
• Do not sit on wrinkles, rivets, or thick seams.

Assistance

• Seek trained and knowledgeable help immediately if you notice reddened areas that do not resolve in less than 24 hours.

Those at Highest Risk

Other, more general features of the person at high risk for pressure ulcers include those who

• lack protective sensation as a result of neuropathy or nervous system disruption, such as cerebrovascular accident (CVA), spinal cord injury, or traumatic brain injury.
• are immobile as a result of neurological deficit, orthopedic involvement, or comatose states.
• are poorly nourished, such as elderly persons, some homebound persons, and those who are living on a low income.
• are incontinent or who have uncontrolled sweating, in whom moisture leads to maceration of the skin.
• have muscle and skin atrophy, making bony prominences even more prominent.

Several groups of individuals are identified as being at the highest risk for pressure ulcer formation. These include the following.

• *Those with SCI or other central nervous system impairments.* Bryant noted that several studies have shown a prevalence rate among SCI of 25% to 40%.[53] Salzberg et al,[54] in a survey analysis, found that 71.5% of 467 spinal cord–injured respondents had experienced at least one pressure ulcer. This concurred with results from their literature survey, which showed prevalence rates of greater than 50% from studies in Brazil, Germany, and Iceland.
• *The elderly.* Bryant also cited several studies reporting prevalence rates of 11.6% to 27.5% in elderly persons.[53] Clarke and Kadhorn found that people younger than 70 years old had a 6% prevalence rate,[55] whereas those at or older than 70 years of age had an 11.6% prevalence rate.
• *Those with orthopedic immobility.* Orthopedic units of acute care hospitals have reported pressure ulcer incidence rates as high as 24%.[53] Those with hip fractures have a 66% chance of ulcer development.[56]

• *Those who are cared for in critical care or intensive care units.* These units typically report incidence rates of 35%, with individual reports ranging from 17% to 56%.[57]

Although pressure is a major contributing element to pressure ulcer formation, these multiple other factors also contribute to the likelihood of a recurrence. Thus, for individuals who are vulnerable to pressure ulcer development, the transdisciplinary wound care team must take the necessary steps to prevent ulcer occurrence and, when necessary, provide the best possible care for ulcers that do develop.

Unavoidable Pressure Ulcers

Even the best care cannot prevent all pressure ulcers from occurring.[58] Skin is the largest body organ and will fail as other organs begin to fail. Patients who are elderly, terminally ill, or in multiple organ failure will often develop pressure ulcers due to many physiological factors at work. Aging and organ failure lead to a decrease in capillary density and blood flow, which slows clearance of toxins and increases risk of pressure ulcers. A flattening of the dermal-epidermal junction decreases the adherence between the epidermis and the dermis and decreases oxygen transfer. The number of pacinian and Meisner's corpuscles decreases, the number and function of the eccrine glands for thermoregulation decrease, subcutaneous fat is lost, skin collagen decreases in amount and elasticity, and capillary walls thin, causing increased ecchymosis. Wound healing is inhibited by a decrease in the number of myofibroblasts.[59]

Clinicians must be able to document that all interventions possible, such as appropriate equipment, frequent position changes, nutrition, hydration, medication modifications, and hygiene, are addressed and that multiple options have been tried before the ulcer is considered "unavoidable."

Features and Locations

Like other types of chronic wounds, pressure ulcers have certain distinguishing features. When a bony prominence bears weight, it exerts localized high pressure on the skin directly below it. This loading profile often results in pressure ulcers with a rounded, craterlike shape with regular edges. Pressure ulcers with irregular shapes are thought to be caused by a combination of normal pressure and shear.

Superficial or deep undermining or tunneling can extend well beyond the edges of the ulcer opening. Undermining is believed to be due to shearing forces exerted parallel to the skin along fascial planes. Undermining is included in the definitions of pressure ulcer staging, and it should be thoroughly documented as to depth and direction, along with the description of the wound itself.

Muscle and soft tissue are more sensitive to pressure than skin; therefore, pressure ulcers typically begin below the skin surface before being manifested on the skin. The common anatomical sites for pressure ulcer development are noted in Figure 19.1. The sites, most frequently subjected to excessive pressure in the pelvic region during sitting and recumbency, include the ischial tuberosities (ITs), sacrum, coccyx, and vertebral spinous processes. The supine and Fowler's positions are implicated in pressure necrosis on the back of the head, the sacrum/coccyx, and the heels. The side-lying position causes most pressure to occur on the lateral aspect of the femoral

trochanter, lateral malleoli, and fibular head that are in contact with the surface. Also, in the side-lying position the uppermost or contralateral leg may incur breakdown on the medial aspect of the first metatarsal head, the medial malleolus, and the medial femoral condyle. Less often, the skin over the ear, the scapula, and the elbow develops pressure ulcers in recumbent positions.

The soft tissues over the sacrum are the most vulnerable to pressure ulcer development. Ulcer formation over the sacrum is usually caused by lying supine with the head of the bed elevated in a position that concentrates more body weight over the sacrum. This is especially true if the head of the bed is elevated higher than 30 degrees.[56] In the sitting position, the sacral area can incur high pressures when the pelvis rotates posteriorly, making the sacrum or coccyx a direct weight-bearing site.

> **PEARL 19•8** The soft tissues over the sacrum are vulnerable to pressure ulcer development. Damaging pressures on the sacrum can result when lying supine in bed with the head of the bed elevated or from sitting in a slouched posture with a marked posterior pelvic tilt.

Several evaluation tools have been developed over the years for the purpose of reporting the severity of a pressure ulcer. In 2007 the National Pressure Ulcer Advisory Panel redefined "pressure ulcer," the four stages of pressure ulcers, and added "deep tissue injury" and "unstageable" categories.[1] These definitions can be found in Table 19.1. The system evaluates only the anatomical depth and amount of tissue destruction of the ulcer; it does not include other wound characteristics, such as exudate, erythema, and odor, which may influence treatment decisions. It is often misused as a method of tracking the healing of a wound as granulation tissue fills in the wound. Because the amount of tissue damaged always remains the same and granulation tissue is not the same as original tissue, a pressure ulcer cannot be reverse-staged. A stage III ulcer will always be a stage III ulcer; it cannot change to a stage II and then to a stage I ulcer. Staging is appropriate only for pressure ulcers. Ulcers of other etiologies should not be documented by pressure ulcer stages.

> **PEARL 19•9** Pressure ulcers are staged according to the depth of tissue involvement. Because ulcers do not heal with the same tissue that was destroyed, ulcers should not be reverse-staged; rather, they retain their highest level of staging. For example, a stage III ulcer that is healing becomes a "healing stage III ulcer with granulation tissue over X% of the wound bed," and when it is closed, its location should be documented as "a closed stage III ulcer".

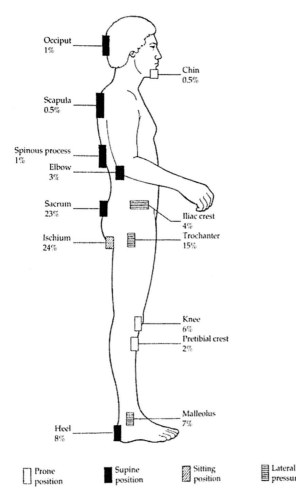

Figure 19•1 *Most common anatomical sites for pressure ulcer development. (From Bryant, R: Acute and Chronic Wounds: Nursing Management. CV Mosby, St. Louis, 1992, with permission.)*

Ideal Positions and Positioning Principles

The human body is not designed to sit or lie in any single posture or position for a long period of time. Instead, people adopt certain positions in sitting and recumbency, with some being

Table 19•1 NPUAP Pressure Ulcer Definitions

Stage I	Intact skin with nonblanchable redness of a localized area, usually over a bony prominence. Darkly pigmented skin may not have visible blanching; its color may differ from the surrounding area. *Further description*: The area may be painful, firm, soft, warmer, or cooler as compared to adjacent tissue. Stage I may be difficult to detect in individuals with dark skin tones. May indicate "at-risk" persons (a heralding sign of risk).
Stage II	Partial-thickness loss of dermis presenting as a shallow open ulcer with a red-pink wound bed, without slough. May also present as an intact or open/ruptured serum-filled blister. *Further description*: Presents as a shiny or dry shallow ulcer without slough or bruising. Bruising indicates suspected deep tissue injury. This stage should not be used to describe skin tear, tap burns, perineal dermatitis, maceration, or excoriation.
Stage III	Full-thickness tissue loss. Subcutaneous fat may be visible, but bone, tendon, or muscle are not exposed. Slough may be present but does not obscure the depth of tissue loss. May include undermining and tunneling. *Further description*: The depth of a stage III pressure ulcer varies by anatomical location. The bridge of the nose, the ear, occiput, and malleolus do not have subcutaneous tissue, and stage III ulcers can be shallow. In contrast, areas of significant adiposity can develop extremely deep stage III pressure ulcers. Bone/tendon is not visible or directly palpable.
Stage IV	Full-thickness tissue loss with exposed bone, tendon, or muscle. Slough or eschar may be present on some parts of the wound bed. Often include undermining and tunneling. *Further description*: The depth of a stage IV pressure ulcer varies by anatomical location. The bridge of the nose, ear, occiput, and malleolus do not have subcutaneous tissue, and these ulcers can be shallow. Stage IV ulcers can extend into muscle and/or supporting structures (eg, fascia, tendon, or joint capsule), making osteomyelitis possible. Exposed bone/tendon is visible and directly palpable.
Unstageable	Full-thickness tissue loss in which the base of the ulcer is covered by slough (yellow, tan, gray, green, or brown) and/or eschar (tan, brown, or black) in the wound bed. *Further description*: Until enough slough and/or eschar is removed to expose the base of the wound, the true depth, and therefore the stage, cannot be determined. Stable (dry, adherent, intact without erythema or fluctuance) eschar on the heels serves as "the body's natural (biological) cover" and should not be removed.
Suspected deep-tissue injury	Purple or maroon localized area of discolored intact skin or blood-filled blister due to damage of underlying soft tissue from pressure and/or shear. The area may be preceded by tissue that is painful, firm, mushy, boggy, warmer or cooler as compared to adjacent tissue. *Further description*: Deep-tissue injury may be difficult to detect in individuals with dark skin tones. Evolution may include a thin blister over a dark wound bed. The wound may further evolve and become covered by thin eschar. Evolution may be rapid, exposing additional layers of tissue even with optimal treatment.

NPUAP, National Pressure Ulcer Advisory Panel.

better for function and tissue health. For example, as mentioned previously, sitting with posterior pelvic tilt can expose the sacrum to damaging pressures. Cushions, support surfaces, and positioning equipment are used to assist users in maintaining functional postures and to protect bony prominences.

Sitting

Correct sitting posture should be considered and encouraged in *any* environment the client is sitting in, whether a wheelchair, a bedside chair, a "geri-chair" (a vinyl surfaced, padded reclining chair found in nursing homes), a living room recliner, a car, or a scooter. Neglecting any of these sitting options may lead to the development of skin breakdown or may inhibit healing of an existing pressure ulcer. When investigating the potential causes of skin breakdown, clinicians should inquire about all of the places an individual sits, since each must be assessed.

The seated posture should be comfortable, stable, and functional. To achieve an erect posture, postural control of the pelvis and trunk are critical requirements. Unfortunately, control of both the trunk and pelvis is often compromised in many wheelchair users so adequate support must be offered by the seating system. In an erect sitting posture, the anatomical curves of the lumbar and thoracic spine are maintained, resulting in an erect head position. In an erect sitting posture, the line of gravity normally lies in front of the thoracic spine over the supporting base, specifically, the ischial tuberosities. (Fig. 19.2A) As a result, a forward or flexion moment is created and must be counteracted by contraction of the posterior trunk musculature to maintain an erect posture. This constant effort is easily experienced when sitting in a seat with a high vertical backrest. In this case, the only way to gain comfortable stability is to slide the buttocks forward on the seat.

Sliding the buttocks forward is exactly what many wheelchair users do to gain stability. This slouched posture is characterized by a posterior pelvic tilt, kyphotic spine, and forward head. (Fig. 19.2B) Posterior rotation of the pelvis results in a more stable base and lower center of gravity, thus some wheelchair users adopt this posture to improve balance. However, the drawback of this posture is that the coccyx and sacrum start to bear weight, and the increased loading on tissue in the sacrococcygeal region increases the risk of pressure ulcers.[60,61] Moreover, this slouched posture can lead to decreased lumbar lordosis, increased thoracolumbar kyphosis, and increased cervical lordosis. Increased thoracolumbar kyphosis can lead to decreased respiratory function; additionally, it stresses the posterior longitudinal ligament and the intervertebral discs, which may lead to increased pain.[60,62]

In sitting, several basic principles should be considered in maintaining correct body posture. These involve seat depth, width, and length; footrest height; back support; and seat and backrest angles.

Seat Depth

The appropriate seat depth is measured as the distance from the point where the user's buttocks touch the backrest of the chair to a point approximately 1 to 1.5 inches from the skin crease in the popliteal fossa of the flexed knee. (Fig. 19.3) This

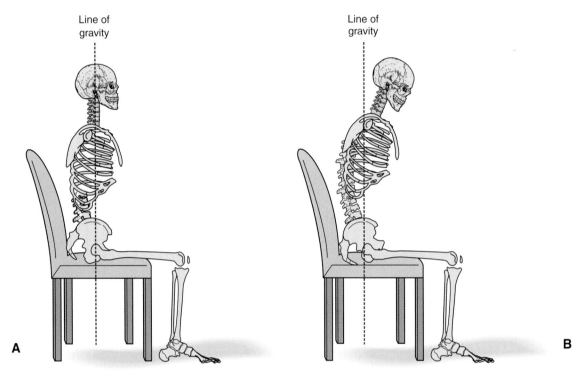

Figure 19•2 *(A) In an erect or upright posture, line of gravity passes through the ear and the acromion process, anterior to the thoracic spine, through the trochanter and behind the ischium. (B) Slouched or kyphotic posture.*

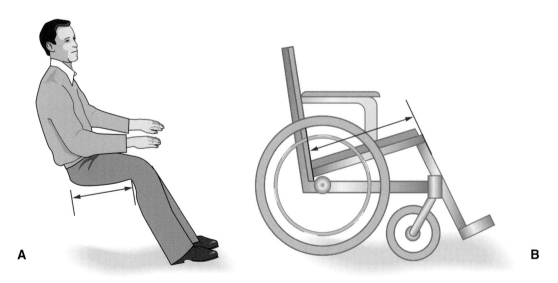

Figure 19•3 *(A) Seat depth measured from posterior aspect of buttocks to 1 to 1.5 inches behind popliteal fossa. (B) Seat depth measured on wheelchair.*

seat depth provides maximum support to both femoral shafts, optimizes weight distribution, and helps hold the body closer to the "ideal" or erect sitting position. If the seat depth is too short, the femoral shafts will not be fully supported. Without this anchoring, the body will tend to slouch and slide out of position. If the seat depth is too long, the seat contacts the back of the person's leg. This pressure can compress the nerves and vessels in the popliteal fossa, causing discomfort or pain. The person will then slide forward on the seat into a slouched kyphotic posture.

Seat Width

The seat width should fit the wheelchair user comfortably, so the greater trochanters are not pressed against the chair side guards or armrests, resulting in pressure against soft tissues. (Fig. 19.4) Excessive space between the person and the side guards results in an unnecessarily wide chair for the user, which can hinder maneuverability and access to push the rims. Ideally, the chair should be narrow enough that a finger can be moved comfortably between the side guard and the person's trochanter. When the wheelchair user is viewed from the front, the top of the push rim of the wheelchair should be easily reached without significant shoulder abduction. This allows the wheelchair user to efficiently propel the wheelchair with the least amount of muscular strain.

Seat Height

The necessary seat height for a wheelchair user is the distance from the floor to the top of the seat cushion. In wheelchair seating, the minimum seat height allows 2 inches of clearance between the footrests and the floor. (Fig. 19.5) Notice that the seat height is measured from the cushion surface, not the wheelchair seat upholstery. This can be a little confusing since the seat height of a wheelchair is measured from the seat upholstery to the ground. Therefore, clinicians must distinguish between the seat height of a wheelchair (used when ordering

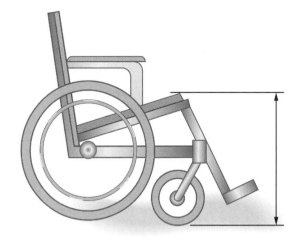

Figure 19•5 *Minimum seat height measured from top of cushion to floor and allowing 2 inches of footrest clearance.*

a wheelchair) and the total seat height for an individual (used when configuring a wheelchair for the user), which includes the height of the cushion. The wheelchair and the seat cushion should be ordered together. Wheelchair seat height should be considered after a seat cushion has been selected. The standard seat height of a wheelchair is 19½ inches, which works well for most users who propel with their upper extremities while using both footrests.

If the wheelchair user propels the chair using one or both feet, then the seat height must be lower to the ground. It is measured from the bottom of the heel to the skin crease in the popliteal fossa minus 1 to 2 inches. This allows the seated person to alternately extend each leg to move the foot forward. It also allows pulling the wheelchair forward with the feet firmly contacting the floor while the body remains in a biomechanically correct position, with the buttocks

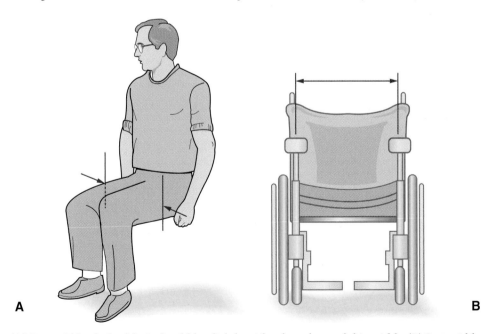

Figure 19•4 *(A) Seat width of wheelchair should be slightly wider than the user's hip width. (B) Seat width measured on wheelchair.*

against the back of the seat and the torso aligned as closely as possible to the upright body position.

Wheelchairs with lower seat heights are available for individuals who propel their chairs with their feet. An alternative is the use of a drop seat to lower the seat height of a standard wheelchair. A drop-seat is a solid board with two hooks on each side of the board. (Fig. 19.6) The seat upholstery is removed from the seat rails, and the hooks of the drop-seat are placed on the rails. The solid board can be adjusted so that the person can sit lower than the seat rails. In effect, this lowers the seat height for the user. There are two drawbacks to drop seats. There is a limit of about $1^{1}/_{2}$ inches that the seat can be dropped, and the insert must be removed before the chair can be folded. Drop seats should be considered only as a last resort for obtaining proper seat height, that is, if no funding is available for the proper wheelchair that is designed with seat upholstery of the correct height. Table 19.2 lists some of the adverse results of using a seat that is too low or too high

Footrest Height

Each footrest should be positioned so the corresponding femoral shaft is parallel to the seat surface of the wheelchair. This distributes sitting pressures along the femoral shafts, redistributes pressure from the pelvic prominences, and offers lower extremity stability. If the footrests are too high, the thighs will not be supported, which can result in abduction and external rotation of the hips and increased pressure placed on the sacrum, coccyx, and ITs. If the footrests are too low, feet will not be well placed and stable on the footrests, and the increased compression of the posterior thigh can lead to decreased comfort and to edema in the lower leg. Moreover, footrests that are too low will encourage the user to slide

Table 19•2 Seat Too High or Too Low	
Seat height too low	• Impairs transfers (sit-stand, lateral transfers to higher surfaces). • Impairs accessibility (to reach table tops or to reach objects overhead). • If lower seat height causes inadequate clearance between footrests and floor, footrests more likely to "bottom out" on uneven terrain or at base of inclines, resulting in tips and falls. • Difficulties in positioning—knees are too high relative to hips—encourages slouched posture.
Seat height too high	• Causes foot propellers to slide forward into a slouched, kyphotic posture in order to reach the ground. • Impairs transfers (sit-stand, lateral transfers from lower surfaces). • Impairs accessibility (eg, too high to get into vans or get the chair under tables). • Elevated center of gravity, with reduced chair stability, increasing risk of tips and falls.

forward on the seat into a slouched kyphotic posture, resulting in shearing forces against the skin of the sacrum and buttocks and poor body alignment.

Back Support

The height of the back support should be as low as possible to encourage upper extremity (UE) range of motion (ROM) and mobility, but high enough to provide adequate trunk support for seated stability. Most back supports in generic chairs and wheelchairs are made of soft upholstery, which provides inadequate support for maintaining the anatomic curves of the thoracic and lumbar spine. Backrests that rise past the apex of the thoracic curve without accommodating the thorax and lumbar curve can push the trunk into flexion; this, in turn, promotes poor posture and increases pressure on the spinous processes, increasing their vulnerability to skin breakdown. The clinician should pay attention to the support of the lumbar spine, alignment of the spinal curves, and protection of the spinous processes. If the user is capable of propelling a wheelchair with his or her UEs, the scapulae and UEs should be uninhibited for freedom of movement. On the other hand, a backrest that is too low will not offer enough trunk stability, and the occupant will constantly fight to stay upright, often using an upper extremity for support. Figure 19.7A shows a backrest height for a typical wheelchair user that supports the trunk without impeding the upper extremity. Figure 19.7B illustrates a low backrest favored by active users with good trunk control.

Seat Tilt, Backrest Recline, and Seat-to-Back Angle

The seat and back surfaces of chairs and wheelchairs are, most often, not horizontal and vertical. Rather, seats and backrests

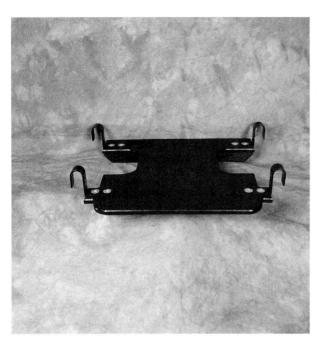

Figure 19•6 *Drop-seat used to lower sitting height closer to the floor to optimize seated position and mobility. (Used with permission of Positioning Solutions, Colorado Springs, CO.)*

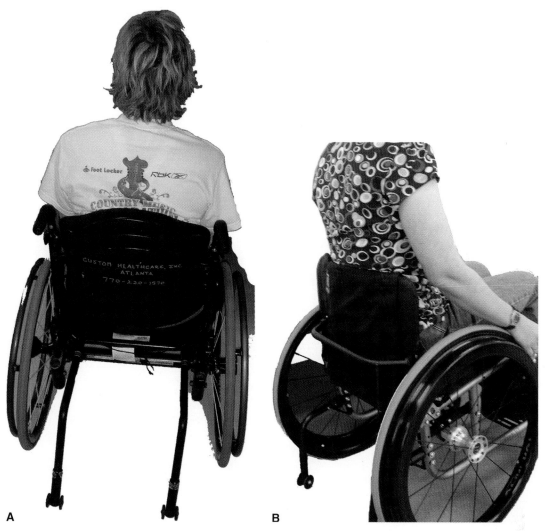

A   **B**

Figure 19•7 *Back supports. (A) Back support slightly inferior to scapula. (B) Low backrest for active users with trunk stability.*

adopt slight angles of tilt and/or recline. *Seat tilt* is the angle between the seating surface and the horizontal, and *backrest recline* is the angle of the backrest with respect to the vertical. (Fig. 19.8) The angle between the seat and the back is called the seat-to-back angle. These angles should be chosen to offer comfort and stability allowed by the extent of the user's hip flexion and spinal mobility, while allowing the head to be upright and eye gaze to be horizontal. Many wheelchairs have a 0- to 7-degree seat angle. A slight seat tilt facilitates seated stability, but can make it harder to transfer out of the seat. Most persons benefit from a seat-to-back angle that is greater than 90 degrees. Backrests should be reclined 10 to 15 degrees with respect to the 90-degree vertical; a 100- to 105-degree seat-to-back angle is another way to describe this. (Fig. 19.9) In a seminal research study, Andersson et al found a large decrease in back muscle electromyogram (EMG) activity from a vertical backrest to one with a 10-degree recline.[63] Certain range-of-motion limitations will necessitate using different seat and back angles. Fixed kyphosis and hip joint mobility restricted to less than 90 degrees flexion (with 0 degrees being straight)

are common indications for a reclined backrest that opens the seat-to-back angle more than that available on many chairs. Wheelchairs with reclining backrests are one option for these clients. (Fig. 19.10) The backrest will need to be reclined so that the seat-to-back angle matches the individual's allowed degree of hip flexion, with the hip as close to 90 degrees as possible and the trunk and femoral shafts fully supported. However, a reclined backrest also increases the forward sliding tendency, so attention must be paid to ensuring that pelvic stability is maintained. A slightly wedged seat cushion can often counteract that sliding tendency when a reclined backrest is indicated. This combination of seat tilt and backrest recline is very effective positioning for many users.

▸ **PEARL 19•10** Wheelchair users cannot sit properly in a chair with a horizontal seat and vertical backrest. A slightly tilted seat and a seat-to-back angle of 100 to 105 degrees offers a more stable, comfortable, and functional seating base.

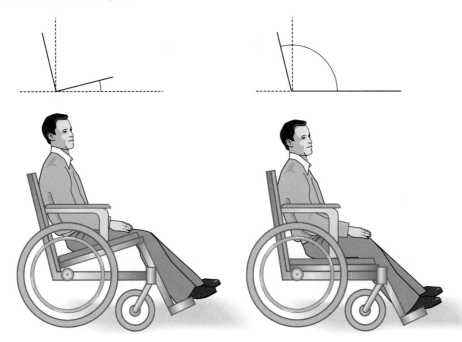

Figure 19•8 *Tilting versus reclining wheelchairs. Tilt: Hip angle does not change. Recline: Hip angle changes as back support reclines.*

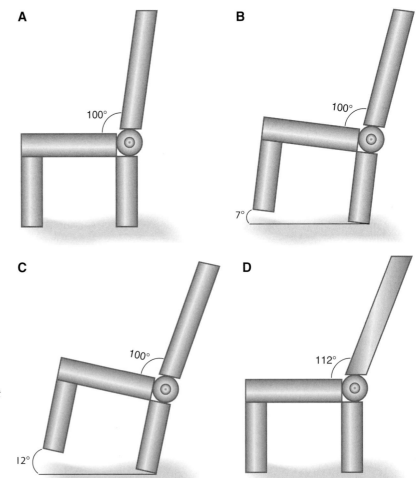

Figure 19•9 *Seat tilt, backrest recline, and seat-to-back angle: (A) 0-degree seat tilt and 100-degree seat-to-back angle; (B) 7-degree seat angle and 100-degree seat-to-back angle; (C) 12-degree seat angle and 100-degree seat-to-back angle; (D) 0-degree seat angle and 112-degree seat-to-back angle.*

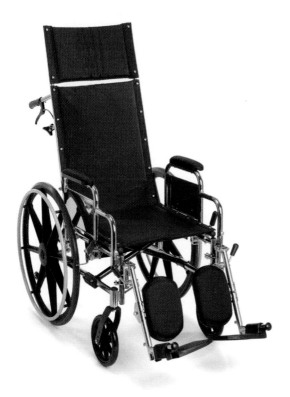

Figure **19•10** *High-backed reclining wheelchair.*

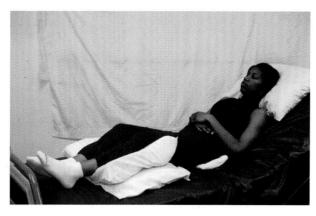

Figure **19•11** *Placing a towel roll between the ischium and trochanter tilts the patient off of the spinous processes of the sacrum and redistributes pressure away from this vulnerable area.*

Recumbent Postures

Supporting the curves of the body and the natural angles of the joints when the client is recumbent is necessary for comfort and for tissue integrity. Frequent position changes of the client, including changing joint angles and weight-bearing surfaces of the body, not just tilting them on rotation mattresses, must be done on a regular schedule and as often as possible. Positioning is critical to ensure that support surfaces can perform as expected, maintaining support and decreased pressure against the skin over bony prominences.

Supine Position

The supine position often encourages caregivers to place pillows under the head, forcing the neck and upper thoracic spine into flexion. Raising the head and upper trunk in this way can increase a developing kyphosis and may cause increased pressure on the sacrum and coccyx. The anatomical resting position of the supine spine is neutral (ie, neither flexion nor extension).[34] If the user's spinal mobility allows it, the use of pillows under the head should be minimized so that the resting or neutral position of the spine can be maintained. A cervical roll or occipital support can be used to protect the occiput and maintain the neck and upper back as close to the neutral position as possible.

Skin over the sacral spinous processes can be protected by placing a small towel roll under one side of the pelvis to redistribute pressures to the ilium rather than to the spinous processes. (Fig. 19.11) The sacrum can also be protected by choosing a support surface that will redistribute interface

pressures away from the sacrum and prevent bottoming out. Bottoming out is determined as follows:

1. The user is positioned comfortably on the surface in the supine position.
2. The clinician attempts to palpate the sacrum by placing a hand under the therapeutic support surface.
3. If the clinician can move the finger less than 1 inch upward through the support surface before touching the sacrum, then the surface is not providing sufficient support or pressure relief to the soft tissues that cover the sacrum. In this case, the user is said to be *bottoming out.*

If the support surface is deemed insufficient, then either the surface must be adjusted or another surface must be evaluated for its pressure-redistributing effectiveness for this individual.

The heels should be protected by elevating them. This can be accomplished with commercially available devices, and there are many designs on the market, some of them shown in Figure 19.12. Alternatively the heels can be elevated completely off the surface by placing pillows under the calf, knee, and thigh. Pillows placed under the heel are not protective because pressure is maintained on the heel. Pillows placed under the heel can also induce hyperextension of the knee, which is likely to become uncomfortable.

The proper resting position of the hip and knee joints in supine position is approximately 25 to 30 degrees of flexion,[34] not full extension as is normally encouraged in this position. A foam leg elevator or pillows that encourage the hip/knee flexion position may be more comfortable for many clients. (Fig. 19.11) This device also accommodates hip and knee flexion contractures while elevating the heel off of the bed. However, as hip flexion is increased in supine, the lumbar spine also flexes, resulting in increased sacral pressures. All clients should spend only limited time in this position.

▶ **PEARL 19•11** The sacrum and the heel are the bony prominences at most risk for skin breakdown in the supine position. These prominences must be protected by unweighting them with positioning and assistive devices.

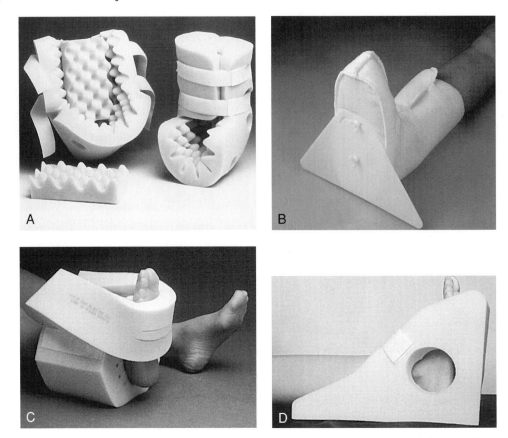

Figure 19•12 *Heel protection. (A) Heelift Suspension Boot (DM Systems Inc., Evanston, IL). (B) Lunax boot with stabilizer (Lunax Boot, Auburn Hills, MI). (C) Foot-drop-stop. (Used with permission of Span-America Medical Systems Inc., Greenville, SC). (D) Cradle boot. (Used with permission of Span-America Medical Systems Inc., Greenville, SC).*

30-Degree Side-Lying Position

The 30-degree side-lying position refers to the angle formed by the horizontal plane of the back, shoulders, and pelvis with the support surface. In contrast to the classic 90-degree side-lying position, the 30-degree side-lying position (Fig. 19.13A) limits pressure on the weight-bearing greater trochanter. A 30-degree foam wedge (Fig. 19.14) is more helpful for maintaining the position than are pillows placed behind the back. Pillows can compress and shift easily, and ensuring that all caregivers will be consistent in using the correct number and proper placement of pillows is almost impossible. The wedge should fully support the shoulders and pelvis in this position. If either the shoulders or pelvis, called the key points of control, are not supported, the body will twist out of position. In addition, the legs must be separated from each other with pillows or a foam device between both the knees and the ankles. If only the knees are separated, the uppermost foot may hang in dependency below the level of the knee, possibly inducing edema and increasing pressure on the medial aspect of the first metatarsal and the medial malleolus of that foot. Foot protection devices, such as those previously mentioned and pictured, may be needed to separate the ankles and protect bony prominences. A wedge or pillow under the uppermost arm helps maintain the shoulder in a comfortable position, that is, abducted about 25 degrees from the body.

150-Degree Side-Lying Position

The 150-degree side-lying position is often underutilized as an alternative to the 30-degree side-lying position for pressure relief. A 30-degree wedge extending from the upper chest to the pelvis is required for this position. (Fig. 19.13B) Another wedge or additional pillows can be placed under the uppermost leg to separate the knees and ankles and to maintain the hip in a slightly flexed and abducted position for comfort. Again, a foot protection device may help protect the malleoli and separate the ankles to prevent skin breakdown between them. This position usually induces a neutral or resting position of the upper shoulder, that is, abducted 55 degrees and horizontally adducted 35 degrees.[34] The shoulder in contact with the bed may incur discomfort, but no more so than when the client is in the 90-degree side-lying position.

> ▶ **PEARL 19•12** Both the 30-degree and 150-degree side-lying positions are useful in alleviating pressures on the sacrum and lateral bony prominences of one lower extremity. However, these positions exert loading on the prominences of the lower, weight-bearing limb. Therefore, regular changing of positions is required to alternate loading from one side of the body to the other.

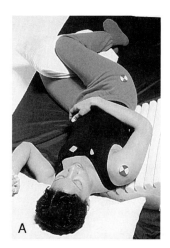
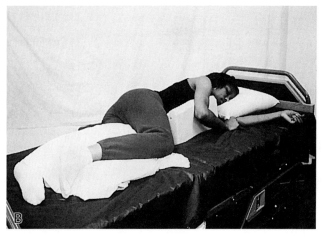

Figure 19•13 *Side-lying positions. (A) The 30-degree side-lying position. Note the 30-degree wedge used to support entire trunk, including pelvis and shoulders, to maintain this position. Also, pillow used between legs to cushion bony prominences at the knees. (B) The 150-degree side-lying position. Note the use of same 30-degree wedge used to support entire trunk again. Another wedge placed between the legs helps to cushion bony prominences and maintain the pelvis in the 150-degree position. (Both photos used with permission of Span-America Medical Systems Inc., Greenville, SC.)*

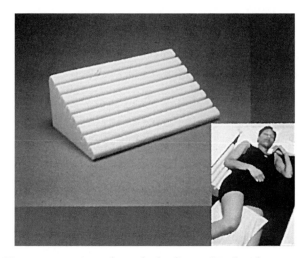

Figure 19•14 *A 30-degree body aligner. (Used with permission of Span-America Medical Systems, Inc., Greenville, SC.)*

Prone Position

This position is uncomfortable for most to attain, let alone to maintain. This is particularly true for elderly persons, especially if they have thoracic kyphosis, and for those who have difficulty breathing when the head is turned to almost 90 degrees. A pillow under the head and upper chest, with the head resting on the edge of the pillow and the face extending over the edge of the pillow can be helpful in facilitating breathing. In this position, the knees and dorsum of the feet need careful monitoring for potential pressure problems. The feet can be elevated on a pillow or, preferably, on a foam block or wedge to allow enough elevation to decrease edema buildup.

Fowler's Position

The Fowler's position is another name for the semireclined supine position in which the head of the bed is elevated relative to the rest of the bed frame. (Fig. 19.15A) Often, this position is overused as a replacement for upright and supported sitting in a chair. The typical Fowler's position requires 30 degrees to 60 degrees of hip flexion. The knees are either flexed with the knee elevated in the bed frame or on pillows, or left in an extended position. As a result, problems may arise because the sacrum bears an excessive amount of weight. The sacrum is exposed to high shearing forces when the body slides toward the foot of the bed because the trunk is unsupported and the feet have nothing to rest or push against to prevent the body from sliding down.[35] Forces on the sacrum caused by shear and weight loading can be reduced in three ways: (1) by selecting an appropriate support surface that redistributes pressure and is designed to reduce shear, (2) by tilting the pelvis with a towel roll under the wing of the ileum so that the spinous processes of the sacrum are not bearing the brunt of the body weight (see below), and (3) by minimizing how high the head of the bed is raised and how long the person remains in that position.

To tilt the sacrum off of the spinous processes, the pelvis is tilted laterally with a bath towel folded several times to achieve a roll shape of 8 to 12 inches long and 4 inches wide. The towel roll is placed under one ilium, between the sacrum and the hip, to tip the pelvis slightly and to reduce direct pressure on the spinous processes. (Fig. 19.15B) Support placed under the plantar surface of the feet in the form of a board, foam wedge, or block will help stabilize the user or help him or her to self-stabilize and prevent sliding. Before elevating the head of the bed, the hip must be aligned with the hinge of the bed frame so that the body and the bed bend at the same point.

> ▶ **PEARL 19•13** A towel roll placed under one side of the pelvis can tilt the weight of the body off the spinous process of the sacrum and provide some protection to this vulnerable site.

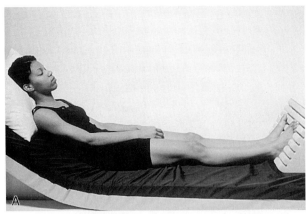

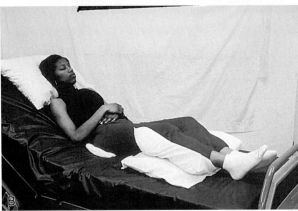

Figure 19•15 *Fowler's position. (A) Hips are aligned with the bend in the bed, knees are extended to decrease pressure on sacrum, and support is placed at the foot to inhibit sliding. (B) Pillows placed under knees for comfort, and towel roll placed under one side of the pelvis to tilt the body weight off of the spinous processes of the sacrum and decrease pressure on this vulnerable point. (Used with permission of Span-America Medical Systems Inc., Greenville, SC.)*

Diagnostic Process

Current teaching by the American Physical Therapy Association (APTA) encourages therapists to follow a diagnostic process when performing an evaluation. The process includes taking a history, performing an examination of body systems, evaluating the information gathered, formulating a diagnosis and prognosis, determining interventions, and evaluating the outcome.[64] This process ensures that the person with a wound is examined as a whole, rather than having the clinician focus only on the wound.

History

Pertinent medical history should include the following:

- Goals of the client and the caregiver, which may not be the same as the clinician's goals.
- Primary diagnosis, such as CVA, SCI, multiple sclerosis, diabetes, neoplasm, renal failure, or AIDS.
- Secondary diagnoses, such as arterial or venous insufficiency, neuropathy, or pressure ulcer.

- Surgical history, including skeletal changes that may cause undue pressures. An ischiectomy, for example, would cause the pelvis to sit unevenly, thus causing increased pressure on the remaining tuberosity.
- Nutritional status, including any swallowing and self-feeding difficulties.
- Medications and medical interventions that could impede the healing process, such as steroids, chemotherapy, radiation therapy, anti-inflammatory drugs, and antiprostaglandins.
- Laboratory and diagnostic test results, including albumin, prealbumin, glucose, and hematocrit.
- Environmental issues, including living arrangements, in-home barriers, and caregiver stability.

Examination and Evaluation

The examination provides the clinician with the clinical signs and symptoms that affect the cause and the treatment of the ulcer. The examination findings should be recorded on a standardized form in a systems review format to ensure thoroughness.

Musculoskeletal Status

ROM, muscle strength, skeletal structure and biomechanical deformities, atrophy, posture, and functional and mobility impairments are examined.

Range-of-Motion Limitations

Contractures limit full range of motion and prevent ideal positioning. Each contracture must be determined to be either *fixed* (immovable or noncorrectable) or *flexible* (movable, or potentially correctable with intervention). A fixed contracture cannot be reduced and will require appropriate support to accommodate for restricted mobility and loss of function. A flexible contracture may be reduced by stretching and positioning; accommodation of flexible contractures with assistive devices and positioning equipment may allow positioning in ideal positions. Thus, restoration of full or partial function may be a reasonable goal. If, for example, maximum hip flexion is determined to be a fixed 75 degrees (with full extension being 0 degrees), then a chair with a 90-degree seat-to-back angle is inappropriate. In this case, the seat-to-back angle must be reduced or laid back to 75 degrees to accommodate the contractures. If, however, hip flexion is found to be 75 degrees, but flexible, and in the clinician's opinion there is the possibility of gaining more hip flexion, then the seat-to-back angle must be adjustable so that the angle can be changed as the ROM improves.

A common error is to mistakenly blame a variety of factors—muscle flaccidity, spasticity, weakness, unintentional loss of motor control—to be a result of malaise, cognitive deterioration, or deliberate intent and to be the reason for the user's inability to keep the hips back on the seat and sit erect. More often, however, the cause of misalignment in sitting is impairment in hip ROM rather than these other factors. In other words, in most cases 90 degrees of true hip flexion is not available, which is a requirement for functional sitting in a standard wheelchair with a 90 degree seat-to-back angle.

True hip flexion is measured with the client relaxed in the supine position. The examiner fully extends one of the client's legs to 0 degree hip flexion and places a thumb on the anterior superior iliac spine (ASIS) and the middle finger of the same hand on the posterior superior iliac spine (PSIS). This allows the examiner to identify the point at which the pelvis begins to rotate posteriorly out of the neutral position. The neutral position of the pelvis is identified by the ASIS being slightly inferior to the position of the PSIS. With the examiner's fingers in position on the ASIS and PSIS, the hip is passively flexed by raising the leg with the knee flexed. At a certain point during hip flexion, the pelvis will begin to rotate posteriorly. That is, the ASIS will move even with and then superior to the PSIS. The contralateral lower extremity will begin to rise off the surface as the pelvis rotates posteriorly. The angle of hip flexion that occurs at the point at which the pelvis begins to rotate is the angle of true hip flexion. (Fig. 19.16) Experienced examiners can determine this measurement with no assistance; inexperienced examiners will benefit from having an assistant mark sites with his or her fingers, hold the leg in position, or take the measurement.

▶ **PEARL 19•14** Limited flexion at the hip, limited extension in the thoracic spine, and fixed contractures are common reasons for poor seated posture. These conditions necessitate equipment that accommodates the limitations, rather than expecting a standard 90-degree seat-to-back angle wheelchair to fit all users.

Muscle Strength

Loss of strength in major muscle groups will compromise the client's ability to maintain correct sitting or recumbent postures and will inhibit independent mobility. If independent bed mobility is limited by muscle weakness, the client will be dependent on others for repositioning to relieve pressure. Those who can reposition themselves are more likely to do so on an as-needed basis and are less likely to incur skin breakdown.

If the paraspinal, abdominal, and other trunk musculature is weak or nonfunctioning, the individual will tend to lean to one side, possibly overweighting the ischium on that side and causing skin breakdown. Furthermore, the undesired tendency is for the person with muscle weakness to sit on the sacrum, slouching the hips forward on the seat: This posture exerts excessive pressures on the coccyx and spinous processes. If poor positioning causes the person to slide his or her hips forward on the seat to reach the floor with the foot, shear and pressure on the coccyx occur, leading to skin breakdown. Weakness in the upper extremities will also impair the ability to perform basic activities of daily living, such as eating, toileting, weight shifting, mobilizing a manual wheelchair, and checking the skin in insensate areas.

Skeletal and Muscular Structure

Part of the evaluation of the skeletal system should include identification of the bony prominences at risk. Some people have spinous processes that are more pointed in shape than others. Those with more pointed prominences are at higher risk, as the pointed shape exerts more pressure over a smaller area of tissue than flatter, smoother prominences. Skeletal deformities can cause some areas that are normally safe from skin breakdown to be at higher risk. For example, a fixed

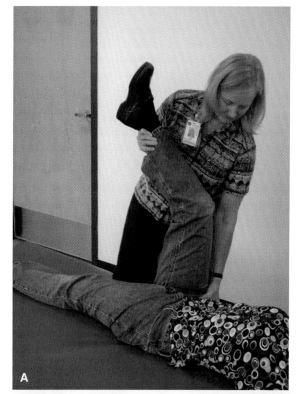

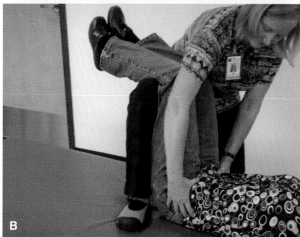

Figure 19•16 *True hip flexion measurement. (A) With one leg straight, passively flex the opposite leg, noting the hip angle at the point that the pelvis begins to posteriorly rotate. (B) Passively flex both legs, and note the hip angle at the point that the pelvis begins to posteriorly rotate.*

scoliosis or kyphosis puts the ribs and spinous processes at higher risk.

Atrophy of the skeletal muscles overlying the bony prominences enhances the risk of pressure ulceration by reducing the cushioning effect of the soft tissues. These sites require attention to client positioning and equipment for protection. Adequate redistribution of pressure with the seat cushion and the support surface will be a key factor in pressure ulcer prevention for these clients.

Postures

The individual's preferred positions in sitting and recumbency should be noted. Additionally, the time spent in each position should be ascertained when evaluating the risk for breakdown. When these postures are not ideal, as described earlier in this text, interventions to protect bony prominences and to assist in achieving close to ideal postures are needed. For example, those who prefer to side-lie must be protected with adequate pressure redistribution support surfaces and supported with wedges to promote 30-degree side-lying rather than the 90-degree position that compromises the trochanter. The most effective pieces of documentation for this change are photographs of the client in the preferred positions before and after intervention. This graphically documents the need for the equipment and the prescribed recommendations to payer sources and shows the improvements attained by the interventions.

▶ **PEARL 19•15** Photographs of postures before and after intervention graphically demonstrate the need for the prescribed equipment and proper use of that equipment.

Functional and Mobility Impairments

Pressure ulcers may be caused by impairments in functional mobility skills, including wheelchair mobility and the ability to self-reposition and attain safe and functional positions in both sitting and in recumbency. Mobility is included as a subscale in the most heavily used risk assessment scales, including Braden, Norton, Waterlow, Gosnell, and Allman. The person who is independent in wheelchair mobility and bed mobility is at lower risk for skin breakdown. A thorough examination of the body systems along with a review of functional impairments will give the therapist the information needed to determine the causes of the impairments and to influence improvements in skills through therapy, positioning, and equipment prescription. Equipment such as support surfaces and seat cushions must be evaluated not just for pressure management, but also for features that improve a user's abilities to move independently.

Neuromuscular Status

Sensation

A thorough assessment of sensation is helpful in determining which anatomical areas of the body are at greatest risk for trauma and pressure ulceration. Cutaneous areas lacking sensation are at the highest risk for skin breakdown from trauma and pressure. For example, those who have loss of protective sensation in their feet caused by LE (lower extremity) distal sensory neuropathy are at great risk for pressure ulcer or trauma-related ulcer development over the weight-bearing surfaces of their feet. Protective footwear is critical for these individuals because they have severely compromised protective sensation. People with sensory loss or deficit in the lower body are at great risk of skin breakdown on the sacrum, coccyx, ITs, greater trochanters, medial femoral condyles, fibular heads, malleoli, and bony prominences of the feet. Caregiver and client education must include attention to protection and daily examination of these sites.

Reflexes and Spasticity

Pathological reflexes and spasticity disrupt positioning in sitting and recumbency by forcing the body into involuntary postures and movement patterns. These abnormal postures can cause excessive interface pressures on bony prominences that do not normally bear weight, such as the medial femoral condyles when hip adductor spasticity is present. When spasticity is present, repetitive and involuntary movements can cause shearing of soft tissues over bony prominences and can significantly limit a person's independent functional mobility. For example, a person with a head injury can have flexor spasticity in the LEs that may result in shear and friction over the heels as they are pressed into the support surface or uncontrollably being moved heavily and repeatedly across the support surface as the muscles contract and relax.

Therapeutic positioning can and should be used as a powerful and dynamic contracture-management strategy. Irreversible, functionally debilitating, and life-threatening contractures will develop in those with pathological reflexes and spasticity unless they are provided with a consistent and aggressive positioning- and contracture-management program.[65-67] Determining if and how the reflexes and spasticity are triggered or inhibited by various positions in recumbency and sitting can assist in establishing the preferred positions for function and safety. For example, facilitating and supporting a chin-tucked position of the head and neck inhibits extensor spasticity of the trunk and extremities, thereby facilitating the person's ability to sit in a functional and erect position in a wheelchair. Thus, whenever possible, reflex-inhibiting positions should be used to inhibit spasticity.

A person with spasticity that causes hip and knee flexion in supine position may be at higher risk for pressure ulcers over the heels and sacrum. The flexion may be inhibited by positioning in a 30-degree side-lying position with separation of the lower extremities. (Figs. 19.17 and 19.18)

Visual Field Deficits

Visual field deficits can impair safe self-mobility for individuals with diagnoses such as stroke and brain injury. For instance, if a person has a left visual field deficit, it is unsafe to allow independent wheelchair propulsion until he or she has learned how to compensate for the visual deficit. An individual's preferred bed-lying position may be affected by a visual field deficit; they will prefer the side that allows them the best field of vision and resist repositioning to the side that limits vision.

Neurovascular Status

The neurovascular system is controlled by the autonomic nervous system (ANS), which innervates all cardiac and smooth muscle and the exocrine glands. The ANS maintains internal homeostasis by affecting circulation (heart rate, ventricular contractile force, vascular resistance, and blood pressure), digestion, kidney function, temperature regulation, and fluid balance (composition, distribution, volume). The ANS controls the vasomotor tone of the arteries and arterioles, thereby controlling blood pressure, tissue perfusion, and vascular space for blood volume. Sweat glands that dissipate heat through evaporation are

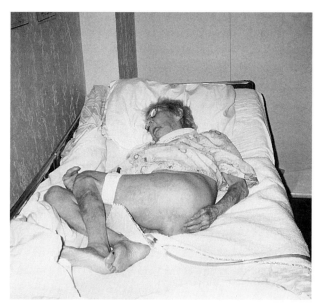

Figure 19•17 *Patient with pathological reflexes and spasticity that inhibit positioning, before intervention. (Used with permission of Positioning Solutions, Colorado Springs, CO.)*

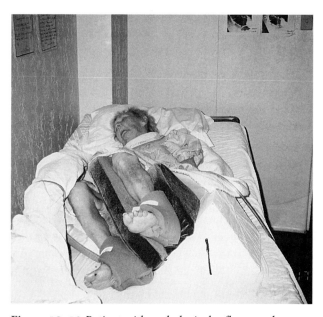

Figure 19•18 *Patient with pathological reflexes and spasticity after intervention to inhibit flexor tone, inhibit the progression of contractures, and eliminate heel pressure (Bedleg Positioning Cushion; used with permission of Positioning Solutions, Colorado Springs, CO.)*

also controlled by the ANS.[51] Because of their lack of autonomic control of vasodilation, vasoconstriction, thermoregulation, and sweating, patients with neurological impairments are at much greater risk for breakdown of the integument.

Cardiopulmonary and Circulatory Status

The ability of the vascular system to deliver blood, oxygen, and nutrients to the integument is directly affected by impairments in the cardiopulmonary and vascular systems. Thus, individuals with compromised small vessel perfusion that occurs in congestive heart failure, atherosclerotic heart disease, chronic obstructive pulmonary disease, and peripheral ischemic vascular disease are at greater risk for pressure ulceration.[68] If sitting and recumbent postures are not corrected, these individuals will require more time to heal because of inadequate perfusion and misaligned positioning.

The cardiopulmonary system may also be impaired by musculoskeletal deformities such as thoracic kyphosis, which can interfere with thoracic expansion and breathing patterns. In addition, weakness of accessory muscles of respiration that impairs diaphragmatic breathing, taken together with immobility that stagnates pulmonary secretion movement, increases the risk for development of pneumonia or respiratory failure.[69] For example, someone with a fixed thoracic kyphosis cannot achieve the ideal upright sitting position, but can achieve an upright position of the head and neck and a fully expanded thorax if accommodation for the kyphosis is made with a reclined back.

The person with a fixed kyphosis cannot achieve a flat supine position without extra head support, unless accommodation is made for the kyphosis with an appropriate bed support surface or with a positioning device such as a foam wedge under the head and upper back. For this person, the interface pressure over the thoracic spinous processes must be evaluated to determine whether skin and soft tissues are at risk for ulceration. Thus, for the person with a thoracic kyphosis, accommodation must be made for the kyphosis so that a fully expanded thorax can be achieved in the seated and recumbent positions and so that gravity can facilitate as much thoracic extension as the deformity will allow. These accommodations will also assist in at least maintaining the kyphotic deformity rather than allowing it to progress.

Some people may have specific head- or foot-elevation requirements. For instance, a person with chronic obstructive pulmonary disease or congestive heart failure may require elevation of the head of the bed to facilitate ease and efficiency of breathing. Raising the head of the bed will increase shear and interface pressures between the support surface and the skin over the sacrum and ITs and will also minimize the ability to be in side-lying position to relieve these tissues. A person with venous insufficiency may need to elevate their feet higher than the heart to improve venous return. Elevating the lower extremities in bed may increase the interface pressures over the sacrum. Once the desired positions are attained, the clinician must evaluate pressure redistribution over the bony prominences to ensure that the client is not at risk for soft tissue breakdown.

Gastrointestinal Status

Examples of medical diagnoses that may be associated with impairments of the gastrointestinal system include dysphagia, esophageal reflux, and malnutrition. Any disturbance in the gastrointestinal system will negatively impact nutritional intake. Pressure ulcers are less likely to develop in individuals who are well nourished.[70,71] Also, for individuals who have existing pressure ulcers, a strong correlation exists between those who are malnourished and those with slower healing rates.[50,71,72] The nutritional status of the individual is directly influenced by the ability to access food and self-feed,[73] and by the specific dietary requirements of that individual.[49] An occupational therapist must be consulted to determine recumbent and seated positions required to provide access to the table, food, and liquids. The consultation should include adaptive equipment necessary for ease and efficiency in self-feeding and the physical assistance and/or supervision needed to ensure success. The expertise of the dietician is important in evaluating and establishing the specific dietary requirements for the individual. A speech and language pathology consultation may be required in order to establish the proper food and liquid consistencies and the correct head and neck positions for safe, unobstructed swallowing to prevent aspiration.

For those individuals who are fed enterally, appropriate head, neck, and trunk positioning is of paramount importance to prevent aspiration of saliva into the lungs and to prevent gastric or esophageal reflux, which could also cause aspiration pneumonia.[74] At least 30 degrees of head elevation is required to prevent gastric reflux.[74] Interface pressures over the sacrum and coccyx should be evaluated to determine the effectiveness of the support surface in this position. The head and neck should be positioned in a slightly flexed and chin-tucked position to avoid aspiration.

Evaluating the person's bowel function, continence, and habits is necessary to determine the seated and recumbent positions that promote function, continence, and independence. For example, if a neuromuscular impairment makes it necessary to perform a bowel program in bed, the support surface and positioning in the recumbent positions should facilitate this process. However, if the program requires that the bowel program be done on the toilet, then it is important to facilitate the ease and safety of the transfer to the toilet and the ease of performing the bowel program, as well as to ensure that the toilet seat is padded and fabricated to avoid pressure ulcer development.

Genitourinary Status

The examination should include whether the client is continent, and if not, what interventions are being used to adapt to incontinence. Incontinence pads and garments add an extra layer between the user and the cushion or support surface and decrease the pressure redistributing properties of the equipment by preventing immersion into the surface.[75,76] If the user is wearing an appropriate incontinence containment product, an additional incontinence pad should not be placed on the chair cushion or bed. If incontinence pads are needed, only one layer should be used to allow as much immersion of the body into the surface as possible. If the individual has urinary incontinence, a support surface or wheelchair cushion cover that is moisture proof should be used to protect the equipment from contamination. The medical record should also note interventions used to cleanse, hydrate, and protect the skin from irritation and breakdown caused by urinary and fecal incontinence.

Positioning equipment associated with the mobility base (wheelchair) should facilitate efficiency, safety, and independence in transfers to the toilet, emptying of the catheter/leg bag, self-catheterization, access to the urinal, personal hygiene, and dressing and undressing.

Sexual functioning should also be discussed with the client and his or her family to assist with suggestions for positions, support surfaces, and positioning aids to facilitate comfort and pleasure for both parties.

> **PEARL 19•16** Positioning and durable medical equipment are commonly known to affect the integumentary and musculoskeletal systems. However, they affect all systems of the body, including neuromuscular, neurovascular, cardiopulmonary, circulatory, gastrointestinal, and genitourinary systems.

Integumentary Status

Examination of the skin, especially the skin subjected to pressure during sitting and recumbency, will identify several qualities and conditions, such as skin turgor, color, texture, elasticity; the presence of wounds or scars, erythema, ecchymosis, dermatitis, areas of excoriation; and palpable differences in skin temperature. Thin, friable skin with poor turgor is vulnerable to skin tears and pressure necrosis and should be protected from insult by appropriate caregiver handling and equipment.

If the history or examination reveals that recurrent skin trauma from pressure or from a surgical procedure has occurred over a bony prominence and has resulted in scarring, ongoing protection of the scar through positioning and equipment is imperative because the reduced tensile strength of the scar renders it particularly vulnerable to breakdown.

Interface Pressures

Interface pressures are the pressures between the support surface (seat or mattress) and the skin. These pressures are not the same as capillary closing pressures, which are at the microscopic level and in the deep tissues of the body. Work by Kosiak based on earlier studies by Landis suggested that capillary closing pressure was 32 mm Hg.[25,77] This value is an average of pressures ranging from 12 to 48 mm Hg and so is not a valid benchmark to use for all people. In addition, since interface pressure is not the same as capillary closing pressure, the value of 32 should not be applied to interface pressure measurements.

Interface pressures are often assessed very subjectively using hand checks. The clinician places his or her hand beneath the mattress or seat cushion, positioning it under the bony prominence in question. If the supporting material has "bottomed out," the therapist will not be able to move his/her fingers more than about 1 inch before encountering the bony prominence. This approach tends to work better on some mattresses and cushion designs than others. For example, a seat cushion made of a firm molded base with a gel bladder for immersion and pressure distribution will require the therapist to place his or her hand beneath the gel bladder rather than the base. For this reason, the use of computerized sensors is an increasingly common objective tool to measure interface pressures.

Sensors range from handheld, single pad sensors to larger pressure-mapping devices designed for use in beds and wheelchairs. (Fig. 19.19) These pressure mats use dozens to hundreds of sensors to provide a quantitative map of pressures across the entire support surface at one time. These objective measures can be a valuable tool in the assessment of the appropriateness of a given support surface for an individual. Of course, interface pressure is but one of many factors that must be considered, such as bed mobility, transfers, posture, stability to maintain body positions, ease of use, and affordability. In other words, interface pressure values should not be the sole determining factor in equipment selection.

To fully evaluate an individual, interface pressure measurements (IPM) should be recorded at all bony prominences in all positions in the seated and recumbent postures. This will identify which prominences may be at most risk for pressure ulcer development and whether the support surfaces are effective in achieving acceptable interface pressures for that person. If the individual is determined to be at high risk

for or currently has pressure ulcers, the interface pressures should be as low as possible and widely distributed across the weight-bearing surfaces of the body. Absolute pressure readings are not good predictors of the vulnerability of the skin to pressure. However, relative pressure comparisons, that is, comparisons of the readings on the same bony prominences of the individual on various surfaces, and an examination of the distribution of the pressures onto more load-tolerant areas of the body yield more useful decision-making information for the clinician. The surfaces of choice are those that best reduce peak pressures for that person.[78] Unfortunately, research has not identified a "safe" interface pressure threshold. Although this might appear to limit the utility of IPM, that is far from true.

Whenever a client presents with postischemic erythema, a cushion and support surface assessment is indicated. IPM can be used to define the individualized threshold for that person and to compare pressure distribution for that client on various products. If they have erythema on the trochanters from sitting, the IPM at the trochanters is unacceptable for that person and other cushion options should be investigated. Another example concerns sites known to be at risk of ulceration. If IPM is performed on a person in bed and the resulting map shows poorly distributed pressures with high peaks at the sacrum and heels, it does not matter what the values are because it is obvious that a better distribution of pressure is needed. Finally, IPM is useful for educating clients and caregivers in positioning and pressure relief. The visual nature of IPM can be useful to show a person exactly how far to lean forward to effectively unweight the buttocks (Fig. 19.20) or to show that a change of position changes pressures; for example, pressure increases on the sacrum when the head of the bed is raised.

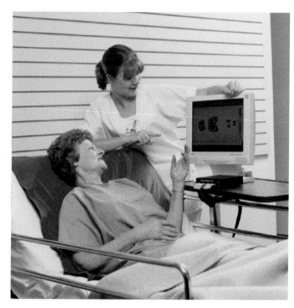

Figure **19•19** *Interface pressure mapping device.*

> **PEARL 19•17** Interface pressure measurements are used to evaluate the same person on many surfaces to demonstrate increases or decreases in pressures during certain movements and to estimate the "safe" pressures for an individual over a specific bony prominence. It is not used to anticipate the efficacy of a surface for all potential users.

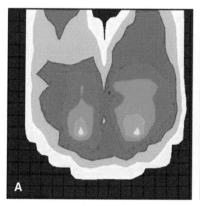
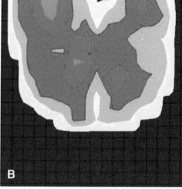

Figure **19•20** *Interface pressure (A) during upright or erect sitting and (B) during forward lean. Note that pressures on the ischials significantly decreases in forward lean position.*

Regardless of whether interface pressure is measured, the effectiveness of a support surface or cushion can only be made through careful assessment of skin over the weight-bearing bony prominences. Skin checks should occur after a person has been positioned on a support surface or seat cushion for some length of time. Localized erythema is indicative of a postischemic response and indicates that the surface was unable to adequately redistribute load over that specific time. If erythema is present, either the support surface must be changed or the turning/repositioning schedule must be increased. Note that erythema is much easier to detect in persons with lightly pigmented skin. Erythema in persons with darkly pigmented skin may be masked by melanin and often does not appear red in color. Good lighting is essential when checking darkly pigmented skin. In addition, if this erythema is persistent and nonblanchable, it may indicate the presence of a stage I pressure ulcer. Erythema due to reactive hyperemia will resolve in one half to three quarters of the time that the tissues were weight bearing.[56,79,80]

▶ **PEARL 19•18** Erythema due to hyperemia will resolve in one half to three quarters of the time period that the tissues were weight bearing. Erythema due to excessive pressure will not resolve in this time, and tissue damage must be considered and addressed.

Positioning When Pressure Ulcers Are Present or Closed

The ideal intervention for treatment of a pressure ulcer is to position the client off the ulcer.[81] Support surfaces and positioning devices are used to achieve these positions and to redistribute pressure off the weight-bearing bony prominences. The need to position off the ulcer site limits the number of available positions and puts the client at high risk for further breakdown. If the ulcer is located over a trochanter, positioning on that side is contraindicated. If the ulcer is located over the sacrum, client should be positioned off that site in the bed and in the chair. If the ulcer is located on the IT, pressure elimination is the best environment to enhance wound closure, whether by the correct seat cushion or by proper positioning on bedrest. If the pressure ulcer is located over the heel, pressure must be eliminated in all positions in bed and in the chair. Even after pressure ulcers are closed, unloading of weight on the scar site must continue to ensure that the wound will not reopen while the newly healed tissues are undergoing maturation and remodeling. Therefore, those who have existing pressure ulcers or ulcers that have been closed for less than 2 years will require constant attention for positioning and will have need of more advanced surfaces that provide the best pressure dispersion possible.

Risk Assessment Score

Most health-care settings use a standardized risk assessment scale to screen all patients for the risk of skin breakdown. Several standardized and validated risk assessment tools are currently in use, each named for their authors. The most common tools include those developed by Braden, Norton, and Gosnell. The Braden scale has the most documentation for reliability and predictive validity.[82] However, risk assessment scales are not designed to inform specific interventions; rather, they are designed to identify those patients who might require individualized intervention plans. For this reason, clinical judgment is needed to evaluate other factors such as specific nutrition needs, skin quality (eg, dryness, fragility), previous skin breakdown, amount of time spent sitting and in bed, available skills and resources, and desires for self-care. A fuller description of risk assessment scales can be found in Chapter 6.

Risk assessment scales have subscales that score factors such as moisture, mobility, and sensation. Mobility is the one subscale that is common to all of the risk assessment scales. For each subscale in which an individual score indicates high risk, there is a need for a prescribed intervention to address prevention. The total score should not lead to a generic plan for wound intervention or equipment selection because this generic plan may not address the specific needs of the individual.[83]

Evaluation of the risk assessment score also assists in selecting the support surfaces and positioning devices used within the wheelchair and bed. Individuals with scores indicating moderate to high risk for pressure ulceration should be evaluated very carefully for support surfaces that most effectively protect the skin. In fact, two studies have been published that demonstrate the utility of risk assessment for prescribing support surfaces. In both cases, the use of specialized surfaces decreased, costs decreased, and positive clinical outcomes increased.[84,85]

Clothing

Evaluating clothing material and fit as well as the fit and effectiveness of appliances is necessary to prevent pressure ulcer development and reoccurrence. Evaluation of the individual's clothing may reveal materials that do not stretch to allow the support surfaces to be effective. Many synthetics do not allow heat loss and can cause the wearer to perspire, predisposing the skin to breakdown from excessive moisture. Wrinkles, pockets, and thick seams can cause pressure points. An ill-fitting prosthesis, orthosis, or shoe can also cause tissue breakdown.

Psychosocial Status

A thorough examination should include gathering psychosocial information, especially symptoms of depression, anxiety, withdrawal, lethargy, passivity, anger, agitation, striking out, and oppositional behavior. Evaluation of the medical record and the client and caregiver responses, in conjunction with relating the current behavior to the current situation, can be very revealing. Many times people are confined to bed when a pressure ulcer exists, the rationale being that complete off-loading of weight from the ulcer, along with the bed support surface, is the therapy that will heal the wound. Bedrest causes social isolation and can lead to anger, withdrawal, loss of appetite, a feeling of helplessness, dependency, low self-esteem, and a decreased will to live, among other responses.[86] It is easy to see why people frequently cannot follow this restrictive and damaging prescription. These behaviors often result in a person's being labeled "noncompliant," implying that they are intentionally refusing to go along with bedrest. Most often they are simply responding to the negative ramifications of bedrest by avoiding it.

When a pressure ulcer is present, much time and energy is spent trying to resolve the wound. Often this occurs at the expense and sacrifice of other activities of daily living. For example, wound care efforts may interfere with the rehabilitation process or the patient's schedule to meet appointments for medical services. Recreational and social activities also may be restricted or eliminated. Additionally, wound-related pain may cause constant distress; complications that may develop, such as infections, can be life threatening and frightening. And bedrest is a total disruption to the lifestyle of the patient and the caregiver(s). Thus, the focus of the medical community on the treatment of the ulcer, instead of on the individual with the ulcer, may be psychologically devastating for all.

Diagnosis and Prognosis

Diagnosis refers to the identification of factors that prevent attainment of the ideal recumbent and seated positions by the client. The diagnosis is based on the information gathered in the examination and evaluation process.

Reimbursement is often driven by functional diagnoses and interventions designed to correct them, rather than by medical diagnoses. An example of a *functional diagnosis* is "Client is bedbound because of loss of skin integrity over the left ischial tuberosity." An example of a *medical diagnosis* is "Client has stage III pressure ulcer over the left ischial tuberosity."

Prognosis refers to a prediction of how close the individual can come to attaining the ideal recumbent and seated positions after intervention. Stated in goal format, the prognosis must

- include the time frame needed to achieve the goal. For example, "In 2 weeks, Ms. X will. . . ."
- be specific and objective. For example, the client will ". . . demonstrate the ability to sit in an upright and supported position in her new seating equipment for 1 hour. . . ."
- emphasize the resulting functional status change. For example, ". . . so that pressure on her IT is decreased and healing of her stage IV pressure ulcer will be measurable."
- be stated in order by body system.[64]

Interventions

Treatment interventions for a pressure ulcer entails direct treatment of the wound with proper dressings and biophysical technologies, choice of support surfaces, and positioning in both sitting and recumbent positions to minimize the pressure on the wound and physical distortion of surrounding tissues.

Treatment of the Wound Site

Guidelines to treat the ulcer site have been presented in Chapters 11 and 12. Pressure ulcers usually occur over bony prominences that are close to the surface of the skin and are susceptible to further injury when weight bearing is inadvertently superimposed on them. Therefore, in addition to the

usual wound treatment guidelines, the clinician should note the following when treating pressure ulcers:

1. Thin, flexible dressings may be preferred when indicated because they conform to bony prominences better and are less likely to fold or curl, causing further damage.
2. Care must be taken to fill undermined or tunneled areas very loosely to prevent undue pressures that can result in further damage or in prevention of wound contraction.
3. Barrier creams may be necessary around the groin and buttocks because urine and feces can irritate the skin, magnify the results of pressure, and cause wound infection.
4. Dressings with smooth slippery outer surfaces are easier to pull clothes over without disturbing the dressing and will stay in place during repositioning.
5. Dressings that adhere well to the skin, but that can be removed without stripping the skin, are preferred.
6. Negative-pressure therapy is often used in large or stalled pressure ulcers. The therapist should be aware that the material inside the wound—whether foam or gauze—becomes very hard when the suction is turned on. Positioning users on a wound while negative-pressure therapy is running can cause extreme pressure on the wound bed and surrounding tissues.

Redistributing Pressure

Pressure exerted over a period of time is the main cause of pressure ulcer development. Therefore, eliminating pressure on the ulcer site is one of the main pillars of ulcer treatment. Pressure can be reduced by many support surfaces and seat cushions and can be eliminated by positioning the person as close to the ideal positions as possible. Table 19.3 summarizes some of the common sites of breakdown as well as some suggested interventions in both the recumbent and sitting positions.

However, the other variable—time—is just as critical. Decreasing time spent on any bony prominence will decrease the risk of tissue breakdown over that prominence. Turning and pressure relief schedules are a typical part of bedside pressure ulcer prevention. The "every 2 hour" rule of thumb may be enough for some people, but may be too often or too little for others. Turning schedules must be individualized, depending on the individual's tissue response to pressure. Pressure relief is also a critical part of prevention for wheelchair users. Education of wheelchair users and their caregivers should include methods and frequency of pressure relief.

Wheelchair users can either perform pressure reliefs independently or use assistance via a caregiver or equipment. Pressure relief for wheelchair users should be done every 15 to 30 minutes.[56,87] In addition to frequency, increasing evidence suggests that relief must last over 1 full minute to allow the tissues to fully reperfuse.[88,89]

Independent pressure relief can be done in a number of ways, including push-up depression lifts, forward lean, and side lean. Push-up depression lifts are done by the user by completely lifting the weight of the body off the seat cushion by pushing off the wheels or armrests. These are beneficial because they completely eliminate pressures on the buttocks. The complication is that they require significant upper body stability and upper extremity strength, and the requirement to

Table 19•3 Suggested Equipment and Positioning Interventions

If ulceration is on the	...then consider the following methods in...	
	Recumbency	Sitting
Sacrum	1. Avoid supine position or place towel roll under one side of pelvis to tip weight off the sacrum. 2. Assess sacral pressures in supine position on the support surface, and minimize. 3. Encourage 30-degree or 150-degree side-lying position following positioning principles. 4. Encourage prone position.	1. If possible, tilt pelvis out of posterior position into neutral. 2. Avoid pressure on sacrum—use cut-out back (see Fig. 13.16B); ensure that back support comes just low enough to support iliac crests. 3. In tilted or reclined position, avoid sacral pressures.
Heel	1. Don't pad under the heel. Elevate it off the surface with protective devices or pillow under the calf and leg. 2. Use support surface that minimizes heel pressures: sloped surface or soft material. Assess pressures with handheld meter. 3. Avoid supine position, encourage 30-degree or 150-degree side-lying. 4. If edema is present, elevate the foot higher than the heart using foam limb elevator.	1. Use protective devices that eliminate heel pressure while positioning the foot in neutral.
Ischial tuberosities (ITs)	1. Avoid Fowler's or elevated position. 2. If bedrest is necessary, use a support surface that will protect remaining skin (assess bony prominences with hand or pressure meter) and be firm enough to allow independent patient movement.	1. Eliminate pressure on ITs. Use seating devices that shift load to femurs and unload ITs (see Fig. 13.16A). 2. Ventilate the IT area. 3. Support patient in the most upright and correct posture. 4. Stabilize the body position to avoid shear with movement.
Malleoli	1. Use protective devices—foam protectors that remove pressure from malleoli—in all positions. 2. Avoid 90-degree side-lying position.	1. Use protective devices. 2. Avoid contact with any part of the wheelchair or other mobility base. 3. Instruct in safe transfer techniques.
Trochanter	1. Avoid all side-lying positions that put pressure on the ulcer. 2. If side-lying cannot be avoided, minimize pressures. Assess pressures on support surface by placing your hand under the trochanter or using a pressure meter.	1. Avoid bed rest; sit as much as possible, only if the wheelchair is fitted correctly, so that lateral trochanters are not in direct contact with side guards or armrests.
Spinous processes	1. Avoid supine position. 2. Encourage 30-degree or 150-degree side-lying position with full support under shoulders and hips to maintain position and to minimize pressures on the spine.	1. Use a back support that eliminates pressure on the ulcer site, or 2. Use a back support that minimizes both pressure and shear on the site with soft, pliable material. 3. Support the body in upright sitting; don't allow the patient to "hang" on the backrest with the spinous processes.

hold an elevated position for more than 60 seconds is simply not possible for many users. Forward leaning has been shown to be effective, reducing pressures on the ischial tuberosities by 78%.[90] Side leaning can be done by hooking the arm on the backrest or armrest and leaning as far to the side as is safe. This approach relieves pressure on one side while elevating it on the other. It also takes twice as long, since the lean must be done in both directions.

Variable-position wheelchairs are available to provide the capability of changing posture to relieve pressure on the buttocks. Both tilt-in-space and recline wheelchairs are available in power and manual versions, with the power versions permitting independent position change by the occupant. The Consortium for Spinal Cord Medicine recommends that users of powered variable-position wheelchairs perform weight shifts every 15 to 30 minutes for at least 1 minute.[87]

Several studies have measured changes in interface pressures using tilt and recline wheelchairs.[90-93] Not surprisingly, all the studies indicate that the reduction in interface pressure is directly related to the magnitude of tilt or recline. This means that users should be encouraged to change position as much as their equipment allows in order to realize maximal relief on the buttocks. If full-range position change is not possible, occupants should be taught to tilt at least 35 degrees or recline 45 degrees. Henderson reported a 27% drop in ischial pressure by tilting the chair back 35 degrees and a 47% drop in ischial pressure by tilting the chair back 65 degrees.[90]

None of these three methods is better than a wheelchair push-up, which results in a full lift off the seat and a 100% drop in ischial pressure. The wheelchair push-up must be a full lift and must be held for at least 1 full minute. The descent back to sitting must be slow and controlled, because a sudden drop can cause damage to tissues.

▶ **PEARL 19•19** Repositioning in bed and frequent pressure relief by one of several methods when sitting are methods necessary to reduce the risk of tissue breakdown. The general rule of thumb that specifies relief every 2 hours in bed or every 15 to 30 minutes when sitting may be adequate for some and not for others.

Bedrest

Persons with pressure ulcers are often confined to bedrest until the ulcers heal. In an extensive literature review, Norton et al specified cognitive and psychosocial complications of bedrest, including depression, learned helplessness, perceptual changes, and fatigue.[86] In addition, their list of physical complications includes osteoporosis, urinary tract infections, decreased cardiac reserve, decreased stroke volume, orthostatic hypotension, pulmonary embolism, deep venous thrombosis, and pneumonia. Other authors note decreased blood volume and hemoglobin concentration, decreased maximum oxygen consumption, fluid stasis in the kidneys that can lead to kidney stones and infection, and increased resting heart rate.[69] Prolonged recumbency and inactivity may also decrease one's appetite, thus resulting in compromised nutritional status.

▶ **PEARL 19•20** Although bedrest can eliminate pressure on an ulcer, it causes numerous negative psychological and physiological complications. The clinician must understand these consequences and work with the client to minimize bedrest.

Appropriate positioning of the head and neck is difficult to achieve in the recumbent position; therefore, the risk of aspiration is greater, not only for food and liquids but also for saliva. Swallowing occurs 24 hours per day, not just during meals. For the bedbound or chairbound individual, appropriate positioning of the head, neck, and trunk to ensure efficient and safe swallowing is an important functional outcome. Consultation with a speech-language pathologist will help identify oral-motor problems and solutions. This is especially important if the client has been examined with a video barium swallow test, and it has been determined that certain positions are required to enhance safe swallowing to avoid aspiration.

Upright positioning for the bedbound or chairbound individual should be initiated as quickly as possible. When appropriate, upright positioning has the following positive benefits: it allows greater diaphragmatic expansion; it improves breathing patterns and depth (improving oxygenation of the blood); and it mobilizes pulmonary secretions.[94] Safe and functional upright positioning in full sitting in a chair (not Fowler's position in bed) for a person who has pressure ulcers on the ITs, sacrum, or coccyx can be achieved by eliminating pressure over the involved bony prominences along with effective postural support with appropriate seat and back support surfaces. By providing a safe and functional sitting position, self-mobility and functional independence are facilitated. Furthermore, cardiac function and perfusion are improved, helping to decrease the time required both to close and to heal the pressure ulcer.

Equipment for Positioning and Support

The goal of pressure ulcer prevention is to protect at-risk tissues by reducing the magnitude and duration of pressure. The goal for a person with a pressure ulcer is wound closure and complete healing, with restoration of functional mobility. To achieve these goals, selected equipment must distribute pressure away from bony prominences at risk, eliminate pressure from sites of existing pressure ulceration, and minimize shear, heat, and moisture. Safe equipment must also allow function and mobility, independent sitting, ambulation, transfers, and proper sitting and recumbent postures.

For pressure management, equipment should reduce or eliminate loading of at-risk sites or pressure ulcer locations. Often, the therapeutic interventions used to prevent pressure ulcers are inadequate for treating an ulcer. The basic goal during pressure ulcer treatment is the removal of pressure. Proper support and positioning is required to remove or greatly minimize external pressure on the ulcer site. Several positioning techniques have already been introduced. In addition, certain seat cushions and back supports that *eliminate* pressure from a pressure ulcer comply with basic wound treatment and can be considered as therapy products for the "treatment" of pressure ulcers.

Equipment used for mobility and support in sitting include wheelchairs, scooters, and seating systems with seat cushions, back supports, and accessory supports for extremities, trunk, head, and neck. Bed equipment includes mattresses, mattress overlays, specialty beds and positioning devices.

Wheelchairs

Proper fitting of the mobility base on which the seat and back are placed is imperative for user function and safety. Many wheelchair options and sizes are available to meet the functional needs of individuals, and many wheelchair cushions are available to ensure adequate skin protection and positioning. These two components must work together to create a wheelchair and seating system tailored to the particular user. This was addressed earlier in this chapter in the section on ideal positions and positioning principles.

Wheelchair Cushions

The wheelchair cushion is one of the most important devices used by wheelchair users because it must protect areas most vulnerable to pressure ulcer formation, that is, ITs, sacrum, and coccyx. Cushions also provide postural support to help position and align users in a functional position.[95] The seat cushion can also help dissipate heat and moisture, limiting two factors that magnify the effects of pressure on the skin.[95] Over 250 cushions are commercially available. Because no single clinician can know every product, a basic understanding of design and performance can assist in selecting an appropriate cushion for wheelchair users. The equivocal nature of wheelchair cushion research means that there is an important principle to remember: No one cushion is best for all people.

▶ **PEARL 19•21** Many wheelchair cushions are commercially available and differ in design and material construction. Proper selection of a cushion is done by a thorough evaluation. While extensive research has been conducted on cushion effectiveness, only one clear conclusion can be drawn: No one cushion is best for all people.

Cushions impact many aspects of functioning during everyday activities, including posture, upper extremity function, comfort, transfers, heat and moisture of the cushion interface, and a host of other factors. In addition, the environment of use, amount of use, and activity level of the user should influence cushion selection. A person who sits in a wheelchair for 16 hours a day and travels in different environments has different needs from a person who sits in a wheelchair for 4 hours a day.

In a general sense, cushions are designed to provide skin protection and positioning for the user. The design and construction of a cushion should reflect its purpose. Wheelchair cushions are made from a variety of materials and reflect many designs. Four material types can be defined: foam/flexible matrix, viscous fluid, air, and gel. Most cushions use a combination of materials to maximize cushion performance by managing the effective and less effective features of each material. Figure 19.21 illustrates the myriad cushions fabricated with different materials.

Skin Protection Cushions

Skin protection is obviously very important for any person at risk of skin breakdown. Decreased mobility and lack of sensation are the most significant contributing factors for pressure ulcer development. Cushions designed for skin protection target loading on the skin and the management of temperature and moisture at the buttock-cushion interface.

In the seated posture, loading on the buttocks represent the greatest risk for tissue damage. Cushions attempt to redistribute

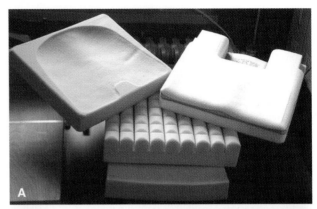
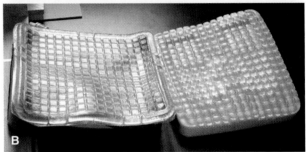
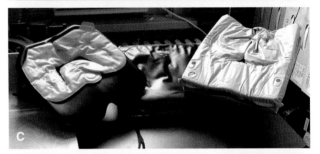
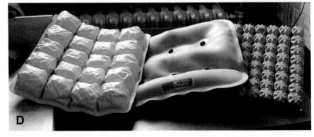

Figure 19•21 *(A) Foam cushions. (B) Gel cushions. (C) Viscous gel cushions. (D) Air-filled cushions.*

pressures away from bony prominences such as the ischial tuberosities and the sacrum/coccyx. Two general techniques are followed: envelopment and redirection or off-loading.

Envelopment is defined as the capability of a support surface to deform around and encompass the contour of the human body.[96] An enveloping cushion should encompass and equalize pressure around irregularities in contour due to buttock shape, objects in pockets, clothing, etc. Cushions that employ envelopment must deflect and deform to immerse the buttocks in the material. Flat cushions must deflect more than precontoured cushions that incorporate a concave sitting surface. Because the ischials are structurally inferior to the trochanters in the sitting position, about 4 to 5 cm of immersion is needed to adequately encompass the buttocks and accommodate the contours of the pelvis. (Fig. 19.22) Simple, flat cushions that are only 2.5 to 4.0 cm thick (1 to 1½ inches) are not able to redistribute pressure adequately. These cushions should be used for comfort rather than skin protection.

Redirection or *off-loading* refers to cushion designs that purposely redirect forces away from bony prominences. Some cushions are designed to partially off-load the ischial tuberosities by putting softer material under them and firmer material under the femurs. Others completely eliminate ischial loading.

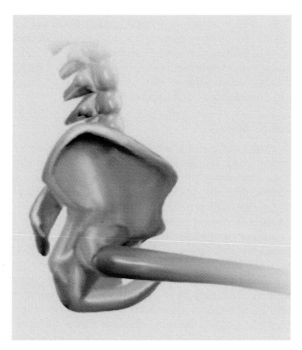

Figure 19•22 *Sagittal view of pelvis. Distance from posterior surface of femurs to tip of ischium is approximately 4.5 cm.*

Cushions accomplish complete off-loading by cut-outs or reliefs in the cushion surface. Cushions that redirect load are often fitted, customized, or individualized to the user to ensure that the person fits the cushion properly. Because the goal is to redirect load away from bony prominences, these cushions generally require the person to sit on the cushion in a specific manner. This requirement should be discussed with the client, who should then be trained in the proper use of the cushion.

Cushions that completely eliminate pressure should be considered for persons with a healing ulcer or who have previously had an ulcer over the ischials. An example is the Isch-Dish® Pressure Relief Seat Cushion (Span-America, Greenville, SC).[75,97] (Fig. 19.23A) The benefits of off-loading the ischial tuberosities for pressure ulcer care and prevention have been well documented.[24,26,75,97-105]

While sitting may be considered by some to be contraindicated during healing, it is sometimes unavoidable, for example, wheeling from bed to bathroom, trips to physician's appointments, or psychological relief from constant bedrest. Refer again to the multiple and serious negative effects of bedrest covered earlier in this chapter.

Interface pressure measurement can be used to judge a cushion's ability to manage pressure on the buttocks. As mentioned previously, interface pressure measurements offer information not readily available through other assessment techniques and can also be quite useful in educating users about posture and pressure relief. While a discussion of seated interface pressure measurement is beyond the scope of this chapter, two important points must be made: no one cushion offers the best interface pressure for all people and no single pressure value has been determined to be the harmful threshold for all people.

Positioning Cushions

Postural support is an important factor in cushion selection since a wheelchair user must perform many activities while seated. Cushions offer a range of positioning features that can enhance postural stability. If positioning is needed, a clinician needs to determine if alignment, accommodation,

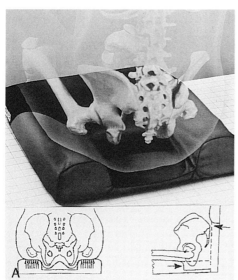

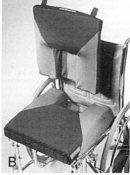

Figure 19•23 *(A) Cut-out, pressure-elimination seat cushion (Isch-Dish®). (B) Sacral cut-out back cushion (Sacral-Dish). (Used with permission of Span-America Medical Systems Inc., Greenville, SC.)*

or correction is needed. Cushions that provide alignment are designed to support the body in a certain position and may include one or all of the following: contouring for the buttocks, lateral pelvic supports, and lateral or medial thigh supports. (Fig. 19.24) Postural accommodation is needed when a client cannot achieve a stable and symmetrical posture, so the cushion is configured to accommodate a deformity. Conversely, if an asymmetry is flexible and correctable, a cushion can be used to position a client and support him or her into a symmetrical posture. Evaluation including ROM, tone, and functional assessment is needed to determine which type of positioning is required.

As one might infer, positioning features of cushions may need to be fitted or individualized to the user. This results in a cushion surface that is site specific, meaning that the user must sit on the cushion correctly. For example, sitting too forward on a cushion may result in the person sitting upon the medial thigh support or pommel. This not only eliminates the positioning ability of the support, it can also adversely impact the cushioning and functionality of the cushion. Clinicians are advised to adequately inform and train users to sit properly on a positioning cushion to ensure proper use. Finally, positioning cushions may have certain features that can hinder transfers and activities such as dressing and undressing. A contoured cushion with a pommel and lateral thigh supports may be needed for positioning, but if the person is independent in transfers, assessment must be made to ensure these positioning features do not pose a barrier to independence.

In summary, many wheelchair cushions are commercially available. Having numerous choices can be helpful for clinicians and clients, but choice can also be confusing.

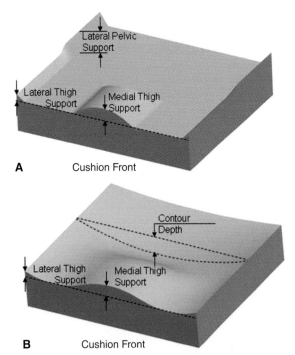

Figure 19•24 *Schematic drawings of flat and contoured cushions. (A) Flat cushion with thigh supports. (B) Contoured cushion with pelvic bucketing.*

Reflecting upon the seating goals with respect to cushion materials and designs allows clients and clinicians to make an informed decision.

Customized Cushions

Customized cushions are shaped specifically to the size and contours of an individual. Because of postural or anatomical anomalies such as fixed pelvic obliquity, fixed scoliosis, dislocated hips, pelvic or femoral malformation, and surgical removal of bone, many people cannot use a generically contoured seat cushion. These customized cushions are molded to the anatomy of the individual, thus providing total contact around the posterior and lateral surfaces of the pelvis, ITs, and thighs. This total contact allows pressure equalization and distribution as long as the user remains in the exact position for which the cushion was molded. Any deviation from this position (eg, sitting on the front of the cushion during a transfer or activities of daily living, turning the head and trunk, causing the pelvis to turn) can change pressure distribution and lead to skin breakdown.

Back Supports

As with the seat cushion, the back support can impact both skin protection and positioning. The skin over prominent spinous processes is vulnerable to breakdown from excessive pressures, especially for users with a kyphotic spine. Poor postural stability can lead to sliding forward on the seat, exposing the tissues to normal pressure, shear, and friction. Padded back cushions and backrests designed for users with a fixed kyphosis or poor trunk stability are available as add-on options for wheelchairs.

The most common backrest is the sling upholstery on a wheelchair. This support is curved from side to side in the frontal plane but does not provide contoured support in the sagittal plane along the spine. Because it is not shaped to the human back, especially the lumbar area, the sling upholstery can induce thoracic kyphosis, especially if worn and stretched out. It puts pressure on the apex of the thoracic curve, flattens the lumbar spine due to inadequate support, and promotes a posterior pelvic tilt because the upper part of the posterior pelvis is unsupported. This generic back "support" may be appropriate for the part-time wheelchair user for short periods of time, but it is not a good long-term intervention for long-term or full-time users.

Add-on back supports are prescribed to offer better trunk support than the sling upholstery. Some back inserts are designed to fit against the sling upholstery to offer additional padding and support. These back inserts offer additional padding and trunk support. One such support, the Sacral Dish® (Span-America, Greenville, SC) eliminates pressure on the sacrum for healing or prevention of a sacral pressure ulcer. (Fig. 19.23B) Another example is the Jay Care® backrest manufactured by Sunrise Medical in Longmont, Colorado that can be configured to reduce loading on the spine due to a fixed thoracic kyphosis. Other backrests are designed to replace the backrest upholstery. These solid backrests can be flat or contoured and typically consist of a rigid frame or shell with a layer of soft support material such as foam, gel, or viscous fluid. (Fig. 19.25) Many contoured backrests are

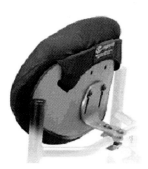
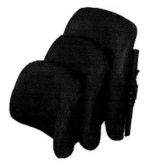

Figure 19•25 *Solid backrests.*

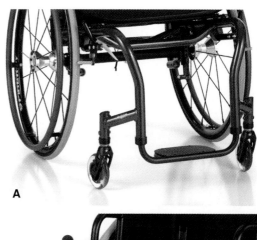

A

designed to offer both lateral stability and support for the lumbar and thoracic spine. Some solid backrests offer angle adjustment to allow the back support to accommodate a kyphotic spine without having to alter the frame of the wheelchair. Add-on back supports must be removed from the wheelchair before folding, so user training is required.

Trunk Supports

Weakness in the trunk musculature as a result of SCI, multiple sclerosis, or fixed thoracic or pelvic deformities may necessitate the use of external supports to maintain an upright sitting position independently. Trunk supports can be attached to the back support or to the wheelchair to assist in lateral trunk stability.

Footrests

Footrests for wheelchairs come in a variety of styles. The most common footrest design is the swing-away, removable footrest. These are height adjustable and can be removed for transfers. (Fig. 19.26B) Because they can be removed, they may be left off the chair under the false impression that they are not essential to the support of the user and therefore expendable. Use of the correctly adjusted footrest must be a rule in all care settings.

Fixed footrests are a permanent part of the chair. Fixed footrests attached to folding chairs are typically selected to ensure that the footrest is not lost. These are the least user-friendly footrests because they may hinder transfers and environmental access in front of the chair. Fixed footrests on rigid frame chairs are a part of the mechanical structure of the wheelchair. They may not have footplates, but they are height adjustable. (Fig. 19.26A) Fixed footrests are not a good option for foot propellers because they will hinder propulsion and maneuverability.

Elevating footrests are cumbersome because they extend out from the chair and make turning difficult and proximity to transfer surfaces hazardous. (Fig. 19.26C) They may be chosen under the mistaken assumption that elevating the LE will reduce edema. However, elevating footrests have never been shown to reduce edema. Elevating footrests may be used in cases when a dependent leg or foot position causes pain or discomfort.

Head and Neck Supports

Special supports may be needed to maintain proper positions of the head and neck, promote adequate visual fields,

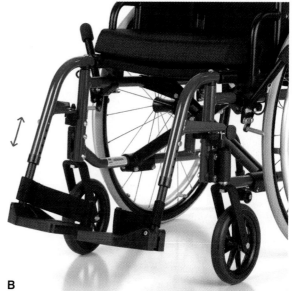

B

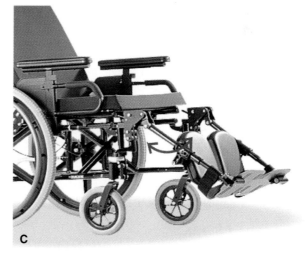

C

Figure 19•26 *Footrests (A) with impact guard on rigid frame chair, (B) adjustable-height, (C) elevating leg rest.*

and help with swallowing and with inhibition of reflex postures. (Fig. 19.27) The prop pictured in Figure 19.27 is a simple head support. Customized supports that wrap around the cranium or neck are also available for more precise positioning, if needed.

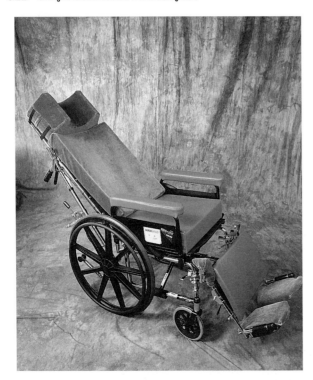

Figure 19•27 *Head support on reclining back chair with trunk guides built in. Twenty-four inch flare-back cushion. Also pictured with seat and head cushion. (Used with permission of Positioning Solutions, Colorado Springs, CO.)*

Ancillary Devices

Ancillary devices include lap and positioning belts and lap trays and are often helpful in positioning a wheelchair user. Lap belts help to maintain pelvic stability, a requirement for good seated posture. Proper positioning of a lap belt is needed to ensure effectiveness and comfort. Lap belts that attach to the rear of the seat and pull down and rearward must contact only the bony pelvis; belts that ride up onto the abdomen cause pain and discomfort and do not perform well. (Fig. 19.28A) Some positioning belts are fastened to the seat rail approximately 6 inches forward of the seat-back junction and pull downward on the proximal thighs. (Fig. 19.28B) These belts do not ride up on the abdomen but are less able to prevent the buttocks from sliding forward in the seat. Lap trays provide a stable surface upon which a user can perform functional activities such as reading or eating. The use of belts and lap trays as restraints is illegal; they are to be used only as positioning or functional devices.

Bed Support Surfaces

The variety of support surfaces on the market has exploded, with literally hundreds of mattresses and overlays to choose from, most without solid research evidence to back up the manufacturers' claims of efficacy. In a systematic review of randomized controlled trials, published or unpublished, that assessed the effectiveness of support surfaces to prevent pressure ulcers, Cullum found the following: (1) the mattresses made of high-specification foam—those with higher manufactured quality specifications, such as indentation load

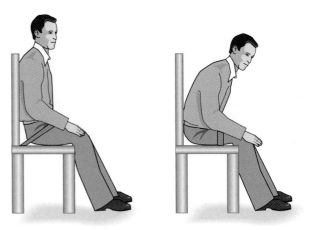

Figure 19•28 *Lap belts can be placed at a standard 45-degree angle (left) or at a 90-degree angle (right).*

deflection and density—reduce the incidence of pressure ulcers compared to standard hospital foam mattresses; (2) the relative merits of alternating pressure and higher-technology constant low-pressure support surfaces are unclear; and (3) the evidence is insufficient to draw conclusions regarding the value of seat cushions, limb protectors, and various constant low-pressure devices for prevention.[104] These conclusions seem to support two earlier literature reviews that summarized published studies on pressure reduction support surfaces. Whittemore and Maklebust both concluded that results were inconsistent among research studies and between research and clinical usage.[105,106] No single support surface has been shown to be superior to the other products in either preventing or helping in the treatment of skin breakdown. Also, while powered surfaces are used clinically in the "treatment" of skin breakdown, studies have shown no statistically significant differences between static and dynamic surfaces in the healing of pressure ulcers.

Thus, the clinician is responsible for making the best choice for the client. The best-informed decision can be made with some basic knowledge of the categories of products, the benefits and drawbacks of each category, the characteristics of clients who have historically used that category of surface, and some objective methods for comparing surfaces. These objective methods should include the quality of component parts, warranty, maintenance requirements, and the ability of the surface to reduce the effects of shear, reduce heat and moisture buildup, and redistribute pressures off bony prominences on a variety of body builds. When comparing powered surfaces, Hasty et al recommended examining the following features: (1) the compliance of the support structure to the individual's anatomy, (2) moisture and temperature control, (3) institutional and convenience factors, (4) individual user comfort, and (5) kinetic factors.[107]

A bed support surface protects the skin and underlying tissues by allowing the user to immerse into the surface and be enveloped by it while externally applied pressure is equalized. It must offer enough support to the body to prevent bottoming out. The firmness provided also gives the user a stable surface for turning and moving in bed, thus equating to functional mobility. The balance of being immersed or enveloped into the surface and supported by it makes a surface both protective and functional. Too much immersion makes a surface too unstable to allow the user to move. However, a firm surface that gives too much support may not be beneficial to body tissue. Foam bolsters around the border of the support surface makes edge-sitting safe for the user. Other considerations when selecting a support surface include (1) ease of consistent use, (2) affordability, (3) ease of cleaning and maintenance, (4) warranty, and (5) accommodation for various body sizes.

The clinician must assess each client individually while he or she is lying on the potential support surface to determine whether pressure redistribution is adequate. Interface pressure mapping has been covered earlier in this chapter, and although it has many limitations, it is the best objective method we have for examining an individual's pressure distribution over the entire support surface. If interface pressure mapping is unavailable, a subjective determination can be made by testing for bottoming out, explained earlier in the discussion of the supine position. If the client does bottom out, other surfaces should be tested until one is found that does not bottom out for this client.

Most often, the selection of a bed support surface is based on the perceived, or manufacturer-suggested, abilities of the product to protect the skin. However, the decision maker must also take into account the user's comfort, functional mobility, and independence. A surface that may assist with the physiological aspects of skin care, but limits these practical factors, only meets a part of the user's health needs. If pressure ulcer

management is to be taken seriously and looked upon as a manifestation of a disease process, then all facets of care, including mobility, comfort, and independence, must be considered in the selection of equipment.

Pressure ulcer treatment usually demands removal of pressure from the ulcer site. Therefore, the effectiveness of a support surface in ulcer treatment is appropriately discussed only when the ulcer is allowed to bear weight. Since a user will have limited choices of position during ulcer treatment, the remaining weight-bearing surfaces of his or her body will require extra protection. Through pressure redistribution and other features described later in this chapter, the support surface can be used to help to prevent breakdown on those remaining weight-bearing body surfaces.

Definitions

In 2007, the Support Surface Standards Initiative of the National Pressure Ulcer Advisory Panel published a new set of definitions to be used in reference to support surfaces. These definitions are shown in Table 19.4.

Of particular note, the terms "pressure reduction" and "pressure relief" have been replaced by the single term, "pressure redistribution." The old definitions for reduction and relief were based on whether a surface could provide less than 32 mm Hg pressure on the body. However, this number has been discredited as a viable number for all people and all tissues, and the ability of a support surface to provide the same interface pressure for all users is unrealistic.

Table 19•4 NPUAP Support Surface Terms and Definitions

Physical Concepts Related to Support Surfaces

Friction (frictional force)	The resistance to motion in a parallel direction relative to the common boundary of two surfaces.
Coefficient of friction	A measurement of the amount of friction existing between two surfaces.
Envelopment	The ability of a support surface to conform, so as to fit or mold around irregularities in the body.
Fatigue	The reduced capacity of a surface or its components to perform as specified. This change may be the result of intended or unintended use and/or prolonged exposure to chemical, thermal, or physical forces.
Force	A push-pull vector with magnitude (quantity) and direction (pressure, shear) that is capable of maintaining or altering the position of a body.
Immersion	Depth of penetration (sinking) into a support surface.
Life expectancy	The defined period of time during which a product is able to effectively fulfill its designated purpose.
Mechanical load	Force distribution acting on a surface.
Pressure	The force per unit area exerted perpendicular to the plane of interest.
Pressure redistribution	The ability of a support surface to distribute load over the contact areas of the human body. This term replaces prior terminology of *pressure reduction* and *pressure relief* surfaces.
Pressure reduction	This term is no longer used to describe classes of support surface. The term is *pressure redistribution*; see above.
Pressure relief	This term is no longer used to describe classes of support surface. The term is *pressure redistribution*; see above.
Shear (shear stress)	The force per unit area exerted parallel to the plane of interest.
Shear strain	Distortion or deformation of tissue as a result of shear stress.

Continued

Table 19•4 NPUAP Support Surface Terms and Definitions—cont'd

Components of Support Surfaces

Air	A low-density fluid with minimal resistance to flow.
Cell/bladder	A means of encapsulating a support medium.
Viscoelastic foam	A type of porous polymer material that conforms in proportion to the applied weight. The air exits and enters the foam cells slowly, which allows the material to respond slower than a standard elastic foam. (Memory foam).
Elastic foam	A type of porous polymer material that conforms in proportion to the applied weight. Air enters and exits the foam cells more rapidly, due to greater density. (Nonmemory foam).
Closed-cell foam	A nonpermeable structure in which there is a barrier between cells, preventing gases or liquids from passing through the foam.
Open-cell foam	A permeable structure in which there is no barrier between cells, and gases or liquids can pass through the foam.
Gel	A semisolid system consisting of a network of solid aggregates, colloidal dispersions, or polymers that may exhibit elastic properties. (Can range from a hard gel to a soft gel.)
Pad	A cushionlike mass of soft material used for comfort, protection. or positioning.
Viscous fluid	A fluid with a relatively high resistance to flow of the fluid.
Elastomer	Any material that can be repeatedly stretched to at least twice its original length; upon release. the stretch will return to approximately its original length.
Solid	A substance that does not flow perceptibly under stress. Under ordinary conditions, it retains its size and shape.
Water	A moderate density fluid with moderate resistance to flow.

Features of Support Surfaces

Air fluidized	A feature of a support surface that provides pressure redistribution via a fluidlike medium created by forcing air through beads as characterized by immersion and envelopment.
Alternating pressure	A feature of a support surface that provides pressure redistribution via cyclic changes in loading and unloading as characterized by frequency, duration, amplitude, and rate of change parameters.
Lateral rotation	A feature of a support surface that provides rotation about a longitudinal axis, as characterized by degree of patient turn, duration, and frequency.
Low-air-loss	A feature of a support surface that provides a flow of air to assist in managing the heat and humidity (microclimate) of the skin.
Zone	A segment with a single pressure redistribution capability.
Multizoned surface	A surface in which different segments can have different pressure redistribution capabilities.

Categories of Support Surfaces

Reactive support surface	A powered or nonpowered support surface with the capability to change its load distribution properties only in response to applied load
Active support surface	A powered support surface with the capability to change its load distribution properties, with or without applied load.
Integrated bed system	A bed frame and support surface combined into a single unit, whereby the surface is unable to function separately.
Nonpowered	Any support surface not requiring or using external sources of energy to operate. (Energy = AC or DC.)
Powered	Any support surface requiring or using external sources of energy to operate. (Energy = AC or DC.)
Overlay	An additional support surface designed to be placed directly on top of an existing surface.
Mattress	A support surface designed to be placed directly on the existing bed frame.

NPUAP, National Pressure Ulcer Advisory Panel.

The terms "active" and "reactive" require further explanation. *Reactive* refers to surfaces that redistribute pressures, but only do so when the client is placed on the surface; they "react" to the load of the body weight. This would describe static surfaces such as foam, nonpowered air and gel, and those powered air mattresses that simply equalize pressure across the surface. *Active* refers to powered surfaces that change their pressure redistribution properties whether a client is on the surface or not. Changes in the characteristics of the active mattress can be seen even when the client is not on the surface. Alternating air mattresses and lateral rotation mattresses are examples of active surfaces.

Overlays

Overlays are support surfaces that are placed on top of a standard commercial or hospital mattress. Usually made of foam, air, or gel, they are typically inexpensive. They must be thin, however, because they add to the overall height of the mattress. This need for thinness necessarily limits the amount of immersion or envelopment that can occur. Thus, bottoming out is common. In addition, the extra height can negate the safety factor of bed rails, and edge sitting is often difficult, especially in short persons whose feet may not reach the floor.

The most common types of overlays are made of vinyl or rubber containing gel or foam. Convoluted (egg crate) foam is considered a product for comfort only. Overlays are generally indicated for the client who requires additional comfort, has good mobility, and has a low to moderate risk of pressure ulceration. Whittemore,[105] citing 19 articles on overlays, concluded that 2-inch foam overlays have almost no pressure-reducing capabilities, whereas 4-inch foam overlays provide significantly better protection, depending on the manufacturer and the physical characteristics of the foam. For a solid, uncut 4-inch foam overlay, Krouskop and Garber recommend a depth of 4 inches, a density of 1.3 pounds per cubic foot, and an indentation load deflection (ILD or IFD—the number of pounds needed to indent a 4-inch sample 25%) of 30 pounds.[108] One randomized controlled trial found a relatively inexpensive foam overlay with a special contoured, cross-cut design to be effective in preventing ulcers in the high-risk client and nearly as effective as low-air-loss mattresses in treating those with ulcers up to stage IV when the there were at least two ulcer-free turning surfaces.[109] (Fig. 19.29)

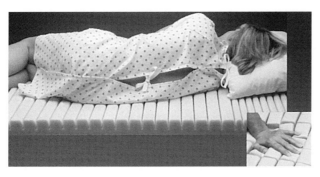

Figure 19•29 *Geo-Matt overlay. (Used with permission of Span-America Medical Systems Inc., Greenville, SC.)*

Reactive Therapeutic Mattress Replacements

Because of the expense of providing a new overlay for each client, many long-term care and acute care facilities are investing in therapeutic mattress replacements. This category of surfaces features mattresses made of various materials, including foam of multilayered densities or one uniform density. (Fig. 19.30A) Also included are air-filled bladders or cylinders in which the amount of air remains constant, those that allow air to shift only within a closed tube (not between tubes or with the outside), gel-filled bladders, and combinations, such as air-filled cylinders surrounded by a foam shell on the top, ends, and sides. (Fig. 19-30B) In this group of surfaces the amount of support material within the system remains the same and reacts to the load placed upon it to redistribute pressure.

These static surfaces and dynamic powered surfaces that equalize pressure must be at least 5 inches thick to be considered therapeutically effective. They are designed to reduce pressure on weight-bearing bony prominences to below the level that occurs on a standard hospital mattress. Most achieve this, as shown by Jester and Weaver.[110] Krouskop found that within 2 to 3 years of use, foam mattresses lose 40% of their stiffness under the two most critical areas of the body: the sacrum and the heel.[111] Foam mattresses are useful in pressure management, but they must be monitored for signs of deterioration, such as lack of resiliency or return to shape after compression, flaking of the foam, change in stiffness or consistency under the weight-bearing areas, and contamination from moisture. Many carry warranties of 5 years or more because the advances in foam manufacturing, as well as

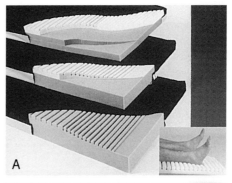

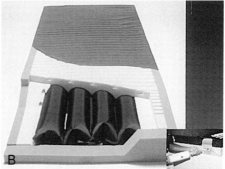

Figure 19•30 *Static mattress replacements. (A) All-foam mattress (Geo-Mattress®). (B) Foam-Air mattress (Pressure-Guard Renew®). (Used with permission of Span-America Medical Systems Inc., Greenville, SC.)*

layering softer foams over firmer foams, have added to the effective life span of foam mattresses.

Reactive surfaces are used to improve user comfort and should be considered part of a program of pressure ulcer prevention for those users who are at moderate to high risk of pressure ulceration,[112] who can be placed into at least three positions, and who can be turned with some frequency throughout the time in bed. In addition, the reactive surface may be appropriate during the treatment of an ulcer if the user can be positioned off the ulcer site and turned frequently. These surfaces may be appropriate to protect the intact skin from breakdown.

In general, pressure-equalizing, reactive static surfaces have been considered as "prevention" mattresses for the moderate- to high-risk client. Patients in critical care units and those in the highest risk groups, such as those who have undergone flap or graft surgeries or are immobile, are commonly placed on active, powered surfaces (see the following section). However, Ooka and coworkers found that reactive static foam mattresses performed as well as active, powered dynamic air mattresses in preventing tissue breakdown in critically ill patients.[113] They reported that instances in which patients who were considered candidates for powered surfaces, but received nonmoving, static surfaces instead, suggested to them the need to look objectively at support surface prescription rather than at what limited protocols or reimbursement schedules say should be used. Although the mattress is an important part of prevention, other standards of good care such as hygiene, a regular turning schedule, and nutrition are equally important. The goal of preventing tissue breakdown cannot be placed solely on the mattress.

▷ **PEARL 19•22** Support surfaces are only one component of pressure ulcer prevention and treatment. The goal of preventing or treating pressure ulcers cannot rely solely on the mattress.

A small group of nonpowered mattresses have been proven to assist in wound healing. These "non-powered advanced pressure-reducing mattresses" are recognized by Medicare as effective and reimbursable for the treatment of stage II to IV pressure ulcers.[114] This group of mattresses provides the convenience of nonpowered surfaces with the outcomes hoped for with powered or active surfaces. Branom showed improved healing rates of stage III to IV pressure ulcers in the elderly when this type of surface was used compared to low-air-loss devices.[115] Ross reported no development of pressure ulcers when this surface was used in intensive care units in place of low-air-loss devices over an 18-month period.[116]

Reactive surfaces generally provide a stable foundation that assists in independent movement of the user, such as turning and repositioning.

Active Powered Mattress Replacements

These active mattress replacements are powered by electric pumps that replace air as it is lost from the system (low-air-loss) or that are programmed to sequentially inflate and deflate alternating compartments beneath the user (alternating pressure and lateral rotation). These surfaces are more expensive than most reactive surfaces

Low-air-loss mattresses are used for removing excessive sweat and heat from the body. Most consist of a large air bladder, or several smaller bladders, with small, laser-made holes permeating the surface. (Fig. 19.31) A vapor-permeable cover is placed on top of the mattress, creating a space or microenvironment between the cover and the mattress. As the user lies on the surface, air leaks out of the laser holes and into the microenvironment from below while vapor from the user permeates the cover and enters the microenvironment from above. Movement of the air removes the vapor from the microenvironment, thus assisting in thermoregulation of the user. The air that leaks out of the laser holes is constantly replaced by the pump, giving the balance of immersion and support required for user care. Some manufacturers have used the term "true" low-air-loss and base this definition on the amount of air supplied by the pump. Some claim the quality of the mattress depends on the size of the blower or pump or the amount of air that is circulated through the mattress. There is no basis for either definition. Figliola showed that removal of moisture from the user can be quantified and that there is a large variance among low-air-loss mattress constructions in this measure, independent of the pump capabilities.[117] Weaver and Jester

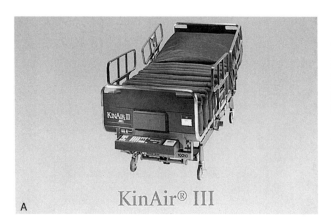
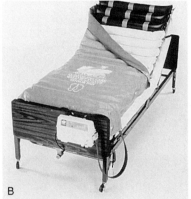

Figure 19•31 *Dynamic powered mattress replacements. (A) Low-air-loss mattress. (Used with permission of KCI, San Antonio, TX). (B) Alternating-pressure mattress. (DFS®; used with permission of Huntleigh Healthcare Inc., Eatontown, NJ).*

showed that low-air-loss mattresses do yield lower interface pressures compared to foam or static mattresses.[118] However, eight studies reviewed by Maklebust indicated that low-air-loss mattresses are effective prevention surfaces, but do not yield significant improvements in healing rates or in the percentage of ulcers that heal completely.[106] They are used to prevent further breakdown of the integument when the client is confined to bed and the number of turning surfaces available to the client is limited by the presence of ulcers on one or more of those surfaces.

Alternating-pressure mattresses are made of multiple individual air tubes linked to a motor and pump. (Fig. 19.31B) At any given time, half of the tubes are more inflated and half are more deflated, and they switch in a programmed, alternating pattern. The constant change in pressures within the tubes yields a surface with constantly changing pressures exerted on a user's body. Although alternating-pressure mattresses are considered to be "treatment" mattresses by third-party payers, no studies have demonstrated that these surfaces yield significant differences in ulcer-healing rates.

Lateral rotation mattresses describe those bed surfaces that can be programmed to periodically tilt the recumbent user between 20 degrees and 40 degrees toward right or left. (Fig. 19.32) Originally used to reduce the negative effects of immobility on body systems (including respiratory, urinary, vascular, and cardiopulmonary systems), these surfaces have been effective in the prevention and treatment of integumentary damage because, like alternating-pressure mattresses, the pressure under the weight-bearing surfaces changes at regular intervals. One study retrospectively showed benefits to lateral rotation surfaces for wound closure.[119] Additionally, rotational surfaces are also effective when manual turning causes pain or when manual assistance for regular turning is not available. However, rotational surfaces should not take the place of manually repositioning the client if at all possible. In a 1995 study, Xakellis et al compared the costs of four pressure ulcer prevention methods: manual turning, pressure-reducing mattresses, chair cushions, and miscellaneous preventive devices.[4] Manual turning was the most costly method by far, with a daily cost

of \$8.83 plus or minus \$1.66. The authors of the study proposed that manual turning is such an expensive method of pressure management that devices for turning should substantially reduce overall costs.

As reimbursement guidelines for bed surfaces were developed in the late 1980s to early 1990s, active surfaces became known as "treatment" surfaces: That is, they were paid for if the person was being treated for a pressure ulcer. Usually, active surfaces are used for those with existing skin ulceration during the period of time required for treatment of the ulcer. However, "treatment" does not imply that a person can bear weight on an ulcer site when placed on one of these surfaces. Although active surfaces are more advanced technologically than are reactive surfaces, pressure ulcer treatment protocols still require positioning the client off the ulcer site as much as possible. Active surfaces are used as prevention in some cases: for example, patients at highest risk of tissue breakdown, such as the nutritionally deficient, bedbound individual with multiple comorbidities.

> **PEARL 19•23** Alternating pressure, low-air-loss, and lateral rotation mattresses are usually prescribed for pressure ulcer treatment or for prevention in the very high-risk individual. However, the patient should not be allowed to lie on the pressure ulcer and must be repositioned as frequently as the skin indicates the need; active mattresses do not relieve the caregiver or the patient of these responsibilities.

Two drawbacks to most of these active surfaces are their instability and expense. The changing dynamics of the support material during operation of these surfaces make self-mobility and maintenance of position more difficult than on more nonmoving surfaces. When the patient pushes off the surface to roll over or sit up, the surface yields rather than supports the body, making mobility difficult. Some patients complain that these surfaces are difficult to sleep on because of the constant movement. A foam layer over the air containers aids in patient stability and mobility. Additionally, these surfaces are more expensive to purchase or to rent than reactive surfaces.

Air-Fluidized Beds

Air-fluidized beds, known for their excellent pressure redistribution, are believed to reduce shearing forces as well. These beds are constructed as a container holding of millions of ceramic beads resembling sand. The surface of the bead containment chamber is a loose-fitting polyester filter sheet that moves with the patient. Air is drawn in through a pump and channeled through these beads, causing them to go into motion below the polyester filter sheet and act as a fluid. The patient in effect "floats" on the sheet, supported by the blowing air and moving beads below. Because rental may be very costly, these beds are usually reserved for patients at highest risk, such as those immediately after flap or graft surgeries or those with dermal ulcers who, because of extremely limited bed mobility, must bear weight on the ulcers in recumbent positions.

This type of bed does have some drawbacks. Maintaining body position is difficult. The side-lying position is especially

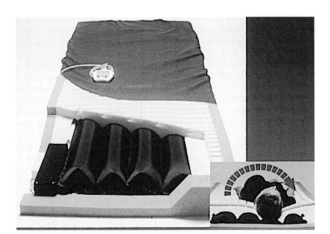

Figure 19•32 *Rotational surface. (PressureGuard Turn Select; used with permission of Span-America Medical Systems Inc., Greenville, SC.)*

difficult because the surface is constantly shifting beneath the "floating" patient due to the air moving through the silicone beads. Also, patient mobility in bed and when getting in and out of the bed safely can be difficult due to the lack of a stable support surface for pushing off when moving or to the high bed edges of some models. Turning patients in these beds may also be difficult for caregivers, especially because of the lack of patient stability in the bed while the air fluidization pump is running. The constant movement of air between the bed surface and the patient's skin may cause dryness of the skin. Also, regular calibration of the warm-air thermostat should be performed so the patient is not subjected to excessive levels of heat, which tend to strain the basal metabolism.

Summary

Treatment of the patient with a pressure ulcer requires a trans-disciplinary approach. The role of physical and occupational therapy or nursing in assessing the patient for the proper seating and mattress equipment, as well as safe postures to heal ulcers or prevent the development of ulcers, influences all other aspects of wound treatment. Money spent on the appropriate equipment and time spent on education of the patient, family, and caregivers in effective positioning are essential to a complete wound care program. In a time of focus on getting the most for every health-care dollar, the proper seating and mattress equipment, properly used, will reap financial benefits many times the cost of this equipment.

▶ Case Study 19•1 Wheelchair and Positioning Needs for an Individual with a Right Ischial Pressure Ulcer and Complex Postural Deviations

History

Mr. B is a 60-year-old man with a chronic right ischial wound with an onset of August 2002. Mr. B had polio as a child. In March 2002 he became a quadriplegic secondary to spinal stenosis, cervical myelopathy, and a spinal stroke. He is a non-insulin-dependent diabetic. He has a suprapubic catheter. Mr. B received in-patient and out-patient wound care in attempts to heal his wound; however, because of the inadequacies of his seating system, he was referred in May 2007 by a vocational rehabilitation specialist for seating and positioning assessment. He sits in his chair about 12 hours a day and works full time. He admits to being inconsistent with performing tilting pressure reliefs.

Abbreviated Systems Review

Musculoskeletal: Mr. B has significant weakness in the upper extremities, absent to little strength in the lower extremities, and poor to fair trunk control. Range of motion in his extremities is significantly limited at most joints, with exception of his wrists. His spinal curvature has cervical, thoracic, lumbar, and sacral deviations convex to the right, which causes a pelvic obliquity (right side lower than left) and a windswept position of the lower extremities to the left. His pelvis is shifted to the left. His scoliosis and pelvic obliquity are somewhat flexible and therefore partially correctable with proper equipment. Mr. B's thorax is large, with a prominent abdomen.

Neuromuscular: His sensation is impaired from his nipple line down to his feet. He is able to perceive pain or discomfort in his buttocks and lower extremities. His visual field is affected by right eye blindness.

Neurovascular: Mr. B has a history of deep venous thromboses and of swelling and pain in his left lower extremity.

Integument: Mr. B has been treated for a right ischial pressure ulcer since August 2002. His wound has been as large as 19 cm × 15 cm × 6 cm deep. At his most recent evaluation, his wound measured 2.7 cm × 1.3 cm × 0.3 cm deep with a 2.4-cm deep undermining at 2 o'clock. The wound is being treated with calcium alginate, periwound barrier, and absorbent cover dressing; dressings are changed daily.

Wheelchair Equipment and Posture

Initial: Mr. B's chair included a custom-molded backrest, a lateral hip guide on the left, an air-filled chambered cushion, an arm trough on the right with a flat arm pad on the left, and a single-piece contoured headrest with adjustable hardware. He placed both feet on the left footrest with a custom-fabricated footplate and had discarded the right footrest in order to gain access to his van. (Fig. 19.33)

Analysis of Mr. B's seated position revealed his trunk was shifted to the right, with the head compensating to the left. His right thigh was adducted in a mild windswept fashion. Pelvic obliquity was lower on the right. The right foot was slightly lower than the left. Shear forces were likely present at the back as well as at the cushion.

At the time of evaluation, he was complaining of pain at his right side and at the right elbow, likely caused by the inadequate lateral thoracic support and excessive weight bearing on the right arm trough because of his postural collapse to the right. Mr. B had removed part of the right lateral component of the thoracic support of his custom backrest because of discomfort. He also complained of sliding in the chair, which can contribute to shearing at his back and buttocks. The shape of his thorax, in addition to his spinal curvature, created a challenge to accommodate for support.

Interventions: It was determined that greater surface contact over the back and right lateral thoracic areas was needed to distribute forces, conform to his asymmetrical spine, improve posture, and relieve pain and discomfort. This was accomplished with a new custom-contoured backrest with a deeper and more contoured right thoracic support with interior reinforcement and variable foam for comfort. A lateral hip guide was also provided to prevent shifting of the pelvis to the left. He did not tolerate attempts to provide an abduction force at the right thigh due to hip discomfort and soft tissue tightness. A center-mounted footplate was found that improved his thigh alignment and permitted the needed access into his van.

His seat cushion was changed to a powered alternating-pressure cushion to aid with healing of his chronic wound. The firmness of this cushion also assisted in leveling his pelvic obliquity.

▶ **Case Study 19•1** **Wheelchair and Positioning Needs for an Individual with a Right Ischial Pressure Ulcer and Complex Postural Deviation—cont'd**

Results: Mr. B sits in a more upright position that decreases pressure over his right ischial area. His pain has significantly decreased. Within 10 weeks his wound measured 1.2 cm × 0.2 cm × 0.2 cm deep, and the undermining had decreased to 1.6 cm. This healing can only be attributed to his positioning and equipment changes; the dressing regimen was consistent from well before equipment delivery to 10 weeks after delivery.

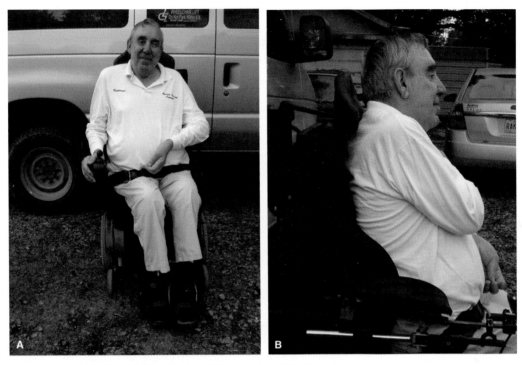

Figure **19•33** *Mr. B's old wheelchair. (A) Front view. (B). Side view.*

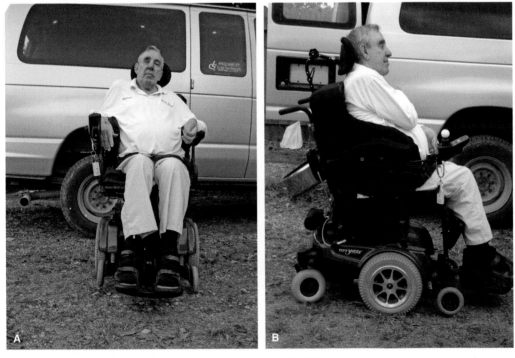

Figure **19•34** *Mr. B's new wheelchair. (A) Front view. (B) Side view.*

Additional Readings on Seated Positioning

Cook A, Hussey S: Assistive Technologies: Principles and Practice. St. Louis, Mosby, 1995.

Engstrom B, Tryck B: *Ergonomics: Wheelchairs and Positioning.* Sweden, Posturalis, 1993.

Rader J, et al: Individualized Wheelchair Seating: For Older Adults. A two-part manual and videotape, published by a not-for-profit institute. Mt. Angel, OR, Benedictine Institute for Long Term Care, 1998. (503) 845-9495.

Falk A, et al: Positioning for Function: Wheelchairs and Other Assistive Technologies. Valhalla, NY, Valhalla Rehabilitation Publications Ltd., 1990.

Trefler E, et al: Seating and Mobility for Persons with Physical Disabilities: Therapy Skill Builders. Memphis, TN, University of Tennessee, 1993.

References

1. National Pressure Ulcer Advisory Panel. Updated staging system: Pressure ulcer stages revised by NPUAP. Available at: http:www.npuap.org/pr2.htm. Accessed on: 10/22/07.

2. Maklebust, J, Sieggreen, M: Pressure ulcers: Guidelines for prevention and nursing management. West Dundee, IL, S-N Publications, 1991.

3. Centers for Medicare and Medicaid Services (CMS): CFR Parts 411, 412, 413, and 489 Medicare Program; Proposed Changes to the Hospital Inpatient Prospective Payment Systems and Fiscal Year 2008 Rates; Final Rule. In: Federal Register 2007; Vol. 72, No. 162, p. 42, 2007.

4. Xakellis, GC, Frantz, R, Lewis, A: Cost of pressure ulcer prevention in long-term care. J Am Geriatr Soc 1995; 43:496–501.

5. National Pressure Ulcer Advisory Panel. Cuddigan, J, Ayello EA, Sussman C (eds): Pressure ulcers in America: Prevalence, incidence, and implications for the future. Reston, VA, 2001.

6. Baker, J: Medicaid claims history of Florida long-term care facility residents hospitalized for pressure ulcers. J Wound Ostomy Continence Nurs 1996; 23:23–25.

7. Brandeis, GH, Berlowitz, DR, Hossain, M, et al: Pressure ulcers: The minimum data set and the resident assessment protocol. Adv Wound Care 1995; 8:18–25.

8. Spector, WD, Fortinsky, RH: Pressure ulcer prevalence in Ohio nursing homes: Clinical and facility correlates. J Aging Health 1998; 10:62–80.

9. Horn, SD, Bender, SA, Bergstrom, N, et al: Description of the national pressure ulcer long-term care study. J Am Geriatr Soc 2002; 50:1816–1825.

10. Xakellis, GC, Frantz, R: The cost of healing pressure ulcers across multiple health care settings. Adv Wound Care 1996; 9:18–22.

11. Whittington, KT, Briones, R: National prevalence and incidence study: 6-year sequential acute care data. Adv Skin Wound Care 2004; 17:490–494.

12. Beckrich, K, Aronovitch, SA: Hospital-acquired pressure ulcers: A comparison of costs in medical vs. surgical patients. Nurs Econ 1999; 17:263–271.

13. Allman, RM, Goode, PS, Burst, N, et al: Pressure ulcers, hospital complications, and disease severity: Impact on hospital costs and length of stay. Adv Wound Care 1999; 12:22–30.

14. Woodbury, MG, Houghton, PE: Prevalence of pressure ulcers in Canadian healthcare settings. Ostomy Wound Manage 2004; 50:22–24, 26, 28, 30, 32, 34, 36–38.

15. Chen, Y, Devivo, MJ, Jackson, AB: Pressure ulcer prevalence in people with spinal cord injury: Age–period-duration effects. Arch Phys Med Rehabil 2005; 86:1208–1213.

16. McKinley, WO, Jackson, AB, Cardenas, DD, et al: Long-term medical complications after traumatic spinal cord injury: A regional model systems analysis. Arch Phys Med Rehabil 1999; 80:1402–1410.

17. Richardson, RR, Mayer, PR: Prevalence and incidence of pressure sores in acute spinal cord injuries. Paraplegia 1981; 19:235–247.

18. Young, K: Transcutaneous oxygen tension measurements as a method of assessing peripheral vascular disease. Clin Phys Physiol Meas 1981; 2:147–151.

19. Salzberg, C: A new pressure ulcer risk assessment scale for individuals with spinal cord injury. Am J Phys Med Rehabil 1996; 75:96–104.

20. Byrne, DW, Salzberg, CA: Major risk factors for pressure ulcers in the spinal cord disabled: A literature review. Spinal Cord 1996; 34:255–263.

21. Disa, JJ, Carlton, JM, Goldberg, NH: Efficacy of operative cure in pressure sore patients. Plast Reconstr Surg 1992; 89:272–278.

22. Evans, GR, Dufresne, CR, Manson, PN: Surgical correction of pressure ulcers in an urban center: Is it efficacious? Adv Wound Care 1994; 7:40–46.

23. Curtin, I: Wound management: Care and cost: An overview. Nurse Manage 1984; 15:22.

24. Zacharkow, D: Wheelchair poster and pressure sores. Springfield, IL, Charles C. Thomas Pub Ltd, 1984.

25. Kosiak, M: Etiology and pathology of ischemic ulcers. Arch Phys Med Rehabil 1959; 40:62–69.

26. Reswick, J, Rogers, JE: Experience at Rancho Los Amigos Hospital with devices and techniques to prevent pressure sores. In: Kenedi, R, Cowden, JM (eds): Bedsore Biomechanics. Baltimore, University Park Press, 1976, pp 301–310.

27. Lassen, NA, Holstein, P: Use of radioisotopes in assessment of distal blood flow and distal blood pressure in arterial insufficiency. Surg Clin North Am 1974; 54:39–55.

28. Holloway, GA, Daly, CH, Kennedy, D, et al: Effects of external pressure loading on human skin blood flow measured by 133Xe clearance. J Appl Physiol 1976; 40:597–600.

29. Ek, AC, Gustavsson, G, Lewis, DH: Skin blood flow in relation to external pressure and temperature in the supine position on a standard hospital mattress. Scand J Rehabil Med 1987; 19:121–126.

30. Sangeorzan, BJ, Harrington, RM, Wyss, CR, et al: Circulatory and mechanical response of skin to loading. J Orthop Res 1989; 7:425–431.

31. Bennett, L, Kavner, D, Lee, BK, et al: Shear vs. pressure as causative factors in skin blood flow occlusion. Arch Phys Med Rehabil 1979; 60:309–314.

32. National Pressure Ulcer Advisory Panel. Support surface standards initiative: Terms and definitions related to support surfaces. Available at: http://www.npuap.org/NPUAP_S3I_TD.pdf. Accessed on: 10/22/07.

33. Trefler, E, Hobson, D, Johnson Taylor, S, et al: Seating and Mobility for Persons with Physical Disabilities. Therapy Skill Builders. a division of Communication Skill Builders, Tucson, AZ, for the University of Tennessee Memphis Rehabilitation Engineering Program, 1993.

34. Magee, D (ed): Orthopedic Physical Assessment. Philadelphia, WB Saunders, 1992.

35. Goossens, RH, Snijders, CJ: Design criteria for the reduction of shear forces in beds and seats. J Biomech 1995; 2:225–230.

36. Fischer, E, Solomon, S: Physiological Responses to Heat and Cold. Baltimore, Waverly, 1965.

37. Hardy, J, Bard, P: Body temperature regulation. St Louis, CV Mosby, 1979.

38. Ruch, R, Patton, HD (ed): Physiology and Biophysics, 19th ed. Philadelphia, WB Saunders, 1965.

39. Patel, S, Knapp, CF, Donofrio, JC, et al: Temperature effects on surface pressure-induced changes in rat skin perfusion: Implications in pressure ulcer development. J Rehabil Res Dev 1999; 36:189–201.

40. Kokate, JY, Leland, KJ, Held, AM, et al: Temperature-modulated pressure ulcers: A porcine model. Arch Phys Med Rehabil 1995; 76:666–673.

41. Lachenbruch, C: Skin cooling surfaces: Estimating the importance of limiting skin temperature. Ostomy Wound Manage 2005; 51:70–79.

42. Visscher, MO, Chatterjee, R, Ebel, JP, et al: Biomedical assessment and instrumental evaluation of healthy infant skin. Pediatr Dermatol 2002; 19:473–481.

43. Buchholz, B, Frederick, LJ, Armstrong, TJ: An investigation of human palmar skin friction and the effects of materials, pinch force, and moisture. Ergonomics 1988; 31:317–325.

44. Egawa, M, Oguri, M, Hirao, T, et al: The evaluation of skin friction using a frictional feel analyzer. Skin Res Technol 2002; 8:41–51.

45. Krouskop, T, van Rijswijk, L: Standardizing performance-based criteria for support surfaces. Ostomy Wound Manage 1995; 41:34–36, 38, 40–45.

46. Fisher, SV, Szymke, TE, Apte, SY, et al: Wheelchair cushion effect on skin temperature. Arch Phys Med Rehabil 1978; 59:68–72.

47. Civelek, A, Ak, K, Kurtkaya, O, et al: Effect of a low molecular weight heparin molecule, dalteparin, on cellular apoptosis and inflammatory process in an incisional wound-healing model. Surg Today 2007; 37:406–411.

48. Pinchofsky-Devin, G: Nutritional Assessment and Intervention. King of Prussia, PA, Health Management Publications, 1990.

49. Pinchcofsky-Devin, GD, Kaminski, MV, Jr.: Correlation of pressure sores and nutritional status. J Am Geriatr Soc 1986; 34:435–440.

50. Pompeo, M: Misconceptions about protein requirements for wound healing: Results of a prospective study. Ostomy Wound Manage 2007; 53:30–32, 34, 36–38.

51. Downey, J, Myers, S: The Physiological Basis of Rehabilitation Medicine. Newton, MA, Butterworth-Heinemann, 1994.

52. Yarkoney, G: Aging Skin, Pressure Ulcerations, and Spinal Cord Injury. New York, Demos, 1993.

53. Bryant, R: Acute and Chronic Wounds. St. Louis, CV Mosby, 1992.

54. Salzberg, CA, Byrne, DW, Cayten, CG, et al: Predicting and preventing pressure ulcers in adults with paralysis. Adv Wound Care 1998; 11:237–246.

55. Clarke, M, Kadhorn, HM: The nursing prevention of pressure sores in hospital and community patients. J Adv Nurs 1988; 13:365–373.

56. U.S. Department of Health and Human Services. Pressure Ulcers in Adults: Prediction and Prevention. Clinical Practice Guideline. Rockville, MD, Public Health Service, U.S. Department of Health and Human Services, Agency for Health Care Policy and Research, 1992.

57. Carlson, EV, Kemp MG, Shott, S: Predicting the risk of pressure ulcers in critically ill patients. Am J Crit Care 1999; 8:262–269.

58. Witkowski, JA, Parish, LC: The decubitus ulcer: skin failure and destructive behavior. Int J Dermatol 2000; 39:892–898.

59. Mulder, GD. Factors influencing wound healing. In: Leaper, DJ, Harding, KG (eds): Wounds: Biology and Management. New York, Oxford University Press, 1998.

60. Sprigle, S, Schuch, JZ: Using seat contour measurements during seating evaluations of individuals with SCI. Assist Technol 1993; 5:24–35.

61. Koo, TK, Mak, AF, Lee, YL: Posture effect on seating interface biomechanics: Comparison between two seating cushions. Arch Phys Med Rehabil 1996; 77:40–47.

62. Samuelsson, K, Larsson, H, Thyberg, M, Tropp, H: Back pain and spinal deformity common among wheelchair users with spinal cord injuries. Scan J Occupational Ther 1996; 3:28–32.

63. Andersson, GB, Murphy, RW, Ortengren, R, et al: The influence of backrest inclination and lumbar support on lumbar lordosis. Spine 1979; 4:52–58.

64. American Physical Therapy Association. Guide to Physical Therapist Practice. A description of patient/client management; Preferred practice patterns. Phys Ther 1997; 77(Pt 1 and 2):1160–1656.

65. Mollinger, LA, Steffen, TM: Knee flexion contractures in institutionalized elderly: Prevalence, severity, stability, and related variables. Phys Ther 1993; 73:437–444; discussion 444–446.

66. Ferguson-Pell, MW: Seat cushion selection. J Rehabil Res Dev Clin 1990; (suppl)(2):49–73.

67. Bridel-Nixon, JA: Pressure sores. In: Morrison, M, Moffat, C, Bridel-Nixon, J (eds): A Color Guide to the Nursing Management of Chronic Wounds. St. Louis, MO, CV Mosby, 1997, pp 160–162.

68. Henson, D, Morrissey, WL: Acute respiratory failure, mechanisms, and medical management. In: Irwin, S, Tecklin, JS (eds): Cardiopulmonary Physical Therapy, ed. 2. St. Louis, CV Mosby, 1990, p 272.

69. Ross, J, Dean, E: Integrating physiological principles into the comprehensive management of cardiopulmonary dysfunction. Phys Ther 1989; 69:255–259.

70. Biena, R, et al: Malnutrition in the hospitalized geriatric patient. J Am Geriatr Soc 1989; 30:433.

71. Ek, AC, Unosson, M, Larsson, J, et al: The development and healing of pressure sores related to the nutritional state. Clin Nutr 1991; 10:245–250.

72. Franson, TR, Duthie, EH Jr., Cooper, JE, et al: Prevalence survey of infections and their predisposing factors at a hospital-based nursing home care unit. J Am Geriatr Soc 1986; 34:95–100.

73. Sullivan, DH, Patch, GA, Walls, RC, et al: Impact of nutrition status on morbidity and mortality in a select population of geriatric rehabilitation patients. Am J Clin Nutr 1990; 51:749–758.

74. Ruder, S, Matassarin-Jacobs, E: Nursing care of clients with cerebral disorders. In: Black, J, Matassarin-Jacobs, E (eds): Luckmann and Sorensen's Medical-Surgical Nursing: A Psychophysiologic Approach, ed. 4. Philadelphia, WB Saunders, 1993, p 720.

75. Rappl, L: Management of pressure by therapeutic positioning. In: Sussman, C, Bates-Jensen, B (eds): Wound Care: A Collaborative Practice Manual for Physical Therapists and Nurses. Gaithersburg, MD, Aspen Publishers, 1998.

76. Fader, M, Bain, D, Cottenden, A: Effects of absorbent incontinence pads on pressure management mattresses. J Adv Nurs 2004; 48:569–574.

77. Landis, E: Micro-injection studies of capillary blood pressure in human skin. Heart 1930; 15:209.

78. Shapcott, N, Levy, B: By the numbers. Team Rehab Report 1999; 11:16–20.

79. Parish, LC, Witkowski, JA, Crissey, JT (eds): The Decubitus Ulcer. New York, Masson Publishing USA Inc, 1983.

80. Sprigle, S, Linden, M, Riordan, B: Characterizing reactive hyperemia via tissue reflectance spectroscopy in response to an ischemic load across gender, age, skin pigmentation, and diabetes. Med Eng Phys 2002; 24:651–661.

81. U.S. Department of Health and Human Services. Pressure Ulcers in Adults: Treatment of Pressure Ulcers. Clinical Practice Guidelines. No. 15. Rockville, MD, Public Health Service, Agency for Health Care Policy and Research, 1994.

82. Langemo, DK: Risk assessment tools for pressure ulcers. Adv Wound Care 1999; 12:42–44.

83. McNees, P, Braden, B, Bergstrom, N, et al: Beyond risk assessment: Elements for pressure ulcer prevention. Ostomy Wound Manage 1998; 44(suppl):51S–58S.

84. Russell, T, Bsn, AL, Lohman, JA: A medical center's experience with managing specialty bed usage. J Wound Ostomy Continence Nurs 2001; 28:274–278.

85. Bergstrom, N, Braden, B, Boynton, P, et al: Using a research-based assessment scale in clinical practice. Nurs Clin North Am 1995; 30:539–551.

86. Norton, L, Sibbald, RG: Is bed rest an effective treatment modality for pressure ulcers? Ostomy Wound Manage 2004; 50:40–42, 44–52, discussion 53.

87. Consortium for Spinal Cord Medicine. Pressure Ulcer Prevention and Treatment Following Spinal Cord Injury: A Clinical Practice Guideline for Health-Care Professionals. Paralyzed Veterans of America, 2000. Available at www.pva.org.

88. Coggrave, MJ, Rose, LS: A specialist seating assessment clinic: Changing pressure relief practice. Spinal Cord 2003; 41:692–695.

89. Makhsous, M, Rowles, DM, Rymer, WZ, et al: Periodically relieving ischial sitting load to decrease the risk of pressure ulcers. Arch Phys Med Rehabil 2007; 88:862–870.

90. Henderson, JL, Price, SH, Brandstater, ME, et al: Efficacy of three measures to relieve pressure in seated persons with spinal cord injury. Arch Phys Med Rehabil 1994; 75:535–539.

91. Aissaoui, R, Lacoste, M, Dansereau, J: Analysis of sliding and pressure distribution during a repositioning of persons in a simulator chair. IEEE Trans Neural Syst Rehabil Eng 2001; 9:215–224.

92. Burns, SP, Betz, KL: Seating pressures with conventional and dynamic wheelchair cushions in tetraplegia. Arch Phys Med Rehabil 1999; 80:566–571.

93. Hobson, DA: Comparative effects of posture on pressure and shear at the body-seat interface. J Rehabil Res Dev 1992; 29:21–31.

94. Gerhart, K, Weitzenkamp, D, Charlifue, S: The old get older: Changes over three years in aging SCI survivors. New Mobility 1996; June:18–21.

95. Boeker, C, Edwards, S: Seating solutions: Choosing the appropriate cushion. Adv Rehabil 1995; 9(4): 9–11.

96. Sprigle, S, Press, L, Davis, K: Development of uniform terminology and procedures to describe wheelchair cushion characteristics. J Rehabil Res Dev 2001; 38:449–461.

97. Rappl, L: A conservative treatment for pressure ulcers. Ostomy Wound Manage 1993; 39:46–55.

98. Key, A, Manley, MT: Pressure redistribution in wheelchair cushion for paraplegics: Its application and evaluation. Paraplegia 1978; 16:403–412.

99. Perkash, I, O'Neil, H, Politi-Meeks, D, et al: Development and evaluation of a universal contoured cushion. Paraplegia 1984; 22:358–365.

100. Peterson, MJ, Adkins, HV: Measurement and redistribution of excessive pressures during wheelchair sitting. Phys Ther 1982; 62:990–994.

101. Mooney, V, Einbund, MJ, Rogers, JE, et al: Comparison of pressure distribution qualities in seat cushions. Bull Prosthet Res 1971; 10:129–143.

102. Ferguson-Pell, MW, Wilkie, IC, Reswick, JB, et al: Pressure sore prevention for the wheelchair-bound spinal injury patient. Paraplegia 1980; 18:42–51.

103. Arakaki, B, Furumasu, J: A pilot study: Factors that influence cushion selection. Presented at: The Thirteenth International Seating Symposium, Pittsburgh, 1997.

104. Cullum, N, McInnes, E, Bell-Syer, SE, Legood, R: Support surfaces for pressure ulcer prevention. Cochrane Database Syst Rev 2004; (3):CD001735.

105. Whittemore, R: Pressure-reduction support surfaces: A review of the literature. J Wound Ostomy Continence Nurs 1998; 25:6–25.

106. Maklebust, J: An update on horizontal patient support surfaces. Ostomy Wound Manage 1999; 45(suppl):70S–77S, quiz 78S–79S.

107. Hasty, JH, Krasner, D, Kennedy, KL: A new tool for evaluating patient support surfaces. A guideline for making practice decisions. Ostomy Wound Manage 1991; 36(Pt 1):51–54, 56–57, 59.

108. Krouskop, T, Garber, SL: The role of technology in the prevention of pressure sores. Ostomy Wound Manage 1987; (16):44–55.

109. Day, A, Leonard, F: Seeking quality care for patients with pressure ulcers. Decubitus 1993; 6:32–43.

110. Jester, J, Weaver, V: A report of clinical investigation of various tissue support surfaces used for the prevention, early intervention, and management of pressure ulcers. Ostomy Wound Manage 1990; 26:39–45.

111. Krouskop, TA, Randall, C, Davis, J: Evaluating the long-term performance of a foam-core hospital replacement mattress. J Wound Ostomy Continence Nurs 1994; 21:241–246.

112. Bates-Jensen, B: Pressure ulcers: Pathophysiology and prevention. In: Sussman, C, Bates-Jensen, B (eds): Wound Care: A Collaborative Practice Manual for Physical Therapists and Nurses. Gaithersburg, MD, Aspen Publishing, 1998.

113. Ooka, M, Kemp, MG, McMyn, R: Evaluation of three types of support surfaces for preventing pressure ulcers in patients in a surgical intensive care unit. J Wound Ostomy Continence Nurs 1995; 22:271–279.

114. Statistical Analysis for Durable Medical Equipment Carriers (SADMERC). Local Coverage Determination (LCD) for Pressure Reducing Support Surfaces Group 2 (L5068). Available at: www.tricenturion.com. Accessed on: 10/22/07.

115. Branom, R, Knox, L: Constant Force Technology vs. Low-air-loss. Presented at: WOCN National Conference, Minneapolis, MN, 1999.

116. Ross, K: Support surface effectiveness in ICU, post-graft, and acute care. Presented at: WOCN National Conference, Minneapolis, MN, 1999.

117. Figliola, RS: A proposed method for quantifying low-air-loss mattress performance by moisture transport. Ostomy Wound Manage 2003; 49:32–42.

118. Weaver, V, Jester, J: A clinical tool: Updated readings on tissue interface pressures. Ostomy Wound Manage 1994; 40:34–36, 38, 40.

119. Anderson, C, Rappl, L: Lateral rotation mattresses for wound healing. Ostomy Wound Manage 2004; 50:50–54, 56, 58.

Acute Burn Management

Kevin Sittig, MD

Kathryn Richardson, MD

Incidence of Burn Injuries

The incidence of burn injuries in the United States and Canada is 1.55 million injuries per year (Box 20.1). Many, including the authors of this chapter, feel that this number is grossly underreported. The majority of the fatalities associated with burn injuries occur before rescue personnel can extricate victims from homes, buildings, or motor vehicles. It has been reported that 75% of burn injuries occur in or around the home. A summary of burn etiologies is presented in Table 20.1.

One disturbing fact is that approximately 70% of all burn injuries remain in the category of accidental and, possibly, preventable. Regardless of how small the area injured, the traumatic events of the accident are branded on the victim's body and in the memory of the responsible party forever.

Burn Care Facilities

The vast majority of minor burn injuries are treated with Neosporin® and an adhesive bandage without evaluation by a licensed health-care professional. Emergency rooms and pediatrician's offices examine and either treat or refer burn injuries to wound care specialists. Those referrals will depend upon the severity of the injury. The American Burn Association

Table 20•1 Etiology of Burns	
Type	**Percentage**
Flame	45.0%
Scald	30.0%
Hot object	7.0%
Electrical	5.0%
Chemical	3.0%
Friction	3.0%
Radiation	0.5%
Inhalation only	0.5%
Other/unknown	6.0%

outlined specific criteria necessitating referral to burn centers as a means to aid the evaluating physician. Box 20.2 lists these transfer criteria.

Anatomy of Skin

Chapter 1 (and other chapters) has already clearly defined the anatomy of the skin. Common sense and science tell us that burn depth is directly related to the temperature of the offending agent and the duration of contact or exposure. Children and the elderly have much thinner skin than adolescents and young adults. Thus, these groups will have different reported burn depths from the same hot bowl of soup spilled onto their laps. To further complicate the situation, the thickness of human skin will vary from one anatomical site to another. The

> **Box 20•1 Burn Incidence in the United States**

There are over 1 million burn injuries and 4500 fire and burn deaths per year.

- 3750 deaths from fires
- 750 deaths from MVC (motor vehicle collisions) and electricity

▶ **Box 20•2** ⬛ **American Burn Association Criteria for Transfer to a Burn Center**

1. Partial-thickness and full-thickness burns greater than 10% of the total body surface area (TBSA) in patients younger than 10 years or older than 50 years of age
2. Partial-thickness and full-thickness burns greater than 20% TBSA in other age groups
3. Partial-thickness burns involving the face, eyes, ears, hands, feet, genitalia, or perineum or skin overlying major joints
4. Full-thickness burns greater than 5% TBSA in any age group
5. Electrical burns, including lightning injury
6. Extensive chemical burns
7. Inhalation injury
8. Burn injury in patients with preexisting illness that could complicate management, prolong recovery, or affect mortality
9. Any burn patient in whom concomitant trauma poses an increased risk of morbidity or mortality treated initially in a trauma center until stable
10. Children with burns seen in hospitals without qualified personnel or equipment for their care
11. Burn injury in patients who will require special social and emotional or long-term rehabilitative support, including cases involving suspected child abuse or neglect

skin of the upper eyelids is obviously thinner than the skin of the back.

Let us take time to review the functions of the largest organ of the human body. The skin primarily functions to (1) provide a barrier to bacteria and (2) assist with thermoregulation. Burn injury and resultant loss of skin integrity allow bacteria direct access to the body. With a significant loss of skin from a burn, the body will be prone to thermoregulatory problems. Prior to the time that reepithelialization occurs by either spontaneous healing or grafting, body temperatures may drop several degrees during short intervals when the skin is exposed (ie, during dressing changes). Patients with grafts to large surface areas will lose the ability to perspire in those areas, making them prone to heat exhaustion.[1]

Burn Depth

The classification of burn depth has evolved over time. While most clinicians are familiar with the terms first-, second-, and third-degree burns, there are some older clinicians who add fourth-degree burns to the categories to indicate an injury that involves all layers of tissue down to and including bone. Current terminology of burn depth stratifies burns into partial-thickness or full-thickness injuries. Partial-thickness burns will include first- and second-degree burns, and full-thickness burns include third-degree injuries. A first-degree burn will injure only the epidermis of the skin and therefore will heal in a few days with little chance of scar and minimal pain. The classic example is a sunburn. A second-degree burn will injure the epidermis and a portion of the dermis and will appear pink and moist with blistering. The depth of dermal injury will determine the length of time to heal and the extent of scarring and pain. The deeper (through the dermis) the injury, the longer the time required to slough nonviable tissue and regenerate new skin. The longer the regeneration time, the greater the probability of scarring and pigmentation disturbances. Superficial second-degree burns whose blisters have been débrided are the most painful burns as the exposed nerve endings have no protective barrier. (Fig. 20.1) Patients with these wounds will complain that even an air current in a room causes an increase in pain when their wounds are open.

Deep second-degree burns will have an increase in pain as the eschar sloughs and exposes nerve endings prior to regeneration of the epidermis. Second-degree burns may take from 1 to 6 weeks to heal, depending on the depth of injury to the dermis. It is well documented that second-degree burns that are unhealed by 3 weeks would likely benefit from excision and grafting to improve cosmetic and functional outcome. Third-degree burns injure both the epidermis and the dermis down to subcutaneous tissue and therefore have no viable basal skin cells to regenerate new skin. Third-degree burn injuries will vary in color on presentation from pale white to dark red, brown, or black, or even transparent. No matter how long or meticulous the wound care of a third-degree burn, the injury will not achieve a new epithelial layer without grafting or protracted time to allow migration of peripheral viable skin. (Fig. 20.2)

Third-degree burns will be dry to the touch and often are described as "leathery." A third-degree burn has destroyed all skin appendages and nerve endings and will be the least painful burn, or it may actually be insensate. (Fig. 20.3) Hair can be pulled out with little to no force and with no pain in this area. The layer of nonviable burned tissue is referred to as *eschar.* When the eschar involves the entire circumference of an extremity, it can potentially result in vascular compromise. Surgical incisions made through this eschar (escharotomies) allow room for edema (much like bivalving a cast to prevent or relieve vascular congestion).

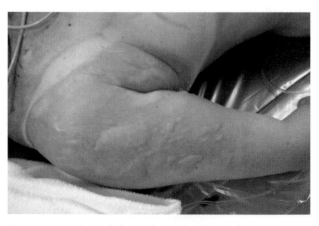

Figure 20•1 *Second-degree burns involving the right shoulder girdle.*

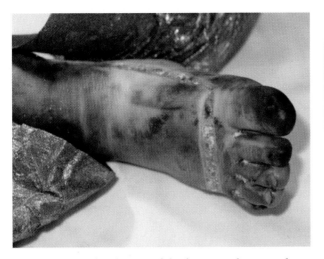

Figure 20•2 *Color changes of the foot secondary to a thermal burn. Note the incisions used to decompress the foot.*

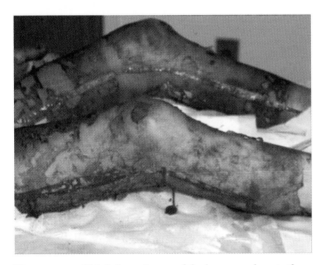

Figure 20•3 *Third-degree burns of the legs secondary to thermal injury. Escharotomies have been performed bilaterally.*

Escharotomy is usually performed at the bedside urgently and, because the burns are full thickness and therefore insensate, general anesthesia is rarely required. Escharotomy may be performed prophylactically, anticipating the total body edema of a large burn volume resuscitation. Escharotomies are generally described as necessary when arterial pulses are markedly diminished or absent. In the acute setting of a burn injury, prior to adequate intravenous resuscitation, vasoconstriction takes place to maintain adequate perfusion to vital organs. Remember that diminished or absent distal pulses could be due to either inadequate resuscitation or need for escharotomy. If there are circumferential full-thickness burns present, then escharotomies will be inevitable and should be performed expeditiously. If the circumferential burns are partial thickness and pliable enough to expand to accommodate the localized swelling, then close observation with frequent pulse checks may be done while resuscitation is ongoing. The reader is referred to Figures 20.4 and 20.5, which depict recommended escharotomy sites. Box 20.3 provides a summary of the pertinent points concerning burn depth.

Box 20•3 Burn Depth

- **First-Degree:** Burns are red and very sensitive to touch. The surface blanches to light pressure; no blisters develop.
- **Second-Degree:** Burns may or may not produce blisters. The bases of the blisters may be erythematous or whitish with a fibrinous exudate. They are sensitive to touch and may blanch to pressure.
- **Third-Degree:** Burns may be white and pliable; black, charred, and leathery; or bright red because of fixed hemoglobin in the subdermal region. They do not blanch to pressure. They are generally anesthetic, and hairs may be pulled easily from their follicles.

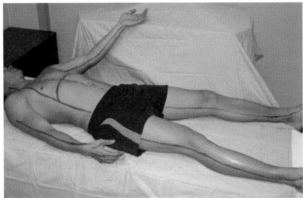

Figure 20•4 *Model demonstrating recommended escharotomy sites.*

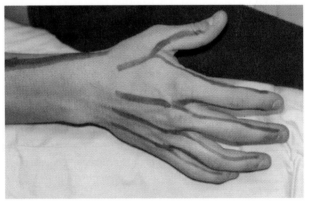

Figure 20•5 *Recommended escharotomy sites on the hand.*

▶ **PEARL 20•1** The determination of the depth of a burn wound is critical to setting the appropriate treatment algorithm into place.

Burn Depth Slide

While physicians with extensive burn care experience downplay the need for color flow Doppler imaging, it is an emerging technology that may provide objective data of documented depth to patients, insurance carriers, and even attorneys.[2] This noninvasive modality could replace the need for invasive full-thickness punch biopsies to determine depth of injury. Burn wounds are complex, and rarely are the depths of injury the same throughout the wound. The center of the wound is generally the deepest, whereas the edges are more superficial. This finding explains why burn wounds tend to heal from the edges toward the center.

Initial Assessment

The initial assessment of a burn wound is done to determine if the client with the wound can be treated as an outpatient or if the wound requires inpatient admission or referral to a burn center. The reasons for such a referral were presented earlier in Box 20.2.

Reasons for admission for burn care include providing intravenous fluid resuscitation for burns involving greater than 10% TBSA (total body surface area) in children and greater than 20% TBSA in adults. Smaller burn injury in patients with associated nausea and poor enteral intake, intolerance to oral pain medications, or inadequate pain control with oral narcotics will justify admission for intravenous pain medication and hydration. Because of the associated local edema in a burn injury, facial and neck or circumferential extremity burns put patients at risk of losing their airway or compromising blood flow to the extremity distal to the circumferential burn. For these reasons, many burns at these sites with less than 20% TBSA injured will need to be admitted, at least for a 24-hour observation. During this critical time, airways can be monitored and intubation performed if required, and distal pulse checks can lead to timely escharotomies if arterial insufficiency develops.

The initial burn injury assessment must correlate with the history of the accident. If the reported event does not match the physical findings, then suspicion dictates further investigation. Such conflicts should alert the clinician to suspect child, adult, or elderly abuse. Admission may be necessary to protect the patient from the perpetrator while the authorities conduct an appropriate investigation.

Types of Burns
Thermal Burns

Anything that is capable of generating heat can cause a burn injury. As stated earlier, the depth of the burn injury will be directly related to the temperature of the offending agent and the duration of contact or exposure to the skin. Thermal injuries may occur as the result of flame burning in direct contact with the skin when clothing ignites or from the intensity of radiant heat from being in close proximity to the flames. By their very nature, flames achieve significant temperatures, even with only brief contact with the skin, and the resultant injuries will likely result in full-thickness injuries. Flames directly contacting the skin will result in destruction of the hair and probable absence of blisters because the heat will cause evaporative loss of the fluid in the injured area. Any intact injured skin that does not have blister fluid beneath it will often peel away when the wounds are being cleansed. Prior to this peeling event, burn injuries of this type may be mistaken for first-degree burns. This dilemma occurs more frequently in darkly pigmented people. Remember, partial-thickness burns should be painful. If cleaning an area of presumed first-degree burn does not illicit pain, then re-examine the wound more closely for a deeper burn injury.

Scald injuries account for the majority of thermal injuries to children and are more likely to occur in the kitchen or bathroom. (Fig. 20.6) As the boiling points of various liquids differ, so will the depth of burn injury. Liquids such as cooking oil or syrup will achieve and maintain a higher temperature at full boil than does water. Their viscosity will also cause longer retention of the heat, and the liquid will stick to the skin. Therefore, boiling oil spilled onto the skin will likely cause a deeper burn than boiling water, as the intensity of the heat and duration of contact will be longer. The kitchen or food preparation area in any home needs to be off-limits to unsupervised children. Hungry children relate pots and pans to food, and when too short to see into them, they will often pull them down. The resultant spills often result in significant burns to their faces and hands.

Scald injuries that occur as a result of contact with water in the bathtub, sink, or shower could all be decreased if hot water heaters were turned down. A recommended setting of 120°F will allow adequate exposure time for most individuals to get out of the water that is too hot with only superficial burns. Children receive significant scald burns when they are left unattended while bathing and turn on the hot water. They may suffer full-thickness burns if the temperature of the water is greater than 130°F and the contact time is prolonged. Accidental scalds will cause burn injury patterns to have irregular borders and associated splash or drip lines. Intentional scald burn patterns are more likely to have clear demarcation of injury from being submerged and held for a period of time. If the physical findings do not correlate with the history of the accident, call protective services.

Tar burns are considered scald injuries and are an occupational hazard for roofers and road construction workers. (Fig. 20.7) These contact burns are difficult to evaluate as the tar must be removed from the injured skin to allow examination. Tar rapidly cools and solidifies when spilled. It cannot be washed off with water or soap and must be dissolved with

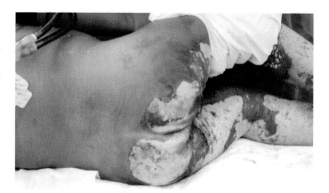

Figure 20•6 *Burns involving the buttocks and posterior legs secondary to a bathroom scald.*

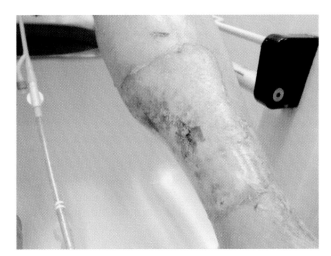

Figure 20•11 *An electrical burn involving the lateral aspect of the leg.*

110 to 220 volts runs through insulated wires, the overhead, uninsulated power lines may carry 100,000 volts. Lightning represents direct current of 100,000,000 volts or more. People who survive lightning injuries have generally been the recipient of an arc of current coming off the object of the direct strike.[26]

The injury from electrical contact is often grossly underestimated by the first responders because the electrical entrance and exit points will be visible, while the extent of deeper tissue destruction may not be visible or obvious. The deeper injury that occurs makes sense when one understands the principles of electricity. Electrical current will travel along pathways with the least resistance to the current. Tissue injury occurs when the current is converted into heat. Human skin provides some resistance to current unless the contact persists. The electrical current will then seek and travel along tissue with the least resistance. Being that our nervous system was designed to conduct electrical currents, the neurovascular bundles in the entrance area will likely serve as the conduits to the deeper structures. Deep muscular structures will be injured from the heat because the electrical current is converted to heat energy. (Fig. 20.12) The classic description of the exit wound is a

"blow out" where the current converges and exits the body. There may be one large exit wound or a collection of multiple smaller wounds. (Figs. 20.13 and 20.14) The visible wounds, unfortunately, are usually the least of the injuries. Managing these wounds generally requires a series of débridements until all nonviable tissue is removed. It may take a few days for tissues to demarcate into clearly viable and nonviable. In electrical injuries that do not require amputation, coverage of the wounds may be as simple as skin grafts, as complex as local flaps, or as extreme as microvascular free flaps.[27]

No discussion of electrical injuries would be complete without devoting some time to fasciotomies. The term *fasciotomy* means to open or incise the fascia. Fasciotomy (like escharotomy) may be done prophylactically if significant swelling is expected. Clinicians readily associate fasciotomy with vascular surgery that has restored blood flow to an extremity that acutely lost inflow. With restoration of blood flow, the muscle swells; fasciotomy allows room for swelling "outward" so there is no vascular embarrassment. If the compartment is not released, venous compression can result, which can eventually lead to impeded arterial inflow. Without reduction of these increased compartment pressures, the muscles are at risk of ischemic

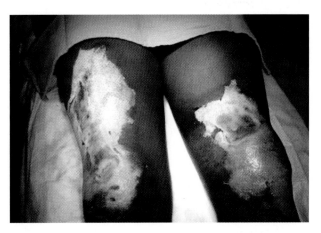

Figure 20•13 *Electrical exit wounds involving the anterior thighs.*

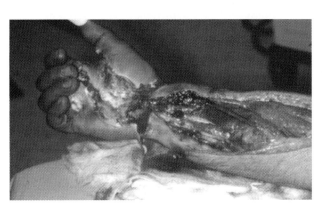

Figure 20•12 *Appearance of the hand and forearm following an electrical burn with subsequent fasciotomy.*

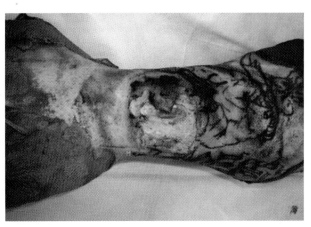

Figure 20•14 *Electrical exit wound involving the wrist of a tattooed individual.*

death. Compartment pressures can be measured by devices using percutaneous needle placement into the compartments. Pressures that exceed capillary pressures (30 mm Hg) should be reduced through fasciotomies.

Resuscitation of the patient with an electrical burn should be sufficient to achieve a urine output of at least 1 ml/kg/hour. Injured muscle tissue will release myoglobin into the circulation, which must be excreted by the kidneys. If large amounts of myoglobin precipitate in the renal tubules, renal failure may occur. To improve the excretion of the myoglobin the patient should be well hydrated, and sodium bicarbonate should be added to the intravenous fluids to alkalinize the urine and to increase solubility of the myoglobin. Diuretic therapy with mannitol is also often used. If myoglobinuria persists after adequate intravenous resuscitation, then one must begin a diligent search for injured muscle tissue and proceed with débridement and/or amputation if required.

In the initial patient assessment of an electrical injury, it is important to order an EKG to rule out cardiac conduction defects and arrhythmias. Even if there is no history of a fall, spinal x-rays should be obtained to rule out any fracture that may have occurred when paraspinous muscles contracted violently in response to the electrical current.[26,27] These considerations are summarized in Box 20.4.

> **PEARL 20•6** A complete neurological exam should be performed on any admission, but it is of greater relevance in patients following significant electrical injury.

Abrasions

Burn centers associated with trauma centers will treat a fair number of patients who have suffered flame injuries related to motor vehicle collisions. They will also treat an equal or greater number of patients referred for wound care of their "road rash." Abrasions to body parts from sliding along roadways results in friction-induced injuries. These wounds are generally contaminated with dirt, glass, clothing debris, and whatever bacteria, molds, and fungi are growing in the area. These abrasion wounds are treated topically with the same antimicrobials and dressing materials that are used on partial or full-thickness flame burns.

Burn Resuscitation

Before it was discovered that intravenous fluids were necessary the first day after the burn, it was not uncommon for

> **Box 20•4** **Management Considerations Following Electrical Injury**

1. Increase resuscitation fluids to achieve 1 ml urine/kg/hour.
2. Perform an EKG.
3. Obtain spinal x-rays.
4. Alkalinize urine if myoglobinuria present.
5. Add mannitol if myoglobinuria persists.
6. Perform surgical débridement of nonviable muscle.

patients with burns greater than 30% TBSA to die from shock and renal failure. Thanks to the efforts of Evans in 1952, burn clinicians understood that the amount of fluid required in acute resuscitation was related to the body surface area of the burn and the patient's body weight.[28,29] The Evans formula of resuscitation remained the standard until Baxter and Shires provided the Parkland formula.[30] This formula provided a guideline for the volume of intravenous fluid administration of lactated Ringer's solution, also based on body surface area burned and body weight. The original formula provided enough fluid to compensate for the ongoing fluid loss from the intravascular space into the interstitial space through the "leaky" vascular endothelium. The leaky endothelium is a global problem in major burn injuries, thus the resultant edema affects the entire body. The length of time that these vessels leak is still being debated, but the general consensus is that the majority of leakage stops within the first 24 hours.

> **PEARL 20•7** The key to successful burn resuscitation is to provide enough intravenous fluid to prevent hypotension and achieve stable urine output without administering excessive fluid that worsens interstitial edema.

The Parkland formula of 4 ml/kg/percentage of total body surface area (TBSA) burn calculates the approximate required intravenous lactated Ringer's solution for the first 24 hours. It is recommended that 50% of this 24-hour volume be administered over the first 8 post-burn hours. The second half of this volume would theoretically then be infused over the remaining 16 hours. The key to this or any other formula is to remember that it is only a guide and that adjustments should be made according to the physiological response of the patient. Urine output continues to be the best clinical indicator of successful resuscitation. While children require 1 ml/kg/hour of urine outflow to achieve renal clearance, adults only require 0.5 ml/kg/hour. Therefore, if a burn patient is making 1 to 2 ml/kg/hour urine during the first 4 hours of resuscitation, then decreasing the infusion rate will likely be tolerated and should be done. On the other hand, if the patient remains oliguric, then he or she likely will require more fluid administered than originally calculated. Burn patients with associated smoke inhalation will often require more fluids than the amount suggested by the Parkland formula. The timing of administration of colloid solutions such as albumin or plasma has changed from not before the second day to anytime after 8 post-burn hours. It has been shown that the administration of colloids can reduce the need for excessive crystalloid infusion and therefore decrease fluid available to leak into the interstitial space.[31-34] Recent publications have suggested that over-resuscitation has resulted in increased numbers of complications, such as compartment syndromes, including abdominal compartment syndromes.[35-38] These complications resurrected attempts to use hypertonic saline solution for resuscitation, which was introduced by Monafo in the 1970s.[39,40] Complications of renal failure and strokes associated with hypertonic saline solution-resuscitated patients is reported in the literature.[41]

The Parkland formula (4 ml/kg/TBSA burn) remains the most commonly used guideline in the resuscitation of a burn patient. To make certain that the reader understands how to use the Parkland formula, the following calculation is provided for the infusion rate of lactated Ringer's solution for a 100-kg patient who sustained deep flame burns to 40% of his body. The calculation would be 4 ml × 100 kg × 40, or 16,000 ml. Remember that this calculation is for the suggested volume of fluid for the first 24 hours, with 50% being given during the first 8 hours. The hourly infusion rate for your patient would therefore be (16,000 × 0.5) ÷ 8 hours, or 1000 ml/hour. Adjustments to this infusion rate will depend upon the patient's physiological response.

Burn Severity

When someone sustains a burn injury, the only questions in that person's mind are usually related to pain and the probability of scarring. The possibility of permanent functional limitations or death is not considered by the patient or the family. This makes perfect sense when one realizes that patients who sustain large burn injuries that are full thickness are relatively pain free and initially have normal cognitive function. The misconception that the more painful the burn, the greater the severity, continues in the mind of the public and personal-injury attorneys. Burn severity should be defined relative to morbidity and mortality. The four factors that have a profound predicative outcome for survival are patient age, total body surface area burn (TBSA), comorbidities, and associated injuries. As one would expect, the younger the patient, the less likely are comorbidities and therefore the lower the mortality rate. The TBSA burn calculation is the most important calculation to make during the initial assessment, along with obtaining an accurate weight. Whether using the rule of nines, variations of the Lund and Browder charts, or computer-based software programs, a clinician is still required to draw the areas injured on a body chart. The percentages of second- and third-degree burns are totaled in order to calculate the total body surface area burn. First-degree burns should be noted but are not considered when calculating the TBSA burn. The importance of calculating the TBSA burn correctly is paramount because that number and the patient's weight will determine the volume of intravenous fluids administered to prevent burn shock, renal failure, and death. When a transfer request is received at a burn center, the clinicians will need to know the amount of the TBSA burn and patient's weight to enable calculating the rate of resuscitation fluids. If a patient tells you he weighs 220 pounds (100 kg) and he actually weighs 280 pounds (127 kg), there is a discrepancy of 27 kg. Assume that this patient has a 60% TBSA burn. Using the Parkland formula of 4 ml/kg/percentage TBSA burn (4 × 100 × 60) with the inaccurate weight would yield the resuscitation need of 24,000 ml of lactated Ringer's solution. The accurate weight would actually require resuscitation fluids (4 × 127 × 60) of 30,480 ml for the first 24 hours. This greater than 6-liter fluid discrepancy could be a significant factor for the patient's survival.

Associated comorbidities such as congestive heart failure, hypertension, coronary artery disease, diabetes, chronic obstructive pulmonary artery disease, obesity, and sleep apnea can make for a real challenge in even a modest size burn of only 30% TBSA. Imagine the fluid shifts and electrolyte and glucose disturbances in a 60% TBSA burn in the 127-kg patient referred to above who just happens to have all of the comorbidities listed. Scenarios such as this are all too common, and the patient will likely have much higher morbidity and mortality than with the same 60% TBSA burn on a healthy 20 year old.

Associated injuries along with the cutaneous burns will also have a significant predictive value on survival. The most important and widely published of these remains smoke inhalation injury.

> ▶ **PEARL 20•8** Despite major advances in wound care, early excision, better antibiotics, and more sophisticated ventilator regimens and critical care, smoke inhalation continues to play a major role in the morbidity and mortality associated with burn patients.[42,43]

Calculate Extent of Body Surface Area Burned

Successful management and resuscitation of a burn patient depends on the accurate assessment of burn depth and the extent of the body surface area injured. A quick estimate of the extent of the injury can be obtained by using the rule of nines. (Fig. 20.15) This practice is widely taught in courses for primary responders such as firefighters and paramedics, as well as in nursing and medical schools. The principle of the rule of nines is based on the premise that the human body can be subdivided into parts that equal 9 or a multiple of 9. The head represents 9%, each arm separately represents 9%, anterior torso equals 18%, the posterior torso and buttocks equal 18%, each leg (thigh and lower leg) represents 18%. The remaining 1% unaccounted for when you add the above is assigned to the genitals. This modality only works when estimating the extent of injury in adults. Children's heads make up from 11% to 19% of their body surface area depending on their age. The younger the child, the greater the surface area assigned to the head. The Lund and Browder chart depicted in Figure 20.16

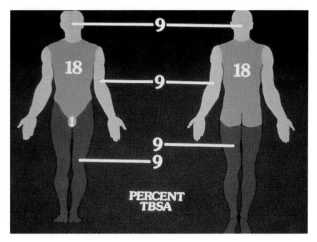

Figure 20•15 *Rule of nines.*

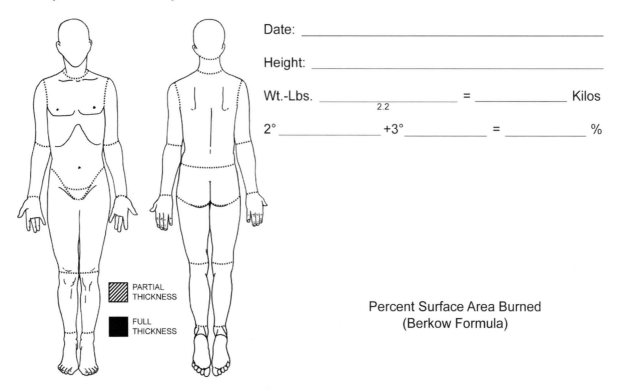

Date: _____

Height: _____

Wt.-Lbs. _____ = _____ Kilos
                        2.2

2° _____ +3° _____ = _____ %

PARTIAL THICKNESS

FULL THICKNESS

Percent Surface Area Burned
(Berkow Formula)

AREA	1 YR.	1-4 YRS.	5-9 YRS.	10-14 YRS.	15 YRS.	ADULT	2°	3°
Head	19	17	13	11	9	7		
Neck	2	2	2	2	2	2		
Ant. Trunk	13	13	13	13	13	13		
Post Trunk	13	13	13	13	13	13		
R. Buttock	2.5	2.5	2.5	2.5	2.5	2.5		
L. Buttock	2.5	2.5	2.5	2.5	2.5	2.5		
Genitalia	1	1	1	1	1	1		
R.U. Arm	4	4	4	4	4	4		
L.U. Arm	4	4	4	4	4	4		
R.L. Arm	3	3	3	3	3	3		
L.L. Arm	3	3	3	3	3	3		
R. Hand	2.5	2.5	2.5	2.5	2.5	2.5		
L. Hand	2.5	2.5	2.5	2.5	2.5	2.5		
R. Thigh	5.5	6.5	8	8.5	9	9.5		
L. Thigh	5.5	6.5	8	8.5	9	9.5		
R. Leg	5	5	5.5	6	6.5	7		
L. Leg	5	5	5.5	6	6.5	7		
R. Foot	3.5	3.5	3.5	3.5	3.5	3.5		
L. Foot	3.5	3.5	3.5	3.5	3.5	3.5		
TOTAL								

Figure **20•16** *Lund and Browder chart.*

further subdivides the body and takes into account changes for all age groups.

When using either the rule of nines or the Lund and Browder chart, one must still make a number of estimates to determine what percentage of each anatomical unit is burned. If only half of an adult arm is burned, then the estimate would be 4.5% by the rule of nines, or 3.5% by the Lund and Browder chart. When burns are scattered about the body, a quick estimate can be performed by using the patient's own palm to represent 1%.

Invasive Lines

With a burn comes the loss of bacterial barrier and a greater likelihood of bacteremia and associated catheter-related infections. The use of invasive lines for monitoring and infusions has routinely been highly selective in most burn centers. While few critical care specialists would administer vast amounts of intravenous crystalloid without central venous pressure monitoring, this is standard practice for burn surgeons.

During the acute resuscitation phase of any burn greater than 30% TBSA, the standard of care would suggest continuous monitoring of cardiac rhythm, oxygen saturation, and hourly vital signs, including heart rate, temperature, blood pressure, and urine output. Blood pressure cuffs may be placed over bandages covering burn wounds when all extremities are burned, but the discomfort to the patient may require placement of arterial lines. These arterial lines provide continuous blood pressure monitoring and easy access for sampling for blood gas analysis and electrolytes.

Indwelling Foley catheters are mandatory for accurate hourly urine output recordings. They will, however, often be left in longer than required as a convenience for the patient and nursing staff. Remember that indwelling urinary catheters can lead to urinary tract infections that result in urosepsis.

Nasogastric tube placement has been recommended during the resuscitation of burn patients. Decompression of the stomach may be required as long as the patient has an ileus. Patients who require intubation will require nasogastric tubes to provide access to administer enteral medications and nutrition.

The use of echocardiography and sophisticated monitors on arterial lines has reduced the need for invasive cardiac monitors such as a Swan Ganz catheter (Edwards Lifesciences, Irvine, CA) catheters.

Airway Management

The decision of when to intubate a patient is not always clear. Physical findings such as use of accessory respiratory muscles, nasal flaring, and tachypnea are clearly indicative of respiratory distress. Couple these findings with a low P_{O_2} and an elevated P_{CO_2}, and no one would argue that urgent intubation should occur to prevent a predictable respiratory arrest. The practice of medicine has clearly moved toward the use of algorithms to guide the practitioner. Most articles, chapters, or books dealing with burn care instruct health-care providers to intubate patients who present with facial and neck burns or smoke inhalation. The logic behind this is that facial and neck burns could lead to edema that could potentially compromise an airway. This degree of edema is unlikely to occur unless the patient has a large TBSA burn requiring administration of large volume of intravenous fluids. Smoke inhalation associated with significant burns is an absolute indication for intubation. Evidence of smoke exposure, such as soot on the skin and in the nasal and oral airway, without associated cutaneous burns and no signs or symptoms of respiratory distress presents a conundrum for the emergency room physician. This patient obviously had exposure to smoke, but has an inhalational injury occurred? Even with a normal chest x-ray, arterial blood gas, and carboxyhemoglobin level, this patient should be admitted for observation.

> **PEARL 20•9** Intubation should occur only if signs or symptoms of respiratory failure develop that are progressing despite administration of supplemental face-mask oxygen.

If intubation is required, and the time and expertise is available to place a nasotracheal tube, it should be considered. The extensive facial and lip edema that occurs and persists for several days in large TBSA burns with facial involvement is impressive to say the least. This massive facial swelling could dislodge an oral endotracheal tube. The nasal route of intubation provides a much more stable tube. It also prevents a patient from using the tongue to self-extubate or causing tube occlusion by biting down on an orally placed one. Performance of dental and mouth care and communication by reading lips is also an advantage of nasotracheal tubes.

Obtaining an airway emergently in a burn patient would follow the same algorithm for any patient. If unsuccessful with either nasal or oral routes of intubation, then proceed with surgical cricothyroidotomy. (Fig. 20.17) If cricothyroidotomy is required, it should be converted to a tracheostomy within 24 hours when possible.

Medical Management of Burn Wounds
Topical Antimicrobials

Partial-thickness burns will heal unless something causes the wounds to convert to a full-thickness injury. The most common cause of this conversion would be infection. Cornified human skin is colonized with bacteria, but provides a barrier to invasion when intact and free from immune deficiencies. Injury to the skin allows bacterial invasion that may result in localized cellulitis or bacteremia and septicemia. (Fig. 20.18)

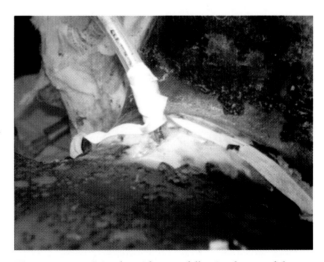

Figure 20•17 *Cricothyroidotomy following burns of the anterior neck.*

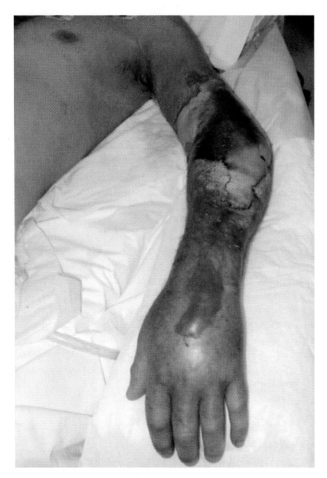

Figure 20•18 *Infected burn of the arm.*

Proper cleansing and application of topical antibiotic to reduce or eradicate the bacterial population in the wound supports a large number of pharmaceuticals. The more common topical antibiotics include silver sulfadiazine, mafenide acetate, Neosporin, Bactroban® acetic acid solution, Dakin's solution, and silver dressings.

Silver sulfadiazine remains the most popular prescribed topical burn antibiotic and is frequently referred to by the brand name Silvadene®(Monarch Pharmaceuticals, Bristol, TN). It provides a relatively large spectrum of coverage against gram-positive and gram-negative bacteria. Because sulfonamides are associated with an increased risk of kernicterus, silver sulfadiazine should not be used on pregnant women approaching term or newborns during their first 2 months. It is water soluble and easy to apply and remove. Neutropenia is listed as a potential side effect when Silvadene is used to cover large burn wounds. There are also controversial reports that Silvadene delays wound healing.[44-46]

Mafenide acetate (Sulfamylon® Mylan Inc., Canonsburg, PA) comes as a cream or in a 5% solution. This topical antimicrobial provides deeper penetration into the burn eschar in addition to penetrating cartilage. It has activity against both gram-positive and gram-negative bacteria (specifically *Pseudomonas*). It is a carbonic anhydrase inhibitor and therefore may cause metabolic acidosis. While the cream is more likely to be applied to burn eschars and ears, the solution is also used over autografts or excised wounds. The solution is unlikely to cause the stinging sensation reported with the cream.[47-49] Sulfamylon is the topical antimicrobial of choice when suspicion or evidence of *Pseudomonas* is present.

Bactroban (GlaxoSmithKline, Philadelphia, PA) cream contains mupirocin and is used as a topical antimicrobial that is selectively against most strains of methicillin-resistant *Staphylococcus*.[50]

Both acetic acid (0.25%) and Dakin's solution (0.25%) are reported to have some activity to reduce colonization with *Pseudomonas*. There are reports, however, that Dakin's solution may be toxic to healthy tissue and could therefore contribute to delayed wound healing.[51-53]

Silver dressings (Fig. 20.19) became a presence in the burn center market several years ago. Early success with the use of silver in such products as Silvadene and Sulfamylon led to the addition of silver to many commercial wound dressings. Silver has antimicrobial activity for both gram-positive and gram-negative bacteria, as well as for yeast and molds. The benefit of these dressings is the ability to continually kill bacteria for up to 7 days with a single application. This concept allows a decreased number of dressing changes and therefore reduces the pain and anxiety associated with dressing changes. The ability to reduce dressing changes has allowed a decrease in length of stay.[54] These silver dressings are being used to control bacteria in partial thickness burns, donor sites, and over skin grafts.[55,56] Fungal colonies and molds may appear in burn wounds. (Fig. 20.20) They are more likely to become apparent after several weeks of broad-spectrum antibiotic use. Aggressive daily débridement and better systemic antifungal therapy has improved survival.

Enzymatic Débridement

Reepithelialization of a second-degree burn cannot occur until the nonviable eschar has separated from the wound bed. Silvadene can form a pseudoeschar that, unless mechanically removed, can delay wound healing. Two enzymatic ointments originally devised to débride pressure ulcers also have been used to débride burn wounds. Collagenase works by degrading collagen in necrotic tissue. It will be inactivated by heavy metals, and therefore silver products should not be

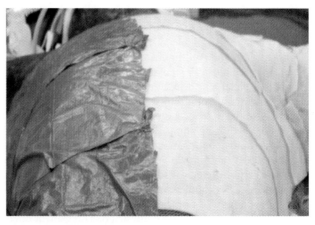

Figure 20•19 *Chest wound with silver-based dressing (Acticoat) in place.*

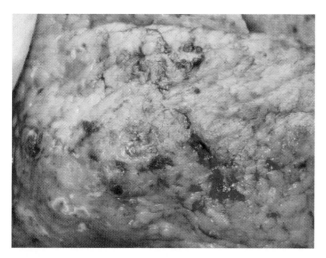

Figure 20•20 *A burn infected with fungal colonies.*

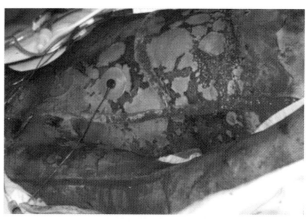

Figure 20•21 *Escharotomy of a burn wound of the chest.*

used concomitantly. A prospective randomized trial comparing collagenase and Silvadene reported faster wound healing with collagenase.[57,58] Papain-urea is another enzymatic débriding agent that works at a wider pH range and is less costly. However, it does not act on collagen and is associated with pain upon application.[59,60] The FDA has banned papain-urea from the market.

Surgical Management of Burn Wounds

When addressing all of the surgical procedures and devices used in management of burn wounds, it is helpful to categorize them based on the time since injury. One method divides them into periods designated acute, early, intermediate, and delayed.

The acute time period covers the first 24 post-burn hours, and the early phase encompasses post-burn days 2 and 3. The intermediate time period includes whatever length of time it takes to achieve wound closure, starting on post-burn day 4. Any reconstructive procedures required to correct or improve scarring are addressed in the delayed period.

The Acute Phase

The acute phase of burn management has been partially addressed in earlier sections of this chapter. Because it is the most critical time, it warrants further discussion. As addressed with discussion of the rule of nines and Parkland formula, the resuscitation during the first 24 hours is a challenging time for the burn team who will often be reevaluating and making critical changes to the ventilator and rate of intravenous fluids every hour. Peripheral pulses in any burned extremity will be monitored and checked hourly. Third-degree burns that are circumferential on any extremity will be unable to expand to accommodate the edema associated with the injury. This burned tissue, referred to as eschar, must be incised (escharotomy) if the pulses are distally absent or diminished. Circumferential, third-degree burns to the chest and abdomen may prevent adequate expansion of the chest during inspiration and lead to problems with proper ventilation. Truncal escharotomy should be performed in this situation. (Fig. 20.21)

The inability of the abdominal wall to expand to accommodate the swelling of the intraperitoneal contents may lead to abdominal compartment syndrome. Edema formation in nonburned soft tissues and muscle, intestine, and lungs is responsible for 50% of the edema associated with large burn injuries.[22,61] Incisions, or escharotomies, in the burns of the chest and abdomen are also performed to relieve the tourniquet effect these burns cause. Escharotomies may also be performed on the neck, hands, fingers, and penis. (Fig. 20.22)

▶ **PEARL 20•10** The key point of the acute phase of surgical management is to maintain perfusion with fluid resuscitation, oxygenation, and decompression with escharotomies and or fasciotomies if required.

Excision of Burn Wounds

At the conclusion of post-burn day 1, it is hoped that the patient will be adequately resuscitated, oxygenated, and therefore hemodynamically stable enough to tolerate surgical removal of third-degree burns planned for post-burn

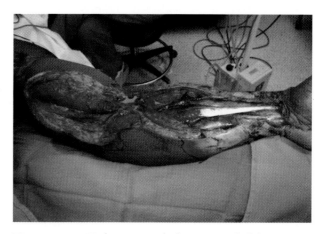

Figure 20•22 *Escharotomy of a burn wound of the forearm.*

day 2 or 3. Seventy-two hours is generally regarded as adequate time for stabilization and a short enough time span to intervene before bacterial overgrowth or invasion occurs. It has therefore been selected by the authors as an end point for the early phase.

It is well accepted that the most important contribution to improving burn survival was the development of early burn excision. Closure of these excised burn wounds with the patient's own skin is the ultimate goal. Depending on the extent and location of the burns, limited donor sites may delay closure or reepithelialization of the wounds for weeks to months. While most burn surgeons will agree that third-degree burns are best managed by early excision, there will be differing opinions on how deep an excision is required and when the patient's own skin should be grafted.

The two types of burn wound surgical excisions commonly used are tangential and fascial. While tangential excisions are routinely performed with a surgical blade, there is a water-driven débriding tool called Versajet (Smith & Nephew, Largo, FL) that employs a hydrosurgical system.[62]

As the term implies, tangential excision is a repetitive layer-by-layer excision. (Fig. 20.23) The depth of the excision will depend upon the type of blade used and the number of passes the surgeon makes over the wound. The principle of tangential burn wound excision is to remove all nonviable or excessively colonized tissue to provide a noninfected, well-perfused wound bed to accept a skin graft. The analogy used to train surgical residents is to view the burn wound as the skin on a potato or apple. The excision performed should remove the burn wound completely. When excising third-degree burns, the excision should remove all injured dermis and fat.

Tangential excisions performed early, when the wound has considerable edema and no microvascular proliferation has occurred, will be associated with markedly less blood loss. This wound bed, however, will have an increase in ongoing fluid loss from the tissues, and unless the grafts are meshed to allow for fluid escape, fluid will accumulate beneath grafts. Any sizeable accumulation will prevent diffusion of oxygen to the graft and result in graft failure.

When excision of large surface areas of third-degree burns is required a surgeon may choose to perform the excision using the electrocautery. This technique usually removes the burned eschar and underlying fat down to fascia in large units.

(Fig. 20.24) The excision is much faster and results in less blood loss than tangential excisions performed with blades. The downside of electrocautery excision down to fascia, however, is the permanent loss of subcutaneous fat. While excessive fat anywhere on the body is generally regarded as unsightly and unhealthy, some fat does have its benefits. Figure 20.25 shows that the thermally injured fat appears red instead of yellow.

Coverage of Excised Burn Wounds

Full-thickness or third-degree burn wounds that undergo surgical excision will ultimately require grafting with the patient's own skin to achieve closure. This self-graft is classified as an autograft and is actually a transplant for which the donor and the recipient are one and the same. These skin grafts may be either split thickness or full thickness. Split-thickness skin grafts comprise epidermis and a thin layer of dermis, and they are harvested with a dermatome. (Figs. 20.26 and 20.27) This instrument allows the surgeon to remove uninjured skin of varying thickness to be used as a graft but leaves behind a

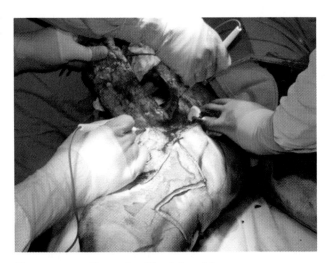

Figure 20•24 *Example of fascial excision.*

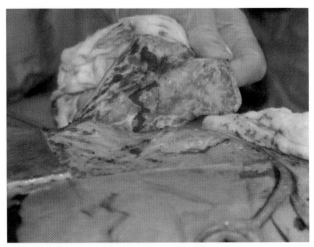

Figure 20•25 *Fat demonstrating red color associated with thermal injury.*

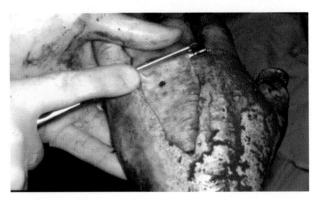

Figure 20•23 *Tangential excision of a burn of the hand.*

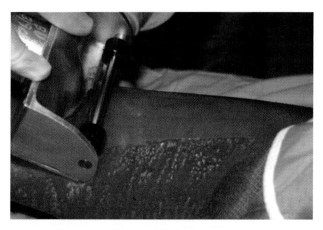

Figure 20•26 *Example of a dermatome used to harvest skin for a graft.*

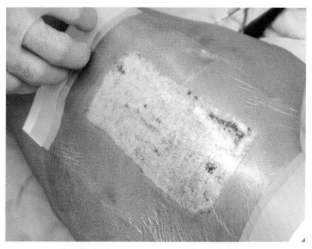

Figure 20•28 *Skin graft donor site on the anterior thigh.*

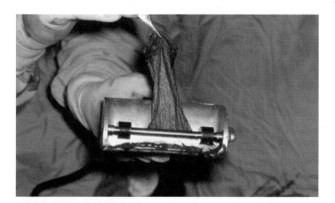

Figure 20•27 *Split-thickness skin harvested with a dermatome.*

donor site wound that must be handled with proper dressings. The length of time this wound will take to reepithelialize will depend on the thickness of the graft harvested. If the donor site skin is too thin or the dermatome is set to harvest too thickly, a full-thickness graft could be inadvertently harvested. Anatomical body locations used for donor sites are chosen for a reason. The skin on the back is one of the thickest areas and therefore serves as a great potential donor site.

Because split-thickness skin grafts are partial-thickness injuries, they can often be more painful than the full-thickness burn wound while they are healing. This fear of pain often results in donor sites being harvested from the anterior thighs or the back. (Fig. 20.28)

Donor site wounds, like partial-thickness burns, will result in some degree of discoloration and scarring. Like a burn, the longer they take to heal, the greater the potential for scarring. While the face has a pink or blush tint, all skin below the neck has a yellow tint. The scalp provides a donor site source that should be strongly considered for all facial grafts.

Patients are reluctant to have their heads shaved. They fear that grafts harvested will grow hair or they will remain bald. They should be informed that split-thickness skin grafts will not transfer hair and their hair will grow back and completely cover any scars. Grafts may be harvested from the same donor

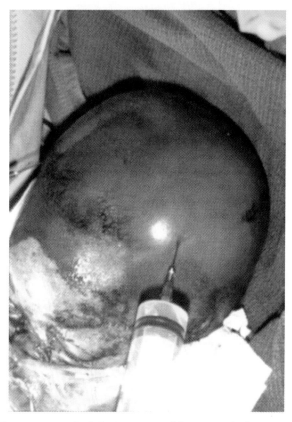

Figure 20•29 *Scalp being prepared for removal of a split-thickness skin graft by clysis (injection of a solution subcutaneously to elevate the tissue).*

sites repeatedly after healing has occurred. (Figs. 20.29 and 20.30)

Split-thickness skin grafts may be placed over prepared wound beds after being meshed or as a smooth unmeshed graft. Meshing occurs by running the skin through a device that creates perforations in the graft in a set pattern. (Figs. 20.31 and 20.32) These perforations may be small or

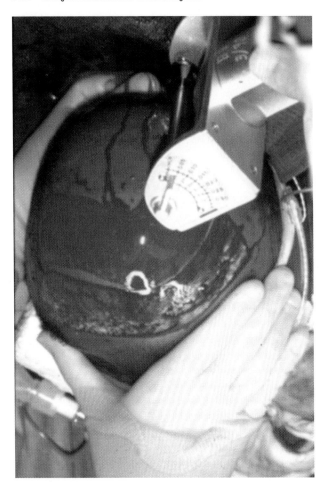

Figure 20•30 *Split-thickness graft being harvested from the scalp.*

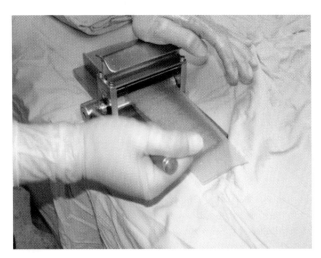

Figure 20•31 *Mesher being prepared for acceptance of graft.*

large, depending on the surgeon's choice. The benefit of the meshed or perforated skin graft is that body fluids drain through the graft and do not accumulate beneath it. Any sizeable collection of fluid or blood beneath a skin graft will prevent passive diffusion of oxygen and result in graft loss. Meshing and

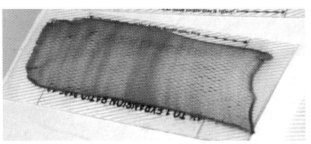

Figure 20•32 *Appearance of the meshed donor graft.*

spreading also allow harvested skin to cover larger areas. The downside of meshed grafts is the permanent cosmetic appearance of the meshed pattern. (Figs. 20.33 and 20.34) Widely meshed grafts also have a higher incidence of contracture formation and therefore need subsequent surgical releases and additional skin grafts. (Fig. 20.35) Split-thickness skin grafts may be secured to the wounds by sutures, staples, or fibrin glue. (Figs. 20.36 and 20.37)

Surgical dressings are generally applied over the grafts to prevent shearing while awaiting vascularization to occur in the grafts. This development of microvascular circulation begins immediately after graft placement and is obvious due to a healthy pink vascularized color in the graft within 24 hours. Clients are generally allowed to actively move grafted body parts within 72 hours. Passive motion directed by the therapist

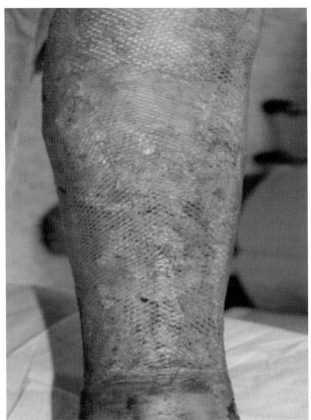

Figure 20•33 *Appearance of the burn tissue following split-thickness grafting with good take.*

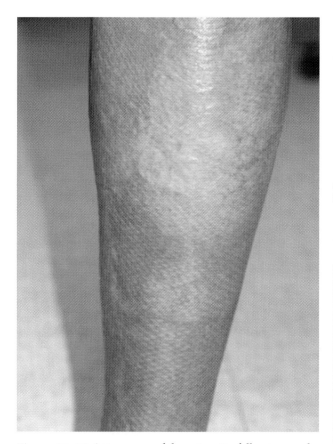

Figure 20•34 *Appearance of the extremity following good graft take and maturation.*

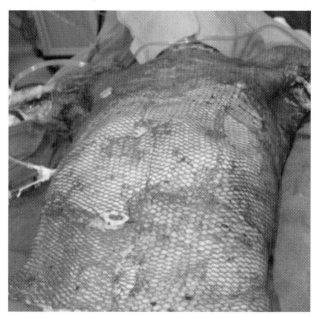

Figure 20•35 *Appearance of a graft that has been meshed at a 3-to-1 ratio.*

to increase range of motion should be delayed for 7 to 10 days after grafting to avoid shearing or avulsion of the grafts.

Full-thickness skin grafts are harvested with a scalpel. (Fig. 20.38) As the name implies, the entire epidermis and

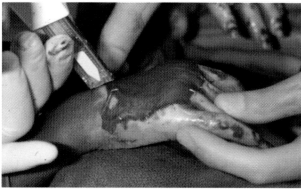

Figure 20•36 *A graft on the dorsum of the hand being secured by staples.*

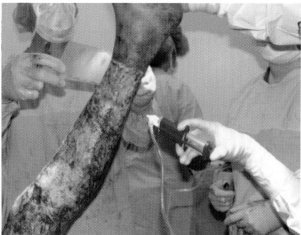

Figure 20•37 *Fibrin glue being used to secure skin graft.*

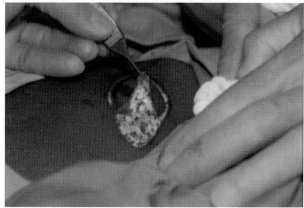

Figure 20•38 *Harvesting of a full-thickness graft.*

dermis are included in the graft. The wound created by harvesting a full-thickness graft is generally closed primarily by undermining the edges of the wound and closing with sutures. The graft itself is generally also secured in place with sutures. (Figs. 20.39 and 20.40) If the wound is too large to allow primary closure, then a split-thickness

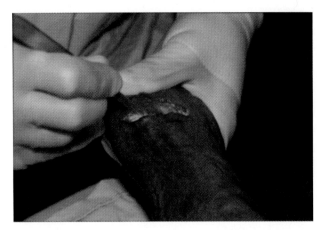

Figure 20•39 *Release of a contracture in preparation for acceptance of a full-thickness graft.*

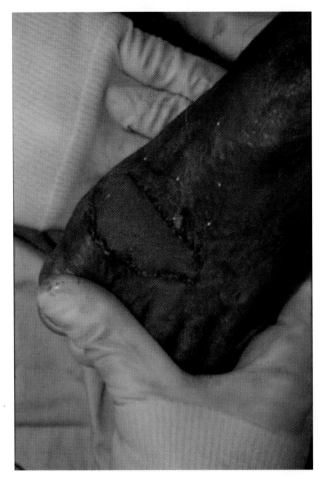

Figure 20•40 *Appearance of released area following placement of a full-thickness graft.*

skin graft may be harvested to graft the full-thickness donor site. Significant shrinkage or primary contracture of the harvested full-thickness skin graft may occur.

After the excision of a full-thickness burn wound, the ideal wound covering is the patient's own skin as a graft or flap. Circumstances may arise that force the surgeon to delay harvesting and placing grafts. Examples would be

▶ **PEARL 20•11** Full-thickness grafts are generally favored over split-thickness skin grafts in areas prone to develop contractures, such as the neck, or in wounds from release of contractures occurring in previous split-thickness skin graft sites.

cardiopulmonary instability forcing termination of the procedure or limited or no available donor sites in the greater than 90% TBSA burn. Even without donor sites, the burn wounds must be excised early to remove the source of the inflammatory response and the impending bacterial overburden the eschar will cause. These wounds are covered with products, tissue, or dressings that are designed to serve as temporary wound closures. The more common products used are cadaver skin (cadaveric allografts), pig skin (porcine xenografts), and to a lesser extent, engineered products such as Integra™ (Integra Lifesciences Corp., Plainsboro, NJ).

Cadaveric allografts (Fig. 20.41) are available for purchase from tissue banks. The storage of this tissue in a –70°C freezer allows the burn center to keep it on hand to be used emergently. The cost fluctuates with availability, but an average would be $1000 per sq. ft. An average adult would require 2 square feet per arm, 4 to 6 square feet for a chest and abdomen, and 5 square feet per leg. These grafts are left in place until autogenous grafts become available or until they spontaneously slough (usually within 2 to 3 weeks). If autogenous grafts must be widely meshed to obtain coverage, cadaveric allografts may be placed over them to provide coverage for the open areas. The autogenous grafts will spread beneath the cadaveric grafts and cause them to lift and slough much like epithelialization beneath a scab.

Because cadaveric allografts are human tissue, the donors are screened like any organ donor and documentation of usage is recorded as such. Pigskin or porcine xenografts (Fig. 20.42) were widely used as a temporary dressing on full-thickness burn excisions prior to the availability of cadaveric allografts. The resurgent use of porcine grafts occurred several years ago because of a shortage of available cadaveric allografts. It has been the experience of the authors that the

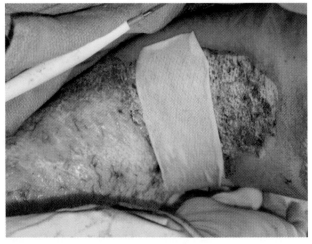

Figure 20•41 *Cadaveric overlay being applied over an extremity burn.*

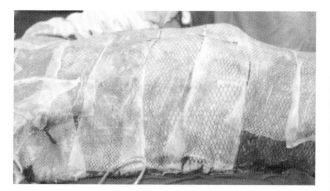

Figure **20•42** *Porcine xenografts applied to the torso.*

porcine xenografts provide acceptable clinical outcomes at roughly one tenth the cost of cadaveric allografts. Porcine grafts are stored on a shelf at room temperature and are approved by the FDA as a medical device and not a tissue. Therefore, the cumbersome record keeping of storing and using the cadaveric allograft is negated.

The commercial product AlloDerm (LifeCell Corp., Branchburg, NJ) is cadaver skin that has been processed to remove the epithelial elements while preserving the dermal matrix and basement membrane.[63] The removal of the epidermal elements render the tissue immunologically inert. This process allows for simultaneous grafting of AlloDerm covered by a very thin split-thickness skin graft. The reported proposed benefit of using AlloDerm is to achieve the benefit of a thicker split-thickness graft while avoiding the scarring associated in the donor site area. The thickness of dermis harvested with the epidermis in a split-thickness skin graft has an inverse relationship to scarring and contracture that occur at the recipient site.[64-68]

Integra was introduced as a temporary wound closure for excised full-thickness burn wounds in 1996. This material is a bilayered product of bovine collagen and glycosaminoglycan covered by silicone. The layer of bovine collagen and glycosaminoglycan were engineered to mimic dermis, and the silicone serves as the epidermis. When Integra is placed on an excised wound bed, the body's tissues grow up and through the matrix of the collagen and glycosaminoglycan. The silicone impedes overgrowth and protects the wound from bacteria and desiccation. The silicone must be removed and an autograft placed in a second operation once the dermal matrix is incorporated and capable of supporting an autograft. The length of time required for the Integra to incorporate is 3 to 4 weeks in adults and 2 to 3 weeks in children and in well-vascularized areas such as scalps and faces. There are reports of further shortening the interval of incorporation by covering the Integra with negative-pressure wound therapy devices such as vacuum-assisted closure (V.A.C.; Kinetic Concepts Inc., San Antonio, TX). The key to successful use of Integra is applying it to excised burn wounds before bacterial colonization has occurred. It is therefore recommended that Integra be placed no later than 72 hours after burn injury. The expense (around $1800 per 4 × 5 inch piece) and infectious vulnerability of Integra have significantly reduced its use in the management of acute full-thickness burns. It continues, however, to provide a valuable tool in the reconstructive area in dealing with burn contractures.[69] Integra is also being used in complex

wounds that have exposed tendons or bones as a means of improving limb salvage without using microvascular free flaps.[70] (Figs. 20.43 through 20.47)

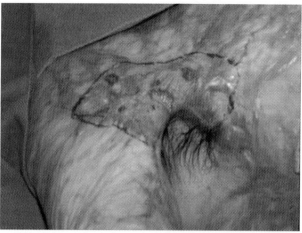

Figure **20•43** *Axillary scar contracture marked for excision.*

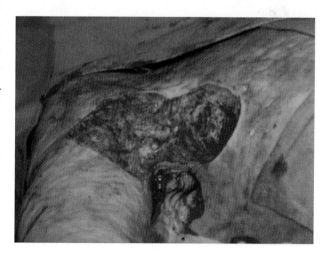

Figure **20•44** *Appearance of axillary region following scar excision.*

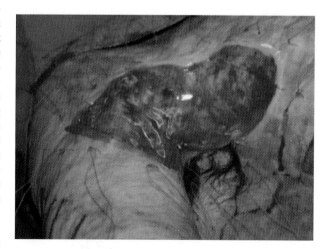

Figure **20•45** *Appearance of axillary region following the suturing of the artificial skin, Integra.*

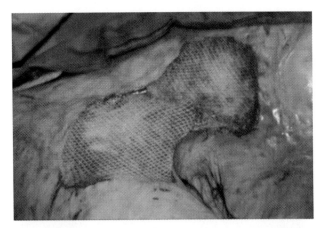

Figure 20•46 *Appearance of axillary region with meshed graft in place.*

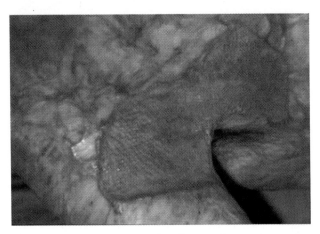

Figure 20•47 *Appearance of axillary graft at postoperative follow-up.*

Intermediate Care

The acute and early phases of burn care addressed assessment and stabilization of a burn as well as early excision of full-thickness burns. While grafting often begins in the early time phase, the majority of grafting occurs after 72 post-burn hours and therefore falls into the intermediate phase of burn care.

After all full-thickness burns have been excised and these wounds have been covered with one of the previously discussed temporary wound coverings, a strategic plan of resurfacing the wounds with autografts must occur. If only limited donor sites are available, then autografts may be maximized by widely expanding (meshing) them. These split-thickness skin grafts should be harvested thin enough to allow for quicker healing and repeat harvesting. If minimal donor sites are available for use, then cultured epithelial autografts (CEAs) are required. CEAs are the patient's own skin cells that are grown in culture. Most burn surgeons obtain two 2 × 6-cm full-thickness biopsy samples of uninjured skin, place them in media, and ship them overnight to Genzyme Corp. (Cambridge, MA) for growth. The samples are processed to obtain only the keratinocytes, which are then grown in culture. The cells will multiply, divide, and ultimately coalesce into a sheet three cell layers thick. The cultured grafts are 10 × 6 cm each, as this is the size of the Petri dish in which they are grown. Each graft costs approximately $1220, and it is generally ready to use 2 to 3 weeks after the tissue is received. An unlimited number of grafts can ultimately be purchased over the next several weeks. These cells may also be placed in freezer storage to allow additional grafts to be produced months or years later. CEAs are the patient's own skin and therefore provide permanent closure of the wounds. The grafted keratinocytes grown in culture are so thin and fragile that the sheet of cells is clipped to Vaseline®(Chesebrough-Ponds, Greenwich, CT) gauze, which will allow the graft to be removed from the carrier dish and placed on the patient. The grafts are secured in place with fibrin glue or staples and covered with meshed gauze. This process is illustrated in Figures 20.48 through 20.50.

Silver dressing materials are placed on the grafts to reduce colonization of bacteria and fungi and improve graft take.

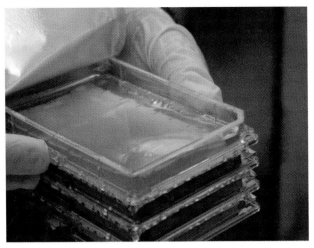

Figure 20•48 *Petri dish holding cultured epithelial autograft.*

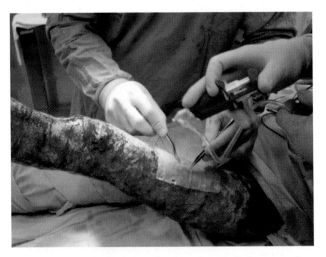

Figure 20•49 *Application of cultured epithelial autograft with gauze to an extremity.*

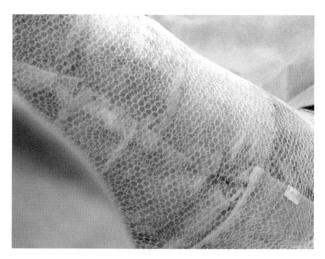

Figure 20•50 *A meshed dressing applied over the extremity grafts to aid in anchoring.*

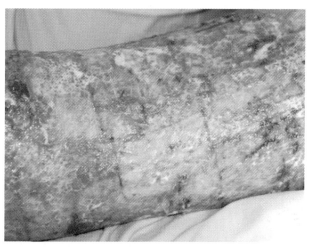

Figure 20•52 *Extremity burn healing following application of cultured epithelial autograft.*

The Vaseline gauze backings are inspected daily and must be removed if evidence of infection appears. If all goes well, the cultured grafts are adherent and able to tolerate removal of the Vaseline backing 1 week later. The presence of these grafts becomes more apparent as the cells dry and cornify. (Figs. 20.51 and 20.52).

These grafts lack the anchoring capabilities that the dermal components of a split-thickness skin graft provide. They therefore are prone to avulsion and blistering for several weeks with the minimal trauma associated with daily wound care and moving or rearranging. These wounds, however, will reheal from residual cells in the wound bed and not require repeat grafting. CEAs are not meshed and therefore heal with a smooth and seamless appearance. (Fig. 20.53) The lack of dermis present, however, results in significant contracture of the wounds, similar to what is seen in widely meshed, very thin split-thickness autografts. Pigmentation of CEAs is also sporadic and much more obvious in darker-pigmented individuals. (Fig. 20.54)

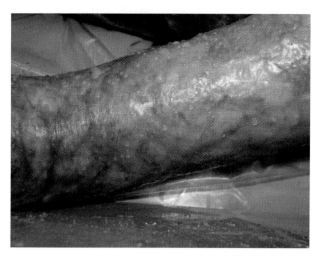

Figure 20•53 *Cultured epithelial autografts heal in a smooth pattern without seams since graft is not meshed.*

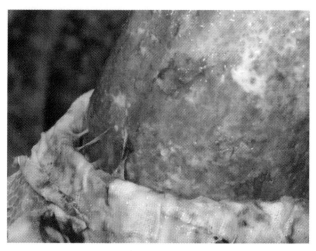

Figure 20•51 *Vaseline gauze being rolled back from an extremity to check for signs of graft infection.*

Attempts at achieving cultured skin that included dermal and epidermal cell lines have failed, but it is hoped that one day it will be the answer to resurfacing full-thickness skin injuries without the morbidity of large donor sites.

The Delayed Phase

Burn survivors must endure the acute pain associated with their wound care, healing donor sites, and grafts. Positions of comfort require human extremities and necks to be in flexion. These positions allow newly healed burn wounds to contract and may require surgical release with repeat grafts. Contracture releases through burn scars benefit from reconstruction with rotational flaps, tissue expanders, microvascular free flaps, or full-thickness skin grafts. When flaps are not an option, then using Integra with delayed placement of split-thickness skin grafts is a viable alternative. (Figs. 20.55 and 20.56) The management of hypertrophic scars that develop in many burn wounds is fully discussed in Chapter 21.

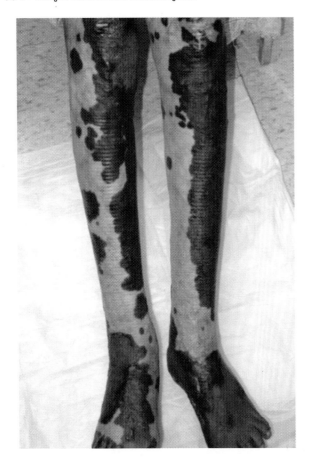

Figure **20•54** *Spotty appearance of extremity due to sporadic pigmentation often seen with cultured epithelial autografts.*

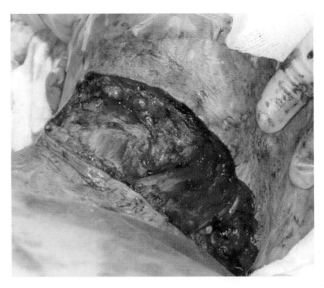

Figure **20•55** *Release of a neck contracture in preparation for artificial skin placement.*

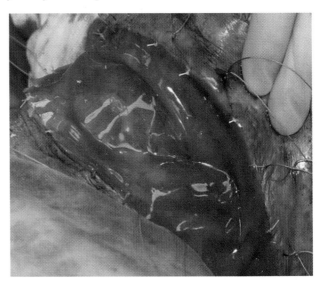

Figure **20•56** *Integra artificial skin being sutured in place on neck wound.*

Summary

In conclusion, burn wounds vary from minor to being a threat to life and limb, with major systemic effects. Optimal management of the wounds and patients is a complex balance of local, surgical, and medical treatments. The best concentration of these efforts occurs in a burn center with its multidisciplinary team approach.

References

1. Davis, S, Shibasaki, M, Low, D, et al: Skin grafting impairs postsynaptic cutaneous vasodilator and sweating responses. J Burn Care Res 2007; 28:435–441.
2. Chatterjee, J: A critical evaluation of the clinimetrics of laser Doppler as a method of burn assessment in clinical practice. J Burn Care Res 2006; 27:123–130.
3. Palmieri, T: Inhalation injury: Research progress and needs. J Burn Care Res 2007; 28:549–554.
4. Birky, M, Clark, F: Inhalation of toxic products from fires. Bull NY Acad Med 1981; 57:997–1013.
5. Prien, T, Draber, D: Toxic smoke compounds and inhalation injury: A review. Burns Incl Therm Inj 1988; 14:451–460.
6. Pitt, R, Parker, J, Jurkovich, G, et al: Analysis of altered capillary pressure and permeability after thermal injury. J Surg Res 1987; 42:693–702.
7. Lund, T, Wig, H, Reed, R: Acute postburn edema: Role of strongly negative interstitial fluid pressure. Am J Physiol 1988; 255:H1069–H1074.
8. Harms, B, Bodai, B, Kramer, G, et al: Microvascular fluid and protein flux in pulmonary and systemic circulations after thermal injury. Microvasc Res 1982; 23:77–86.
9. Isago, T, Noshima, S, Traber, L, et al: Analysis of pulmonary microvascular permeability after smoke inhalation. J Appl Physiol 1991; 71:1403–1408.
10. Teixidor, H, Rubin, E, Novick, G, et al: Smoke inhalation: Radiologic manifestations. Radiology 1983; 149:383–387.
11. Petzman, A, Shires III, G, Teixidor, H, et al: Smoke inhalation injury: Evaluation of radiographic manifestations and pulmonary dysfunction. J Trauma 1989; 29:1232–1238.
12. Agee, R, Long, J, Hunt, J, et al: Use of 133-xenon in early diagnosis of inhalation injury. J Trauma 1976; 16:218–224.

13. Petroff, P, Hander, E, Clayton, W, et al: Pulmonary function studies after smoke inhalation. Am J Surg 1976; 132:346–351.

14. Brown, D, Archer, S, Greenhalf, D, et al: Inhalation injury severity scoring system: A quantitative method. J Burn Care Rehabil 1996; 17:553–557.

15. Masanes, M, Legendre, C, Lioret, N: Using bronchoscopy and biopsy to diagnose early inhalation injury. Macroscopic and histologic findings. Chest 1995; 10:1365–1369.

16. Madnani, D, Steel, N, deVries, E: Factors that predict the need for intubation in patients with smoke inhalation injury. Ear Nose Throat J 2006; 85:278–280.

17. Reske, A, Bak, Z, Samuelsson, A, et al: Computed tomography—A possible aid in the diagnosis of smoke inhalation injury? Acta Anaesthesiol Scand 2005; 49:257–260.

18. Schall, G, McDonald, H, Carr, L: Xenon ventilation-perfusion lung scans. The early diagnosis. JAMA 1978; 240:2441–2445.

19. Lin, W, Kao, C, Wang, S: Detection of acute inhalation injury in fire victims by means of technetium 99m DTPA radioaerosol inhalation lung scintigraphy. Eur J Nucl Med 1997; 24:125–129.

20. Abdi, S, Evans, M, Cox, R, et al: Inhalation injury to tracheal epithelium in an ovine model of cotton smoke exposure. Early phase (30 minutes). Am Rev Respir Dis 1990; 142:1436–1439.

21. Cox, R, Burke, A, Soejima, K, et al: Airway obstruction in sheep with burn and smoke inhalation injuries. Am J Respir Cell Mol Biol 2003; 29:295–302.

22. Carvajal, H, Linares, H, Brouhard, B: Relationship of burn size to vascular permeability changes in rats. Surg Gynecol Obstet 1979; 149:193–202.

23. Ward, P, Till, G: Pathophysiologic events related to thermal injury of skin. J Trauma 1990; 30:575–579.

24. Laffey, J, Kavanagh, B, Ney, L, et al: Ventilation with lower tidal volumes as compared with traditional tidal volumes for acute lung injury and the acute respiratory distress syndrome: The Acute Respiratory Distress Syndrome Network. N Engl J Med 2000; 342:1301–1308.

25. Amato, M, Barbas, C, Madeiros, D, et al: Effect of a protective-ventilation strategy on mortality in the acute respiratory distress syndrome. N Engl J Med 1998; 338:347–354.

26. Hemmat, M, Adyani, Y, Ahmadian, N: Electrical and lightning injuries. J Burn Care Res 2007; 28:256–261.

27. Cancio, L, Jimenez-Reyna, J, Barillo, D, et al: One hundred ninety-five cases of high-voltage electric injury. J Burn Care Rehabil 2005; 26:331–340.

28. Evans, E, Purnell, O, Robinett, P, et al: Fluids and electrolyte requirements in severe burns. Ann Surg 1952; 135:804–817.

29. Greenhalgh, D: Burn resuscitation. J Burn Care Res 2007; 28:555–565.

30. Baxter, C: Fluid volume and electrolyte changes in the early post-burn period. Clin Plast Surg 1974; 1:693–703.

31. Engrav, L, Colescott, P, Kemalyan, N, et al: A biopsy of the use of the Baster formula-resuscitate burns or do we do it like Charlie did it? J Burn Care Rehabil 2000; 21:91–95.

32. Pruitt Jr, B: Protection from excessive resuscitation: Pushing the pendulum back. J Trauma 2000; 49:387–391.

33. Shah, A, Kramer, G, Grady, J, et al: Meta-analysis of fluid requirements for burn injury. J Burn Care Rehabil 2003; 24:S118.

34. Fredrich, J, Sullivan, S, Engrav, L, et al: Is supra-Baxter resuscitation in burn patients a new phenomenon. Burns Incl Therm Inj 2004; 30:464–466.

35. Greenhalgh, D, Warden, G: The importance of intra-abdominal pressure measurement in burned patients. J Trauma 1994; 36:685–690.

36. Latenser, B, Kowal-Vern, A, Kimball, D, et al: A pilot study comparing percutaneous decompression with decompressive laparotomy for acute abdominal compartment syndrome in thermal injury. J Burn Care Rehabil 2002; 23:190–195.

37. Hobson, K, Young, K, Ciraulo, A, et al: Release of abdominal compartment syndrome improves survival in patients with burn injury. J Trauma 2002; 53:1129–1134.

38. Oda, J, Inoue, K, Harunari, N, et al: Resuscitation volume and abdominal compartment syndrome in patients with major burns. Burns 2006; 32:151–154.

39. Monafo, W, Halverson, J, Schechtman, K: The role of concentrated sodium solutions in the resuscitation of patients with severe burns. Surgery 1984; 95:129–135.

40. Monafo, W: The treatment of burn shock by the intravenous and oral administration of hypertonic lactated saline solution. J Trauma 1970; 10:575–586.

41. Huang, P, Stucky, F, Dimick, A, et al: Hypertonic sodium resuscitation is associated with renal failure and death. Ann Surg 1995; 221:543–547.

42. Saffle, J, Davis, B, Williams, P: Recent outcomes in the treatment of burn injury in the United States: A report from the American Burn Association patient registry. J Burn Care Rehabil 1995; 16:219–232.

43. Tredgett, E, Shankowsky, H, Aerum, T, et al: The role of inhalation injury in burn trauma. A Canadian experience. Ann Surg 1990; 212:720–727.

44. Stern, H: Silver sulfadiazine and the healing of partial thickness burns: A prospective clinical trial. Br J Plast Surg 1989; 42:581–585.

45. Maitre, S, Jaber, K, Perrot, J, et al: Increased serum and urinary levels of silver during treatment with topical silver sulfadiazine. Ann Dermatol Venereol 2002; 129:217–219.

46. Silvadene cream 10% [product information insert]. Bristol, TN, Monarch Pharmaceuticals Inc., 2005.

47. Shuck, J, Thorne, L, Cooper, C: Mafenide acetate solution dressing: An adjunct in burn wound care. J Trauma 1975; 15:595–599.

48. Kucan, J, Smooth, E: Five percent mafenide acetate solution in the treatment of thermal injuries. J Burn Care Rehabil 1993; 14:158–163.

49. Maggi, S, Soler, P, Smith, P, et al: The efficacy of 5% Sulfamylon solution for the treatment of contaminated explanted human meshed skin grafts. Burns 1999; 25:237–241.

50. Physicians' Desk Reference, ed 61. New York, Thomson Healthcare, 2007, p 1394.

51. Goforth, H, DeLullo, J, Miller, S, et al: Preliminary in vitro sensitivity testing of burn wound associated bacteria to various concentrations of acetic acid solutions. J Burn Care Rehabil 1998; 19:178–187.

52. Heggers, J, Sazy, J, Stenberg, B, et al: Bactericidal and wound-healing properties of sodium hypochlorite solutions: The 1991 Lindberg Award. J Burn Care Rehabil 1991; 12:240–244.

53. Kozol, R, Gillies, C, Elgebaly, S: Effects of sodium hypochlorite (Dakin's solution) on cells of the wound module. Arch Surg 1988; 123:420–423.

54. Peters, D, Verchere, C: Healing at home: Comparing cohorts of children with medium-sized burns treated as outpatients with in-hospital applied Acticoat to those children treated as inpatients with silver sulfadiazine. J Burn Care Res 2006; 27:198–201.

55. Tredgett, E, Shankowsky, H, Groenweld, A, et al: A matched-pair, randomized study evaluating the efficacy and safety of Acticoat silver-coated dressing for the treatment of burn wounds. J Burn Care Rehabil 1998; 19:531–537.

56. Demling, R: The burn edema process: Current concepts. J Burn Care Rehabil 2005; 26:207–227.

57. Soroff, H, Sasvary, D: Collagenase ointment and polymyxin B sulphate/Bacitracin spray versus silver sulfadiazine cream in partial-thickness burns: A pilot study. J Burn Care Res 1994; 15:13–17.

58. Hansbrough, J, Achauer, B, Dawson, J, et al: Wound healing in partial-thickness burn wounds treated with collagenase ointment versus silver sulfadiazine cream. J Burn Care Rehabil 1995; 16:241–247.

59. Shapira, E, Giladi, A, Neuman, Z: Use of water-insoluble papain (WIP) for debridement of burn eschar and necrotic tissue: Preliminary report. Plast Reconst Surg 1973; 52:279–281.

60. Starley, I, Mohammed, P, Schneider, G, et al: The treatment of pediatric burns using topical papaya. Burns 1999; 25:636–639.

61. Brouhard, B, Carvajal, H, Liares, H: Burn edema and protein leakage in the rat: Relationship to size of injury. Microvas Res 1978; 15:221–228.

62. Granick, M, Jacoby, M, Noruthrun, S, et al: Clinical and economic impact of hydrosurgical debridement on chronic wounds. Wounds 2006; 18:35–39.

63. Callcut, R, Schurr, M, Sloan, M, et al: Clinical experience with Alloderm: A one-staged composite dermal/epidermal replacement

utilizing processed cadaver dermis and thin autografts. J Inter Soc Burn Inj 2006; 32:583–588.

64. Wainwright, D: Use of an acellular allograft dermal matrix (Alloderm) in the management of full-thickness burns. Burns 1995; 21:243–248.

65. Walden, J, Garcia, H, Hawkins, H, et al: Both dermal matrix and epidermis contribute to an inhibition of wound contraction. Ann Plast Surgery 2000; 45:162–166.

66. Rennekampff, H, Kiessig, V, Griffey, S, et al: Acellular human dermis promotes cultured keratinocyte engraftment. J Burn Care Res 1997; 18:535–544.

67. Sheridan, R, Choucair, R: Acellular allogenic dermis does not hinder initial engraftment in burn wound resurfacing and reconstruction. J Burn Care Res 1997; 18:496–499.

68. Tsai, C, Lin, S, Lai, C: The use of composite acellular allodermis-ultrathin autograft on joint area in major burn patients. One year follow-up. Kaohsiung J Med Sci 1999; 15:651–658.

69. Jeng, J, Fidler, P, Sokolich, J, et al: Seven years' experience with Integra as a reconstructive tool. J Burn Care Res 2007; 28:120–126.

70. Yowler, C, Mozingo, D, Ryan, J, et al: Factors contributing to delayed extremity amputation in burn patients. J Trauma 1998; 45:522–526.

chapter 21

Rehabilitation of the Burned Individual

Carla M. Saulsbery, LOTR, CHT

Shannon B. Abney, LOTR

There have been major advances in the medical, surgical, and rehabilitative treatment of burn injuries over the past several decades.[1] Burns over more than 30% of a patient's total body surface area (TBSA) were uniformly fatal approximately 25 to 30 years ago. Today, about 12% of those who sustain burns of this magnitude die. With current methods of burn care, patients are increasingly surviving larger and more debilitating burns. The main objective and primary measure of success in the quality of burn care has shifted from survival per se to restoration of the patient's preinjury level of function, with the best possible cosmesis. Achieving this objective requires involvement of an entire burn care team, including highly trained and knowledgeable physical and occupational therapists. Of all the different and challenging processes that a burn patient undergoes, rehabilitation lasts the longest because it begins on the day of injury and never truly ends.[2]

The rehabilitation program's objectives change over time. In the acute care stages, rehabilitation focuses on restoring baseline cardiopulmonary status and preventing musculoskeletal dysfunction. In the later stages, rehabilitation focuses on regaining and restoring baseline function, returning to employment or school, and adjusting to possible aesthetic and psychological changes. This ever-changing focus ultimately underscores the need for an integrated burn care team approach.[2]

Each year an estimated 1 million people sustain burn injuries, and there are several at-risk populations in the United States that include a number of underserved groups. These include children under the age of 4 (for whom burn injury represents one of the leading causes of disability), adults over 65 years of age, African Americans and Native Americans, the poor, and people living in rural areas and substandard housing. In addition, national disasters represent a significant source of burn injuries. Approximately one third of the people injured in recent terrorist attacks sustained major burn injuries. Military personnel also sustained injuries from explosions, fires, and accidents.[2]

An estimated 500,000 people with burn injuries receive medical treatment per year. Treatment is received in hospital emergency departments and outpatient clinics, free-standing urgent care centers, and private physician's offices. There are approximately 4000 fire and burn deaths per year. This total includes an estimated 3500 deaths secondary to residential fires and 500 from motor vehicle and aircraft crashes, electricity, chemicals or hot liquids and substances, and other sources of burn injury. About 75% of these deaths occur at the scene or during the initial transport.[3] A total of 40,000 people with burn injuries are hospitalized per year, with 25,000 admissions to the 125 hospitals with specialized burn centers. Burn centers average 200 admissions a year, while the other 5000 U.S. hospitals average less than 3 burn admissions per year.[3]

Selected statistics on admissions to burn centers for 1995 to 2005 include a 94.4% survival rate. Over one third of admissions (38%) exceeded 10% TBSA, and 10% exceeded 30% TBSA. Most injuries involve 70% male and 30% female patients, and the vital body areas include the face, hands, and feet. Ethnicity includes 62% Caucasian, 18% African American, 12% Hispanic, and 8% other. Causes of burn injuries are 46% fire/flame, 32% scalding, 8% hot object contact, 4% electrical, 3% chemical, and

6% other. Forty-three percent of burn injuries occur in the home, 17% on the street or highway, 8% are occupational, and 32% are other. Thirty-one percent of burn patients are uninsured, underinsured, or private or self-pay; 25% are insured by government programs.[3]

Better acute care management of patients with massive injuries has been one of the major advances in burn care over the past few decades. It is not surprising that patients with larger burn injuries have longer hospital stays, incur more expenses, and usually require years of rehabilitation and reconstruction. It is reasonable to consider that a person who sustains massive burn injuries may suffer irreparable loss of function, but can have a good quality of life after recovery. Unfortunately, data are scarce comparing the perceived quality of life of severely burned individuals to that of unburned healthy individuals. Most major burn injuries have both physical and psychological consequences. These consequences include pain, itching, loss of function, and psychological issues. The psychological consequences include, but are not limited to, depression, anxiety, loss of self-esteem, and inability to socialize.[2]

Less than 50% of patients who experience a major burn injury return to the same job or employer without accommodations or restrictions. Most health insurance is connected with the patient's employment, and prolonged time off for recovery can cause significant hardships to patients and their families. Little information is available on the variety of factors that influence return to employment after burn injury. Overall, quality of life after a burn injury is difficult to measure. Several studies indicate that many burn survivors are able to return to their preinjury functional status. The chances of the patient achieving a positive outcome is enhanced and affected by the comprehensive multidisciplinary burn care team approach, aftercare, and supportive and healthy family dynamics.[2]

Anatomy and Physiology of the Skin and How It Relates to a Burn Injury

The skin is the largest organ of the human body and comprises 15% of the total body weight. Its thickness varies from 1.5 mm to 4 mm. The thickest areas of the skin include the scalp, back, palms, and soles of the feet. It is vitally important that the burn therapist be intimately familiar with the normal structures and functions of the skin and the abnormal anatomy and physiology of the skin after a burn injury. The skin is divided into two principle layers: the external covering called the *epidermis* and the deeper layer called the *dermis*.[4] The dermis is primarily composed of collagen and fibrous connective tissue.[5]

Epidermis

The epidermis consists of stratified epithelium. It is avascular and very thin, ranging from 0.07 mm to 0.12 mm. Its purpose is protection, water proofing, and regeneration.[4] The epidermis is composed of four distinct layers: (1) stratum corneum, or horny layer; (2) stratum granulosum, or granular layer; (3) stratum spinosum, or spinous layer; and (4) stratum basale, or basal cell layer. A fifth layer, the stratum lucidum, is located on the soles of the feet and palms of the hands. It is a thin eosinophilic band that is located at the base of the stratum corneum.[5]

The stratum corneum is 15 to 20 layers thick and is the outermost covering.[4] It is also composed of dead cells, and they are easily sloughed. The stratum corneum is water repellent and maintains the body's vapor barrier.[5] The second layer, stratum granulosum, consists of flattened nucleated cells containing distinctive cytoplasmic inclusions called keratohyalin granules. This stratum is a transitional layer between the stratum corneum and the lower layers of the epidermis that produce keratinocytes.[4] The next layer is the stratum spinosum, and these cells synthesize proteins but are no longer able to reproduce.[5] The innermost layer, stratum basale or basal cell layer of keratinocytes, is the germinative layer of the epidermis. The basal keratinocytes are cuboidal or low columnar in shape.[4] This layer is in intimate contact with the basement membrane. It is bonded and conforms to the dermis by fingerlike projections of the papillary dermal tissue.[5] The basal keratinocytes contain various cytoplasmic structures and organelles, such as mitochondria, endoplasmic reticulum, rosettes of ribosomes, Golgi complexes, and prominent nucleoli.[4]

Epidermal Structures

There are a variety of cellular structures other than keratinocytes found in the epidermis. These structures function within the epidermis and in combination with the cutaneous epidermal structures that make the entire epidermis a metabolically active and essential component of the skin.[4] The four major cell types are melanocytes, keratinocytes, Merkel's cells, and Langerhans' cells.

Melanocytes are pigment-producing cells that are responsible for the inherent skin color. These cells produce pigment in response to ultraviolet radiation.[5] Melanocytes are located at the dermal-epidermal junction, although some are located in the dermis. The distribution of these cells varies throughout the body and changes with age.[4] Keratinocytes produce the protein called keratin, which waterproofs the cells of the stratum corneum. Merkel's cells are thought to increase the skin's strength, and Langerhans' cells provide nonspecific immune protection from invading microorganisms.[5]

Cutaneous Appendages of the Epidermis

Several other structures that are epidermal in origin and significantly affect the function and physiology of the skin are the hair follicles, sebaceous and apocrine glands, and the eccrine sweat glands.[4] (Fig. 21.1)

Hair Follicles

Hair follicles are composed of "pockets of epithelium" and are continuous with the superficial epidermis. The hair follicle is divided into three portions: (1) infundibulum, (2) isthmus, and (3) inferior portion. The infundibulum is the most superficial and is primarily epidermal. The isthmus comprises the tissue between the entry into the follicle of the sebaceous gland and the insertion of the arrector pili muscle. The inferior portion gives rise to the hair bulb, including the hair

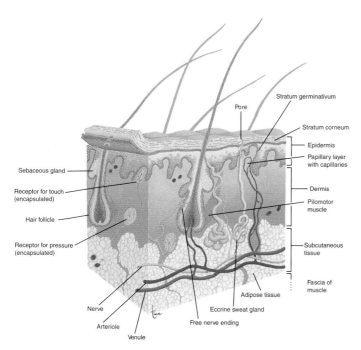

Figure 21•1 *Skin. Structure of the skin and subcutaneous tissue. From Scanlon, V:* Essentials of Anatomy and Physiology, *ed 5. Philadelphia, FA Davis, 2007, Fig. 5-1, pp 88–103.*

papilla and matrix. The hair follicle is primarily composed of epidermal tissue and has a significant function in the reepithelialization of the burn wound. Unless the burn wound is a deep partial- or full-thickness injury, the epidermal tissue will be present in the wound site from which epidermal skin buds will generate new epithelium.[4]

One of the physiological functions of the hair is that it participates in the sensory system of the skin due to nerve endings connected to the hair follicles. Air is trapped by the hair, and this serves as a source of insulation, which is primarily effective on the scalp. Hair also combats infection by trapping infectious organisms and keeping them distanced from the surface of the skin.[4]

Sebaceous Glands

The sebaceous glands arise from an epithelial bud from the outer hair root sheath and the junction of the infundibulum and isthmus. They are distributed throughout the entire body, except the plantar and dorsal surfaces of the feet and the palms of the hand. The role of the sebaceous gland is to secrete sebum, which assists in keeping the skin moist and supple. If a burn injury damages or destroys the sebaceous glands, the new skin may not have the ability to secrete enough sebum to keep the skin moist, therefore requiring frequent applications of moisturizing creams.[4]

Apocrine Sweat Glands

The apocrine sweat glands are primarily located in the axilla and pubic region. They consist of a coiled secretory gland located in the lower portion of the dermis and a straight excretory duct that empties onto the infundibular portion of the hair follicle. This is typically adjacent to the sebaceous gland. The apocrine sweat is continuously secreted. It also consists of an excretion that occurs when a reservoir of apocrine secretion is propelled upward. The quantity of apocrine sweat produced daily is generally small, sterile, and odorless within the duct. However, when the apocrine secretion combines with bacteria on the skin's surface, the bacteria degrade the apocrine sweat, which results in body odor.[4]

Eccrine Sweat Glands

The eccrine sweat glands are composed of epidermal skin layers and are located throughout the body. The highest concentrations are located on the forehead, axilla, and palms of the hands and soles of the feet. The lowest concentrations are located on the arms and legs. At birth there are approximately 3 million eccrine glands present, and no additional ones are formed throughout the rest of the life span.[4]

The eccrine glands consist of a coiled body and three sections of eccrine ducts. This coiled duct and gland lie in the dermis and give rise to a straight duct. This straight duct connects with the spiral duct and then exits to the skin surface. The eccrine sweat gland is innervated extensively by unmyelinated nerve fibers and responds to sympathetic and parasympathetic stimulation. Sweat is a colorless and odorless hypotonic solution that is approximately 99% water by weight. The remaining 1% contains various solutes of electrolytes, lipids, minerals, and amino acids.[4]

The most effective way for the body to dissipate heat is through sweating. Due to internal or external factors, the body temperature rises and the hypothalamus initiates the sweating mechanism. After prolonged exposure to a heated environment, the body will begin the process of acclimation. To effectively cool the body temperature, the sweat must evaporate. Evaporation will cool the skin's surface and create a thermal gradient to dissipate the heat from the core of the working muscles and tissues out to the skin. The loss of the thermal gradient from the core to the skin creates an increase in an individual's core temperature. This could reach dangerous levels, even with minimal exertion, especially in those with deep partial-thickness and full-thickness burn injuries. If a significant percentage of eccrine sweat glands are destroyed in a burn injury, the patient must rely on the remaining sweat glands for thermoregulation. Consequently, the patient is further compromised by the lack of evaporative sweating, which can also result in an even greater rise in core temperature. The ability to sweat and the amount of skin that has the capacity to sweat are very important considerations in the rehabilitation of burn patients sustaining deep partial-thickness and full-thickness injuries.[4]

Dermis

The dermis comprises primarily extracellular proteins and a dense fibroelastic connective tissue made of collagen, elastic fibers, and an interfibrillar gel substance.[4] It is 2 to 5 mm thick and composed of two layers: the *reticular dermis,* forming the base, which is thicker and interfaces with the subcutaneous tissue, and the *papillary dermis,* which is thinner, more superficial, and lies directly beneath the basement membrane of the epidermis.[4,5]

Papillary Dermis

The papillary dermis is molded against the overlying epidermis and conforms to basal layer ridges, grooves, and appendages. It is composed of smaller, loosely distributed elastic and collagen fibrils. The papillary dermis contains a substantially greater proportion of interfibrillar gel and connective tissue. It also supports and encloses the superficial portions of the microcirculation and the lymphatic network.[4]

Reticular Dermis

The reticular dermis is the deeper and thicker component. It is more acellular and avascular and contains elastic fibers and dense collagen bundles. The collagen bundles are arranged primarily at the surface of the skin, with some collagen arranged in a perpendicular orientation. The function of this arrangement is to provide the skin with a preferential direction of extensibility. When the reticular dermis is injured, the collagen fibers will return to their original state and become aligned parallel to the direction with the least amount of extensibility. This functional orientation will play a significant role in the healing and possible hypertrophic scarring that may occur after sustaining a burn injury.[4]

Dermal Structures

There are several different types of structures contained within the dermis. These structures include the smooth muscle of the arrector pilorum, blood vessels, lymphatics, and a network of nervous structures and organs. The arrector pilorum muscles insert on the hair follicle below the sebaceous duct and cause the hair follicle to elevate when contracted. This contraction results in an increase in metabolic rate of the skin and assists in maintaining the thermoneutral environment the body needs when exposed to cold.[4]

The skin's blood supply is derived from the cutaneous branches of the subcutaneous musculocutaneous arteries. The cardinal function of the cutaneous vasculature is providing thermoregulation and nutrition to the skin. It also plays a major role in the inflammatory process. The amount of damage to the microcirculation and vascular network can be a limiting factor in the healing of a burn wound. Partial-thickness burn injuries that do not involve the deeper layers of the dermis and the majority of the vascular bed have potential to heal rapidly because the integrity of the microvascular circulation remains intact. As the burn wound heals, it is extremely important during dressing changes, débridement, splinting, and exercise activities to protect the microcirculation from damage because it supplies the reepithelialization process.[4]

One of the major sensory organs of the body is the skin, and it provides constant feedback to the nervous system about the nature and stress of human environment. It contains all the principle sensations of touch, pain, warmth, cold, itch, tickle, and pressure.[4]

Functions of the Skin

The primary functions of the skin are the following: protection, thermoregulation, immunological function, fluid and electrolyte balance, metabolism, neurosensation, and social and interactive functions.[5]

The skin is one of the most active and dynamic organs of the body. It has a direct impact on the ability of the other organ systems to function normally and to adapt to the environment. When the skin is subjected to a burn injury, it has the ability to adapt to this stress; however, the nature, extent, depth, and condition of the burn can greatly be affected by the healing process of the skin.[4]

Burn Wound Classification, Depth, and Clinical Signs

The traditional classification of burn wounds are superficial, superficial partial-thickness, deep partial-thickness, full-thickness, and subdermal burns. Various clinical criteria include cause of the burn, wound appearance, sensation (pinprick test), blanching under pressure, and hair follicle integrity, all of which are used in the assessment of burn depth. Initially, burn depth can be difficult to determine and may change to a deeper injury secondary to desiccation, mechanical injury, and infection. If the burn wound changes to a deeper classification, longer healing time is expected with greater scar formation and possible functional impairment. The burn therapist should think in terms of burn wound dynamics rather than just classification to understand the actual damage the burn injury has caused.[6]

A superficial burn involves the epidermis only. The skin is erythematous, dry with no blisters, painful and tender, exhibits minimal edema, and heals spontaneously in 3 to 7 days with no scarring.[6] (Fig. 21.2)

A superficial partial-thickness burn involves damage to the epidermis and some of the papillary dermis. It is characterized by moderate edema, intact and weeping blister formation, erythema, and significant pain. It typically heals spontaneously by reepithelialization with minimal scarring and possible slight pigmentation changes.[6,7] (Fig. 21.3)

A deep partial-thickness burn damages the tissue that extends into the reticular layers of the dermis and may include fat domes of the subcutaneous layer. It may be mottled white

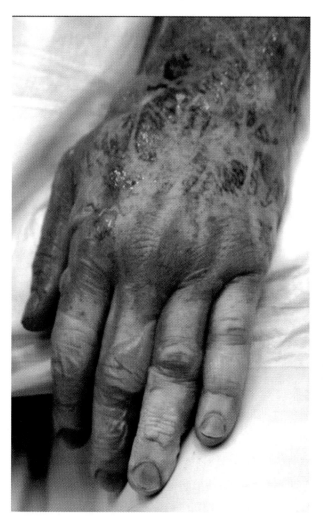

Figure 21•2 *Superficial burn wound.*

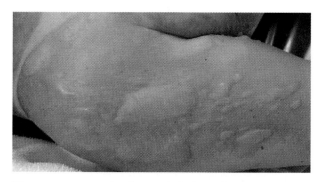

Figure 21•3 *Superficial partial-thickness burn wound.*

(pale) or bright pink to cherry red. It consists of thick-walled large blisters and a very wet surface with marked edema. Healing is slow (21 to 35 days) if no infection is present; however, it may convert to full thickness if infection occurs. Excessive hypertrophic scarring and contractures may develop and result in functional deformities if healing takes longer than 3 weeks.[6] (Fig. 21.4)

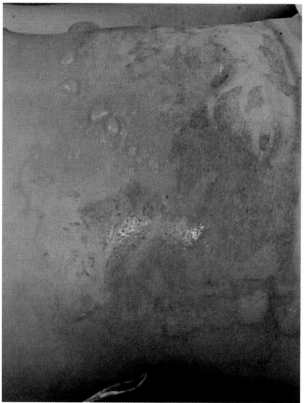

Figure 21•4 *Deep partial-thickness burn wound.*

A full-thickness burn involves the entire thickness of the skin down to and including the subcutaneous tissue. It is mixed waxy white, tan, or charred, with thrombosed blood vessels. Full-thickness injuries are dry, leathery, and rigid, with little or no pain present. Large areas require skin grafting or may need many months to heal, which can result in severe hypertrophic scarring and major deformities. Full-thickness burns also result in altered pigmentation and sensation, decreased elasticity, and decreased sweating.[6] (Fig. 21.5)

A subdermal burn injury extends beyond all skin layers and may include the fascia, muscle, tendon, nerves, or bone. It is dry; charred; mottled brown, white, or red; with no sensation. A subdermal injury requires skin grafting or, possibly, amputation of the involved extremities or digits.[6,8]

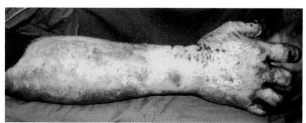

Figure 21•5 *Full-thickness burn wound. Note the white-yellow eschar.*

Burn Wound Healing and Scar Formation

The process of wound healing includes three stages: (1) inflammatory, (2) migration and proliferation of connective tissue cells and blood vessels, and (3) maturation and deposition of new connective tissue matrix.[7]

The ultimate goal of wound management is to allow a wound to close as rapidly as possible, to resemble the original tissue as much as possible, and to produce the least amount of scarring.[9]

Inflammatory Phase

The inflammatory phase of wound healing involves the initial response to trauma, beginning at the time of injury and lasting 3 to 5 days. It has been noted that burn wounds have a lag period before entering the inflammatory phase.[10] The first part of the inflammatory phase is a vascular response, where the main task is to stop hemorrhage. Platelets aid in hemostasis and also initiate the release of the platelet-derived growth factor (PDGF).[10] Damaged cell membranes then activate enzymes that stimulate synthesis of prostaglandins and leukotrienes.

The cellular response is the second phase of inflammation. Growth factors, a subclass of cytokines, stimulate cells to divide and proliferate. Fibrin and another protein, fibronectin, act as a "glue" to hold the wound together until the appearance of collagen; however, if too much fibrin is deposited, cells have difficulty entering the wound. The white "cheesy" layer commonly seen on the surface of a burn wound is actually a combination of fibrin and the topical antimicrobial agent silver sulfadiazine. The fibrinous layer of chronic wounds or burns requires débridement to assist in cellular migration and to improve wound healing.[9]

The inflammatory phase may actually be repeatedly induced surgically in large burn injuries. Therapeutic interventions during the inflammatory stage would include edema reduction, wound care, early range of motion, positioning and splinting, ambulation, and functional activities.[11]

Proliferative Phase

The proliferative phase begins once fibroblasts arrive and collagen production begins to improve the strength of the wound. Reepithelialization occurs at the surface of the wound and deeper granulation tissue, which consists of macrophages that provide the scaffold for cell migration. The red and moist granulation tissue seen in the bottom of wounds open for a period of time acts as a precursor to the formation of scar tissue. Collagen synthesis and angiogenesis lead to an attempt by the wound to contract and close.[9]

In partial-thickness burns, there are still viable skin adnexa from which new epithelium can grow. Typically, deep partial-thickness burns, which will take longer than 3 weeks to heal, are grafted to minimize the development of hypertrophic scarring. During scar formation, altered regulation of the reparative process can lead to abnormal healing. A wound that fails to heal, or requires prolonged healing time, continues to have an inflammatory response; therefore, these wounds are more prone to develop thicker and more erythematous scars. The thickening of "hypertrophic" scars appears to result from an imbalance of collagen synthesis and degradation, but the cause of hypertrophic scarring is unknown.[9] In full-thickness burns, contraction is an important part of wound healing. Contraction begins soon after wounding and peaks at 2 weeks.[10] A large full-thickness burn injury, however, will require grafting to close the wound and to minimize scarring. Therapeutic interventions appropriate for this stage of healing include those performed during the inflammatory phase with the addition of stretching and strengthening exercises. Wound edema at this stage may become chronic and will impact both wound healing and range of motion.[11]

Maturation Phase

In this final phase wound strength continues to improve, but actual collagen content does not change. The scar flattens and becomes less erythematous, appearing to "mature." This phase begins after a few weeks and may last for years until there is no further change in scar appearance. Wound tensile strength continues to increase because collagen fibers are aligned along lines of stress.[9,11] Scar maturation generally takes 6 to 18 months. Race, genetic predisposition, burn depth, type of graft, burn size, patient age, and anatomical location are all factors that influence scar formation. Very fair skinned and black individuals typically demonstrate a higher likelihood of forming a hypertrophic scar.[12] The resulting mature burn scar will never regain the appearance of uninjured dermis, nor will it regain the tensile strength of uninjured tissue. Therapeutic interventions should include range-of-motion exercise, strengthening and reconditioning, functional activities, biophysical technologies, and scar management techniques. During the early maturation phase, the therapist must be careful to avoid mechanical trauma that may damage the newly healed tissue and scar.

Initial Evaluation and Treatment Planning

Evaluation of the burn patient and treatment planning is continuous and changes daily. The initial evaluation is typically performed within 24 to 48 hours of patient admission. Initially, most limitations are due to pain, edema, and constricting eschar.[13] In the instance of an electrical injury, the therapist will also need to perform an in-depth motor and sensory evaluation to document any neuropathy. The results of this evaluation will provide the surgeon with information about any suspected neurological involvement secondary to the passage of electrical current through the body.[13] (Box 21.1)

The burn wound assessment should include the total percentage of the body surface area burned (TBSA), location of the burn, and the depth of the burn. The TBSA and the depth of the burn wound will have an effect on the development of scar contractures. Superficial partial-thickness burns usually heal within a few days to 2 weeks, with minimal to no scarring. Therapeutic interventions involve maintaining the patient's functional status and mobility.[13]

Deep partial-thickness burns often require more than 21 days for healing, presenting a challenge to the therapist due to the resultant scar tissue and surgery required to heal

▶ **Box 21•1** **Acute Burn Evaluation**

- Date of burn and cause
- Associated injuries
- Past medical history
- Age, gender
- Total body surface area burned
- Burn depth
- Edema
- Range of motion
- Sensation
- Family support

- Functional mobility, ambulation
- Neurological status, cognition
- Self-care skills
- Hand dominance
- Hand involvement
- Occupation and educational level
- Leisure activities
- Strength
- Psychological status
- Insurance coverage

these wounds.[13] Full-thickness burns (third degree) will require skin grafting and have been noted to have a four times greater risk to develop increased scar contracture with subsequent loss of motion. Full-thickness burns (fourth degree) from an electrical current or prolonged contact with flame often result in amputation of involved extremities or digits.[8] Muscle paralysis may also occur due to permanent nerve damage.[14]

The anatomical location of the burn wound is an important consideration to anticipate contracture development and to appropriately focus treatment.[13] Contractures interfere with skin and graft healing and are a common problem after burn injury, with reported incidence of 28% to 42%. Contractures of the upper extremity may affect activities of daily living, and lower-extremity contractures interfere with transfers and ambulation. The shoulder is the most frequently contracted joint, followed by the elbow, hand, and knee. TBSA and burn depth have been associated with contracture development, along with a prolonged hospital stay.[15] Limitations in any joint range of motion are noted for treatment-planning purposes. Hand dominance should be recorded for functional and patient self-assessment purposes. If the burn injury involves a single upper extremity, it typically involves the dominant hand. Burns to the hand, especially the palmar surface, will limit grasp during activities of daily living, such as feeding, and in the ability to grasp a walker for ambulation.[13]

Mobility and ambulation are often limited by edema, bandages, and the patients' hesitancy to move due to pain at the time of evaluation. Cardiovascular endurance should be noted and is often limited from the overall systemic and catabolic effects of the burn injury. The initial evaluation should also document family support and the psychological aspect of the burn patient. Additional information of value to the therapist evaluating a burn on an outpatient would be contracture location, limitations in joint range of motion, and scar assessment. The focus of treatment for the therapist is the preservation of joint range of motion, improving function, and the minimization of contractures and scars.

Treating patients during dressing changes allows the therapist to see the burn and to observe the impact that motion has on the wound; however, performing range-of-motion exercises at this time can lead to increased pain because of exposed

nerve endings. Bedside treatments offer an advantage if the dressings are not adherent to the wound because they act as padding for the therapist's hand placement during passive or active-assistive range-of-motion exercises.[13] The importance of bed mobility and positioning change must not be overlooked. Instructing the patient or nurse about frequent bed position changes assists in preventing further tissue damage.[13]

Permission to ambulate is a medical decision. The current tendency is to begin out-of-bed activities and ambulation much earlier than was previously the case because prolonged bedrest will affect the patient's overall endurance.[13] Pain and hypotension secondary to lower-extremity burns often interfere with ambulation. If the posterior surface of the lower extremity is involved, patients assume the position of ankle plantar flexion, with either extreme knee flexion or knee extension and trunk flexion.[13]

Transporting patients to the rehabilitation department will depend on hospital policy. Treatment outside the protective environment of the patient's room encourages interaction with other patients and provides a sense of progress in burn recovery. The accomplishments of basic tasks such as feeding, grooming, and personal hygiene add to the patients feeling of accomplishment, and assistive devices or adaptations should be provided.[13]

Whenever possible, patient treatment should coincide with pain medication administration. Analgesics and intramuscular narcotics require approximately 20 to 30 minutes before they are effective. Frequency, duration, and intensity of treatment are all governed by patient tolerance, pain, and progress.[13] Splinting and proper positioning should be adjuncts to treatment in the prevention of burn scar contracture and the regaining of functional independence. Resumption of exercise after grafting will depend on the protocol of the treatment facility. Typically, with grafts that are fixated with sutures or staples, an immobilization period of 5 to 7 days is observed. Fibrin sealant has been found effective in the fixation of grafts by providing wounds with a scaffold for the ingrowth of fibroblasts and capillary endothelial cells.[16] The use of fibrin glue graft fixation and earlier mobilization has been found to provide better functional results in the treatment of hand burns.[17] Some burn surgeons advocate gentle range-of-motion exercise on postoperative day 1 when fibrin sealant is used for graft adherence.

When a burn patient experiences a limitation in motion due to pain, the therapist needs to ask, "Is it stretching pain or pinching pain?" Stretching pain results from the attempted elongation of tissue and is concentrated to the focused area of treatment. When treating an area of circumferential burns, pain that limits motion occurs on the surface opposite that being stretched. The tender tissue may be folding upon itself and causing a "pinching" pain.[13]

In the treatment of contractures, a retrospective study by Richards compared patients treated with a multimodal approach (massage, exercises, pressure) with those treated with a progressive treatment program (static or dynamic splints, serial casting). Results found significantly fewer days were required to correct the contractures in the progressive treatment group.[18,19]

Positioning the Burn Patient

Positioning focuses on decreasing edema, preventing tissue destruction, and maintaining tissue in an elongated state. Positioning must also focus on preventing localized neuropathies of the ulnar or peroneal nerves. Should a patient have difficulty maintaining range of motion between exercise sessions, then positioning may be required at all times, except for dressing changes and exercise. Conversely, should a patient be able to maintain gains made in range of motion, then positioning would be appropriate at night only.[20] (Fig. 21.6)

Neck

The use of pillows should be avoided with anterior neck burns to prevent chondritis of the ears. Eighty-three percent of burn centers position the patient's neck in neutral or slight hyperextension during the emergent phase and continue until wound closure.[21] Care should be taken to avoid respiratory compromise. The use of a towel roll placed under the patients' shoulders will provide neck extension. If a neck burn is asymmetrical, a lateral flexion contracture may develop. The neck should be positioned with the head in midline using towel rolls, rolled sheets, or IV bags placed lateral to the head on the same side as the burn.[11,20]

Trunk

Lateral trunk burns, if left untreated, can lead to scoliosis. Foam wedges or blanket rolls can be used while the patient is in bed to maintain proper trunk alignment.

With an anterior chest burn, the shoulder girdle will protract, resulting in a rounded shoulder posture. Having the patient lie supine on a rolled sheet that is positioned along the length of the spine provides sustained stretch to the anterior chest and trunk.

Shoulder

Burns involving the anterior axilla can lead to the development of a posture of shoulder adduction and internal rotation. Therefore, shoulder abduction and external rotation is the position of choice.

Axillary burns are positioned with the shoulder in 90 degrees of abduction with 15 to 20 degrees of horizontal adduction to avoid stretch and compression of the brachial plexus.[20] Some therapists feel that shoulder flexion of 130 to 150 degrees with external rotation for short time periods can be done without damaging the brachial plexus.[20]

Arm slings or Murphy slings are made of stockinet and attached to an IV pole. These slings provide both extremity elevation and shoulder abduction.[20] (Fig. 21.7) Foam abduction wedges or abduction troughs can be purchased commercially or fabricated by the therapist. A high-density foam abduction airplane splint has been found to be less time consuming to fabricate and provides ideal positioning in either the supine or prone position.[22] The abduction angle can be easily increased with the addition of a second wedge piece versus remolding of

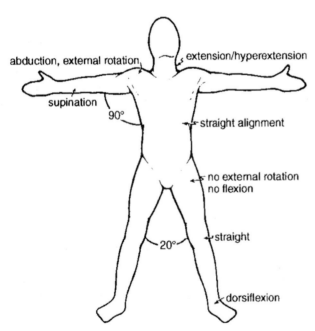

Figure 21•6 *Positioning for the prevention of contractures. From: Apfel, L, Irwin, C, Staley, M, et al: Fig 10-1. In: Richards, R, Staley, M (eds): Burn Care and Rehabilitation. Philadelphia, FA Davis, 1994.*

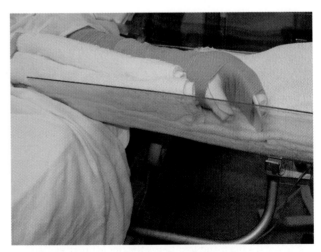

Figure 21•7 *Bedside abduction troughs for upper-extremity positioning.*

the thermoplastic conformer. The foam is sealed in plastic so the collection of exudate is not an issue.[22] Positioning of the shoulders while the patient is sitting can be accomplished using a lap tray, bedside table, or blanket rolls. When tissue integrity permits, figure eight clavicle straps can be used to pull the shoulders into retraction. Shoulder range of motion of 135 degrees has been considered to be a good functional outcome since most patients are able to perform their activities of daily living with this range.

Elbow

Antecubital fossa burns and circumferential burn to the upper extremity can lead to a combined elbow flexion and forearm pronation contracture.[20] Elbow extension is often more difficult to regain than is elbow flexion. Devices that are used for shoulder positioning can be used for the elbow so that the elbow is extended and the forearm is positioned in supination or in neutral. Thermoplastic elbow splints are used at night to maintain elbow extension.

Forearm, Wrist, and Hand

Volar surface burns predispose the patient to wrist flexion and forearm pronation contractures, while dorsal surface burns may cause wrist extension contractures.[20] The forearm is generally positioned in supination with the wrist extended, except when there is an isolated dorsal wrist burn. The recommended functional position of the wrist is from neutral to a 30-degree extension. Initially, a small towel or gauze roll placed in the palm of the hand can be used to position the wrist into extension.[20]

The hand must be elevated to decrease edema and minimize dense, soft tissue fibrotic contracture formation. The use of foam wedges and blanket or sheet rolls provides an effective method to elevate the extremity.

Lower Extremity

Lower-extremity burns are positioned with the hips in neutral rotation with slight abduction. Patients will tend to position themselves in the "frog position" of external rotation and knee flexion, which increases the risk for peroneal nerve palsy and resultant foot drop. Towel or blanket rolls, foam wedges, or lower-extremity abduction wedges all effectively position the lower extremities. (Fig 21.8) Prone positioning, if the patient can tolerate it, is excellent for stretching tight hip flexors. Burns to the posterior aspect of the leg can lead to a flexion contracture of the knee.

Posterior knee conformer splints, custom molded to position the knees in full extension, are often the most effective way to manage posterior knee burns should contractures develop.

Plantar flexion contractures are common, and a footboard can be used to maintain neutral ankle position; however, a splint is preferable to a footboard, especially in the noncompliant patient.[20]

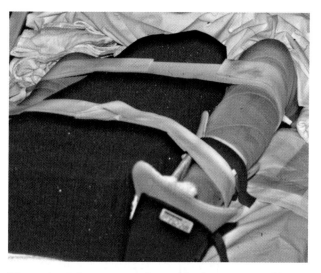

Figure 21•8 *Lower-extremity positioning to prevent hip external rotation and knee flexion using AFOs and foam abduction wedge.*

Splinting the Burn Patient

Splints have been used in burn care to support and protect the burn, maintain joint position, and prevent or correct deformity. In the acute phase, splinting is used to immobilize and decrease edema. During the wound-healing phase, splints may prevent the development of contracture; however, special care is required to ensure the splints do not interfere with healing as the result of improper placement or fit. In the rehabilitation phase, splinting is used to reduce contractures, prevent deformity, maintain natural body contours, and complement pressure therapy. Splints typically immobilize a joint at its end range and are adjusted as increases in range of motion are made. Following reconstructive procedures, splints are used for restoring function and maintaining gains made due to surgical contracture release. Splints applied following reconstructive procedures are usually molded directly to the site and should be monitored closely for evidence of wound maceration or breakdown.[23] Splints can be static, dynamic, or serial static. According to Colditz, the stage of healing will determine the type of splinting used.[24] Static splints are used during the acute or inflammatory phase, while dynamic and serial static splints are used during the proliferative stage of healing. Serial static splints, casting, or dynamic splints are best used during the maturation phase. Initially, most dynamic splints are worn for 20 to 30 minutes, but it is important to monitor the splint and check for pressure point areas. The timing of splint application to the hand requires a sound understanding of the healing tissue.[24]

When a burn injury extends to involve either the joint or tendon, the goal of splinting would be to stabilize the joint or to immobilize the tendon in a slack position to prevent rupture.

Often, the position of comfort is the position of deformity. Splints applied to prevent such deformities are used as a means to maintain gains in range of motion and to apply a sustained stretch to contracting scar tissue. Serial splints or

> ▶ **PEARL 21•1** The position of comfort is the position of contracture. Positioning should focus on the prevention of deformity. Positioning should also focus on preventing compression neuropathies.

serial casting can be used to restore function by providing sustained stretch to scar contractures and are used to maintain gains following treatment. Effective splinting applies a sustained force for an extended period of time, resulting in tissue elongation.[24]

Splinting material is constructed as either perforated or solid. Splints fabricated from solid materials are occlusive and can cause maceration unless there is an absorbent dressing covering the wound or adequate skin hygiene is performed.

> **PEARL 21•2** A broad variety of splinting options exist for the management of burn injury. A listing of several of these are included in this chapter, along with associated advantages and disadvantages.

Common Burn Splints
Neck
Soft Cervical Collar

Circumferential foam neck orthosis is generally used when tissue is fragile.[23]

Advantages
- Commercially available and simple to apply
- Can be used in any phase of healing
- Maintains neutral extension

Disadvantages
- Absorbent; requires replacement cover
- Used more for positioning than compression

Molded Neck Splint

A molded splint provides total-contact rigid neck support.[23] (Fig. 21.9)

Advantages
- Rigid definitive pressure with exact contour of surface
- Low-temperature material molded directly onto the patient; can be used for serial splinting

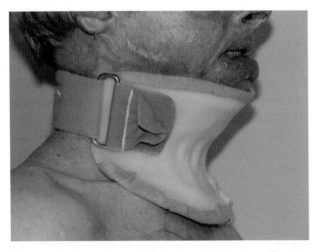

Figure 21•9 *Custom-molded thermoplastic neck-conforming orthosis.*

- High-temperature silicone-lined material molded over a positive mold of the patient's neck
- Maintains exact position

Disadvantages
- Occlusive, with the potential for skin breakdown
- Potential for skin breakdown over bony areas, chin, or clavicle

Dynamic Antitorticollis Strap and Neck Splint

The dynamic anticorticollis strap is applied while the patient is in bed to gently rotate the head and neck toward the neutral position.[25]

Advantages
- Can be applied immediately after burn without compromising wound healing
- In combination, provides 24-hour neck positioning
- Adjustable and low cost

Disadvantages
- Must monitor frequently for potential pressure areas

Watusi Collar

This flexible neck orthosis allows neck range of motion and provides circumferential pressure to the neck.[26]

Advantages
- Made from items available in hospital and fabric stores
- Applied 2 weeks after grafting; can be worn 23 hours a day
- Life span of collar reportedly 3 months

Disadvantages
- Patients possibly sensitive to silicone or have skin breakdown
- Used primarily in children

Mouth/Oral Commissure

Microstomia caused by facial burns can result in a decrease in the ability to open the mouth and is typically treated with oral appliances.[18] A review by Dougherty and Ward discussed 37 devices listed by the type of stretch provided: horizontal, vertical, and circumoral.[27] Serghiou and colleagues surveyed the management of facial burns and reported that during the acute phase, 84% of therapists initiate splinting with microstomia devices.[18,21]

The Microstomia Prevention Appliance® (MPA; MPA Co., Dallas, TX) is a prefabricated oral orthosis used to preserve horizontal mouth opening. The splint consists of two acrylic sections fitted onto two curved stainless-steel bars, with a set screw used to secure the device. (Fig. 21.10)

Advantages
- Commercially available in three sizes, easily applied and fitted
- Adjusted for progressive stretch

Disadvantages
- Must be removed for eating; drooling a problem
- Must be monitored for pressure necrosis in corners of mouth

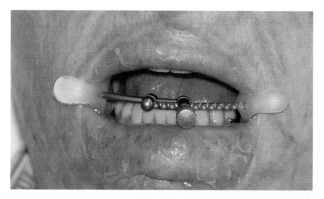

Figure 21•10 *Microstomia device (MPA) for horizontal commissures contracture.*

External Traction Hooks

Thermoplastic "hooks" that fit in the oral commissures and attach to elastic that encircles the head are used for stretching horizontally.[23] (Fig. 21.11)

Advantages
- Can be fabricated using low- or high-temperature plastic; easily applied
- Tension easily adjusted by patient

Disadvantages
- Must be monitored for pressure necrosis

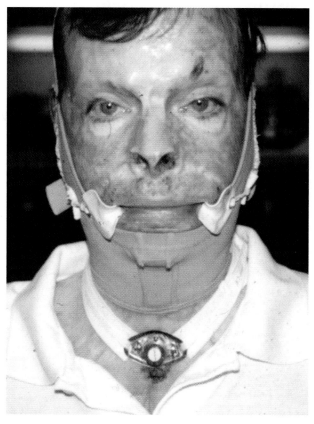

Figure 21•11 *External traction hook for horizontal microstomia contracture.*

Vertical Microstomia Splints

Modified dynamic mouth splints provide vertical stretch. Only four vertical stretching devices are described in the literature.[27] Two recent studies described the use of thermoplastic splinting material and either a coiled helix spring or a long-thread screw.[28,29]

Advantages
- Patients report comfortable and easy to use
- Threaded screw orthosis can be made by therapist; low cost

Disadvantages
- The coiled helix spring orthosis made by a dentist
- Skin or lip breakdown a possible complication of either splint

No orthosis will be ideal for every patient, and success depends on patient compliance. Most of the appliances described in the literature are to be worn continuously for an average of 6 months, then changing to night wear only.[27]

Axilla and Anterior Chest

Airplane Splint, Thermoplastic Conformer

Early extended grafting, postoperative splinting, and intensive range-of-motion exercises beginning 5 days after grafting have been found to be effective in the treatment of axillary burns and the prevention of contracture.[30]

Advantages
- Formed on the patient; used in any phase of burn treatment
- Made as conforming splint or open frame joined by a connecting bar that supports the extremity and attaches to piece at the hip[31,32]

Disadvantages
- Must strap securely to avoid migration and pressure points
- Reinforcement may be required to support the arm

Clavicle Strap

A figure eight clavicle strap can be used early in the posthealing phase. An early version consisted of semilunar S-shaped foam pads retained with a figure eight elasticized wrap.[33] Modifications of the figure eight strap have been used after axillary contracture release.[34] In a study by Obaidullah and colleagues, the use of a figure eight sling proved beneficial after axillary contracture release and skin grafting in preventing the recurrence of an axillary contracture. The sling was worn continuously for the first 3 months and then only during the day. The patient was able to continue with daily activities, and compliance was improved.[34] (Fig. 21.12)

Advantages
- Commercially available and adjustable
- Can be made by the therapist
- Minimizes protraction of the shoulders

Disadvantages
- Can cause chaffing or irritation of the anterior axilla
- Can constrict circulation in the upper extremities
- Can be difficult to apply

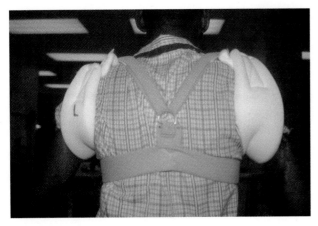

Figure **21•12** *Figure eight clavicle strap.*

Elbow and Knee

Elbow or Knee Conformer

A conforming splint is applied to the extensor or flexor surface of the arm or leg.[23]

Advantages

- Formed directly on patient; distributes pressure along length of the splint
- Used in serial splinting; can be remolded to accommodate increases in range of motion (ROM)

Disadvantages

- Potential for ulnar or peroneal nerve compression; flare splint over area to avoid pressure

Dynamic Supination Splint

Used to increase forearm supination. The latest splint design is a "corkscrew" about the axis of the forearm rotation that pulls the forearm towards a supinated position.

Advantages

- Dynamic splint that does not limit elbow flexion and extension, therefore the patient can perform activities of daily living
- Provides for a low load prolonged stretch to burn scar contracture

Disadvantages

- Technically requires advanced splinting skills
- Must be monitored for migration and pressure areas

Hip

Abduction Brace

Thermoplastic cuffs are applied to the medial and posterior aspects of the thighs and separated with a thermoplastic bar.[23]

Advantages

- Used to preserve hip extension and abduction and to prevent internal rotation, adduction, and hip flexion

Disadvantages

- Can only be used while patient lying down

Ankle

Posterior Ankle-Foot Splint

The conforming construction makes the splint useful for serial splinting.[23] (Fig. 21.13)

Advantages

- Maintains functional position of the ankle; prevents shortening of the Achilles tendon
- Commercially available or custom fabricated from low-temperature thermoplastic
- Can be lengthened to include the knee

Disadvantages

- Heel area must be flared to minimize pressure necrosis of heel
- Not used in ambulation

Foot

Toe Conformer

The toe conformer is applied to the dorsum of the foot to prevent or correct a hyperextension toe deformity.[23]

Advantages

- Can be used under soft shoes to apply pressure to the contracting scar

Disadvantages

- Shearing may be a problem during ambulation

Casting the Burn Patient

Casts are used for postoperative immobilization to prevent graft movement and to minimize scar formation. Casting is also used when traditional splinting methods fail. Casts maintain a static position while providing constant stretch and pressure to the contracted burn scar. Indications for use include patients nonadherent with traditional splinting, failure of gains with traditional splinting, or with children. Serial

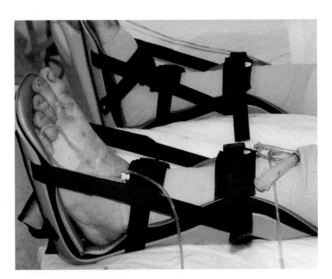

Figure **21•13** *Ankle-foot orthosis to prevent heel cord tightening and plantar flexion contracture.*

plaster casting has been found to be effective for increasing range of motion and is effective in both the inpatient and outpatient setting. Casting provides low-force, long-duration stretch that results in realignment of collagen fibers into an elongated state.[35,36,37] Serial casting was found effective in increasing range of motion in the elbow and knee joints versus wrist and ankle.[36] (Fig. 21.14)

Casting materials can be either plaster bandage or synthetic fiberglass casting tape. Before casting, the therapist needs to discuss the plan of treatment with the patient, assess joint range of motion, and assess skin integrity and presence of wounds. Plaster casting is best used over wounds as the plaster permits wicking of drainage. A cast change every 1 to 2 days is recommended for large open wounds. If the wound is small, casts can be left on up to 1 week.[35] The use of range-of-motion exercises prior to casting is important. The therapist should also consider the potential for nerve compression from the cast and monitor distal circulation. Contraindications to casting are heterotopic ossification, excessive edema, poor medical or social situation, and an agitated patient.[35] Casts can be bivalved so they can be removed for hygiene, skin lubrication, and range of motion.

Plaster, a gypsum-impregnated cloth bandage, is the most common casting material and is usually applied in four to six layers (<¼ inch thick). Setting time for extra-fast-setting plaster is 2 to 4 minutes, and 5 to 8 minutes for fast-setting and elastic plaster.[23]

Advantages of Plaster Casting

- Easy to mold with low cost
- Good conformity/contouring
- Low incidence of allergic reaction
- Can be removed without cast cutter by soaking and cutting off
- Allows for air circulation, which decreases the chance of skin maceration

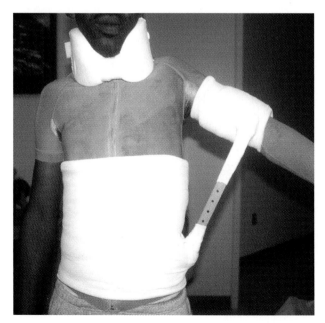

Figure 21•14 *Airplane axillary cast for axillary contracture.*

Disadvantages of Plaster

- Increased weight, messy, and longer drying time
- Prone to indentations that may cause skin breakdown[35]
- Sensitivity to water exposure

Synthetic casting tape consists of polyester or fiberglass fabric impregnated with polyurethane resin. Fiberglass casting material is usually applied in three to four layers and has a setting time of 2 to 8 minutes.

Advantages of Fiberglass

- Lightweight with shorter drying time, less mess
- Strong, with minimal layers

Disadvantages of Fiberglass

- Decreased ease of molding/contouring
- Higher cost versus plaster
- Higher peak curing temperature than plaster
- Must wear gloves when applying and must use a cast cutter to remove
- Abrasive outer surface[35]

Tubular stockinet and Webril® padding (Kendall Co., Mansfield, MA) are recommended under both types of casting materials due to the burn patient's fragile skin. Padding should be kept to a minimum to prevent cast slippage. Cast felt can be used to pad over bony prominences. Appropriate skin care, standard wound care treatment, and scar management (compressive wraps, silicone) can be used under the cast.

> ▶ **PEARL 21•3** The phase of wound healing determines the type of splint used. Static splints are used in the acute or inflammatory phase. Serial static and dynamic splints are used in the proliferative phase. Serial static and dynamic splints or casts are used in the maturation phase.

Exercise

Exercise, in conjunction with positioning and splinting, is an essential part of a burn patient's rehabilitation program.[38] Therapists often feel uneasy exercising a burn patient due to the large extensive areas of burn, pain experienced by the patient, and the fear of causing further tissue damage. Burn patients and their families may not understand why such exercises and painful treatments are important in the rehabilitation process.[38]

The ultimate goal of a burn rehabilitation program is to assist the patient to return into society at the most optimal functional level as possible compared to his or her preinjury status. Therapeutic exercise is used to prevent contracture development, increase range of motion, and increase function. Most burn units will perform exercises two times daily. It may take only 1 to 4 days for a burn scar contracture to develop. Exercise should focus on those areas most likely to contract, with attention to contiguous areas of scar tissue that cross multiple neighboring joints.[38] The longer a fibrotic contracture exists, the more difficult it will be to regain optimal mobility of soft tissue due to nonextensible adhesion and scar tissue formation.[39]

Immediately following a major burn injury, there is a great demand placed on the cardiovascular system as a result of fluid shifts and hemodynamic changes. Avoid strenuous exercise of patients with preexisting cardiac or pulmonary problems.[38] The burn patient will often have an increase in resting heart rate resulting in lower cardiac reserves for any range-of-motion or mobility training. When exercising the burn patient in the intensive care unit, the therapist must monitor both the patient's heart rate and blood pressure. Cardiac dysrhythmias are common after electrical injuries.[14] Initially, exercise will focus on reducing edema. If the patient is alert and can assist, then active exercises are performed. As edema decreases, the focus of exercise then becomes preserving range of motion and functional strength. Patients of all ages should exercise more frequently for shorter periods of time; however, as the depth of burn injury increases, so should the emphasis on exercise.[38]

Contraindications to exercise include exposed joints, tendon exposure over the proximal interphalangeal joints of the finger, thrombophlebitis, deep vein thrombosis, and compartment syndrome. Depending on the surgeon's postoperative policy, exercise to areas following skin grafting may not be permitted. Typically, an immobilization period of 5 to 7 days is observed. Exercise continues for all other joints not grafted. When cultured skin is used for graft coverage, exercise therapy is discouraged by the manufacturer for 10 days.[38] Active range-of-motion exercises are preferred to minimize stress to the new graft.

Passive range of motion (PROM) is frequently used to maintain joint and connective tissue mobility and as a method to obtain full joint range of motion. PROM is used to minimize the formation of contractures and should be performed gently and slowly, with precautions taken to avoid overstretching joint structures.[39]

Active-assistive ranges of motion (A-AROM) exercises are performed when a patient has difficulty completing full range of motion. A-AROM also aids in decreasing the physiological energy demands placed on a patient during times of high metabolic stress.[38] The use of overhead pulleys and or static weight can be used to elongate scar tissue. Slow, prolonged sustained stretch is the preferred method of elongating tissue and is very effective when preceded by a heat modality. Forced joint motion, which pushes the scar tissue well beyond blanching, may damage the joint and induce heterotopic ossification.[11]

Active range of motion (AROM) is often less painful and is used when a patient can achieve full range of motion. AROM should be encouraged for any body area not burned to preserve joint ROM, prevent muscle atrophy, or to strengthen weakened muscles.[38] When performing A-AROM or AROM exercises, the patient must be taught proper motions and not be allowed to substitute with trunk side bending or shoulder shrugging.[39]

Stretching interventions are designed to elongate the contractile elements and increase extensibility of soft tissues. Soft tissue structures are taken beyond their available length to increase ROM during stretching exercises. Stretching can be performed manually by the therapist or performed independently by the patient after careful instruction. There are many types of stretching exercises, including manual, mechanical, and self stretching. Effective stretching techniques require proper positioning of the patient and adequate stabilization. Most stretching techniques are performed with the patient supine. Contraindications to stretching are bony block, acute inflammatory processes, or when there is sharp acute pain with joint motion. A low-load, long-duration stretch is considered the safest and yields the most changes in soft tissue and scar. Studies have shown low-intensity, prolonged mechanical stretching using a cuff weight or a weight-pulley system to be effective, particularly in long-standing contractures. Mechanical stretch duration reported in the literature ranges from 30 minutes to as long as 8 to 10 hours. The latter stretch duration would be provided by serial casts or splints.[40]

Proprioceptive neuromuscular facilitation (PNF) patterns of movement may be used in PROM, A-AROM, or AROM.[39] PNF pattern stretching techniques can be used as an adjunct to manual stretching or self-stretching, but were found to be less appropriate for stretching fibrotic contractures. Integrating functional activities into a stretching program uses the gained range of motion to perform activities of daily living. The application of superficial heat (paraffin) is used primarily for small areas and may be applied before or during the stretching procedure. Soft tissue friction massage is often used prior to stretching to increase the mobility of scar tissue.[40]

Therapists must be aware of any breakdown or self-release of tissues with repetitive stretch. A fine balance exists between collagen tissue breakdown and repair. Continued low-grade inflammation from repetitive stress can cause excessive collagen formation and hypertrophic scarring.[40]

Conditioning exercises include both strengthening and endurance and should be started after complete ROM has been achieved consistently. Burn injury results in severe deconditioning and fatigue that can impact function. A 3-year outcome study performed at Harborview Medical Center revealed an almost universal complaint of fatigue as a major barrier in return to work or other daily activities.[41] When implementing a strengthening program, the muscles opposing scar tissue contractures should be strengthened. For example, if the antecubital space of the elbow is burned, then exercises designed to strengthen the triceps should be emphasized.[38] Conditioning exercises are started during the maturation phase of healing.[11] Exercise programs consisting of up to 30 minutes of treadmill walking have demonstrated a favorable effect on the aerobic capacity of participants.[41] (Figs. 21.15 and 21.16)

Functional exercise can begin early in the patient's hospital recovery course and serves to increase self-esteem and satisfaction.[11,38] Functional activities such as personal hygiene and eating should become a focus of treatment. These activities also provide movement patterns and use joint ROM. An example would be eating hand to mouth, using elbow flexion and forearm supination, some shoulder flexion, abduction, and lateral rotation.[39] (Fig. 21.17)

Newly healed scars and grafts are fragile and can blister easily. Compression garments may need to be removed during exercise until the skin integrity permits exercise with the compression garments.

There are various early ambulation protocols, with times ranging from 3 days to 7 days. Patients begin ambulation when

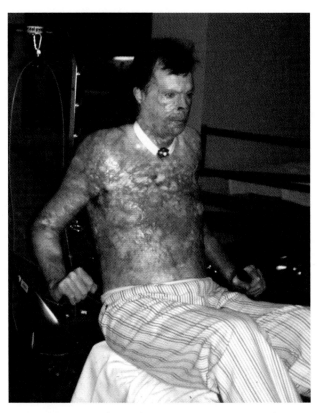

Figure 21•15 *Total gym for upper-extremity strengthening.*

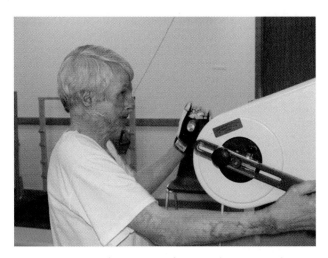

Figure 21•16 *Cycle restorator for reconditioning and upper-extremity strengthening.*

vital signs are stable and they are able to bear weight on the lower extremities. Partial- or full-thickness burns to the lower extremities will require elastic bandage wrapping prior to ambulation or whenever the lower extremities are in a dependent position. Elastic wraps are applied in a figure eight pattern and provide vascular support to help control edema and pain from dependency.[42] Compression wraps will also reduce the risk of deep vein thrombosis.[14]

The benefits of early ambulation are known, but it is often difficult to mobilize a previously bedridden patient with

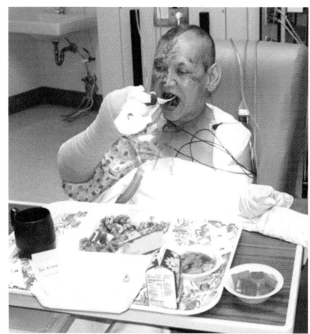

Figure 21•17 *Functional exercise.*

major burns. An alternative method is to place the patient on a tilt table and gradually tilt the patient to an upright position. This is an effective treatment for orthostatic hypotension, but does little to improve lower-extremity strength or mobility. Trees and colleagues reported use of a modified tilt table that allowed patients to perform weight-bearing exercises, such as an inclined squat in a gravity-reduced environment. They found patients demonstrated greater knee flexion and the patients were able to progressively strengthen their lower extremities.[43]

Some facilities advocate the use of video documentation to assist patients in retaining the information they receive during therapy sessions.[44] Video documentation assists both the patient and caregiver in the performance of the patient's home program.

Exercises for Specific Areas

Face

Facial exercises focus on the prevention of ectropion (contracture of the eyelid) and microstomia (narrowing of the oral orifice) contractures.[38] Some of the exercises suggested include the following:

- Tightly close and open eyes
- Open mouth as wide as possible, smile, say "EEE"
- Place fingers in the commissures of the mouth and pull laterally
- Blow bubbles

Neck

- Look up to the ceiling, keeping the mouth closed, while sitting in a chair
- Keeping mouth closed, turn chin toward each shoulder
- Laterally flex neck so ear moves toward the shoulder

Trunk

- Side-lie over a bolster
- Reach, while twisting trunk, to grasp objects; can be performed sitting or standing

Upper Extremity

- PNF patterns using cane exercises
- Pulleys, wall climbing, or finger ladder; catching and throwing a ball; wand or T-bar

Note: Assistive pulley exercises are easily misused by the patient, resulting in compression of the humerus against the acromion process. Proper shoulder mechanics should be stressed to the patient.

- Activities of daily living such as combing hair, eating
- Shooting baskets, throwing Velcro® darts
- Reciprocal exercise unit; upper or lower body ergometer[39]

Hand

- Pegs into pegboard, molding putty
- Differential tendon glide, full fisting
- Wringing a washcloth

Lower Extremity

- Total gym, bicycle
- Kicking a ball, marching games
- Laying prone with weight applied at ankle to stretch posterior knee contracture

▶ **PEARL 21•4** Due to the great demand placed on the cardiovascular system as a result of fluid shifts and hemodynamic changes, caution should be taken to avoid strenuous exercise of patients with preexisting cardiac or pulmonary problems.

Heterotopic Ossification

Heterotopic ossification (HO), a periarticular bone formation, has been reported to occur in 1% to 23% of burn patients. The onset is usually insidious, and the etiology in burn patients is unknown. Therapists are usually the first to suspect HO, with common findings of a sudden decrease in range of motion, pain, and localized edema. The elbow is the most common joint involved, and there can be entrapment of the ulnar nerve with associated sensory and motor deficit. A study by Hunt and colleagues reported that 95% of joints that developed HO had either adjacent or overlying partial- or full-thickness burns, and there was prolonged closure of the overlying area.[45] Overzealous manipulation has been suspected. Once a diagnosis of HO is confirmed by x-ray, passive stretching and active-assistive range of motion exercises beyond the range of pain-free motion should be avoided. Therapy will require modification, but range of motion within a pain-free range should continue.[46]

Surgical excision is considered when the patient's ROM decreases to the point of interfering with activities of daily living (ADLs), there are signs of ulnar nerve entrapment, or the patient is unable to perform therapy. Surgery is successful in improving ROM, and the use of continuous passive motion (CPM) has been used postoperatively. Injury to the ulnar nerve is the most significant complication, and the therapist will need to manage this deficit with appropriate splinting and therapy.[45]

▶ **PEARL 21•5** Once heterotopic ossification is confirmed, passive stretching and active-assistive range-of-motion exercises beyond the range of pain-free motion should be avoided.

Biophysical Technologies

Therapists involved in burn care use biophysical energies as an adjunct to treatment, although there is little supportive evidence in the literature. Paraffin has been used in treating burn scar contractures in combination with sustained stretch, and it can increase collagen extensibility, make the skin more pliable, decrease joint discomfort, and increase joint ROM.[7] Paraffin has been used in other patient populations where skin tightness and musculoskeletal problems occur.[47] Paraffin is used in burn rehabilitation as a superficial heat modality to increase tissue extensibility prior to stretching. Some therapists find it useful to apply paraffin to a joint surface area while the joint is placed in a stretch position. The mineral oil found in paraffin lowers the melting point that provides the lower specific heat, allowing paraffin to be used on the newly healed skin of the burn patient.[48] If the patient can not tolerate the "dip and wrap" technique, the paraffin can be painted on the area.[7] A modified method for paraffin application has been described using pieces of mesh gauze dipped in paraffin and applied to the scar area. Plastic wrap and a towel are applied over the area, and a gentle, long stretch is applied.[7] Caution should be taken when using paraffin on fragile skin or areas of decreased sensation.[7] Moist heat with adequate padding can be used for applying heat to larger surface areas during stretching. (Fig. 21.18) The use of ultrasound for scar management is inconclusive. An early study by Ward et al found the effect of ultrasound on range of motion and pain was not predictable.[49]

Management of Hand Burns

Burns to the hands are common due to their exposed position. It has been reported that 50% of hand burns occur in the work environment.[18,50] Although each hand represents less that 3% of the TBSA, burns to the hands can result in deformities that are devastating. The ultimate goal of hand burn management should be to maximize and restore function. Range of motion and grip strength are important, but the individual's ability to use his or her hands in daily tasks must not be overlooked.[50]

Deep second- and third-degree burns of the hand are excised and grafted, which achieves reduced hospital stay and lower costs.[51] Deeper fourth-degree hand burns involve tendon, bone, and joints and requires débridement of nonviable tissue. Surgical management includes flaps, K-wire, or amputation, and there is often moderate to severe long-term hand impairment with this type of burn.[51] (Fig. 21.19)

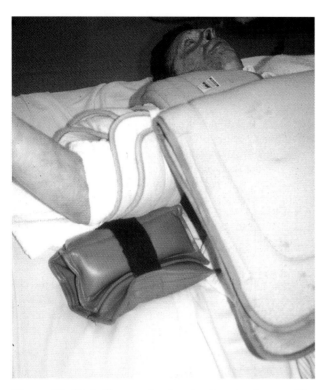

Figure 21•18 *Axillary contracture treatment using paraffin, moist heat, and positional stretch.*

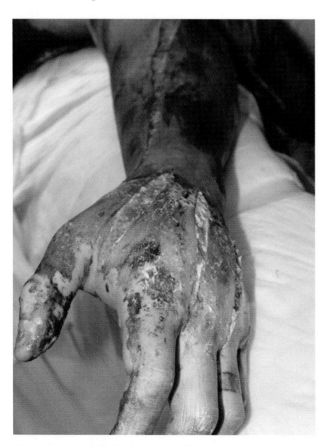

Figure 21•19 *Full-thickness hand burn after escharotomies. Note claw deformity of the hand.*

The three most common deformities seen in the burned hand are thumb web-space contracture, proximal interphalangeal joint flexion contractures, and fifth-digit boutonniere deformities.[52] Burns of the dorsum of the hand, edema, and later the force of the contracting scar can pull the metacarpophalangeal (MP) joints into hyperextension with the interphalangeal (IP) joints flexed or hyperextended, resulting in a claw hand deformity. Flattening of the transverse and longitudinal arches occurs, and the fifth digit may be ulnarly rotated. The thenar web is contracted, and the thumb is pulled into extension and adduction. Scarring in the interdigital web spaces pulls the digits together.[7] Burns of the extensor surface of the hand, where the skin is thinner, can result in an exposed tendon and in either a boutonniere or mallet deformity. A boutonniere deformity involves the extensor apparatus at the proximal IP (PIP) joint and can be the result of direct thermal injury or of tendon ischemia. Exposed tendons should be covered with a moist protective dressing to prevent desiccation prior to splinting. Other causes of a boutonniere deformity occurs at the PIP joint secondary to volar scar banding or remodeling of the volar plate and collateral ligaments in combination with shortened oblique retinacular ligaments. Dorsal hooding or syndactyly is the loss of the dorsal digital web spaces and can result from inadequate positioning following a dorsal hand burn. Splinting should position the MCP (metacarpophalangeal) joints in flexion of at least 65 to 70 degrees, which preserves the length of the collateral ligaments.[53]

Palmar hand burns can result in loss of the palmar web and loss of thumb and finger extension and abduction. A 1-cm scar contracture in an adult hand may cause little loss of motion, whereas that same contracture in a child's hand may cause a more significant loss of motion.[7]

Sensory impairment can be functionally devastating with permanent sensory deficits following thermal injury regardless of burn depth. Although the information is far from conclusive, the therapist should anticipate the probability of impaired sensation in all hand burns involving the dermis.[7,53] Rehabilitation of the burned hand includes edema reduction, range-of-motion exercises, splinting, and compression.

Edema

In superficial partial-thickness hand burns, edema is usually minor, whereas in deep partial-thickness or full-thickness burns edema is more severe and prolonged.[53] Intervention is necessary to prevent fibrosis and ischemic necrosis of the intrinsic muscles of the hand.[7] Treatment of hand edema can be accomplished by elevation, manual massage, external elastic support, and range-of-motion exercises. A combination of compression wrap with continuous retrograde massage was found effective in reducing hand and finger edema.[54]

Exercise

With deep dorsal hand burns, repeated flexion and extension or forced composite flexion should be avoided to prevent possible rupture of the extensor mechanism. Isolated active or passive MCP joint range with the IPs extended, followed by hook fist exercises, will impose less stress on the fragile extensor tendon.[53] Should the wound be considered superficial, or once adequate tissue coverage is obtained, then gentle ROM exercises to increase flexion may begin.[38] Overly aggressive passive range-of-motion exercises constantly injure the fragile new tissue, resulting in an increase of collagen deposition and, consequently, more scarring.[7] Brand and Hollister recommend short, frequent periods of light and repetitive active ROM exercises to prevent joint stiffness.[53,55]

Once there is graft adherence or wound closure, range of motion focuses on regaining total joint motion. A composite flexion fist with associated wrist flexion will stretch dorsal contractures. Functional use of the hand in daily activities should be encouraged, and resistive exercises should be increased in pace with the patient's tolerance.[7]

Splinting

Generally, superficial hand burns are treated with positioning and range-of-motion exercises only. Acute splinting of the deep partial- or full-thickness hand burn requires custom splinting and should be as follows: (1) wrist extension of 20 to 30 degrees, (2) metacarpophalangeal joint flexion of 80 to 90 degrees, (3) interphalangeal full joint extension, and (4) thumb palmar abduction. (Fig. 21.20) Preservation of the first web space is important for grasp and the performance of ADLs. The flexor pollicis longus, a powerful muscle of the thumb, should be placed in an elongated position.[7]

If the hand is extremely edematous, it must not be forced into the above-described position, but the splint remolded as edema subsides. During this acute phase of burn management, the digits should be dressed individually to promote range of motion and the splint applied with elastic wrap. The splint must be checked for fit and correct application. An ill-fitting splint or one applied incorrectly can lead to deformity. As the patient's range of motion improves and wound status changes, the splinting program may change from continual to wearing a splint only at night.

If the central slip of the extensor tendon to the PIP joint has ruptured, the involved joint can be splinted using a gutter splint or circumferential X-lite splint for 6 weeks. This position inhibits the lateral bands from sliding volarly and resulting in the classic burn boutonniere deformity.[7] A pseudoboutonniere deformity is treated by splinting the MCP and IP joints, typically using a serial cast or static progressive splint to restore MP flexion and IP joint extension.

Palmar burns of the hand and wrist may result in a cupping deformity. A palmar extension splint that places the wrist and hand in maximum extension, applying sustained stretch to the healing wound or contracting scar is used. Exercises to maintain collateral ligament length should be balanced with splinting.[53] When the hand burn involves both the dorsal and volar surfaces, the therapist should closely evaluate the direction of the deforming forces and splint accordingly.[7]

Serial static splinting works effectively to stretch a thumb web space contracture. The splint is molded from low-temperature thermoplastic and holds the thumb and index finger in full extension with abduction of the first and second metacarpal.[56] Casting can be effective in correcting contractures in the burned hand. (Fig. 21.21)

Dynamic or serial static splints are used to correct scar contracture in the burned hand. Low-force, prolonged stretch is recommended to allow an adequate amount of time for tissue elongation. Serial static extension splints are used for PIP joint flexion contractures greater than 45 degrees initially to minimize dorsal pressure of the PIP joint. Once the contracture is less than 45 degrees, then a dynamic Capener splint may be used.[57]

Compression

Self-adherent elastic compression wrap applied in a spiral fashion to each individual digit and continued onto the hand and forearm is used before full wound closure is achieved.[53] Once wound closure has been achieved or grafts are adherent, interim compression wraps or gloves are used until the patient's skin can tolerate the commercially made gloves. Open-fingertip design is recommended for use during the day to allow sensory input to the patient's fingertips and to monitor circulation.[7] Inserts may be required to provide scar management and apply compression to the web spaces or the palm of the hand.

Outcome

Individuals with the deepest hand burns requiring grafting appear to demonstrate the greatest loss of function in ROM,

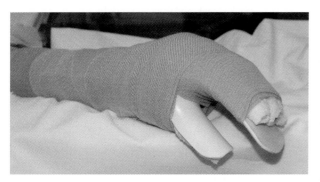

Figure 21•20 *Splinting the acutely burned hand.*

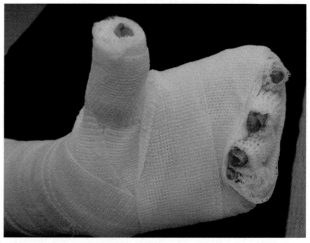

Figure 21•21 *Casting for burn hand palmar contracture.*

grip strength, and coordination. These patients may require up to 1 year or more for function to return.[7] Sheridan and coworkers reported normal function in 97% of those with superficial hand burns and 81% of those with deep dermal and full-thickness injuries requiring surgery. Ninety percent were able to independently perform activities of daily living.[58] There are nine hand-function assessment instruments commonly used in hand therapy, including the Michigan Hand Outcomes Questionnaire, Jensen Test of Hand Function, and TEMPA (Test d'Evaluation des Membres Supériers des Personnes Agées).[50] There is not, however, a clear set of functional assessment tools that are valid for persons with hand burns.[59]

> **PEARL 21•6** Excessive edema of the hand can lead to fibrotic muscle changes and result in claw hand deformity.

Hypertrophic Scarring

Hypertrophic scarring and scar management is the responsibility of the entire burn team and is an essential concern and challenge for the burn therapist. Poor cosmesis, contractures, severe itching, and pain associated with hypertrophic scars can interfere and often impair a burn survivor's ability to return to functional activities of daily living in work, play, and leisure.[60] As more people survive severe burn injuries, the focus of therapeutic intervention has shifted from survival to optimizing the burn survivor's functional and cosmetic outcome. To achieve these outcomes, the burn therapist must use a variety of prophylactic and therapeutic methods to control the development of hypertrophic scarring and hasten scar maturation.[61]

Hypertrophic scarring is generally considered common after a burn injury; however, published data on the prevalence of hypertrophic scarring is relatively scant.[2] Deitch et al studied the occurrence of hypertrophic scars in spontaneously healed burns and found approximately 30% of burn sites in African Americans and approximately 15% in Caucasians developed hypertrophic scars. McDonald and Deitch also studied grafted sites in both pediatric and adult patients. This study demonstrated over 75% of burned areas in children (African American and Caucasians) became hypertrophic and approximately 50% in African American adults and only 7% in Caucasian adults. Spurr and Shakespeare examined pediatric patients in two different time periods in 1968 and 1984. Despite the changes in clinical practice, introduction of pressure therapy, and the increase in the number of children requiring skin grafts, the prevalence of hypertrophic scarring for both time points was 65%. Dedovic and colleagues reported that in children up to 5 years of age, the prevalence of hypertrophic scarring was approximately 30%. Between 6 and 15 years of age, the prevalence was approximately 50%. This report did not stratify by race, origin, or whether the area healed spontaneously or required skin grafting. The most recent study by Bombaro concluded the prevalence of hypertrophic scarring was 67%. The prevalence was more than 75% in non-Whites and over 60% in Caucasians.[62] Overall, the prevalence of hypertrophic scarring after a burn injury varies between 7% and 68% in Caucasians and 30% and 75% for survivors of non-Caucasian descent.[63]

A hypertrophic scar is a raised, erythematous, pruritic, nonpliable mass of tissue that remains within the boundaries of the wound.[2] A keloid scar extends beyond the original wound boundaries. It remains controversial that hypertrophic scars vary from keloids only quantitatively and that keloids represent the most severe degrees of hypertrophic scars.[60] A hypertrophic scar consists of large amounts of extracellular matrix whose composition and organization are altered from those of the normal dermis. Collagen fibers form nodular whorl-like patterns, with an abundance of immature connective tissue and prolonged chronic inflammatory reaction.[2] The etiology of hypertrophic scars is largely unknown, but well-established associations are infection, delayed or prolonged healing, burns, wound tension, and, possibly, bacterial colonization.[64] Other possible causes of hypertrophic scar formation include granulation tissue, chronic inflammatory processes, increased blood flow, genetics, increased serum protein, and altered ground substance.[60]

Clinical signs or characteristics of an immature (active) hypertrophic scar include the following:

- Increase in vascularity (hyperemia)—red, raised or elevated, and rigid
- Increase in fibroblasts, myofibroblasts, collagen, and granulation tissue
- Reduced interstitial spaces
- Abundant and altered ground substance[60] (Figs. 21.22 and 21.23)

Clinical signs of hypertrophic scarring may not be evident until 6 weeks or more after healing; however, the scar's eventual appearance is probably dependent upon the initial wound healing process. As the hypertrophic scar matures, vascularity as well as the number of fibroblasts decreases. The whorl-like pattern of collagen becomes oriented in a more parallel condition, and there are a diminished number of capillaries and fibroblasts in the scar. Clinically, the mature scar is described as pale, planar, and pliable and may take up to 2 years or longer to achieve complete maturation.[60]

Deitch and associates indicated a number of factors and variables that affect scar formation. The following

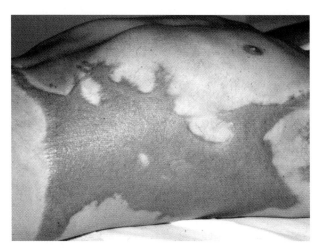

Figure 21•22 *Hypertrophic scar formation following a spontaneously healed burn.*

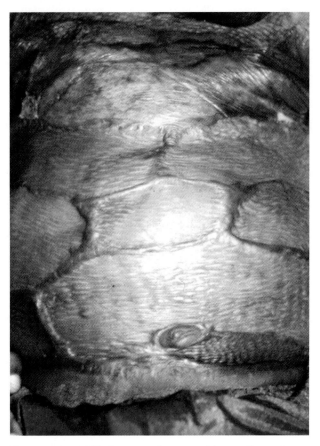

Figure 21•23 *Window pane hypertrophic scar formation along graft edges.*

greater skin tension, and an increased rate of collagen synthesis.
- *Location.* Certain areas of the body that are predisposed to scar formation are the sternum, upper back, shoulder, buttocks, and dorsal aspects of the feet.
- *Depth.* Deeper burns that involve the reticular dermis have an increased incidence of scarring due to the formation of granulation tissue and have prolonged healing time.
- *Tension.* Increased scarring is frequently seen in high tension areas such as the shoulder and upper back.
- *Gender.* Sex does not appear to be a predictor of scar formation as male/female ratios are approximately equal.[60]

Other predisposing factors to note when monitoring for signs of hypertrophic scarring are nonadhering skin grafts, infection, persistent presence of necrotic tissue, or excessive motion of the skin graft edges during the healing process. All of these factors may play a role in determining the outcome of the scar; however, the most significant variable for prediction of hypertrophic scarring is the time from injury to complete wound closure.[60]

> **PEARL 21•7** The longer it takes a wound to heal and the greater the depth of the wound, the greater the risk of hypertrophic scar development.

guidelines will assist burn therapists in identifying high-risk individuals:

- If healing occurs in *less than 10 days*, usually hypertrophic scarring does not develop—*no compression therapy is required.*
- If healing occurs *between 10 and 14 days,* monitor for hypertrophic scarring—*recommended compression for African Americans only.*
- If healing occurs *between 14 and 21 days,* hypertrophic scarring usually develops—*compression strongly recommended.*
- If healing takes *longer than 21 days,* skin grafting is required and *compression is mandatory.*[12]

Additional factors that may affect hypertrophic scar formation include the following:

- *Race.* Generally, darker-pigmented populations, such as African Americans and Asians, are more susceptible to hypertrophic scarring. Deitch and associates noted African Americans have two times greater incidence of scarring when compared to Caucasians.
- *Age.* Although Deitch noted age was not a predictor, younger people scar more than older people, as they are thought to be more susceptible to trauma, have

Scar Assessment

To determine the effectiveness of various treatment methods of hypertrophic scarring, the burn therapist needs a reliable, valid, and clinically useful outcome measure. To date, such an outcome measure has not been found; however, a variety of methods and techniques have been used with varying degrees of reliability and validity. These include photography, ultrasound, elastometers, extensometers, tonometers, pneumatonometers, durometers, infrared thermometers, biopsy, laser Doppler flowmetry, cutometers, three-dimensional molds, and patient-rating scales. Most of these are clinically impractical as they are costly, time-consuming, highly technological, and often nonportable.[61]

In 1990, Sullivan and associates developed a rating scale for evaluating and assessing burn scar maturation as previous scales were highly subjective.[65] They developed the first tool, the Vancouver Scar Scale (VSS), which attempted to rate scar pliability, vascularity, pigmentation, and height. In general, the higher the total score, the more immature or active the scar, as opposed to the scores returning to zero as the scar becomes more mature or inactive. The rating scale is clinically practical and economical, but the major disadvantage of this tool continues to be the subjectivity of the rating for the subtests. Although the Vancouver Scar Scale is widely used and frequently cited in the literature, few studies have been conducted to determine its reliability and validity.[60,61] Table 21.1 shows the original Burn Scar Index.

At the Shriners Burn Institute in Cincinnati, a modification is used to monitor scar maturation in the outpatient setting. Scar characteristics include vascularity, pliability, and height.

Table 21•1 Burn Scar Scale (VSS)

Pigmentation	Vascularity
0 Normal: Color that closely resembles the color over the rest of the body	0 Normal: Color that closely resembles the color over the rest of the body
1 Hypopigmented	1 Pink
2 Hyperpigmented	2 Red
	3 Purple

Pliability	Height
0 Normal	0 Normal
1 Supple: Flexible with minimal resistance	1 <2mm
2 Yielding: Giving way to pressure	2 <5 mm
3 Firm inflexible: Not easily moved, resistant to manual pressure	3 >5 mm
4 Banding Ropelike tissue that blanches with extension of scar	
5 Contracture: Permanent shortening of scar, producing deformity or distortion	

Pigmentation was removed from consideration as it was not believed to offer useful information regarding the maturation process of a scar. Patients are evaluated on monthly intervals and at discharge. A grafted area and a donor site are assessed each visit, and photographs are taken for visual comparison. The patient's compliance with the compression therapy program is recorded as the number of hours a compression device is worn each day. This method demonstrates to the caregiver and the patient the importance of the pressure program to enhance scar maturation. Regardless of whether a formal assessment tool is used to monitor scar maturation, photographs taken at various intervals can provide the clinician, patient, and family members a visual representation of the scar's progression.[60]

Burn therapists continue to be interested in accurate measurements of scar characteristics over time to quantify research and note clinical progress. Photographs and clinical notes are difficult to quantify, and results can be variable when several therapists are assessing the patient's scars.[66] In an attempt to improve the ease of administration, aid in scoring, and increase staff compliance in use of the Vancouver Scar Scale, Baryza and Baryza developed a pocket-sized Plexiglas tool to be used for pigmentation, vascularity, pliability, and height subtests.[61] The areas of pigmentation and height were amended slightly from the original Vancouver Scar Scale. Mixed pigmentation was added, and the height subtests changed to the following numerical scores: 1, >0 to 1 mm; 2, >1 to 2 mm; 3, >2 to 4 mm; and 4, >4 mm. See Figure 21.2 for the original Burn Scar Assessment-Vancouver Scar Scale. The Plexiglas tool is 2 mm thick to allow for comparison of height measurements. The amended scar scale with the numerical scores is printed on the tool and placed 5 mm from the end to give the therapist a convenient comparison for

thicker scars. The larger end of the tool is used to blanch the scar to determine the vascularity score. The tool can be sterilized for use in the operating room; however, for most clinical situations, it can be cleaned with alcohol or soap and water.[66] An ideal measuring tool has content validity, interrater reliability, test-retest reliability, ease of administration, low cost, and is noninvasive.[66] Baryza reported high interrater reliability with the Plexiglas tool, but did not provide details of the methodology.[61]

Authors have used photographs and numeric scales to assess scar parameters, such as irregularity, pliability, disfigurement, thickness, height, and color. A major limitation is the questionable validity of the assessment of the three-dimensional components of scars (texture, height, and thickness) from a two-dimensional photograph. The quality and reproducibility of photographs for assessing scar maturation is questionable. Another modification to the Vancouver Scar Scale was developed by Forbes-Duchart and associates. They developed a color scale to aid with vascularity rating. Two modifications were made to the existing VSS in an effort to decrease subjectivity and improve for ease of rating. The first modification included two pictorial scales, one for Caucasian clients and one for Aboriginal clients. The second modification adopted the Plexiglas tool developed by Baryza and Baryza for the use of the height and pigmentation subtests. The resultant tool is referred to as the Modified Vancouver Scar Scale (MVSS).

A study by Forbes-Duchart and associates measured the interrater reliability of the MVSS. All subtests showed significant correlations, except for the pigmentation subtest. Results indicated that only total scores of the MVSS should be used to determine burn scar outcomes because individual subtest scores appear to have little reliability. Further modifications such as reclassifying the color scales as "light," "medium," and "dark"; omitting the pigmentation subtest; and additional research with a greater number of subjects is warranted. Scar maturation assessment in a reliable cost-effective, user-friendly manner is an ongoing challenge for the burn therapist and the entire burn team. This study is an important step for burn therapists in the evolution of scar maturation assessment.[61]

Treatment and Management of Hypertrophic Scars

Burn scarring is minimized through the use of various prophylactic and therapeutic methods, thereby creating the most optimal functional and cosmetic outcome. There are limited methods available to control hypertrophic scar formation; however, physical intervention is based on attempts to alter the mechanical and physical properties of the scar by using pressure therapy, silicone products, and scar massage. A few of the treatment approaches used by a physician may include altering collagen metabolism or removing the scar altogether.[60] Others may include intralesional steroids, topical application of retinoic acid, intralesional hyaluronidase, topical zinc and vitamin E, topical putrescence, surgical excision or revision, radiation therapy, compression therapy, cryotherapy, and laser treatments. The results of these treatments have not produced entirely satisfactory results.[67]

Compression Therapy

Pressure has been used successfully in the treatment of keloids since 1835. This has included the use of unna boots, sponge fixation, and vascular support garments. The use of compression therapy for burn scar control has become a widely accepted therapeutic intervention.[60]

Pressure therapy, usually noted as compression or pressure garments, has been used by therapists for at least three decades and has been the standard line of therapy to affect the maturation rate and modify the appearance of hypertrophic scars.[68] There are no studies to confirm the mechanism by which pressure alters the structure of the scar; however, pressure has been known to have a thinning effect on the dermis. Mechanical compression of a scar causes blanching or decreased blood flow through the scar, which leads to tissue hypoxia and resultant reduction in the proliferation of cells. The number of collagenase inhibitors is reduced, the rate of collagen lysis is enhanced, and an improved balance between collagen synthesis and lysis of a scar is established. Compression therapy on burn scars produces the following:[60]

- Decreased edema
- Decreased deposition and change in ground substance
- Absent or fewer scar nodules
- Collagen bundle realignment parallel to epidermal surface
- Increased scar pliability and flattening of scars
- Gradual decrease in myofibroblasts
- Possible decreased itching and pain

Overall, compression therapy appears to accelerate the scar maturation process by inducing changes in the physical properties of scar tissue. These changes occur in a period of months to years.[60]

Guidelines for Compression Therapy and Application

The amount of compression necessary to induce scar maturation remains controversial; however, many researchers have recommended approximately 25 mm Hg capillary pressure to produce changes in scar tissue. This number has not been proven absolute, and good clinical results, such as better appearance of the scar and less itching, have been reported with compression levels as low as 5 to 15 mm Hg pressure.[60,68] Accelerated remodeling of scars may occur with pressures less than 10 mm Hg, and scars treated with greater than 15 mm Hg have been noted to have flatter, smoother, and less erythematous scar characteristics. Clinically, positive results may be achieved with lower pressures over time, but higher pressures, ranging from 25 to 35 mm Hg, may induce more rapid maturation of hypertrophic scars.[60] Pressures above 40 mm Hg could possibly cause complications, such as maceration and paresthesia.[68] In general, hypertrophic scarring begins shortly after injury; therefore, the earlier the pressure is applied, the better the results.

Compression therapy or pressure garments are recommended to be worn 22 to 23 hours a day and removed only for personal hygiene, moisturizing the skin, and stretching with scar massage. They are generally required for up to 2 years or until signs of complete scar maturation, such as pale, planar, and pliable scar characteristics, are noted by the burn therapist and physician.[60]

There are mixed reports on long-term compliance with compression garments; however, it remains significant that effectiveness of scar maturation seems to be related directly to the duration of pressure. Evidence supporting the speed of scar maturation and enhancement of cosmetic outcome is variable.[69]

Complications with Pressure Garments

Despite the clinical effectiveness of custom-made pressure garments, several complications and hindrances may occur. These include the following: (1) continuous wear of the garments continuously for months to years, (2) equal pressure is not applied to all areas of the body and face, (3) frequent alterations or remeasurements secondary to weight gain or loss and growth spurts, (4) difficulty in donning and doffing, (5) feeling uncomfortable and hot, (6) problems with skin irritation or scar breakdown, (7) retardation of bone growth or alteration of bony architecture, and (8) retardation of soft tissue growth.[60]

Other specific complications caused by pressure garments may include the following:

- *Scar maceration.* Maceration may occur with application of the garment or movement, tightness of the garment over joints, excessive perspiration, poor hygiene, or skin sensitivity.
- *Friction.* Shearing forces may be caused by application of pressure garments or friction between the garment

and skin that occurs with movement. If recurrent open areas and breakdown becomes a persistent problem, some garment companies will add inserts or soft material to specific areas.

- *Tight fit over joints.* The garment's fit should be monitored closely to prevent excessive pressure over joints, which can lead to skin irritation and breakdown, especially with increased activity.
- *Hygiene.* Proper hygiene is necessary while wearing pressure garments, splints, or inserts as they retain heat. Excessive perspiration, buildup of creams or moisturizers, and poor hygiene could cause scar maceration, possible infection, and increased healing time.
- *Skin sensitivity.* Some burn patients develop a rash or dermatitis while wearing pressure garments, and the physician should examine and diagnose this accordingly.[60]
- *Skeletal and soft tissue growth.* Leung and associates reported regressed skeletal growth of the chin and thoracic region in four children wearing pressure garments.[60,70] Leung et al also noted narrowing of the transverse arch of an adult's hand due to wearing a compression glove with an insert. They recommended padding to distribute the pressure more evenly, face masks for children to be worn no more than 12 hours per day, and no transparent or hard face masks for children under 1 year of age. To assist with minimizing skeletal and soft tissue complications, it is recommended to (1) monitor the fit of the pressure garments or masks so that they are not applying excessive pressure or causing potential skin breakdown; (2) remeasure or replace garments frequently, as needed; (3) remold, recast, or remeasure face masks, especially during growth spurts; and (4) discontinue pressure garments and face masks as soon as complete maturation of scars is achieved.[60]

Various Materials Used for Compression Therapy

There are multiple materials and different techniques available for burn therapists to use for compression and pressure therapy on burn scars. Pressure materials used begin with those creating the least amount of shearing forces and end with custom-made garments. These materials include (1) elastic bandage/ACE® wraps, (2) self-adherent elastic wrap (cohesive bandage), (3) elastic tubular support bandage, (4) ready-made elastic pressure garments, and (5) custom-made elastic pressure garments.[60]

Elastic Bandage/ACE® Wraps

Elastic bandages are often used for pressure therapy in the early stages of burn recovery as they can be applied over burn dressings without creating shearing forces. They control edema, enhance venous and lymphatic drainage, and provide early vascular support for recently spontaneously healed burn wounds or skin grafts. They are inexpensive, washable, and reusable. Elastic bandages provide adequate pressure; however, if applied improperly, they can cause several complications. If wrapped too tightly or unevenly, they can cause increased edema, compromised circulation,

neuropathy, or pressure areas or sores. Proper application includes

- wrapping distal to proximal, with more pressure applied distally,
- overlapping one half of the bandage width with each successive turn,
- applying tension of the bandage on the upstroke turn, and
- avoiding circular wraps on the extremities.

The two most common techniques are the figure eight technique and the spiral wrap. Whitmore and associates reported that the figure eight technique provides more pressure than the spiral wrap and should be used for compression on the lower extremities.[60,71] The spiral wrap or figure eight can be used with the upper extremities, using the figure eight pattern over the elbow joints to allow for greater freedom of movement. Pressure of the elastic bandage is determined by the tension applied. Parks and associates reported that each layer of wrap provides approximately 10 to 15 mm Hg pressure on the extremities and 2 to 5 mm Hg on the thorax.[60,72] It is recommended to double wrap the lower extremities of burn patients to prevent venous pooling and provide greater comfort.[60]

Self-Adherent Elastic Wrap (Cohesive Bandage)

Self-adherent elastic wrap, also known as *cohesive bandage,* is typically used on the hands or feet in the early stages of wound healing to prevent or control edema, provide vascular support, and minimize scar formation. They have multiple trade names and come in a variety of widths and colors. The cohesive bandage can be applied over thin dressings and on fragile tissue that cannot tolerate shearing forces. These bandages can interfere with movement somewhat; therefore, it is recommended to minimize the dressings underneath them. Cohesive bandages should be applied distal to proximal, normally using a spiral wrap.

Elastic Tubular Support Bandage

Tubular support bandages are used for compression on spontaneously healed burn wounds or grafts that are ready to tolerate minimal shearing forces. They may be used for definitive compression therapy; however, they are typically used as interim pressure therapy *after* elastic bandages and *before* custom-made pressure garments. They are cotton based and are available in a variety of tubular sizes and prefabricated garments.[60] Rose and Deitch reported the size chosen by the therapist can achieve low tension (5 to 10 mm Hg), moderate tension (10 to 20 mm Hg), or high tension (20 to 30 mm Hg).[60,73] Other studies by Rose and colleagues demonstrated tubular support bandages are effective in suppressing hypertrophic scar formation, in satisfactory patient compliance, and for reduced cost. They are easy to apply and can effectively be used on the upper and lower extremities and trunk. The extremities are tapered; therefore, it is recommended to double the tubular support bandage distally or use a prefabricated shaped support to assist with equalizing the pressure by providing a graduated distal-to-proximal compression to the limb.[60,73-75]

Ready-Made Elastic Pressure Garments

Several companies manufacture "off-the-shelf" elastic garments in a variety of sizes and styles. They can be stocked in the burn center and fitted with a few quick measurements. Ready-made garments can be used as the definitive garment or as interim compression therapy until the custom-made garment arrives.

Custom-Made Elastic Pressure Garments

Dr. Paul Silverstein, a surgeon at Brooke Army Hospital in the late 1960s, was treating a patient with a vascular support for postphlebitic syndrome. As the bilateral lower-extremity burn wounds healed, Dr. Silverstein noted the uncovered leg developed the typical raised hypertrophic scarring. The scars on the leg covered with the vascular support remained relatively smooth and flat. About the same time, Dr. Duane Larson, at the Shriners Burn Institute in Galveston, Texas, observed minimized hypertrophic scarring when using pressure splints at burned areas. The vascular supports used by Dr. Silverstein were fabricated by the Jobst Institute Inc. (Toledo, OH). Follow-up discussions with Jobst were initiated, and research was conducted by Larson and coworkers.[76,77] The results of this study led the Jobst Institute to develop the first line of pressure garments for the management of hypertrophic scarring. A variety of other companies have followed the Jobst Institute's lead in manufacturing custom-made pressure garments, offering multiple colors and options. Despite the burn clinician's preference in manufacturer, continuous pressure for the treatment of minimizing hypertrophic scar formation is well accepted.[76]

It is recommended to measure a patient for pressure garments when the following occurs:

- A burn wound or graft takes longer than 14 days to heal.
- A burn wound or graft is almost healed.
- Only a few unhealed areas less than the size of a quarter or 1 inch in diameter are present.
- A donor site has delayed healing and signs of hypertrophic scarring.
- Edema is completely resolved.[60]

Most companies provide detailed instructions and forms for measuring all body parts of the patient. Measurements should be taken directly over the skin and not the bandages for proper fit. If the face, hand, or foot is complicated to measure, it is recommended that a positive plaster mold of the area be fabricated and sent to the pressure garment company to ensure accurate fit. The first set of garments should be assessed for proper fit by the therapist and a second set ordered so the patient will have an alternative garment to wear while washing the other.

Garments should last approximately 2 to 3 months before requiring replacement. For active patients, such as those returning to work and wearing gloves, garments may require more frequent replacement. Children may also need to be remeasured for new garments during growth spurts and adults remeasured secondary to weight gain or loss. Generally, garments need to be replaced when they lose their resilience, fail to hold their shape, are very oily to touch, and have irreparable holes, or problems with zippers or Velcro.[60]

Inserts

Inserts are sometimes useful and necessary in certain areas, especially in concave surfaces, to achieve adequate pressure for burn scars. Inserts can be made of a variety of materials, such as foams, felt, silicone elastomer, and putties. To increase pressure in finger web spaces and reduce further problems with syndactyly, materials such as strips of gauze, elastic strips, splinting materials, or pliable rubber tubing are often used. Silicone elastomer inserts are easy to fabricate, they apply even pressure over scars, and they are beneficial for thick rigid scars that are not located over joints. Silicone elastomer putty has a putty base and catalyst that are combined to provide a smooth, flexible insert. The putty is easier and less time consuming to fabricate than the regular silicone elastomer. The putty works well for finger and toe web spacers, over the dorsum of foot and toes, in the palm of the hand, or for smaller, rigid scars that require increased pressure to assist in the progression of scar maturation.[60]

Silicone Gel Sheeting

Silicone is a synthetic polymer generally based on the element silicon or the dimethylsiloxane monomer.[78] Silicone gel pads or sheeting are inert, clear, and flexible and have been used since the early 1980s as an effective modality in burn scar management to soften and reduce hypertrophic scars in a shorter time than in traditional pressure therapy.[79] Reports by Perkins and Wessling indicate silicone gel sheeting is beneficial in increasing range of motion, minimizing pain, preventing the shrinkage of skin grafts, minimizing hypertrophic scarring, assisting with softening and smoothing of scars, and providing increased pressure over movable areas where pressure is difficult to maintain.[80,81] The mechanism of action of the silicone gel is not yet known, and other possibilities such as pressure, temperature, oxygen transmission, water vapor transmission, and silicone absorption do not appear to be factors.[60] Quinn and associates found hydration of the skin was altered when silicone sheets are used, and there was evaporative water loss of normal skin. They concluded the possibility that the stratum corneum provided a reservoir for fluid.[78,82] Katz and others reported silicone might act by altering scar hydration,[83,84] and Davey and associates postulated action by the reduction of water vapor loss to decrease capillary activity, collagen deposition, and hypertrophic scar formation.[85] Ahn and colleagues showed that silicone placed on hypertrophic scars for a minimum of 12 hours daily and a duration of only 2 months were effective in increasing scar elasticity, flattening established hypertrophic burn scar formation, and preventing large scar volume of surgical scars.[86] The patient's skin should be monitored closely as the silicone gel sheeting may cause skin irritation if left in place for prolonged periods. Wearing time should gradually be increased from 12 to 24 hours, as tolerated.[60] The silicone gel sheeting can be secured with elastic wraps or bandages, cohesive wraps, adhesive tape, or pressure garments.

▷ **PEARL 21•8** Compression therapy is recommended 22 to 23 hours a day and is generally required for up to 2 years or until signs of complete scar maturation are seen.

Management of Facial Scars—Transparent Face Mask

The face is one of the most frequently burned areas of the body, especially due to flash burns.[60] Burns to the head, face, and neck can be devastating and have a considerable impact on a patient's functional, cosmetic, emotional, and psychological recovery.[21] The formation of hypertrophic scars and deforming contractures may lead to immense facial disfigurement and functional problems. The burn patient may experience problems with the function of the eyes or eyelids, vision, speech and communication, hearing, and feeding and eating, along with the significant increase in the psychological and social stressors associated with the entire common complication of severe burn injury and trauma.[87] The patient's self-image may be altered, leading to considerable psychological problems with self-esteem and self-confidence. It is commonly acknowledged that the face is a large part of our self-image and our perception of how we are viewed by others.[21]

Nonsurgical, postsurgical, and reconstructive management of facial scarring creates challenging and difficult problems for burn therapists who work to obtain the best possible functional and cosmetic outcomes for the patient. Various treatment techniques used to minimize hypertrophic scarring include custom-made elastic face masks and hoods with foam, silicone, or elastomer inserts and transparent face masks.[87] It is recommended to maintain pressure on the face until complete scar maturation occurs to assist in preventing or reducing hypertrophic scar formation and contractures, such as eyelid ectropion or lower lip eversion. Due to the contours of the face, the elastic face mask does not provide adequate pressure on the nasolabial folds, adjacent cheek areas, or under the lower lip. Foam inserts, silicone gel sheeting, elastomer, or splinting material can be used under the elastic mask in the contoured areas to assist in delivering pressure required for scar remodeling. In general, elastic face masks are not well accepted by patients due to its objectionable appearance.

Rigid transparent face masks made of cellulose acetate butyrate were reported by Rivers and associates to improve patient compliance and facial scar management.[88] The transparent face mask involves fabricating a negative mold of the patient's face and/or neck by using dental alginate and plaster strips. This is carefully removed from the patient's face, and plaster is then poured into the negative mold to form a positive impression of the patient's face and/or neck. The high-temperature transparent material is heated in a convection oven and vacuum molded or manually stretched over the positive mold. Once cooled, a dremel is used to trim and smooth the edges of the rigid transparent mask as needed. Straps are riveted to the mask to secure it to the patient's head using Velcro or other strapping techniques. The rigid transparent face mask is fitted to the patient's face and properly secured. Once optimal fit is achieved, the patient should be seen monthly so that the therapist can increase pressure in areas as needed. The vascular blanching of the facial scars beneath the transparent face mask allows the therapist to ensure an accurate fit and pressure on facial scars and to adjust the mask as indicated. Patients with facial scarring appear to accept the appearance of the transparent face mask over the elastic face masks as it is more socially acceptable and exposes the facial features in public. A random survey distributed at the American Burn Association Conference in 2001 reported that 81% of therapists use the transparent face mask to treat and manage facial scars. A few disadvantages of the transparent face mask are lack of flexibility around the mandible and chin, the length of time it takes to fabricate it, and the skills required of a therapist or technician to construct it.[87] The burn patient may not require a full face mask; therefore, a partial rigid mask for the upper or lower face can be fabricated. A rigid insert may also be used directly on the scarred areas of the face and/or neck and secured with an elastic open face mask or chin strap. It is recommended that the mask be worn at all times except during bathing, meals, and facial massage or stretching. Some therapists recommend wearing elastic face masks with the appropriate inserts at night and the rigid, more socially acceptable transparent face masks during the day.[60]

An alternative method of using the dental alginate and plaster strips to fabricate the negative impression of the burn patient's face is used at Louisiana State University Health Sciences Center Regional Burn Center in Shreveport, Louisiana. This method involves the burn physician, occupational therapist, and anesthesiologist working together to appropriately sedate the patient in the operating room in order to fabricate the negative impression. This alternative method is typically used during a surgical procedure and on very young children or high-anxiety, claustrophobic patients. One disadvantage is slight distortion of the impression or mold around the mouth if the patient has to be orally intubated for the procedure. (Figs. 21.24 through 21.26)

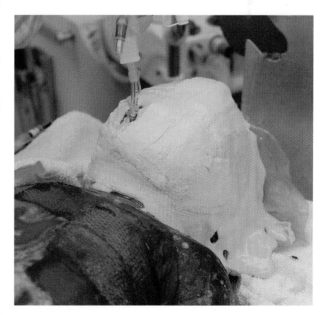

Figure 21•24 *Obtaining a negative facial mold using calcium alginate and plaster cast strips for reinforcement.*

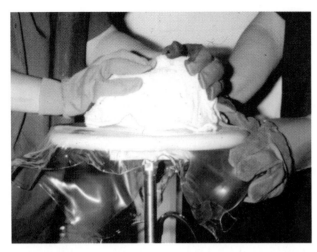

Figure 21•25 *Silon STS® being vacuum molded over the positive face mold.*

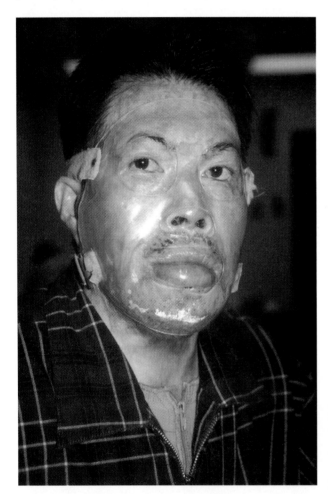

Figure 21•26 *Silon STS facial orthotics.*

A commonly used material for the transparent face mask is called Silon-STS®, or silicone thermoplastic splinting (Biomed Sciences Inc. Allentown, PA). To our knowledge, it is the first product to combine the molding attributes of a high-temperature thermoplastic splinting material with a therapeutic surface of silicone, thereby applying both pressure and topical silicone therapy in one convenient step.

Jennifer Whitestone, a biomedical engineer, developed a new concept for creating burn masks. Since that time, other companies have used the process to produce positive forms using a production method called *image science*, or *non-contact surface scanning*. The scanning process captures a burn patient's facial contours in less than 20 seconds. The data from the scan is formatted into a 3D STL file and a positive mold can then be produced. Silon-STS is then vacuum-formed over the form, producing the final transparent face mask.

Another material known as Silon-LTS®, or low-temperature splinting (Biomed Sciences Inc.), is the first developed low-temperature splinting material that also offers the silicone adherent technology; however, it is opaque rather than transparent. It functions much like the Silon-STS but is softened in water at approximately 160°F and can be molded directly to the patient's skin, thereby eliminating the time-consuming step of taking an impression and making a plaster mold. It offers great versatility because it expands the usefulness of composite splinting technology and scar management at the same time. It can be used in a variety of ways, such as in conformers, lower partial face masks, or chin/neck conformers.

Scar Massage

Scar massage is a method used in the postacute and rehabilitation phase after a patient sustains a burn injury and begins showing signs of hypertrophic scarring. Massage has been recommended to elongate, soften, and increase the immature scar's pliability.[89] Although no studies identify the exact mechanisms by which massage works, it has been reported that massage assists with softening scar tissue by possibly freeing restrictive fibrous bands and increasing circulation. Through tactile stimulation, massage with lubrication aids in stretching the scars and desensitizes the tissue.[60] (Figs. 21.27 and 21.28) Theoretically, the mechanical effect of the massage may loosen the scars from underlying tissue and increase movement when used in conjunction with range-of-motion exercises.[89]

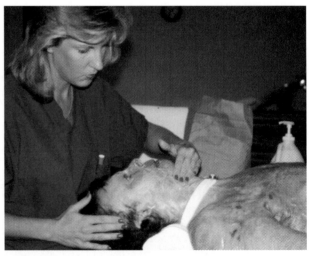

Figure 21•27 *Scar massage with passive stretching.*

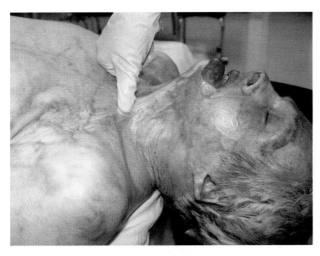

Figure 21•28 *Scar massage with lubrication aides in softening the hypertrophic scar.*

Therapists, patients, and caregivers should massage the rigid, thick hypertrophic scars by pressing and mobilizing the tissue to make the scars blanch. It is recommended to massage with lubrication three to six times daily for 5 to 10 minutes per session and for each scar area.[60]

Itching

One of the most reported complications of burn injuries and recovery is the patient's complaint of itching (pruritus). The incidence of severe itching has been reported to be as high as 87%, and most of the burn patient's complaints of itching are for wounds located on the extremities. Itching can remain a quality of life issue for the burn survivor if it interferes with sleeping, eating, working, playing, or leisure activities. It has been reported to be one of the most distressing postburn issues that a burn patient may experience. Standard treatment to manage and minimize the effects of pruritus has been the use of oral antihistamines and topical lotions.[90]

Neuropathy

Generalized peripheral neuropathy has been described when there is distal sensory loss and weakness in a symmetrical pattern. Mononeuropathies are diagnosed when weakness and sensory loss fit a pattern of a specific peripheral nerve distribution.[91] Mononeuropathy was found in patients who had sustained an electrical injury or had a history of alcohol abuse.

Polyneuropathy is most common among patients who have burns that are greater than 15% full thickness, who are older than 40 years of age, and who stay in the ICU for more than 20 days.[91] Positioning is important to avoid nerve compression due to external compression. This includes avoiding prolonged elbow flexion, avoiding the frog-leg position in the lower extremities, and avoiding prone position with the arms overhead.[91]

Electrical Injuries

Electrical burn injuries account for 3% to 6% of burn injuries admitted yearly to major burn units and will usually have con-comitant musculoskeletal dysfunction, including fractures and muscle necrosis. The severity of an electrical injury depends on the type of current, its duration, and the voltage.[92] Mechanisms of injury involve thermal, electrical, and vascular components.[93]

Contact with electrical current produces tetanic muscle contractions, making release of an electrified object more difficult and prolonging contact time. Low-voltage injuries (120 to 240 volts) typically result from household accidents, with women and children usually involved. High-voltage injuries, voltage greater than 1000 volts, typically occur from power lines or lightning strikes. Tissue damage is greater, and almost 80% of high-voltage victims will require at least one amputation. Most high-voltage injuries involve the upper extremities.[14,94]

High-voltage currents may arc and can often cause associated flame burn.[14] Patients with high-voltage injuries have the most associated injuries consisting of traumatic brain, spinal cord, and orthopedic injuries. Neurological complications have been reported to be as high as 67%, with some symptoms having a delayed presentation as late as 2 years after injury.[92,94] Range-of-motion exercises may be contraindicated in cases of cardiovascular instability.[93] Individuals with electrical injuries also complain of cognitive problems (50%), paresthesias (49%), muscle twitching, difficulty walking, and balance problems.[18] Amputation rates from electrical burns can vary from 24% to 44%, making prosthetic fitting and training a significant part of the rehabilitation process.[92]

Areas covered by skin graft or burns that are allowed to heal spontaneously will be intolerant to shear and pressure, which will delay prosthetic fitting and training. The fitting or fabrication of a functional prosthesis will require ingenuity by the therapist. Patients with a transradial amputation can be fitted with universal cuffs to allow attachment of utensils. A clamshell design can be used over wound dressings and serves as an attachment device to allow the patient to perform functional activities.[92]

Pediatric Burns

Mortality in children sustaining extensive burns has dramatically decreased in the past 20 years.[95] Severely burned children (>40% TBSA) will experience long-term physical impairment, and the rehabilitative process may take years to complete.[96] Abnormal changes, such as loss of muscle and bone mass, are common and lead to decreased ADLs. Long-term sequelae can include changes in skeletal development and a decrease in bone density.[97] It has been noted that children are more prone to scar contracture development than are adults.[13]

Children are more difficult to position and splint than adults, presenting a unique challenge. Positioning older children can be accomplished by having the child lie prone while playing a game or watching TV to increase neck extension. With younger children, mobiles can help encourage neck rotation or extension. Securing a splint with cohesive wrap reduces the problem of removal or slippage, while covering a hand or foot splint with a large sock decorated by the child may encourage compliance.

The exercise goals for children should take into consideration the appropriate level of development. Frequently, an exercise approach needs to be in the form of play activities to stimulate the child's participation. (Fig. 21.29) The therapist will need to be flexible and creative, using therapeutic activities that can be easily graded in complexity and be adapted for use in bed, while sitting, or for the ambulatory patient.[98] The effects of a supervised exercise program consisting of an aerobic and resistance-training component have been found to be effective in reducing the number of scar releases and also lead to increased muscular strength and functional outcome in children.[95,96] In addition to conventional therapy, caregiver education is important. Toddlers and children are unable, or too unreliable, to actively participate in an independent exercise program. Outside assistance from the parents or other persons is important to supplement the therapy program provided by the therapist.[23]

Psychological Considerations and Adjustment To Recovery

When a person sustains a burn injury, it can be one of the most aesthetically devastating, traumatic events ever experienced. The severely impaired and disfiguring appearance can be socially incapacitating, and burn patients often feel that they lose control of their lives upon arrival at the burn center. Accordingly, it is not surprising that psychological problems are identified in a significant number of burn patients. It is very important to provide psychiatric services so that early and effective interventions can support and treat the patient through this traumatic injury.[2]

A person's coping skills after sustaining a burn injury are strongly influenced by their preinjury psychological status. If a person typically displays highly dysfunctional behavior before sustaining major burn trauma, this dysfunction is likely to be amplified during the recovery process. The causes of many burn injuries indicate that many individuals were psychologically impoverished prior to the traumatic event. For example, a substantial number of burn injuries are

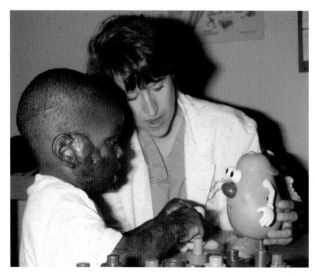

Figure 21•29 *Using play with pediatric patients.*

the result of attempted suicide, assault, and arson. Estimations of preexisting psychiatric disorders are significantly higher than normal population standards, and the most common diagnoses include depression, antisocial personality disorder, organic brain syndromes, and alcohol and drug abuse. In summary, the relationship between burn injury and prior psychiatric disorders is complex. There is an intricate interaction between personal characteristics and environmental factors, and the best indicator of a burn survivor's coping skills is often related to how they were functioning in life prior to the burn injury.[99]

Three basic stages of burn recovery consistently have been identified for burn survivors. They are the early, intermediate, and long-term stages of recovery. These stages also correspond to the level of physical recuperation the burn patient is experiencing, such as intensive critical care, acute rehabilitative care, and long-term outpatient adjustment. The duration of each stage varies, depending on the burn patient's individual personality and temperament factors, extent of the burn injury, and the treatment environment.[99]

Early Stage of Recovery

The early stage of recovery is the period in which the patient is being treated in the intensive care unit and experiencing significant physiological changes and repeated medical procedures. The most frequent complaints during this stage of recovery are delirium, anxiety, sleep disturbance, intense pain, and confusion. Supportive psychological interventions that focus on immediate concerns and strengthening the patient's existing coping strategies are effective approaches during this stage.[99]

Intermediate Stage of Recovery

The intermediate phase of recovery begins when the patient has begun to stabilize physically and issues of healing take precedence over the issues of survival. The patient is typically out of the intensive care unit, surgical procedures are less frequent, physical status is improving, sleep patterns may be becoming more regular, and clarity of thought is beginning to return. The patient frequently experiences a considerable degree of intense pain and endures a series of painful procedures, such as dressing changes, wound care and débridement, positioning, splinting, exercising, and functional tasks. Despite their improved physical status, the patient usually copes during this stage by remaining in a state of psychological shock. This usually will diminish with time, gradually giving way to coping with pragmatic concerns. The most common psychological problems during the intermediate stage of recovery are depression and posttraumatic stress disorder (PTSD). Other concerns the patient may experience include nightmares, anxiety, and regression of behaviors, with such interpersonal difficulties as hostility, dependence, or inappropriate sexual behavior. Brief psychological counseling is often helpful for depression, but in the more severe depressive episodes medications may be necessary. PTSD is relatively common with burn patients; the course is usually brief, and symptoms rarely extend beyond discharge from the hospital. However, a combination of counseling and medication is helpful when symptoms do not subside after a short period. Burn patients potentially exhibit a number of problematic behavioral patterns. The consistent application of behavioral modification techniques is often helpful to reduce these complications. Techniques that are particularly effective in minimizing these behaviors include behavioral contracting, assertiveness training, selective ignoring of negative communication or behaviors, and limit setting. A combination of psychological and pharmacological treatments, brief supportive therapy, behavior modification strategies, and continued intervention with the patient's family are often effective in alleviating these difficulties and offer the burn patient optimal levels of support during this stage.[99]

Long-Term Stage of Recovery

The long-term stage of recovery begins when the patient is discharged from the hospital and reintegrates back into society. Only a minority of burn survivors report adjustment difficulties, and the first year following discharge is usually the most difficult. The patient often continues to have vivid memories of the accident and experiences changes in family and occupational roles. Common problems the first year after discharge are associated with vocational and emotional adjustment. Emotional problems such as anxiety and depression are most frequently reported and may be prolonged if the burn injury was quite severe or involved facial disfigurement or loss of hand function. Additional problems in the long-term adjustment stage that may persist past the first year of recovery usually involve perceptions of diminished quality of life and lowered self-esteem. One of the strongest buffers against these problems is to receive high levels of social support from family and friends. In summary, the burn survivor's adjustment to the burn injury is determined by a complex interaction of personality, environment, extent of injury, and preexisting coping skills.[99] (Fig. 21.30)

Special Considerations for Pediatric Burn Injuries and Recovery

Children who sustain burn injuries also pass through early, intermediate, and long-term stages of recovery. Their long-term adjustment is usually satisfactory; however, children and adolescents, in particular, who have sustained visible and disfiguring burns to the face and hands, have a greater incidence of adjustment problems and depression. Providing resources for brief psychological counseling or support groups, a strong degree of social support from caregivers, and sensitivity on the part of medical staff to provide high levels of reinforcement and consistency may offer adequate adjustment for the patient after sustaining a burn injury.[99]

School Reentry Programs

Returning to school is an important indicator of functional aptitude and emotional adjustment in school-aged burn survivors. School reintegration after sustaining a burn injury

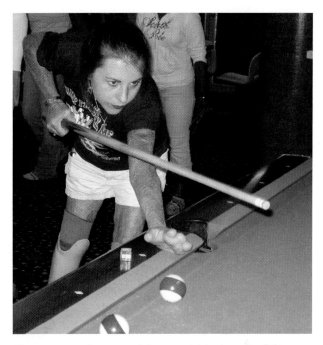

Figure 21•30 *Return to leisure activities is part of the psychological healing process for this woman after losing both lower extremities and partial amputation of the digits of the right hand secondary to her burn injury.*

provides school-aged children with a sense of normalcy and routine. School reentry programs have become a critical component of discharge planning for the pediatric burn patient because returning to home, and subsequently back to school, can be a significant source of anxiety and stress. These programs provide the burn-injured child, their parents and family, school teachers and fellow students with a level of understanding and emotional support to make the transition from hospital to back to school occur as smoothly as possible.[100]

Burn Camps

Burn centers have actively been searching for ways to help with the transition from the status of *burn victim* to that of *burn survivor*, especially in terms of self-esteem. Psychiatrists, psychologists, and social workers assist the burn team in helping survivors and their families with interventions during hospitalization, through discharge, and with the transition back into society. Pediatric burn camps are one such program and have grown in popularity during the last 15 years.[101]

The original children's burn camp started in 1983, conceptualized and directed by Marion Doctor, LCSW, and sponsored by Denver Children's Hospital Burn Center. The goal of the camp and program was to provide a safe summer camping experience and to facilitate the burn survivor's rehabilitation process and recovery after experiencing a serious burn injury. The concept was successful, and the word of its merit spread quickly. As of 2006, there were more than 40 burn camps in the United States and similar camps in Canada and other countries. The purpose of these camps is to give burn-surviving children the opportunity to experience success and enhance their self-esteem.[101] (Fig. 21.31)

Summary

Rehabilitation of the burned patient encompasses positioning, splinting, ROM, and scar management, along with psychological support. Preventing contractures, managing the hypertrophic scar, and assisting the return to maximal independence in daily living skills, school, or work will be the goal of the therapist. Therapists working with burn patients must understand the complications that may arise during treatment as the rehabilitation of the burn patient is an ever-changing process.

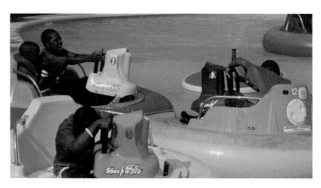

Figure 21•31 *Burn camps provide a safe summer experience for the pediatric burn survivor.*

▶ Case Study 21•1 | Second and Third Degree Burn

History

Mr. D.S. is a 59-year-old male with a past medical history of gastrointestinal ulcer disease. He sustained 45% TBSA second- and third-degree burns to the face, neck, chest, bilateral upper extremities, hands, and bilateral thighs on November 3, 2005. The patient is married, a mechanic, and sustained the burn injury while working on the engine of a truck that ignited and caused an explosion. Upon admission to the regional burn center, Mr. D.S. was electively intubated, escharotomies were performed to bilateral upper extremities, and fluid resuscitation initiated. He underwent approximately nine operative procedures of tangential excision and split-thickness skin grafts to bilateral upper extremities and hands, face, neck, chest, and bilateral thighs. Donor sites included the lower abdomen and the entire back. He received both occupational and physical therapy while hospitalized.

Mr. D.S. was extubated and discharged to a rehabilitation facility on December 9, 2005, for continued wound care, occupational therapy, physical therapy, and psychiatric intervention and treatment.

Mr. D.S. was discharged from rehabilitation to home on December 29, 2005, to begin outpatient therapy three to four times weekly. He attended outpatient occupational therapy three to four times weekly until December 2006 and continues to be followed quarterly in the outpatient burn clinic for compression therapy, scar management, and surgical reconstruction. He was also followed by the psychiatry department for treatment of post-traumatic stress disorder (PTSD). As an outpatient, Mr. D.S. underwent several reconstructive procedures from February 2006 to April 2007, which included the following:

- Contracture release of anterior neck with full-thickness skin graft 2/06
- Contracture release of left anterior axilla with split-thickness skin graft and negative-pressure wound therapy placement postoperatively for 4 days 2/06

- Contracture release of anterior neck and right axilla with placement of Integra 8/06
- Removal of Integra with split-thickness skin graft to neck and right axilla; contracture release of lower lip with full-thickness skin graft 9/06
- Contracture release of lower lip with full-thickness skin graft; contracture release of right small finger with full-thickness skin graft 4/07

Initially, as an outpatient, Mr. D.S. ambulated into clinic independently in a slightly forward flexed posture of neck and trunk. AROM was limited in all joints as follows:

- Mouth opening 1¼ inches
- Neck extension 25 degrees
- Neck rotation bilaterally 45 degrees
- Right shoulder flexion/abduction 130 degrees
- Left shoulder flexion/abduction 110 degrees
- Right elbow—minus 24 degrees extension to 140 degrees flexion
- Left elbow—minus 12 degrees extension to 100 degrees flexion
- Forearm supination and pronation bilaterally 75 degrees
- Wrist extension bilaterally 30 degrees
- Wrist flexion bilaterally 50 degrees
- Right hand composite fist 75%
- Left hand composite fist 50%
- Slight limitations of extension of all digits bilaterally secondary to palmar scarring

Strength: Overall, strength is within functional limits.

Grip Strength:
- Right 30# (norms 59–154)
- Left 12# (norms 43–128)

Pinch Strength:
- Right lateral 13# (norms 18–34)
- Left lateral 6# (norms 13–31)

▶ **Case Study 21•1** **Second and Third Degree Burn—cont'd**

- Right tip 7# (norms 16–34)
- Right tripod 11# (11–24)
- Left tripod 4# (10–26)

Endurance: Endurance is fair. The patient demonstrates independent ambulation without an assistive device for short distances, but needs a wheelchair for community distances.

ADLs: He requires minimal to moderate assistance with dressing, bathing, hygiene, and feeding tasks.

Adaptive Equipment Issued: Patient uses adaptive feeding utensils, long-handled bath sponge, and sock aid.

Splinting/Orthotics: He uses bilateral elbow conformers, chin/neck conformer, soft collar, and microstomia prevention appliance. Serial casting was applied to both elbows to increase elbow extension prior to placement of bilateral elbow conformers.

Wound/Scar Assessment: All skin grafts, donor sites, and spontaneously healed wounds are completely healed. Scars are hypertrophic throughout face, mouth, neck, chest, bilateral upper extremities, and hands. Scars are red in vascularity, elevated 2 to 3 mm, are firm/nonyielding, and hyperpigmented. Contractures are at oral commissures, with lower lip eversion, significant anterior neck contracture scar bands, bilateral anterior axillary contractures, anterior chest scar band, and slight flexion contractures of digits, with the left hand greater than the right. Scars are hypersensitive and painful, especially at the mouth and lips, lower face and jaw, neck, chest, and bilateral hands.

Psychological: He reports feelings of depression, with occasional problems of flashbacks and nightmares. Patient complains of scar pain at rest and during stretching activities, with hypersensitivity of scars, especially on face, neck, chest, and hands.

Recommended Interventions

Management of ROM Limitations and Contractures: Patient will perform active-assistive ROM exercises with incorporated scar massage into stretching program for mouth and face, neck, bilateral upper extremities and hands (all joints and planes of movement); AROM and strengthening exercises for total body will be as follows:

- Reciprocal overhead pulleys
- Wand exercises while supine on mat, with stretching and scar massage with lotion
- Stretching of neck into extension/hyperextension while supine on mat with scar massage
- Restorator, Thera-Band®, and total gym strengthening exercises
- Resistive weight well activities

- Resistive grip and pinch strengthening exercises
- Functional tasks in ADLs

Management of Contractures with Splinting Devices: Neck conformer alternating with soft cervical collar, microstomia prevention appliance, and elbow conformers are indicated to prevent further contracture formation and increase ROM. Splints were adjusted and remolded as indicated.

- Neck conformer worn daily except during exercise, hygiene, and self-care tasks
- Soft cervical collar worn at night
- Microstomia prevention appliance worn progressively to 20 minutes three to four times daily
- Bilateral elbow conformers worn for nighttime and rest periods during the day

Management of Hypertrophic Scarring: Interim compression therapy is initiated upon complete wound healing, then is progressed to long-term custom-made compression garments. Compression therapy is indicated to decrease hypertrophic scar formation and maximize complete scar maturation and cosmesis. Patient is to wear compression garments 23 hours daily, as follows:

- Tubigrip® to bilateral upper extremities
- Isotoner® gloves for bilateral hands
- Custom-made Jobst garments—vest, gloves, and modified chin strap with silicone insert inferior to lower lip and chin
- Low-temperature thermoplastic sheeting (Silon-LTS) for lower face, chin, and neck conformer

Management of Scar Pain and Hypersensitivity: Scar massage and stretching with lotion to all areas of face, neck, and upper body are completed two to three times daily. Patient wears silicone inserts to scars on chest, lower face, jaw, and chin under compression garments for nighttime wear only. Vibration massage is performed on hypertensive scars on lower face and chest two to three times daily.

Management of Psychological Issues: Patient is followed by psychiatrist for counseling and medical management of depression, posttraumatic stress disorder (PTSD), and pain. Medications include the following:

- Trazodone
- Seroquel
- Lexapro
- Fentanyl patch
- Lortab/Percocet

Patient and wife attend the annual Louisiana Burn Camp, "I'm Still Me," as volunteer camp counselors to assist in burn injury recovery, and the patient assists and offers support to other adult and pediatric burn survivors.

References

1. Palmieri, TL, Klein, MB: Burn research state of the science: Introduction. J Burn Care Res 2007; 28:544–545.
2. Faucher, LD: Rehabilitation of the burn patient, trauma, and thermal injury. In: ACS Surgery: Principles and Practice. WebMD, Inc., 2004, pp 1–7. Available at www.acssurgery.com.
3. American Burn Association. Burn Incidence and Treatment in the US: 2007 Fact Sheet. Available at: http://www.ameriburn.org/resources_factsheet.php. Accessed 8/26/2007.
4. Falkel, JE: Anatomy and physiology of the skin. In: Richard, RL, Staley, MJ (eds): Burn Care and Rehabilitation: Principles and Practice. Philadelphia, FA Davis, 1994, pp 10–28.
5. Rutan, RL: Physiologic responses to cutaneous burn injury. In: Carrougher, GJ (ed): Burn Care and Therapy. St. Louis, Mosby, 1998, pp 1–33.
6. Johnson, C: Pathologic manifestations of burn injury. In: Richard, RL, Staley, MJ (eds): Burn Care and Rehabilitation: Principles and Practice. Philadelphia, FA Davis, 1994, pp 29–48.
7. deLinde, LG, Miles, WK: Remodeling of scar tissue in the burned hand. In: Hunter, JM, Mackin, EJ, Callahan, AD (eds): Rehabilitation of the Hand: Surgery and Therapy, ed. 4. St. Louis, Mosby, 1995, pp 1267–1294.
8. Carrougher, GJ: Burn wound assessment and topical treatment. In: Carrougher, GJ (ed): Burn Care and Therapy. St. Louis, Mosby, 1998, pp 133–165.
9. Greenhalgh, DG, Staley, MJ: Burn wound healing. In: Richard, RL, Staley, MJ (eds): Burn Care and Rehabilitation: Principles and Practice. Philadelphia, FA Davis, 1994, pp 70–102.
10. Kirsner, RS, Bogensberger, G: The normal process of healing. In: Kloth, LC, McCulloch, JM (eds): Wound Healing: Alternatives in Management, ed. 3. Philadelphia, FA Davis, 2002, pp 3–34.
11. Ward, SR: Physical rehabilitation. In: Carrougher, GR (ed): Burn Care and Therapy. St. Louis, Mosby, 1998, pp 293–327.
12. Deitch, EA, Wheelahan, TM, Rose, MP: Hypertrophic burn scars: Analysis of variables. J Trauma 1983; 23:895–898.
13. Richard, RL, Staley, MJ: Burn patient evaluation and treatment planning. In: Richard, RL, Staley, MJ (eds): Burn Care and Rehabilitation. Philadelphia, FA Davis, 1994, pp 201–220.
14. Myers, BA: Wound Management: Principles and Practice, ed. 1. Upper Saddle River, NJ, Prentice Hall, 2004, pp 323–348.
15. Schneider, JC, Holavanahalli, R, Helm, P, et al: Contractures in burn injury: Defining the problem. J Burn Care Res 2006; 27:508–514.
16. Gibran, N, Luterman, A, Herndon, D, et al: Comparison of fibrin sealant and staples for attaching split-thickness autologous sheet grafts in patients with deep partial—or full—thickness burn wounds: A phase 1/2 clinical study. J Burn Res 2007; 28:401–408.
17. Currie, LJ, Sharpe, JR, Martin, R: The use of fibrin glue in skin grafts and tissue-engineered skin replacements: A review. Plast Reconstr Surg 2001; 108:1713–1726.
18. Esselman, PC, Thombs, BD, Magyar-Russell, G, et al: Burn rehabilitation, state of the science. Am J Phys Med Rehabil 2006; 85:383–413.
19. Richards, R, Miller, S, Staley, M, et al: Multimodal versus progressive treatment techniques to correct burn scar contracture. J Burn Care Rehabil 2000; 21:506–512.
20. Apfel, LM, Irwin, CP, Staley, MJ, et al: Approaches to positioning the burn patient. In: Richard, RL, Staley, MJ (eds): Burn Care and Rehabilitation. Philadelphia, FA Davis, 1994, pp 221–241.
21. Serghiou, MA, Holmes, CL, McCauley, RL: A survey of current rehabilitation trends for burn injuries to the head and neck. J Burn Care Rehabil 2004; 25:514 –518.
22. Chown, GA: The high-density foam aeroplane splint: A modified approach to the treatment of axilla burns. Burns 2006; 32:916 –919.
23. Daugherty, MB, Carr-Collins, JA: Splinting the burn patient. In: Richard, RL, Staley, MJ (eds): Burn Care and Rehabilitation. Philadelphia, FA Davis, 1994, pp 242–323.
24. Colditz, JC: Therapist's management of the stiff hand. In: Hunter, JM, Mackin, EJ, Callahan, AD (eds): Rehabilitation of the Hand: Surgery and Therapy, ed. 4. St. Louis, Mosby, 1995, pp 1141–1159.
25. Serghiou, MA, McLaughlin, A, Herndon, DN: Alternative splinting methods for the prevention and correction of burn scar torticollis. J Burn Care Rehabil 2003; 24:336–340.
26. Foley, KH, Doyle, B, et al: Use of an improved Watusi Collar to manage pediatric neckburn contractures. J Burn Care Rehabil 2002; 23:221–226.
27. Dougherty, ME, Warden, GD: A thirty-year review of oral appliances used to manage Microstomia, 1972 to 2002. J Burn Care Rehabil 2003; 24:418–431.
28. Wurst, KJ: A modified dynamic mouth splint for burn patients. J Burn Care Res 2006; 27:86–92.
29. Davis, S, Thompson, JG, Clark, J, et al: A prototype for an economical vertical microstomia orthosis. J Burn Care Res 2006; 27:352–356.
30. Vehmeyer-Heeman, M, Lommers, B, Van den Kerckhove, E, et al: Axillary burns: Extended grafting and early splinting prevents contractures. J Burn Care Rehabil 2005; 26:539–542.
31. Kim, D, Wright, S, Morris, R, et al: Management of axillary burn contractures. Techniques in hand and upper extremity Surg 2007; 11:204–208.
32. Manigandan, C, Gupta, AK, Venugopal, K, et al: A multi-purpose, self-adjustable aeroplane splint for the splinting of axillary burns. Burns 2003; 29:276–279.
33. Parks, DH: Prevention and correction of deformity after severe burns. Surg Clin North Am 1978; 58:1279–1289.
34. Obaidullah, HU: Figure-of-8 sling for prevention of recurrent axillary contracture after release and skin grafting. Burns 2005; 31:283–289.
35. Staley, M, Serghiou, M: Casting guidelines, tips, and techniques: Proceedings from the 1997 American Burn Association PT/OT casting workshop. J Burn Care Rehabil 1998; 19:254–269.
36. Bennett, GB, Helm, P, Purdue, GF, et al: Serial casting: A method for treating burn contractures. J Burn Care Rehabil 1989; 10:543–545.37.
37. Johnson, J, Silverberg, R: Serial casting of the lower extremity to correct contractures during the acute phase of burn care. Phys Ther 1995; 75:262–266.
38. Humphrey, C, Richard, RL, Staley, MJ: Soft tissue management and exercise. In: Richard, RL, Staley, MJ (eds): Burn Care and Rehabilitation. Philadelphia, FA Davis, 1994, pp 324–360.
39. Kisner, C, Colby, LA: Range of motion. In: Kisner, C, Coly, L : Therapeutic Exercise: Foundations and Techniques, ed. 5. Philadelphia, FA Davis, 2007, pp 43–65.
40. Kisner, C, Colby, LA: Stretching for impaired mobility. In: Kisner, C, Coly, L: Therapeutic Exercise: Foundations and Techniques, ed. 5. Philadelphia, FA Davis, 2007, pp 65–104.
41. Helm, P, Herndon, DN, deLateur, B: Restoration of function. J Burn Care Res 2007; 28:611–614.
42. Schmitt, M, Richard, RL, Staley, MJ: Lower extremity burns and ambulation. In: Richard, RL, Staley, MJ (eds): Burn Care and Rehabilitation. Philadelphia, FA Davis, 1994, pp 361–379.
43. Trees, DW, Ketelsen, CA, Hobbs, JA: Use of a modified tilt table for pre-ambulation strength training as an adjunct to burn rehabilitation: A case series. J Burn Care Rehabil 2003; 24:97–103.
44. Malic, C, Phipps, A, Botea, D, et al: The virtual physiotherapist for burn patients. Burns 2007; 33:S29–S30.
45. Hunt, JL, Arnoldo, BD, Kowalske, K, et al: Heterotopic ossification revisited: A 21 year surgical experience. J Burn Care Res 2006; 27:535–540.
46. Crawford, CM, Varghese, G, Mani, MM, et al: Heterotopic ossification: Are range of motion exercises contraindicated? J Burn Care Rehabil 1986; 7:323–327.
47. Sandqvist, G, Akesson, A, Eklund, M: Evaluation of paraffin bath treatment in patients with systemic sclerosis. Disabil Rehabil 2004; 26:981–987.

48. Shamus, E, Wilson, S: The physiologic effects of therapeutic modality intervention on the body systems. In: Prentice, WE, Quillen, WS, Underwood, F (eds): Therapeutic Modalities in Rehabilitation, ed. 3. New York, McGraw-Hill, 2005, pp 551–565.

49. Ward, RS, Hayes-Lundy, C, Reddy, R, et al: Evaluation of topical ultrasound to improve response to physical therapy and lessen scar contracture after injury. J Burn Care Rehabil 1994; 15:74–79.

50. Umraw, N, Chan, Y, Gomez, M, et al: Effective hand function assessment after burn injuries. J Burn Care Rehabil 2004; 25:134–139.

51. Nuchtern, JG, Engrav, LH, Nakamura, DY, et al: Treatment of fourth-degree hand burns. J Burn Care Rehabil 1995; 16:36–42.

52. Torres-Gray, D, Johnson, J, Mlakar, J: Rehabilitation of the burned hand: Questionnaire results. J Burn Care Rehabil 1996; 17:161–168.

53. Howell, JW: Management of the burned hand. In: Richard, RL, Staley, MJ (eds): Burn Care and Rehabilitation. Philadelphia, FA Davis, 1994, pp 531–575.

54. Flowers, KR: String wrapping versus massage for reducing digital volume. Phys Ther 1988; 68:57–59.

55. Brand, PW, Hollister, A: Postoperative stiffness and adhesion. In: Brand, PW (ed): Clinical Mechanics of the Hand, ed. 2. St. Louis, Mosby, 1985, pp 163–178.

56. Colditz, J: Anatomic considerations for splinting the thumb. In: Hunter, JM, Mackin, EJ, Callahan, AD (eds): Rehabilitation of the Hand: Surgery and Therapy, ed. 4. St. Louis, Mosby, 1995, pp 1161–1172.

57. Kwan, MW, Kennis, WY: Splinting program for patients with burnt hand. Hand Surg 2002; 7:231–241.

58. Sheridan, RL, Hurley, J, Smith, M, et al: The acutely burned hand: Management and outcome based on a ten-year experience with 1047 acute hand burns. J Trauma 1995; 38:406–411.

59. Kowalske, KJ, Greenhalgh, DG, Ward, SR: Hand burns. J Burn Care Res 2007; 28:607–610.

60. Richard, RL, Staley, MJ: Scar management. In: Richard, RL, Staley, MJ (eds): Burn Care and Rehabilitation: Principles and Practice. Philadelphia, FA Davis, 1994, pp 380–418.

61. Forbes-Duchart, L, Marshall, S, Strock, A, et al: Determination of inter-rater reliability in pediatric burn scar assessment using a modified version of the Vancouver Scar Scale. J Burn Care Res 2007; 28:460–467.

62. Bombaro, KM, Engrav, LH, Carrougher, GJ, et al: What is the prevalence of hypertrophic scars following burns? Burns 2003; 29:299–302.

63. Corica, GF, Wigger, NC, Edgar, DW, et al: Objective measurement of scarring by multiple assessors: Is the tissue tonometer a reliable option? J Burn Care Res 2006; 27:520–523.

64. Baker, RH, Townley, WA, Mckeon, S, et al: Retrospective study of the association between hypertrophic burn scarring and bacterial colonization. J Burn Care Res 2007; 28:152–156.

65. Sullivan, T, Smith, J, Kermode, J, et al: Rating the burn scar. J Burn Care Res 1990; 11:256–260.

66. Bryza, MJ, Baryza, GA: The Vancouver Scar Scale: An administration tool and its interrater reliability. J Burn Care Rehabili 1995; 16:535–538.

67. Musgrove, MA, Umraw, N, Fish, JS, et al: The effect of silicone gel sheets on perfusion hypertrophic burn scars. J Burn Care Rehabil 2002; 23:208–213.

68. Van den Kerckhove, E, Stappaerts, K, Fieuws, S, et al: The assessment of erythema and thickness on burn related scars during pressure garment therapy as a preventative measure for hypertrophic scarring. Burns 2005; 31:696–702.

69. Teot, L: Scar evaluation and management: Recommendations. —J Tissue Viability 2005; 15(4):6–14.

70. Leung, KS, Cheng, JCY, Ma, GFY, et al: Complications of pressure therapy for post-burn hypertrophic scars. Burns 1984; 10:434–438.

71. Whitmore, JJ, Burt, MM, Fowler, RS Jr, et al: Bandaging the lower extremity to control swelling: Figure-8 versus spiral technique. Arch Phys Med Rehabil 1972; 53:487–490.

72. Parks, DH, Larson, DL, Houssaye, AJ: Hypertrophic scarring: Pressure dressings. In: Fellar, I, Grabb, WC (eds): Reconstruction and Rehabilitation of the Burned Patient. National Institute of Burn Medicine, 1979, pp 20–27.

73. Rose, MP, Deitch, EA: The effective use of tubular compression bandage, Tubigrip, for burn scar therapy in the growing child. J Burn Care Rehabil 1983; 4:197–201.

74. Judge, JC, May, SR, DeClement, FA: Control of hypertrophic scarring in burn patients using tubular support bandages. J Burn Care Rehabil 1984; 5:221–224.

75. Kealy, GP, Jensen, KL, Laubenthal, KN, et al: Prospective randomized comparison of two types of pressure therapy garments. J Burn Care Rehabil 1990; 11:334–336.

76. Ward, RS: Pressure therapy for the control of hypertrophic scar formation after burn injury. A history and review. J Burn Care Rehabil 1991; 12:257–262.

77. Larson, DL, Abston, S, Evans, EB, et al: Techniques for decreasing scar formation and contractures in the burned patient. J Trauma 1971; 11:807–823.

78. Van den Kerckhove, E, Stappaerts, K, Boeckx, W, et al: Silicones in the rehabilitation of burns: A review and overview. Burns 2001; 27:205–214.

79. Bradford, BA, Breault, LG, Schneid, T, et al: Silicone thermoplastic sheeting for treatment of facial scars: An improved technique. J Prosthodont 1999; 8:138–141.

80. Perkins, K, Davey, RB, Wallis, KA: Silicone gel: A new treatment for burns scars and contractures. Burns 1983; 9:201–204.

81. Wessling, N, Ehleben, CM, Chapmanet, V, et al: Evidence that use of a silicone gel sheet increases range of motion over burn wound contractures. J Burn Care Rehabil 1985; 6:503–505.

82. Quinn, KJ: Silicone gel in scar treatment. Burns 1987; 13:S33–S40.

83. Eishi, K, Bae, SJ, Ogawa, F, et al: Silicone gel sheets relive pain and pruritus with clinical improvement of keloid: Possible target of mast cell. J Dermatolog Treat 2003; 14:248–252.

84. Katz, BE: Silicone gel sheeting in scar therapy. Cutis 1995; 56:65–67.

85. Davey, RB, Wallis, KA, Bowering, K: Adhesive contact media—An update on graft fixation and burn scar management. Burns 1991; 17:313–319.

86. Ahn, ST, Monafo, WW, Mustoe, TA: Topical silicone gel for the prevention and treatment of hypertrophic scar. Arch Surg 1991; 126:499–504.

87. Rogers, B, Chapman, T, Rettele, J, et al: Computerized manufacturing of transparent face masks for the treatment of facial scarring. J Burn Care Rehabil 2003; 24:91–96.

88. Rivers, EA, Strate, RG, Solem, LD: The transparent face mask. Am J Occup Ther 1979; 33:108–113.

89. Silverberg, R, Johnson, J, Moffat, M: The effects of soft tissue mobilization on the immature burn scar: Results of a pilot study. J Burn Care Rehabil 1996; 17:252–259.

90. Hettrick, H, O'Brien, K, Laznick, H, et al: Effect of transcutaneous electrical nerve stimulation for the management of burn pruritus: A pilot study. J Burn Care Rehabil 2004; 25:236–240.

91. Kowalske, K, Holavanahalli, R, Helm, P: Neuropathy after burn injury. J Burn Care Rehabil 2001; 22:353–357.

92. Huang, ME, Nelson, VS, Flood, KM, et al: Limb deficiency and prosthetic management. 3. Complex limb deficiency. Arch Phys Med Rehabil 2006; 87(suppl 1):S15–S20.

93. Selvaggi, G, Monstrey, S, Van Landuyt, K, et al: Rehabilitation of burn injured patients following lightning and electrical trauma. NeuroRehabilitation 2005; 20:35–42.

94. Arnoldo, BR, Purdue, GF, Kowalske K, et al: Electrical injuries: A 20-year review. J Burn Care Rehabil 2004; 25:479–484.

95. Celis, MM, Suman, OE, Huang, TT, et al: Effect of a supervised exercise and physiotherapy program on surgical interventions in children with thermal injury. J Burn Care Rehabil 2003; 24:57–61.

96. Cucuzzo, NA, Ferrando, A, Herndon, DN: The effects of exercise programming versus traditional outpatient therapy in the rehabilitation of severely burned children. J Burn Care Rehabil 2001; 22:214–220.

97. Mayes, T, Gottschlich, M, Scanlon, J, et al: Four year review of burns as an etiologic factor in the development of long bone fractures in pediatric patients. J Burn Care Rehabil 2003; 24:279–284.

98. Reeves, SU, Warden, G, Staley, MJ: Management of the pediatric burn patient. In: Richard, RL, Staley, MJ (eds): Burn Care and Rehabilitation. Philadelphia, FA Davis, 1994, pp 499–530.

99. Moss, BF, Everett, JJ, Petterson, DR: Psychologic support and pain management of the burn patient. In: Richard, RL, Staley, MJ (eds): Burn Care and Rehabilitation: Principles and Practice. Philadelphia, FA Davis, 1994, pp 475–498.

100. Christiansen, M, Carrougher, GJ, Engrave, LH, et al: Time to school re-entry after burn injury is quite short. J Burn Care Res 2007; 28:478–481.

101. Rimmer, RB, Fornaciari, GM, Foster, KN, et al: Impact of a pediatric residential burn camp experience on burn survivors' perception of self and attitudes regarding the camp community. J Burn Care Res 2007; 28:334–341.

chapter 22

Managing Wound-Related Pain

Marie K. Hoeger Bement, PT, PhD

Carol G.T. Vance, PT, MA

Kathleen A. Sluka, PT, PhD

Introduction and Definitions

Pain is defined as an unpleasant sensory and emotional experience associated with actual or potential tissue damage or is defined in such terms as those set forth by the International Association for the Study of Pain (IASP).[1,2] Inherent in the definition of pain is its multidimensional nature. There are three dimensions of pain, which are defined as the sensory discriminative, motivational affective, and cognitive evaluative.[3] The sensory discriminative component of pain mediates the quality, intensity, duration, and location of the pain. The motivational affective component is concerned with the emotional aspects and the unpleasantness associated with pain. Lastly, the cognitive evaluative dimension of pain modulates both of the previous two dimensions and puts pain in the context of past experiences and current state of the individual. This chapter will discuss the basic science mechanisms of pain, the assessment of pain, and the management of wound-related pain. When possible, reviews, books, or book chapters are referenced to provide additional information for the reader. For a more in-depth review of the basic science mechanisms and an evidence-based approach for management of a variety of pain conditions, the reader is referred to "Pain Mechanisms and Management for the Physical Therapist."[1]

Spontaneous pain, or pain at rest, is very common and can be a substantial part of the pain associated with wounds. Referred pain is pain felt outside the area of injury and is not associated with a response to an applied stimulus. The most common example of referred pain is that of pain in the left shoulder and down the left arm during a heart attack (angina pain from cardiac ischemia). Pain can occur in response to externally applied stimuli and may be referred to as evoked incident pain. Hyperalgesia is an increased pain response to a normally noxious (painful) stimulus. When this increased pain response occurs at the site of injury, it is termed *primary hyperalgesia*. Hyperalgesia also may occur outside the site of injury and is called *secondary hyperalgesia*. (Fig. 22.1) Primary hyperalgesia is thought to reflect changes in the peripheral nervous system, whereas secondary hyperalgesia is thought to be mediated by changes in the central nervous system (more on secondary hyperalgesia will be covered below in the section Central Pain Pathways). *Allodynia,* on the other hand, is defined as pain in response to a normally innocuous (nonpainful) stimuli or activities.[2] Allodynia is thought to be mediated by changes in the central nervous system where activation of a peripherally located non-nociceptor is perceived as painful. An example of allodynia is a painful response to gentle touching of the skin after wounding from a burn injury.

Pain can be acute or chronic. Acute pain is protective and serves as a warning sign that the body is experiencing actual or potential tissue damage. Clinically, acute pain is usually the result of an injury that can be pinpointed to time and place, such as suffering a burn injury. Acute pain occurs immediately at the time of injury and usually goes away once healing is completed. On the other hand, chronic pain is non-protective and serves no biological purpose. Pain can be considered chronic if (a) pain outlasts normal tissue-healing time, (b) pain is greater than would be expected from the extent of the injury, and (c) pain occurs in the absence of identifiable tissue damage.[2] Thus, the concept of pain as a symptom, as occurs with acute pain, changes to the concept of pain as a disease, as occurs with chronic pain. Regardless of whether pain is acute or chronic, all patients have a right to pain treatment. For wounds, pain can be quite severe at rest and can be further increased during treatments, including débridement, dressing changes, or mobility. Thus, treatment of wound pain will focus not only

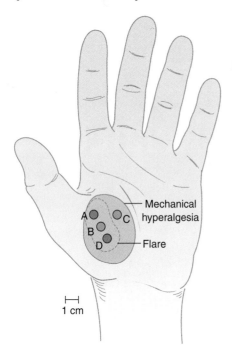

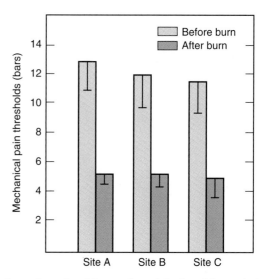

Figure 22•1 *Primary and secondary hyperalgesia. Two burns were formed on the glabrous skin of the hand (A and D). Mechanical pain thresholds for pain were recorded at sites A, B, and C. Mechanical pain threshold decreased at all three of the recorded sites. Primary hyperalgesia developed at the area of injury (ie, flare) and secondary hyperalgesia developed outside of the area of injury. Used with permission from Raja, SN, Campbell, JN, Meyer, RA: Evidence for different mechanisms of primary and secondary hyperalgesia following heat injury to the glabrous skin. Brain 1984; 107:1179–1188.*

on the pain at rest that is associated with the injury, but also on controlling the pain during and after treatment.

▸ **PEARL 22•1** Pain is an unpleasant sensory and emotional experience associated with actual or potential tissue damage. Acute pain is protective and serves as a warning sign that the body is experiencing actual or potential tissue damage, whereas chronic is pain nonprotective and serves no biological purpose.

Pain from a wound can occur as a result of direct injury to the nociceptive nerve endings innervating the area, activation of excitatory receptors on nociceptive nerve endings, or from wound treatment itself. Inflammation and infection will release substances that can activate and sensitize nociceptors, which results in increased transmission to the central nervous system and thus increased pain. These substances include prostaglandins and inflammatory cytokines, as well as neuropeptides such as substance P and calcitonin gene-related peptide (CGRP). Furthermore, mechanical activation of nociceptors that occurs with débridement or compression of the wound from dressings also will activate nociceptors.

Pain Pathways
Peripheral Pain Pathways

Pain is transmitted from the peripheral site of injury (ie, wound) to the spinal cord and on to the cortex where it is

perceived as pain. This pain pathway is typically described as a three-neuron pathway that includes the nociceptor, the spinothalamic tract, and the thalamocortical tract.[4,5] (Fig. 22.2) The first-order neurons are nociceptors that are activated in the peripheral tissue by damaging or potentially damaging (ie, noxious) stimuli. In the skin, free nerve endings of nociceptive primary afferent fibers are located at the dermal-epidermal junction. (Fig 22.3) Nociceptors also innervate deeper tissues, including the fascia, the connective tissues surrounding muscle, and the joint capsule and synovium.[4] Nociceptors include both thinly myelinated Aδ and unmyelinated C fibers. Polymodal nociceptors are generally activated by mechanical and thermal stimuli as well as by chemical stimuli that trigger pain associated with acute and chronic wounds. There are also "silent" nociceptors that do not respond to mechanical or thermal stimuli applied to the peripheral receptive field.[6,7] These silent nociceptors are only activated after tissue injury. Inflammation, which may be induced by infection, causes silent nociceptors to be activated by noxious stimuli resulting in hyperalgesia.

▸ **PEARL 22•2** Nociceptors are activated by mechanical, thermal, and/or chemical stimuli.

The central terminals of this unipolar first-order neuron terminate in the spinal cord dorsal horn where they synapse with a second-order neuron. The second-order neuron is typically referred to as the spinothalamic tract neuron, which sends axon projections supraspinally to the ventroposterior

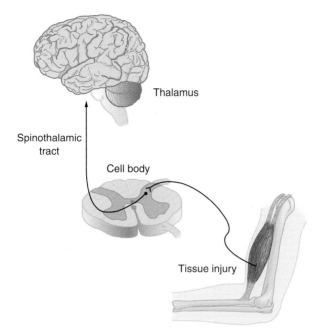

Figure 22•2 *Pain pathway. Tissue injury activates a nociceptor, which sends information to the spinal cord. The signal continues along the spinothalamic tract, which sends projections to the thalamus. This information is then sent to the somatosensory cortex where pain is perceived.*

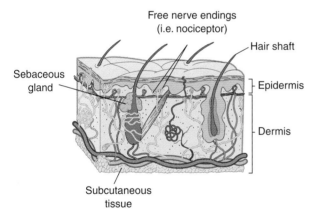

Figure 22•3 *Nociceptor located at the dermal-epidermal junction.*

lateral nucleus of the thalamus. In the thalamus, the second-order neuron then synapses with a third-order neuron, which in turn projects to somatosensory cortex.[4,5] Importantly, perception of the location and nature of pain occurs when the nociceptive signals reach the cortex. Thus, if there is a dysfunction anywhere along the pathway that would prevent the transmission of the pain signal to the cortex, pain would not be experienced.

The sensitivity of nociceptors to painful stimuli is modifiable, increasing in response to tissue injury.[7] Following tissue injury, sensitization of primary afferent fibers can occur.[8] Sensitization of a neuron is characterized by increased spontaneous activity, a decrease in threshold of response to noxious stimuli, an increase in responsiveness to the same noxious stimuli, and/or an increase in receptive field size.[8] Following tissue injury, silent nociceptors begin to respond to noxious stimuli and will spontaneously fire. Taken together, there is a general increase in activity of nociceptors after tissue injury. An increase in nociceptor activity will increase the number of afferents firing following a peripheral insult, which in turn increases input to the central nervous system. This sensitization increases the responsiveness of primary pain afferent nociceptors to noxious stimuli and hence constitutes an explanation for hyperalgesia at the site of injury (ie, primary hyperalgesia).

▶ **PEARL 22•3** Tissue injury sensitizes pain neurons causing increased spontaneous activity, a decrease in threshold of response to noxious stimuli, an increase in responsiveness to the same noxious stimuli, and/or an increase in receptive field size. This may be demonstrated clinically by an increase in pain reports, including spontaneous or nonevoked pain, and spreading of pain.

Sensitization of nociceptors occurs in response to peripheral inflammatory mediators that are released or present at the site of injury.[8,9] (Fig. 22.4) These substances are released from non-neuronal cells and include serotonin, bradykinin, prostaglandins, and cytokines. Serotonin, released from platelets, activates muscle nociceptors and causes pain in

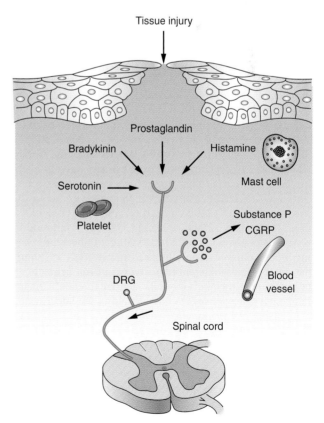

Figure 22•4 *Inflammatory mediators.*

humans.[10,11] Bradykinin is released from plasma after tissue injury, is present in inflammatory exudates, sensitizes nociceptors, and produces pain and hyperalgesia in humans.[12-14] Prostaglandins are metabolites of the arachidonic acid cascade and are produced in response to tissue injury. Importantly, prostaglandins E_2 and I_2 directly excite and sensitize afferent fibers.[15] The NSAIDs produce their effects by reducing prostaglandin production through inhibition of the enzyme cyclooxygenase, which is involved in the breakdown of arachidonic acid.

During inflammation, macrophages release cytokines that include interleukins (IL1β, IL-6) and tumor necrosis factor (TNF-α; for a review on cytokines see Gosain and Gamelli).[16] Cytokines mediate the inflammatory process and sensitize primary afferent nociceptors, thus producing mechanical and thermal hyperalgesia.[17-21] These inflammatory cytokines are increased in the synovial fluid of patients with arthritis.[20,21] In patients with chronic venous leg ulcers, there is a significantly higher concentration of proinflammatory cytokines in the wound fluid of nonhealing ulcers compared with healing ulcers.[22] Blocking TNF- α receptors or available TNF- α reduces hyperalgesia in animal models of inflammation and neuropathic pain.[23,24] Additionally, decreases in pH occur, with inflammation causing activation of acid-sensing ion channels on nociceptors, which results in increased nociception and hyperalgesia.[25,26] While the actions of each of these inflammatory mediators is described individually, many mediators act together to enhance the inflammation or hyperalgesia, producing a potentiated response.[27] This helps to explain why individuals report pain associated with the acute inflammatory process (eg, acute burns or trauma-induced wounds) and with chronic wounds (eg, pressure ulcers).

Although blood borne factors are considered to be the major initiator of inflammation, a substantial amount of literature beginning at the turn of the century is devoted to the involvement of the peripheral nervous systems in this process.[28,29] Neurogenic inflammation is a term used to describe the role of the nervous system in the development and maintenance of peripheral inflammation. Neuropeptides such as substance P and calcitonin gene-related peptide (CGRP) are contained in small-diameter afferents (group III and IV) and, when released from primary afferent fibers in the periphery, produce an inflammatory response.[30,31] These substances intensify the inflammatory events in the periphery, producing plasma extravasation and vasodilatation.[30,32,33] In fact, substance P and CGRP are also found in inflammatory exudate and primary afferent fibers innervating inflamed tissue in both humans and animals.[34,35] Elimination of primary afferent fibers by peripheral neurectomy or capsaicin (which kills group IV afferents) reduces the inflammatory response.[36-38] Interestingly, the neurogenic component of inflammation involves the central nervous system, specifically dorsal root reflexes generated in the spinal cord.[29] Thus, the inflammatory pain response associated with acute and chronic wounds involves both the peripheral and central nervous system.

The release of neuropeptides peripherally has been shown to promote wound healing.[39-42] For example, peripheral application of substance P or CGRP speeds wound healing in animal models.[39,42] In contrast, blockade of substance P or CGRP receptors, or removal of nociceptive afferents with capsaicin, reduces wound healing.[40,43,44] In people with diabetic neuropathy, this is particularly relevant as there is loss of pain sensation, loss of nociceptors in the periphery, and, therefore, loss of the normal protective function of nociceptors. Furthermore, topical application of morphine for pain control in a cutaneous wound also impairs wound healing.[45] Opioids work peripherally at the site of injury to reduce activation of nociceptors and thus reduce peripheral release of substance P and CGRP. Interestingly, this impairment of wound healing by morphine can be prevented by application of substance P in combination with the morphine.

The processing of nociceptive information and pain in the central nervous system is complex, involving multiple anatomical pathways and brain sites. The responses to nociceptive information are coordinated within the spinal cord, ascending nociceptive pathways, descending facilitatory pathways, and descending inhibitory pathways. All of these are interrelated and control the level of pain at a given time. Thus, pain processing is plastic and modifiable. Although it is not feasible to describe in detail all of the pain systems involved in nociceptive processing, the more major and well-studied pathways will be highlighted.

Central Pain Pathways

The spinal cord is the first termination site of nociceptors in the central nervous system integrating incoming information that is subject to both local spinal and supraspinal modulation. In the spinal cord, laminae I to VI constitute the dorsal horn where the majority of sensory afferents terminate. In general, the fine sensory fibers conveying noxious information from the skin terminate in the most superficial layers, laminae I, II, and V. The terminals of larger fibers conveying tactile information are dispersed between laminae III and IV. Many of these fibers terminate on spinal interneurons that relay information to cells deeper in the spinal cord. Primary afferent fibers from several peripheral structures (cutaneous, joint, muscle, and viscera) converge on one neuron. This convergence is thought to be the basis for referred pain and secondary hyperalgesia. Thus, pain felt in one muscle is referred to another muscle or skin that sends projections to the same dorsal horn neuron.

Neurons in the dorsal horn of the spinal cord are classified as high threshold, wide dynamic range, and low threshold. High-threshold neurons respond only to noxious stimulation. Low-threshold neurons respond only to innocuous stimuli. Wide dynamic range neurons respond to both noxious and innocuous stimuli. Thus, transmission of nociceptive information through the dorsal horn activates high-threshold and wide dynamic range neurons. Following tissue injury (eg, acute and chronic wounds), sensitization of both high-threshold and wide dynamic range neurons occurs. This is manifested as an increase in receptive field size, increased responsiveness to innocuous or noxious stimuli, or decreased threshold to noxious stimuli.[46-48] These changes in spinal neurons are commonly referred to as central sensitization. Sensitization of wide dynamic range neurons to innocuous mechanical stimuli may underlie allodynia, a painful response to an innocuous stimulus. The underlying basis of secondary hyperalgesia, pain outside the site of injury, is hypothesized to result from expansion of receptive fields and increased sensitivity to noxious stimuli.

> ▸ **PEARL 22•4** Following tissue injury, in addition to peripheral sensitization, central sensitization occurs, causing increased receptive field size, increased responsiveness to innocuous or noxious stimuli, or decreased threshold to noxious stimuli to neurons located in the central nervous system. In the clinical setting, this may be demonstrated through a spreading of pain and an increase in pain behaviors, such as allodynia.

From the spinal cord, nociceptive information is transmitted through the spinothalamic tract neurons in the ventroposterior lateral (VPL) and medial thalamic nuclei. From here, the VPL projects to the somatosensory cortex (SI and SII), and this pathway is thought to be involved in the sensory-discriminative component of pain (ie, location, duration, quality, and intensity). Neurons in the VPL receive convergent input from the dorsal column pathway that transmits information regarding touch sensation and the spinothalamic tract conveying information regarding pain and temperature sensation.[49,50] The ascending projections from the medial thalamic nuclei and the posterior complex are more diffuse and include areas such as the anterior cingulate and insular cortices. Thus, this pathway is thought to be the basis for the motivational-affective component of pain (ie, unpleasantness).

Pain Assessment

The biopsychosocial model is a philosophy of clinical care and a practical clinical guide that is commonly used for the treatment of pain. It involves understanding the disease through multiple levels of organization that extend from the societal to molecular mechanisms. Clinicians must evaluate and treat not only the biological component of the disease but also the psychological and social dimensions. Treatment for pain is diverse and involves a multidisciplinary approach that includes pharmacology, psychology, physical therapy, activity modifications, and in selected cases, surgery.

Assessment of pain is critical for effective restoration of function due to the negative effect pain has on healing, function, sleep, and mood. Understanding the severity of pain and how it is affected by peripherally applied stimuli is necessary in order to determine treatments. For wound pain, in particular, many of the treatments themselves are painful. These treatments should be assessed separately from the pain at rest so that effective therapy can be given during the treatment.[51]

There are a number of methods to measure pain, most of which involve self-report. The use of self-report is imperative because there is a definite contrast in how patients and staff perceive a patient's pain levels.[52] The most commonly used methods are number scales, which include the verbal rating scale, the numerical rating scale, or the visual analog scale. These scales are generally quick, valid, and easy to use. The verbal rating scale asks people to verbally give a number between 0 and 10, with 0 as no pain and 10 as the worst pain imaginable. (Fig. 22.5) With the visual analog scale, people are asked to mark on a 10-cm line, with or without numbers, where there pain is according to the same anchors: no pain and worst pain imaginable. (Fig. 22.5) These types of scales make the assumption that pain is unidimensional and thus do not take into account the multidimensional nature of pain. However, these scales are easy to use and beneficial in assessing rapidly changing wound pain, such as with procedures that are known to induce pain. Thus, rating scales are useful and important for conveying the intensity of the pain experience.

> ▸ **PEARL 22•5** The numerical rating and visual analog scales are unidimensional. These scales used independently of other pain assessment tools provide a narrow view of the entire pain experience, specifically pain intensity.

The use of a body diagram in pain assessment allows the patient to draw the location of his or her pain on outlines of the human body, both the front and back. This type of diagram is useful in understanding the area of the body that is affected by pain. Consistent use of the body pain diagram can

Visual Analog Scale (VAS)

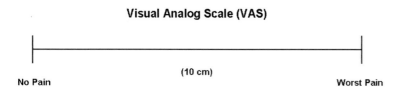

(10 cm)

No Pain   Worst Pain

Numerical Rating Scale

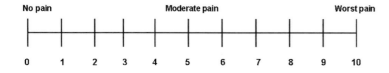

No pain   Moderate pain   Worst pain

0   1   2   3   4   5   6   7   8   9   10

Figure 22•5 *Numerical rating scale and visual analog scales. Both of these scales are used frequently in pain management to assess pain intensity.*

also help the clinician to distinguish changes in pain behaviors, such as the spreading of pain.

There are numerous pain questionnaires used to assess wound pain. We will discuss two here: the Brief Pain Inventory (BPI) and the McGill Pain Questionnaire (MPQ). These two questionnaires are useful to assess functional impact and multidimensional nature of pain, respectively. To examine the affect of pain on mood, physical activity, work, social activity, and sleep, the BPI uses a 0 to 10 numeric rating scale, with 0 being pain "does not interfere with function" and 10 being "pain that completely interferes with function."[53] There are also numerical rating scales of pain that are graded as worst, best, and average. The Brief Pain Inventory has been modified for the use in patients with diabetic peripheral neuropathy (BPI-DPN), which has been validated by Zelman and colleagues.[54] For both the BPI and the BPI-DPN, caution should be used because memory for pain intensity is poor, whereas memory for functional limitations as a result of pain is excellent.[55]

The McGill Pain Questionnaire assesses the three dimensions of pain using a bank of descriptor words.[51,56] (Fig. 22.6) A numerical intensity scale and a pain drawing are incorporated into the questionnaire. The descriptor words are grouped into 20 categories and are weighted. The 20 categories include adjectives that are associated with the sensory-discriminative (descriptors 1–10), the motivational-affective (descriptors 11–15), and the cognitive-evaluative (descriptor 16) dimensions of pain. Subjects are asked to circle all the words that best describe their pain, but are allowed to pick only one in each of the 20 categories. It is scored by counting the number of words chosen and a pain rating index that weights the word in the list. There is also a short form of the MPQ that includes 15 words that encompass all 3 categories, and the patient rates them as 0 (none), 1 (mild), 2 (moderate), or 3 (severe). The MPQ, both full length and the short form, is reliable and valid. Its most useful benefit is to measure the multidimensional nature of the pain experience. The MPQ has been used extensively in the assessment of many types of wound pain, including burns, vascular insufficiency, pressure ulcers, and neuropathies.

> **PEARL 22•6** The McGill Pain Questionnaire is more sensitive in assessing chronic wound pain than a single rating of pain intensity using the numerical rating scale.[53]

Similar to assessment, there are different models of wound pain. Krasner's model of wound pain defines three types of wound pain: noncyclic acute wound pain (ie, drain removal), cyclic acute wound pain (ie, daily dressing changes), and chronic wound pain (ie, persistent nonevoked pain).[57] (Fig. 22.7) This model is based on the timing of pain and does not take into account psychosocial issues. Treatment strategies are recommended for each type of pain. Another model is the Wound Pain Management Model, which defines six dimensions of pain, including location, duration, intensity, quality, onset, and impact on activities of daily living.[58] This model assumes that all wounds are painful until further assessment proves differently. Both of these models assist the clinician in the assessment and development of appropriate wound care.

Types of Wound Pain
Neuropathic Pain

Injury to the peripheral and/or central nervous system causes neuropathic pain. Patients describe neuropathic pain as sharp, burning, and lancinating. Other potential symptoms include altered sensation and autonomic changes. If large fibers are damaged, in addition to small fibers that transmit pain and temperature, patients also present with muscle weakness. The prevalence of neuropathic pain is difficult to estimate due to the broad classification, which includes traumatic injury or disease conditions that affect the nervous system.

Neuropathic pain may be present in any wound that involves damage to the nervous system. With wounds, tissue trauma negatively impacts the peripheral nervous system. Specifically, damage to the peripheral nervous system may cause the formation of neuromas, which are bundles of nerve tissue that fire spontaneously. Furthermore, as discussed in the introduction, tissue damage causes peripheral sensitization. These changes in the peripheral nervous system alter the pain signals to the central nervous system, which can lead to central sensitization. Thus, tissue damage associated with wounds may cause additional damage to the peripheral and central nervous systems, which helps to explain why patients with neuropathic pain report hyperalgesia, allodynia, spontaneous pain, and the spreading of pain.

> **PEARL 22•7** Individuals with wounds that cause damage to the peripheral and/or central nervous systems are at risk for the development of neuropathic pain. For example, tissue trauma in the periphery (ie, wound) may damage nociceptors and their primary afferent fibers, which send signals to the spinal cord. This wound damage would sensitize the peripheral nervous system (ie, peripheral sensitization).

Diabetic neuropathy is the most common type of peripheral neuropathy. With diabetes, there is selective small fiber loss resulting in pain and paresthesia that is frequently described as burning, although pain may also be reported as deep, aching, sharp, and/or shooting. Pain frequently increases at night or with stressful conditions.[59] In addition to painful neuropathy, individuals with diabetes experience pain secondary to arterial insufficiency (see vascular disorders). Thus, pain associated with diabetes may be due to changes in the vascular and nervous systems.

In a survey of patients with type 2 diabetes, 64% of participants reported pain.[60] A follow-up neurological examination found that 37% had nonneuropathic pain and 26% had neuropathic pain. It is estimated that painful diabetic neuropathy affects 20% to 24% of individuals with diabetes mellitus, with pain worsening, improving, or remaining the same with the progression of the disease.[61] The presence of pain is not dependent on intact sensation. Patients with no or little sensation may still experience severe neuropathic pain due to the changes in the areas of the nervous system that modulate pain.

Glucose levels may or may not affect pain perception in individuals with diabetes. Morley and colleagues found

Where Is Your Pain?

Part 1.

Please mark, on the drawings below, the areas where you feel pain. Put E if external, or I if internal, near the areas which you mark. Put EI if both external and internal.

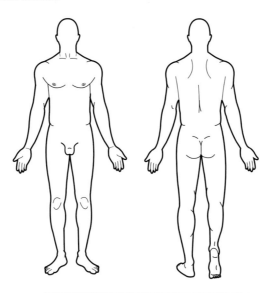

What Does Your Pain Feel Like?

Part 2.

Some of the words below describe your ***present*** pain. Circle ***ONLY*** those words that best describe it. Leave out any category that is not suitable. Use only a single word in each appropriate category – the one that applies best.

1		2		3		4
Flickering		Jumping		Pricking		Sharp
Quivering		Flashing		Boring		Cutting
Pulsing		Shooting		Drilling		Lacerating
Throbbing				Stabbing		
Beating				Lacinating		
Pounding						

5		6		7		8
Pinching		Tugging		Hot		Tingling
Pressing		Pulling		Burning		Itchy
Gnawing		Wrenching		Scalding		Smarting
Cramping				Searing		Stinging
Crushing						

Figure 22•6 *McGill Pain Questionnaire. This figure is used with permission from: The McGill Pain Questionnaire: Major properties and scoring methods. Pain 1975: 1(3):277–299. Copyright Elsevier.*

Continued

9		10		11		12	
Dull		Tender		Tiring		Sickening	
Sore		Taut		Exhausting		Suffocating	
Hurting		Rasping					
Aching		Splitting					
Heavy							
13		**14**		**15**		**16**	
Fearful		Punishing		Wretched		Annoying	
Frightful		Grueling		Blinding		Troublesome	
Terrifying		Cruel				Miserable	
		Vicious				Intense	
		Killing				Unbearable	
17		**18**		**19**		**20**	
Spreading		Tight		Cool		Nagging	
Radiating		Numb		Cold		Nauseating	
Penetrating		Drawing		Freezing		Agonizing	
Piercing		Squeezing				Dreadful	
		Tearing				Torturing	

How Does Your Pain Change With Time?

Part 3.

1. Which word, or words, would you use to describe the **pattern** of your pain?

1		2		3	
Continuous		Rhythmic		Brief	
Steady		Periodic		Momentary	
Constant		Intermittent		Transient	

2. What kind of things **relieve** your pain?

3. What kind of things **increase** your pain?

How Strong Is Your Pain

Part 4.

People agree that the following 5 words represent pain of increasing intensity. They are:

1		2		3		4		5
Mild		Discomforting		Distressing		Horrible		Excruciating

To answer each question below, write the number of the most appropriate word in the space beside each question.

1. Which word describes your pain right now?   _____

2. Which word describes it at its worst?   _____

3. Which word describes it when it is least?   _____

4. Which word describes the worst toothache you've ever had?   _____

5. Which word describes the worst headache you've ever had?   _____

6. Which word describes the worst stomach ache you've ever had?   _____

Figure 22•6 McGill Pain Questionnaire.

The Chronic Wound Pain Experience (CWPE)

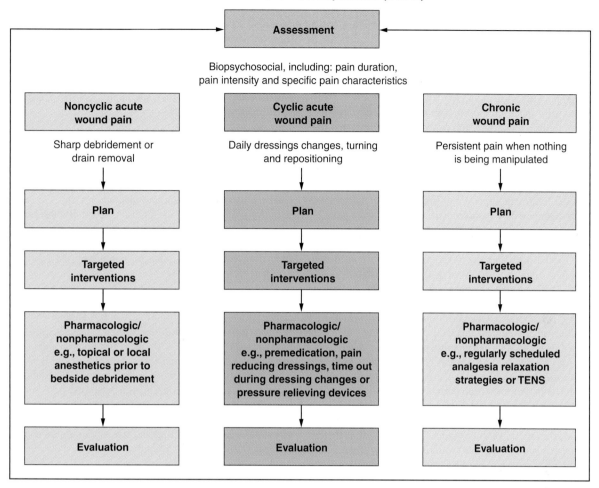

Figure **22•7** *Krasner's model of the chronic wound pain experience. Used with permission from Krasner, D: The chronic wound pain experience: A conceptual model. Ostomy Wound Manage 1995; 41:20–25.*

that diabetic individuals with elevated glucose levels were more sensitive to a noxious stimulus than individuals without diabetes.[62] In contrast, Chan and colleagues found that rapid changes in blood glucose concentrations did not affect heat pain thresholds in patients with diabetes with and without painful peripheral neuropathy.[63] Good blood glucose control is imperative for the management of diabetes but may not influence pain perception in this population.

Another condition that has a strong neuropathic component is phantom pain. Phantom pain is that which is felt in an area of the body that has been amputated. The majority of patients with amputations report phantom pain, with 72% and 67% of patients reporting phantom limb pain at 8 days and 6 months after amputation, respectively.[64] The cause of the amputation may be a factor in the prevalence of phantom pain. Phantom pain in patients with peripheral vascular disease was reported 79% of the time at 6 months following the amputation. In individuals with amputations secondary to cancer, 60% and 32% reported phantom pain at 1 month and 2 years, respectively. It is very difficult to

compare the presence of phantom pain across populations due to the broad range of medical management. For example, the lower prevalence in the oncology patients could be due to their treatment protocol, which incorporates the World Health Organization analgesic ladder. Not enough studies have been conducted to fully assess the relationship of the development of phantom limb pain with the cause of amputation; however, it is important to note that regardless of the cause of the amputation, a significant number of individuals report long-lasting phantom pain.

Phantom pain may change with time, with fewer individuals reporting phantom pain in the later stages following an amputation than the acute stages. However, if phantom pain is still present after 6 months, the pain will likely remain.[67] The qualitative descriptors of pain also change over time, with knifelike reports in the acute stage and squeezing and burning reported in the later stages.[64]

The presence of phantom limb pain is related to pain reports prior to surgery. Patients who had pain prior to their amputation were more likely to develop phantom pain than were patients without pain.[64] Similarly, preamputation pain predicted phantom pain at 24 months, whereas acute phantom limb pain (4 to 5 days after surgery) predicted the presence of phantom limb pain at 6- and 12-month follow-ups.[68] Furthermore, phantom limb pain in patients with peripheral vascular disease was related to preamputation coping skills, which supports the use of the biopsychosocial model for assessing pain.[65] These studies indicate the necessity for a thorough pain assessment and management protocol to be established prior to amputation to help prevent the development of phantom limb pain. Bach and colleagues demonstrated that patients who received preoperative lumbar epidural blockade for 72 hours were less likely to have phantom pain at a 6-month follow-up than were patients who did not receive the epidural.[69] Subsequent research studies both supported and refuted the treatment approach of preoperative pain management to decrease the incidence of phantom limb pain.[70,71] Regardless of these mixed results, pain management should be addressed both before and after surgery.

The mechanisms behind phantom limb pain continue to be explored. Experiments showing that manipulation of the residual limb influences phantom limb pain sensations demonstrate that peripheral neural mechanisms are involved, including peripheral sensitization and neuroma formation.[72] In addition to the central mechanisms that were previously discussed in relation to neuropathic pain, there is likely reorganization of the somatosensory cortex.[73] Thus, both the peripheral and central nervous systems are involved in the presentation of phantom limb pain.

Vascular Related Pain

Both the arterial and venous systems are important in the development of specific types of wounds as well as in their pain characteristics. In a survey of leg and foot ulcer patients, the most common cause of the ulcer was venous insufficiency, with patient ulcer pain reported by the staff in 47% of the cases.[74] There is considerable variability in the prevalence of venous leg ulcer pain, with studies reporting 28% to 93% (summarized by Nemeth et al).[75] With venous insufficiency, the lower extremity is edematous, which can cause mechanical activation of nociceptors. Furthermore, inflammation is frequently present, resulting in chemical activation of nociceptors. In both arterial and venous insufficiency, neuropathic pain is likely a component due to the close association between the nerves and vascular system as well as the tissue destruction that affects the nervous system.

There are several qualitative descriptors for how individuals with venous leg ulcers describe their pain, which include the following: dull, aching, heavy, stabbing, sharp, and tiring. These pain reports increase when the lower extremity is placed in dependent position, such as sustained sitting or standing. Thus, pain management includes elevation of the limb and/or compression. Nemeth and colleagues assessed pain levels in individuals with venous leg ulcers receiving care in the home or clinical setting during the first 5 weeks of compression therapy.[75] The majority of patients reported leg ulcer pain (85%). The intensity tended to decrease with time; although 81% of the patients continued to report pain at the end of the 5 weeks. Despite the standard care of using compression to treat venous leg ulcers, there is limited research to support or refute this intervention for pain suppression.

Dysfunction of the arterial system can also cause pain. Arterial insufficiency decreases tissue perfusion, causing ischemic conditions. Two types of pain, intermittent and resting, are associated with arterial insufficiency. Intermittent pain is caused by exercise or with lower extremity elevation causing a local ischemic event. Pain while walking (intermittent claudication) is one of the most common complaints and is predictable by nature, with pain occurring in the same location of the lower extremity at the same distance walked.[76] This type of pain is frequently reported as sharp, burning, and cramping, with an anatomical distribution dependent on the artery involved.[77] The pain will cease with the discontinuation of walking and/or by placing the lower extremity in a resting dependent position. If the arterial insufficiency is severe, then resting pain may also be reported. For example, with the progression of peripheral arterial disease, individuals may complain of pain at night while supine in bed due to a decrease in blood pressure.[78] Thus, patients may sleep with their foot resting off the bed in dependency as a pain management technique.

Caution should be assessed when managing wounds caused by vascular conditions because wounds may have both arterial and venous dysfunction. Compressing a wound with mixed arterial and venous involvement would help to control pain caused by venous insufficiency but increase pain by making the arterial insufficiency worse. This is another reason why pain should be continually assessed throughout the wound management program. Furthermore, pain may continue once the wound has healed because the underlying vascular pathology remains. With all types of wounds, if reports of pain change, then further assessment should be completed to identify and manage the cause.

Pressure Ulcers

The mechanism for the development of pressure ulcers involves prolonged compression of tissue between a bony prominence and underlying support surface. Pain may be present before visual identification of a pressure ulcer is possible due to the mechanical activation of nociceptors and tissue injury that is occurring to structures below the skin surface. Chemical activation of nociceptors also occurs due to the inflammation process and ischemic changes that occur with tissue injury, further increasing pain reports.

There is a considerable amount of variability regarding the prevalence and characteristics of pressure ulcer pain, which is summarized as follows: 12% to 41% report no pain, 12% to 80% report continuous pain, and 54% to 100% report occasional pain.[79-82] Unfortunately, despite the majority of patients reporting pain, two of the studies found that only 2% to 6% of those individuals reporting pain received some type of pain medication.[79,80]

The variability of pain reports associated with pressure ulcers is likely due to a number of factors, including the use of more than one type of pain assessment tool as well as the presence of verbal and cognitive impairments. For example, Dallam and colleagues reported that one third of their subjects were not able to respond to the pain evaluation tools, and of those subjects who did respond 48% were found to have a cognitive impairment.[79] Furthermore, there were several types of pain assessment tools used. The studies that used the McGill Pain Questionnaire reported the greatest prevalence of pressure ulcer pain, thus the McGill Pain Questionnaire may be more sensitive than other pain assessment tools in identifying pressure ulcer pain.

Similar to burns, the depth of tissue damage that occurs with pressure ulcers may help explain pain severity. Pressure ulcers that involve greater tissue destruction may also damage nociceptors, causing an increase in pain, or destroy nociceptors, causing an absence of pain. This relationship has not been well studied. Alternatively, Rastinehad concluded that pressure ulcers are extremely painful, regardless of the depth of tissue damage.[83]

Even though the relationship between the amount of tissue damage and pain severity is inconclusive, the type of tissue that is damaged may help explain pain behaviors. It is important to recall that pain characteristics are specific to the tissue that is damaged. For example, cutaneous pain has the following characteristics: sharp, easy to localize, and rarely refers. However, muscle pain is described as dull, burning, difficult to localize, and frequently refers.[84] Periosteal pain is difficult to localize and is frequently described as dull, deep, and boring. This relationship between pain characteristics and the type of tissue damaged may be applied to all types of wound pain.

Burn Pain

Burn pain occurs from tissue trauma secondary to a thermal, chemical, or electrical insult. Burn pain can be very intense, with the majority of patients reporting severe or excruciating pain, with pain occurring daily.[85] Furthermore, typical burn wound management produces frequent and intense nociceptive stimulation causing procedural pain. Several studies demonstrate that the greatest amount of pain occurs during therapeutic procedures, such as wound débridement and dressing changes.[85-87] Furthermore, approximately half of burn patients reported little or no pain relief from medication during a therapeutic procedure.[88]

The depth of tissue injury that occurs with a burn trauma is related to pain behaviors. As discussed in Chapter 21, there are different degrees of burns. With first-degree burns, tissue injury is localized to the epidermis. The majority of individuals with this type of burn experience mild to moderate pain, such as with sunburn.[89] With second-degree burns, pain can be quite severe due to the injury to the epidermis and dermis. This causes damage and potential exposure of free nerve endings (ie, nociceptors; refer to Fig. 22.3). Allodynia is frequently reported for this degree of burn, with patients complaining of pain with minimal amount of stimulus, such as air currents. With a deep second-degree burn, the pain receptors may or may not be intact, resulting in pain hypersensitivity or absence, respectively. Third-degree burns are considered full-thickness wounds, with damage occurring to the subcutaneous tissue that results in the destruction of cutaneous nerve endings. Pain may not be reported due to the destruction of the free nerve endings. Thus, greater tissue damage does not necessarily result in greater pain reports because with a full-thickness injury pain may be absent. However, if deeper tissue is damaged, pain may be quite severe due to the location of nociceptors in deeper structures, such as muscle and periosteal tissue.

> **PEARL 22•8** The amount of tissue damage is not correlated with pain behaviors due to the location of nociceptors. For example, wounds that damage both the epidermis and dermis may cause significant pain reports due to damage to the nociceptors; however, if nociceptors are destroyed, then pain is no longer transmitted to the cortex.

Significant pain may be reported as healing occurs and nerves regenerate. Furthermore, it is important to note that frequently a burn injury is more than just one depth. For example, a burn may be third degree in the center of the wound but be considered second degree around the perimeter of the wound. Therefore, in this case the patient would complain of pain on the wound perimeter where there is less tissue damage. (Fig. 22.8)

Despite the relationship between tissue depth and pain behaviors, caution should be used when evaluating this relationship. The amount of tissue damage is just one of many factors involved with how patients report burn pain, and these two events may not be related. For example, several studies have demonstrated that pain behavior is not associated with burn severity, size, location, or length of time since injury.[85,90]

Appropriate management of burn pain is vital for restoration of function and quality of life. Patient reports of procedural pain during hospitalization were significantly related to psychological adjustment up to 2 years after discharge.[91] Furthermore, long-term ongoing burn pain was reported in 35% to 52% of individuals, with more than 50% of these people reporting that it interfered with function and their rehabilitation.[92,93] Thus, burn pain should be frequently and consistently assessed and appropriately managed.

In addition to assessing pain, health-care professionals should be aware of the psychological distress that burn

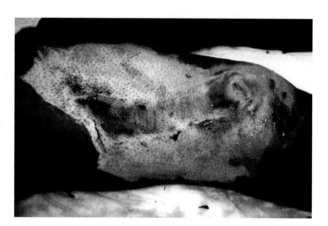

Figure 22•8 *Burn pain in relation to tissue damage. The amount of tissue damage does not equate to an increase in pain reports. This burn injury located on the lower extremity has very deep third-degree central burns and thick eschar but second-degree burns on the periphery. This patient would likely complain of intense pain around the periphery due to the damaged nociceptors, but have no pain in the center due to the absence of nociceptors.*

patients frequently report, which reiterates the importance of using the biopsychosocial model. For example, anxiety of individuals hospitalized with burn injuries was associated with pain reports.[94] Patterson and colleagues, in their review of psychological functioning in burn patients, found that there is a higher incidence of premorbid psychopathological disorders than typically demonstrated in the general population.[95] Thus, preinjury and acute injury psychological status may be an important factor in how individuals manage, including their pain behaviors.

Interventions

When approaching the subject of treatment for wound pain, several general concepts should be mentioned. First, if an intervention for wound pain is to be administered in an effective manner, proper and continuing wound assessment is essential. As mentioned previously, determining the extent of peripheral and central sensitization will guide the clinician in determining the best mode of action. Secondly, even when wound pain is assessed, often treatment of pain is inadequate or nonexistent. For wounds associated with moderate to maximal pain, there is no substitute for aggressive pharmacological management. Third, there are few, if any, randomized controlled trials to date outlining clear parameters for nonpharmacological interventions for wound pain. However, research from animal models and human subjects involving inflammatory pain, neuropathic pain, and chronic musculoskeletal pain may be of assistance in treating wounds.[96-98] Lastly, the clinician should realize that in treating the underlying cause of the wound by administering techniques that facilitate the normal inflammation and repair process they will secondarily reduce pain associated with the wound. For example, lifestyle modifications for arterial wounds, compression and reduction of interstitial edema for ulcers of venous origin, and monitoring and controlling blood sugars in the diabetic population will directly affect tissue healing, resulting in a decrease in wound pain.

Pharmacological Intervention

The cornerstone of effective management of acute pain is administration of opioids, especially for moderate to severe pain. This pain management method is applicable in wounds associated with burns, trauma, and those following surgical procedures. Opioids are commonly used regardless of the amount of tissue trauma.[99,100] Providing an accurate opioid dose is essential to providing relief of pain and suffering, particularly for those with burns. Compelling evidence is available for the importance of controlling acute wound pain. Burn pain during hospitalization is significantly correlated with psychological adjustment at 1 month, 1 year, and 2 years after burn injury.[91] Unfortunately, in some instances this powerful class of drugs is withheld or an insufficient dose is given. For instance, therapeutically insufficient opioid doses are often prescribed to geriatric patients and in 95% of patients with less-severe burns.[101] Burn patients typically require more than the average dose to appropriately address their pain levels at rest, particularly during procedures.[102]

The tendency to underprescribe and underdose is related to the adverse central effects of opioids, as well as the fear of tolerance and addiction (summarized by Choiniere).[102] Tolerance

may be specifically addressed by careful dosing increases over time in concert with ongoing pain assessment. Dosing and careful monitoring are also important in assessing the adverse side effects of opioids, such as depression of respiration, nausea, and constipation. Choiniere recommends carefully monitoring adverse side effects and prescribing drugs such as fentanyl and alfentanyl for procedural pain of débridement and dressing changes since these drugs act rapidly, have a shorter duration of action, and oversedation following the intervention is reduced.[102] Perry and Heidrich conducted a nationwide survey of burn centers, totaling over 10,000 treatments, and found not a single case of iatrogenic effects when opioids were prescribed for pain relief.[103] The majority of research on opioids and acute wound pain has been conducted on burns; however, the use of opioids may be applicable to a broad spectrum of wound pain management. The clinician should be aware of potential side effects of this class of drugs as well as the usefulness of opioids in management of pain to allow for functional exercises and wound débridement and dressing.

> ▶ **PEARL 22•9** Opioids are the cornerstone to affective pharmacological wound management. Careful dosing and monitoring can help prevent the onset of adverse side effects, including respiratory depression, nausea, and constipation.

Other classes of drugs, besides opioids, are beneficial in providing pain relief. NSAIDs can be used alone or in conjunction with opioid medication. NSAIDs are frequently used in the management of leg ulcer pain.[104] These drugs work both peripherally and centrally to reduce inflammation and pain and have relatively few side effects; thus, they are effective for mild to moderate pain conditions. Prolonged use of NSAIDS, however, is not recommended due to adverse side effects, especially for elderly patients because of the possibility of gastrointestinal bleeding and the potential to impair wound healing.

In addition to oral and intravenous drug administration, the use of topical analgesics in the form of liquids, gels, foams, and creams are an important component of a comprehensive pain management program. Careful examination, with particular regard to wound size and wound pathology, will decrease the potential side effect of toxicity. Topical analgesics have been used with success in intervening in wound procedural pain for wounds typically less than 50 cm^2 and of venous and pressure origin. A Cochrane review of six independent trials of topical 5% EMLA (lidocaine/prilocaine cream) applied prior to débridement of venous ulcers provided pain relief when compared to placebo cream.[105] Even though the largest ulcer treated was 100 cm^2, the authors recommend caution when using local anesthetic application in venous wounds greater that 50 cm^2. Of note, one of the indications for use of EMLA cream is analgesia of intact skin. Local application of benzydamine gel, which is a NSAID, to 30 pressure ulcers in 17 subjects provided pain relief in the first 24 hours following application in 29 of the 30 wounds, and all 30 wounds were pain free after 48 hours.[106]

Several studies have assessed topical opioid use. Specifically, dimorphine and morphine gels are effective in the management of pressure ulcers. Double-blinded placebo controlled trials found significant reduction in pain scores, with only one episode of adverse effects of opioid toxicity.[107,108] Twillman and colleagues assessed the use of topical opioids in the management of painful skin ulcers.[109] Nine patients with wounds of varying etiologies were treated with topical morphine-infused dressings; eight subjects demonstrated reductions in pain scores. The only patient who did not respond favorably was most likely an inappropriate candidate due to the absence of inflammation.[109] This finding may be explained by the work of Stein and colleagues,[110] which shows that upregulation of opioid receptors in the peripheral terminals occurs as a result of tissue injury and inflammation; thus, the inflammatory process makes more opioid receptors available to inhibit pain. However, caution should be used since topical application of morphine in an animal model of wound healing shows impaired healing.[45] Research indicates that the use of topical analgesics is beneficial in the management of wound pain, especially with procedural pain.

Many protocols exist for the use of topical agents for procedural and persistent wound pain. Unfortunately, little data exist for these regimens used concurrently with traditional pharmacological intervention. Overall, topical opioids and other analgesics can be used to minimize the central effects of nausea, constipation, and respiratory depression, which can occur when using opioids systemically.[111] When using more than one medication in wound management, a thorough understanding of the mechanisms and effects is important to avoid potential interactions between the medications. For a general review of pharmacology in pain management refer to Loeser and Bonica or Hedderich and Ness.[112,113]

Nonpharmacological Intervention

Judicious clinical practice recommends that all patients receive patient education as part of their clinical treatment experience. Patient education regarding wound pain can be addressed by informing patients about their specific diagnosis and the expected course of their pain experience. Research demonstrates the importance of patient education as part of a pain management program, although this is not specific to wound healing. For example, successful postoperative pain management is related to receiving preoperative information.[114,115] Patient education would also include positioning advice, such as leg elevation to decrease venous pain. Future research is needed to assess patient education and pain management specific to wounds.

Another important nonpharmacological intervention is the appropriate choice of wound dressings. Making the correct selection of a primary and secondary wound dressing to provide a moist wound environment and facilitate autolytic débridement and wound repair is outlined in Chapter 12. The proper choice of wound dressing is related to patient comfort.[116,117] Recognizing that dressing changes are one of the most pain-inducing events in wound care, the clinician should take proper care not only in dressing selection but in the removal of dressings. Many of the modern moisture-retentive dressings are indicated for 3 to 7 days of continuous use. Refraining from daily changes will decrease the overall pain experience for patients. Dressing removal that

incorporates factors such as direction of hair growth, proper skin stabilization, and use of sprays or liquid film products to decrease dressing adherence to the skin will diminish procedural pain and patient anxiety. There is also evidence for having the patient involved in their dressing changes as a method to decrease procedural pain.[117] Thus, establishing a wound dressing protocol that incorporates pain control is an important issue in successful wound management. (Fig. 22.9)

In addition to education and dressing options, there are several biophysical technologies that may be included in wound pain management. One such example is electroanalgesia (EA) or electrical stimulation for pain suppression, which is frequently used in a broad spectrum of pain control. EA, often referred to as TENS (transcutaneous electrical nerve stimulation), can be used at either high or low frequencies and is generally applied around the site of injury to reduce pain at rest or during procedures. For people with wounds, care should be taken to apply electrodes to intact areas of the skin with good circulation, although electrodes may also be applied proximal to the site of injury or to the contralateral limb for pain reduction.[118] EA reduces chronic hyperalgesia induced by muscle inflammation. Sensory level EA at high and low frequencies produced a hypoalgesic response to experimentally induced mechanical pain.[119] Electrical stimulation clearly reduces pain and hyperalgesia through central mechanisms that involve activation of endogenous inhibitory pathways (for a review see Sluka).[120-123] Specifically, low frequencies activate μ-opioid, serotonin, and GABA receptors and high frequencies activate δ-opioid and GABA receptors to reduce pain, hyperalgesia, and central sensitization.[120,121,124]

Previous animal work shows that EA is effective for reduction of hyperalgesia associated with acute and chronic inflammation as well as neuropathic injury.[122,125] Similarly, in human subjects electrical stimulation is effective in reducing pain associated with acute postoperative pain and chronic musculoskeletal pain.[98,126-128] Furthermore, in patients with painful diabetic neuropathy, electrical stimulation using the H-Wave® stimulator (Electronic Waveform Lab Inc., Huntington Beach, CA) decreased pain scores when performed daily for 4 weeks.[129] Overall research indicates that electrical stimulation will reduce acute pain associated with procedures such as débridement and dressing changes, more ongoing pain associated with the inflammation and repair process, and neuropathic pain.

> ▶ **PEARL 22•10** Electroanalgesia may be used in the management of the following types of pain: acute procedural, ongoing inflammatory, and neuropathic. Depending on the wound characteristics, the electrodes may bracket the site of injury, be placed proximal to the site of injury, or be applied to the contralateral limb.

Light therapy is another biophysical technology used for wound pain management. Monochromatic infrared therapy (MIT) is a noninvasive light energy that is topically applied, and infrared energy is absorbed through the skin. In 1994 the FDA approved its use for temporary increases in local circulation and reduction of pain. This form of light therapy

Suggested strategies for the relief of pain at dressing changes

Avoid any unnecessary noxious stimuli to the wound, such as drafts from open windows, prodding, poking, friction and shear forces.

Handle wounds gently, being aware that any slight touch or contact can cause pain

---

Select a dressing that

- is appropriate for the type of wound
- maintains moist wound healing and prevents desiccation
- reduces friction at the wound surface
- minimizes pain and trauma on removal
- remains *in situ* for a longer period to reduce the need for frequent dressing changes

---

Reconsider dressing choice if:

- removal is causing a problem with pain or bleeding/trauma to the wound or surrounding skin
- soaking is required for removal

Reduce patient's anxiety

- Educate the patient on the procedure.
- Identify what the patient recognizes to be pain triggers and reducers.
- Invite the patient to be involved as much as possible (e.g. assist with dressing removal).
- Encourage slow rhythmic breathing.
- Pace the procedure to the patient's preference. Offer the patient "time out". Negotiate a signal for "time out", such as clap hands or raise a finger.

Modified and used with permission from Briggs and Torra I Bou, 2002 (EWMA Position Document: Pain at wound dressing changes)

Figure 22•9 *Strategies to decrease pain during dressing changes.*

has been investigated for therapeutic effect in patients with diabetic peripheral neuropathy (DPN) and has been reported to improve many clinical parameters.[130-132] Improvements were noted with sensation thresholds, balance, and wound healing, along with decreased falls, fear of falling, and neuropathic pain. Many of these studies are funded in part or supported by manufacturers of a particular monochromatic light system and did not include placebo or control groups.[130-133] Specific results show that treatment with light therapy reduces pain associated with diabetic neuropathy in a sham-controlled double-blind protocol.[134] In contrast, several studies do not show reductions in pain following the application of MIT. Two randomly controlled trials investigating MIT concluded there was no decrease in pain.[135,136] There were no significant differences in quality of life, neuropathy, vibration or sensory perception threshold, or nerve conduction velocities between active or sham treatment groups.[136] Thus, clinicians should recognize that there is limited and somewhat low-level evidence supporting pain reduction with MIT in patients with DPN and that no evidence exists for pain reduction in wounds. Additional

research detailing wavelength, frequency, area of irradiation, dose of incidental or absorbed radiation, treatment time, and inclusion criteria for subjects is warranted.

Biophysical technologies that have an impact on wound healing such as compression, conductive and inductive electrical stimulation, ultrasound, ultraviolet light, hyperbaric oxygen, negative-pressure wound therapy, and diathermy can also produce positive affects in pain management. These technologies are reviewed in Part 5 of this text. If an intervention facilitates the process of normal inflammation and repair, it will likely decrease wound pain due to the resulting decrease in activation of nociceptors that occurs with tissue injury.

Thermal agents, such as heat and cold, have limited application for wound pain. Gentle warming of the affected area may be indicated to increase blood flow, although this would not be the modality of choice for pain reduction in acute wounds for obvious reasons of accentuation of the hemodynamic response of inflammation (reviewed in Chapter 2). There is a physiological basis for pain reduction accomplished with application of heat therapy in subacute and chronic conditions, but noticeably absent is any detailed information to support its application specifically for wound pain.

Application of heat abstraction (ie, cooling) can decrease acute, subacute, and chronic pain, although cooling of tissues may have a negative impact on healing.[7,137] In rabbits, healing rates were significantly slower in animals housed in a cool environment following induced surgical lesions, and excessive prolonged cooling of burned tissue in rats via massage with an ice cube resulted in deeper tissue injury in comparison to soaking in tap water.[138,139] Thermal agents, both heating and cooling, are frequently used in general pain management; however, their role specific to wound pain is not known at this time.

If compression therapy using a mechanical pump or ambulatory garments reduces edema, a resultant decrease of neuron firing and a decrease in pain can be accomplished while simultaneously facilitating normal inflammation and repair of wounds. A pilot study of compression of upper-extremity vascular wounds used the medical records of 27 patients who used intermittent pneumatic compression (IPC). Although their focus was on limb salvage, they also reported 25 of 26 patients experienced reduction in pain with IPC treatments.[140] Likewise, reducing the forces of pressure and shear in patients with compromised mobility via pressure-relieving devices may result in favorable pain reduction due to the decrease in mechanical activation. Use of pressure-relieving devices and compression therapy are reviewed in Chapters 19 and 30, respectively.

Alternative Interventions

Many complementary and alternative interventions have been used and described in the literature to reduce pain associated with wounds. These interventions include hypnosis, relaxation and breathing exercises, percutaneous electrical neuromuscular stimulation (PENS), therapeutic touch therapy, and most recently, virtual reality (VR) distraction. Some of the techniques have strong literature support (ie, hypnosis), while others are more speculative in nature (ie, therapeutic touch therapy).[141] In the case of extreme pain, these interventions may be used as an adjunct to opioid therapy.

A review of the literature offered mixed results. Hypnosis decreases procedural pain of débridement in burn patients when compared to standard treatment of delivery of information prior to débridement sessions. Wright and Drummond reported that rapid induction analgesia (RIA), which is a form of hypnosis, decreased the sensory and affective components of pain, analgesic intake, and anticipatory anxiety.[142] In contrast, Frenay and colleagues found that anxiety scores decreased during patient dressing changes,[143] but VAS pain scores and patient satisfaction were not significantly different when comparing use of a hypnotic technique to stress-relieving strategies.

Several research studies have assessed relaxation to control wound pain. Slow, rhythmic breathing in combination with jaw relaxation shows promise according to a literature review addressing the question of effectiveness of breathing exercises for procedural pain in wound care.[144] The authors suggest, however, that although breathing exercises are simple to implement, there is a lack of clear evidence at this time upon which to base decisions with regard to procedure and patient type.

Music used as a form of distraction did not demonstrate a significant difference in pain and anxiety scores when compared to sham in 11 burn patients.[145] However, several other studies of virtual reality (VR) systems report that it is a promising analgesic technique for concurrent use with standard pharmacological care when addressing procedural pain in burn patients.[146-148] The VR helmets used offer visual, auditory, and in some instances, tactile sensory input. They simulate games and are operated by head motion, and they completely block the subject's vision of the real world. In healthy normal subjects, VR decreased thermal pain by 30% or greater in the majority of subjects.[149] Hoffman offers a case report of a water-friendly VR helmet that could increase the number of burn patients' access to this distraction intervention for clinicians who use hydrotherapy or other water-based settings for procedures.[148] A review of nonpharmacological interventions by de Jong,[141] which focused on the promotion of psychological comfort in burn patients, concluded that the best evidence was found for hypnosis and distraction relaxation. Furthermore, clinicians should be aware of the factors that contribute to the pain experience. For instance, if a client has high anxiety and/or stress, then distraction or relaxation may be good options to employ due to their influence on the affective component of pain.

▶ **PEARL 22•11** Ongoing research indicates that alternative therapies that incorporate hypnosis, distraction, and relaxation may be good options in the management of wound pain.

Summary

The treatment of pain is very complex and frequently mismanaged. To combat patients' pain, clinicians should be aware of the peripheral and central factors that contribute to pain processing. Furthermore, appropriate pain assessment tools should be continuously used to capture the multidimensional and dynamic nature of pain. This will help the wound care team to establish a protocol that incorporates both pharmacological and nonpharmacological interventions to best manage pain.

▶ **Case Study 22•1** Neuropathic Pain Management

History

Dori is a 65-year-old female with a 27-year history of type 2 diabetes mellitus. Dori is receiving treatment in an outpatient clinic for a plantar ulcer over the first and second metatarsal heads of her right foot. Dori complains of chronic neuropathic pain described as a burning ache in both of her feet that increases at night. During ulcer débridement, Dori complains of sharp pain. Physical examination reveals decreased sensation in bilateral lower extremities.

Pain Mechanisms

Dori presents with two types of pain, chronic neuropathic pain and acute procedural pain. The chronic neuropathic pain is due to changes in the peripheral and central nervous system that modulate pain. Changes in the central nervous system do not require peripheral input to cause pain. The acute pain caused by débridement is due to mechanical activation of nociceptors. This type of pain does require input from the peripheral nervous system.

Pain Assessment

A visual analog scale (VAS) may be used to assess the pain intensity for the acute and chronic pain that Dori is experiencing.

The VAS scale is beneficial for pain that is dynamic, as with acute procedural type pain, because it allows the clinician to frequently assess Dori's pain intensity. Additional pain assessment tools should be incorporated because the VAS does not give a good perspective on the entire pain experience; specifically, the VAS is unidimensional and assesses only pain intensity. The Brief Pain Inventory (BPI) and the McGill Pain Questionnaire (MPQ) are both good options to use in addition to the VAS.

Pain Management

Pharmacological intervention is indicated in the management of chronic neuropathic pain. Additional pharmacological management, such as topical analgesics, may be used for the procedural pain. There are several nonpharmacological interventions that may be employed in conjunction with the pharmacological interventions. Some examples include patient education, application of electroanalgesia, and distraction exercises.

References

1. Sluka, KA: Mechanisms and Management of Pain for the Physical Therapist. International Association for the Study of Pain. Seattle, IASP Press, 2009, pp. 3–18.
2. Merskey, H, Bogduk, N: Classification of chronic pain: Descriptions of chronic pain syndromes and definitions of pain terms. International Association for the Study of Pain, ed. 2. Task Force on Taxonomy, Seattle, IASP Press, 1994.
3. Melzack, R, Casey, KL: Sensory, motivational, and central control determinants of pain: A new conceptual model. In: Kenshalo, D (ed): The Skin Senses. Springfield, IL, Thomas, 1968. pp 423–443.
4. Willis, WD, Coggeshall, RE: Sensory Mechanisms of the Spinal Cord, ed. 2. New York, Plenum Press, 1991.
5. Kandel, ER, Schwartz, JH, Jessell, TM: Principles of Neural Science, ed. 4. New York, McGraw-Hill, 2000.
6. Schaible, HG, Schmidt, RF: Effects of an experimental arthritis on the sensory properties of fine articular afferent units. J Neurophysiol 1985; 54:1109–1122.
7. Hoeger Bement, MK, Sluka, KA: Pain: Perception and mechanisms. In: Magee, DJ, Zachazewski, JE, Quillen, WS (eds): Scientific Foundations and Principles of Practice in Musculoskeletal Rehabilitation. St. Louis, Elsevier, 2007, pp 217–237.
8. Meyer, RA, Ringkamp, M, Campbell, JN, et al: Peripheral mechanisms of cutaneous nociception. In: McMahon, SB, Koltzenburg, M (eds): Textbook of Pain. London, Churchill Livingston, 2006, pp 3–34.
9. Julius, D, Basbaum, AI: Molecular mechanisms of nociception. Nature 2001; 413:203–210.
10. Fock, S, Mense, S: Excitatory effects of 5-hydroxytryptamine, histamine, and potassium ions on muscular group IV afferent units: A comparison with bradykinin. Brain Res 1976; 105:459–469.
11. Richardson, BP, Engel, G: The pharmacology and function of 5-HT3 receptors. Trends Neurosci 1986; 9:424–428.
12. Manning, DC, Raja, SN, Meyer, RA, et al: Pain and hyperalgesia after intradermal injection of bradykinin in humans. Clin Pharmacol Ther 1991; 50:721–729.
13. Koltzenburg, M, Kress, M, Reeh, PW: The nociceptor sensitization by bradykinin does not depend on sympathetic neurons. Neuroscience 1992; 46:465–473.
14. Petho, G, Derow, A, Reeh, PW: Bradykinin-induced nociceptor sensitization to heat is mediated by cyclooxygenase products in isolated rat skin. Eur J Neurosci 2001; 14:210–218.
15. Schaible, HG, Schmidt, RF: Excitation and sensitization of fine articular afferents from cat's knee joint by prostaglandin E2. J Physiol 1988; 403:91–104.
16. Gosain, A, Gamelli, RL: A primer in cytokines. J Burn Care Rehabil 2005; 26:7–12.
17. Ferreira, SH, Lorenzetti, BB, Bristow, AF, et al: Interleukin-1 beta as a potent hyperalgesic agent antagonized by a tripeptide analogue. Nature 1988; 334:698–700.
18. Cunha, FQ, Poole, S, Lorenzetti, BB, et al: The pivotal role of tumour necrosis factor alpha in the development of inflammatory hyperalgesia. Br J Pharmacol 1992; 107:660–664.
19. Watkins, LR, Wiertelak, EP, Goehler, LE, et al: Characterization of cytokine-induced hyperalgesia. Brain Res 1994; 654:15–26.
20. Kaneko, S, Satoh, T, Chiba, J, et al: Interleukin-6 and interleukin-8 levels in serum and synovial fluid of patients with osteoarthritis. Cytokines Cell Mol Ther 2000; 6:71–79.
21. Kaneyama, K, Segami, N, Nishimura, M, et al: Importance of proinflammatory cytokines in synovial fluid from 121 joints with temporomandibular disorders. Br J Oral Maxillofac Surg 2002; 40:418–423.
22. Trengove, NJ, Bielefeldt-Ohmann, H, Stacey, MC: Mitogenic activity and cytokine levels in non-healing and healing chronic leg ulcers. Wound Repair Regen 2000; 8:13–25.

23. Sorkin, LS, Xiao, WH, Wagner, R, et al: Tumour necrosis factor-alpha induces ectopic activity in nociceptive primary afferent fibres. Neuroscience 1997; 81:255–262.

24. Sommer, C, Schmidt, C, George, A: Hyperalgesia in experimental neuropathy is dependent on the TNF receptor 1. Exp Neurol 1998; 151:138–142.

25. Reeh, PW, Steen, KH: Tissue acidosis in nociception and pain. Prog Brain Res 1996; 113:143–151.

26. Sluka, KA, Radhakrishnan, R, Benson, CJ, et al: ASIC3 in muscle mediates mechanical, but not heat, hyperalgesia associated with muscle inflammation. Pain 2007; 129:102–112.

27. Steen, KH, Steen, AE, Kreysel, HW, et al: Inflammatory mediators potentiate pain induced by experimental tissue acidosis. Pain 1996; 66:163–170.

28. Rees, H, Sluka, KA, Westlund, KN, et al: The role of glutamate and GABA receptors in the generation of dorsal root reflexes by acute arthritis in the anaesthetized rat. J Physiol 1995; 484(Pt 2):437–445.

29. Sluka, KA, Rees, H, Westlund, KN, et al: Fiber types contributing to dorsal root reflexes induced by joint inflammation in cats and monkeys. J Neurophysiol 1995; 74:981–989.

30. White, DM, Helme, RD: Release of substance P from peripheral nerve terminals following electrical stimulation of the sciatic nerve. Brain Res, 1985; 336:27–31.

31. Yaksh, TL, Bailey, J, Roddy, DR, et al: Peripheral release of substance P from primary afferents. In: Gebhart, GF, Bond, MR (eds): Proceedings from the Fifth World Congress on Pain. Amsterdam, Elsevier, 1988, pp 51–54.

32. Levine, JD, Clark, R, Devor, M, et al: Intraneuronal substance P contributes to the severity of experimental arthritis. Science 1984; 226:547–549.

33. Brain, SD, Williams, TJ: Inflammatory oedema induced by synergism between calcitonin gene-related peptide (CGRP) and mediators of increased vascular permeability. Br J Pharmacol 1985; 86:855–860.

34. Marshall, KW, Chiu, B, Inman, RD: Substance P and arthritis: Analysis of plasma and synovial fluid levels. Arthritis Rheum 1990; 33:87–90.

35. Larsson, J, Ekblom, A, Henriksson, K, et al: Immunoreactive tachykinins, calcitonin gene-related peptide and neuropeptide Y in human synovial fluid from inflamed knee joints. Neurosci Lett 1989; 100:326–330.

36. Levine, JD, Moskowitz, MA, Basbaum, AI: The contribution of neurogenic inflammation in experimental arthritis. J Immunol 1985; 135(suppl):843s–847s.

37. Lam, FY, Ferrell, WR: Inhibition of carrageenan induced inflammation in the rat knee joint by substance P antagonists. Ann Rheum Dis 1985; 48:928–932.

38. Sluka, KA, Lawand, NB, Westlund, KN: Joint inflammation is reduced by dorsal rhizotomy and not by sympathectomy or spinal cord transection. Ann Rheum Dis 1994; 53:309–314.

39. Kjartansson, J, Dalsgaard, CJ: Calcitonin gene-related peptide increases survival of a musculocutaneous critical flap in the rat. Eur J Pharmacol 1987; 142:355–358.

40. Kjartansson, J, Dalsgaard, CJ, Jonsson, CE: Decreased survival of experimental critical flaps in rats after sensory denervation with capsaicin. Plast Reconstr Surg 1987; 79:218–221.

41. Dalsgaard, CJ, Jonsson, CE, Haegerstrand, A, et al: Sensory neuropeptides contribute to oedema formation in experimental burns. Scand J Plast Reconstr Surg Hand Surg 1987; 21:291–292.

42. Delgado, AV, McManus, AT, Chambers, JP: Exogenous administration of substance P enhances wound healing in a novel skin-injury model. Exp Biol Med 2005; 230:271–280.

43. Khalil, Z, Helme, R: Sensory peptides as neuromodulators of wound healing in aged rats. J Gerontol A Biol Sci Med Sci 1996; 51:B354–361.

44. Smith, PG, Liu, M: Impaired cutaneous wound healing after sensory denervation in developing rats: Effects on cell proliferation and apoptosis. Cell Tissue Res 2002; 307:281–291.

45. Rook, JM, McCarson, KE: Delay of cutaneous wound closure by morphine via local blockade of peripheral tachykinin release. Biochem Pharmacol 2007; 74:752–757.

46. Schaible, HG, Schmidt, RF, Willis, WD: Enhancement of the responses of ascending tract cells in the cat spinal cord by acute inflammation of the knee joint. Exp Brain Res 1987; 66:489–499.

47. Palecek, J, Dougherty, PM, Kim, SH, et al: Responses of spinothalamic tract neurons to mechanical and thermal stimuli in an experimental model of peripheral neuropathy in primates. J Neurophysiol 1992; 68:1951–1966.

48. Hoheisel, U, Mense, S, Simons, DG, et al: Appearance of new receptive fields in rat dorsal horn neurons following noxious stimulation of skeletal muscle: A model for referral of muscle pain? Neurosci Lett 1993; 153:9–12.

49. Jones, SL, Light, AR: Serotonergic medullary raphespinal projection to the lumbar spinal-cord in the rat: A retrograde immunohistochemical study. J Comp Neurol 1992; 322:599–610.

50. Willis, WD, Westlund, KN: Neuroanatomy of the pain system and of the pathways that modulate pain. J Clin Neurophysiol 1997; 14:2–31.

51. Melzack, R, Katz, J: Pain measurement in persons in pain. In: Wall, PD, Melzack, R (eds): Textbook of Pain. New York, Churchill Livingston, 1999, pp 409–426.

52. Whipple, JK, Lewis, KS, Quebbeman, EJ, et al: Analysis of pain management in critically ill patients. Pharmacotherapy 1995; 15:592–599.

53. Cleeland, CS, Ryan, KM: Pain assessment: Global use of the Brief Pain Inventory. Ann Acad Med Singapore 1994; 23:129–138.

54. Zelman, DC, Gore, M, Dukes, E, et al: Validation of a modified version of the Brief Pain Inventory for painful diabetic peripheral neuropathy. J Pain Symptom Manage 2005; 29:401–410.

55. Dawson, EG, Kanim, LE, Sra, P, et al: Low back pain recollection versus concurrent accounts: Outcomes analysis. Spine 2002; 27:984–993, discussion 994.

56. Melzack, R: The McGill Pain Questionnaire: Major properties and scoring methods. Pain 1995; 1:277–299.

57. Krasner, D: The chronic wound pain experience: A conceptual model. Ostomy Wound Manage 1995; 41:20–25.

58. Price, P, Fogh, K, Glynn, C, et al: Managing painful chronic wounds: The wound pain management model. Int Wound J 2007; 4(suppl):4–15.

59. Galer, BS, Gianas, A, Jensen, MP: Painful diabetic polyneuropathy: Epidemiology, pain description, and quality of life. Diabetes Res Clin Pract 2000; 47:123–128.

60. Davies, M, Brophy, S, Williams, R, et al: The prevalence, severity, and impact of painful diabetic peripheral neuropathy in type 2 diabetes. Diabetes Care 2006; 29:1518–1522.

61. Schmader, KE: Epidemiology and impact on quality of life of postherpetic neuralgia and painful diabetic neuropathy. Clin J Pain 2002; 18:350–354.

62. Morley, GK, Mooradian, AD, Levine, AS, et al: Mechanism of pain in diabetic peripheral neuropathy. Effect of glucose on pain perception in humans. Am J Med 1984; 77:79–82.

63. Chan, AW, MacFarlane, IA, Bowsher, D: Short term fluctuations in blood glucose concentrations do not alter pain perception in diabetic-patients with and without painful peripheral neuropathy. Diabetes Res 1990; 14:15–19.

64. Jensen, TS, Krebs, B, Nielsen, J, et al: Phantom limb, phantom pain, and stump pain in amputees during the first 6 months following limb amputation. Pain 1983; 17:243–256.

65. Richardson, C, Glenn, S, Horgan, M, et al: A prospective study of factors associated with the presence of phantom limb pain six months after major lower limb amputation in patients with peripheral vascular disease. J Pain 2007; 8:793–801.

66. Mishra, S, Bhatnagar, S, Gupta, D, et al: Incidence and management of phantom limb pain according to World Health Organization analgesic ladder in amputees of malignant origin. Am J Hosp Palliat Care 2007; 455–462.

67. Jensen, TS, Krebs, B, Nielsen, J, et al: Immediate and long-term phantom limb pain in amputees: Incidence, clinical characteristics, and relationship to pre-amputation limb pain. Pain 1985; 21:267–278.

68. Hanley, MA, Jensen, MP, Smith, DG, et al: Preamputation pain and acute pain predict chronic pain after lower extremity amputation. J Pain 2007; 8:102–109.

69. Bach, S, Noreng, MF, Tjellden, NU: Phantom limb pain in amputees during the first 12 months following limb amputation, after preoperative lumbar epidural blockade. Pain 1988; 33:297–301.

70. Jahangiri, M, Jayatunga, AP, Bradley, JW, et al: Prevention of phantom pain after major lower limb amputation by epidural infusion of diamorphine, clonidine, and bupivacaine. Ann R Coll Surg Engl 1994; 76:324–326.

71. Nikolajsen, L, Ilkjaer, S, Christensen, JH, et al: Randomised trial of epidural bupivacaine and morphine in prevention of stump and phantom pain in lower-limb amputation. Lancet 1997; 350:1353–1357.

72. Jensen, TS, Nikolajsen, L: Phantom pain and other phenomena after amputation. In: Wall, PD, Melzack, R (eds): Textbook of Pain, ed. 4. Edinburgh, Churchill Livingston, 1999, pp 799–814.

73. Flor, H, Elbert, T, Knecht, S, et al: Phantom-limb pain as a perceptual correlate of cortical reorganization following arm amputation. Nature 1995; 375:482–484.

74. Ebbeskog, B, Lindholm, C, Ohman, S: Leg and foot ulcer patients. Epidemiology and nursing care in an urban population in south Stockholm, Sweden. Scand J Prim Health Care 1996; 14:238–243.

75. Nemeth, KA, Harrison, MB, Graham, ID, et al: Understanding venous leg ulcer pain: Results of a longitudinal study. Ostomy Wound Manage 2004; 50:34–46.

76. Holloway, GA, Jr: Arterial ulcers: Assessment and diagnosis. Ostomy Wound Manage 1996; 42:46–48, 50–41.

77. Johansen, KH: Pain due to vascular disease. In: Loeser, JD (ed): Bonica's Management of Pain. Philadelphia, Lippincott Williams & Wilkins, 2001, pp 587–612.

78. Sieggreen, MY, Kline, RA: Arterial insufficiency and ulceration: Diagnosis and treatment options. Nurse Pract 2004; 29:46–52.

79. Dallam, L, Smyth, C, Jackson, BS, et al: Pressure ulcer pain: Assessment and quantification. J Wound Ostomy Continence Nurs 1995; 22:211–215, discussion 217–218.

80. Szor, JK, Bourguignon, C: Description of pressure ulcer pain at rest and at dressing change. J Wound Ostomy Continence Nurs 1999; 26:115–120.

81. Eriksson, E, Hietanen, H, Asko-Seljavaara, S: Prevalence and characteristics of pressure ulcers. A one-day patient population in a Finnish city. Clin Nurse Spec 2000; 14:119–125.

82. Quirino, J, de Gouveia Santos, VL, Quednau, TJP, et al: Pain in pressure ulcers. Wounds 2003; 15:381–389.

83. Rastinehad, D: Pressure ulcer pain. J Wound Ostomy Continence Nurs 2006; 33:252–257.

84. Coda, BA, Bonica, JJ: General considerations of acute pain. In: Loeser, JD, Butler, SH, Chapman, CR, et al (eds): Bonica's Management of Pain. Philadelphia, Lippincott Williams & Wilkins, 2001, pp 222–240.

85. Perry, S, Heidrich, G, Ramos, E: Assessment of pain by burn patients. J Burn Care Rehabil 1981; 2:322–326.

86. Byers, JF, Bridges, S, Kijek, J, et al: Burn patients' pain and anxiety experiences. J Burn Care Rehabil 2001; 22:144–149.

87. Weinberg, K, Birdsall, C, Vail, D, et al: Pain and anxiety with burn dressing changes: Patient self-report. J Burn Care Rehabil 2000; 21:155–156, discussion 157–161.

88. Choiniere, M, Melzack, R, Girard, N, et al: Comparisons between patients' and nurses' assessment of pain and medication efficacy in severe burn injuries. Pain 1990; 40:143–152.

89. Montgomery, RK: Pain management in burn injury. Crit Care Nurs Clin North Am 2004; 16:39–49.

90. Klein, RM, Charlton, JE: Behavioral observation and analysis of pain behavior in critically burned patients. Pain 1980; 9:27–40.

91. Patterson, DR, Tininenko, J, Ptacek, JT: Pain during burn hospitalization predicts long-term outcome. J Burn Care Res 2006; 27:719–726.

92. Choiniere, M, Melzack, R, Papillon, J: Pain and paresthesia in patients with healed burns: An exploratory study. J Pain Symptom Manage 1991; 6:437–444.

93. Dauber, A, Osgood, PF, Breslau, AJ, et al: Chronic persistent pain after severe burns: A survey of 358 burn survivors. Pain Med 2002; 3:6–17.

94. Ptacek, JT, Patterson, DR, Doctor, J: Describing and predicting the nature of procedural pain after thermal injuries: Implications for research. J Burn Care Rehabil 2000; 21:318–326.

95. Patterson, DR, Everett, JJ, Bombardier, CH, et al: Psychological effects of severe burn injuries. Psychol Bull 1993; 113:362–378.

96. Sluka, KA, Walsh, D: Transcutaneous electrical nerve stimulation: Basic science mechanisms and clinical effectiveness. J Pain 2003; 4:109–121.

97. Sluka, KA, Wright, A: Knee joint mobilization reduces secondary mechanical hyperalgesia induced by capsaicin injection into the ankle joint. Eur J Pain 2001; 5:81–87.

98. Johnson, M, Martinson, M: Efficacy of electrical nerve stimulation for chronic musculoskeletal pain: A meta-analysis of randomized controlled trials. Pain 2007; 130:157–165.

99. Carr, DB: Preempting the memory of pain. JAMA 1998; 279: 1114–1115.

100. Coderre, TJ, Choiniere, M: Neuronal plasticity associated with burn injury and its relevance for perception and management of pain in burn patients. Pain Res Manag 2000; 5:205–213.

101. Honari, S, Patterson, DR, Gibbons, J, et al: Comparison of pain control medication in three age groups of elderly patients. J Burn Care Rehabil 1997; 18:500–504.

102. Choiniere, M: Pain of burns. In: Melzack, R, Wall, PD (eds): Handbook of Pain Management: A Clinical Companion to Textbook of Pain. New York, Churchill Livingstone, 2003, pp 591–601.

103. Perry, S, Heidrich, G: Management of pain during debridement: A survey of U.S. burn units. Pain 1982; 13:267–280.

104. Goncalves, ML, de Gouveia Santos, VL, de Mattos Pimenta, CA, et al: Pain in chronic leg ulcers. J Wound Ostomy Continence Nurs 2004; 31:275–283.

105. Briggs, M, Nelson, EA: Topical agents or dressings for pain in venous leg ulcers. Cochrane Database Syst Rev 2003; 1:CD001177.

106. Jepson, BA: Relieving the pain of pressure sores. Lancet 1992; 339:503–504.

107. Flock, P: Pilot study to determine the effectiveness of diamorphine gel to control pressure ulcer pain. J Pain Symptom Manage 2003; 25:547–554.

108. Zeppetella, G, Paul, J, Ribeiro, MD: Analgesic efficacy of morphine applied topically to painful ulcers. J Pain Symptom Manage 2003; 25:555–558.

109. Twillman, RK, Long, TD, Cathers, TA, et al: Treatment of painful skin ulcers with topical opioids. J Pain Symptom Manage 1999; 17:288–292.

110. Stein, C: The control of pain in peripheral tissue by opioids. N Engl J Med 1995; 332:1685–1690.

111. Stein, C: Peripheral mechanisms of opioid analgesia. Anesth Analg 1993; 76:182–191.

112. Loeser, JD, Bonica, JJ: Bonica's Management of Pain, ed 3. Philadelphia, Lippincott Williams & Wilkins, 2001.

113. Hedderich, R, Ness, TJ: Analgesia for trauma and burns. Crit Care Clin 1999; 15:167–184.

114. Niemi-Murola, L, Nieminen, JT, Kalso, E, et al: Medical undergraduate students' beliefs and attitudes toward pain: How do they mature? Eur J Pain 2007; 11:700–706.

115. Sjoling, M, Nordahl, G, Olofsson, N, et al: The impact of preoperative information on state anxiety, postoperative pain, and satisfaction with pain management. Patient Educ Couns 2003; 51:169–176.

116. Lloyd Jones, M: Minimizing pain at dressing changes. Nurs Stand 2004; 18:65–70.

117. Briggs, M, Torra i Bou, JE: Pain at wound dressing changes: A guide to management. In: Moffatt, C (ed): European Wound Management Association Position Document. London, Medical Education Partnership, 2002, pp 12–17.

118. Ainsworth, L, Budelier, K, Clinesmith, M, et al: Transcutaneous electrical nerve stimulation (TENS) reduces chronic hyperalgesia induced by muscle inflammation. Pain 2006; 120:182–187.

119. Chesterton, LS, Barlas, P, Foster, NE, et al: Sensory stimulation (TENS): Effects of parameter manipulation on mechanical pain thresholds in healthy human subjects. Pain 2002; 99:253–262.

120. Sluka, KA, Deacon, M, Stibal, A, et al: Spinal blockade of opioid receptors prevents the analgesia produced by TENS in arthritic rats. J Pharmacol Exp Ther 1999; 289:840–846.

121. Kalra, A, Urban, MO, Sluka, KA: Blockade of opioid receptors in rostral ventral medulla prevents antihyperalgesia produced by transcutaneous electrical nerve stimulation (TENS). J Pharmacol Exp Ther 2001; 298:257–263.

122. Vance, CG, Radhakrishnan, R, Skyba, DA, et al: Transcutaneous electrical nerve stimulation at both high and low frequencies reduces primary hyperalgesia in rats with joint inflammation in a time-dependent manner. Phys Ther 2007; 87:44–51.

123. Sluka, KA: Neurobiology of pain and foundations of electrical stimulation for pain control. In: Robinson, AJ, Snyder-Mackler, L (eds): Clinical Electrophysiology: Electrotherapy and Electrophysiological Testing, ed. 3. Baltimore, Lippincott Williams and Wilkins, 2008, pp 104–149.

124. Radhakrishnan, R, King, EW, Dickman, JK, et al: Spinal 5-HT(2) and 5-HT(3) receptors mediate low, but not high, frequency TENS-induced antihyperalgesia in rats. Pain 2003; 105:205–213.

125. Somers, DL, Clemente, FR: Transcutaneous electrical nerve stimulation for the management of neuropathic pain: The effects of frequency and electrode position on prevention of allodynia in a rat model of complex regional pain syndrome type II. Phys Ther 2006; 86:698–709.

126. Bjordal, JM, Johnson, MI, Ljunggreen, AE: Transcutaneous electrical nerve stimulation (TENS) can reduce postoperative analgesic consumption. A meta-analysis with assessment of optimal treatment parameters for postoperative pain. Eur J Pain 2003; 7:181–188.

127. Neary, JM: Transcutaneous electrical nerve stimulation for the relief of post-incisional surgical pain. AANA J 1981; 49:151–155.

128. Richardson, RR, Siqueira, EB: Transcutaneous electrical neurostimulation in postlaminectomy pain. Spine 1980; 5:361–365.

129. Kumar, D, Marshall, HJ: Diabetic peripheral neuropathy: Amelioration of pain with transcutaneous electrostimulation. Diabetes Care 1997; 20:1702–1705.

130. Volkert, W, Hassan, A, Hassan, MA, et al: Effectiveness of monochromatic infrared photo energy and physical therapy for peripheral neuropathy: Changes in sensation, pain, and balance—A preliminary, multi-center study. Phys Occup Ther Geriatr 2006; 24:1–18.

131. Powell, MW, Carnegie, DE, Burke, TJ: Reversal of diabetic peripheral neuropathy and new wound incidence: The role of MIRE. Adv Skin Wound Care 2004; 17:295–300.

132. Powell, MW, Carnegie, DH, Burke, TJ: Reversal of diabetic peripheral neuropathy with phototherapy (MIRE) decreases falls and the fear of falling and improves activities of daily living in seniors. Age Ageing 2006; 35:11–16.

133. DeLellis, SL, Carnegie, DH, Burke, TJ: Improved sensitivity in patients with peripheral neuropathy: Effects of monochromatic infrared photo energy. J Am Podiatr Med Assoc 2005; 95:143–147.

134. Leonard, DR, Farooqi, MH, Myers, S: Restoration of sensation, reduced pain, and improved balance in subjects with diabetic peripheral neuropathy. Diabetes Care 2004; 27:168–172.

135. Clifft, JK, Kasser, RJ, Newton, TS, et al: The effect of monochromatic infrared energy on sensation in patients with diabetic peripheral neuropathy: A double-blind, placebo-controlled study. Diabetes Care 2005; 28:2896–2900.

136. Lavery, LA, Murdoch, DP, Williams, J, et al: Does anodyne light therapy improve peripheral neuropathy in diabetes? A double blind, sham controlled randomized trial to evaluate monochromatic infrared photo energy. Diabetes Care 2007; 316–321.

137. Benson, TB, Copp, EP: The effects of therapeutic forms of heat and ice on the pain threshold of the normal shoulder. Rheumatology 1974; 13:101–104.

138. Lundgren, C, Muren, A, Zederfeldt, B: Effect of cold vasoconstriction on would healing in the rabbit. Acta Chir Scand 1959; 118:1–4.

139. Sawada, Y, Urushidate, S, Yotsuyanagi, T, et al: Is prolonged and excessive cooling of a scalded wound effective? Burns 1997; 23:55–58.

140. Pfizenmaier, DH, 2nd, Kavros, SJ, Liedl, DA, et al: Use of intermittent pneumatic compression for treatment of upper extremity vascular ulcers. Angiology 2005; 56:417–422.

141. de Jong, AE, Middelkoop, E, Faber, AW, et al: Non-pharmacological nursing interventions for procedural pain relief in adults with burns: A systematic literature review. Burns 2007; 33:811–827.

142. Wright, BR, Drummond, PD: Rapid induction analgesia for the alleviation of procedural pain during burn care. Burns 2000; 26:275–282.

143. Frenay, MC, Faymonville, ME, Devlieger, S, et al: Psychological approaches during dressing changes of burned patients: A prospective randomised study comparing hypnosis against stress reducing strategy. Burns 2001; 27:793–799.

144. de Jong, AE, Gamel, C: Use of a simple relaxation technique in burn care: Literature review. J Adv Nurs 2006; 54:710–721.

145. Ferguson, SL, Voll, KV: Burn pain and anxiety: The use of music relaxation during rehabilitation. J Burn Care Rehabil 2004; 25:8–14.

146. van Twillert, B, Bremer, M, Faber, AW: Computer-generated virtual reality to control pain and anxiety in pediatric and adult burn patients during wound dressing changes. J Burn Care Res 2007; 28:694–702.

147. Hoffman, HG, Doctor, JN, Patterson, DR, et al: Virtual reality as an adjunctive pain control during burn wound care in adolescent patients. Pain 2000; 85:305–309.

148. Hoffman, HG, Patterson, DR, Magula, J, et al: Water-friendly virtual reality pain control during wound care. J Clin Psychol 2004; 60:189–195.

149. Hoffman, HG, Seibel, EJ, Richards, TL, et al: Virtual reality helmet display quality influences the magnitude of virtual reality analgesia. J Pain 2006; 7:843–850.

chapter 23

Surgical Considerations in Wound Care

David E. Mahon, MD, CWS, FACCWS, FACS

The most effective modality for chronic wound care remains surgical débridement. The goal of any wound care, acute or chronic, is always the same: closure and reepithelialization of the wound. Thus, the wound care practitioner must be familiar with some surgical wound techniques and procedures. This chapter presents wound care management from a surgical perspective. The patterns of wound healing, the preparation of the wound care bed, and advanced débridement and closure techniques are discussed. Some remarks concerning plastic and vascular surgical considerations conclude the chapter.

Types of Wound Closure

Acute wounds are defined as wounds that are expected to close primarily, as in simple suturing of a laceration. The normal, orderly process of wound closure occurs after an injury and requires only basic wound care (ie, clean and close wounds). The physiology of wound closure, both acute and chronic, was previously discussed in Chapter 2. Before discussing complex wound closure techniques, a primer on wound closure and care is in order.

All wounds heal in three distinct patterns: primary, secondary, and tertiary intention. Primary intention refers to the direct closure or approximation of a wound, usually with sutures or closure devices, but it may also involve placement of grafts or flaps.[1] While up to 6 hours after injury has been previously thought to be the ideal time for closure for primary intention healing, current studies have challenged this period of time, and, provided gross contamination has not occurred, wounds may be cleaned, débrided, and closed after longer periods. There is growing evidence that wounds, especially well-vascularized wounds such as facial injuries, may be closed within 24 hours.[2]

> **PEARL 23•1** All wounds heal in three types of patterns: primary, secondary, or tertiary (or delayed primary).

Suturing involves a stitch or series of stitches working to appose the edges of a surgical or traumatic wound. The technique involves the use of needles of variable size and shape, for instance, a cutting needle, which has a razorlike triangle designed to be placed through tissue such as skin. A circular or noncutting needle is used to approximate delicate tissue such as bowel or blood vessels. Other types of needles may be used depending on the tissue traversed, including reverse cutting needles and blunt needles.[3]

The type of stitch used in closure of the wound is usually divided into categories: absorbable versus nonabsorbable, monofilament versus braided, natural versus synthetic. Advantages and disadvantages are noted in all suture materials, and there is no perfect material for all cases. For example, absorbable suture heals with a more pronounced inflammatory reaction but does not need to be removed. Monofilament is usually less strong than braided multifilament but has the advantage of not allowing bacteria to reside between the braids. Natural suture material, such as silk, is generally easier to work with, whereas synthetic material is more available and nonabsorbable. For skin closures, skin staples or nylon sutures are the most common closure instruments due to their strength and resistance to infection.[4] Table 23.1 provides a listing of various types of suture material.

The length of time that sutures remain in place is determined by many factors, including anatomical location. Table 23.2 provides a listing of standard suture removal times for uncomplicated wounds.

Other forms of skin closure are now available. There are derivatives of cyanoacrylate that act as a form of skin glue. One example of this type of product would be Dermabond® (Ethicon, Johnson & Johnson, Somerville, NJ), which is a 2-octyl cyanoacrylate formulation. This product may also be used to approximate skin edges and facilitate closure.[1,4]

Many other products are marketed for closure of wounds, specifically chronic wounds. These products all rely on applying tension to the skin edges; the skin may then be expanded over a period of time in order to reepithelialize the area. Examples of these products include Dermaclose RC® (Wound Care Technologies, Chanhassen, MN) (Fig. 23.1), which applies consistent radial tension to the open wound, and Wound Bullet® (Boehringer Labs, Norristown, PA), which places a cylinder and stitches in the healing wound and may

Table 23•2 Suture Removal Times for Uncomplicated Wounds	
Face	3–5 days
Scalp	7 days
Chest	7–10 days
Abdomen	7–10 days
Extremities	7–10 days
Ear	10–14 days
Back	12–14 days
Foot	12–14 days

Table 23•1 Suture Material Chart			
Suture Types			
Absorbable		**Nonabsorbable**	
Gut		Nylon	
Chromic gut		Silk	
Polyglycolic acid (Dexon)		Polypropylene (Prolene)	
Polyglactin 910 (Vicryl)			
Monofilament		**Multifilament**	
Nylon		Silk	
Polydioxanone (PDS)		Polyglycolic acid (Dexon)	
Natural		**Synthetic**	
Silk		Nylon	
Gut		Polyglactin 910 (Vicryl)	
Suture Sizes			
Larger	1	1	Skin
	0	0	
	0.00	2-0	Fascia
	0.000	3-0	
	0.0000	4-0	Bowel
	0.00000	5-0	
Smaller	0.000000	6-0	Vessels

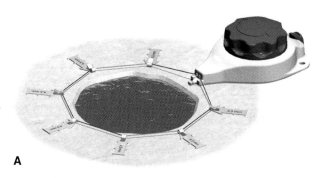

A

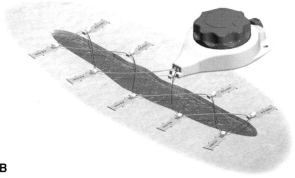

B

Figure **23•1** *The DermaClose™ RC Continuous External Tissue Expander being used on a (A) circular and (B) longitudinal wound. Courtesy of Wound Care Technologies, Chanhassen, MN.*

be adjusted to pull together the skin edges. These devices all rely on the elasticity of the skin in order to provide a primary intention closure.

Secondary intention, sometimes called spontaneous healing, occurs when a wound is allowed to heal by contraction and reepithelialization. An example of secondary intention would be the drainage of an abscess and subsequent healing.[5] This process takes more time and requires a prolonged inflammatory phase. With abscess draining, secondary intention minimizes the risk of trapping bacteria in the wound resulting in a second abscess. Chronic wounds, such as the focus of the wound care specialist, typically heal by secondary intention.

Tertiary intention, also known as delayed primary healing, is a management technique that allows closure of the wound in a delayed fashion. This closure style, commonly used for ruptured appendix treatment, involves leaving the wound open for 4 to 5 days. At this point, bacterial contamination of the wound is minimal due to body defenses, thus sutures may be placed to close the wound. This has the advantage of minimizing bacterial contamination of the infected wound while also allowing cosmetic and functional closure of the tissues.[1,2,6,7] (Fig. 23.2)

Wound Bed Preparation

Débridement is considered the most desirable modality to facilitate wound closure and healing. The goal of débridement is to remove devitalized and necrotic tissue while leaving and promoting the ingrowth of healthy granulation tissue. The act of débridement has been demonstrated to remove not only tissue that delays healing and may incite infection, but also acts as a catalyst for growth and stimulus of fibroblasts and other healing cells. Débridement changes chronic nonhealing wounds into acute wounds that may then undergo the normal stages of healing.[2,8-10]

The technique of surgical débridement may be done either bluntly or sharply. Blunt débridement includes using materials and instruments to push or pull devitalized tissue from the wound bed. An example would be using a gauze sponge to sweep the adherent slough from a wound. The dirty wound, which may have stringy slough or slime on its superficial surface, will be cleared of these substances in order to perform other forms of débridement, such as pulsatile lavage. While easy to perform, this form of débridement does not adequately stimulate the wound bed to promote capillary ingrowth nor usually adequately remove the adherent slough.

Sharp débridement involves the use of instruments to more precisely remove slough or devitalized tissue from the superficial and deep wound bed. Figure 23.3 shows several

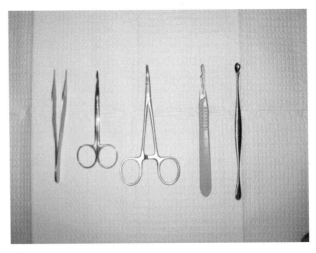

Figure 23•3 *Instruments typically used in wound débridement from left to right: Adson forceps, Iris scissors, hemostat, #15 blade/scalpel, curette.*

commonly used débriding tools. This is a preferred method of débridement, although the patient's and wound care specialist's level of comfort performing this form of débridement may be an issue.[10,11] The steps to perform surgical or sharp débridement follow in Box 23.1.

Besides surgical or sharp débridement, there are other forms of débridement that should be mentioned. Mechanical, enzymatic, autolytic, and biotherapy forms of débridement are available. Briefly, mechanical débridement includes such modalities as wet-to-dry dressings, which are of questionable benefit, or such therapies as the Versajet® (Smith & Nephew, Largo, FL). This hydrosurgery system uses a high-speed saline jet to mechanically débride the wound, with high-powered water being used to remove nonviable tissue. Also used is MIST® Ultrasound Therapy (Celleration Inc., Eden Prairie, MN), which involves noncontact ultrasonic energy that kills bacteria and facilitates wound débridement and healing.[17] These techniques allow removal of tissue without sharp instrumentation, but the therapy usually involves purchase or leasing of the units and availability of the disposable kits. Additionally, multiple therapy sessions may be required to achieve desired débridement.[10]

Enzymatic débridement involves the use of the enzyme collagenase which provides chemical débridement by breaking cross-linking of collagen. The collagenase product available is Santyl® (HealthPoint Ltd., Fort Worth, TX), which contains the collagenase enzyme commercially derived from the bacterium *Clostridia histolyticum.* This enzyme will digest collagen in devitalized tissues.

Autolytic débridement relies on the body's ability to use serous fluid and enzymes, which are present in wound exudates, to loosen and débride necrotic tissue. Inflammatory cells that are drawn to the wound help to soften and débride the eschar; this method is slower than other methods and may pose a somewhat increased risk of promoting infection by allowing nonviable tissue to remain sequestered under the dressing. A variety of synthetic dressings may be used, including the hydrocolloids and semipermeable dressings to facilitate autolytic débridement.[10,15,16]

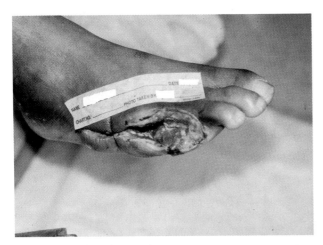

Figure 23•2 *Wound in an individual after amputation for a diabetic foot infection. Note the single suture being used to assist wound contraction while local care is being performed to clear up infection and prepare wound for delayed primary closure.*

▶ **Box 23•1** **Steps in Performing Surgical or Sharp Débridement**

1. Obtain an informed consent. Institutional protocols and procedural time-outs should be followed.[10]
2. Significantly irrigate the wound with water or saline in order to grossly clean the area. This helps to remove superficial slough in order to facilitate placement of anesthetic cream.[11]
3. If not performed under general anesthesia or conscious sedation, place anesthetic cream (ie, lidocaine gel) on the wound with the gloved finger or a tongue blade. The wound bed is not sterile so sterile preparation is not necessary. Gloves are worn to prevent cross-contamination. The longer the cream is left in contact with the wound, the more anesthetic effect is obtained.[12]
4. Lidocaine or bupivacaine may also be used to inject the wound in an intradermal and subcutaneous pattern. This does require sterile technique in order to minimize infection. The skin wheal is started in the peripheral area of the wound and injected circumferentially around the wound. The advantage of this approach includes the fact that a deeper level of anesthesia may be obtained, but since the injection itself is painful, patient comfort and compliance may be an issue.[2,13]
5. Beginning at the periphery of the wound, an instrument is used to cut away necrotic or nonviable tissue. Many instruments may be used, including scissors or scalpels. This author prefers the curette because the instrument is convenient, may be reused after sterilization, and is easily mastered. With a sweeping motion, the curette is dragged across the wound from the periphery to the center. The wound, regardless of the instrument used, is débrided from the superficial to the deep tissues. When capillary bleeding ensues or all necrotic tissue is removed, the débridement is complete.[10,14,15]
6. Deeper débridement should generally be avoided unless in an infected area or a deep form of anesthesia is used. If tissue is questionably viable, it should be left in place. Serial débridements are safer and provide better removal of nonviable tissue than one deep and large débridement. Likewise, if the patient experiences significant discomfort, the procedure should be abandoned and no other forms of anesthetic should be considered.[16]

Biotherapy, also referred to as MDT or maggot débridement therapy, is very effective in removing necrotic tissue. The débridement provided by the maggots is selective as the insects feed on the debris collected in nonviable wounds. Commercially available under the product name Medical Maggots™ (Monarch Labs, Irvine, CA), the *Phaenicia sericata* larvae are nontoxic. First described by Dr. William Baer at Johns Hopkins in the 1930s, the therapy has been shown to be effective by leaving the maggots in place for 2 to 3 days under a special dressing. However, there are cost issues with the purchase and transportation of the larvae as well as significant patient anxiety about their use.[10,19]

Factors That Impair Wound Healing

There are obvious factors that will impede wound healing and negate surgical débridement. These include malnutrition, advanced age, osteomyelitis, and poor oxygenation.

Malnutrition

Malnutrition is a leading reason that surgical wound débridement fails. A patient who is malnourished cannot mount the proper immune response to heal a wound. Generally, the serum albumin is a reliable and easily available blood test to quantify the degree of malnutrition. Albumin levels lower than 2.0 imply severe nutritional deficiency that will impair wound healing.[18-20] Furthermore, vitamin deficiencies are also associated with poor wound healing. These vitamin deficiencies include vitamins A, B, C, and trace metals. Vitamin C deficiency causes a deficient production of collagen as well as the lysis of stable collagen, resulting in defective wound healing.[21] Vitamin A deficiency occurs because of the relative increase in the need for this vitamin during tissue injury.[15] Vitamin B deficiencies result in decreased collagen formation and cross-linking, whereas the need for trace metals such as copper and zinc results in poor collagen formation.[22] All chronic wound patients should be considered for vitamin supplementation because of the ease of administration and its availability.[23] The role of nutrition in wound healing is addressed further in Chapter 4.

Aging

Advanced age will impact a healing wound; as one ages, structural and functional changes place the aged at risk for trauma and ulcers. Furthermore, skin integrity and thickness diminish with age. Surgical débridement should be conservative in this population so as to not cause further damage to the granulation bed.[15]

Osteomyelitis

Osteomyelitis, an infection of the bone, is a major cause of nonhealing after appropriate débridement. Surgical débridement of patients with osteomyelitis should generally include débridement of the underlying bone as well as a bone biopsy in order to ascertain the causative organism.[14] The bone biopsy may be done with either a needle or an open surgical method. Classification of osteomyelitis is varied; different classification systems have been developed but the traditional system involves the duration of the disease: acute (within 2 weeks), subacute (weeks to months), and chronic (greater than 3 months).[24] The Cierney-Mader system classifies infection by anatomic extent. This system is presented in Box 23.2.

Acute osteomyelitis is usually not an issue for the wound care specialist, whereas chronic osteomyelitis is much more prevalent. Chronic osteomyelitis is an infection that has been present several months and is associated with an area of bone necrosis called a *sequestrum*.[24] Furthermore, the most common organisms that infect osteomyelitis are *Staphlococcus aureus* and *Pseudomonas* species; however, mycobacteria and fungi have also been reported in immunocompromised patients.[25] One should realize that healing of an osteomyelitic wound is difficult and that the treatment relies on both the use of appropriate antibiotics and bony and wound débridement, which includes unroofing of the sequestrum and removal of all necrotic and nonviable tissues. The treatment may also involve the use of antibiotic beads placed into the surgical site to treat the involved bone as well as the use of hyperbaric oxygen, which has been demonstrated to increase oxygen tension in the wound thereby aiding wound healing and augmenting antibiotic efficacy.[24]

> **PEARL 23•2** The most accurate radiological imaging technique to determine osteomyelitis is magnetic resonance imaging (MRI); the gold standard for diagnosing osteomyelitis is the bone biopsy.[26]

Tissue Oxygenation

Poor oxygenation of wounds will obviously delay and prevent wound healing. While wounds are dependent on both the macrovasculature and microvasculature, blood flow studies are necessary in order to assess the macrovasculature (ie, large blood vessels such as the femoral artery); specialized tests such as transcutaneous oxygen measurement may be necessary to evaluate the microvasculature. For example, patients with previous radiation to the wound area most likely will have microvasculature problems, while the larger vessels are normal.[8,15] Evaluation of the wound for adequate vascularity is paramount before wound débridement. No instrumentation should be considered until blood flow studies have been considered.[15] Arterial blood flow is easily assessed with arterial Doppler studies, which demonstrate the ankle-brachial index

(ABI) as well as any segmental stenoses or occlusions. If the ABI is less than 0.8, then a revascularization procedure should be considered.[27]

Treatment of Osteomyelitis

Osteomyelitis involving chronic wounds occurs when the overlying ulcer or wound penetrates to involve the bone. (Fig. 23.4) The cortex of the bone is relatively resistant to infection, but bacteria that are in chronic contact with the bone may penetrate the bony barrier and lead to a smoldering infection of the bone. Furthermore, this may lead to sinuses, abscesses, and nonhealing wounds. The clinical evaluation of probing bone at the base of a nonhealing wound is a reliable clinical sign of osteomyelitis.[28] The palpation of a rough edge, or fracture line of the bone, also verifies the clinical impression of osteomyelitis.

The radiological diagnosis of osteomyelitis is made in a number of ways. Plain film radiographs of the bone suggest osteomyelitis when periosteal reaction is seen or when fracture is seen below an ulcer. Destruction of bone, loss of cortex, and cortical or medullary lucencies also are consistent with the diagnosis of osteomyelitis. However, most plain films are normal in the case of early osteomyelitis; osteomyelitis of greater than 1 month will usually present with some radiological abnormality.[29] Other radiological modalities to diagnose osteomyelitis include nuclear medicine studies such as bone scans. The injection of technetium-99 will demonstrate abnormality in the affected bone. However, the bone scan may be falsely positive because of uptake by the overlying wound. The overlying ulcer will "light up" and signify inflammation within the wound and not the bone.[30] Computerized tomography (CT) scanning has also been used, but the most reliable radiological imaging for osteomyelitis is magnetic radiological imaging (MRI).[9,30] This imaging modality is generally considered to be the most accurate radiological test to confirm a clinical diagnosis of osteomyelitis and offers the surgeon an anatomical approach to the diseased bone. The role of imaging in diagnosis of osteomyelitis is discussed in greater detail in Chapter 9.

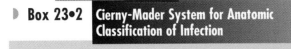

> **Box 23•2 Cierny-Mader System for Anatomic Classification of Infection**

Anatomic extent of infection

1. Medullary
2. Superficial cortex
3. Localized (cortex and medullary, mechanically stable)
4. Diffuse (cortex and medullary, mechanically unstable)
5. Subtype by physiologic status
   A Healthy
   Bs Compromised due to systemic factors
   Bl Compromised by local factors
   Bls Compromised by local and systemic factors
   C Treatment worse than disease[24]

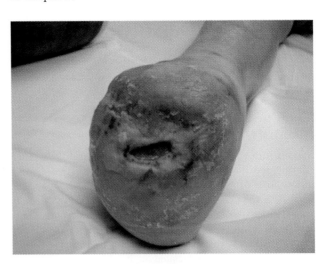

Figure 23•4 *Chronic osteomyelitis in the residual limb of a patient with type 2 diabetes mellitus.*

The surgical bone biopsy remains the gold standard for diagnosing osteomyelitis. An approach to performing a bone biopsy is outlined in Box 23.3. This procedure must be performed in the operating room.

The débridement of bone is considered the essential step in obtaining a good healing result. Studies that compared wide resection of necrotic bone with little resection of bone strongly favored aggressive débridement as the hallmark of success.[30]

Grafts

Grafts are considered a primary intention closure technique. They are used when granulating wounds are large and not expected to close in a timely manner. Considering that fibroblasts in healing wounds are known to converge at approximately 1 mm per day, a 5-cm wound can take nearly 2 months to close. A skin graft, which uses the patient's own skin to patch the defect, relies on the underlying wound's ability to supply nutrients and repopulate the epidermis. During the first days after grafting, nutrients are provided to the graft by plasma circulation whereby plasma cells proliferate into the graft from the dermis and provide nutrients to it.[31] The new skin graft will heal provided adequate circulation to the site is maintained.

There are different types of skin grafts. The split-thickness skin graft is epidermis with a small amount of underlying dermis that is removed from the patient.[32] A defect, which consists of dermis, is left at the donor site. The skin graft is then placed on the chronic wound, and the epithelial cells migrate together to close the wound.

The full-thickness graft is epidermis and dermis taken together to cover a chronic wound. These grafts leave full-thickness defects at the donor site but have the advantage of better skin coloring and texture and have less contraction than do split-thickness grafts.

Another form of graft is the composite graft, which involves skin and underlying tissues, most commonly muscle. These grafts are used in cosmetically sensitive areas and provide more rigidity.[33]

▸ **PEARL 23•3** Skin grafts include split-thickness, full-thickness, and composite grafts.

In order to facilitate the skin graft "taking" or growing into the surrounding tissues, pressure must be applied directly to the graft after placement. This pressure helps to allow capillary ingrowth and subsequent revascularization. The pressure also limits motion and shear forces that can tear a graft from its anchoring bed. Traditionally, the method of providing pressure and reducing shear has been to suture bolster dressings to the graft after fixating the graft to the surrounding skin using staples or sutures.[34] The direct pressure from the bolsters compresses the graft and limits motion. Vacuum-assisted closure (V.A.C.®; Kinetic Concepts Inc., San Antonio, TX) has been used to perform both these functions and has the added benefit of removing the serous drainage from the wound that can build up and lead to graft separation and loss.

Grafts, by their nature, are operative cases. The graft should be harvested and placed only by qualified surgeons. The technique of graft placement is presented in Box 23.4.

▸ **Box 23•3   Procedure for Performing a Bone Biopsy**

1. Obtain an informed consent. Institutional protocols and procedural time-outs should be followed. Antibiotics should be stopped 48 hours prior to the procedure. This will prevent a false-negative biopsy result as the antibiotics can mask growth of an organism.
2. Don personal protective gear.
3. Unlike a wound débridement, this procedure is invasive and should be performed using sterile technique.
4. Anesthetize the patient using local anesthesia, making sure to inject the periosteum (or outer layer) of the bone. Conversely, regional or general anesthetic can be used. A chlorhexidine or povidone-iodine preparation of the skin, deep tissue, and bone should be performed as the biopsy will be done through this wound bed.
5. All overlying necrotic and nonviable tissue should be removed with sharp surgical débridement (see débridement notes).
6. Once the bone is encountered, palpation of the bone should reveal some abnormality of the cortex, such as a rough edge or fracture line. The biopsy should be attempted at this abnormal area. Preparation of the bone with a chlorhexidine or povidone-iodine solution should be performed. This will

minimize contamination of the specimen with the bacteria present within the wound tissues.
7. A thin needle may be used to aspirate the bone. The aspirate is then sent to the microbiology laboratory for culture and sensitivity. The thick connective tissue surrounding the cortex should not be mistaken for bone. This tissue may need to be removed prior to biopsy. Advanced surgical techniques may include using an osteotome to elevate the diseased bone or a rongeur to remove devitalized bone. A deeper medullary infection should be managed by bivalving the bone and removing marrow as well as cortex.[24]
8. All bone that is removed is placed in a sterile specimen container to be sent to the microbiology lab for culture and sensitivity. Most departments require a fresh specimen in a sterile container, but each department should be queried before biopsy to determine specific handling requirements.
9. Once the biopsy and débridement are complete, a rasp is used to smooth the remaining bone so that sharp spicules of bone will not remain. Antibiotic beads may be placed into the resulting defect. Conversely, a muscle or myocutaneous flap may be used to cover the site.[24]

▶ Box 23•4   Technique of Graft Placement

1. A suitable donor site is chosen. Usually, because chronic wounds involve the lower extremities, the ipsilateral thigh is a suitable donor site. This site is prepped and draped in a sterile fashion. Since this is an operative case, informed consent and hospital policies should be followed.[34]

2. The recipient site is likewise prepared in a sterile fashion. The recipient site is débrided in order to remove devitalized tissue and to help recruit fibroblasts and other cells to migrate to the site.

3. A dermatome is usually used to remove the recipient graft. This device, which will remove epidermis and a portion of dermis, is set to remove a certain thickness of tissue. (Fig. 23.6) The graft should be thin enough to allow durability but not so thick as to preclude tissue ingrowth.[35]

4. Once the donor graft has been harvested via the dermatome (the graft may also be taken "free hand," which means removal by the surgeon's scalpel only), the graft is placed in saline solution to prevent desiccation.[36]

5. The graft is then put through a mesher that makes holes in the graft, thus allowing egress of fluid from the graft site and preventing loss of the graft. (Fig. 23.7) Likewise, holes may be made by hand in the donor graft so that the graft has a Swiss cheese appearance.

6. Once meshed, the graft is placed on the donor site and immobilized. Sutures may be used to secure the graft to the skin edges of the recipient site or devices such as the V.A.C. may be used. The graft is dependent upon the recipient site's blood supply in order to provide nutrients to the graft. Immobilization of the graft for the first 5 days is necessary. Any disruption of the graft during this time frame will cause loss of the graft.

7. The V.A.C.® may be used to secure the graft to the recipient site and has the added advantage of removing serous fluid from the site. This helps prevent fluid build-up under the graft that may lead to the graft pulling away from its blood supply and, ultimately, loss of the graft. Vacuum therapy usually is set at −75 mm Hg in a continuous mode.[37]

8. The graft is then dressed sterilely and left intact for 5 days. On the fifth day, the site is undressed and the graft is examined to assess the presence or absence of infection as well as vascularity and graft integrity.[34]

9. The graft is further immobilized for another 5 days and then reassessed. In general, graft immobilization is continued until day 10; a successful graft will be adherent to the underlying capillary bed by that point. Once adherent, epidermal growth will continue until fully healed.

10. The donor site is covered with absorptive dressings such as absorptive Tegaderm.

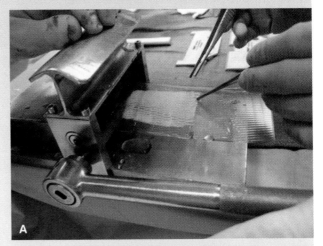

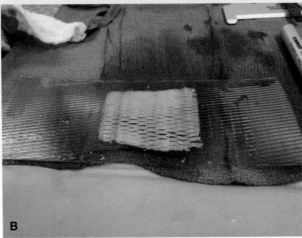

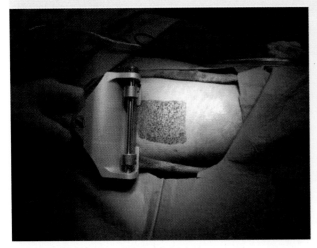

Figure 23•6 *Dermatome being used to harvest tissue for a split-thickness graft.*

Figure 23•7 *(A) Split thickness skin graft being removed from the mesher. (B) Appearance of graft following meshing.*

Flaps

Another method of primary wound closure is by placement of a flap. A flap is tissue and its blood supply that is transferred from one site to another site. The classification of flaps is based on either the blood supply to the flap or the type of tissue used to create the flap.[34] For example, a random cutaneous flap includes the blood supply from a subdermal plexus artery to an epithelialized segment of skin. Examples of random cutaneous flaps include rotational flaps and skin advancement flaps such as Z-plasties.

▸ **PEARL 23•4** Tissue flaps are classified according to their blood supply source or the type of tissue transferred.

Classification of tissue flaps also can be made based on the type of tissue transferred. Cutaneous flaps include the full-thickness layer of the skin as well as underlying fat. Fasciocutaneous flaps include skin, subcutaneous tissue, and underlying fascia; muscle flaps include muscle as well.[34]

One of the advantages of flaps over other methods of wound closure is that layered tissues may be used, thus providing permanent and durable closures. Furthermore, cosmesis is optimized as the native patient tissue is used to cover the defect. Infected and radiated wounds are also amenable to flaps as the adjacent tissues will help to fight infection and revascularize ischemic areas.[38]

The disadvantages of flap reconstruction include the availability of specialized plastic surgeons as well as the length and complexity of the operations. Operative times may be lengthy, which may be risky to the patient's general medical conditions. Furthermore, if a flap is reliant on a single blood vessel, injury or insult to that vessel may compromise the entire graft. Nonetheless, success rates for flap closure have been reported to be around 90%.[26]

Vascular Insufficiency Compounding Wound Healing

A major factor in the inability to heal chronic wounds is the deficiency of oxygen at the wound bed. The development of tissue hypoxia involves compromise of the macrovascularity or microvascularity to the wound site.[8] The evaluation of the chronic wound necessitates quantification of the degree of hypoxia and its possible correction. The factors and determination of the causes of vascular insufficiency are summarized further in Chapter 17. This discussion will center on the surgeon's role in treatment of vascular insufficiency.

Occlusive arterial disease is a leading cause of lower-extremity chronic wounds. A diagnosis of chronic ischemia is made based on the patient's history (such as diabetes mellitus or concomitant history of other vascular compromise such as coronary artery disease) and/or the physical examination (absent pulses, diminished ankle-brachial indices). Patient symptoms include the five P's (pain, pallor, paresthesias, pulselessness, and paralysis) and are present in acute ischemia but may be lacking in chronic ischemia.

▸ **PEARL 23•5** The hallmark symptoms of arterial insufficiency include the five P's: pain, pallor, paresthesia, pulselessness, and paralysis.

Radiological studies such as arterial Dopplers or angiography may be necessary to substantiate the diagnosis.[39] Transcutaneous oxygen measurements have also been used to determine microvasculature ischemia.[40]

▸ **PEARL 23•6** The vascular status of a chronic wound should be determined before débridement; an arterial Doppler study with ankle-brachial index is the optimal screening study.

Indications for surgical therapy for chronic arterial insufficiency generally fall into three categories: the deterioration of a wound despite optimal local wound care, cellulitis or an infected wound unresponsive to local wound treatment and antibiotics, or incapacitating pain and/or impending limb loss. If any of these indications are present, surgical therapy should be considered.[40]

Open surgical therapy includes a host of bypass procedures wherein the stenosed or occluded segment of artery is bypassed with another vessel or artificial conduit (such as Gore-Tex®; W.L. Gore and Associates, Flagstaff, AZ). For example, a high-grade stenosis, or blockage, of the femoral artery may be bypassed by using the patient's saphenous vein in a femoral-popliteal bypass. This allows blood and its oxygen to be carried around the blockage to the tissues of the lower leg.[39] Other surgical interventions include endarterectomies, whereby arterial blockage is improved by removing a piece of plaque from the vessel lumen.[39,41]

Newer techniques to facilitate blood flow include endovascular surgery. Endovascular approaches to treatment of arterial disease include using angioscopy, angioplasty, or stenting in order to open the vessel. Angioscopy is the use of a small camera or scope to view the inside of the blood vessel; angioplasty may be used to dilate the narrowed vessel much as coronary angioplasty opens the heart vessels. The plaque that is blocking the vessel is forcibly dilated, allowing an increase in the blood flow distal to that point.[42] A metal or plastic stent will be placed across a narrowed area to provide rigidity and prevent reocclusion of the stenosed blood vessel. Angioplasty and stenting have shown promising short-term results, but their long-term results still lag behind bypass procedures. In the chronic wound patient, improvement of blood flow, even temporarily, may lead to healing.[43]

A last consideration for operative intervention in the chronic vascular insufficiency patient is amputation. The indications for amputation are unremitting pain in a nonhealing wound and a limb-threatening infection. If either of these conditions exists despite optimal medical and surgical treatment, amputation may be considered. An amputation is done at a level above the wound at which adequate perfusion exists to heal the wound. The determination of adequate perfusion has been debated; the level is most often determined clinically, where all infected or nonviable tissue is removed while preserving as much limb as possible.[39] Transcutaneous oxygen measurements have been suggested as the best modality to determine adequate perfusion but have not been substantiated in large trials.[40]

Summary

The best wound is the one that never happens. Unfortunately, wounds are a fact of medical practice. When faced with wounds, acute or chronic, the desire is to obtain an effective closure as rapidly as possible. This chapter has presented several surgical options to speed wound resolution, including primary and delayed closure through suturing and a variety of grafts. The importance of wound bed preparation was also presented.

> ### ▶ Case Study 23•1   Traumatic Lower Extremity Wound Treated with Split Thickness Grafting

A 46-year-old male with type 2 diabetes mellitus is involved in a motorcycle accident. He suffers a full-thickness skin loss in the right lower leg along with a comminuted open right tibial fracture. There is gross contamination of the wound, with road debris being tattooed into the wound. There are no other life-threatening injuries. The orthopedic surgeon and the trauma surgeon bring the patient to the operating room where an external fixator is placed on the tibia and the wound is débrided and washed out. (Fig. 23.5A) Postoperatively, the wound is treated with a silver alginate dressing as moderate slough is noticed at the base of the wound. The arterial Doppler that is performed shows a diminished arterial-brachial index of 0.7. A follow-up arteriogram demonstrates a high-grade stenosis of the left external artery.

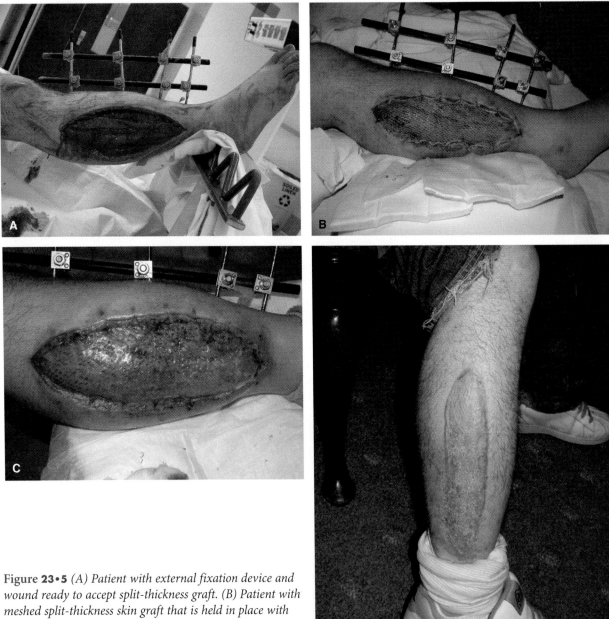

Figure 23•5 *(A) Patient with external fixation device and wound ready to accept split-thickness graft. (B) Patient with meshed split-thickness skin graft that is held in place with staples at day 4. (C) Appearance of meshed split-thickness graft as epithelialization progresses at day 14. (D) Appearance of limb following full graft take and maturation at 6 months.*

▶ **Case Study 23•1** | **Traumatic Lower Extremity Wound Treated with Split Thickness Grafting—cont'd**

Diabetic control is deemed to be good based on the patient's blood sugars. A vascular surgeon is consulted, and a balloon angioplasty was performed on the iliac artery stenosis and a stent placed in the iliac artery.

The wound develops healthy granulation tissue at the base, and the silver alginate is continued. The patient is scheduled for placement of a split-thickness skin graft after the wound continues to improve.

A split-thickness skin graft is taken from the right thigh and placed over the wound on the right lateral leg. The graft is meshed 3:1 after a dermatome was used to remove the epidermis and portion of the dermis from the thigh. An absorptive Tegaderm® (3M Company, St. Paul, MN) is placed over the

donor site in the thigh, and negative-pressure wound therapy is instituted with V.A.C. to secure the graft to the right leg. The V.A.C. setting is −75 mm Hg in the continuous mode.

The V.A.C. is removed on day 5, and the graft is noted to be adherent to the wound bed without evidence of infection. (Fig. 23.5B) A new V.A.C. dressing is placed.

The V.A.C. is again removed on postoperative day 10, and the graft is noted to be viable, adherent, and without infection. (Fig. 23.5C) A silver hydrogel dressing is again used.

Three weeks after grafting the recipient site at the right lateral leg is reepithelialized, and the donor site in the right thigh has healed as well. The patient goes on to do well and at 6 months presents with a well-matured graft. (Fig. 23.5D)

References

1. Lawrence, W, Lowenstein, A: Plastic surgery. In: Norton, J, Bollinger, R, Chang, A, et al: Surgery: Basic Science and Clinical Evidence. New York, Springer, 2001, pp 1993–2105.
2. Hunt, T: Wound Healing: Current Surgical Diagnosis and Treatment. New York, McGraw-Hill, 2006.
3. Fuller, J: Surgical Technology: Principles and Practice. Philadelphia, WB Saunders, 1994.
4. Autio, L, Olson, K: The four S's of wound management: Staples, sutures, steri-strips and sticky stuff. Holist Nurs Pract 2002; 16:80–88.
5. Lewis, R, Whiting, P, ter Riet, G, et al: A rapid and systematic review of the clinical effectiveness and cost-effectiveness of debriding agents in treating surgical wounds healing by secondary intention. Health Technol Assess 2001; 5:11–33.
6. Tsang, T, Tam, P, et al: Delayed primary closure using skin tapes for advanced appendicitis in children. Arch Surg 1992; 127:451–453.
7. Cohn, S, Giannotti, G, Ong, AW, et al: Prospective randomized trial of two wound management strategies for dirty abdominal wounds. Ann Surg 2001; 233:409–413.
8. Hunt, T, Hopf, H, West, JM, et al: Physiology of wound healing. Adv Skin Wound Care 2000; 13(suppl):6–11.
9. Attinger, C, Janis, J, Steinberg, J, et al: Clinical approach to wounds debridement and wound bed preparation including the use of dressings and wound healing adjuvants. Plast Reconstr Surg 2006;117(suppl):72S.
10. Stephen-Hayes, J, Thompson, G: The different methods of wound debridement. Brit J Nurs 2007; 16:S6–S16.
11. Blanke, W, Hallern, B: Sharp wound debridement in local anaesthesia using EMLA cream: 6 years experience in 1084 patients. Eur J Emerg Med 2003; 103:229–231.
12. Williams, D, Enoch, S, Miller, D, et al: Effect of sharp debridement using curette on recalcitrant nonhealing venous stasis ulcers: A concurrently controlled, prospective cohort study. Wound Rep Reg 2005; 13:131–137.
13. Derksen, D, Pfenninger, J: Local anesthesia. In: Pfenninger, J, Fowler, GC: Procedures for Primary Care Physicians. St. Louis, Mosby, 1994, pp 135–140.
14. Mathes, S, Nahai, F: Reconstructive Surgery: Principles, Anatomy and Technique. New York, Churchill Livingstone, 1997.
15. Myers, WT, Leong, M, Phillips, LG, et al: Optimizing the patient for surgical treatment of the wound. Clin Plast Surg 2007; 34:607–620.
16. Baranoski, S, Ayello, E: Wound Care Essentials: Practice Principles. Philadelphia, Lippincott Williams and Wilkins, 2004.
17. Ennis, W, Valdes, W, Foremann, P, et al: Evaluation of clinical effectiveness of MIST ultrasound therapy for the healing of chronic wounds. Adv Skin Wound Care 2006; 19:437–446.
18. Sibbald, R, Williamson, D, Schultz, GS, et al: Preparing the wound bed—debridement, bacterial balance, and moisture balance. Ostomy Wound Manage 2000; 46:14–35.
19. Milne, C, Corbett, L, Dubuc, L: Wound, Ostomy, and Continence Nursing Secrets. Philadelphia, Hanley & Belfus, 2004.
20. Pompeo, M: Misconceptions about protein requirements for wound healing: Results of a prospective study. Ostomy Wound Manage 2007; 53:30–44.
21. Colins, N: Adding vitamin C to the wound management mix. Adv Skin Wound Care 2004; 17:109–112.
22. Zagoren, A, Johnson, D, Amick, N, et al: Nutritional assessment and intervention in the adult with a chronic wound. In: Krasner, D, Rodeheaver, G, Sibbald, G: Chronic Wound Care: A Clinical Source Book for Healthcare Professionals. King of Prussia, PA, Health Management Publications, 2007, p 760.
23. Ord, H: Nutritional support for patients with infected wounds. Brit J Nurs 2007; 16:1346–1348, 1350–1352.
24. Skinner, H: Current Diagnosis and Treatment in Orthopedics. New York, Lange Medical Books, 2003.
25. Chapman, M: Chapman's Orthopaedic Surgery. Philadelphia, Lippincott Williams and Wilkins, 2000.
26. Lewis, VL, Jr., Bailey, MH, Pulawski, G, et al: The diagnosis of osteomyelitis in patients with pressure sores. Plast Reconstr Surg 1988; 2:229–232.
27. Dean, S: Leg ulcers causes and management. Aust Fam Physician, 2006; 35:480–484.
28. Treiman, G, Oderrich, G, Ashrafi, A, et al: Management of ischemic heel ulceration and gangrene: An evaluation of factors associated with successful healing. J Vasc Surg 2000; 31:1110–1118.
29. Butt, W: The radiology of infection. Clin Orthop 1973; 96:20–30.
30. Cunha, B, Dee, R, Klein, NC, et al: Bone and joint infections. In: Dee, R, Hurst, L, Gruber, M, et al: Principles of Orthopedic Practice. New York, McGraw-Hill, 1997, p 1522.
31. Schwartz, SI: Principles of Surgery. New York, McGraw-Hill, 1989, p 2087.
32. Stueber, K, Goldberg, N: Wound coverage: Grafts and flaps. In: Dagher, FJ (ed): Cutaneous Wounds. Mt. Kisco, NY, Futura Publishing, 1985.
33. Vasconex, HC, Ferguson, REH, Vasconez, LO: Plastic and Reconstructive Surgery. Current Surgical Diagnosis and Treatment, ed 12. New York, McGraw-Hill, 2006, pp 1209–1222.
34. American College of Surgeons: ACS surgery. New York, WebMD, 2002, pp 973–990.
35. James, MI, McGrouther, DA: Delayed exposed skin grafting: A 10-year experience of the technique. Brit J Plast Surg 1985; 38:124.

36. Georgiade, GS, Riefkohl, R, Levin, LS, et al: Plastic, maxillofacial, and reconstructive surgery. Plast Reconst Surg 1997; 100:15–17.

37. Scherer, L, Shiver, S, Chang M, et al: The vacuum assisted closure device: A method of securing skin grafts and improving survival. Arch Surg 2002; 137:930–933.

38. Gosain, A, Chang, S, Mathes, S, et al: A study of the relationship between blood flow and bacterial inoculation in musculocutaneous and fasciocutaneous flaps. Plast Reconst Surg 1990; 86:1152–1162.

39. Moore, W: Vascular and Endovascular Surgery: A Comprehensive Review. Philadelphia, Saunders Elsevier, 2006.

40. Hopf, H, Uenon, C, Aslam, R, et al: Guidelines for the treatment of arterial insufficiency ulcers. Wound Rep Reg 2006; 14:693–710.

41. Edwards, W: Composite reconstruction of the femoral artery with saphenous vein after endarterectomy. Surg Gynecol Obstet 1960; 111:651–653.

42. Johnston, K: Iliac arteries: Reanalysis of results of balloon angioplasty. Radiology 1993; 186:207–212.

43. Wagner, J, Klose, K: Infrapopliteal angioplasty for limb salvage: A 4-year experience. J Vasc Interv Radiol 1997; 8(suppl):247–249.

chapter 24

Surgical Management of the Neuropathic Foot

Robert J. Snyder, DPM, FACFAS, CWS, FACCWS

Jason Hanft, DPM, FACFAS

Howard B. Petusevsky, DPM, FACFAOM

Epidemiology of the Neuropathic Foot

In the United States, 1.3 million new cases of diabetes are diagnosed annually in people aged 20 and over.[1] The prevalence of diabetes in the United States for all ages is 6.3%. In the Medicare population (aged 65 and over), persons with diabetes incur 1.7 times the health-care expenditures of those without diabetes. Individuals with diabetes who are enrolled in private health insurance through their employers incur higher mean annual costs; $132 billion was spent in 2002, with direct medical expenditures of $91.8 billion and indirect costs of $23.2 billion. Inpatient days accounted for 43.9% of direct medical expenditures. Patients in this group incurred costs that were approximately 2.4 times higher than a similar group without diabetes ($7,778 versus $3,367).[2]

Neuropathic foot ulcers are a serious complication of diabetes.[3] Of the over 20 million patients in the United States with this disease, 15% will develop foot ulcers, and 6% will be hospitalized with this condition.[4,5] Vascular disease is 20 times more prevalent in this group, and impaired blood flow impedes healing.[6] Functional microangiopathy leads to many sequelae, including neuropathy; this condition is the most important factor leading to ulceration and is present in more than 80% of patients with diabetes and ulcerative lesions.[7] Williams et al proved that neuropathy and microvascular complications increased the annual cost of care by 70%. Among the millions of patients in the United States with diabetes, there are an estimated 1200 amputations performed each week; 84% of these surgeries are preceded by a foot ulcer.[8,9] The direct costs of lower-extremity amputations in patients with diabetes range between $20,000 and $60,000[10]; however, when expenditures relating to rehabilitation and failed vascular procedures are coupled with the indirect cost of lost productivity, these amounts exceed these cited costs.[11]

> **PEARL 24•1** It is estimated that up to 15% of the 20 million persons with diabetes in the United States will develop a neuropathic foot ulcer.

In a retrospective review of 186 amputations performed on 146 patients with diabetes, Van Damme et al determined that an aggressive control of infection and distal revascularization of calf or foot arteries,[12] when feasible, could improve the results of foot surgery in this patient group. Additionally, the poor functional recovery after major amputation (only 63% had autonomic gait with limb prosthesis) argued for foot-sparing surgery whenever possible. A retrospective study by Apelqvist et al involving treatment of patients with diabetes who had foot ulcers indicated the potential cost savings of preventative and multidisciplinary foot care.[13]

> **PEARL 24•2** Limb amputation in patients with diabetes is associated with a 5-year mortality rate of 39% to 68%, increasing with more proximal amputation.

Persons with diabetes often develop a triad of neuropathy, including the sensory, autonomic, and motor systems. Insensate feet coupled with dry, cracked skin and muscle imbalance create a recipe for disaster; contracted digits and plantar-flexed metatarsals in tandem with pressures and insidious foot trauma lead to ulcerations, frequently resulting in bone infections.

Surgical Planning: Primary Closure versus Staging and Management of Dead Space

The importance of blood flow and oxygen delivery to a wound bed cannot be overstated[14]; despite heroic efforts by wound care specialists, ulcerations will not heal in the presence of pronounced peripheral vascular disease. Vascularity, therefore, remains of prime importance when evaluating a patient for an operative intervention.

The detection of significant arterial compromise is vital to the prevention and treatment of foot disease and the success of surgical procedures.[15] In a prospective study of 162 patients, Yeager et al concluded that in individuals requiring toe or partial forefoot amputation, success of revascularization was the primary predictor of initial healing and freedom from major amputation.[16] Poor prognosis is often related to necrosis and ischemia.[17]

> ▸ **PEARL 24•3** For those patients at risk for amputation, successful revascularization of the affected segment is the primary predictor of initial healing and prevention of major amputation.

The palpation of foot pulses, calculation of the ankle-brachial index (ABI), and/or the toe-brachial index (TBI), among others, are commonly employed techniques for determining vascularity; however, the reliability of these tests remains controversial. Patients with diabetes exhibit arterial "stiffness," referred to as medial calcinosis.[18] This rigidity, coupled with edema and tissue glycosylation, may alter the clinician's ability to accurately palpate pedal pulses. Tanembaum et al demonstrated that the average foot pressure in the diabetic was 20 mm Hg greater than the pressure in a nondiabetic control subject.[19] Peripheral arteries in this group may, therefore, be relatively incompressible,[20] thus complicating the use of segmental pressures alone for assessing lower-extremity perfusion; in extreme cases, occlusive compression is not even possible at 300 mm Hg.[21] The International Consensus on the Diabetic Foot (ICDF) guidelines suggest that an ABI of 1.15 represents the upper limit above which measurements are deemed unreliable.[22]

> **PEARL 24•4** Medial calcinosis often results in uncompressible peripheral arteries, thus requires further studies to determine the available blood supply.

In summary, there is no single noninvasive parameter will reliably predict healing, and a palpable pulse does always indicate appropriate vascularity.[23,24] It therefore

remains imperative to have vascular and endovascular consultation.

Surgical patients may be classified as emergent, elective, or palliative. In the two latter scenarios, vascular workup and intervention when necessary should be performed before surgery commences. However, emergent cases often require life- and limb-saving intervention before vascular issues are addressed.

Patients who develop deep infections, for example, often require urgent surgical débridement to remove all necrotic and nonviable tissue. This results in the creation of a large space that could fill with blood or hematoma, thus delaying healing and establishing a medium for reinfection. Additionally, removal of bone (ie, metatarsal head) for a nidus of chronic osteomyelitis may lead to similar sequelae. Primary closure is usually not advocated in a setting of infection unless a more definitive amputation is planned. Usually the wound is observed postoperatively to ensure viability and revascularization before an attempt is made to fill the void. It is therefore imperative to manage this "dead space" so that further complications are avoided and healing progresses unencumbered.

Gauze/Iodoform Gauze

When a large cavity is created after surgery, one simple method of filling dead space that has been used over the years is to pack it with saline-soaked gauze or iodoform packing. Deep retention sutures may be of assistance. However, this packing must be changed frequently and does not allow for primary wound closure. In addition, it goes against principles of moist wound healing, which advise against the use of gauze. Usually, secondary closure (delayed primary closure) is attempted 7 to 10 days after initial débridement; however, wound edges begin to contract, making delayed primary closure more difficult. (Some clinicians may tack the wound edges to the adjacent tissue to prevent this.) Additional surgical procedures may therefore be required over time.

Penrose Drain

A Penrose drain(s) may be used to remove blood and other fluids from the wound cavity; however, this method does nothing to decompress the space and is predicated on gravity. Often, patients are placed in a dependent position to facilitate drainage. Additionally, the drain can act as a source of reinfection and should not be used for more than several days; thus, a long-term solution remains elusive.

Jackson-Pratt Drain

Use of a Jackson-Pratt drain creates decompression of dead space while facilitating removal of fluids. The device is not predicated upon gravity and therefore can be placed anywhere on the foot or leg; it will continue to function with the patient in any position. However, these drains are not meant for long-term use as they may create a potential for suprainfection and the need for additional surgery.

Negative-Pressure Wound Therapy

Negative-pressure wound therapy (NPWT) removes stagnant wound fluid while decreasing periwound edema and increasing circulation to the area. These devices work actively to create wound contraction while stretching the underlying cells, thereby changing their genetic signals. This therapy remains very effective in controlling dead space while slowly closing the tissue defect. This results in complete wound healing or creates a scenario for which a less invasive surgical procedure will be required to produce complete closure. NPWT is discussed in detail in Chapter 30.

Soft Tissue Transfers

The use of soft tissue transfers (ie, muscle flaps, composite flaps, and microvascular free muscle transfers) represent additional alternatives for managing dead space. Although technically more difficult to perform, these procedures bring additional blood supply to the wound and potentiate host defense, antibiotic delivery, and overall healing potential.

Bone Grafting

Bone grafting can successfully manage dead space and is predicated upon vascularity of the donor site. Cancellous bone is preferred over cortical grafts for filling osseous voids and can be used with or without further stabilization with external fixation. Autologous cancellous bone graft revascularizes rapidly and allows the host the enhanced ability to resist infection.

Polymethylmethacrylate Beads

Polymethylmethacrylate beads (PMMA) can be used to fill dead space while delivering local antibiotics at levels up to 200 times higher than the therapeutic systemic dose. This technique requires that PMMA be impregnated with antibiotic, molded into beads, and strung onto 28-gauge monofilament wire. The beads are inserted into the wound after thorough débridement in an operating room setting. For the antibiotic to work locally, it must be thermostable, eluted in reasonable quantity, and located in a liquid medium. The wound should therefore be tightly closed or a "pouch" created with an occlusive film dressing such as OpSite (Smith & Nephew, Largo, FL) or a cadaveric allograft to prevent antibiotic loss. Although the beads may be left in the wound permanently, in most cases they are subsequently removed. Some disadvantages to using PMMA beads may include impaired local immune response, antibiotic resistance, and the need for a second surgery to remove the beads. Some clinicians place the end of the wire holding the beads at the surface of the skin so that they may be removed without additional operating room procedures.[25]

> **PEARL 24•5** PMMA beads deliver antibiotic locally at a level up to 200 times higher than the therapeutic systemic dose.

Bone Graft Substitutes

Graft substitutes include a number of products ranging from allogenic to autogenous materials. They may be used separately or in tandem. Bone graft incorporation occurs through a process called "creeping substitution," whereby the graft material is replaced by new bone. This complex event is based on three underlying processes: osteoconduction, osteoinduction, and osteogenesis.[26] Osteoconductive materials include the inorganic bioceramics, calcium phosphate, calcium sulfate, and

hydroxyapatites. Calcium sulfate represents a substrate that hardens to dense filler and can readily be used to fill defects and support purchase of fixation devices. This material resorbs completely and rapidly.[27] This substrate may be used effectively to pack débrided bone defects and dead space and may be useful in the treatment of osteomyelitis when combined with antibiotics. Examples of calcium sulfate osteoconductors include OsteoSet® beads and Allomatrix® (Wright Medical Group, Arlington, VA).

Wound Débridement

One of the central tenets of healing neuropathic diabetic foot wounds is appropriate aggressive surgical débridement and off-loading. Débridement should include removal of all necrotic and devitalized tissue from the wound. The goal is to convert a chronic wound into an acute one.[28,29]

> **PEARL 24•6** The key to wound débridement is to remove all necrotic and devitalized tissue, thus converting a chronic wound into an acute one.

Digital Procedures

Digital contracture deformities (claw toes) associated with motor neuropathy often lead to ulcerations distally and dorsally. In these areas skin and bone are almost contiguous, and infected wounds frequently lead to osteomyelitis. Bone may be "shelled out" distally, leaving a skin envelope that may be packed and left to granulate or be closed with sutures. However, it is often necessary to perform a distal Syme's amputation. After the distal phalanx is removed, flaps are created dorsally and plantarly and fashioned so that the toenail and contiguous structures are excised in toto. The plantar flap is cut long in order to close the defect. It is sometimes necessary to remove a portion of the middle phalanx as well.

Claw toe deformities that are flexible may be treated with percutaneous flexor tenotomies. This simple procedure may correct the deformity and off-load the ulcer, resulting in rapid healing and prevention of recurrence.[30]

When dorsal ulcerations are present at the joints of the proximal or distal phalanges, wound excision and arthroplasty are often required. However, these procedures may create defects that are not easily closed, and digital amputations (partial or full) may therefore be required. After these procedures, if portions of phalangeal or metatarsal joints are left intact, cartilage must be denuded from the heads of the bones to prevent necrosis and foreign body reactions.

In patients requiring toe or partial amputation, a prospective study involving 162 patients found that success of revascularization was the primary predictor of initial healing and freedom from major amputation. Unfortunately, neuropathic ulceration predicted the need for repeat forefoot surgery following healing.[31]

Nehler et al performed a retrospective analysis of 92 patients with diabetes with 97 forefoot infections[32]; this cohort included patients with forefoot sepsis requiring immediate hospitalization for digital amputations and were deemed to have adequate arterial circulation for healing based upon noninvasive and clinical assessment. The study concluded that patients who had diabetes coupled with forefoot sepsis requiring acute hospitalization and primary digital amputation had a high incidence of intermediate-term, persistent, and recurrent infection leading to a modest rate of limb loss, despite having apparently salvageable lesions and noninvasive evidence of presumed adequate forefoot perfusion.

In light of these statistics, it is clear that excision of all infected soft tissue and bone followed by reconstruction of the toes and forefoot should be attempted whenever possible in patients with diabetes.[33] Rosenblum et al concluded that complex neuropathic ulcers in patients with diabetes could be successfully treated by an aggressive surgical approach involving removal of infected bone and ulcerations and correction of underlying structural abnormalities, provided arterial insufficiency was corrected first.[34]

Medial plantar ulcerations with underlying osteomyelitis of the great toe and adjacent plantar integument may be treated with "fillet-flaps" of the hallux. Using a medial incision, the ulcerations and toenail are completely excised, all bone removed from the hallux, and the cartilage from the first metatarsal head denuded. This creates a large, well-vascularized flap that can be rotated to close the surgical defect as well as any adjacent areas medially or plantarly under the first metatarsal head. Similar procedures can be performed at the lesser digits to cover adjacent plantar ulcers. Unfortunately, despite these heroic efforts, additional surgical intervention may be inevitable. Murdoch et al showed that following amputation of the great toe, 36 out of 48 patients (75%) underwent a more proximal amputation at a mean of 9.6 months.[35]

Resection of Metatarsals

Positional deformities of metatarsals often create plantar ulcerations that may not heal with conservative care. Wounds may become infected and seed to bone, causing osteomyelitis. In this scenario, surgical excision of metatarsal heads and shafts are frequently required. These procedures are traditionally performed through dorsal incisions; however, they may also be facilitated through the ulcer site plantarly using two semielliptical incisions. In each case, the bone should be cut at an angle that creates a beveled edge plantarly to prevent new lesions from forming.

In a retrospective study involving 25 patients with diabetes exhibiting plantar neuropathic ulcerations undergoing 34 metatarsal head resections, Griffiths and Weiman observed a mean healing rate of 2.4 ± 1.6 months postoperatively; none recurred during the mean follow-up time of 13.8 ± 11.0 months, thus these investigators recommended such procedures in an effort to achieve healing of chronic neuropathic foot ulcers under the metatarsals in this patient group.[36] However, when metatarsal heads are removed for the treatment of osteomyelitis, for example, the metatarsal parabola becomes skewed, often leading to transfer lesions, new ulcerations, and subsequent infections. Off-loading often remains challenging.

▶ **PEARL 24•7** Conservative off-loading procedures are of great importance to bedridden patients, who are at a high risk for developing pressure ulcerations over bony prominences.

This is particularly relevant when two or more metatarsal heads are excised. Many clinicians opt for either pan-metatarsal head resections (removal of all the metatarsal heads) or transmetatarsal amputations. However, in a preliminary retrospective study on 10 patients by Hamilton et al,[37] success using combinations of therapies such as gastrocnemius resection, peroneus longus-to-peroneus brevis tendon transfer, and resection of second through fifth metatarsal heads while preserving the first ray proved successful. Increased risk of ulceration under the first metatarsal head remained absent. None of the patients exhibited skin breakdown in this area, and all cohorts achieved a healed plantar grade foot without recurrence, transfer callus development, or contralateral breakdown at a mean follow-up of 14.2 months. Due to the small sample size, additional research is required to further determine the validity of this technique.

▶ **PEARL 24•8** Pan metatarsal head resection is recommended when two or more metatarsal heads are to be removed in an attempt to maintain the normal parabola of the foot and prevent transfer lesions.

Transmetatarsal Amputation

The transmetatarsal amputation (TMA) represents a functional forefoot/midfoot amputation. The procedure involves removal of bones in the forefoot/midfoot extending behind the metatarsal heads or shafts and fashioned so an appropriate metatarsal parabola is established. Dorsal and plantar flaps are created. The plantar flap is cut longer than the dorsal flap to facilitate closure; additionally, the plantar flap usually has a better blood supply.

In a retrospective study conducted by Stone et al,[38] functional ambulation was achieved in 23 of 25 (92%) limbs with healed midfoot amputations. Overall limb salvage for TMA/midfoot procedures was estimated to be 73%, 68%, and 62% at 1, 3, and 5 years, respectively.

Lengthening of Achilles Tendon for Treatment of Forefoot Ulcers and Stabilization of Amputations Such as Transmetatarsal Amputation

Lengthening of the Achilles tendon (TAL) for the treatment of plantar forefoot ulcers and stabilization of amputations remains a highly effective adjunctive therapy. Many retrospective, prospective, and clinical studies prove that the pressure on the plantar aspect of the forefoot is significantly reduced as a result of this procedure.[39,40]

Limited ankle dorsiflexion in conjunction with sensory neuropathy is one of the main contributing factors causing plantar ulcerations of the forefoot in patients with diabetes mellitus.[41,42] Additionally, glycosylation of the soft tissues contribute to tightening and contracture of the Achilles tendon, which causes a decrease in elasticity and tensile strength.[43] Muscular imbalances occur secondary to diabetic polyneuropathy, allowing the posterior muscle groups to gain a mechanical advantage over the weak anterior muscles.[44] All of these factors contribute to an increase in peak plantar pressures on the forefoot resulting in ulceration.[32,33]

> **PEARL 24•9** Achilles tendon lengthening is often performed in conjunction with more proximal amputations such as transmetatarsal amputation to significantly reduce pressure on the forefoot.

TAL is one of the oldest procedures performed; a review of the literature revealed that Delpech described a multilevel percutaneous lengthening in France in 1823.[45] The preferred method for TAL is a percutaneous triple hemisection first described by Hoke in 1931.[46,47] The procedure has been modified several times over the years.[48] A commonly used technique involves triple hemisectioning of the Achilles tendon through a percutaneous approach, thereby lengthening both the soleus and gastrocnemius components of the Achilles tendon. After sectioning, a dorsiflexion force is applied to the foot. The extremity should be maintained in a dorsiflexed position in a posterior splint, short leg cast, or removable cam walker. However, surgeons must be aware that extreme care must be taken in performing this procedure because there is a risk of overlengthening the Achilles tendon. If this occurs, the patient may develop a calcaneal gait, which may result in a difficult-to-treat plantar calcaneal ulceration.[34]

TAL is also extremely important in the stabilization of amputations. Patients who have had transmetatarsal, Lisfranc's, or Chopart's amputations can develop an equinovarus foot deformity.[49] Tendon imbalance occurs, resulting in significant gait alteration and altered function of the foot.[50,51]

In summary, TAL is a very useful adjunctive procedure in treating and reducing the recurrence of neuropathic ulcerations of the plantar aspect of the forefoot in patients with diabetes mellitus and equinus. A recent review of the literature, however, suggests that the procedure be used judiciously. Surgeons must address the underlying biomechanical and structural causes of the ulceration.[52]

Cadaveric Allograft and Human Skin Equivalents and Skin Grafts

Cadaveric allograft appears to be superlative for coverage of complicated wound pathologies; benefits remain particularly noteworthy when applied to wounds exhibiting exposed bone and tendon.[53] In a retrospective study, Snyder and Simonson observed that granulation tissue often completely covered bone and tendon after allograft slough or incorporation.[54] The study concluded that cadaveric allograft may prevent desiccation while controlling infection and substantially reducing pain.

Although the precise mechanism of action is unknown, it is hypothesized that living human skin equivalents (HSEs) fill the wound with extracellular matrix and induce the expression of growth factors and cytokines that contribute to wound healing.[55] Apligraf® (Organogenesis, Canton, MA) is a bilayered living skin substitute that, like human skin, contains both an epidermis and dermis; living keratinocytes and fibroblasts are derived from human neonatal foreskin.[56] The living fibroblasts are anchored in a bovine type-1 collagen lattice, and living keratinocytes form a stratified epidermis.[57]

> **PEARL 24•10** Apligraft is a bilayered skin substitute containing both an epidermis and dermis and delivers living keratinocytes and fibroblasts to the wound.

Veves et al performed a 24-center prospective, randomized, controlled trial (RCT) involving 208 patients comparing Apligraf plus conventional therapy (débridement, saline dressings, and total off-loading) to conventional therapy alone.[58] This pivotal study concluded that Apligraf may be a very useful adjunct for the management of diabetic foot ulcers that were resistant to the currently available standard of care and that accelerating wound healing could have a positive effect on reducing costs.

Dermagraft® (Advanced BioHealing, Inc., Westport, CT), is another dermal matrix human skin equivalent populated with fibroblasts. It has been shown to have clinical efficacy and cost benefit in the management of neuropathic ulcers in patients with diabetes.[59]

As a secondary endpoint of a prospective RCT concerning the effectiveness of human skin equivalent in noninfected neuropathic diabetic foot ulcers, Veves et al noted that patients using bilayered living cell therapy had a lower incidence of osteomyelitis.[60] Patients receiving Apligraf had a statistically significant ($P < 0.05$) lower incidence of osteomyelitis at the study site (2.7% versus 10.4%) when compared to patients treated with conventional therapy at 6 months; these data compare with 8.9% versus 3.1%, respectively, at sites other than the study ulcer. All patients were screened at baseline and underwent x-ray evaluation for clinical signs of infection. Most importantly, Apligraf patients required significantly fewer amputations of the study limb at 6 months (6.3% versus 15.6%; $P < 0.5$) compared to patients treated with conventional methods.

Limb amputation in patients with diabetes is associated with an increased risk of further amputation and a 5-year mortality rate of 39% to 68%.[61] Clearly, these data correspond with a significant cost benefit. Patients with lower infection rates require less frequent hospitalizations, and decreased amputation leads to substantial cost reduction. Apligraf may substantially decrease mortality and morbidity in this patient group. Once the wound is prepared with healthy granulation tissue, the use of split-thickness skin grafts may be feasible.

Infection and Limb Salvage

In diabetic and neuropathic patients, delays in healing of chronic wounds are often related to underlying osteomyelitis. Other causes such as severe peripheral vascular disease and/or improper off-loading can also lead to chronic ulcerations. The most common etiology is the loss of sensation due to neuropathy. Repeated pressures lead to skin breakdown, causing a typical neuropathic ulcer. As a wound remains open for a greater duration of time, infection has an increased opportunity to spread and devastate the limb. The evolution is often insidious and leads to amputation or bone resection.[62] There are a multitude of surgical procedures used to address infection and osteomyelitis. This section attempts to describe some of those procedures.

> **PEARL 24•11** The greater the duration of time that a wound remains open, the greater the risk for infection and possible limb loss.

Midfoot

The selection of a procedure is based on many factors, including surgeon preference as well as the pattern and the extent of infection. Infection must be treated aggressively in the neuropathic foot. The development of an open wound, abscess, or fungal or bacterial infection at the distal aspect of the foot can track along tissue planes and produce a deep-space infection.[63] This infection spreads rapidly along the long flexor tendons within the midcompartment of the foot and produces a raging fulminate infection within the midfoot. Incision and drainage with aggressive débridement of all devitalized tissue and infected bone is performed in order to stop the progression of the infection.[64] (Fig. 24.1) Local antibiotic therapy such as antibiotic-impregnated polymethylmethacrylate beads is sometimes used alone or in conjunction with system antibiotic therapy.[65] (Fig. 24.2)

Amputation may be performed at several distinctive levels within the midfoot. These include the transmetatarsal amputation (TMA), Lisfranc's joint disarticulation (involving the tarsometatarsal joint), and Chopart's joint disarticulation (disarticulation of tarsal bones from the talus and calcaneus). Amputations that are proximal to the midshaft level of the metatarsals require tendon-balancing procedures to offset the functional loss of the peroneal tendons and tibialis anterior tendon.[65] This procedure is performed to prevent an equinovarus position of the foot that would result in a foot that has abnormal pressure distribution. It may be necessary to further protect and augment the function of the extremity with bracing to significantly reduce the possibility of future ulceration and further limb loss.

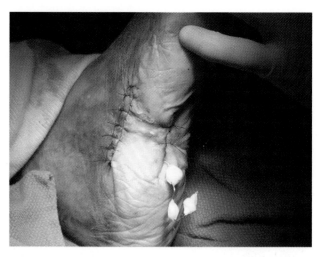

Figure 24•2 *This patient was treated for osteomyelitis of the cuboid. The procedure consisted of partial débridement of the cuboid in conjunction with PMMA antibiotic-impregnated beads to deliver high levels of antibiotic locally for a sustained period of time.*

The tarsectomy procedure, resection of tarsal bones of the foot, is reserved for patients with extensive infection of the tarsal bones. Excision of all the tarsal bones, however, leaves the patient with a nonfunctional foot. This procedure is sometimes used as a limb-sparing procedure. (Fig. 24.3)

One of the most common foot deformities seen in the neuropathic foot is the development of a rocker-bottom deformity of the midfoot. Midfoot ulcerations tend to extend along the tarsometatarsal (LisFranc's) joints and may require removal of one or more of the tarsal bones, including the cuneiforms and/or the cuboid, to reduce significant points of pressure. Exostectomy, resecting the bony prominence, is indicated when there is a fixed and stable deformity.[66] (Fig. 24.4) This procedure may yield a large dead space if a large amount of

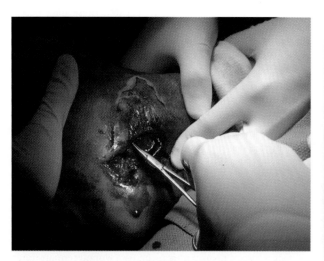

Figure 24•1 *Deep-space infection localized to the tarsal tunnel area. Incision and drainage with débridement of devitalized tissue is performed and care is taken to avoid the posterior tibial neurovascular bundle.*

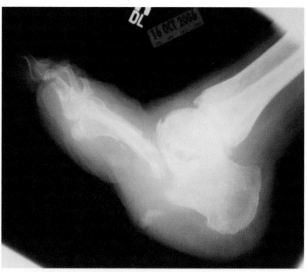

Figure 24•3 *Lateral view of an x-ray depicting a patient with history of previous tarsectomy procedure.*

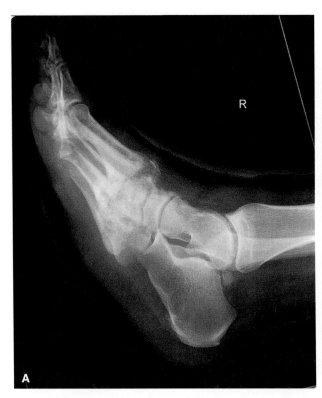

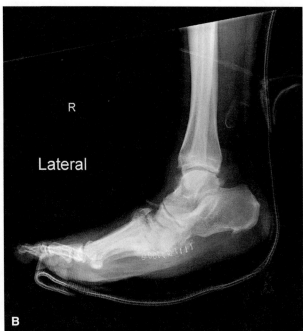

Figure 24•4 *(A) Lateral view of an x-ray revealing a rocker-bottom foot deformity secondary to Charcot's neuroarthropathy. The calcaneal cuboid joint is subluxed with a prominent cuboid plantarly. The patient has a history of recurrent plantar ulceration secondary to the bony prominence. (B) Plantar exostectomy procedure was performed to remove the plantar prominence.*

bone is resected. Exostectomy with a flap is sometimes employed to fill the void and provide adequate soft tissue coverage between the bone and skin. Many types of flaps can be used; however, the discussion of the risks and benefits of each type of flap is beyond the scope of this text.

> ▌ **PEARL 24•12** Exostectomy is indicated when there is a fixed and stable deformity.

Calcaneus and Cuboid

In the hindfoot, superficial and deep infection or abscesses should be treated aggressively with incision and drainage, débridement of all devitalized tissue, and proper antibiotic therapy. Generally, these wounds are left open to allow for continued drainage after surgery and healed by delayed primary closure, secondary intention, or negative-pressure wound therapy. (Fig. 24.5)

Bedridden patients are especially prone to developing pressure ulcerations at pedal bony prominences such as the posterior heel, lateral midfoot, and malleoli. These wounds can progress to become ulcerations that can compromise the underlying osseous structures and place the patient at risk for limb loss. (Fig. 24.6)

Calcanectomies, partial or complete, are salvage procedures by which part or the entire calcaneus is excised due to either osteomyelitis or chronic ulceration. This is usually a limb salvage attempt to avoid below-the-knee amputation.[67]

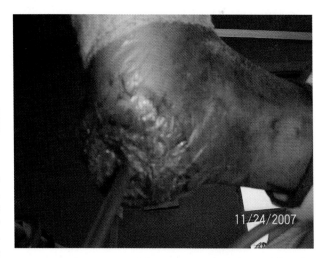

Figure 24•5 *Extensive débridement was performed for all nonviable tissue and bone to the posterior lateral aspect of the heel. Negative-pressure V.A.C.® therapy was instituted postoperatively to facilitate closure of the wound.*

All ulcerated and necrotic tissue is resected, as well as the involved bone, and the wound is closed primarily if possible. Sometimes, in order to achieve this, additional bone is resected to achieve closure. Crandall et al showed that the rate of failure of this type of procedure in patients with

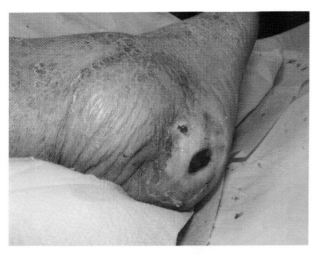

Figure 24•6 *Pressure ulceration to posterior lateral aspect of heel. Aggressive off-loading with good sound wound care principles are instituted to prevent further progression of the wound.*

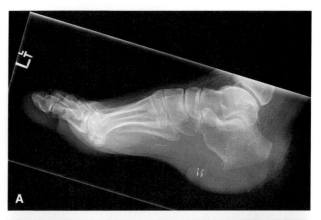

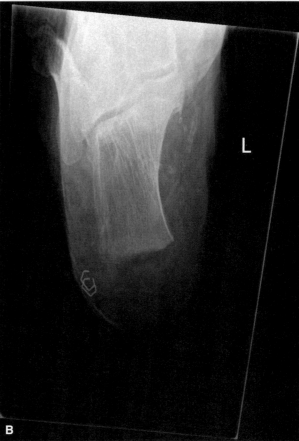

diabetes was as high as 65% in a 10-year study.[68] In spite of the risks associated with these complications, this remains a viable alternative to limb loss. (Fig. 24.7)

Talus, Tibia, and Fibula

Limb salvage of the ankle is often performed via partial or total ostectomy. If complete resection of the ankle joint is mandated, then below-the-knee amputation should be a consideration. (Fig. 24.8)

Partial resections are the simplest method of salvage and require first that the offending prominence be readily identified through imaging studies. Once the prominence is isolated, the surgical approach is often dictated by the depth of ulceration. Superficial ulcers can be directly incised and the bony prominence resected.[69] Deeper ulcerations often require the approach to be away from the ulceration in order to prevent contamination of noninfected tissue. External fixation may also be applied to provide stability to the resected area and allow for some weight bearing to the affected extremity postoperatively. (Fig. 24.9)

Reconstruction and Charcot Arthropathy

Preserving function with restoration of alignment and joint stability are the goals of reconstructive surgery of the neuropathic limb. Maintaining a weight-bearing axis of the lower extremity and preventing amputation are also important. It is always important to keep in mind that a successful intervention is one that leads to a foot and ankle suitable for proper footwear and bracing.

▶ **PEARL 24•13** Reconstructive procedures are implemented when bracing and custom-molded shoe gear have failed to improve the patient's outcome.

Figure 24•7 *A portion of the calcaneus was resected secondary to osteomyelitis. The patient presented with a long history of pressure ulceration to the area that progressed to infect the underlying bone. (A) Lateral view of an x-ray revealing the amount of bone resected for the partial calcanectomy. (B) Calcaneal axial view of the same foot.*

Physicians should attempt major reconstructive interventions when bracing and custom-molded shoe gear has failed to improve the patient's function and symptoms. It is paramount to evaluate possible outcomes when performing surgical reconstructive procedures and to assess whether further nonsurgical means can allow proper ambulation.

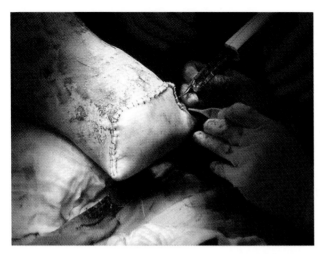

Figure 24•8 *A below-the-knee amputation was performed, and the flap was reapproximated with skin staples.*

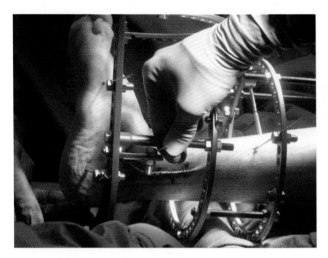

Figure 24•9 *An example of a patient who underwent arthrodesis of the ankle joint using a circular external fixator to compress the tibia and talus together while also providing stability to the fusion site. A portion of the distal fibula was also removed for exposure to the ankle joint.*

Midfoot

The most common location in the foot affected by Charcot's joint affliction are the tarsometatarsal joints. Instability to these joints leads to a rocker-bottom foot deformity. Depending on the location of the primary deformity, plantar ulcerations may be located medially, centrally, or laterally. Arthrodesis or fusion of a joint is indicated when there is instability within the midfoot that would result in further collapse and continuation of the deforming force even if exostectomy were to be performed. These surgical procedures would be performed during the nonactive phase of the disease.[70]

Medial column fusion is indicated when instability of the medial column is present and there is significant bone loss, subluxation, joint dislocation, or compromise. This procedure is preferably performed when there is no ulceration in

order to reduce the postoperative incidence of infection. (Fig. 24.10)

Correction of midfoot deformities may also be performed by osteotomies to correct angular deviations of bony segments. Midfoot osteotomies are directed at reducing the resultant deformity secondary to Charcot's neuroarthropathy. These may employ internal fixation, external fixation, or a combination of both. (Fig. 24.11)

Calcaneus and Cuboid

Surgical management of the neuropathic hindfoot is always challenging. Indications for reconstructive surgical procedures of major tarsal bones include recurrent ulceration,

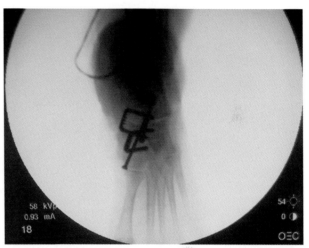

Figure 24•10 *Intraoperative x-ray view demonstrating fusion of the medial column encompassing the medial cuneiform, navicular, and talus articulations.*

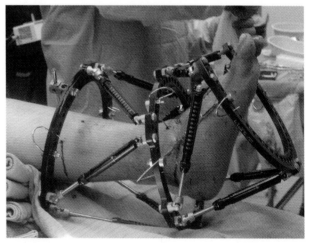

Figure 24•11 *A Talar Spatial Frame® from Smith & Nephew was employed to perform a gradual correction of a Charcot's foot deformity. A transverse midtarsal osteotomy and soft tissue release of the talar navicular joint were also completed to allow for the correction. (Photo courtesy of Ira Fox, DPM)*

chronic pain, acute fractures, and misalignment with joint instability.

Reconstructive surgical procedures of the rear foot can be divided into osseous and soft tissue procedures. Osseous procedures include those directed to restore alignment with arthrodesis of major joints such as the subtalar joint, talonavicular joint, and calcaneocuboid joints to obtain a rectus foot that redistributes plantar forces more evenly. (Fig. 24.12) Soft tissue procedures include those directed to maintain dynamics of the foot by means of tendon transfers and lengthening.

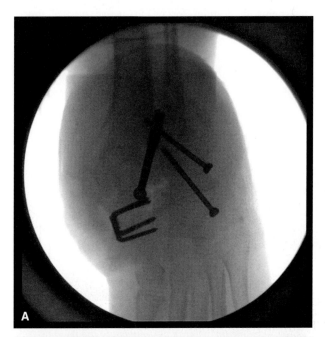

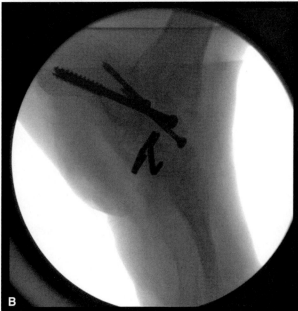

Figure 24•12 *(A) Intraoperative anterior-posterior x-ray view of a triple arthrodesis procedure. (B) Lateral x-ray view of same foot.*

Desirable alignment of the foot after these procedures would be with 5 to 10 degrees of hindfoot valgus and slight external rotation. There are various methods of fixation, all of which have their various dynamics, and they are used based on the surgeon's preference.[70]

Adjunctive soft tissue procedures include tendon transfers of anterior or posterior muscle groups as well as out-of-phase tendon transfers to obtain equally distributed forces across the plantar aspect of the foot. Percutaneous Achilles tendon lengthening is recommended when equinus is present.

Talus, Tibia, and Fibula

Neuroarthropathy of the ankle is a complicated condition to manage, no matter what stage the Charcot's deformity presents, even if adequate immobilization with internal or external fixation is accomplished. This is mainly due to the risk of a worsening prognosis of the deformity. The focus of correcting the deformity is to maintain the weight-bearing axis of the ankle. The axis needs to be centered over the subtalar joint. When there is bone fragmentation, this axis can be medial or lateral to the weight-bearing axis. This can lead to many complications, such as a bony prominence that frequently leads to ulceration. (Fig. 24.13) The deformity may not only cause wound problems but also cause infection, loss of limb, sepsis, failure of fixation, and death.

Reconstruction of the ankle in the presence of neuroarthropathy is technically challenging. Indications for surgery should include gross instability, recurrent ulcerations, and infections not manageable with bracing or casting. Bone fragmentation may cause the talus to dislocate anterior to the tibia, and more than likely the deformity is a varus or valgus complication. The surgeon must plan the best procedure for the insensate patient with either internal or external fixation. External fixation should be the treatment of choice in the presence of an infected open wound. This would be a complication secondary to the deformity of a boney prominence. The external fixator may be used to stabilize the limb until the infection is cleared. Negative-pressure wound therapy may also be placed over the wound as an adjuvant therapy even if the infection is not yet cleared. The surgeon should also consider the potential for healing from the surgical incision. External fixators may be employed for various procedures involving reconstruction of the ankle. Some afford weight bearing of the extremity and others only provide support to the involved area and do not allow for additional weight bearing. In general, some of these techniques can be done through small incisions when using external fixation in order to minimize postoperative complications.[71] (Fig. 24.14)

▶ **PEARL 24•14** External fixation is the preferred treatment in the presence of an open wound when further stability of the affected segment is required.

During the nonactive phase of Charcot's deformity, internal fixation provides an alternate means of completing arthrodesis of the ankle. Internal fixation is accomplished

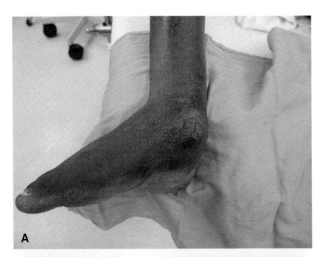

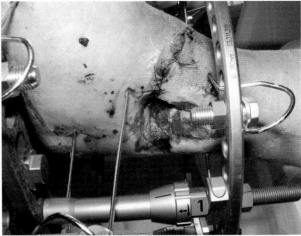

Figure 24•14 *A clinical photograph showing the lateral view of the ankle. The distal portion of the fibula was infected and a large portion was resected. The ankle was then fused, and a large circular external fixator was applied to compress and stabilize the fusion site. A local flap is planned to cover the defect.*

for ensuring that the foot will be able to purchase the ground and offer a stable platform during ambulation.[69]

Summary

Neuropathic ulcers are a serious complication usually associated with diabetes mellitus. Peripheral vascular disease often complicates this condition and leads to greater patient morbidity. Patient mortality is significantly increased with more proximal amputations; therefore, when possible, limb sparing procedures should target the foot. It is imperative that the physician recognize an ischemic limb event prior to managing this complex scenario.

Emergent cases address infection and lead to the development of a large dead space in the foot once all necrotic and devitalized tissue is débrided. This space is managed with several modalities such as drains, PMMA antibiotic-impregnated beads, NPWT, and soft tissue and bone grafts. Primary closure is not performed until it can be ascertained that the site is free of infection. Amputation of a segment of the foot may also be performed due to the extent of the infection. Often, if an amputation exceeds the transmetatarsal level proximally, tendon balancing procedures will also be incorporated in order to prevent an equinovarus deformity of the remaining foot and ankle by either resecting a bony prominence or realigning bones and fusing their associated joints. Their function is to remove pressure from an area, dispersing pressure more evenly throughout the foot, or to transfer it to an adjacent area. Bracing is often combined with surgical off-loading procedures to further assist with redistributing pressure throughout the foot. This creates a more functional and plantigrade foot for weight bearing, reducing the recurrence of ulcerations and further patient morbidity.

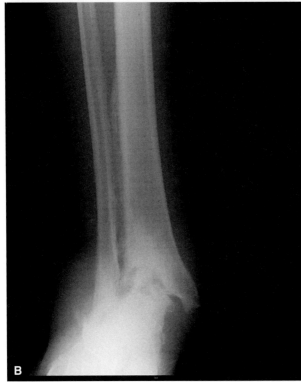

Figure 24•13 *(A) Clinical picture of a patient with Charcot's neuroarthropathy of the ankle. Note the prominence at the medial aspect of the ankle with overlying hyperkeratotic changes of the skin. (B) Anterior-posterior x-ray view of the same ankle. Note the extensive bony destructive changes of the ankle. The fibula is also seen directly contacting the calcaneus laterally.*

with cannulated screws, an intramedullary rod, or plates. The goal with internal or external fixation is to maintain good alignment, with the ankle in 0 to 5 degrees of dorsiflexion and the hindfoot in 5 to 10 degrees of valgus with a slight external rotation. The position of the ankle is critical

▸ **Case Study 24•1** ▕ **Evaluation and Management of a Patient with Osteomyelitis**

Subjective Findings

The patient is a 58-year-old male with type 2 diabetes initially seen for a complaint of dorsal right foot ulceration following incision and drainage with continued drainage and redness from the ulceration site. He was febrile with nausea, chills, and stomach cramps at the time of presentation and was immediately admitted to the hospital for further evaluation and treatment.

History of Previous Illness: The patient was admitted to another facility 1 month ago and received a week-long course of intravenous antibiotics, and he was subsequently discharged. He was readmitted 2 days later and received emergency incision and drainage with further intravenous antibiotic administration. He was discharged to home on intravenous antibiotics and subsequently went on to develop *Clostridium difficile* colitis that was treated with Flagyl®. X-rays taken at admission revealed bony destructive changes to the midfoot with gas in the tissues.

Past Medical History: Patient has a history of uncontrolled diabetes mellitus with HgA$_{1c}$ >9, peripheral neuropathy, *C. difficile* colitis, nonobstructive coronary artery disease, and hypertension.

Past Surgical History: Patient has had cardiac catheterization and tonsillectomy.

Current Medications: Patient currently takes metoprolol, 75 mg; Vytorin®, 10/40 mg; NovoLog®, mix 70/30

Social History: Patient denies any tobacco, alcohol, or illicit drug use.

Allergies: Patient has no known drug allergies.

Review of Systems: Patient has nausea, fever, and chills but denies vomiting. He has a known history of diarrhea and some diffuse abdominal discomfort. The remainder of the exam was negative.

Objective Findings

Patient was alert and oriented to person, place, and time.

Vital Signs: Temperature 100.4°F; pulse rate, 94; respiratory rate, 20; blood pressure 110/52.

Laboratory Values: WBC, 21.8; hemoglobin, 12; hematocrit, 35.2; platelet count, 434,000; sodium, 131; potassium, 3.9; chloride, 95; carbon dioxide, 26; BUN, 12; creatinine, 0.93.

Blood Cultures: Culture was positive for OSSA (oxacillin-sensitive *Staphylococcus aureus*).

Wound Cultures: Culture was positive for OSSA.

Radiographic Findings: There was soft tissue swelling overlying the dorsal and lateral aspect of the right foot. Also present was an associated lucency within the soft tissues, likely soft tissue gas interposed between the fourth and fifth metatarsal interspaces and projecting along the dorsal aspect of the foot. There was irregularity along the cortex of the base of the fourth and fifth metatarsals, with patchy sclerosis in the intermedullary portions of the bases of the fourth and fifth metatarsals. Findings were compatible with underlying osteomyelitis at this level. (Fig. 24.15)

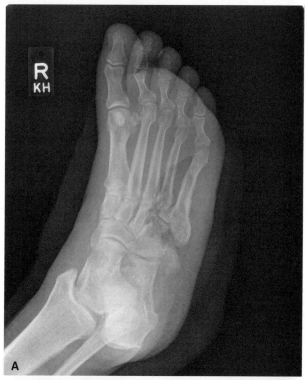
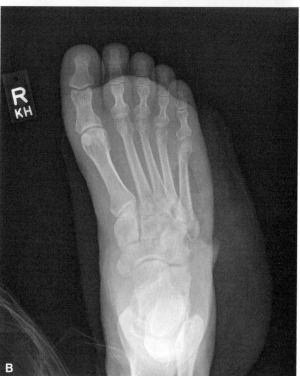

Figure 24•15 *Right foot x-rays with medial oblique (A), and dorsal plantar (B) views. Bony destructive changes are noted at the cuboid articulation with the fourth and fifth metatarsal bases. Extensive soft tissue edema is also seen.*

▶ **Case Study 24•1** ▕ **Evaluation and Management of a Patient with Osteomyelitis—cont'd** ▏

MRI Findings: Extensive subcutaneous edema was present consistent with cellulitis of the midfoot and forefoot, with a large ulceration site along the dorsal and lateral aspects of the foot. Fluid is seen tracking from the defect down to the third through fifth metatarsal bases. There is osteomyelitis involving the bases of the second through fifth metatarsals, cuboid, and second and third cuneiforms. The changes at the first cuneiform and the navicular are likely due to osteomyelitis; however, reactive edema cannot be excluded. (Figs. 24.16 and 24.17)

Dermatological Assessment: There is a full-thickness ulceration measuring approximately 10 cm × 4 cm with 70% granular and 30% fibrotic base with exposed bone overlying the dorsal lateral right foot. Copious brown serous drainage was noted, with extensive periwound erythema and warmth. No malodor is noted. No other open lesions or macerations were noted. (Fig. 24.18)

Vascular Assessment: Posterior tibial and dorsalis pedis pulses are palpable +2/4, and capillary fill time is less than 3 seconds for all toes of both feet. Skin temperature is noted to be warm to cool from proximal to distal of the lower extremity bilaterally, except for localized warmth of the right foot ulceration site. No digital hair growth is observed.

Orthopedic Assessment: Moderate amount of fluctuance was palpable over the lateral margin of the right foot ulceration site. Compression of the anterior ankle proximal to the ulceration

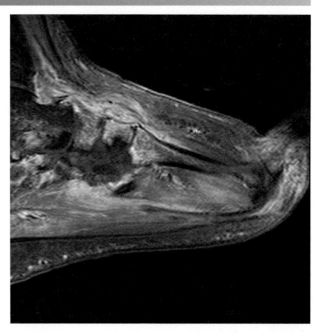

Figure 24•17 *T2 MRI image taken in sagittal plane revealing extensive cellulitis and bony destructive changes seen along the medial column of the foot.*

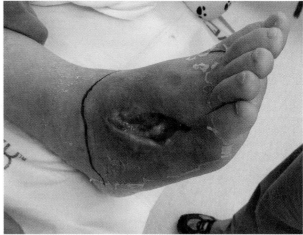

Figure 24•18 *Clinical presentation of right foot prior to surgical intervention. There is an extensive ulceration overlying the dorsal and lateral right foot with surrounding cellulitis and suspected underlying abscess.*

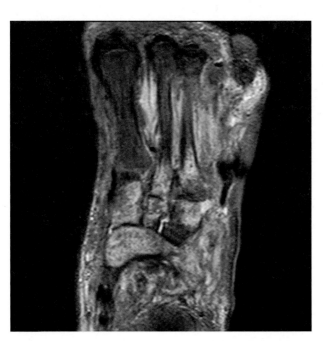

Figure 24•16 *STIR MRI image in axial plane demonstrating extent of osteomyelitic involvement. Note the increased uptake in the affected bones such as the metatarsal bases, cuneiforms, and navicular.*

produced approximately 10 to 15 ml of purulence into the wound site. No crepitus was palpated at the right foot wound site. Manual muscle strength testing and range of motion tests were not performed.

Neurological Assessment: Epicritic sensation was grossly absent per Semmes-Weinstein 5.07 (10 g) monofilament ascending to midcalf level of the lower extremity bilaterally.

Continued

▶ Case Study 24•1   Evaluation and Management of a Patient with Osteomyelitis—cont'd

Assessment:

1. Sepsis
2. Status post incision and drainage, right foot with remaining dorsal lateral ulceration, secondary cellulitis, and probable underlying osteomyelitis
3. Diabetes mellitus
4. Peripheral neuropathy

Plan:

1. Control infection by performing incision and drainage with débridement of devitalized and necrotic soft tissue and bone to include multiple bone biopsies to verify infected bones.
2. Infectious diseases consultation and administration of broad-spectrum intravenous antibiotic therapy.
3. Negative-pressure wound therapy to wound site after intervention.

Results: Patient's vital signs and laboratory findings stabilized after incision and drainage. Osteomyelitis was confirmed per bone biopsy in metatarsals 2 to 5, lateral cuneiform, and cuboid.

Treatment Options

1. Treatment would include further débridement of all infected bone with implantation of antibiotic-impregnated beads to fill the dead space and deliver high concentrations of antibiotic locally. Wound should be covered with a flap and application of external fixation to provide stability to the foot during the recovery process. The patient remains at risk for further progression of infection. A nonfunctional foot is the result of further débridement and places the patient at risk for further ulceration and morbidity. Secondary complications due to the flap, such as donor site morbidity and flap failure, and those risks associated with external fixation are also possible. The patient requires further long-term IV antibiotics, which may interfere with normal flora and place him at risk for future resistant infections. The recovery process is long. There is an increase in the cost associated with care; however, the patient maintains his foot with questionable function.

2. Treatment would consist of below-the-knee amputation and fitting of the extremity for prosthesis. The recovery period would be shorter; however, the patient's cardiovascular demand is increased and he is placed at greater risk for mortality within 5 years. Extensive physical therapy is also required to encourage ambulation with the prosthesis. All infected bone is guaranteed to be removed, and there is no need for further long-term IV antibiotics.

References

1. Centers for Disease Control, National diabetes fact sheet, 2005, http://www.cdc.gov/diabetes/pubs/estimates.htm, Date accessed: Jan. 20, 2010.
2. Kaczander, B, Kushlak, P, Hokawala, et al: Alternative modalities in wound healing. Podiatry Management 2007; 26:81–90.
3. Weiman, JT, Smiell, JM, Su, Y: Efficacy and safety of a topical gel formulation of recombinant human platelet derived growth factor-BB (becaplermin) in patients with chronic neuropathic diabetic ulcers: A phase III randomized placebo-controlled double-blind study. Diabetes Care 1998; 21:822–827.
4. Jiwa, F: Diabetes in the 1990's: An overview. Stat Bull Metrop Insurance Co 1997; 78:2–8.
5. National Institutes of Health, National Institute of Diabetes and Digestive and Kidney Diseases (NIDDM): Prevention and early intervention for diabetes foot problems: Research Review: 1998 Bethesda, MD.
6. Gibbons, GW, Marcaccio, EJ, Habershaw, GM: Management of the diabetic foot. In: Callow, AD, Ernst, CD (eds): Vascular Surgery: Theory and Practice. Stamford, CT, Appleton and Lange, 1995.
7. Levin, ME: Preventing amputation in the patient with diabetes. Diabetic Care 1995; 18:1383–1395.
8. Williams, R, Van Gaal, L, Lucioni, C: Assessing the impact of complications on the costs of type 2 diabetes. Diabetologia 2002; 45:S13–S17.
9. Percoraro, RE, Reiber, GE, Burgess, EM: Pathways to diabetic limb amputation. Diabetes Care 1990; 13:513–521.
10. Eckman, MH, Greenfield, S, Mackey, WC, et al: Foot infections in diabetic patients: Discussion and cost effectiveness analysis. JAMA 1995; 273:712–720.
11. Brem, H, Balledux, J, Bloom, T, et al: Healing diabetic foot ulcers and pressure ulcers with human skin equivalent. Arch Surg 2000; 135:627–634.
12. Van Damme, H, Rorive, M, Martens, BM, et al: Amputations in diabetic patients: A plea for foot-sparing surgery. Acta Chir Belg 2001; 101:123–129.
13. Apelqvist, J, Ragnarson-Tennvall, G, Persson, U, et al: Diabetic foot ulcers in a multidisciplinary setting: An economic analysis of primary healing and healing with amputation. J Intern Med 1994; 235:463–471.
14. Ennis, WJ, Mensese, P: Factors impeding wound healing. In: Kloth, L, McCulloch, J (eds): Wound Healing: Alternatives in Management. Philadelphia, FA Davis, 2002.
15. Williams, DT, Harding, KG, Price, P: An evaluation of the efficacy of methods used in screening for lower-limb arterial disease in diabetes. Diabetes Care 2005; 28:2206–2210.
16. Yeager, RA, Moneta, GL, Edwards, JM, et al: Predictors of outcomes of forefoot surgery for ulceration and gangrene. Am J Surg 1998;175:388–390.
17. Horta, C, Vilaverde, J, Mendes, P, et al: Evaluation of diabetic foot amputation rate. Acta Med Port 2003; 16:373–380.
18. Emanuele, MA, Buchanan, BJ, Abraira, C: Elevated leg systolic pressure and arterial calcification in diabetic occlusive vascular disease. Diabetes Care 1981; 4:289–292.
19. Tenembaum, MM, Rayfield, E, Junior, J, et al: Altered pressure flow relationship in the diabetic foot. J Surg Res 1981; 31:307–313.
20. Gundersen, J: Segmental measurements of systolic blood pressure in the extremities including the thumb and great toe. Acta Chir Scand Suppl 1972; 426:1–90.
21. Hu, MY, Allen, BT: The role of vascular surgery in the diabetic patient. In: Bowker, JH, Pfeiffer, MA (eds): The Diabetic Foot. St. Louis, Mosby, 2001.
22. Apelqvist, J, Bakker, K, van Houtum, WH, et al: International consensus and practical guidelines on the management and the prevention of the diabetic foot: International working group on

the diabetic foot. Diabetes Metab Res Rev 2000; 16(suppl 1): S84–S92.

23. Bloomgarden, ZT: Diabetic retinopathy and neuropathy. Diabetes Care 2005; 28:963–970.

24. Snyder, R: Controversies regarding vascular disease in the patient with diabetes: A review of the literature. Ostomy Wound Manage 2007; 53:26–34.

25. Snyder, RJ, Cohen, MM, Sun, C, et al: Osteomyelitis in the diabetic patient: Diagnosis and treatment. Medical, surgical, and alternative treatments. Ostomy Wound Manage 2001; 47(Pt 2):24–41.

26. Malay, DS: Feature: A closer look at bone graft substitutes. Podiatry Today 2005; 18:28–34.

27. Alexander, DI, Manson, NA, Mitchell, MJ: Efficacy of calcium sulfate plus decompression bone in lumbar and lumbosacral spinal fusion: Preliminary results in 40 patients. Can J Surg 2001; 44:262–266.

28. Steed, D, Donohoe, D, Webster, M: Effect of extensive debridement and treatment of healing of diabetic foot ulcers. J Am Coll Surg 1996; 183:61–64.

29. Attinger, C, Bulan, E, Blume, P: Surgical debridement: The key to successful wound healing and reconstruction. Clin Podiatr Med Surg 2000; 17:599.

30. Daniels, T, Tamir, E: Surgical treatment of diabetic foot complications: Clinical review. Geriatr Aging 2006; 9:499–504.

31. Yeager, RA, Moneta, GL, Edwards, JM, et al: Predictors of outcome of forefoot surgery for ulcerations and gangrene. Am J Surgery 1998; 175:388–390.

32. Nehler, MR, Whutehill, TA, Browers, SP, et al: Intermediate-term outcome of primary digit amputations in patients with diabetes mellitus who have forefoot sepsis requiring hospitalization and presumed adequate circulatory status. J Vasc Surg 1999; 30:509–517.

33. Roukis, TS, Zgonis, T: Modifications of the great toe fibular flap for diabetic forefoot and toe reconstruction. Ostomy Wound Manage 2005; 51:30–42.

34. Rosenblum, BI, Pomposelli, FB, Jr, Giurini, JM, et al: Maximizing foot salvage by a combined approach to foot ischemia and neuropathic ulceration in patients with diabetes: A 5 year experience. Diabetes Care 1994; 17:983–987.

35. Murdoch, DP, Armstrong, DG, Ducas, JB, et al: The natural history of great toe amputations. J Foot Ankle Surg 1997; 36:204–208.

36. Griffiths, GD, Weiman, TJ: Metatarsal head resection for diabetic foot ulcers. Arch Surg 1990; 125:832–835.

37. Hamilton, GA, Ford, LA, Perez, H, et al: Salvage of the neuropathic foot by using bone resection and tendon balancing: A retrospective review of 10 patients. J Foot Ankle Surg 2005; 44:37–43.

38. Stone, PA, Back, MR, Armstrong, PA, et al: Midfoot amputations expand limb salvage rates for diabetic foot infections. Ann Vasc Surg 2005; 19:805–811.

39. Lin, SS, Lee, TH, Wapner, KL: Plantar forefoot ulceration with equinus deformity of the ankle in diabetic patients: The effect of tendo-Achilles lengthening and total contact casting. Orthopedics 1996; 19:465–475.

40. Claxton, M, Armstrong, D: Addressing tendon balancing concerns in diabetic patients. Podiatry Today 2003; 16:63–70.

41. Boulton, A, Veves, A, Young, M: Etiopathogenesis and management of abnormal foot pressures. In: Levin, ME, O'Neal, LW, Bowker, JH (eds): The Diabetic Foot. St. Louis, Mosby, 1993, pp 199–233.

42. Van Gils, C, Roeder, B: The effect of ankle equinus upon the diabetic foot. Clin Podiatr Med Surg 2002; 19:391–409.

43. Grant, WP, Sullivan, R, Sonenshine, DE: Electron microscopic investigation of the effects of diabetes mellitus on the Achilles tendon. J Foot Ankle Surg 1997; 36:272–278.

44. Van Gils, C, Roeder, B: The effect of ankle equinus upon the diabetic foot. Clin Podiatr Med Surg 2002; 19:391–409.

45. Schwentker, E: Toe Walking—Orthopedic Surgery E-Medicine Clinical Reference 2007. Available at: http://emedicine.medscape.com/article/. Accessed: February 3rd, 2009.

46. Hoke, M: An operation for the correction of extremely relaxed flat feet. J Bone Joint Surg 1931; 13:773–783.

47. Hatt, R, Lamphier, T: Triple hemisection: A simplified procedure for lengthening the Achilles tendon. N Engl J Med 1947; 236:166–169.

48. Sanders, L: Transmetatarsal and midfoot amputations. Clin Podiatr Med Surg 1997; 14:741–761.

49. Stuck, RM, Sage, R, Pinzur, M, et al: Amputations in the diabetic foot. Clin Podiatr Med Surg 1995; 12:141–155.

50. Catanzariti, A, Mendicino, R, Haverstock, B: Considerations for protection of the residual foot following transmetatarsal amputation. Wounds 1999; 11:13–20.

51. Lieberman, J, Jacobs, R, Goldstock, L: Chopart amputation with percutaneous heel cord lengthening. Clin Orthop 1993; 296:86–91.

52. Kim, P, Steinberg, J: Diabetes watch: Tendo-Achilles lengthening: Friend or foe in the diabetic foot? Podiatry Today 2007; 20:20–26.

53. Snyder, RJ: Treatment of non-healing ulcers with allografts. Clin Dermatol 2005; 23:388–395.

54. Snyder, RJ, Simonson, DA: Cadaveric allograft as adjunct therapy for non-healing ulcers. J Foot Ankle Surg 1999; 38:93–101.

55. Eaglstein, WH, Iriondo, M, Laszio, K: A composite skin substitute (Graftskin) for surgical wounds: A clinical experience. Dermatol Surg 1995; 21:839–843.

56. Eaglstein, WH, Alvarez, OM, Auletta, M, et al: Acute excisional wounds treated with tissue-engineered skin (Apligraf). Dermatol Surg 1999; 25:195–201.

57. Schmid, P: Immunohistologic characterization of Graftskin (Apligraf). Wounds 2000; 12(suppl A):4A–11A.

58. Veves, A, Akbari, CM, Primavera, J, et al: Endothelial dysfunction and the expression of endothelial nitric oxide synthetase in diabetic neuropathy, vascular disease, and foot ulceration. Diabetes 1998; 47:457–463.

59. Hanft, JR, Surprenant, MA: Healing of chronic foot ulcers in diabetic patients treated with a human fibroblast-derived dermis. J Foot Ankle Surg 2002; 5:291–299.

60. Veves, A, Falanga, V, Armstrong, D, et al: Graftskin, a human skin equivalent, is effective in the management of noninfected neuropathic diabetic foot ulcers. Diabetes Care 2001; 24:290–295.

61. Reiber, GE, Boyko, EF, Smith, DG: Lower extremity foot ulcers and amputations in diabetes. In: Harris, MI, Cowie, CC, Reiber, G, et al (eds): Diabetes in America. Washington DC, US Government Printing Office, 1995, pp 409–428.

62. Tan, JS, Friedman, NM, Hazelton-Miller, C, et al: Can aggressive treatment of diabetic foot infections reduce the need for above-ankle amputation? Clin Infect Dis 1996; 23:286–291.

63. Kravitz, S, McGuire, J, Sharma, S: The treatment of diabetic foot ulcers: Reviewing the literature and a surgical algorithm. Adv Skin Wound Care 2007; 20:227–237.

64. Murali, NS: Limb conservation in severe diabetic foot infection—A new technique. Int J Diabetes Dev Ctries 1994; 14:55–59.

65. Guirini, JM, Rosenbaum, BI: Surgical treatment of the diabetic foot. McGlamery's Comprehensive Textbook of Foot and Ankle Surgery, ed. 3. Baltimore, MD, Williams & Wilkins, 2001, pp 1595–1616.

66. Brodsky, JW, Rouse, AM: Exostectomy for symptomatic bony prominences in diabetic Charcot feet. Clin Orthop 1993; 296:21–26.

67. Smith, DG, Stuck, RM, Ketner, L, et al: Partial calcanectomy or the treatment of large ulcerations of the heel. J Bone Joint Surg 1992; 74:571–576.

68. Crandall, RC, FW, Wagner, FW: Partial and total calcanectomy: A review of thirty-one consecutive cases over a ten year period. J Bone Joint Surg 1981; 63:152–155.

69. Rosenblum, BI, Guirini, J, Miller, LB, et al: Surgical treatment of the ulcerated foot. In: Veves, A, Giurini, J, LoGerfo, F (eds): The Diabetic Foot, ed. 2. Totowa, NJ, Humana Press, Inc., 2006, pp 335–362.

70. Garapati, Rajeev, Weinfeld, S: Complex reconstruction of the diabetic foot and ankle. Am J Surg 2004; 187:81s–86s.

71. Sanders, LJ, Frykberg, RG: Diabetic neuropathic arthropathy of feet: The Charcot foot. In: Frykberg, RG (ed): The High Risk Foot in Diabetes Mellitus. New York, Churchill-Livingstone, 1990, pp 297–338.

The authors wish to thank Drs. Manuel Rodriquez, Pedro Abrantes, Maxime Savard, Kennedy Legel, Bryan Calvo, and Tanisha Smith for contributing to the development of this manuscript.

chapter 25

Neonatal and Pediatric Issues in Wound Care

Mona Mylene Baharestani, PhD, APN, CWOCN, CWS, FACCWS

Introduction

To health-care professionals, the mere mention of the word "wound" almost reflexively elicits images of chronic, traumatic, or surgical wounds occurring in profiled subsets of adult and geriatric individuals. As though nonexistent, or of lesser significance, wound care in neonatal and pediatric populations is rarely discussed in textbooks and curricula.

Integumentary vulnerability is not typically associated with youth, but rather the converse.[1] (Fig. 25.1) In fact, expectations

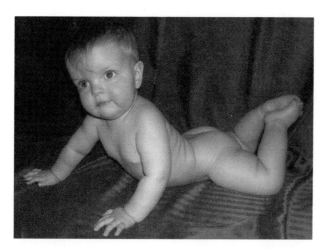

Figure 25•1 *Integumentary vulnerability is not typically associated with youth.*

of innate integumentary resiliency and rapid, uneventful healing based purely on chronology have, in part, perpetuated a lack of wound care knowledge transfer to pediatrics.[1] Despite major technological and surgical advances having increased survival rates among critically and chronically ill neonates and children, wound care practices delivered to this vulnerable population remain antiquated.[2-4] Ethical and litigious issues involved in carrying out research in this vulnerable population further convolute this problem, leaving practitioners without evidence on which to base care.[3] Most papers on wound care in neonates and children are either anecdotal or are discussions of wound healing principles and clinical practice guidelines for adults.[5] Safety and clinical efficacy research-based data for wound care dressings, drugs, and adjunctive treatments in neonates and children are desperately needed.[6-9]

Pediatric Skin and Wound Care Practices

There is a paucity of pediatric wound care research upon which to guide clinical practice, with few interventions having been studied in this population.[5-7] By default, wound and skin care regimes are commonly based on individual or institutional preference and routine rather than science.[8] Illustratively, the Pieper et al study of 13 home care agencies reported that while children represented 3% of all visits and 17% of children had wounds, basic wound care principles were not implemented.[5] In fact, open surgical wounds and pressure ulcers among this pediatric population were often cleansed with hydrogen peroxide, household soap, or povidone-iodine. Forty-four percent were treated with dry gauze and 19% with gauze moistened with normal saline.[5] Despite these practices, over 90% of the home care nurses interviewed described the pediatric wound care as appropriate.[5] Similarly, Munson et al found that among 104 neonatal intensive care units (NICUs), fewer than 25% had wound care protocols.[10] A survey of 13 NICUs in the United Kingdom found wound care practices to be widely varied, with no written policy or guidelines available for staff. In fact, 32% of wounds were either left open to air, to desiccate, or were covered with dry dressings, with the prevailing view that plastic surgery would "cure" the wound at a later time.[11] Despite 8 of the units surveyed having access to wound specialists, only 1 unit reported using this specialty.[11] A U.S. survey of 305 NICUs by Baker et al also reported a lack of skin care practice consensus with less than 30% of those interviewed agreeing on how to treat skin breakdown in micropreemies.[12] Consequentially, wounds were treated with hydrogen peroxide, exposure to air, or "allowed to heal" without intervention.[12]

Wound Healing in Neonates and Children

As with adults, wound healing in critically and chronically ill neonates and children can be compromised by infection, malnutrition, hypotension, edema, and physiological instability preventing safe pressure redistribution. Neonates are at especially high risk for overwhelming life-threatening sepsis secondary to bacterial proliferation and overgrowth within the wound bed as they possess minimal to no antigen exposure.[14,15] Several factors place neonates at significantly increased risk for epidermal stripping, infection, increased transepidermal water loss with resultant heat loss, and toxicity from percutaneous absorption.[11,14,16] These factors include their decreased epidermal-to-dermal cohesion, deficient stratum corneum, impaired thermoregulation, high body surface area-to-weight ratio compared to adults, and immature immune system and hepatic and renal function.

▶ **PEARL 25•1** Wounds in neonates and children follow the same healing trajectory as that in adults, although they typically exhibit faster rates of closure.[13]

Integumentary Development

Intact skin provides physical and thermoregulatory protective barrier functions, preventing fluid and electrolyte losses and invasion by microorganisms.[1]

▶ **PEARL 25•2** Knowledge of integumentary developmental milestones in the premature neonate is critical when selecting skin and wound care cleansers, protective barrier films and ointments, adhesives, dressings, devices, and topical drugs, as barrier function is directly influenced by gestational age.[3]

At 24 weeks gestation, premature neonates have minimal stratum corneum, and the rete ridges are attenuated. Their skin is red, wrinkled, translucent, and gelatinous in appearance. (Fig. 25.2) Subcutaneous tissue has not developed, therefore the dermis is lying directly over muscle.[17] At this early stage of development, skin stripping secondary to adhesive dressing and/or tape removals often results in full-thickness tissue loss.

Subcutaneous fat deposition begins between 26 and 29 weeks gestation, and wrinkling of the skin lessens. The barrier function of the skin remains poor, such that at 26-weeks gestation, as much as 110 ml of water can be lost in 24 hours.[18] Subcutaneous tissue is evident, and the stratum corneum is two to three cell layers thick at 30 weeks, compared to 40 weeks when it reaches 30 layers thick.[17] (Fig. 25.3) Functional integumentary maturity occurs at 33 weeks. Despite achieving full epidermal keratinization and increased dermal/epidermal junctional strength, the skin remains fragile and easily damaged. (Fig. 25.4)

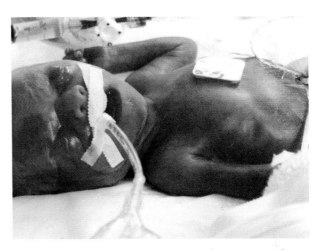

Figure 25•2 *Premature neonate 24 weeks gestation. Photo courtesy of P. Palmer, RN, BSN.*

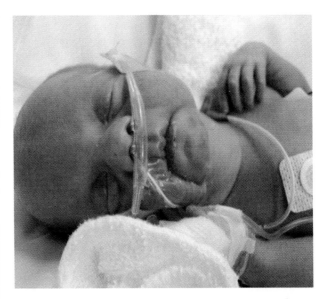

Figure 25•3 *Premature neonate 30 weeks gestation. Photo courtesy of P. Palmer, RN, BSN.*

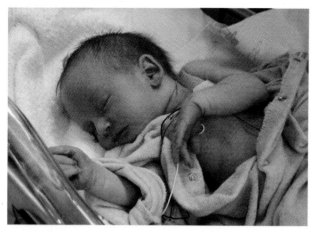

Figure 25•4 *Premature neonate 36 weeks gestation. Photo courtesy of P. Palmer, RN, BSN.*

> ▶ **PEARL 25•3** Once neonates reach full term (36 weeks), the skin becomes structurally similar to that of the adult. The epidermal and dermal layers are up to 60% as thick as adult skin.[18]

Common Wound Types Among Neonates and Children

Based on epidemiological studies and empirical evidence, the most commonly encountered wound types among hospitalized and chronically ill neonates and children are epidermal stripping, extravasation injuries, incontinence-associated perineal dermatitis, chemical and thermal injuries, wounds secondary to congenital abnormalities, and pressure ulcerations.[3]

Epidermal Stripping

Epidermal stripping is most commonly seen in neonates born before 27 weeks of gestation secondary to tape and adhesive dressing removal.[7] Given neonates' attenuated rete ridges, adhesive products characteristically bond more aggressively to the epidermis than the epidermis does with the dermis. In very low birth weight neonates and those who are immunocompromised, epidermal stripping results not only in increased discomfort, but can also lead to increased morbidity.[3]

Preventive Points

1. Use an alcohol-free liquid skin barrier on the skin under adhesive dressings in neonates over 30 days of age.[19]
2. Use clear film dressings to secure intravenous sites.[20]
3. Pad splints and use padded straps over splints rather than tape.[19]
4. Use tubular latex-free stretchy gauze netting instead of tape.
5. Remove adhesives gently using the horizontal stretch method.[21,22]
6. Avoid adhesive removers and bonding agents in the neonatal population as these products can potentiate the risk of epidermal stripping and result in toxic percutaneous absorption.
7. Handle neonates and those with edematous skin with extreme care.[20]
8. Mepiform® or Mepitac® (Molnlycke Health Care Inc., Norcross, GA) soft silicone dressing may be used as a tape in those with blistering disorders (eg, epidermolysis bullosa).[20]

Treatment Options

1. Use soft silicone dressings to treat denuded areas.
2. Secure dressing with tubular latex-free stretchy gauze netting.

Extravasation Injuries

Extravasation injuries occur as a result of inadvertent vesicant fluid leakage from a vein or cannula into surrounding soft tissue.[21-24] (Fig. 25.5) Extravasation injuries occur at an estimated rate of 0.1% to 15% and are most commonly seen in neonates of 26 weeks gestation or less.[24-26] Infiltration/extravasation staging is described in Table 25.1.[27]

Preventive Points

1. Sterile transparent dressings should be used to secure intravenous lines to allow for at least hourly site inspections.[21]
2. Periwound skin protection from maceration can be provided by using an alcohol-free liquid skin barrier in neonates older than 30 days of age.

Treatment Options

1. Treatment of wounds secondary to extravasation include the following:
   • Application of a hydrogel-filled glove or boot to the affected site. Potential problems in using the hydrogel-filled glove or boot include periwound maceration, infant's inability to move the affected

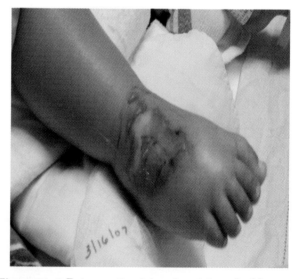

Figure 25•5 *Extravasation injury in a 3.5-week-old newborn.*

Stage	Characteristic
Table 25•1 Staging of IV Infiltrates/ Extravasation	
0	Absence of redness, warmth, pain, swelling, blanching, mottling, tenderness, or drainage Flushes with ease
1	Absence of redness, swelling Flushes with difficulty Pain at site
2	Slight swelling at site Presence of redness Pain at site Good pulse at site 1- to 2-second capillary refill below site
3	Moderate swelling above or below site Blanching Pain at site Good pulse below infiltration site 1- to 2-second capillary refill below infiltration site Skin cool to touch
4	Severe swelling above or below site Blanching Pain at site Decreased or absent pulse Capillary refill greater than 4 seconds Skin cool to touch Skin breakdown or necrosis

Intravenous Nursing Society. From Flemmer, L, Chan, J. A pediatric protocol for management of extravasation injuries. Pediatr Nurs 1993; 19:355–358, 424.

extremity secondary to the gel weight, and trauma upon removal of securing tapes/film dressing.[22]
- Use of a hydrofiber covered by a thin hydrocolloid.[22,28]
- Application of hydrogels covered with silicone dressings.

2. In the presence of necrotic tissue, surgical consultation should be obtained, coupled with use of autolytic débridement.

Surgical Wounds

In a 2005 prevalence audit (*N* = 252) by Noonan and colleagues, 43% of hospitalized children were found to have an open surgical wound and/or closed incision.[29] Seventy-one percent of patients required daily nursing observations, 22% received twice-daily dressings, 5% received complex dressing care, and 2% received negative-pressure wound therapy.[29]

Prevention Points

1. Monitor for signs and symptoms of infection.
2. Protect periwound skin of children and neonates over 30 days of age with a liquid barrier film.[19]

Treatment Options

1. While antimicrobial dressings containing cadexomer iodine and sustained-released silver have been successfully used in adult populations in the management of malodor and reduction of bacterial load, similar neonatal and pediatric data are lacking.[1] However, a case series of burn wounds and a dehisced surgical wound were safely and successfully treated with silver dressings.[14,30] Simon et al similarly reported positive clinical outcomes over a 3-year period in which Manuka Medihoney™ (Derma Sciences, Princeton, NJ) was used on dehisced surgical wounds and infected port-explantation sites in pediatric patients receiving chemotherapy.[31]
2. In full-thickness wounds with large amounts of wound drainage, ostomy pouches and wound drainage collectors, or negative-pressure wound therapy, may be appropriate.
3. Hydrogels, hydrofibers, foams, and soft silicone dressing use in the management of noninfected open surgical wounds have been reported anecdotally in neonatal and pediatric populations.

Incontinence-Associated Dermatitis (Diaper Dermatitis)

The prevalence of diaper dermatitis among neonates and children has been reported to be between 16% and 42%.[26,29] In fact, diaper dermatitis is one of the most common dermatological conditions encountered among neonates and children who are diapered.[29] Diaper dermatitis can be staged according to the integrity of the epidermis and presence or absence of *Candida albicans* skin infection.[29] (Box 25.1; Fig. 25.6)

Prevention Points

1. Change diapers at least every 3 to 4 hours, or sooner if needed.[32]
2. Use diapers containing absorptive gels.[32]
3. Cavilon™ No Sting Barrier (3M, St. Paul, MN) is approved for infants over 30 days of age.[19]

Treatment Options

1. Follow recommendations regarding diapering as described under Prevention Points.
2. Avoid use of commercial diaper wipes in neonates.[32]
3. Use clear petrolatum-based ointments or zinc oxide-based barriers.[32]

> **Box 25•1 Types of Diaper Dermatitis[29]**
>
> - *Type 1.* Epidermis intact and no candidal infection present
> - *Type 2.* Epidermis intact and candidal infection present
> - *Type 3.* Epidermis not intact and no candidal infection present
> - *Type 4.* Epidermis not intact and candidal infection present

From Noonan, C, Quigley, S, Curley, MAQ: Skin integrity in hospitalized infants and children—A prevalence survey. J Ped Nursing 2006; 21:445–453.

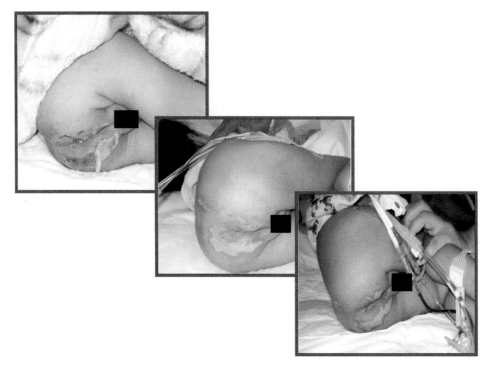

Figure 25•6 *Incontinence associated perineal dermatitis type 4.*

4. If *Candida albicans* is present, treat with an antifungal ointment. Avoid the use of powders in the nursery.[32]
5. Avoid products containing dyes and fragrances.[32]

Chemical Burns

Chemical injuries may occur secondary to the application of adhesive removers, bonding agents, Betadine® (Purdue Pharma L.P., Cranbury, NJ), and alcohol-based preparation solutions.[21]

Prevention Points

1. If Betadine or alcohol-based preparation agents are used prior to procedures or insertion of lines and drains, limit the amount used and rinse immediately with sterile water.[21]
2. Always check under the patient to ensure that they are not lying on linens soaked in solution.
3. Avoidance of these agents and use of aqueous-based skin preparations is best.[21]
4. In preterm neonates there is the additional concern of percutaneous toxicity from alcohol- and Betadine-based solutions.[33]

Treatment Options

1. If there is no wound drainage, or minimal drainage, apply a hydrogel and cover with a silicone dressing.
2. In the presence of moderate to heavy drainage, apply a hydrofiber covered with a silicone dressing, or consider use of a transferent dressing, such as Mepilex® Transfer (Molnlycke® Health Care Inc., Norcross, GA).
3. In the presence of necrotic tissue, surgical consultation should be obtained, coupled with use of autolytic débridement.

Thermal Injuries

Thermal injuries among neonates may occur secondary to heat from monitoring electrodes or less commonly from use of a cold light for the identification of veins and arteries for line insertions.[21] Among children in the community, the most common cause of thermal injuries is fire.

Preventive Points

1. To prevent neonatal burns from heat, reduce monitoring device temperatures and limit the application time as is feasible.[21]
2. To prevent neonatal burns from cold light, minimize exposure time and use a protective guard.[21]

Treatment Options

1. Use of Biobrane® (Smith & Nephew, Largo, FL), a biosynthetic dressing consisting of a layer of peptides derived from porcine dermal collagen incorporated into silicone and nylon, has demonstrated clinical efficacy over conservative treatment in terms of pain control, wound healing, and hospital length of stay in children with partial-thickness burns.[34] Further randomized controlled trials are required to examine the incidence of hypertrophic scarring and to compare clinical outcomes to other skin substitutes.[34]
2. In a prospective, randomized study of 63 children with partial-thickness scald burns in which the efficacy of Mepitel® (Molnlycke Health Care, Norcross, GA), a silicone dressing, was compared to silver sulfadiazine, statistically significant differences were noted.[35] The wounds of children treated with Mepitel not only healed faster, but also exhibited less eschar formation

and less pain, required less analgesics, and had lower hospital and dressing charges.[35]

3. Select an age-appropriate wound-cleansing agent and topical dressing to address wound needs. (See section on Wound Care Principles in Pediatrics below.)

Wounds Secondary to Congenital Conditions

Aplasia cutis congenital, which occurs in 0.03% of births, is a defect of the skin manifested by absent areas of the epidermis and subcutaneous tissue.[1] Wounds are partial- or full-thickness, with 80% occurring on the scalp.[22] Life-threatening bleeding and infection have been reported.

Treatment Options

1. Lesions of the skull require imaging to assess the depth of involvement.[1]
2. Small partial-thickness areas (<1 cm^2) usually reepithelialize well with use of atraumatic moisture-retaining dressings and topical antibiotics.[1]
3. Larger or full-thickness wounds require dermatology, plastic surgery, and neurosurgery intervention.[1]

Epidermolysis bullosa (EB) is a heterogeneous, genetic group of mechanobullous disorders characterized by skin and mucosal blistering in response to minor friction or trauma.[1,36] (Fig. 25.7) Inherited EB is grouped into three major types

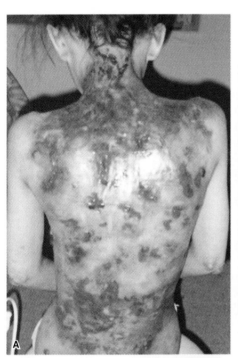
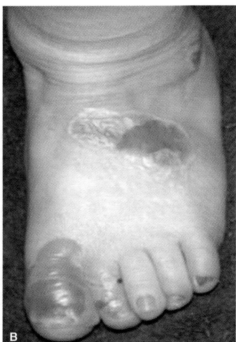
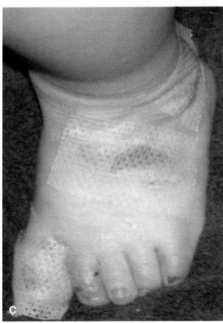

Figure 25•7 *Epidermolysis bullosa (EB). Photos courtesy of Molnlycke Health Care.*

based on the depth of blister formation: simplex, junctional, or dystrophic.[36]

Preventive Points

1. Use gentle handling techniques to minimize friction and shear forces to the skin.[22]
2. Avoid adhesives and tapes.
3. Secure dressings by stretchy nonlatex tubular gauze netting.[1]
4. Use only flat-seamed clothing or clothing that is turned inside out.[22]
5. Avoid tight clothing and nonpadded shoes.[36]
6. Secure cardiac monitoring and pulse oximetry devices with nonadhesives.[22]
7. Decrease humidity and heat as they can result in increased blistering.[22]
8. Exert caution with use of diapers as they can cause blistering.

Treatment Options

1. Dressings can be secured by stretchy nonlatex tubular gauze netting.[1]
2. Each finger and toe should be individually wrapped with nonadherent dressings to prevent fusion of digits.[36]
3. In the presence of minimal drainage, use nonadherent moisture-retentive dressings.[1]
4. Tailor use of absorptive dressings when exudates are high.[1]
5. Soft silicone dressings provide an excellent atraumatic option.
6. Large blisters must be lanced or aspirated with a sterile hypodermic needle without removing the roof.[1]
7. Apligraft® (Organogenesis Inc., Canton, MA) has been shown to induce rapid healing in children with acute and chronic wounds without side effects. Controlled studies with larger sample sizes and longer follow-up is needed before greater widespread use is advocated.[37]
8. After surgical correction of pseudosyndactyly, mitten deformity of the hand, a biological tissue matrix, Integra™ Bilayer Matrix Dressing (Integra LifeSciences Corp., Plainsboro, NJ), may be used to cover the wound followed by Apligraft for epidermal coverage.[38] Further controlled studies are needed.

Pressure Ulcerations

Although commonly believed to be a problem only among immobilized geriatric populations, pressure ulcer rates are as high as 27% in pediatric intensive care units, 23% in neonatal intensive care units, and 20% to 43%, reportedly, among outpatients with spina bifida.[39-42] (Fig. 25.8) Lack of pressure redistribution and friction/shear-related forces result in microvascular soft tissue damage and result in partial- to full-thickness pressure ulcers among neonates and children, similar to adults. However, in children, unlike adults, greater than 50% of pressure ulcers are related to sustained pressure from equipment and devices.[42]

Stage I to IV, unstageable, and suspected deep tissue injuries should be documented in accordance with the National Pressure Ulcer Advisory Panel's (NPUAP's) updated definitions (Box 25.2).[43]

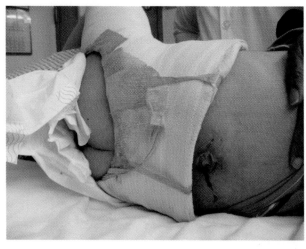

Figure 25•8 *Pressure ulcer in an 8 year old secondary to a plaster cast.*

Prevention Points

1. Perform risk assessments at least daily, using an age-appropriate, valid, and reliable pressure ulcer risk assessment scale.[2] (Table 25.2)
2. Provide preventive skin care.
3. Perform frequent skin assessments under blood pressure cuffs, pulse oximetry devices, tracheostomy plates, oral and nasal gastric tubes, nasal prongs and mask, continuous positive airway pressure (CPAP) masks, arm boards, traction boots, and plaster cast edges.[44]
4. Provide protective padding under devices as feasible (eg, thicker silicone dressings or foam dressings).[1,45]
5. Address pressure redistribution by using only support surfaces on cribs, isolettes, incubators, and beds that are age and weight appropriate. Turn and reposition patients at least every 2 hours as is medically feasible. Unique to the neonatal and infant population, being held by health-care professionals and parents also serves to off-load pressure.
6. Loosen tapes, hats, and clothing in the presence of edema.[20]
7. Minimize friction and shear forces.
8. Maximize nutritional status as is consistent with overall goals of care.
9. Maintain a quality monitoring program.

Treatment Options

1. Perform wound cleansing as needed (refer to section on Wound Care Principles in Pediatrics below).
2. Address pressure redistribution as described above under Prevention Interventions.
3. Débride necrotic tissue as is consistent with overall treatment goals.
4. Manage bacterial colonization and infection.
5. Maximize nutritional status as is consistent with overall goals of care.
6. Select appropriate local care (refer to section on Wound Care Principles in Pediatrics below).

▶ Box 25•2 Pressure Ulcer Staging System

- *Suspected deep tissue injury.* Purple or maroon localized area of discolored skin due to damage of underlying soft tissue as a result of ischemia from pressure and/or shear. This area initially presents as intact skin or a blood-filled blister and may rapidly evolve to expose additional layers of tissue, even with optimal treatment. Variations in skin pigmentation may change visual presentation, and thus early deep tissue injury may be difficult to discern. Other characteristics of the area may include pain, firmness, softness, or a difference in temperature as compared to adjacent tissue.
- *Stage I.* Persistent redness of a localized area of intact skin, usually over a bony prominence. Other characteristics of the area may include delayed capillary refill, pain, firmness, softness, or a difference in temperature as compared to adjacent tissue. It is usually a minor and resolvable condition. Variations in skin pigmentation may change visual presentation.

- *Stage II.* Partial-thickness loss of epidermis or dermis presenting as a shallow open ulcer without slough. It may present as an intact or open/ruptured serum-filled blister.
- *Stage III.* Full-thickness tissue loss. Subcutaneous fat may be visible, but bone, tendon, or muscle are not exposed. Slough may be present, but it does not obscure the depth of tissue loss. Other characteristics may include undermining and tunneling. Rolled edge of dermis may be seen.
- *Stage IV.* Full-thickness tissue loss with exposed bone, tendon, or muscle. Slough or eschar may be present on some parts of the wound bed. Other characteristics often include undermining and tunneling.
- *Unstageable.* Full-thickness tissue loss in which actual depth of the ulcer is completely obscured by slough (yellow, tan, gray, green, or brown) and/or eschar (tan, brown, or black) in the wound bed. Blood blisters are not débrided and therefore placed in the deep tissue injury group.

From Black, J, Baharestani, MM, Cuddigan, J, et al: National Pressure Ulcer Advisory Panel: Updated staging system. Adv Skin Wound Care 2007; 20:269–274.

Wound Care Principles in Pediatrics

Knowledge of product safety and manufacturer's recommended use data in the neonatal and pediatric populations is essential.[2]

▶ **PEARL 25•4** Selection of wound care dressings, drugs, or adjunctive therapies for use in neonatal and pediatric populations requires consideration of the goals of therapy, the practice environment, resource availability, patient age, integumentary maturity, skin condition, product concentration and adherence, potential for skin sensitization, impact of product absorption, and need for avoidance of products containing dyes, fragrances, and preservatives.[2,8,46]

Patient Assessment

A thorough assessment should include, but is not limited to the following factors[1]:

- Current medical issues
- Clinical stability
- Age (including gestational and conceptional)
- Medical history
- Surgical history
- Allergies and skin sensitivities
- Medication history
- Review of laboratory and diagnostic tests
- Height and weight
- Social history

- Family support systems
- Pain status (using a valid and reliable tool such as CRIES, CHIPPS, NIPS)[47]
- Nutritional history
- History of previous wounds, treatment, and healing outcomes
- Pressure ulcer risk assessment score (using a valid and reliable tool such as Braden Q, Braden, Glamorgan)[2]
- Targeted physical examination

Dressing Selection Criteria

Ideally the dressing should do the following[21]:

- Protect the wound, while being atraumatic
- Be easy to apply
- Not require frequent changes
- Stay in place in a humidified environment
- Be cut to the correct size, or have the capability to be cut

Commonly Used Wound Care Products

Soft silicone
- Given their atraumatic nature, soft silicone dressings are becoming more commonly used in neonatal and pediatric preventive skin care and wound management.
- Silicone dressings are available as contact layers, exudate transferents, absorbents, antimicrobials, fixation tapes, and gel sheets for scar management.
- Avoid use of soft silicone in those with known silicone allergy.

Table 25-2 Neonatal and Pediatric Pressure Ulcer Risk Assessment Tools

Tool	Based on	N	Setting	Age	Sensitivity	Specificity
Barnes	Literature review	None	Pediatric acute care	Not specified	Not performed	Not performed
Bedi	Adult Waterlow	None	PICU Progressive care unit	Neonate to age 12	Not performed	None
Cockett	Literature review	None	PICU	Not specified	Not performed	None
Garvin	Not specified	None	PICU	Not specified	Not performed	None
NSRAS	Adult Braden	32	NICU	26 to 40 weeks gestation	83%	81%
Pattold Pressure Scoring System	Literature review Key components for maintaining skin	None	PICU	Not specified	None	None
Derbyshire	Medley and Adult Waterlow	None	Not stated	Not specified	No	None
Braden Q	Adult Braden Expert panel	322	PICU	21 days to age 8 yr	88% (Modified version 92%)	58% (Modified version 59%)
Pediatric Waterlow	Pediatric pressure ulcer risk factor identification and incidence study (Waterlow)	302	Pediatric acute care	Neonate to age 16 yr	None	None
Glamorgan	Literature review Expert panel Pediatric pressure ulcer risk factors study (Willock)	336	Pediatric acute care	Birth to age 18 yr	98.4%	67.5%

NICU = Neonatal Intensive Care Unit; PICU = Pediatric Intensive Care Unit; NSRAS = Neonatal Skin Risk Assessment Scale.
Reproduced with permission from Baharestani; M.M. Pressure ulcers in special populations: neonates and pediatrics. In S. Baranoski; E. Ayello (eds), Wound Care Essentials: Practice Principles, ed. 2. Philadelphia, Lippincott Williams & Wilkins, 2007.

Liquid barrier films. Liquid barrier films that do not contain alcohol are applied to the skin to prevent epidermal stripping secondary to adhesive removal and to protect against chemical erosion from wound fluid.[1] Cavilon No Sting Barrier film is approved for neonates over 30 days of age to prevent skin stripping due to adhesive removal.[19]

Hydrocolloids

- Multiple references to the successful use of hydrocolloids in maintaining wound bed moisture by providing autolytic débridement, as a waterproof and bacterial barrier, and as a barrier to other adhesives have been reported in neonatal and pediatric literature.[32,48-53]
- Thin hydrocolloids possess multiple inherent benefits in the treatment of neonatal and pediatric wounds, including the following[54]:
  1. Reduction of epidermal water loss
  2. Allowance of full limb range of motion
  3. Easy application to small body surfaces
  4. Sterile dressing delivery
  5. Suitability for use in incubators and humidified environments
  6. Barrier to viral and bacterial transmission
- Given the adherence of hydrocolloids, caution must be used to prevent epidermal stripping, especially among neonates. Use of silicone dressings in this population provides a less traumatic alternative.

Hydrogels

- Hydrogels come in two basic forms, amorphous gels and semisolid sheets. The primary components of hydrogels are cross-linked polymers and water.
- Neonatal and pediatric case studies describing use of hydrogels have been described in the management of toxic epidermal necrolysis, wound dehiscence, extravasation injuries, pressure ulcers, fungating lesions, and burns.[28,30,54-56]

Foams. Foam dressings are polymeric materials with hydrophilic contact layers and hydrophobic outer layers. These dressings vary in thickness and may be impregnated with surfactants, glycerin, charcoal, or silver. Successful use of these products has been reported anecdotally in pediatric case studies.[1]

Composites. Composite dressings are multilayered superabsorbent dressings designed for the management of moderately to heavily draining wounds. Successful use of composite dressings was reported anecdotally in the management of an extravasation injury in a 27-week gestational age neonate.[57]

Semipermeable films. Semipermeable films are versatile, transparent, thin, polyurethane moisture-vapor-permeable dressings designed to maintain a moist environment. These dressings facilitate epithelialization of minimally exuding partial-thickness wounds and provide autolysis of noninfected wounds. Film dressings can also be used to secure primary dressings, while promoting a moist environment.

Hydrofibers. Comprised of carboxymethylcellulose, hydrofibers are highly absorbent dressings that transform into solid sheet gels once in contact with fluid.

Their success has been reported anecdotally in pediatric case studies.[7]

Alginates. Alginates are seaweed-based dressings designed for the management of moderately draining wounds. In adults, light bleeding can usually be controlled by using these dressings, although this has not been studied in pediatrics.[1] Calcium alginates are not recommended for use in neonates secondary to calcium absorption concerns.[22]

Negative-pressure wound therapy (NPWT). Application of sterile hydrophobic (V.A.C.® GranuFoam® or GranuFoam Silver®, KCI Inc., San Antonio, TX) or hydrophilic (V.A.C. WhiteFoam Dressing, KCI Inc.) cut to the appropriate wound geometry, covered with a transparent film drape, and fitted with a T.R.A.C.® Pad (KCI Inc.) attached to a computerized, calibrated microprocessor unit delivers controlled negative-pressure wound therapy. Patient age, exposed structures within the wound, bacterial load, and treatment goals influence selection of dressing type, pressure setting, dressing change frequency, and use of interposing layer(s). Clinical series of neonates and children with acute and chronic wounds successfully treated with V.A.C. NPWT have been reported.[58-60] Baharestani's series of 24 neonates and children treated with V.A.C. NPWT recommends the need for close monitoring for fluid loss and dehydration, age-specific pressure settings and individualized dressing change frequencies.[59] Recommended age and wound specific pressure settings are recommended by Baharestani and others.[59,60] (Table 25.3)

Topical Enzymes

While the safety and efficacy of topical enzymes in the pediatric population has not been studied, there are anecdotal reports of successful use in the management of pediatric burns and extravasation injuries.[61,62] The manufacturer's recommended use of these drugs is only for those over the age of 18 years.[1]

Hyperbaric Oxygen Therapy

Hyperbaric oxygen therapy (HBOT) can be used for pediatric patients from birth through adolescence.[63] The pediatric incidence of HBOT-related side effects and complications is approximately 1.7%, the same as for adults.[63] The three most common problems encountered are middle ear barotraumas (6%); central nervous system oxygen toxicity (0.7%) in unconscious, ventilator-dependent critically ill patients; and pneumothorax and potential air embolism in those with undiagnosed, congenital lung malformation.[63] A chest x-ray is recommended for infants and children prior to HBOT as clinical presentation of a congenital lung malformation may be delayed.[63]

Preterm infants and neonates must be monitored for the following[64]:

- High risk for bronchopulmonary dysplasia among those receiving mechanical ventilation in the treatment of respiratory distress syndrome.
- Need for retinal exam to assess the degree of vascular maturity in assessing risk for retrolental fibroplasia.

Table 25•3 Recommended V.A.C. Negative-Pressure Wound Therapy Settings for Pediatric Patients

Pediatric Subgroup	Approximate Age Range	Recommended Negative-Pressure Setting
Newborn (neonate)	Birth to 1 month of age	−50 to −75 mm Hg
Infant	Greater than 1 month but 2 years or less	−50 to −75 mm Hg
Child	Greater than 2 years but 12 years or younger	−75 to −100 mm Hg (Sternal −50 to −75 mm Hg)
Adolescent	Greater than 12 years but 21 years or younger	−75 to −125 mm Hg (Sternal −50 to −75 mm Hg)

From: Baharestani, MM. Use of negative pressure wound therapy in the treatment of neonatal and pediatric wounds: A retrospective examination of clinical outcomes. Ostomy Wound Manage. 2007; 53:75–84; Baharestani, MM, Amjad, I, Bookout, K., et al. V.A.C therapy in the management of paediatric wounds: clinical review and experience. International Wound Journal 2009;6:1–26.

- A sudden and catastrophic decrease in cardiac output in those with ductal-dependent congenital heart disorders (although rare). Physical exam, chest x-ray, and, if indicated, echocardiography should be performed prior to HBOT if cardiac anomalies are suspected.[63]
- Increased risk of gastric barotraumas, regurgitation, and aspiration in crying children.[63] Infants can suck on pacifiers or bottles during compression to equalize the ears, and stimulation of burping must be performed prior to decompression.[63] If gastric gas is not expelled, regurgitation may occur.[63] Nasogastric tube insertion can also be performed to vent gastric distention.[63]

Successful outcomes have been reported in the treatment of pediatric degloving injuries,[65] osteomyelitis, reoperative flap repair of hypospadias,[66] and necrotizing fascitis in neonates.[67] Use of HBOT in the treatment of pediatric sickle-cell ulcers has been met with variable success.

Dressing Changes

Dressing changes can illicit significant fear among pediatric patients. Stress-reducing techniques which can be employed include:

- Have two people present for neonates and small children (one to provide comfort and one to change the dressing).[21]
- Involve family members as appropriate, assisting with dressing changes, observing, or cuddling and holding their child.[21]
- Involve the child life specialist so that he or she may suggest patient distraction techniques.
- Decrease patient and family stress by decreasing noise, bright lights, and too much handling.[21]
- Keep dressing change frequency to a minimum consistent with the needs of the wound, the need for monitoring, and the manufacturer's recommendations. This will further decrease patient distress, pain, and anxiety.
- Prepare dressings prior to uncovering the wound in order to limit wound exposure time, given the thermoregulatory stress and pain receptor exposure implications.[21]

Irrigation

- Use only warm fluids, as cold irrigants will increase patient stress and decrease wound bed temperature, thus ceasing polymorphic and macrophagic activity until restoration of normotherapy occurs.[19]
- Maintain aseptic technique.[21]
- Use sterile water and normal saline cleansing agents for pediatric wounds,[68] with sterile water being preferred for neonates.[32] For neonates, these cleansers should be warmed to body temperature and normal saline diluted 1:1 with sterile water.[32,50]
- Use a 20-ml syringe with a blunt needle or a polytetrafluoroethylene (Teflon®) catheter to gently flush away wound exudates.[32]
- Avoid antiseptics, given their potential for tissue damage and absorption.[32,50]

Pain Assessment and Management

- Integral to every wound assessment should be a comprehensive assessment of pain.[68]
- Assess behavioral characteristics (crying, facial expressions, motor response, restlessness, or undue quietness).[69-70]
- Use a valid and reliable pain assessment scale (eg, CRIES, CHIPPS, NIPS) in conjunction with patient assessment.[21,47,69]
- Follow institutional pain management guidelines.[21]
- Use of soft silicone-based dressings, hydrocolloid pastes, hydrocellular foams, and hydrogels coupled with analgesics, distraction, and guided imagery may be beneficial in pain management.[1]
- Autolytic débridement, where clinically appropriate, can be facilitated through the use of hydrogels, hydrocolloids, foams, and preactivated polyacrylate with Ringer's solution dressings.[6]
- Use of securement devices such as tubular stretchy latex-free gauze netting can securely maintain dressing

placement while allowing for atraumatic nonadhesive dressing removals.[6]

Dressing Securement

- Avoid using tape on premature infants' skin as feasible.
- When needed, secure dressing with latex-free stretchy tubular gauze netting materials.
- When a wound is over a joint, ensure proper positioning to prevent contracture development during wound healing.[70]

Support Surfaces

Children are typically placed on support surfaces designed for adults; however, the clinical efficacy and safety of this practice raises serious concerns.[71] Programmable low-air-loss beds designed for adults do not possess settings to accommodate heights or weights of infants and small children.[72] Small children and infants often sink into and between cushions.[72] When adult specialty beds are placed in the turn mode, the occiput of small children may pivot on the same pressure point, potentially increasing shear and friction and not redistributing pressure.[73] If a low-air-loss bed or alternating overlay is clinically indicated for an infant or child, only those that are age appropriate, clinically efficacious, and safe should be used in accordance with manufacturers' recommendations.[2] Products currently available in these categories are the Nimbus® Pediatric System (Huntleigh Healthcare LLC, Eatontown, NJ), an alternating overlay for patients weighing between 13 and 55 lbs, and the PediDyne® (KCI Inc.), a low-air-loss bed for children ages 6 months through 5 years and weights of 15 to 60 lb.

According to the findings of Solis et al,[74] pressure redistribution devices effective for children are significantly different from those used for adults. In their study of 13 healthy children aged 10 weeks to 13.5 years, the highest interface pressure readings were noted under the occiput (average 59 mm Hg).[74] In older, larger children ages 10 to 14, the highest pressures were in the sacral area.[74] Two-inch to 4-inch convoluted foam was effective in decreasing these interface pressures.[74] Similarly, a McLane et al study of 54 children ranging from infancy to age 16 found the highest interface readings were at the occiput from infancy to age 6 and at the occiput, coccyx, and heels in ages 6 to 18.[72] For children less than 2 years of age, using the Delta® foam overlay (Span America, Greenville, NC) resulted in the lowest interface occiput pressures.[72] For children older than 2 years of age, using Delta foam overlay and a Gel-E Donut® pillow (Children's Medical Venture, Norwell, MA) significantly lowered occipital pressure and provided pressure redistribution similar to that of a low-air-loss bed (Hill-Rom Inc., Batesville, Indiana).[72]

Coupled with the selection of appropriate support surfaces and positioning devices is manual off-loading whenever medically feasible. In an examination of the occurrence of pressure ulcers over the occiput and ears of 59 children undergoing cardiovascular surgery, Neidig et al reported a 3.4-fold decrease in incidence with repositioning of the head every 2 hours.[75]

Cultural and Religious Considerations

Ensure consistent cultural and religious sensitivity when selecting dressings (eg, some dressings contain animal-derived products), establishing collaborative treatment goals, and when evaluating wound healing outcomes (eg, higher incidence of hypertrophic or keloid formation in those with darkly pigmented skin).[70]

Education

- Recognize each child's uniqueness, the developmental characteristics of each age group, and the psychological and psychosocial factors that they face.[76]
- Involve children in care as is feasible, allowing for choices (eg, what they want to eat, selection of special stickers on their dressings).
- Maintain peer-related activities as feasible.
- Use play therapy as is age and developmental stage appropriate.[76]
- Provide the child returning to school with resources, education, and contact information for teachers and the school nurse.[2]
- Use age-appropriate language for the learner.
- Educate teenagers on a one-on-one basis with respect for their privacy. Educational materials that are concise and focused are best received.[76]
- Assess how much the patient, parent(s), and/or caregiver want to know.
- Involve the family as is feasible and consistent with their wishes and that of their child.
- Assess the patient, parent(s), and/or caregiver level of understanding, expectations, coping skills, and access to sources of support.[76]
- Assess for possible feelings of guilt associated with the cause of the wound and level of anxiety.[21]

Wound Assessment Documentation

Thorough, comprehensive wound assessment documentation includes, but is not limited to the following:

- Etiology
- Phase of healing
- Type (acute or chronic)
- Location/distribution
- Dimensions (length, width, depth) measured in centimeters of the total body surface area (TBS) affected
- Presence of tunneling, undermining, sinus tracts measured in centimeters
- Tissue types (granulation, slough, eschar, epithelialization)
- Status of surrounding skin (intact, erythema, hyperkeratotic, indurated, fluctuant, crepitant, candida overgrowth, denudation secondary to adhesive stripping)
- Exudate (amount, color, consistency, odor)
- Previous treatments and outcomes
- Level of pain

- Presence of infection
- Overall goals of care
- Patient and family goals

Summary

While wound care practices developed for adult and geriatric populations provide a rudimentary foundation for neonatal and pediatric wound care, they do not negate the need for developmentally specific evidence-based guidelines.[1] Given the wide variation in percutaneous toxicity potential and developmental and integumentary maturity spanning from the very low birth weight premature infant through adolescence, clinicians desperately need age-appropriate products, educational tools, and research-based guidelines from which to deliver safe and effective wound care practice.[1]

References

1. Baharestani, MM, Pope, E: Chronic wounds in neonates and children. In: Krasner, D, Rodeheaver, GT, Sibbald, GT (eds): Chronic Wound Care: A Clinical Source Book for Healthcare Professionals, ed. 4. Malvern, PA, HMP Communications, 2007, pp 679–693.
2. Baharestani, MM: Pressure ulcers in special populations: Neonates and pediatrics. In: Baranoski, S, Ayello, E (eds): Wound Care Essentials: Practice Principles, ed. 2. Philadelphia, Lippincott Williams & Wilkins, 2007, pp 427–435.
3. Baharestani, MM: An overview of neonatal and pediatric wound care knowledge and considerations. Ostomy Wound Manage 2007; 53:34–55.
4. Baharestani, MM: Neonatal and pediatric wound care: Filling voids in knowledge and practice. Ostomy Wound Manage 2007; 53:6–7.
5. Pieper, B, Templin, T, Dobal, M, et al: Prevalence and types of wounds among children receiving care in the home. Ostomy Wound Manage 2000; 46:36–42.
6. Siegfried, EC, Shah, PY: Skin care practices in the neonatal nursery: A clinical survey. J Perinatol 1999; 19:31–39.
7. Irving, V: Caring for and protecting the skin of pre-term neonates. J Wound Care 2001; 10:253–256.
8. Malloy-McDonald, MB: Skin care for high risk neonates. J Wound Ostomy Continence Nurs 1995; 22:177–182.
9. Irving, V: Skin problems in the pre-term infant: Avoiding ritualistic practice. Prof Nurse 2001; 17:63–66.
10. Munson, K, Bare, D, Hoath, S, et al: A survey of skin care practices for premature low birth weight infants. Neonatal Netw 1999; 18:1–5.
11. Irving, V: Neonatal iatrogenic skin injuries: A nursing perspective. J Neonatal Nurs 1999; 5:10–14.
12. Baker, SF, Smith, BJ, Donohue, PK, et al: Skin care management practices for premature infants. J Perinatol 1999; 19:426–431.
13. Bale, S, Jones, V: Caring for children with wounds. J Wound Care 1996; 5:177–180.
14. Rustogi, R, Mill, J, Fraser, JF, et al: The use of Acticoat™ in neonatal burns. Burns. 2005; 31:878–882.
15. Keener, KE: The surgical neonate. In: Wise, BV, McKenna, C, Garvin, G, et al (eds): Nursing Care of the General Pediatric Surgical Patient. Aspen Publishers, Gaithersburg, MD, 2000.
16. Lund, CH, Tucker, JA: Adhesion and newborn skin. In: Hoath, SB, Maibach, HI (eds): Neonatal Skin Structure and Function, ed. 2. New York, Marcel Deckker, 2003.
17. Eichenfield, L, Hardaway, C: Neonatology dermatology. Curr Opin Pediatr 1999; 11:471–479.
18. Campbell, JM, Banta-Wright, SA: Neonatal skin disorders: A review of selected dermatologic abnormalities. J Perinat Neonat Nurs 2000; 14:63–83.
19. 3M Cavilon No-Sting Barrier Film [brochure]. St Paul, MN, 3M Health Care, 2000.
20. Report from an independent advisory group. Issues in neonatal wound care minimizing trauma and pain. The Tendra Academy. Norcross, GA, Molnlycke Health Care Inc., June, 2005.
21. Irving, V, Bethell, E, Burton, F: Neonatal wound care: Minimizing trauma and pain. Neonatal Advisory Group. Wounds UK 2006; 2:33–41.
22. Irving, V: Wound care for preterm neonates. Infant 2006; 2:102–106.
23. McCullen, KL, Pieper, B: A retrospective chart review of risk factors for extravasation among neonates receiving peripheral intravascular fluids. J Wound Ostomy Continence Nurs 2006; 33:133–139.
24. Wilkins, C, Emmerson, A: Extravasation injuries on regional neonatal units. Arch Dis Child Fetal Ed 2004; 89:F274–275.
25. Shenaq, SM, Abbase, EH, Friedman, JD: Soft-tissue reconstruction following extravasation of chemotherapeutic agents. Surg Oncol Clin N Am 1996; 5:825–845.
26. McLane, KM, Bookout, K, McCord, S, et al: The 2003 national pediatric pressure ulcer and skin breakdown prevalence survey. J Wound Ostomy Continence Nurs 2004; 31:168–178.
27. Flemmer, L, Chan, J: A pediatric protocol for management of extravasation injuries. Pediatr Nurs 1993; 19:355–358, 424.
28. Thomas, S, Rowe, HN, Keats, J, et al: The management of extravasation injury in neonates. Available at: www.worldwidewounds.com/1997/october/Neonates/NeonatePaper.html Accessed 1/11/2006.
29. Noonan, C, Quigley, S, Curley, MAQ: Skin integrity in hospitalized infants and children—A prevalence survey. J Ped Nursing 2006; 21:445–453.
30. McCord, S, Bookout, K, McLane, K, et al: Use of silver dressing with neonatal abdominal evisceration. Poster presentation at: 36th Annual Conference for Wound, Ostomy, Continence Nurses (WOCN), Tampa, FL, June 2004.
31. Simon, A, Sofka, K, Wiszniewsky, G, et al: Wound care with antibacterial honey (Medihoney) in pediatric haematology. Support Care Cancer 2006; 14:91–97.
32. Association of Women's Health, Obstetric and Neonatal Nurses (AWHONN): Neonatal skin care. Evidence-based clinical practice guideline. Washington DC, AWHONN, 2001.
33. Linder, N, Davidovitch, N, Reichman, B, et al: Topical iodine-containing antiseptics and subclinical hypothyroidism in preterm infants. J Pediatr 1997; 131:434–439.
34. Mandal, A: Pediatric partial-thickness scald burns: Is Biobrane the best treatment available? Int Wound J 2007; 4:15–19.
35. Gotschall, CS, Morrison, MI, Eichelberger, MR: Prospective, randomized study of the efficacy of Mepitel® on children with partial-thickness scalds. J Burn Care Rehabil 1998; 19:279–283.
36. Bello, YM, Falabella, AF, Schachner, LA: Epidermolysis bullosa and its treatment. Wounds 2001; 13:113–118.
37. Valencia, IC, Fallabella, AF, Schahner, LA: New developments in wound care for infants and children. Pediatr Ann 2001; 30:211–218.
38. Rottman, SJ, Glat, PM: The use of a biologic tissue matrix (Integra Bilayer Matrix Wound Dressing) in the treatment of recessive dystrophic epidermolysis bullosa pseudosyndactyly deformity. Wounds 2006; 18:315–321.
39. Curley, MAQ, Razmus, IS, Roberts, KE, et al: Predicting pressure ulcer risk in pediatric patients—the Braden Q scale. Nurs Res 2003; 52:22–31.
40. Baharestani, M, Vertichio, R, Higgins, MB, et al: A neonatal and pediatric evidence-linked pressure ulcer and skin care performance improvement initiative. Poster presentation at: Symposium on Advanced Wound Care and Medical Research Forum on Wound Repair, San Diego, CA, April 21–24, 2005.
41. Okamoto, GN, Lamers, JV, Shurtleff, DB: Skin breakdown in patients with myelomengocele. Arch Phys Med Rehab 1983; 64:20–23.

42. Willock, J, Hughes, J, Tickle, S, et al: Pressure sores in children—The acute hospital perspective. J Tissue Viability 2000; 10:59–62.

43. Black, J, Baharestani, MM, Cuddigan, J, et al: National Pressure Ulcer Advisory Panel: Updated staging system. Adv Skin Wound Care 2007; 20:269–274.

44. Baharestani, MM, Ratliff, C: Pressure ulcers in neonates and children: An NPUAP white paper. National Pressure Ulcer Advisory Panel. Adv Skin Wound Care 2007; 20:208–220.

45. Smith, ZK: Adapting a soft silicone dressing to enhance infant outcomes. Ostomy Wound Manage 2006; 52:30–32.

46. Hoath, SB, Narendran, V: Adhesives and emollients in the preterm infant. Semin Neonatol 2000; 5:289–296.

47. Suraseranivongse, S, Kaosaard R, Intakong P, et al: A comparison of postoperative pain scales in neonates. Br J Anaesth 2006; 97:540–544.

48. Quigley, SM, Curly, MAQ: Skin integrity in the pediatric population: Preventing and managing pressure ulcers. J Spec Pediatr Nurs 1996; 1:7–18.

49. Darmstadt, GL, Dinulos, JG: Neonatal skin care. Ped Clin NA 2000; 47:757–782.

50. Taquino, LT: Promoting wound healing in the neonatal setting: Process versus protocol. J Perinat Neonatal Nurs 2000; 14:104–118.

51. Lund, C: Prevention and management of infant skin breakdown. Nurs Clin NA 1999; 34:907–920.

52. Hagelgans, NA: Pediatric skin care issues for the home care nurse. Pediatr Nurs 1993; 19:499–507.

53. Packard, S, Douma, C: Skin care. In: Cloherty, JP, Eichenwald, EC, Stark, AR (eds): Manual of Neonatal Care. ed. 5. Philadelphia, Lippincott Williams & Wilkins, 2004.

54. Atkins, J, Irving, V, Young, T: Development of a wound care policy for neonates. Poster presentation at: the Wound Care Society Conference in Harrogate, UK, in 1996.

55. Harris, AH, Coker, KL, Smith, CG: Case report of a pressure ulcer in an infant receiving extracorporeal life support: The use of a novel mattress surface for pressure reduction. Adv Neonatal Care 2003; 3:220–229.

56. Moushley, R, Meadows, L: Burn care of children. In: Wise, BV, McKenna, C, Garvin, G, et al (eds): Nursing Care of the General Pediatric Surgical Patient. Gaithersburg, MD, Aspen Publishers, 2000.

57. Fell, J: Versiva dressing in the management of a severe extravasation injury in a premature baby. Poster, dated 2002.

58. Caniano, DA, Ruth, B, Teich, S: Wound management with vacuum-assisted closure: Experience in 51 pediatric patients. J Ped Surg 2005; 40:128–132.

59. Baharestani, MM: Use of negative pressure wound therapy in the treatment of neonatal and pediatric wounds: A retrospective examination of clinical outcomes. Ostomy Wound Manage 2007: 53:75–84.

60. Baharestani MM, Amjad I, Bookout K., et al. V.A.C therapy in the management of paediatric wounds: clinical review and experience. International Wound Journal 2009;6:1–26.

61. Hansbrough, JF, Hansbrough, W: Pediatric burns. Pediatri Rev 1999; 20:117–123.

62. Spooner, J: Use of a papain, urea enzymatic debriding ointment on a pediatric patient with an intravenous infiltrate burn. Poster

63. Norvell, H, Land, C: Age-specific considerations. In: Larson-Lohr ,V, Norvell, HC (eds): Hyperbaric Nursing. Flagstaff, AZ, Best Publishing, 2002, pp 166–180.

64. Thomas, P, Borer, R, Martorano, F: Hyperbaric medicine in pediatric practice. In: Kindwall, E, Whelan, H (eds): Hyperbaric Medicine Practice, ed. 2. Flagstaff, AZ, Best Publishing, 1999.

65. deVincentis, G, Caracciolo, G, Anselmi, A, Andriessen, A: An adhesive hydrocellular dressing in the treatment of paediatric patients with extensive soft tissue trauma Poster presentation at: Symposium on Advanced Wound Care, April 18–22, 1998, Miami, FL.

66. Anderson, C, Myer, E, Perdrizet, G, et al: Complex hypospadias repair: The use of adjunctive hyperbaric oxygen therapy. Presented at: 20th Annual Symposium on Advanced Wound Care, Tampa, FL, April 28–May 1, 2007.

67. Hsieh, WS, Yang, PH, Chao, HC, et al: Neonatal necrotizing fasciitis: A report of three cases and review of the literature. Pediatrics 1999; 103:e53–e60.

68. Samaniego, I: Developing a skin care pathway for pediatrics. Derm Nursing 2002; 14:393–396.

69. Royal College of Nursing. Clinical practice guidelines: The recognition and assessment of acute pain in children. London, Royal College of Nursing, 2002.

70. Report from an independent multidisciplinary advisory group. Issues in paediatric wound care: Minimizing trauma and pain. The Tendra Academy®. Norcross, GA, Molnlycke Health Care Inc., April 2004.

71. Law, J: Transair paediatric mattress replacement system evaluation. Br J Nurs 2002; 11:343–346.

72. McLane, KM, Bookout, K, McCord, S, et al: The 2003 national pediatric pressure ulcer and skin breakdown prevalence survey. J Wound Ostomy Continence Nurs 2004; 31:168–178.

73. McCord, S, McElvain, V, Sachdeva, R, et al: Risk factors associated with pressure ulcers in the pediatric intensive care unit. J Wound Ostomy Continence Nurs 2004; 31:179–183.

74. Solis, I, Krouskop, T, Trainer, N, et al: Supine interface pressure in children. Arch Phys Med Rehabil 1988; 69:524–526.

75. Neidig, JRE, Kleiber, C, Oppliger, RA: Risk factors associated with pressure ulcers in the pediatric patient following open-heart surgery. Prog Cardiovascular Nurs 1989; 4:99–106.

76. Hickey, K, Vogel, LC, Anderson, CJ, et al. Pressure ulcers in pediatric spinal cord injury. Top Spinal Cord Inj Rehabil 2000; 6(suppl):85–90.

chapter 26

Endogenous and Exogenous Electrical Fields for Wound Healing

Luther C. Kloth, MS, PT, CWS, FACCWS, FAPTA
Min Zhao, MD, PhD

Since the mid-1960s, considerable research has been directed at evaluating the effects of exogenous electrical currents on healing of chronic wounds, which, unlike acute wounds, do not heal spontaneously within a predictable time frame and are frequently unresponsive to many standard treatment interventions. Currently, treatments available to patients with chronic wounds are mostly influenced by federal and regional insurance authorities who more and more base reimbursement decisions on treatment effectiveness, which they in turn establish by determining the strength of evidence derived from basic science and clinical research trials.

The objectives of this chapter are to (1) describe the endogenous bioelectric system of the integument and its influence on wound repair; (2) define basic terminology related to the use of exogenous, conductively (capacitively) coupled electrical currents (CCECs) for enhancing chronic wound healing; (3) review basic science research and discuss reputed mechanisms by which CCEC accelerates wound healing; (4) review clinical research evidence that supports the use of CCEC as an efficacious intervention for healing chronic wounds; (5) describe clinical methods of applying CCEC to facilitate wound healing; and (6) identify precautions and contraindications for the use of CCEC for wound healing.

Endogenous Electrical Currents

Several organs of the body that play vital roles in preserving or protecting life generate natural bioelectric currents that may be measured and analyzed to determine if the organ is functioning normally. Examples of these endogenous currents include the transmembrane voltages found in cell membranes and the action potentials and electrical impulses carried along peripheral nerves to synapses in skeletal muscle and along the vagus nerve to facilitate cardiac muscle contraction. Measurable currents are also found in the skin (the largest organ of the body) and wounds, as well as in the cells that facilitate wound repair. This section discusses the biologically inherent currents that are associated with healing.

Naturally Occurring Electric Fields in Wounds—Endogenous Wound Electric Fields

A Brief History of "Animal Electricity"

Animal electricity was among the most important scientific discoveries in the 18th and 19th centuries. In 1794 Luigi Galvani demonstrated that when the cut end of a frog sciatic nerve from one leg touched the muscles of the opposite leg, muscles in that leg contracted.[1,2] In the same year, an anonymously written paper reported that when the excised leg of a frog was brought into contact with an exposed spinal cord, the other leg twitched.[3] We now know that the muscular contraction occurred as a result of the electrical currents of injury from the damaged nerve and skinned leg. Galvani thus provided evidence for "animal electricity." In 1831, Carlo Matteucci was able to confirm Galvani's findings.[4] He showed that an injured muscle released a small electric current and that, in Galvani's demonstration, it was this electric current that induced the muscle contraction in the dissected frog leg without the aid of metallic or atmospheric electricity.[1,2,4] Those experiments had demonstrated the existence of the injury electric currents. It is now known that when part of the cell membrane is damaged, the cell membrane potential becomes negative and electric current flows from the outside into the cell through the damage site. This is due to the steady, long-lasting voltage gradient within the extracellular and intracellular spaces. It is this voltage that drives the flow of electric charges into and around injured wound tissues and severed cutaneous nerves (Fig. 26.1). This discovery predated that of the better-known action potential, which is a rapid, self-regenerating voltage change localized across the cell membrane.

Galvani is credited with having laid the foundations of a new science, electrophysiology, by hypothesizing that animal tissues had intrinsic electricity, which was believed to be involved in fundamental physiological processes such as nerve conduction and muscle contraction. However, during his time and for some years thereafter, animal electricity and its apparent association with the philosophy of "vitalism" was criticized by Alessandro Volta, who demonstrated that inorganic matters (such as metals) without any animal parts could also be used to generate "electricity" and induce muscle contraction.[5] The next conceptual breakthrough in "bioelectricity" occurred in 1868, when Julius Bernstein postulated that the nerve cell membrane was able to selectively pass certain kinds of ions, thereby producing membrane potentials.[6] Thus, the

A. Measurement of endogenous wound electric currents

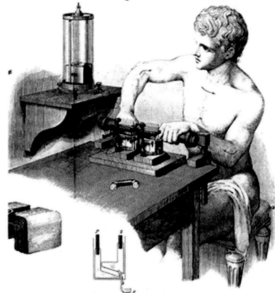

B. Injury electric currents at a nerve cut

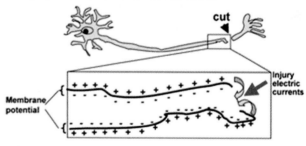

Figure 26•1 *Measurement of endogenous wound electric fields by Du Bois Reymond in mid 1800s. (A) Du Bois Reymond, a founder of modern electrophysiology measured approximately 1 μA flowing out of a cut in his own finger using a galvanometer. (From Du Bois-Reymond, E: Untersuchungen uber thierische Elektricitat, Zweiter Band, Zweite Abtheilung (Erste Lieferung). Berlin, Georg Reimer, 1860, pp 1–387.) (B) Schematic diagram of injury currents at a severed nerve. Plasma membrane maintains a membrane potential inside negative, outside positive. When a cut is made, positive ions flow into and negative ions flow out at the opening, resulting in a net inward electric current (flow of positive charges) into the cut (red arrow).*

concept of the nerve impulse, previously thought of as a flow of electric "particles" along the nerve fiber, became understood simply as a localized region of "depolarization" that traveled down the nerve fiber, with the membrane potential being immediately restored behind it.

Through the work of many scientists such as Hodgkin and Huxley,[7] and more recent work on molecular and genetic studies of ion channels and transporters on the plasma membrane, we know that electrophysiology underlies many fundamental biological activities. Historically, "animal electricity" does have a scientific basis and warrants reconsideration, reevaluation, and exploitation to a greater extent in medicine and biology. There are excellent published resources about the plasma membrane potentials and action potentials of cells. However, to begin this chapter we will only describe endogenous electric fields at the skin and other epithelia associated with wounds.

Discoveries of Electricity Associated With Injury and Wounds

In the 18th and 19th centuries, when Galvani and Matteucci made preparations of cut sciatic nerve and muscle tissues, electric currents were generated at the cuts. (Fig. 26.1) The electric potentials associated with the cuts are called *injury potentials*. Electric currents resulting from those potentials can be detected and measured by a galvanometer and by using muscle preparation, which is a way of setting up the muscle.[8] Contemporary counterparts of those experiments made on severed nerve and muscles confirmed that there are indeed injury electric potentials, at the severed spinal cord, for example.[8,9] The German physiologist Emil Du-Bois Reymond is credited with having made the first scientific recording of endogenous electric currents at a wound.[10] In 1860, using a galvanometer, he measured direct current (DC) flow out of a cut in his own finger.[11] (Fig. 26.1) He and others also observed disappearance of the currents when wounds healed.[10-13]

Where Are Steady Electrical Fields Found?

Spatial segregation of ion channels and pumps carrying inward current from those carrying outward current maintain a transcellular current flow, as well as trans-cell membrane current flow. A wound creates a low-resistance pathway in which the transepithelial potential (voltage) drives current out of the wound. Endogenous steady electric fields at wounds have been confirmed and studied with modern techniques, such as micro-glass electrodes, and vibrating probes, and self-referencing electrodes.[14-16] Electric fields have been detected at wounds of amputated amphibian limbs, human fingertips, corneal and ocular lens epithelia, and skin wounds.[17-27] These steady currents have also been detected at damaged bone and the transected site of spinal cord.[8,28] Similar steady-state ionic currents have also been measured during development and regeneration, and disruption of these currents alters normal development, regeneration, and wound healing.[14,24,29-31]

> ▶ **PEARL 26•1** In our body or organs surrounded by epithelia, wound electric currents are typically found wherever the integrity of the epithelium has been breached.

Physiological Basis of Endogenous Wound Electric Fields

Transepithelial Potential Difference

Skin and corneal epithelia act as batteries and have electric potentials. Well-orchestrated directional ion transport is the basis of transepithelial potential differences (TEPs) in cornea and skin. Corneal epithelium, for example, possesses a sophisticated system of ion and water transport using channels and pumps. (Fig. 26.2) "Pump" is used here to denote the

commonly used terms of cell membrane pumps and ion transporters. The main source of the electric potential across the corneal epithelial layer is the directed epithelial transport of cations (Na^+-K^+) inward to the basal side and of anion (Cl^-) out apically into tear fluid. The basolateral membrane uptakes Cl^- into the cells via Na^+-K^+-$2Cl^-$ cotransporter, and the anion is released into the apical milieu via Cl^- channels. Na^+ is actively transported from the tear to the stroma.[32,33] The

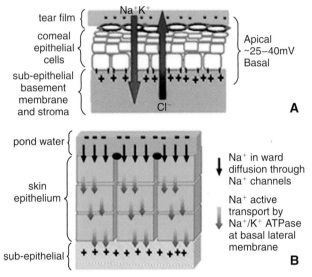

Figure 26•2 *Epithelium is a battery. Skin and other epithelia maintain an electric potential difference across them due to active ion transport. (A) Epithelium of the cornea pumps Na^+ to the basal side and Cl^- to the apical side. The transport of those ions generates an electric potential difference, positive at the basal side relative to the apical side. (Modified from Levin, MH, Kim, JK, Hu, J, et al: Potential difference measurements of ocular surface Na^+ absorption analyzed using an electrokinetic model. Invest Ophthalmol Vis Sci 2006; 47:306–316.) (B) Diagram of Na^+ transporting syncytial epithelium in frog skin. Sodium ions enter the outer cells (top) of the epithelium via Na^+ channels in the outer membranes of these cells, migrating along a steep electrochemical gradient. Once in the cell, they can diffuse to other cells of the epithelium via gap junctions that link the cells of the epithelium, and they can be actively transported from all of these cells via electrogenic pumps that are in all of the plasma membranes of the epithelium except the outer membrane with the Na^+ channels. This results in a transport of Na^+ from the water bathing the epithelium to the internal body fluids of the animal and the generation of a 50-mV potential across the epithelium. Tight junctions between cells at the outer edge of the epithelium minimize the escape of the positive charge transported inward and therefore minimize the collapse of the potential generated by the epithelium's electrogenic Na^+ transport. (Modified from Vanable, JW, Jr: Integumentary potentials and wound healing. In: Borgans, RB, et al (eds): Electric Fields in Vertebrae Repair. New York, Alan R. Liss, 1989.)*

outer cells of corneal epithelium are connected by tight junctions and form the major electrical resistive barrier. Directional ion transport coupled with a resistive barrier establishes the TEP of around +25 to 40 mV (inside positive).[34-36A]

Since 1945, several investigators have reported measuring electropositive voltages from the dermis of superficial wounds and electronegative voltages from the surface of intact skin.[20,26,27] These measurable TEPs are known to be present as a result of Na^+ channels in the apical membrane of the skin's mucosal surface that allow Na^+ to diffuse from the outside of epidermal cells to the inside. (Figs. 26.2 and 26.3) Thus, human skin maintains a variable level of negative electrical charge on its outer surface that results, in part, from the flux of Na^+ from the skin surface to the interior of epidermal cells. Further experimental evidence supporting the existence of the skin battery has been demonstrated by applying amiloride (a compound that blocks Na^+ channels in the outer epidermal membrane) to the skin. This results in inhibition of the skin battery so that bioelectric current flow cannot be detected.

> ▶ **PEARL 26•2** Foulds and Barker measured TEPs of human skin and reported values ranging from 10 mV to almost 60 mV, depending on the region measured.[27] In addition, they demonstrated the presence of a skin battery in normal human volunteers by placing a reference electrode in electrical contact with the dermis and a mobile electrode at multiple positions on the skin. They found the average negative potential for all skin sites of all subjects to be –23.4 mV.

Disruption of the Skin Barrier—Generation of Injury Current and Wound Electric Fields

When a wound occurs in the skin, the TEP provides the electromotive force needed to drive a steady, measurable current outward through the moist low wound resistance provided by the absence of skin. (Fig. 26.4) Essentially, an electrical leak occurs that short-circuits the skin battery at the wound site,

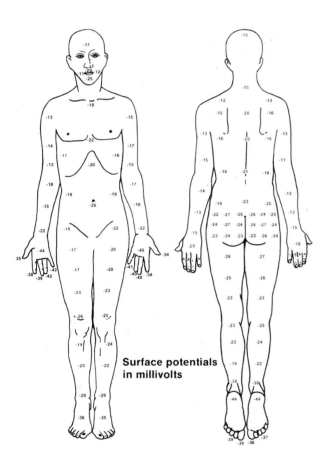

Figure 26•3 *Average human skin battery potential measured on a typical person aged 29 years. The exterior of the skin was found to be electronegative with respect to the inside of the body, and the measurable voltages (mV) are comparable to those measured in animal skins. (From Foulds, IS, Barker, AT: Human skin battery potentials and their possible role in wound healing. Br J Dermatol 1983; 109:515–522, with permission.)*

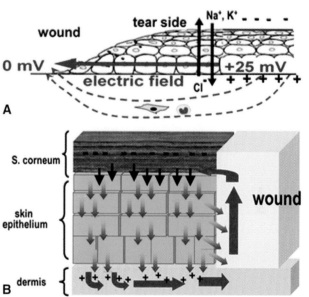

Figure 26•4 *Wounds breach the tight sealing between epithelial cells and short-circuit the transepithelial potential difference at the wound, thus generating laterally orientated endogenous wound electric signals. (A) Cornea wound. Wounding disrupts the epithelial barrier and short-circuits transepithelial potential at the wound. Ions and charged particles flow out from the wound edge and form endogenous wound electric currents; the red solid arrow is pointing toward the wound. Black arrows indicate active transport of ions maintained in intact cells, which serves as a battery that sustains the electric current flow. (B) The path of electric currents with wound made through the stratum corneum in guinea pig skin. The schematic graph shows that the skin battery drives positive charges inward (small red arrows). The ions escape through the wound and return between the stratum corneum and the layers of live epidermis, resulting in wound electrical current flow (big red arrows).*

allowing current to flow out of the wound.[26] Using a self-referencing electrode, Reid et al demonstrated endogenous wound electric fields (EF) with high spatial resolution at cornea and skin wounds.[22,24,25] At a corneal epithelial wound, a large outward current of 4 $\mu A/cm^2$ immediately appears at the wound edges. This current gradually increases to 10 $\mu A/cm^2$ and persists at 4 to 8 $\mu A/cm^2$. Detailed mapping of electric current flow at cornea wounds shows that the strongest currents flow at the wound edge. (Fig. 26.5A). In a circular epithelial wound of the cornea with a diameter of approximately 1.8 mm, the largest outward currents are measured at 0.9 mm from the wound center.[36,37] (Fig. 26.5B) Barker et al demonstrated transepithelial potential difference (blue line) and electrical potential difference (red line) with a microelectrode in a mammalian skin wound.[26] When the resistance of the wound is low, as when the wound is kept moist, current

driven by the epidermal TEP flows out of the wound and returns to the battery via the route between the dead cornified layer and live epithelium. As the currents return to the epidermal battery, a steep drop in the lateral voltage potential occurs near the edge of the wound. (Fig. 26.5C) At a fingertip wound of a human subject, the endogenous electric current is readily measured with a vibrating probe. (Fig. 26.6) Wound-induced lateral EFs at skin and cornea last much longer than injury currents measured from single cells.

> **PEARL 26•3** Conversely, in the skin immediately bordering a wound, there is a steep, lateral voltage gradient that decreases from a high of 140 mV/mm at the wound edge to 0 mV/mm just 3 mm lateral to the wound edge. (Fig. 26.5C)

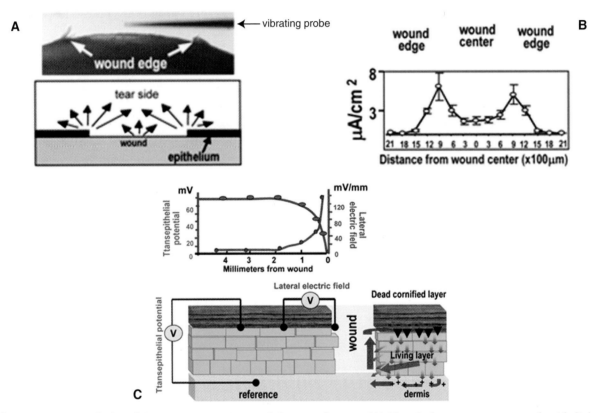

Figure 26•5 *Wound edges drive strong currents toward the wound center. (A) Electrical currents at a corneal epithelial wound measured with a vibrating probe. The lower panel shows the direction and size of the currents represented with the length of the arrows. (B) The wound electrical currents are strongest at the wound edge. (From Reid, B, Song, B, McCaig, CD, et al: Wound healing in rat cornea: The role of electric currents. FASEB J 2005; 19:379–386.) (C) Lateral electric potentials in the vicinity of a wound made in the mammalian skin. Schematic graphs illustrate the transepithelial and lateral electric potentials and the corresponding measurement methods. Transepithelial potentials in the vicinity of the wound were measured as shown on the left. Data obtained from such a measurement are shown as the blue curve. (For actual data, see Barker et al, Am J Physiol Regul Integr Comp Physiol 1982; 11: R248.) The resistance at the wound decreased due to the short-circuitry at the wound. When the wound is kept moist, the current driven by the epidermal TEP flows toward the wound and returns to the "epithelial battery" via the route between the dead cornified layer and the live epithelial layers. The lateral field in the vicinity of the wound, plotted as a function of distance from the wound edge, is shown as the red curve. As the currents return to the epidermal battery, the lateral voltage potential drops gradually (the red curve). (Modified from Vanable, JW Jr: Integumentary potentials and wound healing. In: Borgans, RB, Robinson, K, Vanable, J, McGinnis, M, et al (eds): Electric Fields in Vertebrate Repair. New York, Alan R. Liss, 1989, p 187.)*

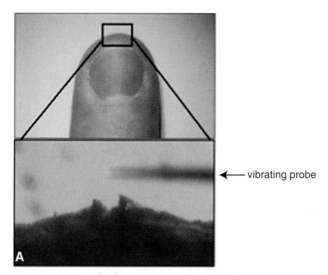

Skin wound current

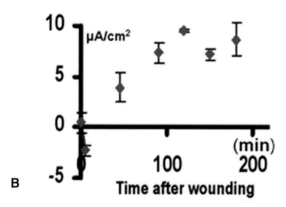

Figure 26•6 *Endogenous electric signals at a small wound on the fingertip. (A) Vibrating probe measurement at a tiny lancet wound at the fingertip. (B) Large and steady rising electric currents from the small cut. (From Reid, B, Nuccitelli, R, Zhao, M: Non-invasive measurement of bioelectric currents with a vibrating probe. Nat Protoc 2007; 2:661–669 . [First published in Nature Protocols, 3, 2, 2007, doi:10.1038/nprot.2007.91.] ©Nature Publishing Group, a division of Macmillan Publishers Limited.)*

Interestingly, during a 4-day study, Cheng and associates, using a porcine (pig) model,[38] demonstrated that an occlusive wound dressing maintained a measurable postwounding EF of the injury at 29.6 ± 8.6 mV, compared to a significantly reduced field strength of 5.2 ± 12.6 mV recorded from wounds exposed to air over the same time period. Their study provides evidence that the wound current of injury can be sustained with occlusive, moisture-retentive dressings, which may contribute to the accelerated healing that occurs under occlusion.[39,40] Occlusive and other types of dressings that trap transudate or serous fluid consisting of 0.9% sodium chloride (NaCl) provide a wound environment that is friendly to cells. With a deficiency of the wound's own "physiological saline," the sterile commercial substitute known as "normal" saline may be used to mimic transudate fluid

(water and electrolytes), thereby maintaining a moist wound environment that also provides a conductive medium for maintaining the flow of the biological injury current.

▶ **PEARL 26•4** If the wound is allowed to dry, the resistance of the desiccated scab (eschar) blocks the current flowing out of the wound, eliminating the measurable lateral voltage gradient.[26]

Wounds closed by new epithelium do not have a measurable current of injury. McGinnis and Vanable have shown that currents escaping through wounds and their accompanying lateral voltage gradients were reduced and ultimately became nonexistent owing to the resistance created by the epithelium.[41] Whether the Na+ current of injury actually contributes to wound healing has as yet not been fully established.[42,43] This may be attributed to the involvement of multiple ions and the complexity of control of wound electric fields by various ion channels and pumps. (Fig. 26.7)

This endogenous bioelectrical system of the human body and the bodies of mammals and amphibians has been shown to contribute to tissue healing in many experimental studies.[17,20,24,26,27,36B,44-46]

Biological Effects—Role of the Endogenous Electric Fields in Wound Healing

The measurable current of injury that flows outward from hydrated wounds has a positive polarity at the epithelial wound edge surface. However, within the strata granulosum, spinosum, and basale of the skin, the flow of electric currents is directed into the wound, with the wound edge negative and periwound underskin positive. (Figs. 26.4, 26.5) Thus, in a three-dimensional structure of the skin wound, the intact skin

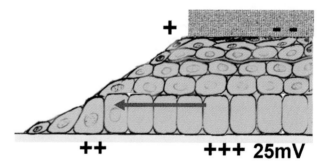

Figure 26•7 *Flow of the electric current and potentials at a skin wound. Electrically negative intact skin surface is shown on the right. When the epithelial layer is damaged, the wound site becomes short-circuited. As a result, the surface of the wound edge becomes more positive in relation to the negative potential of the normal skin surface (upper part of the diagram). Consequently, the wound edge becomes less positive (thus negative) relative to the periwound in the epidermis after wounding. The potential difference in the epidermis provides directional signals for the healing epithelial cells to migrate into the wound. The resultant intraepidermis electric signal is shown by the red arrow and the signs at the lower part of the diagram.*

will maintain a negative skin surface potential as demonstrated by Foulds and Barker.[27] When the skin is wounded, which short-circuits the normal transepithelial potential, the surface of the wound edge becomes positive relative to the intact skin surface farther away from the wound. After wound closure by reepithelialization, collagen remodeling occurs despite the fact that the current of injury and the lateral voltage gradient no longer exist. Therefore, there is little reason to expect that endogenous wound currents affect the remodeling phase of healing. Open wounds are obviously closed following resurfacing with new, delicate epithelium, but they are not healed until remodeling and maturation of all tissues have occurred.

▸ **PEARL 26•5** In the regenerating epithelial layer, the wound side becomes negative relative to the periwound underskin. (Fig. 26.7) It is the cells within those layers that actively contribute to epithelialization. The field strength measured is sufficient to promote cell migration during the healing events of inflammation, fibroplasia, contraction, and reepithelialization.[36B]

Galvanotaxis/Electrotaxis

Galvanotaxis or electrotaxis is the directional migration of cells in an electric field (EF). Investigators have observed that some types of cells, when adhered to the substratum, migrated actively to a specific pole. When they became detached, they moved toward the opposite pole through electrophoresis effect. Many studies have reported migration of cells involved in tissue repair toward the anode or cathode created by an electrical field delivered into a tissue culture.[14,29,37,45-61]

▸ **PEARL 26•6** Electrotaxis is not explained by simple physics in that live organic cells behave as positively or negatively charged dead, inorganic particles (eg, ions) and therefore move toward an EF of opposite polarity.

Human epithelial cells from skin and cornea respond to applied EFs of physiological strength by directional cell migration. Other types of cells, such as neutrophils, macrophages, fibroblasts, endothelial cells, and nerve cells, are also responsive to small applied EFs.

Both human keratinocytes and bovine corneal epithelial cells migrate directionally toward the cathode in an EF as low as approximately 25 mV/mm (0.5 mV across a cell of 20 μm in diameter), well within the physiological range.[24,62] Again, it is important to note that not all cell types migrate in the same direction. Corneal epithelial cells and osteoblasts migrate cathodally, and corneal stromal fibroblasts and osteoclasts migrate anodally.[63,64] Other cells, such as human skin fibroblasts and melanocytes, appear to take a longer time or do not respond at the same EF strengths.[65,66] Several investigators have reported enhanced motility of different cells to either the anode or cathode in vitro (see Table 26.1).

Electric Fields as an Overriding Signal to Direct Migration of Epithelial Cells in Wound Healing

For the cells surrounding the wound to heal the defect, they have to proliferate and migrate directionally into the wound. It is well accepted that the following cues guide migration of cells into the wound.[24]

1. *Chemical substance release.* Chemical substances released by cells in the wounds may attract cells into the wound by chemotaxis or directional cell migration in response to chemical gradients.
2. *Contact inhibition release.* Cells immediately next to the wound do not have neighbor cells at the side facing the wound center. These cells, therefore, know to move in the wound direction.
3. *Wound cavity (empty space).* Simply because of the availability of space and no impediment to movement, cells move toward the wound.
4. *Population pressure.* Growth of adjacent surviving cells may push cells along the leading edge into the wound.
5. *Injury stimulation.* Injury stimulation per se, such as mechanical stimulus from the wounding, may induce various intracellular and intercellular signaling to

Phase of Healing	Biological Effects	Cells	Cells ↑ Motility to:	Investigator
Inflammatory	Phagocytosis and autolysis	Macrophage	DC (+)	Orida, Feldman[54]
		Neutrophil	DC (+)	Fukushima et al[51]
		Neutrophil	PC (+)	Eberhardt et al[77]
		Activated neutrophil	DC (−)	Dineur[49]/Monguio[53]
Proliferative	Fibroplasia	Fibroblast	PC (−)	Bourguignon, Jy, Bourguignon[47]
		Fibroblast	DC (−)	Erickson, Nuccitelli[50]
		Fibroblast	DC (−)	Yang et al[58]
		Keratinocytes	DC (−)	Fang et al[59]
		Keratinocytes	DC (−)	Sheridan et al[61]
Remodeling	Wound contraction	Myofibroblast	PC (−)	Stromberg[56]
	Epithelialization	Epidermal	DC (−)	Cooper, Schliwa[48]

Table 26•1 In Vitro Studies of Enhanced Cellular Motility/Electrotaxis in DC and PC Electric Fields

activate cells to move into the wound. Injury induces signals such as intracellular calcium, ERK1/2, and p38 MAP kinases,[67] and *c-fos* and *c-jun*.[68-70]

▶ **PEARL 26•7** Compared with the five well-accepted directional cues, how important are the endogenous wound EFs? When external (exogenous) EFs of physiological strength are applied into the wound, corneal epithelial cells and skin keratinocytes follow the direction of the EFs to migrate significantly faster into the wound to enhance healing.[24] Remarkably, when exogenous EFs of physiological strength are applied against those well-accepted directional guidance cues, corneal epithelial cells and skin keratinocytes migrate in the direction of the EFs and *ignore* the other cues.[24]

In a monolayer wound healing model, application of direct current electric fields of physiological strength has an "overriding" effect in directing cell migration. Electric fields less than half the strength of measured in vivo signals are able to direct cells to migrate against the other cues listed above.[24] (Fig. 26.8) See the published video at: http://www.nature.com/nature/journal/v442/n7101/extref/nature04925-s2.mov

Knowing that wound healing of skin and cornea requires migration of stratified multilayered epithelial cells, investigators have examined the guidance effect of EFs on migration of stratified epithelium.[24] When physiological, endogenous EFs are applied to a wound on an organ-cultured cornea, migration of stratified epithelium on the wound is predominantly guided by those electric signals.[24] The cells could be directed to move against the previously mentioned, well-accepted directional guidance cues; however, when the EFs are applied into the default healing direction, migration of stratified epithelium is significantly enhanced.[24] (Fig. 26.9) See the published video at: http://www.nature.com/nature/journal/v442/n7101/extref/nature04925-s5.mov

Results from these experiments demonstrate that endogenous wound EFs do not merely contribute to guiding cell migration, but rather play a far more significant and perhaps a more predominant role than currently believed.

Other Effects of Endogenous Currents—Cell Division, Nerve Sprouting, and Angiogenesis

In addition to cell migration, cell metabolism and many other cell behaviors may be affected by endogenous EFs. This is especially important for those cells within approximately 500 µm from the wound edge where the endogenous EFs are maximal. (Fig. 26.5) Cell migration, cell proliferation, leukocyte infiltration, and nerve sprouting within this distance from the wound edge will inevitably happen in the presence of the endogenous wound EFs. (Figs. 26.4, 26.5)

Much less is known about the effects of endogenous EFs on wound healing responses. However, a pharmacological approach to modulate endogenous wound EFs has been developed, and that approach will be discussed next. This may prove to be an easier, more practical and useful way of exploiting the effects of exogenous electrical stimulation on wound healing by delivery of current into the wound via direct electrode contact or by inducing current with pulsed

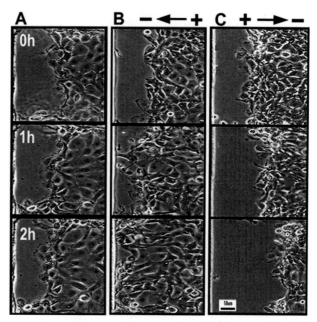

Figure 26•8 *Electric signals are a predominant guidance cue for directional cell migration in wound healing in corneal epithelial monolayer. (A) No applied electric fields, cells at the wound edge migrate toward the left. (B) When a physiological electric field is applied with polarity in the default healing direction, cells at the wound edge migrate into the wound with significantly increased speed. The cathode is at left. (C) When the electric field is applied with the polarity against the default healing direction, cells at the wound edge migrated away from the wound, toward the cathode on the right. The cells do so ignoring other directional signals, such as wound cavity, contact inhibition release, etc. (From Zhao, M, Song, B, Pu, J, et al: Electrical signals control wound healing through phosphatidylinositol-3-OH kinase-gamma and PTEN. Nature 2006; 442:457–460.).*

radiofrequency fields (PRFs). The latter method is presented in Chapter 27.

As discussed at the beginning of this chapter, the physiological basis of endogenous wound EFs is directional ion transport. (Figs. 26.3, 26.4) There are a battery of chemicals and pharmacological agents available to enhance and inhibit transport of specific ions. Increasing TEP pharmacologically would increase the endogenous wound EFs. Research has shown that Cl^- is the major component of endogenous electric currents at a cornea wound.[22] Reid et al tested six drugs and demonstrated that four of them increased Cl^- and Na^+ transport, while two decreased Cl^- and Na^+ transport. These six chemicals produced diverse pharmacological effects, but share one common effect: They change ion transport across cornea epithelium. Four of the six drugs consistently and significantly enhanced Cl^- transport, which subsequently increased the transcorneal electric potential difference and increased wound edge current. The other two drugs inhibited ion transport, which significantly decreased transcorneal electric potential difference and the wound edge currents.[22] As seen in Figure 26.10, silver nitrate ($AgNO_3$) increases, whereas

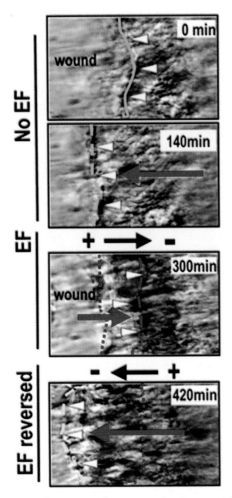

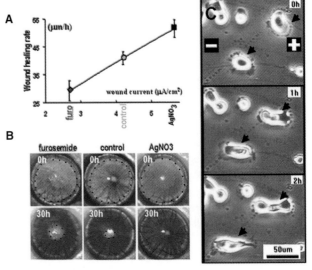

Figure 26•9 *Electric signals are a predominant guidance cue for directional cell migration in wound healing of stratified epithelium: 0–140 min, stratified epithelium migrates into the wound in the absence of an applied electric field; 140–300 min, an applied physiological electric field directs cells to migrate away from the wound; 300–420 min, when the polarity of the applied electric field is reversed, the electric signal now guides cells to migrate into the wound. Dotted lines represent the wound edge at the beginning; dashed lines represent the wound edge after indicated period of time. White arrowheads indicate wound edges, and red arrow the directions of cell migration. See video at http://www.nature.com/nature/journal/v442/n7101/extref/ nature04925-s5.mov (From Zhao, M, Song, B, Pu, J, et al: Electrical signals control wound healing through phosphatidylinositol-3-OH kinase-gamma and PTEN. Nature 2006; 442:457–460.)*

Figure 26•10 *Pharmacological modulation of endogenous wound electric fields modulates corneal epithelial wound healing in vivo (A and B). An applied electric field oriented cell division (C). (A) Treatment with $AgNO_3$, which enhances ionic transport of the epithelium, increased the endogenous wound electric fields at a corneal wound. By contrast, furosemide (furo) treatment, which inhibits ionic transport, resulted in a marked decrease of the endogenous wound electric fields at the wound edge. This in turn directly correlated with wound healing rates of rat cornea in vivo. (B) Photos show that manipulation of endogenous wound electric currents using $AgNO_3$ or furosemide directly affect wound healing in vivo. For clarity, the wound edge is marked with dots. (From Zhao, M, Song, B, Pu, J, et al: Electrical signals control wound healing through phosphatidylinositol-3-OH kinase-gamma and PTEN. Nature 2006; 442:457–460.) (C) Two human corneal epithelial cells (arrows) dividing in an applied electric field of 150 mV/mm. The field vector is horizontal, and cleavage occurred roughly perpendicular to the applied EF. (Modified from Zhao, M, Forrester, JV, McCaig, CD: A small, physiological electric field orients cell division. Proc Natl Acad Sci U S A 1999; 96:4942–4946.)*

furosemide inhibits, transport of Na^+ and Cl^-. Correspondingly, the wound electric currents are enhanced and decreased, respectively. The rate of wound healing was directly proportional to the size of the TEP and to the size of the endogenous wound EFs.[22,24,71] In corneal wounds of isolated bovine eyes, reducing the endogenous EFs with the Na^+ channel blocker benzamil or with Na^+-free saline decreased wound electric currents and slowed wound healing. External injection of electric currents to restore and amplify the natural EFs at wounds in Na^+-free medium enhanced wound healing.[44]

Corneal epithelial cells near the lesion divide in response to wounding. Enhancing the endogenous wound EF with two ion transport-enhancing drugs, PGE_2 (prostaglandin E_2) or aminophylline, resulted in a 40% increase in cell divisions within 600 μm of the wound edge, and suppressing the EFs with ouabain caused a 27% suppression of mitoses.[71] Interestingly, corneal epithelial cells divide in an applied EF in culture with the cleavage plane forming perpendicular to the field vector.[72] (Fig. 26.10C) The same striking phenomenon occurs in vivo and appears to be regulated by the endogenous EFs. In corneal wounds, the mitotic spindles lie roughly parallel to the EF vector, with cleavage occurring perpendicular to the field lines. Enhancing the endogenous wound EFs with PGE$_2$ nearly doubled the proportion of dividing cells with cleavage planes orientated perpendicular to the field vector.[71]

Nerves sprout to reinnervate regenerating skin and cornea epithelium. When the endogenous electric field was enhanced with PGE$_2$, aminophylline, AgNO$_3$, or ascorbic acid, neurite growth toward the wound was significantly enhanced, with more and earlier sprouts oriented toward the wound edge. Decreasing the endogenous electric fields with ouabain or furosemide prevented directional nerve sprouting toward the wound edge.[73]

The latter results support a role for endogenous electric fields not only in directing cell migration, but also in regulating the frequency and direction of cell division and directional nerve sprouting in wound healing. These in vitro studies demonstrate the galvanotaxis/electrotaxis theory, which may be used as the basis for selecting the anode or cathode in the clinical treatment of wounds with electric stimulation.

Endothelial cells and leukocytes also respond to applied EFs in vitro.[24,74,75] It is likely that their behaviors and functions in wound healing will be affected by endogenous wound EFs. However, as they are not immediately adjacent to the wound edge where the endogenous EFs are strongest, they may experience less strong electric signals. Nevertheless, considering the existence of much longer-lasting endogenous wound EFs farther away from the wound edge, the lower strength may be compensated by longer exposure. Indeed, long time exposure of vascular endothelial cells to weak applied EFs (approximately 100 mV/mm) does induce alignment and migration of the cells.[75,76] (Fig. 26.11) It is important to note that the weak EFs used to cause galvanotaxic/electrotactic migration and other cellular responses in culture may well be generated in vivo as described in the previous section.

A review of the literature revealed one human study that analyzed the effect of direct contact ES on the cell composition in skin exudate. In 10 wounds treated with ES for 30 min, Eberhardt et al found that 69% of 500 cells counted 6 hours after ES were neutrophils compared to 45% found for control

wounds.[77] The authors suggested that the 24% difference in neutrophil percentage occurred because of the galvanotaxic effect created by the exogenously applied currents. Mertz et al assessed epidermal migration macroscopically for 7 days after two 30-min sessions of monophasic pulsed-current ES delivered to induced wounds in pigs.[78] They observed that wounds treated with negative polarity on day 0, followed by positive polarity on days 1 to 7, demonstrated enhanced epithelialization by 20% compared to those receiving treatment with either positive (+9%) or negative (–9%) alone. In addition, they observed that alternating positive and negative polarity daily inhibited epithelialization by 45%. Thus, evidence indicates that cells involved in the different phases of wound healing are partly dependent on endogenous bioelectrical signals to facilitate their migration and proliferation. Later in the chapter, the types and characteristics of electrical currents that have been reported to facilitate healing of chronic wounds will be described.

How Cells Sense and Transduce the Electric Signals–Signaling Mechanisms

Apparently, there are multiple signaling pathways underlying the mechanisms that explain how polarity of the physiological EFs influence cell migration and other responses. The first targets of EFs (membrane receptors) are likely on the plasma membrane because of the high electric resistance of the cellular membrane.

> **PEARL 26•8** Since most biomolecules, such as growth factors, are charged, gradients of those molecules may form in EFs. Such chemical gradients may contribute to directional cell migration. Using genetic manipulation, Zhao et al found that EF-induced directional cell migration can be decoupled from chemotactic response.[79] Therefore, electrotactic and chemotactic responses may exert their effects separately, but orchestrate in directing cell migration to further wound healing.

Membrane Receptors

An EF may physically move charged receptor molecules in the plasma membrane and create receptor asymmetry between cathodal and anodal facing sides. For example, receptor asymmetries for polysaccharide-binding plant lectins, concanavalin A, and for neurotransmitter acetylcholine (AchR) have been demonstrated.[80,81] Growth factor receptors are distributed and activated asymmetrically in skin keratinocytes and corneal epithelial cells in direct current EFs.[59,74,82,83] Application of an EF upregulates epidermal growth factor receptors (EGFRs) and causes redistribution of the receptors toward the cathodal side of cells.[84] A downstream signaling molecule ERK1/2 (extracellular signal-regulated kinase 1/2) is activated and becomes highly colocalized with F-actin at the leading lamellae of cells migrating cathodally.[83] (Fig. 26.12)

PI3 Kinase and PTEN Are Key Molecules in Electrotactic/Galvanotactic Migration

PI3 kinases (phosphoinositide-3 kinases) are important downstream molecules of epidermal growth factor receptors

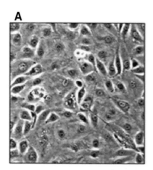 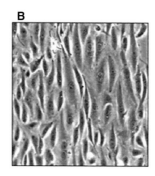

Figure 26•11 *Electric signal-induced alignment and elongation of human vascular endothelial cells. (A) Human umbilical vein endothelial cells without application of an electric field orient randomly. (B) When an electric field is applied for longer than 8 hours, cells elongate and orient perpendicular to the electric field direction (the electric field lines run horizontal to the left in B).*

and many other receptors. When being activated, PI3 kinases (PI3Ks) produce PIP3 (phosphatidylinositol(4,5)-bisphosphate), which binds and activates protein kinase B, also known as Akt, a serine/threonine kinase. Akt activation plays roles in diverse cellular processes such as cell migration, cell proliferation, and apoptosis.[44] The tumor-suppressor gene *Pten* codes for protein PTEN (phosphatase and tensin homolog) that is a key negative regulator of PI3K signaling through dephosphorylating PIP3.

> ▷ **PEARL 26•9** Recent research highlighted important roles for PI3K/PTEN molecules in cell polarization and directional cell migration, suggesting a significant role for PTEN in wound healing where spatially organized tissue growth is essential.[44]

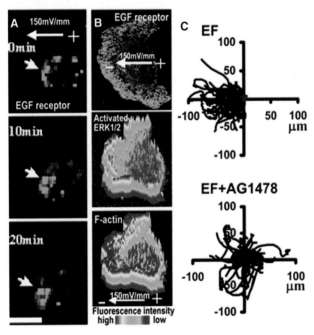

Figure 26•12 *Applied electric fields induce polarized signaling of epidermal growth factor receptors, which are required for electrotactic migration. (A) Epidermal growth factor receptors redistribute to the cathode side of a live cell subjected to an applied electric field. (B) Epidermal growth factor receptors, activated ERK1/2, and actin polymerization redistribute to the cathode facing side of the cells, and cells migrate toward the cathode. ERK1/2 (extracellular signal-regulated kinase 1/2) provides downstream signaling of epidermal growth factor. (Modified from Zhao, M, Pu, J, Forrester, JV, et al: Membrane lipids, EGF receptors, and intracellular signals colocalize and are polarized in epithelial cells moving directionally in a physiological electric field. FASEB J 2002; 16:857–859.) (C) Inhibition of epidermal growth factor receptors abolished electric field directed cell migration. From Pu, J, McCaig, C, Cao, L, et al: EGF receptor signalling is essential for electric field-directed migration of breast cancer cells. J Cell Sci 2007; 120:3396–3403.*

Application of exogenous EFs of physiological strength (100–150 mV) activates Akt in skin keratinocytes and corneal epithelial cells within minutes. (Fig. 26.13) When cells are made to express green fluorescence protein-tagged Akt (Akt-GFP), the location of Akt-GFP represents where PI3 kinases are being activated. Application of an EF distributes the location of PI3 kinase activation toward the direction of migration. When the polarity of the EF is reversed, PI3 kinases are being activated at the front of

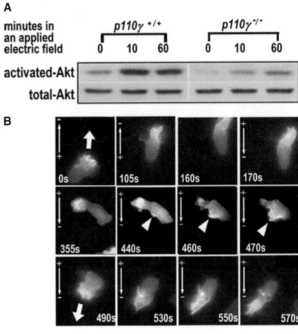

Figure 26•13 *An applied electric field induces polarized activation of PI3 kinase. (A) An applied electric field activates PI3 kinases (phosphatidylinositol-3-OH kinase), which leads to activation of Akt, as indicated by an increase in phosphorylation of Akt shortly after an electric field is switched on. Total Akt is the control. Akt, or protein kinase B, is a serine/threonine kinase. Upon binding to PI3 kinase product PIP3, Akt translocates to the plasma membrane, where it is activated. Akt activation plays important roles in diverse cellular processes such as glucose metabolism, cell proliferation, apoptosis, transcription, and cell migration. Primary cultures of mouse keratinocytes in serum-free medium (200 mV/mm). Deletion of a gene (p110γ) encoding a catalytic subunit of PI3 kinase significantly attenuated activation of Akt because there are no active PI3 kinase to produce PIP3. γ110γ[+/+] are from cells with the gene deleted. (B) Dynamic distribution of Akt-GFP (Akt tagged with green fluorescence protein) as a probe for PI3 kinase activation to the leading edge (arrows) of HL-60 cell (a human promyelocytic leukemia cell line). When polarity of the EF is reversed, Akt-GFP redistributes toward the new leading edge (arrowheads at 440 sec). (From Zhao, M, Song, B, Pu, J, et al: Electrical signals control wound healing through phosphatidylinositol-3-OH kinase-gamma and PTEN. Nature 2006; 442:457–460.)*

the cells facing the new cathode to which the cells become oriented and migrate.[24,45] (Fig. 26.13). (See published video at: http://www.nature.com/nature/journal/v442/n7101/extref/nature04925-s6.mov). Therefore, electric signals activate PI3 kinases, and more importantly, the activation is spatially controlled within the cells.

PI3 kinase inhibition or genetic disruption of PI3 kinase (γ-phosphatidylinositol-3-OH kinase) in mice decreases EF-induced signaling and abolishes directed cell migration. Deletion of the tumor suppressor gene *Pten* (the negative regulator of PI3 kinase signaling) enhances the signaling and electrotactic response.[24] Taken together, these results identify two important genes and molecules in mediating EF-induced cellular responses. (Fig. 26.14)

Other Signaling Mediators

Membrane potential perturbation has been suggested as one very initial step needed for inducing cellular response. The plasma membrane facing the cathode depolarizes, whereas the membrane facing the anode hyperpolarizes, which may affect ion flow in and out of cells and directional cell migration.[85,86] In many types of cells, such as keratinocytes, extracellular Ca^{++} depletion or Ca^{++} channel blockage abolishes directional cell migration. However, this is not the case for fibroblasts because two lines of fibroblast cells exhibit cathode-directed motility in the absence of extracellular calcium and electric fields cause no detectable elevations or gradients of cytosolic free calcium.[59,87-94] cAMP regulates electrotaxis in keratinocytes and nerve crest cells, and Rho small GTPases are also implicated in electrotactic response.[74,95-98] These signals result in cytoskeletal reorganization and are important for the responses in an EF.[99] Better understanding of these signaling mechanisms will offer possibilities of combining pharmacological intervention with electric stimulation.

In summary, naturally occurring wound EFs are an intrinsic property of wounds. Electric fields activate multiple cellular-signaling pathways, of which PI3K/PTEN are two key mediators for electrotaxis/galvanotaxis response. More importantly, EFs could be a dominant guidance signal directing cell migration in wound healing. Since cells possess signaling systems for EFs, exogenous application of "therapeutic" currents used clinically for wound healing is expected to have diverse effects on tissue healing responses. Therefore, the in vivo situation may be very complicated and presently relies on best practice based on clinical research outcomes to determine its clinical effectiveness.

> ▶ **PEARL 26•10** Cell migration and cell proliferation are the two aspects critical for wound healing. ES provides a directional vector as well as a nonvector instigating mechanism to activate cells in wound healing by targeting different types of cells.

Using pharmacological agents to enhance endogenous wound EFs, together with exogenous delivery of ES via direct electrode contact may prove to be a new promising avenue for exploiting electric signaling in wound healing. One important point that needs to be mentioned is that when drugs such as furosemide are administered, they may affect ion transport systems and decrease endogenous wound EFs. As the endogenous EFs are important for wound healing, usage of such

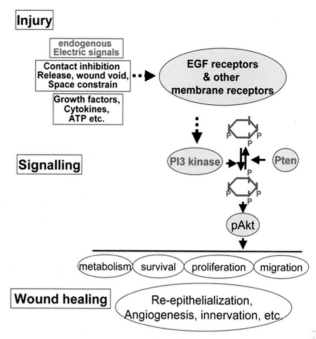

Figure 26•14 *Electric signaling in wound healing. Injury generates endogenous wound electric fields. Together with other signals, physiological electric fields may activate multiple intracellular signaling pathways. Two key signaling molecules that are required for electric field-induced intracellular signaling have been identified.[24] Electric fields, of strength equal to those detected endogenously, activate PI3 kinase, which activates Akt and increases its activated form – pAkt through production of PIP3. Akt activation is critical for many cellular responses following wounding, such as cell migration, survival, and proliferation. PTEN (tumor suppressor phosphatase and tensin homolog) dephosphorylates the second messenger PIP3 and converts it back to the precursor PIP2, antagonizing the action of PI3K. Genetic disruption of p110 the catalytic subunit of PI3 kinase γ (one major isoform of PI3 kinases) decreases electric field-induced signaling and abolishes directed movements of healing epithelium in response to electric signals. Deletion of the Pten enhances signaling and electrotactic responses. Therefore, these two genes play an essential role in electrical signal-induced wound healing and control electrotaxis. Dashed arrows omit many links.*

drugs in patients with chronic, refractory wounds may need to be investigated. If detrimental effects are found, use of these types of drugs as diuretics should be avoided.

Exogenous Electrical Currents for Wound Healing–Electrical Terminology

Reviewers and readers of literature that addresses wound healing with ES have indicated that they are sometimes baffled by the different types of EF currents and stimulation parameters reported in the clinical research studies. A primary reason for this confusion may arise from the lack of standardization of ES terminology. To mitigate the reader's bewilderment as to how EF signal parameters of amplitude, frequency, and duration affect wound treatment dosage and healing, terminology related to ES and the types and characteristics of therapeutic electrical currents are presented here.[100]

Charge

Electrical charge (Q) is a fundamental property of matter. Matter can be electrically neutral or negatively or positively charged. *Electrons* are negatively charged particles. When an electrically neutral atom is acted upon by an outside force such as a magnetic field, it gains or looses electrons, thereby altering its neutral charge and causing it to take on electrical properties. An atom that is no longer in its neutral state is called an ion. A negative ion is an atom that has gained one or more electrons to become negatively charged (–); a positive ion is an atom that has lost one or more electrons to become positively charged (+). Charge is measured in units called coulombs (C), representing a specific quantity of electrons (e–). One coulomb contains 6.25×10^{18} electrons. The amount of charge delivered into wound tissues through a treatment electrode to enhance healing is in the microcoulomb (μC) range, which will be discussed later.

Charge Density

Charge density is a measure of the electrical charge per unit of the cross-sectional area of a treatment electrode, expressed as electrical charge per square centimeter (Q/cm^2). However, because the magnitudes of charge delivered to wounds in clinical practice are relatively small, charge densities for ES electrodes are more likely to be expressed as microcoulombs per square centimeter ($\mu C/cm^2$). Charge density is inversely related to treatment electrode size. Thus, for a given current level (eg, 5 mA) delivered to a small and large electrode, the intensity of stimulation perceived will be greater at the smaller electrode. Phase and pulse charge represent the total charge or dosage of electrical current within each phase of each electrical pulse.

Conductive (Capacitive) Coupling of Electrodes to Patient

Exogenous (externally applied) delivery of electrical currents into wound tissues may be conducted via two electrodes placed in direct contact with wound and periwound tissues (conductive coupling).[101] (Fig. 26.15A, left) Both direct current (DC) and pulsed current (PC) are delivered to wound tissues via conductive coupling. Alternatively, electric current may be transmitted by pulsed electromagnetic field (PEMF) waves into wound tissues by contact or noncontact of periwound tissues with a coil that emits an electromagnetic field that in turn induces an electric current in the wound tissues (inductive coupling).[102] (Fig. 26.15B, right) Although both methods are intended to mimic the normal endogenous

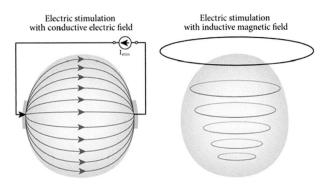

Figure 26•15 *Exogenous electrical currents may be delivered into wound tissues either by (A) Conductive coupling, in which electrodes are placed in direct contact with the wound and/or periwound skin, or (B) inductive coupling, using pulsed electromagnetic field energy (PEMF) to induce currents in wound tissues either by contact or noncontact of the PEMF coil with the periwound skin.*

currents that facilitate wound healing, additional research is needed to reveal the possible mechanisms by which this occurs. In this chapter we will cover the conductive coupling method. The inductive method will be covered in Chapter 27.

Electrodes

Electrodes are the conductive elements of an electrical circuit that are applied to the body to transfer electrical charge into the tissues. For delivery of current into tissues, a minimum of two electrodes are required. The negative electrode or cathode (–) attracts positive ions (cations, eg, Ca^+, Na^+, K^+), while the positive electrode or anode (+) attracts negative ions (anions, eg, Cl^-) in the tissues. Electrodes consist of carbonized silicon, conductive polymers, gel, silver-plated polymeric fabric, or aluminum foil placed in contact with saline moist gauze.

Electrode-Tissue Interface: Wound Treatment Electrodes and Polarity

With the conductively coupled method of delivering exogenous electrical currents to wound tissues, the electrode-tissue interface is the site of electron-to-ion and ion-to-electron exchange. Living tissue is a plentiful source of ions that serve as the conductive electrolyte in the interface. At any electrode-electrolyte junction, electrodes tend to release ions into solution (tissue fluid), while electrolytes tend to combine with the electrode. To create ionic current flow in living tissue, the electrodes must have opposite charges (opposite polarities). The cathode (negative [–] electrode), which has the greater concentration of electrons, attracts positive ions from the underlying tissues. The anode (positive [+] electrode), which has a relative deficiency of electrons, attracts negative ions from the tissues.[103] At any given time while current is flowing, one electrode is relatively more positive while the other is relatively more negative. When the cathode and anode associated with direct current have sufficient charge, they may cause undesirable electrochemical burning of tissues due to pH changes of sodium hydroxide (NaOH) and hydrogen chloride (HCl), respectively.

Electrical Circuit

An electrical circuit used for wound healing treatment consists of at least two lead wires, one of which is connected to the cathode terminal and the other connected to the anode terminal of an ES device. The patient end of each lead is connected to an electrode that is applied to the patient. Electrodes placed in contact with the tissues of the body are described as being conductively coupled.

Voltage

Voltage (V) refers to the electron moving force or the electrical force capable of moving charged particles (ions across cell membranes in wound tissues) that lie between two or more electrodes applied to the body. The volt is a measure of electrical pressure (analogous to water pressure) and is the EMF (electron or ion moving force in metal conductors and tissues respectively) needed to drive a current of 1 ampere through a resistance of 1 ohm. The relationship between voltage and amperage is expressed as Ohm's law: $V = IR$, where V is voltage, I is current, and R is resistance.

In order to produce directed current flow, there must be a source of free electrons from the ES device delivered to the patient via conductive electrodes positioned to distribute the flow of charge into wound and periwound tissues. The electrical force capable of moving the charge between two electrodes applied to the body is the voltage or potential difference between the two electrodes. The voltage between the two electrodes contacting the wound and periwound skin is created by the separation of charges between them, such that one electrode has an excess of negatively charged electrons or ions compared with the other. With direct and monophasic pulsed current, the two electrodes are polarized with respect to each other, one being negative and the other positively charged.

Recall that endogenous, measurable electric fields (currents) are created by transmembrane voltages found in cell membranes and that when the epithelium of human skin is wounded, a low-resistance pathway is created where the transepithelial potential (voltage) drives current out of the wound. After wounding, and in a moist wound environment, there is a lateral voltage gradient of 140 mV/mm at the wound edge that decays to 10 mV/mm at 500 to 1000 μm from the wound edge.[36,37]

Low-Voltage and High-Voltage Devices

Low-voltage devices deliver either monophasic or biphasic waveforms of longer durations (milliseconds to seconds) and therefore require lower driving voltages (clinically usually between 20 and 35 V). All commercially available conductively coupled ES devices (except high-voltage pulsed current devices) fall into this category. High-voltage devices have a monophasic waveform with phase durations less than 100 microseconds that require a high driving voltage (clinically usually between 75 and 150 V).

> **PEARL 26•11** Conductively coupled electrical stimulation devices are classified according to the voltage range delivered to treatment electrodes.

Current

The directed flow of charge from one place to another within matter (ie, tissues) is called current. The charge may consist of free electrons or ions. An electrical current (I) is defined as the rate of flow of charged particles (electrons or ions) past a specific point in a specific direction. Current flow in a metal wire conductor occurs as a result of the flow of electrons, whereas current flow in tissues is carried by ions (eg, Na^+, K^+, Cl^-). The unit of measure of current is the ampere (A), which is defined as the rate at which charge flows past a fixed reference point in a conductor, or mathematically as $I = C/t$, where I = amps; C = coulombs; and t = time (in seconds, sec). An ampere is equal to 1 C per second. Coulombs indicate the number of electrons, whereas amperes indicate the rate of electron flow. Exogenous currents delivered to wounds that are intended to mimic the physiological tissue currents have an order of magnitude that may be 1000 to 1,000,000 times less than 1.0 A, which places them in the milliampere (mA) to microampere (μA) range.

> **PEARL 26•12** When a unidirectional current—direct current (DC) or pulsed current (PC)—is delivered into soft tissues of a wound via contact electrodes, active cells that participate in the phases of healing (eg, neutrophils, macrophage, fibroblasts, keratinocytes) may become more motile or they may be upregulated to synthesize soluble mediator proteins (eg, growth factors, cytokines) that enhance tissue repair.

Resistance

As electrons and ions (charged particles) flow in metallic and biological conductors, respectively, their movement is impeded by collisions with other charged carriers and by the inherent properties of the substance. Thus, resistance is the opposition to the flow of current.

A conductor's resistance is 1 Ω if a potential difference of 1 V causes 1 A to flow through it. This is one form of Ohm's law, which states $R = V/I$. The skin provides the greatest opposition to current flow because it is composed primarily of keratin and contains very little fluid.[104] Skin lesions such as open wounds can significantly lower skin resistance at the wound site. Techniques that can be used to decrease electrical resistance of periwound skin include hydration and skin warming. In addition, the use of high-voltage currents of approximately 100 V can cause spontaneous breakdown in skin resistance. Following the initial resistance drop, a slower decrease in skin resistance continues.[105,106] This occurs because skin resistance is proportional to duration of the electrical pulse or phase. In other words, the shorter the phase duration, the lower the skin resistance.

Waveforms

Direct current has no waveform because once it leaves the zero baseline it continues to flow in one direction for 1 second or longer (for as much as 48 hours for wound dressings that deliver microamperage, continuous direct current). (Fig. 26.16)

Waveforms are visual representations of voltage or current on an amplitude-time plot. They represent pictures of either

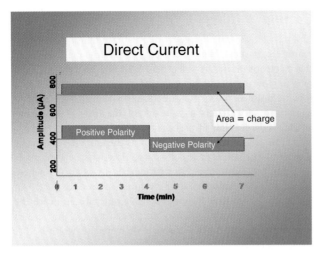

Figure 26•16 *Direct current flows continuously and therefore has no waveform, but it has distinct positive or negative polarity. DC that flows for sufficiently high current levels for significant periods of time may cause electrochemical injury to the skin and wound tissues. At sufficiently low microampere levels, exogenous DC current may be used to mimic the endogenous DC current of injury.*

monophasic or biphasic current flow as an electrical event that begins when the current or voltage leaves the zero (isoelectric) baseline in one direction, then after a finite time either returns to and stops at the same baseline (monophasic waveform) (Fig. 26.17A) or crosses the baseline in the opposite direction.

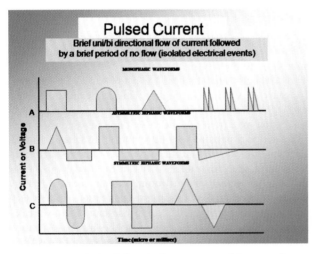

Figure 26•17 *Pulsed electrical currents used in wound healing are either monophasic or biphasic. In baseline A, examples of monophasic pulses above (or below) the zero baseline. When they are above the baseline, they have positive polarity. When they are below the baseline, they have negative polarity. Baselines B and C are examples of biphasic pulses, one phase above and one phase below the zero baseline. Their shape may be asymmetrical (as for baseline B) and charge unbalanced with polarity or symmetrical (as in baseline C) and charge balanced without polarity.*

It ends when the voltage or current returns again to the baseline (biphasic waveform). (Fig. 26.17B, C)

Phase

A phase is an electrical event that begins when the current (or voltage) leaves the isoelectric line and ends when it returns to the baseline. A waveform depiction of current or voltage over time may be monophasic or biphasic.

Phase/Pulse Duration

Phase duration is the time in microseconds or milliseconds between the beginning and the end of one phase of a pulse. Pulse duration is the time in microseconds or milliseconds between the beginning of the first phase and the end of the second phase that may include the interphase interval within one pulse. (Fig. 26.18)

Pulse Frequency

Pulse frequency describes the number of pulses per second (pps) for a pulsed current or the number of cycles (Hertz, or Hz) per second for alternating current.

Types of Electrical Currents

Two types of electrical current are generally described as direct current (DC) and alternating current (AC). However, the majority of clinical trials that have studied the effects of ES on wound healing have used "pulsed" waveforms or pulsed current (PC), as described by the American Physical Therapy Association.[100] The use of the term PC is not meant to imply that there is an additional type of basic current (there are still only two, DC and AC). Figures 26.16 and 26.17, respectively, show graphic representations of continuous DC (CDC) and PC that have been used in wound healing studies and practice. Low-frequency AC (1 to 1000 Hz) shown in Fig. 26.19 has not been used in wound healing clinical trials for reasons that will be discussed next.

Alternating Current

Alternating current, or AC, is the continuous bidirectional flow of charged particles in which a change in direction of flow occurs at least once every second. An AC sine waveform is represented by one cycle that describes an electrical event beginning when the current or voltage leaves the zero (isoelectric) baseline in one direction then crosses the same baseline in the opposite direction and ending when the current or voltage returns again to the baseline. When available from an electrical stimulation device, the AC waveform is the sine wave in which both phases of the cycle are charge balanced so there is no electrode polarity.[36,37] (Fig. 26.19)

> ▶ **PEARL 26•13** Unlike PC, AC has no off time interval between phases of adjacent cycles, and because it has no polarity, AC cannot be used to mimic the steady endogenous physiological DC currents that exist in mammalian skin bordering the wound. These currents produce a steep, lateral voltage gradient that falls from a high of 140 mV/mm at the wound edge to 0 mV/mm just 2 mm lateral to the wound.

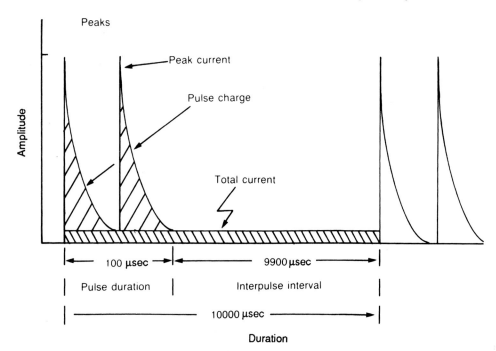

Figure 26•18 *Waveform of high-voltage monophasic pulsed current (HVMPC). Clinical voltage levels used to deliver low levels of current to wound tissues (~3.2 μC/pulse) will not cause tissue injury from electrochemical pH changes. (From Nelson, RM, Currier, DP: Clinical electrotherapy. Norwalk, CN, Appleton and Lange, 1987, p 63, with permission.)*

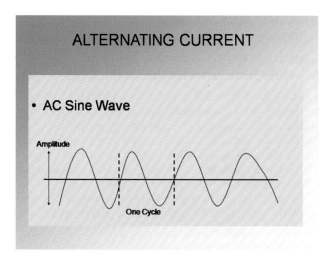

Figure 26•19 *Waveform of alternating current (AC) that, unlike the endogenous wound current, has no polarity. Thus, of the three types of electrotherapeutic currents, DC, PC, and AC, the latter type of current is least likely to be able to mimic the endogenous DC bioelectric current associated with wound injury and healing.*

Some authors have incorrectly indicated that current delivered by transcutaneous electrical nerve stimulation (TENS) devices represents AC.[107-114] Actually, ES devices classified as TENS units by the U.S. Food and Drug Administration deliver trains of isolated electrical events (pulses) that are either monophasic or biphasic PC, not AC.[102] Since only DC and PC have been used in clinical wound healing studies, AC will not be discussed in this context.

Direct Current

Direct current is the continuous, unidirectional flow of charged particles for 1 second or longer. (Fig. 26.16) When delivered to wound tissues, the direction of current flow is determined by the polarity selected, with positively charged ions moving toward the negative electrode (cathode) and negatively charged ions moving toward the positive electrode (anode).[102] Continuous DC has no pulses and subsequently no waveform. However, because DC flows for 1 second or longer, when it is delivered through anode and cathode electrodes to a solution containing electrolytes (eg, NaCl) or to tissues that contain electrolytes, the current causes the charged ions of Na^+ and Cl^- to migrate toward the cathode and anode, respectively. At the cathode, Na^+ reacts with H_2O to form NaOH and H_2, while at the anode Cl^- reacts with H_2O to form HCl and O_2. Thus, when therapeutic dosages of DC are delivered to the body, the caustic products that form at the electrode-tissue interface may create alkaline and acid pH changes at the cathode and anode, respectively. If the dosage of DC (current amplitude in milliamperes or microamperes multiplied by time) is allowed to flow in the skin and subcutaneous tissues at sufficiently high amplitude over a long enough time period, the pH changes at the electrode-tissue interface will cause observable tissue irritation. The irritation may manifest itself as erythema observed in light skin tones or as blistering from electrochemical burning secondary to a much greater acidic or alkaline pH change on the skin. These undesirable responses to DC may be diminished by delivering less than 1 mA (1–1000 μA) to the electrodes. Although CDC and pulsed DC between 50 and 1000 μA have been reported to have positive wound healing outcomes in six clinical studies, it is no longer used, largely because of practitioner concern regarding the risk of causing electro-chemical skin irritation.[115-120] Interestingly, a new wound dressing that delivers microamperage CDC and is being mar-keted in the United Kingdom may be marketed in the United States pending FDA clearance. Later in this chapter results will be discussed for several clinical trials that reported accel-erated healing of chronic wounds treated with CDC at 50 to 1000 μA. Since the endogenous physiological currents de-scribed earlier in the chapter are steady DC currents that are measurable in humans along the wound edge, exogenous microamperage DC (see Fig. 26.16) or monophasic PC (see Figs. 26.18 and 26.20) may be the best choices for mimicking the endogenous physiological electrical signals.

Pulsed Current

PC is the brief unidirectional or bidirectional flow of charged particles (electrons or ions) in which each pulse is separated by a longer off period with no current flow. Thus, each pulse is an iso-lated electrical event separated from each of a series or train of pulses by a finite off time. PC is described by its waveform, am-plitude, duration, and frequency. PC can have two waveforms: monophasic or biphasic. A monophasic pulse represents a very brief movement of electrons or ions away from the isoelectric line, returning to the zero line after a finite period of time (less than 1 sec). (Fig. 26.18) When the duration of a monophasic pulse is less than 1 msec, the current is not DC because it does not cause electrochemical changes in the tissues.

Monophasic PC waveforms described in the clinical wound healing literature include the rectangular waveform of low-voltage monophasic PC and the twin-peaked waveform of high-voltage monophasic PC.[57,121-128] High-voltage PC (HVPC) typically has very short-duration (20–60 μsec) twin triangular pulses that have single-phase charges on the order of 1.6 μC.[125-128] (Fig. 26.18)

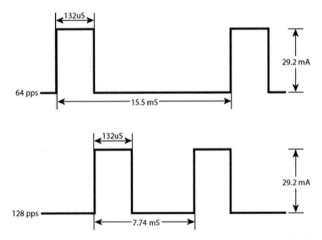

Figure 26•20 *Waveform of low-voltage monophasic pulsed current (LVMPC) used in six clinical trials that reported positive healing outcomes following treatment of chronic wounds in conjunction with standard care.*[57,121-124,229]

> ▶ **PEARL 26•14** Because HVPC is unidirectional, one may incorrectly assume that this type of current is "galvanic" or DC, which may cause caustic skin and wound tissue damage secondary to pH changes. However, investiga-tors have demonstrated that pH changes do not occur in human skin following 30 min of HVPC stimulation.[129]

The biphasic PC waveform also represents a very brief duration of movement of electrons or ions. However, in this case the pulse is bidirectional and consists of two phases. One phase leaves the isoelectric line and after a finite time returns to baseline. Without delay (or in some waveforms, a few microseconds delay), the second phase leaves the isoelectric line in the opposite direction and after a brief time returns to baseline. The biphasic waveform may be asymmetrical or symmetrical about the isoelectric line. (See Fig. 26.17B and C). In the symmetrical biphasic wave-form, the phase charges of each phase are electrically equal or balanced; therefore, there is no polarity. Asymmetrical biphasic waveforms may be electrically balanced or unbal-anced. The use of biphasic symmetrical (charge balanced) and asymmetrical (charge unbalanced) waveforms have been described in clinical wound healing literature dis-cussed later.[130-132]

Review of the Evidence—Basic Science Research

In Vitro Research—Effects of Conductively Coupled Electric Stimulation on Tissue Cells

Substantial experimental research has contributed to the ex-panding body of knowledge that provides insights into the cellular and physiological mechanisms by which exogenous EFs enhance wound healing. Numerous studies have investi-gated how cells respond when exposed to electrical currents of different amplitudes and frequencies. Other studies have reported changes in cell synthesis and metabolism.

In vitro research is reported to increase DNA and protein synthesis by fibroblasts, upregulate insulin receptors on fibroblasts, upregulate receptors for transforming growth factor-β (TGF-β) on human dermal fibroblasts, and increase ATP concentration in the skin. Bourguignon et al stimu-lated healthy human fibroblasts in cell cultures with high-voltage pulsed current (HVPC).[133,134] They observed that the fibroblasts were perturbed to increase their rate of DNA and protein synthesis, the latter of which increased by 160% over controls. Maximum synthesis occurred with commonly used clinical stimulus parameters of 50 and 75 V and 100 pulses per second (pps), with the cells in close proximity to the cathode. Voltages greater than 250 V inhibited both protein and DNA synthesis. Within the first minute of fibroblast stimulation using the same stimulus parameters cited in the previous study, Bourguignon et al reported an increase in Ca^{2+} uptake followed by upregulation of insulin receptors on the fibroblast membrane during the second minute of stimulation.[47] When insulin was added to the electrically stimulated cultures, there was an immediate second increase in Ca^{2+} uptake and significant increases in both protein and DNA synthesis compared to nonstimulated cells. The significance of the latter finding is that during ES treatment of wounds, if insulin is available to bind the additional receptors, the fibroblasts will significantly increase both protein and DNA synthesis.

TGF-β is also known to play an important role in collagen synthesis. Falanga et al have shown that ES upregulates receptors for TGF-β on human dermal fibroblasts in culture.[135] Fibroblasts that were exposed to 100 V and 100 pps had receptor levels of TGF-β that were sixfold greater than those of control fibroblasts.

Cheng et al assessed the effects that occurred in rat skin following microampere levels of DC stimulation.[136] They reported that 10 to 1000 µA applied to skin strips 0.5 mm thick at 500 µA for 2 hours in vitro increased ATP concentration in the skin fivefold. They also found that 100 to 500 µA of DC increased amino acid uptake 30% to 40% above control levels and that 50 µA was required to obtain a maximum stimulation effect on protein synthesis. Other investigators noted that fibroblasts in a three-dimensional collagen matrix exposed to an electric field responded by increasing the intake of 3H-thymidine.[137]

Based on the findings of these in vitro studies, a possible mechanism by which ES enhances soft tissue healing is by triggering the opening of voltage-sensitive calcium channels in the fibroblast plasma membrane. Subsequently, upregulation of insulin and TGF-β receptors on the cell surface may trigger increased rates of collagen and DNA synthesis, the latter of which suggests that fibroblasts are stimulated to propagate.

In Vitro and In Vivo Research–Antibacterial Effects of Electrical Stimulation

In the management of chronic wounds, reducing the bacterial burden, thereby allowing chronic inflammation to subside and avoiding infection, is clearly recognized as an important prophylactic objective.

The antibacterial effects of ES have been investigated both in vitro and in vivo, and the results summarized in Table 26.2 point out that such currents may impose a bacteriostatic or bactericidal effect on microorganisms that commonly colonize or infect wounds.

Using milliampere levels of AC and microampere (<1.0 mA) and milliampere levels of cathodal DC delivered through platinum electrodes, Rowley noted that, as would be expected, in vitro growth rates of *Escherichia coli* were affected very little or not at all by AC while a significant bacteriostatic effect occurred with DC.[138] Rowley indicated that the decrease in growth rate with DC was not due to a pH change since the cells were kept in a buffered condition. Wolcott et al observed that human wounds initially colonized with *Pseudomonas* and/or *Proteus* organisms were pathogen free following several days of treatment with microampere levels of cathodal DC.[139] Prompted by these findings, Rowley et al demonstrated a bacteriostatic effect after delivering 1 mA of cathodal DC for 72 hours to rabbit

cutaneous wounds infected with *Pseudomonas aeruginosa*.[140] Barranco et al stimulated cultures of *Staphylococcus aureus* with DC at amplitudes of 0.4, 4, 40, and 400 µA with stainless steel, platinum, gold, and silver electrodes.[141] They determined that the silver anode electrode had excellent growth inhibitory capacity on *S. aureus* at 0.4 and 4 µA, with negligible toxic effects from electrode corrosion, gas production, or pH changes. Marked growth inhibition occurred with the other three electrodes at 400 µA, but at this amplitude, undesirable pH shifts, electrode corrosion, gas formation, and media discoloration occurred. In an in vivo study, Chu et al found that silver-coated nylon fabric applied via the anode at currents between 0.4 and 40 µA for 4 or 24 hours was therapeutically more effective ($P < 0.001$) on *P. aeruginosa* than when silver-coated nylon fabric was applied without the anode.[142] Following this report, numerous investigations established that antibacterial activity occurred in the presence of silver cations deposited in vivo or in vitro by low levels of DC.[143-150] In other in vitro studies, investigators found that 100 µA of DC delivered to cell cultures via a silver wire anode had a bacteriostatic effect on gram-positive bacteria, whereas the same current amplitude and polarity produced a bactericidal effect on gram-negative bacilli.[151,152] The authors suggested that differences in cell wall composition may have been a determining factor in the effectiveness of the electrically mediated silver antisepsis. Other investigators have compared in vitro antibacterial effects of HVPC and DC and found that HVPC applied at 50 to 800 mA and 100 pps for 30 min had no inhibitory effects on *S. aureus*, whereas both anodal and cathodal continuous DC applied at 1, 5, and 10 mA did inhibit *S. aureus* growth.[153] The findings from the latter study suggest that the mechanism by which DC kills bacteria is through electrochemical pH changes that occur at both poles, specifically an alkaline pH at the cathode and an acid pH at the anode.

Electrochemical pH changes have not been shown to occur at the anode or cathode when HVPC is applied to human tissues for 30 min.[129] However, when Kincaid and Lavoie evaluated antibacterial effects of HVPC in vitro, they observed pH changes only at the cathode at a dosage of 500 V and at both the anode and the cathode at 250 V.[154] Szuminsky et al attempted to identify the mechanisms by which HVPC applied at 500 V causes bacterial killing in vitro.[155] They observed bactericidal effects at both poles but were unable to conclude whether the killing effect was due to the direct action of the current on the organisms, electrophoretic recruitment of antimicrobial factors, local heat generation, or pH changes. Although both of the latter studies demonstrated antimicrobial effects in vitro, it is unlikely that the high voltages used would be tolerated if applied to wounds of human subjects.

To determine the efficacy of common types of electrical currents on bacterial growth in vitro, Merriman et al applied each current type (µADC [microamperage direct current]; monophasic, mAPC [milliamperage pulsed current][156]; biphasic, mAPC and HVPC) to culture plates containing *S. aureus* for 1 hr at 37°C on 3 consecutive days. From the zone of inhibition measurements they found significant growth inhibitory effects for µADC and HVPC ($P < 0.05$), but not for monophasic and biphasic PC. There were also no differences

Table 26•2 In Vitro, In Vivo, and Clinical Studies on the Antibacterial Effects of Conductive Electrical Stimulation

Reference	Study Type	Pathogens	Current Type	ES Parameters	Polarity/Effect	Electrode Type	Growth Rate
Rowley[138]	In vitro	Escherichia coli	DC	mA = 1.0, 14, 140	Cathode; None	Platinum	Bacteriostatic
			AC	Frequency = 1, 10, 30, 60	Not applicable	Platinum	No effect
Wolcott et al[139]	Clinical	Pseudomonas aeruginosa Proteus	DC	μA = 200, 400, 600, 800	Cathode	Carbon/rubber on saline gauze	Bactericidal
Rowley et al[140]	In vivo	P. aeruginosa	DC	mA = 1.0	Cathode; None	Copper mesh in gauze	Bacteriostatic
Baranco et al[141]	In vitro	Staphylococcus aureus	DC	μA = 40 and 100	Anode (negligible gas and pH change)	Silver, platinum, gold, stainless steel	Bacteriostatic
Chu et al[142]	In vivo	P. aeruginosa	DC	μA = 0.4 and 40	Anode	Silver-coated nylon fabric	Anode plus Ag+ nylon more effective than Ag+ nylon alone
Ong et al[151]	In vitro	S. aureus P. aeruginosa	DC	μA = 26, 100, 300, 500, 800	Anode	Silver wire	Bactericidal
Laatsch et al[152]	In vitro	Gram (+) bacteria Gram (−) bacilli	DC	μA = 100	Anode Anode	Silver wire Silver wire	Bacteriostatic Bactericidal
Kincaid et al[154]	In vitro	S. aureus E. coli P. aeruginosa	HVPC	V = 150, 200, 250, 500 F = 120 pps	Cathode (toxic end products) Anode (toxic end products)	Stainless steel Stainless steel	Bacteriostatic No effect
Szuminsky et al[155]	In vitro	E. coli Klebsiella P. aeruginosa S. aureus	HVPC	V = 500 F = 120 pps	Anode (gas and pH change) Cathode (gas and pH change)	Stainless steel Stainless steel	All inhibited at both poles
Merriman et al[156]	In vitro	S. aureus	μADC	μA = 500	Anode: Corrosion and discoloration of medium Cathode: Gas	Stainless steel	Bacteriostatic
			M mA PC	mA = 30 @ 128 pps	No electrode effects	Stainless steel	No effect
			B mA PC	mA = 30 @ 128 pps			No effect
			HVPC	V = 250 @ 100 pps	Anode: Corrosion and discoloration of medium Cathode: Gas		Bacteriostatic
Daeschlein et al[157]	In vitro	E. coli P. aeruginosa Klebsiella S. aureus S. epidermidis E. faecium	M mA PC	mA = 42 F = 128 pps	Anode and cathode: No electrode effects	Cotton patches contained bacteria	All bacteria significantly reduced Anode greater log 10 bacterial reduction than cathode

AC, alternating current; B mA PC, biphasic milliamperage pulsed current; DC, direct current; F, frequency; HVPC, high-voltage pulsed current; μADC, microamperage direct current; M mA PC, monophasic milliamperage pulsed current; pps, pulses per second.

between anodal and cathodal polarity. They concluded that for infected wounds, µADC and HVPC may have an initial antibacterial effect that is unchanged with subsequent treatments. Daeschlein et al have also evaluated the antibacterial effects of monophasic, mAPC polarity (positive and negative) on wound pathogens in vitro.[157] They exposed three gram-negative (*E. coli, P. aeruginosa, Klebsiella pneumonia*) and three gram-positive (*S. aureus, Staphylococcus epidermidis, Escherichia faecium*) bacteria to monophasic square waves with a duration of 140 µsec, at a frequency of 128 pps and an intensity of 42 mA, for 30 min. Control cultures of the same bacteria were set up in the same manner, except the current was not activated. Unlike other in vitro studies that used culture plates, these investigators used cotton patches containing the bacteria to simulate wounds and to eliminate possible contamination from electrode corrosion and toxic end products. In contrast to the study by Merriman et al, who reported no bacterial growth inhibitory effects between positive and negative polarity,[156] Daeschlein et al found that positive polarity had a greater antibacterial effect than negative polarity and that bacterial reductions differed significantly between positive polarity and control and negative polarity and control,[157] with the highest log 10 reduction factor achieved with positive polarity.

Interestingly, an emerging antimicrobial technology designed for wound applications contains a matrix of 25 microbatteries per square inch embedded into a polyester fabric layer containing a biocompatible, proprietary silver formula that is held in position on the polyester with a biocompatible binder. The wireless product known as Procellera™ (Vomaris,Wound Care, Inc., Chandler, AZ) has been approved by the FDA for professional use as an antimicrobial barrier for partial-thickness and full-thickness wounds, including pressure ulcers, venous and diabetic ulcers, first- and second-degree burns, surgical incisions, and graft donor sites. The dry dressing is electrically inactive and may be cut to size prior to placing it into a wound. (Fig. 26.21A) When moistened with wound exudates or by saline, its batteries are activated to generate a sustained voltage (2–10 mV) for up to 7 days on the surface of the dressing making contact with the wound surface. (Fig. 26.21B)

> **PEARL 26•15** The antimicrobial activity of the Procellera device is enhanced by the synergistic action of the bioelectric field and the silver embedded in the dressing.

Gram-negative microbes have a net negative charge. Gram-positive microbes have a lipopolysaccharide coating that carries a negative charge. All microbes, therefore, are attracted to the anode containing silver. Silver then binds the sulfhydryl groups and denatures the proteins that destroy the respiratory system of the microbe as well as other essential proteins within it. Silver kills viruses and fungi in a similar manner by binding with sulfhydryl groups and denaturing other proteins. The development of resistance to silver in a bioelectric environment would be exceptionally rare because an organism would have to undergo multiple mutations of essential cellular functions within a single generation. In addition, in vivo porcine studies evaluated the effects of Procellera

on deep and full-thickness wounds. Histological and chemical analyses found that the millivoltage stimulation significantly increased the rate of wound epithelialization ($P < 0.001$), increased epithelial thickness, decreased crust formation, and decreased white blood cell infiltration of the wounds. The investigators also found that stimulated wounds had reduced levels of interleukin-1α levels in the early phases of healing. Reduced interleukin-1α levels are correlated with diminished pain and inflammation.[158]

In summary, numerous in vitro and in vivo studies have demonstrated that microampere or millivoltage levels of DC kill or at least inhibit proliferation of common wound pathogens. Currently, there are many silver-impregnated dressings available that passively deliver silver ions to wounds with the intention of controlling the bacterial burden. Thus, one might speculate that the efficacy of such dressings could be enhanced by actively repelling the silver ions into the wound with microamperage, anodal DC. (Fig 26.22)

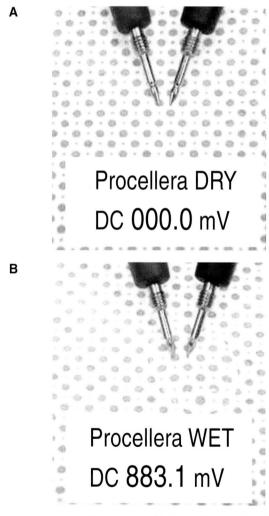

Figure 26•21 *The antimicrobial Procellera DC device contains 25 microbatteries and a silver formulary. (A) Dry inactive dressing with 0 mV measured. (B) Moist active dressing showing millivolts measured (Vomaris Innovations, Chandler, AZ).*

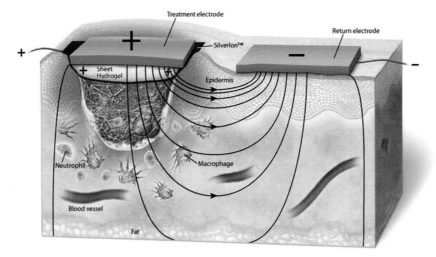

Figure 26•22 *Illustration showing the potential use of microampere DC to aid in the delivery of silver ions by placing the anode (+) on a commercial silver dressing.*

In Vitro Research–Electrical Stimulation Enhances Antibiotic Effectiveness Against Biofilm and Cancer Cells

Interesting research has shown that antibiotic effectiveness against biofilm cells is increased in the presence of a weak DC electrical field.[159,160]

> ▶ **PEARL 26•16** When investigators passed 1 mA of DC through a chamber containing a biofilm and an antibiotic, an increase in the killing of the bacteria of about 8 log orders was observed after 24 hours compared with the control that was exposed to the same amount of antibiotic but no current.

Recently, researchers reported that drug-resistant rat and human tumor cells lose their drug resistance when exposed for 3 days in vitro to 7.5 µA, 50 Hz AC pulses with a 10-second interval.[161] The researchers found that treating drug-resistant tumor cells with electric pulses restores the cells' ability to take up the anticancer drug doxorubicin. Such electrical stimulation is known not to damage cells but to decrease the proliferation of tumor cells. The tumor cell lines used overexpress the MDR1 protein, which makes them resistant to anticancer drugs such as doxorubicin. Following the 3 days of electrical stimulation, the cells were exposed to increasing concentrations of doxorubicin for 3 hours, resulting in their increased uptake of the drug, causing them to die, even at low doxorubicin concentrations. Exposing the cells to an electric current was more effective than treating the cells with an MDR1 inhibitor.[161] These findings suggest the potential application of electrical stimulation to improve the efficacy of existing chemotherapeutic treatments.

Review of the Evidence: Animal Research

Effects of Electrical Stimulation on Wound Tensile Strength, Collagen Deposition, and Epithelialization

Many animal studies have evaluated several tissue and cellular responses following delivery of ES into traumatically induced wounds or their periwound tissues. The most notable response reported is an increase in tensile strength following treatment with cathodal DC at current levels frequently less than 1.0 mA.[162-166] Other studies demonstrated fibroblast proliferation in the wound along with collagen deposition.[167-171] Investigators have also reported that anodal HVPC enhanced epithelialization more rapidly than the cathode, but had no effect on wound tensile strength.[172-174]

Effects of Electrical Stimulation on Edema

Three other studies on frog and rat hind limbs showed that sub-motor levels of cathodal HVPC limited acute traumatic edema development by blocking macromolecular leakage from microvessels.[175-177] The effects of ES have also been assessed on edema associated with burns in rats. Matylevich et al evaluated the effect of 40 mA DC on plasma albumen extravasation following partial-thickness burns in Sprague-Dawley rats. In the treatment group,[178] DC from the anode was delivered to burns via silver nylon wound dressings while control burns were treated with silver nylon dressings without current. They performed confocal fluorescence microscopy with fluorescein thiocyanate (FITC) to quantitatively assess albumen leakage and its accumulation in tissues. During treatment with DC, leakage decreased 30% to 45% and approached normal rates at 4 hours after the burn. At that time, FITC-albumen concentration peaked, but was 18% to 48% less than in the control burns and neared the level of nonburned controls by 18 hours after the burn. The investigators concluded that DC has a beneficial effect in reducing plasma protein extravasation following burn injury. In a subsequent study, Chu et al used the same research design as Matylevich et al on wound edema after full-thickness burns in the same rat species.[179] They reported that DC decreased burn edema by 17% to 48% at different time periods up to 48 hours after the burn. While polarity and current density had no effect on treatment results, beginning treatment during the first 8 postburn hours resulted in the least edema accretion. They also observed significant edema reduction when DC treatment was applied 36 hours after the burn.

Although the findings from the latter two animal studies can not be generalized to humans, in view of complications from excessive leakage of plasma proteins from burn and traumatic wounds in humans, there is a need for clinical research to ascertain whether the results from the animal studies can be replicated in humans.

Effects of Electrical Stimulation on Skin Grafts, Donor Sites, and Flaps

Several studies have looked into the effects of ES on skin grafts and donor sites and flaps in animal models. Chu et al examined the effects of weak anodal DC (20–40 µA) delivered through silver nylon dressings for 5 days in a guinea pig model on (1) healing of partial-thickness scald burns,[180] (2) split-thickness grafts taken from these wounds when healed, and (3) the resulting donor sites. Scald wounds in 180 animals treated with weak DC reepithelialized by 12 postburn days, whereas only 20 of 40 animals with control wounds that received sham DC had reepithelialized by 16 postburn days. Split-thickness grafts taken from the healed scald wounds showed more rapid revascularization with DC treatment than did control grafts. Grafts and donor sites treated with DC showed more rapid reepithelialization, decreased contraction, improved hair survival, and decreased dermal fibrosis compared to controls not treated with DC. Only donor wounds treated with DC could be repeatedly harvested as donor sites for successful split-thickness autografts. The authors suggested that DC treatment might limit the extent of tissue damage as evidenced by DC-treated wounds having less inflammation, granulation tissue, and fibrosis than control wounds. During wound healing by secondary intention, mast cells regulate the extent of scar fibrosis that, when excessive, is represented by keloid and hypertrophic scar formation. Interestingly, in related research involving four human subjects, investigators evaluated the effect of anodal PC on the thickness of donor site scars and found that ES reduced scar thickness and hypertrophic scar formation.[57]

Failure of "take" of grafts and flaps is a major concern shared by plastic surgeons. Politis et al used µADC to establish whether ES could improve the posttraumatic quality of dermis and epidermis in full-thickness skin grafts in rats.[181] They delivered 4.5 µA of DC to skin grafts for 3 days to study the effects of three surgically implanted electrode configurations: anode on top of the graft, cathode on top of the graft, and an inactive electrode on top of the graft. Quantitative and histological evaluations on postoperative day 7 revealed the presence of

necrotic skin in 80% to 90% of graft surface areas in animals treated with cathodal stimulation and control animals that received no current. In animals treated with anodal DC, only 50% of the graft area was necrotic, and the significantly thicker dermis had multilayered patches of intact epidermis. Two other studies investigated the effect of ES on the survival of ischemic skin and musculocutaneous flaps.[182,183] Im et al stimulated the ischemic central portion of bipedicle skin flaps in pigs with a monophasic pulsed current (PC) at 35 mA, 128 pps, and a pulse duration of 140 µsec for 30 min twice daily for 9 days following skin flap elevation.[182] The skin flaps were stimulated with the cathode on postoperative days 1 to 3, with the anode on days 4 to 6 and the cathode on days 7 to 9. Two control pigs received sham ES treatment, and two others received no treatment. The length of viable flap and the extent of skin necrosis were measured on postoperative day 21. The mean area of skin flap necrosis was 28% in control animals and 13.2% in ES-stimulated animals ($P < 0.001$). The authors suggested that the initial 3 days of cathodal treatment might have prevented severe ischemia by hampering sympathetic vasoconstriction and also might have counteracted ischemia reperfusion that could have occurred in the transition zones of the skin flap. They also suggested that anodal stimulation of the flap in the later stages of tissue repair might have prevented tissue injury by scavenging superoxide radicals.

The other study that assessed the effect of ES on flaps used a PC device (transcutaneous electrical nerve stimulation) with an unspecified waveform and parameters that are customarily used to suppress musculoskeletal pain.[183] In that study, 10 groups of rats received different current amplitudes (mA) and pulse frequencies for postoperative treatment of musculocutaneous flaps. A highly significant difference ($P < 0.001$) was noted between the group with the highest percentage of flap survival (94.6%) that received high-intensity (20 mA), high-frequency (80 pps) stimulation delivered to the base of the flap for 3 days and the other groups. Also, a significant difference ($P < 0.001$) in flap survival occurred when high-intensity (20 mA) treatment was compared with low-intensity (5 mA) treatment. Flap survival was not related to the ES frequency used. In conclusion, the evidence cited from animal studies suggests that ES facilitates survival of failing skin grafts and musculocutaneous flaps.

Effects of Electrical Stimulation on Blood Flow

The U.S. Food and Drug Administration indicates enhancement of blood perfusion as the main label (indication) for ES muscle stimulation devices used to treat wounds. Two studies have demonstrated increased blood flow following treatment of wounds with PC, which may explain the positive outcomes of ischemic skin and flap survival reported in previous studies.[124,182-184] In a pilot study, Greenberg et al used the same pulsed ES device used by Junger et al to evaluate the effects of polarity on epithelialization and angiogenesis in burn wounds of pigs.[124,184] They observed prominent neovascularity on day 10 in wounds treated with negative versus positive polarity. Conversely, Mohr et al reported that negative polarity from HVPC produced greater blood flow in rats than did positive polarity.[185]

Not only did blood flow volume increase instantly at pulse frequencies of 2, 20, 80, and 120 pps, but flow also increased steadily with increasing current amplitude, up to the onset of muscle contraction, and continued to be elevated up to 20 min following stimulation. Mehri et al found there to be an age-related waning in skin vascular reactivity by sensory nerves that was associated with a decrease in wound repair efficacy.[186] Using laser Doppler flowmetry they compared blood flow following 1 min of low- or high-frequency stimulation. They found that compared to younger control rats, the vascular response in old rats was significantly reduced (46%) at the high frequency, but there was no difference in vascular response between the two groups at the lower frequency. This suggests that enhancement of cutaneous blood flow by stimulation of sensory nerves occurs best at lower stimulation frequencies.

As previously mentioned, endothelial cells respond to applied electric fields (EFs) in vitro, and it is likely that their behaviors and functions in wound healing will be affected by endogenous wound EFs.[24,74,75] Kanno et al and Patterson et al showed that weak pulsed ES caused significant increases in blood flow and capillary density in rat ischemic limbs secondary to stimulating vascular endothelial growth factor (VEGF) secretion from muscle cells in vitro and in vivo, and muscle contraction was not required.[187,188]

> **PEARL 26•17** Recent work shows that electrical stimulation induces significant angiogenesis in vivo through enhanced vascular endothelial growth factor (VEGF) production by muscle cells.

Zhao et al have reported that applied EFs of small physiological magnitude directly stimulate VEGF production by endothelial cells in culture without the presence of any other cell type.[74] EFs as low as 75 to 100 mV/mm (1.5–2.0 mV across an endothelial cell) directed the reorientation, elongation (Fig. 26.11) and migration of endothelial cells in culture, all of which are precursors to blood vessel formation. Some clinical studies are presented later in the chapter regarding the use of ES to enhance blood flow in ischemic lower extremities.

Review of the Evidence—Human Research

Research on human subjects, designed to answer questions pertaining to the mechanisms responsible for wound healing or questions related to the efficacy of a particular wound treatment, are highly desirable to clinicians and patients who want the most effective treatment options and to third-party payers who base reimbursement for services on evidence-based clinical studies. This section addresses human subject studies designed to answer several questions related to the clinical effects of ES.

Effects of Electrical Stimulation on Cutaneous Arterial (Microcirculatory) Blood Flow with Sensory or Motor Level Stimulation

Several studies have evaluated the effect of ES on cutaneous microcirculatory blood flow in the extremities. In some of these studies, investigators applied ES to the skin of the distal extremity while indirectly measuring changes in microcirculatory blood flow as reflected by skin temperature changes in the same or in other extremities. In these studies blood flow was measured by placing thermistors on the skin to measure warming brought about by ES-induced cutaneous vasodilation.[189-193,195,197,199]

Kaada successfully treated 10 patients with 19 leg ulcers of various etiologies using the burst mode from a monophasic PC device.[189] He delivered 15 to 30 mA of pulsed DC via the cathode for 30 to 45 min, three times daily, to the web space between the first and second metacarpals of the ipsilateral hand. The anode was positioned at the ulnar border of the ipsilateral wrist. All of the leg ulcers, which had resisted treatment for several months to 4 years, healed completely in response to the remote pulsing stimulation of muscles underlying the electrodes on the hand and wrist. Kaada suggested that the remote ES of hand muscles improved cutaneous microcirculation of the ipsilateral lower extremity (LE), as evidenced by increased temperature of the toes and healing of the leg ulcers.[189] He further proposed three mechanisms by which remote ES of hand muscles may cause vasodilation of small vessels in the ipsilateral LE: (1) activation of a central serotonergic link that inhibits sympathetic vasoconstriction, (2) activation and release of vasoactive intestinal polypeptide into the plasma, and (3) activation of a segmental axon-reflex leading to vasodilation. The finding that serotonin inhibitors block the vasodilation response, whereas the opiate antagonist naloxone and antagonists of humoral vasodilators do not affect the responses, provides supportive evidence for the first proposed mechanism.[110,189-193]

Other investigators have also reported cutaneous vasodilation responses of hand and digital vessels to remote transcutaneous stimulation of the skin over the spinal cord or ulnar nerve at μADC levels of ES[194,195]; however, not all studies using such levels agree with these findings. One study reported a reduction in digital temperature, suggesting vasoconstriction of digital vessels after sensory and motor excitation elicited by noninvasive stimulation of acupuncture points.[196] Ernst and Lee applied pulsed μADC levels of ES to the dorsal web space of the hand with a monophasic pulse duration of 800 μsec delivered below the pain threshold at 1 pps.[197] They reported an increase in sympathetic constrictor tone with subsequent vasodilation after 50 min. In a controlled study, no change in sympathetic tone was noted after sensory stimulation in patients with chronic pain.[198] Skudds et al found that pulsating contractions of hand muscles in asymptomatic individuals increased local cutaneous blood flow evidenced by a measurable increase in hand skin temperature.[199]

There are equivocal research findings related to the use of pulsed mA and μADC levels of ES and its remote effects produced on cutaneous circulation in the distal extremities. However, with additional clinical research, this approach to treatment of hand, foot, and digital ulcerations may prove effective in facilitating increased perfusion and wound repair in patients with primary diagnoses of Raynaud's disease, reflex sympathetic dystrophy, and pain associated with diabetic polyneuropathy.

Effects of Electrical Stimulation on Muscle and Skin Arterial Blood Flow with Pulsed Motor Level Stimulation in Healthy Subjects

Other human studies have confirmed that ES applied at sufficient amplitude to elicit a continuous series of pulsating (nontetanizing) muscle contractions increases regional arterial blood flow in asymptomatic individuals. In these studies described next, blood flow in larger arterial vessels was measured more directly with Doppler flowmeter and photoplethysmography.[200-203]

Currier et al used pulsed motor level stimulation to elicit isometric contractions from the calf muscles of healthy subjects equal to 10% and 30% of maximum voluntary contraction using 2500 Hz AC with a 50% duty cycle.[200] Using a Doppler flowmeter to measure blood flow delivered to the leg through the popliteal artery, they reported a significant increase in blood flow to the stimulated leg during the 9 min of ES and during the 5-min poststimulation period. In 30 healthy subjects, Tracy et al used a directional Doppler probe to measure significantly increased blood flow through the femoral artery as a result of pulsed contractions of the quadriceps at frequencies of 10, 20, and 50 pps, but not at 1 pps.[201] Hecker et al monitored upper extremity digital blood flow with photoplethysmography during 1 hour of submotor ES with five different pulse frequencies (2, 8, 32, 64, 128 pps) of monophasic PC applied over the brachial and radial arteries of 10 healthy subjects.[202] They showed a trend toward an increase in arterial blood flow (nonsignificant) only at 32, 64, and 128 pps, without significant skin temperature changes. Using laser Doppler flowmetry, Cramp et al assessed forearm skin temperature and blood perfusion response to PC at low (4 pps) and high (110 pps) frequencies in 30 healthy subjects.[203] Subjects were randomly assigned to control and two treatment groups. Under a double-blind proviso, biphasic PC was applied to skin over the median nerve for 15 min. Skin temperature and blood flow readings were recorded before and during ES and for 15 min after ES had been terminated. While no significant changes were observed in skin temperature, significant increases in skin blood flow during the treatment period did occur in the low-frequency group compared to the other two groups ($P = 0.0106$; ANOVA).

Effects of ES on Wound and Periwound Skin Blood Flow

Several studies have evaluated the effects of ES on wound blood flow and blood flow in periwound skin. In these studies investigators used laser Doppler imaging to assess macrovascular flow and intravital video microscopy, together with computerized image analysis, to measure microvascular blood flow.[204-208]

Petrofsky et al spanned wounds of 18 subjects with ES electrodes to assess whether wound blood flow would be enhanced by delivering a rectangular, biphasic, balanced pulse with a duration of 250 μsec and a frequency of 30 pps for 5 min across the wounds.[204] Ten patients with or without type 2 diabetes with wounds of mixed etiology, location, and duration and 8 control subjects with no wounds participated. The stimulation amplitude was set to sensory threshold for sensate subjects and to

15 mA if subjects were insensate. Blood flow within the wound and the periwound skin was measured with laser Doppler flow imaging (LDI) before and after stimulation. In subjects with wounds, average blood flow increased 53% over prestimulation and was sustained for a brief period after stimulation. Petrofsky et al also demonstrated with LDI that in patients with wounds, skin blood flow increased significantly more during ES administered in a warm room compared to a cool room.[205,206]

Wikstrom et al enrolled nine nonsmoking, healthy volunteers to participate in two studies in which blood flow changes induced by PC were quantified by two different methods.[207] In one study, nine subjects with intact skin received ES at different frequencies (2 pps, 100 pps, and sham) to the left distal leg for 60 min in each of three sessions. They assessed changes in blood flow by LDI every 5 min and found that mean blood flow increased by 40% during low-frequency stimulation and by 12% during high-frequency stimulation. No change in blood flow occurred during sham stimulation. In the second study, PC stimulation was used to alter blood flow in capillaries of blister wounds induced on the lower legs of the nine subjects. The investigators used intravital video microscopy and computerized image analysis to study microcirculatory blood flow, measured as red blood cell velocity (RBC-V) in 5 to 14 individual capillaries in each wound before and during 45 min of PC stimulation at 2 and 100 pps. Mean RBC-V increased 23% during low-frequency PC ($N = 6$) and by 17% during high-frequency PC ($N = 8$). Their findings show that PC stimulation at 2 and 100 pps enhances peripheral wound blood flow and that LDI and intravital video microscopy can be used to study the microcirculation.

Cosmo et al also used LDI to investigate the effects of ES on arterial blood flow in and around chronic leg ulcers of various etiologies in 15 older adult patients.[208] Mean age of the patients was 73 (range 38 to 85) and ulcer age ranged from 3 months to 16 years. While stimulating the ulcers and periwound areas with low-frequency PC (2 pps at 10–45 mA for 60 min), they measured wound and periwound skin blood flow every 5 min. After 60 min of ES, mean blood flow to the wounds and periwound skin increased 35% and 15%, respectively. Fifteen minutes after terminating the ES, there was still a mean blood flow increase of 29% in the wounds and 9% in the periulcer skin. These results and the results of Petrofsky et al and Wikstrom indicate that ES with PC enhances blood flow in chronic ulcers and periulcer skin.[203-207]

Enhancement of Wound Angiogenesis by Electrical Stimulation

As previously mentioned, Greenberg et al observed that ES augmented angiogenesis in burn wounds of pigs.[183] Junger et al published findings for humans indicating that blood flow increased secondary to increasing capillary density in wounds treated with ES.[124] They reported a mean increase of 43.5% in capillary density in the venous leg ulcers of 15 patients whose wounds had not improved after several months of standard care. They treated the wounds with monophasic PC for 30 min daily for a mean of 38 days. The monophasic PC with a140-μsec pulse duration delivered a weak DC component having an average current of 630 μA at 128 pps or 315 μA at

64 pps. For the first 7 to 14 days, they delivered 630 μA of current to the wounds via the cathode. They then switched the wound treatment electrode polarity to positive for 3 to 10 days. After this time, the polarity was changed back to negative. When the wound had made significant clinical progress toward healing, they reduced the current amplitude to 315 μA. Capillary density, as observed by light microscopy, improved from a prestimulation baseline of 8.05 capillaries/mm^2 to 11.55 capillaries/mm^2 after stimulation ($P < 0.039$). In addition, they also measured the transcutaneous partial pressure of oxygen (TcPO$_2$, or oxygen tension) in the periwound skin before and after the ES treatments. They found that TcPO$_2$ increased from 13.5 to 24.7 mm Hg, respectively (normal mean is 65 mm Hg),[209] and that skin perfusion increased as determined by laser Doppler fluxmetry. They attributed these measured changes to stimulation of capillary regrowth into the patient's wounds.

Additional Evidence of Electrical Stimulation Enhancement of Human Cutaneous Blood Flow–Elevation of Tissue Oxygenation

It is commonly known that cells involved in tissue repair require oxygen to function most efficiently. Cells become ineffectual in hypoxic tissue environments and die in anoxic environments. While oxygen is needed for the survival of cells involved in wound healing, bacterial cells, which have detrimental effects on wound healing processes, are adversely affected by elevated levels of tissue oxygen. Indeed, a reduction in tissue oxygen partial pressure decreases resistance to infection by impairing oxidative killing of bacteria by neutrophils.[210] There is increasing evidence from human studies that ES facilitates a temporary increase in local cutaneous tissue oxygen tension.

The transcutaneous partial pressure of oxygen (TcPO$_2$, or oxygen tension) is related to cutaneous oxygen delivery, which in turn is dependent upon local arterial perfusion. TcPO$_2$, measured in millimeters of mercury (mm Hg), indicates oxygen available to tissues and can be used to assess actual and potential wound sites for likelihood of healing. Gagnier et al assessed the effects of ES on TcPO$_2$ in 30 individuals with spinal cord injury (SCI).[211] Ten patients were assigned to each of three groups that received ES either by a positive or negative monophasic paired spiked waveform or by a symmetrical biphasic square waveform. All three groups received submotor stimulation. Thirty minutes before ES, during 30 min of ES, and 30 min after ES was terminated, the TcPO$_2$ was recorded and compared with the prestimulation baseline. The TcPO$_2$ increased considerably compared with prestimulation values in each of the three groups both during and after ES. However, the differences in TcPO$_2$ changes found among the three different ES waveform groups were not statistically significant. The authors proposed that all three waveforms and the protocol they employed could be used with SCI individuals to increase local TcPO$_2$ to facilitate wound healing.

Dodgen et al further investigated the effects of ES on cutaneous oxygen levels.[212] They enrolled 10 patients with diabetes and 20 age-matched normal subjects to participate in three sessions of ES. They delivered current from monophasic paired spikes through the cathode placed over the gastroc-soleus muscle group at submotor stimulus amplitude. They also delivered an asymmetrical biphasic (balanced) waveform via the cathode placed over the gastroc-soleus with the amplitude set just below muscle contraction or adequate enough to elicit a 1+ level contraction. TcPO$_2$ levels were measured by oximetry for 30 min prior to ES, during a 30-min ES session, and for 30 min after the session. The older normal subjects showed increased TcPO$_2$ following 30 min of ES regardless of the waveform or level of stimulation used. This increase continued for 30 min after ES ended. On the other hand, diabetic subjects showed no significant increases in TcPO$_2$ following 30 min of ES, but did show significant increases in TcPO$_2$ 30 min after ES ended. Possibly, the delayed response in the diabetic subjects could be attributed to neuropathic changes having compromised sympathetic vasomotor control and/or to sensory nerve dysfunction compromising conduction of sensory afferent impulses.

In a study by Peters et al, 11 of 19 diabetic patients were found to have impaired lower extremity (LE) perfusion based on TcPO$_2$ baseline readings of less than 40 mm Hg.[213] The 11 patients received subsensory ES applied to the lateral aspect of the leg for four 60-min periods on 2 consecutive days. Oximetry and LDF were used to assess perfusion before and after the ES sessions. On day 1 of the experiment, measurements were recorded from the dorsum of the foot and at the base of the great toe, bilaterally. Unlike the results of Dodgen et al, who showed a delayed response to an increase in TcPO$_2$, patients in the Peters et al study showed a significant increase in perfusion in the HVPC-stimulated extremity, reflected by a significant increase in TcPO$_2$ after 5 min of ES.[212,213] However, after the ES sessions, the stimulated feet did not show any significant increase in perfusion over control feet. The investigators concluded that subsensory ES elicits a transient increase in cutaneous perfusion in individuals with diabetes and impaired LE perfusion. Thus, ES may be useful in enhancing wound healing in diabetic and other patient populations, such as the elderly and persons with SCI, known to have difficulty healing chronic wounds such as pressure ulcers and leg ulcers due to vascular compromise.

The effect of ES on TcPO$_2$ in patients with SCI has been studied. It is widely recognized that SCI patients have an altered autonomic nervous system below the level of the cord lesion. Some evidence also suggests that a decrease in the number of adrenergic receptors in the skin may occur below the level of the cord lesion.[214] The reduction of adrenergic receptors could in turn cause abnormal vascular responses in the skin below that level. Other investigators have determined that the TcPO$_2$ in the skin over the sacrum in the supine position and the tibia is lower in persons with SCI than in able-bodied individuals.[215-217] This evidence indirectly suggests that the abnormal vascular responses in the skin below the level of the spinal cord lesion may reduce cutaneous blood flow, thereby lowering tissue oxygenation and predisposing the tissues to pressure ulcer formation.

Mawson et al specifically investigated the effect of ES on TcPO$_2$ in the sacral skin of SCI patients at high risk of pressure ulcer development in this area.[216] The objective of their four-part study was to determine whether HVPC stimulation could increase sacral skin TcPO$_2$ in SCI persons lying prone and supine, thereby possibly preventing pressure ulcers. The normal range for TcPO$_2$ is 60 to 100 mm Hg.[215] In one group of three subjects (two incomplete quadriplegic subjects and one complete paraplegic subject), they applied ES with subjects lying prone for two 60-min sessions a few days apart. The cathode was placed at spinal level T6, and the anode was placed at L2. During the first session for each subject, ES parameters were set at 50 V and 10 pps. During the second session, parameters were set at 75 V and 10 pps. Following a 5-min baseline recording, TcPO₂ was recorded at 5-min intervals during each 60-min stimulation period and during a 20-min poststimulation period.

For all three subjects lying in the prone position, they found that stimulation with HVPC led to a sustained, dose-related increase in TcPO₂ at the sacrum. The increase was more dramatic in two subjects with baseline TcPO₂ values at or below the lower end of the normal range. The authors noted that stimulation with 100 V had no additional incremental effect on TcPO₂ levels above that achieved with 75 V. In a second group of 29 SCI subjects lying supine, HVPC was applied with the cathode (polarity assumed) positioned at spinal level T6 and the anode at T12. Prior to ES, TcPO₂ was recorded from sacral skin at the end of a 15-min baseline period. The ES parameters used included 75 V, 10 pps, delivered for 30 min followed by a 15-min poststimulation period of 15 min.

After 30 min of ES, TcPO₂ increased 35%, from a baseline of 49 mm Hg to 66 mm Hg ($P < 0.00001$). This level fell slightly to 63 mm Hg by the end of the 15-min poststimulation period. The investigators hypothesized that ES may be able to prevent development of pressure ulcers by restoring sympathetic tone and vascular resistance below the level of the cord lesion, resulting in an increase in perfusion to the cutaneous capillary beds.

In another study Mawson et al investigated whether cutaneous oxygenation at the sacrum is reduced secondary to reduced perfusion in people with spinal cord injury.[218] They compared TcPO₂ levels in 21 subjects with spinal cord injury and 11 able-bodied controls lying prone and supine on egg-crate mattresses. TcPO₂ levels of SCI individuals were lower than those of controls in the prone position (65.3 ± 16 mm Hg vs 76.4 ± 13 mm Hg; $P = 0.053$) and markedly lower in the supine position (49.1 ± 26 mm Hg vs 74.2 ± 10 mm Hg; $P = 0.004$). Examination of mean TcPO₂ levels over time showed that those of the controls fell slightly after lying supine but returned to the previous level within 15 min. In contrast, those of the spinal cord injured fell rapidly by 18 mm Hg and stabilized after 15 min at a level 27 mm Hg below that of the controls. Five of the 10 (50%) SCI subjects with TcPO₂ levels below the median supine TcPO₂ level had a pressure ulcer compared to 1 among the 11 (9%) SCI subjects with TcPO₂ levels above the median ($P = 0.055$, by Fisher's exact test). These results suggest the need for further studies on the role of reduced cutaneous tissue oxygenation in the etiology and prevention of pressure ulcers.

Bactericidal Effect of Microampere Direct Current on Intact Human Skin

Only one study was found that investigated the antibacterial effect of DC on humans. Via nonmetallic carbon electrodes measuring 10 cm², Bolton et al delivered 5 μA or more

of constant DC per square centimeter for 4 or 18 hours to 29 intact skin sites inoculated with 10⁷ CFUs of *Staphylococcus epidermidis* on the backs of 13 human volunteers.[219] They found that due to a bactericidal effect the numbers of CFUs per square centimeter recovered from sites beneath the anode decreased with increasing stimulation time up to 20 hours and with increasing current density over 50 μA of total DC. When they varied total current and current density independently on 16 sites on the backs of eight subjects, the effect was dependent on current density, not on total current. Additionally, on three subjects they found that when they used the same voltages on electrodes that prevented electrochemical reactions from occurring on the inoculated sites, the electrodes failed to reduce the numbers of CFUs compared with those from control sites. This showed the bactericidal effect to be caused by the electrochemical reactions beneath the anode that produced local acidity in the range of pH 3 or less. In contrast, no significant antibacterial effect of DC stimulation was observed after any duration of current flow or any current density beneath the cathode, beneath which an alkaline pH of 9 or more occurred. Two in vitro studies described earlier agree with the anodal bactericidal effect reported in this study.[153,157]

Clinical Wound Healing with Different Electrical Stimulation Devices and Stimulation Parameters

A review of the clinical research related to treatment of human wounds with ES shows that virtually all research is designed to compare healing of wounds treated with active ES plus standard care to healing of control wounds treated with placebo ES plus standard care. In these studies, both the active and placebo ES treatment was applied to wounds for only 30 to 60 min, 5 to 7 days per week. During the remaining 23 or 23.5 hours of each protocol day, investigators were ethically bound to provide wound treatment, which consisted of standard wound care alone. The clinical trials that provide evidence-based support for ES as an efficacious treatment of chronic wounds are reviewed next according to whether the type of therapeutic current used in the study was DC or PC.

As indicated earlier in the section on electrical terminology, ES may be delivered to wounds to promote wound healing using a variety of stimulation parameters, including current types (DC and PC) and waveforms (monophasic and biphasic, the latter of which may be symmetrical and charged balanced or asymmetrical and charge unbalanced). Other ES parameters for low- and high-voltage ES devices include voltage and current amplitudes, pulse frequencies, and pulse durations as seen in Table 26.3.

Clinical Studies Performed with Conductive Direct Current

In three case series and two randomized controlled trials (RTCs), investigators report using 200- to 800-μA levels of DC (referred to as low-intensity direct current, or LIDC)

Table 26•3 **Conductive Electrical Stimulation Parameters for Wound Healing With Low- and High-Voltage, Monophasic Pulsed Current**

Stimulation Parameters	LVPC Devices (voltage range)	LVPC Devices (wound voltage treatment range)	HVPC Devices (wound voltage treatment range)	HVPC Devices (wound voltage treatment range)	DC Devices (continuous)
Voltage (V)	0–150	25–50	150–500	50–150	0.001–10
Current (mA)	0–100	30–35	0.1–1.0	0.3–0.6	0.2–0.8
Pulse frequency (pps)	0–5000	50–130	0–100	50–100	NA
Pulse duration (μsec)	0–10,000	130	10–100	20–60	NA

DC, direct current; HVPC, high-voltage pulsed current; LVPC, low-voltage pulsed current; NA, not available.

to treat chronic wounds of various etiologies. In three of these studies, wounds were initially treated with the cathode followed by periodic polarity reversal.[116-118] In the other two studies, the cathode and the anode were used solely as the treatment electrodes.[115,218] These studies are summarized in Table 26.4. In the three studies that initially used the cathode, polarity selection was not arbitrary. Instead, polarity selected was based on the finding that initial application of the cathode to the ulcer slowed healing but had an antibacterial effect, while application of the anode enhanced healing but allowed bacterial replication.[116,140] As previously mentioned, in vitro studies have shown that cathodal DC has an antibacterial effect on select wound pathogens.[138,140] Hence, in the study of Wolcott et al,[116] the cathode was applied over the ulcer for 3 days or until the wound was clinically noninfected, then the anode was applied to stimulate healing. They reported that for 75 patients each with one ulcer, 34 (45%) wounds closed completely over 9.6 weeks at a mean healing rate of 18.4% per week. The mean healing rate of the other 41 wounds was 9.3% per week, and these wounds closed an average of 64.7% over 7.2 weeks. Results were also provided for eight patients with bilateral size-matched ulcers of the same etiology. One ulcer on each of these patients was treated with ES and the other control ulcer received standard care alone. Of the eight wounds treated with ES, six closed completely, and the other two closed to 70% of their original size. The eight control wounds healed less well, with three showing no healing, three others healed less than 50%, and the remaining two healed less than 75%. Remarkably, 71% of all the patients in this study were paraplegics whose rate of tissue repair was about 40% slower than that for patients with other primary diagnoses. Despite the overall slower rate of wound healing for the spinal cord-injured patients, the ES protocol was successful in producing an 81.8% wound volume decrease at a healing rate of 13.4% per week for the 75 treated ulcers combined. In this study, if a growth plateau occurred at any time, investigators reversed the electrode polarity, which, based on the results, appears to have had a beneficial effect. However, since there are no reports of multiple polarity reversals during the healing process in nonregenerating

species, there appears to be no scientific explanation for reversal of polarity when wound healing progression stops.

In a parallel study with similar results, Gault and Gatens treated 76 patients with 106 ischemic skin ulcers with the same ES device and protocol used by Wolcott et al.[116,117] Six patients with 12 bilateral size-matched ulcers served as the control group. The six control ulcers that received standard wound care healed at a rate of 14.7% per week compared with 30% per week for the six ES-treated ulcers. Three of the six ES-treated ulcers healed completely, whereas two of the control wounds increased in size during the 4-week treatment period. For the 100 single ulcers in the study, the healing rate was 28.4% per week, with complete healing of 48% of the ulcers in 4.7 weeks, which is an improvement over the single wound results reported by Wolcott et al.[116]

The RCT of Carley and Wainapel was modified from the previous two studies, so patients received 20 hours of ES per week rather than 42 hours.[116-118] They enrolled 30 patients with chronic dermal ulcers and paired them according to age, diagnosis, wound location, etiology, and size. One member of each pair was randomly assigned to have his or her wound treated with 300 to 700 μADC plus standard care; the control member received only standard care. As in the previous two studies described, for the first 3 days ES was applied directly to the wound via the anode following cathodal stimulation. Polarity was reversed for 3 days if measurable healing stopped. The healing rate of wounds treated with ES increased from 1.5 to 2.5 times faster than control wounds over weeks 3, 4, and 5 of the study. In all three of these cathode first studies, ES combined with standard wound care promoted faster rates of healing than standard care alone.

Another case series involved eight venous leg ulcers that were unhealed from 8 months to 5 years, and treated them with 50 to 100 mA of cathodal DC only.[115] All wounds closed in an average of 30 days, and none recurred over a 3-year follow-up period. Note that the use of cathode polarity alone in this latter study does not agree with the polarity protocol used in the three studies that used polarity reversal. On the other hand, healing may have advanced secondary to a reduction in wound bacterial burden owing to the antibacterial effects of cathodal DC or to enhanced fibroblast motility due

Table 26-4 Clinical Wound Healing Studies With Direct Current

Author and Reference	Study Design (N)	Wound Diagnosis	Dressing Type, ES Parameters, Protocol	Current Type and Patient Study Groups	Number of Patients or Wounds	% Patients or Wounds Healed/Time (wks)	Other Information Provided by Authors
Assimacopoulos[115]	Case series	Venous	50–100 µA/cathode	DC	8	100/4 wks	Biopsy 1 year after closed showed dense hyalinized collagen
Wolcott et al[116]	Case series Embedded RCT	Mixed	200–800 µA, 6 hr/day for 0.8–15.4 weeks; switched polarity: cathode, anode, cathode	DC DC Control	75 Bilateral wounds: 8 8	40/9.6 wks 95/15.3 wks 32/15.4 wks	Healing rate/wk: 53 paraplegics = 9.3% 5 venous disease = 14.4 % Other = 100% 13.4% 5.0%
Gault and Gatens[117]	Case series Embedded RCT	Mixed	Protocol similar to Wolcott et al except polarity changes only once	DC DC Control	100 Bilateral wounds: 6 6	48/4.7 wks 50/4 wks 0/4 wks	Healing rate/wk: 28.4% 30.0% 14.7%
Carley and Wainapel[118]	RCT	Not mentioned	300–700 µA, 4 hr/day for 5 weeks; polarity switching same as Wolcott et al	DC Control	15 15	Not mentioned	Healing rate/wk: 18.0% 9.0%
Katelaris et al[221]	Comparative controlled	Venous	20 µA/cathode	DC + povidone Povidone DC + saline Saline	4 11 5 4	Not mentioned	Heal time (mean days) 85. 3 49.2 45.9 46.1
Cukjati et al[218]	RCT	Mixed	600 µA DC, 0.5 hr, 1.0 hr, or 2 hr/day via anode or 15–20 mA PC, 1 hr or 2 hr/day until wound closure	DC or balanced biphasic PC/standard care Sham ES	42 181 54 23	90/60 wks 72/60 wks 70/60 wks	Healing rate/wk not reported Healing rate/wk not reported
Hampton et al[224]	Descriptive, nonblinded	Mixed	µA DC 24 hr/day via cathode w/dressing change every 48 hr; two cycles of 3 wks separated by 1 wk of standard care	All received DC and standard care	18 patients with 21 wounds	3/16 wks	Healing rate/wk for 8 wks = 5.25%

DC, direct current; ES, electrical stimulation; RCT, randomized controlled trial; PC, pulsed current.

to the electrotaxic influence of the cathode, which would favor connective tissue formation in the proliferative phase.

In a RCT of Cukjati et al, patients with 300 wounds were enrolled.[220,214] The most frequent primary diagnosis was spinal cord injury (71.7%). The majority of wounds were pressure ulcers (82.7%) but included wounds of other etiologies: arterial insufficiency (1%), diabetic neuropathy (6.3%), trauma (6.1%), and venous insufficiency (3.9%). Wounds were randomly assigned to be treated with standard wound care ($N = 54$ controls), sham ES ($N = 23$), charge-balanced biphasic PC ($N = 181$), and anodal DC ($N = 42$). Wounds treated with DC either had the anode applied over the wound surface with the cathode placed on healthy skin, or both the anode and cathode were placed on healthy skin on opposite sides of the wound along its margin. Their rationale for using both electrode placements and pooling the resulting data was based on the fact that both methods have been shown to accelerate wound healing.[111,118,126,131,132] The DC was delivered at 600 µA for 0.5, 1, or 2 hours per day until wound closure. Both electrode placement methods were also used for PC that was delivered at 15 to 20 mA for 0.5, 1, or 2 hours daily until wound closure. Results from the pooled ES data showed that over 90% of ES-treated wounds closed within 60 weeks, whereas during the same time period only 70% of sham-treated wounds and 72% of wounds treated with standard care closed. The investigators also found that wounds treated with PC healed significantly faster than wounds treated with sham ES or standard care. Despite the fact that there was no significant difference in the healing rates between wounds treated with PC and DC, the difference in healing rates between the DC-treated wounds and wounds treated with sham ES and standard care was highly in favor of DC, but was not statistically significant.

In a comparative controlled study, Katelaris et al assessed the effect of four different treatments on healing of venous leg ulcers.[221] Their wound treatments consisted of applications of povidone-iodine (PI) or normal saline with and without 20 µA of cathodal DC. They made no mention of treatment duration or frequency. They found no statistical differences in healing times between PI alone and normal saline alone or for normal saline with and without DC stimulation. Needless to say, they found that when PI was used with the cathode, the mean healing time was statistically longer (85.3 days) than the other three treatments; they proposed that this may have been due to cathodal ionization of iodine that lead to cellular toxicity.

Recently, a bioelectric wound dressing called POSiFECT® RD (Biofisica, Odiham, Hampshire, UK, and Atlanta, GA) has been developed to enhance wound healing by augmenting the natural current of injury. The disposable dressing contains a miniature electric circuit that delivers a DC microamperage current to the wound bed for a minimum of 48 hours. The current that comes from two built-in lithium nonrechargeable coin cell batteries is conveyed to a circuit that consists of an anode and cathode. The anode is a flexible metal ring embedded into hydrogel in the dressing, and the cathode is a dime-sized electrode embedded in hydrogel that is applied directly to the wound bed. (Fig. 26.23) For small wounds the anode ring is positioned so it encircles the

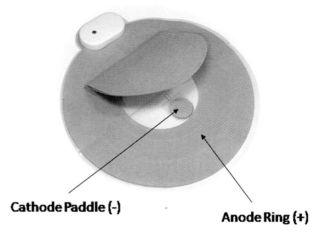

Cathode Paddle (-)   **Anode Ring (+)**

POSiFECT® RD

Figure 26•23 *The POSiFECT RD DC device, with anode ring and cathode tab (BioFisica, Odiham, Hampshire, UK, and Atlanta, GA).*

wound, whereas for large wounds a portion (eg, one third) of the anode ring may be removed so the remaining large part of the ring can be placed with the anode applied to intact skin along a portion of the wound edge. Once the cathode is in place on the wound bed, an appropriate secondary absorptive dressing may be placed over it to absorb excessive exudates. An initial pilot study by Feldman et al showed that pressure ulcer healing was initiated during weeks 1 to 3 of POSiFECT RD treatment.[222] This observation led to a treatment protocol used in subsequent clinical studies in which two cycles of 3 weeks of active treatment were separated by 1 week of standard wound treatment. This treatment regime was used in three separate single case studies involving patients with an intractable heel pressure ulcer, a painful, highly exudating leg ulcer infected with *P. aeruginosa*, and a venous leg ulcer of 2 years duration containing bacterial biofilms.[223-225] In these cases the microamperage ES treatment led to heel ulcer closure in 13 weeks, infected leg ulcer closure in 18 weeks, and enhanced granulation tissue growth in 2 weeks. One other preliminary study with the electric wound dressing, a prospective, descriptive, evaluative, nonblinded clinical trial with a sample of 18 patients with 21 recalcitrant wounds was completed in 2005.[226] Prior to enrolling these patients into the study, all of their wounds had been nonhealing for 6 months. The nine pressure ulcers, 11 venous leg ulcers, and one traumatic wound were treated daily with POSiFECT RD for two cycles of 3 weeks separated by 1 week of standard care alone. All wounds were assessed at 8 weeks and 16 weeks. During the first 8 weeks of the study, the mean surface area of the wounds decreased 7.65 cm^2 from 18 cm^2 to 10.3 cm^2. After 16 weeks, six wounds had closed and six others were almost closed. The remaining nine wounds also showed some improvement (see Table 26.4 Hampton Study). At a 1-year follow-up, 10 wounds had closed and none of the previously healed wounds had recurred. The authors concluded that the outcomes represented clinical effectiveness of the bioelectric dressing and demonstrated the capability for activating chronic wound healing.

Effects of Conductive Direct Current on Biofilms

Biofilms are bacterial communities that live within an extracellular polysaccharide matrix synthesized by bacteria following adhesion to a suitable surface. Bacterial biofilms are resistant to biocides and antibiotics and contribute to wound chronicity. As previously mentioned, data from a few in vitro studies have shown that biofilm killing is significantly enhanced when biocides and antibiotics are exposed to weak electric fields from microamperage levels of DC. (Fig. 26.24) Clinically, only a case study has been reported in which it was concluded that a biofilm was responsible for delayed healing of a venous leg ulcer of 2 years duration in an 83-year-old female.[225] The patient was not able to tolerate compression therapy, but after 6 days of treatment with POSiFECT RD, slough was reduced and the ulcer had decreased in size by 50%. Following 17 additional days of electrical dressing treatment, the wound bed consisted of 100% granulation tissue. The authors presumed that since DC electric fields have been reported to disrupt bacterial biofilms, perhaps the bioelectric dressing interfered with the biofilm viability, allowing healing to proceed.

▶ **PEARL 26•18** Investigators have reported that low-intensity DC electric fields (field strengths of 1.5 to 20 V/cm and current densities of 15 µA/cm2 to 2.1 mA/cm2) can totally override the intrinsic resistance of biofilm bacteria to biocides and antibiotics.[158,159,227,228]

Clinical Studies Performed with Conductive Pulsed Current

Based on voltage levels and pulse durations, PC devices are divided into two voltage ranges. *Low-voltage* PC (LVPC) devices deliver either monophasic or biphasic waveforms with pulse durations up to 1 sec and require lower driving voltages between 0 and 150 V.[100] *High-voltage* PC (HVPC) devices deliver only a twin-peaked monophasic waveform, with phase durations that are typically 5 to 50 µsec long and therefore require higher driving voltages between 150 and 500 V.[100]

Low-Voltage Monophasic Pulsed Current

Between 1989 and 1997, five human subject wound healing studies were published that used the same low-voltage monophasic PC (LVMPC) device (Varipulse®, formerly manufactured by Staodyn Inc., Longmont, CO) with a 140-µsec pulse duration, a peak pulse amplitude of 30 to 35 mA, and a pulse frequency of either 64 or 128 pps.[57,121-124] In these studies summarized in Table 26.5, the accumulated pulse charge was between 250 and 500 µQ/sec, which equates to dosages between 0.89 and 1.78 Q/day delivered to the wound. Calculations of these dosages that have been used clinically to enhance rates of healing with low- and high-voltage PC are shown in Figures 26.25 and 26.26, respectively.

The Varipulse device, upgraded and renamed Dermapulse®, by Staodyn, Inc. was acquired by GerroMed GMBH (Hamburg, Germany), which has developed a device called Wound EL™ that has the same stimulus parameters as the former Dermapulse.

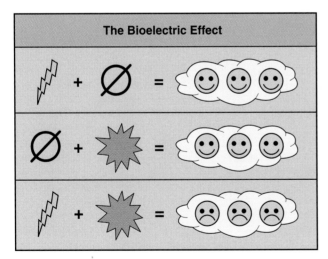

Figure 26•24 *The bioelectric killing effect of biofilms. Killing effects are significantly enhanced when biocides and antibiotics are exposed to weak electric fields from microampere levels of DC.*[158,159,227,228]

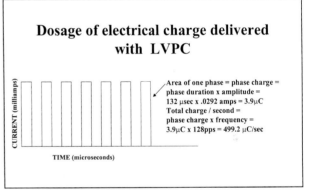

Figure 26•25 *Calculation of exogenous EF dosage that has been used in five clinical studies to enhance rates of wound healing with LVMPC.*[57,121–124]

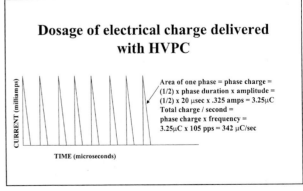

Figure 26•26 *Calculation of exogenous EF dosage that has been used in seven clinical studies to enhance rates of wound healing with HVMPC.*[126,127,236–240]

Table 26•5 Clinical Wound Healing Studies With Low Voltage, Monophasic Pulsed Current

Author and Reference	Study Design (N)	Wound Diagnosis	Dressing Type, ES Parameters, Protocol	Current Type and Patient Study Groups	Number of Patients or Wounds	% Patients or Wounds Healed/Time (wks)	Other Information Provided by Authors
Weiss et al[57]	Case series N = 4	Surgical: Donor sites both anterior thighs	SWC both thighs. PD: 150 μsec PF: 128 pps mA: 35 P: (+) WF: rectangular	LVMPC; one thigh tx 30 min BID for 7 days; other thigh = control	Four females ages 44–68 with chronic venous leg ulcers tx with skin grafts	Donor scars tx with ES were softer and flatter. Control scars were hypertrophic. Thickness of ES tx scars 46% less than control scars	2–3 postoperative months, 3/4 patients agreed to punch biopsies of ES and control donor sites. Two patients tx with ES had marked ↓ in mast cells compared to controls
Feedar et al[121]	Double-blind, placebo controlled N = 50	Mixed: 70% pressure ulcers, 18% surgical, 2% vascular, 10% traumatic	SWC plus ES: PD: 132 μsec PF: 128 pps mA: 29.2 P: (−) for 3 days after wound débrided then change every 3 days until wound reached stage II, at which time PF was changed to 64 pps WF: rectangular	LVMPC; Wounds tx 30 min BID for 4 wks Control: SWC plus placebo ES, 30 min BID for 4 wks Placebo crossover wounds	26 24 14	0/4 0/4 0/4	Healing rate/wk: Active ES: 14%/wk to 44% of initial size Sham ES: 8.25%/wk to 67% of initial size Sham ES: 2.9%/wk to 88% of initial size Active ES: 12.8%/wk to 49% of size after crossover
Gentzkow et al[122]	Double-blind, placebo controlled N = 40	Pressure ulcers stages II–IV	SWC plus ES: PD: 132 μs PF: 128 pps mA: 35 P: (−) until ulcer débrided, then changed every 3 days until wound reached stage II, at which time PF was changed to 64 pps WF: rectangular	LVMPC; Wounds tx 30 min BID for 4 wks Control: SWC plus placebo ES Placebo crossover wounds	21 19 15	0/4 0/4 0/4	Healing rate/wk: Active ES: 12.5%/wk to 49.8% of initial size Sham ES: 5.8%/wk to 23.4% of initial size Sham ES: Healed 13.4% of initial size Active ES: Healed 47.9% f initial size
Gentzkow et al[123]	Prospective, baseline controlled N = 61	Pressure ulcers stages III and IV	SWC first 4 wks. Second 4 wks: SWC plus ES; PD: 1 40 μs PF: 128 pps mA: 35	LVMPC; Wounds tx 30 min BID for 4 wks or longer All patients served as their own controls	61	23% closed in a mean of 8.4 wks (13.2% of stage IV and 34.8% of stage III)	Improvement of 2 or more wound characters: Week 2 = 60.7% Week 4 = 80.4% Last week = 82.0%

Study	Design	Wound Type	ES Parameters	Protocol	N	Outcomes
			P: (–) until wound débrided then alternated +/– if wound condition worsened WF: rectangular	Criteria for wound improvement were: Improvement of two or more wound characters Improvement of one or more wound stages		Improvement of 1 or more wound stages: Week 2 = 27.9% Week 4 = 58.8% Last week = 73.8%
Junger et al[124]	Open prospective pilot study N = 15	Venous leg ulcers	Previous tx of compression therapy failed to show clinical progress over a mean of 6.5 yr. ES plus compression therapy consisted of: PD: 140 μsec PF: 128 pps mA: 42 P: (–) until wound granulated then (+) and 64 pps during epithelialization WF: rectangular	LVMPC; Wounds tx 30 min/day for 38 days	15 / 0/8	6.5 years of compression therapy of 15 ulcers failed to show significant evidence of healing After a mean of 38 days of ES ulcer area ↓ 63% (P <0.01) from 16 to 6 cm² and wound capillary count ↑ 8.05/mm² to 11.55 mm² (+43.5%)
Barczak et al[229]	Double-blind, placebo controlled N = 24	Pressure ulcers, grade 3-5 [Daniel 230] In patients with spinal cord injury	SWC plus ES: PD: 140 PF: 128 pps mA: 38 P: (–) until wound granulated, then +/– change every 3 days WF: rectangular	LVMPC; ES group Placebo group	24/33 10/16 14/17	First 28 days: ↓/day = 1.1% ↓/day = 2.0% Median healing 73% faster for ES group (P = 0.028)
Wood et al[119]	Double-blind RCT N = 74	Pressure ulcers Stage II and III	SWC (assumed) plus 3, 1-min ES tx/wk of 300 μA at 0.5 pps and 3, 3-min tx of 600 μA at 0.5 pps to wound edge. P: Not reported. WF: Not reported	LVMPC; ES group Placebo group	74 43 31 / 58/8 3/8	Plastic surgery after 28 days: 86/12 wks 69/12 wks; Decrease wound size >80%: 73% 13%
Kaada[109]	Case series N = 10	Mixed	Dressing not reported. ES 3/day, 30–40 min PD: Not reported PF: 100 pps mA: 15–30 P: Not reported WF: Not reported	LVMPC; (TENS)	10 / 70/22	None reported

BID, twice daily; ES, electrical stimulation; LVMPC, low-voltage monophasic pulsed current; P, polarity; PD, pulse duration; PF, pulse frequency; pps, pulses per second; RCT, random controlled trial; SWC, standard wound care; tx, treatment; WF, waveform.

This device has produced a greater antibacterial effect with positive polarity than negative polarity and has demonstrated that bacterial reductions differed significantly between positive polarity and control and negative polarity and control, with the highest log 10 reduction factor achieved with positive polarity.[157] (Fig. 26.27; see Table 26.2) Please note that the characteristics of this PC do not fit the definition of DC; therefore, it would be misleading to refer to it as pulsed low-intensity direct current.

In the first of five studies mentioned, Weiss et al found that 1 month after 7-day treatment of four human subject partial-thickness donor sites with positive polarity ES from the Varapulse,[57] the surgically induced wounds had softer and flatter scars compared with hypertrophic contralateral control scars. Histological findings from punch biopsies verified that electrically treated scars were reduced in thickness by a mean of 46% compared with control scars. Biopsy results also established that the ES-treated scars had a marked reduction in mast cells, which suggests that ES can limit fibrosis, possibly by reducing the number of mast cells.

In another study with the Varipulse, investigators reported the results of a 4-week prospective, randomized, double-blind multicenter trial in which 26 chronic dermal ulcers of mixed etiologies were treated with standard wound care and 30 min twice daily of active cathodal ES at an initial pulse frequency of 128 pps and a peak amplitude of 29.2 mA (500 µQ/sec).[121] Thirty-five (70%) of the wounds were stage II, III, and IV pressure ulcers. When the ulcer was débrided or exuded serosanguinous drainage, the treatment electrode polarity was reversed every 3 days until the wound progressed to a partial-thickness ulcer. Maintaining the same amplitude, the pulse frequency was then reduced to 64 pps (250 µQ/sec), and the polarity of the treatment electrode was changed daily until the wound closed. The 24 patients randomized to the control group were treated with standard wound care 24 hours a day and sham ES 30 min twice daily. After 4 weeks, wounds in the treatment and control groups averaged 44% and 67% of their initial size ($P < 0.02$). The weekly healing rates were 14% and 8.25%, respectively. None of the wounds treated with ES increased in size, compared to five wounds in the control group. After being assigned to the control group for 4 weeks, 14 wounds were crossed over to the ES protocol. After 4 weeks of sham ES treatment, the mean wound size reduction was 11.3% at a healing rate of 2.9% per week. After 4 weeks of active ES, these wounds were 49% of their size at crossover and had healed at a rate of 12.8% per week. The authors concluded that the results of the study support the use of low-voltage monophasic PC as an effective intervention for enhancing the healing of chronic dermal ulcers.

Using the same low-volt PC device (Dermapulse, formerly called Varapulse) and the parameters and protocol used in the study just described, Gentzkow et al conducted a double-blind, randomized multicenter trial on 37 patients with 40 pressure ulcers.[122] Nineteen ulcers were treated with standard wound care plus sham ES, and 21 were treated with standard care plus active ES. After 4 weeks, the ES-treated wounds had healed more than twice the rate as that of sham-treated ulcers (49.8% vs 23.4%, $P = 0.042$), at weekly healing rates of 12.5% and 5.8%, respectively. At the end of the 4-week study period, 15 patients who had received sham ES received active ES. In the 15 crossover patients, 4 weeks of active ES produced 3.5 times as much healing as had occurred during the 4 weeks of sham treatment (47.9% vs 13.4%, $P = 0.012$). Not surprisingly, the average healing after 4 weeks of active ES for the 15 crossover ulcers (49.9%) was almost identical to the healing after the first 4 weeks of the 21 ulcers in the active ES group (49.8%), which indicates a reliable treatment effect.

In a subsequent study, Gentzkow et al again used the same ES device (Dermapulse), ES parameters, and protocol in a prospective, baseline-controlled study on pressure ulcers in three health-care facilities over a mean of 8.4 weeks.[123] In this study, a cohort of 61 stage III or IV pressure ulcers served as their own control. As in the previous study, the first 4 weeks were a controlled phase during which all wounds received carefully documented standard wound care, consisting of dressings that maintained a moist wound environment, a 2-hour turning and repositioning schedule, a pressure-reducing bed surface, infection control, and nutritional support. Only wounds that did not demonstrate measurable progress toward closure or regressed during the control period were enrolled in the second phase of the study.

After 4 weeks of optimal standard wound care, 61 wounds in 51 patients met the inclusion criteria for phase-two enrollment in which patients continued to receive the same standard wound care. In addition, 30-min sessions twice daily of active ES were added to their daily wound care program. With this research design, the authors assumed that subsequent changes in wound measurements and select healing characteristics could be attributed to the effects of ES. Progress toward wound healing as defined by the authors was a reduction of at least one wound stage or two wound characters (necrosis, purulence, exudates, covered by eschar). In the last week of the study (mean 7.3 weeks), 50 of 61 wounds (82.0%) had improved two or more wound characters and 45 of 61 wounds (73.8 %) had improved one or more stages toward wound closure.

In the fifth study in which the Dermapulse was used, Junger et al investigated the effect of ES on wound healing and angiogenesis.[124] They treated 15 venous leg ulcers that had failed to show significant evidence of healing with standard compression therapy over a mean period of 79 months. After

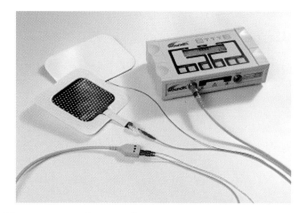

Figure 26·27 *The woundEL LVMPC device delivers the same signal previously used in clinical wound healing studies performed in the United States and Germany that reported positive healing outcomes (GerroMed Pflege, Hamburg, Germany).*[57,121-124,229]

a mean of 38 days of wound treatment with daily ES for 30 min, the mean ulcer area decreased by 63% ($P < 0.01$) from 16 to 6 cm². Prior to starting ES treatment, when they examined these wounds with light microscopy to determine capillary density, they counted a mean of 8.05 capillaries per square millimeter compared with 11.55 capillaries per square millimeter after ES ($P < 0.039$). The latter findings agree with those of other investigators who used the same ES device and observed prominent neovascularity following stimulation of burn wounds in pigs.[181] In summary, three of the five studies described above showed statistically significant decreases in the surface areas of wounds treated with ES over an average of 4.6 weeks.[119,121,122]

Dermapulse was also used in a German study to determine the therapeutic effectiveness of ES in paraplegic patients with pressure ulcers.[229] In this randomized, double-blind, placebo-controlled trial, 24 SCI patients were enrolled with 33 stage III to V pressure ulcers.[230] Fourteen patients with 17 ulcers were assigned to the control group, and 10 patients with 16 ulcers were assigned to the ES group. Wounds of both groups were surgically débrided prior to starting the study protocol, and all wounds were subsequently treated with standard care. In addition, the ES group received active ES, and the control group received inactive ES. The Dermapulse parameters were set to deliver the dosage described for the five studies mentioned above.[57,121-124] The study protocol was carried out for 30 min twice daily, 7 days per week, for 28 days. The primary outcome measure was percentage of wound size decrease per day over 28 days. At 28 days ES-treated wounds decreased 2% per day and control wounds decreased 1.1% per day. Median wound healing after 28 days was 73% faster for the ES group ($P = 0.028$). After 28 days, plastic surgery was performed to close 13 of 17 control wounds and 14 of 16 ES wounds. At 12 weeks 86% of ES-treated wounds were closed compared with 69% of control wounds (nonsignificant).

In an additional study that used low-voltage PC, authors described the current as "pulsed low-intensity direct current" that was delivered to the periwound tissue at 0.5 pps.[119] The investigators referred to the current as being DC; thus, the assumption is that it was monophasic, but not DC, because the definition of DC is the continuous flow of charged particles for 1 sec or longer. That means the current used in the study, which was delivered at 0.5 pps and a pulse duration of 500 μsec, falls into the monophasic PC category. The authors described the trial as a multicenter, double-blind placebo study in which 71 patients with 74 chronic stage II and III pressure ulcers were treated with either an active or a sham "pulsed DC" device after showing no significant improvement after 5 weeks of standard wound care. Active devices were used to treat 43 ulcers and sham devices were used to treat 31 ulcers, three times a week for 8 weeks. Neither the patient nor the clinician knew the identity of active or sham devices. Both groups also received standard wound care. The active devices initially delivered 300 μA of PC at 0.5 pps through negatively charged probe electrodes for 1 min to each of three different periwound sites on opposite sides of the ulcer, followed by 600 μA for 3 min at each site. After 8 weeks, 25 of the 43 ulcers (58%) closed in the active device group, whereas only 1 of

31 ulcers (3%) closed in the sham (placebo) group. A statistical analysis revealed a highly significant difference for the decrease in ulcer surface area of the 43 wounds treated with the active device compared with the 31 wounds treated with the sham device ($P < 0.0001$).

In another study, Kaada reported results from a case study that 7 of 10 chronic wounds of mixed etiologies healed in 22 weeks following treatment with LVMPC from a TENS device.[109]

Low-Voltage Biphasic Pulsed Current

The two phases of biphasic PC may be symmetrical and charge balanced, which means the charge of each phase is equal and there is zero net DC (no electrochemical effect on tissues). Alternatively, the two phases may be asymmetrical and either charge balanced or unbalanced. If the two phases are charge balanced, there is also zero net DC, but if they are charge unbalanced, there will be some net DC effect on tissues. Studies that report using biphasic PC do not always indicate whether the pulse phases are charge balanced or charge unbalanced. Transcutaneous electrical nerve stimulators (TENS) are ES devices that are labeled for pain suppression applications by the FDA. Most of these devices are intentionally designed to deliver biphasic charge-balanced pulses, so there is zero net DC to eliminate the possibility of electrochemical skin irritation. Several clinical studies have investigated the effects of TENS (ie, LV biphasic PC, or LVBPC) on wound healing. These studies summarized in Table 26.6 will be reviewed next in this section.

Many studies have reported the effects of LVBPC on wound healing. Six of the studies used solely the indirect electrode or bipolar placement method of applying the treatment electrodes on the periwound skin adjacent to the wound edge.[110,111,114,130,131,220] (Fig 26.28) One study used both the direct or monopolar placement method of applying the treatment electrode directly over the wound and the indirect

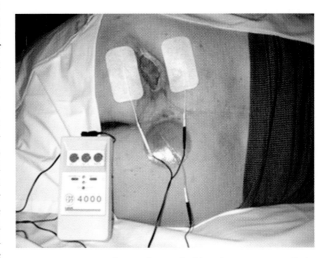

Figure 26•28 *Conductively coupled bipolar treatment electrodes of opposite polarity positioned on opposite sides of a wound. This electrode placement approach has been used to deliver LVBPC in six clinical studies.*[110,111,114,130,131,220]

Table 26•6 Clinical Wound Healing Studies With Low-Voltage, Biphasic Pulsed Current

Author and Reference	Study Design (N)	Wound Diagnosis	Dressing Type, ES Parameters, Protocol	Current Type and Patient Study Groups	Number of Patients or Wounds	% Patients or Wounds Healed/Time (wks)	Other Information Provided by Authors
Kaada et al[110]	Case series	Hanson's disease ulcers	Dressing not reported. ES 30 min BID, 5–6/wk PD: Not reported PF: 100 pps mA: 25 Polarity: (−) WF: Symmetrical	LVBPC	32	59/12	Mean healing time 5.2 wks
Karba et al[111]	Case series	Pressure ulcers Vascular Traumatic	Dressing not reported. ES 60 min/day PD: 250 μs PF: 40 mA: 15–20 W: Symmetrical	LVBPC	14 82 17	107/113 (time not reported)	100% of pressure ulcers healed in 5.5 wks. 90% of vascular ulcers healed in 10 wks. No report
Lundeberg et al[112]	Double-blind RCT	Diabetic ulcers	SWC plus ES: 20 min BID ES PD: 1 ms PF: 80 pps mA: Submotor Controls: Moist wound care alone	LVBPC (ES active) No ES	32 32	42/12 15/12	% ulcers healed: 2 wks: 0% ES vs. 4% sham 4 wks: 12% ES vs 7% sham 8 wks: 25% ES vs 11% sham 12 wks: 42% ES vs 15% sham
Stefanovska et al[114]	Case series	7 SCI with 9 pressure ulcers	Dressing not reported. ES 20 min BID to wound edge PD: 250 μsec PF: 40 pps mA: <50 WF: Not reported	LVBPC	9	8/9 healed in mean of 14.4 wks	Mean healing rate = 0.07 cm²/day
Baker et al[130]	RCT	80 SCI patients with 185 pressure ulcers	SWC plus ES: 30 min TID to wound edge 1. WF = asymmetrical PD: 100 μsec PF: 50 pps mA: Submotor On/off =7:7 sec 2. WF: Symmetrical PD: 300 μsec PF: 50 pps mA: Submotor	LVBPC 1. 2. 3. 4. Controls	35 32 18 19	Not reported	Mean wound area % decrease/wk → 63.7 50.6 38.5 29.2

Reference	Design	Wound population	Protocol / Parameters	ES type	Sample size	Outcome	Results / Conclusions
Baker et al[131]	RCT	Diabetic ulcers	3. Microcurrent PD: 10 μs PF: 1 pps mA: 4, submotor On/off: 7:7 4. Controls SWC plus ES: Parameters and protocol as above study by Baker et al[131]	LVBPC 1. 2. 3. 4.	29 24 20 20	Not reported	27.0 16.4 17.2 17.3 Wounds treated with asymmetrical biphasic increased healing rates by 60% over controls.
Debrecini et al[132]	Prospective, historic controls	24 ischemic LEs; 10 diabetic	SWC plus vascular drugs and ES: PD: Not reported PF: 1–2 pps mA: 15–30, 20 min/day for 1 yr	LVBPC	12 ischemic ulcers; 6 LE gangrene	After 1 yr, 20/24 reported ↓ ischemic pain; halted progress of gangrene or healed ulcers	For 5–6 yr prior, all patients treated with pentoxifylline and vasodilator or antiplatelet drugs, none of which had positive effects.
Frantz[231]	Double-blind RCT	Pressure ulcers	SWC plus ES: (parameters not reported). ES for 30 min TID for 8 wks. Controls tx with SWC.	LVBPC (TENS) (ES active) Control	19 15	42/8 20/8	All ulcers in ES group healed by 20 wks.
Sumano et al[232]	Historical controls	Mixed wounds and burns	Dry dressing reported for 34 nonburn wounds. Saline dressing for 10 burn wounds. ES to all wounds via acupuncture needles in skin around wound edge daily or every other day. ES parameters: PD: Not reported PF: 67 pps mA: 0.04 delivered charge density of 0.4 to 0.8 C/cm².	Modified biphasic wave	44 wounds 34 wounds 10 burns	Not reported	Healing reported to have proceeded in an organized manner
Adunsky et al[233]	Double-blind RCT	Pressure ulcers	SWC plus ES: (parameters not reported) 20 min TID for 2 wks then BID. Controls received placebo ES plus standard moist care. 8-week study with 12-wk follow-up	LVBPC (ES active) Control	35 28	Not reported	Ulcer area decrease and rate of healing better in active ES than control group through day 45. Between days 46 and 57, there were no differences between groups. Time needed for wound closure 52% longer for control group.

BID, twice daily; ES, electrical stimulation; LE, lower extremity; LVBPC, low-voltage biphasic pulsed current; P, polarity; PD, pulse duration; PF, pulse frequency; RCT, random controlled trial; SCI, spinal cord injury; SWC, standard wound care; TID, three times daily; tx, treatment; WF, waveform.

or bipolar electrode application method.[220] (Figs. 26.28 and 26.29) In the latter study, the rationale for using both electrode placements and pooling the data from both was based on the authors' realization that both methods have been shown to enhance wound healing.[118,111,126,131,132] An additional study was a case series and another was a nonrandomized-controlled trial.[111,114] In two other studies that used only the indirect electrode placement method, the authors stated they purposely wanted to stimulate cutaneous nerves rather than deliver current directly into the wound tissue where there are no cutaneous nerves, as has been done in previous studies.[130,131] They reasoned that stimulation of the cutaneous nerves near the wound could enhance wound healing through activation of the peripheral nervous system.

In these two randomized controlled studies, the same low-voltage PC device (Ultrastim; Henley International, Houston, TX [no longer in business]) and ES parameters were used.[130,131] In both studies the investigators treated wounds with one of four ES interventions: biphasic asymmetrical waveform (charge balanced), biphasic symmetrical waveform (charge balanced), microcurrent stimulation, or an ES sham protocol. Because the patients in these studies had impaired protective sensation in periwound skin secondary to spinal cord injury or diabetes, the authors stated that one purpose of both studies was to evaluate the efficacy of ES in enhancing wound healing in patients with neurologically impaired skin, while minimizing adverse electrochemical effects of the stimulation on the skin.[130,131] In the 4-week study involving dermal ulcers in patients with spinal cord injury, wounds were treated to closure. Thirty-five wounds treated with the biphasic asymmetrical waveform closed, 32 treated with the biphasic symmetrical waveform closed, 18 with microcurrent closed, and 19 treated with sham ES closed. A statistically significant difference was found between the group that received the biphasic asymmetrical waveform and the combined microcurrent and sham ES groups that served as controls. No significant difference was found between the combined

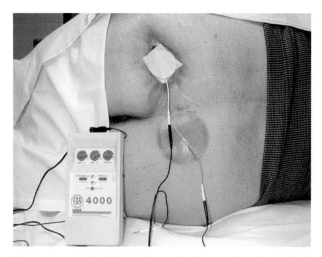

Figure 26•29 *Conductively coupled monopolar electrode placement with treatment electrode placed on a conductive saline, moist gauze, or on a wafer hydrogel dressing. The return electrode is applied to intact skin.*

groups treated with microcurrent and sham ES and the group treated with the symmetrical biphasic waveform. No adverse electrochemical effects were observed on the skin of patients in this study. Interestingly, 11 control patients treated with standard wound care for 4 weeks had a mean weekly healing rate of 9.7%. When these 11 patients were crossed over to be treated with active ES, their mean healing rate was statistically greater during the ES protocol (43.3% per week), and 7 of the 11 wounds closed during that time. The findings of this study agree with those of Stefanovska et al and Cukjati et al, who also compared wounds treated with biphasic asymmetrical ES with DC-stimulated and control wounds.[114,220] In the second study by Baker et al, the increased healing rate of diabetic foot ulcers treated with the biphasic asymmetrical waveform plus standard wound care enhanced healing by almost 60% over control wounds treated only with standard wound care, but there was no statistical difference between the group treated with symmetrical biphasic ES and the group treated with asymmetrical biphasic ES.[131]

In six other clinical studies that investigated the effects of ES on wound healing, TENS devices were used to deliver biphasic PC. One of these studies was a case report and two were uncontrolled case series in which ulcers of various etiologies, including neuropathic lesions, were treated by placing the electrodes over cutaneous nerves in the periwound skin.[108,109,113] As in other studies, the rationale for using the indirect stimulation method was based on the premise that a neuronally triggered mechanism would augment wound healing.[109,111,113,114,119,130,131] Kaada and Emru also reported using TENS (biphasic PC) in a case series to treat 32 patients with leg ulcers secondary to Hansen's disease that had failed to heal during extended periods of standard care.[110] Using the indirect method, ES was delivered to the wounds at 25 mA and 100 pps, with pulse durations of 200 to 300 µsec for 30 min twice daily, 5 to 6 days a week. Twelve weeks after the study terminated, 59% of the wounds closed, and wounds of all those who completed therapy closed in a mean of 5.2 weeks. In a randomized controlled trial, Lundeberg et al evaluated the effect of TENS (biphasic asymmetrical PC) on wound healing.[112] Sixty-four patients with chronic diabetic foot ulcers were randomized to either receive active ES (parameters not given) or sham ES (controls) for 20 min twice daily for 12 weeks in addition to standard wound care. Polarity of the treatment electrode was changed each session. After 12 weeks, there was a statistically significant treatment effect based on closure of 42% of wounds in the active ES group compared to 15% of the controls ($P < 0.05$). In a randomized, double-blind clinical trial, Frantz used a TENS device to deliver biphasic PC to chronic wounds.[231] Thirty-four patients, each with one pressure ulcer that had been resistant to healing for at least 3 months, were randomized to one of two wound treatment groups. All ulcers in both groups were treated with saline-moist gauze that was changed TID and remoistened at 4-hour intervals. In one group this was combined with active ES applied to the wound for 30 min TID. The same protocol was used on the second group, except they received sham ES. During the 8-week protocol, eight wounds closed with active ES compared with three that closed with sham ES; however, all wounds treated with active ES closed by 20 weeks.

In summary, several of the studies that evaluated the effect of low-voltage biphasic PC on wound healing have demonstrated statistically significant enhancement of both healing rate and number of wounds closed compared to controls.[112,130,131]

In 34 chronic wounds of mixed etiologies and 10 burn wounds, investigators delivered modified biphasic PC to the wounds by inserting acupuncture needles subcutaneously into periwound skin surrounding the wounds daily or every other day.[232] The authors reported using an ES device that delivered a charge density between 0.4 and 0.8 C/cm² to the wound edge perimeter. Although the authors did not report the healing rates or incidence of wound closure, they did indicate a statistical correlation ($r = 0.98$) between wound severity and the number of treatments needed for wound closure.

Adunsky and Ohry describe the use of DC in the treatment of stage III pressure ulcers (decubitus direct current treatment) to evaluate rates of ulcer closure and wound area reduction.[233] However, specifications for the device (Lifewave Hi-Tech Medical Devices Ltd., Tel Aviv, Israel) indicate that the Lifewave™ BST unit delivers symmetrical, biphasic, rectangular pulses with zero net DC along with stochastic (random) pulses. (Fig 26.30) During the trial, the device is said to have determined wound size measurements and recorded the bioelectrical activity around the wound before and after each treatment. Although the authors made no mention of the ES treatment parameters used, the device specifications indicate that the current output is limited to 10 mA, the pulse duration is 4 ms, and pulse frequency is fixed at 2 pps. The study is described as a multicenter, randomized, double-blind, placebo-controlled trial that included 63 patients allocated to an active ES treatment group ($N = 35$) and an inactive ES placebo control group ($N = 28$). The study lasted 8 consecutive weeks, followed by a 12-week follow-up period. At the end of treatment (day 47) and at the end of the follow-up period (day 147), there was no difference between the groups with respect to rates of complete closure of ulcers ($P = 0.28$ and 0.39, respectively),

as well as for the mean time required to achieve complete wound closure ($P = 0.16$). However, the authors reported that absolute ulcer area reduction and rate of wound area reduction (reflected by change from baseline ulcer area percentage) were better in patients allotted to the ES treatment group until day 45 (standardized estimate for trend of healing speed ≥0.44 and –0.14 for treatment and control groups, respectively). From day 45 to day 57, there were no differences between the two groups. A logistic regression analysis favored complete healing in the treatment group, compared with the control group (odds ratio 1.6, CI 0.4–4.73). Analysis of data from protocol patients disclosed that time needed for wound closure was 52% longer in the control group ($P = 0.03$) compared with the treatment group. The results presented in this study suggest that the charge-balanced biphasic ES signal used for treatment of stage III pressure ulcers in addition to standard wound care may be useful in accelerating the healing process during the initial period of care.

Both LVMPC and LVBPC have been used in several clinical studies on pressure ulcers. Those studies are summarized in Table 26.7.

High-Voltage Monophasic Pulsed Current

High voltage monophasic PC (HVMPC; frequently referred to as HVPC) is characterized by its "twin pulses" of short duration (typically, 20 to 60 μsec) and a voltage range of 150 to 500 V. (See Fig. 26.17) Because of the assumption that all monophasic pulses are DC, HVMPC is frequently referred to as HVPGC (G for galvanic), which implies that there is a DC component that will create electrochemical effects on tissues. However, research has shown that HVMPC does not cause pH changes that lead to undesirable polar effects (eg, blistering and burning) on human skin.[129] Thirteen publications from clinical studies,[126,127,236-246] including an experimental animal study, three case reports, one small noncontrolled comparative trial, one case series, and seven clinical trials, have evaluated the effects of HVMPC on wound healing. These studies are summarized in Table 26.8. Interestingly, 10 of these 12 studies evaluated the effects of HVMPC on vascular or diabetic ulcers of the lower extremity. These studies are summarized in Table 26.9, which is modified after a table by Kloth in a review of lower-extremity wounds.[234]

The use of HVPC to enhance tissue healing dates back to 1966 when a veterinarian applied this type of current to the hind limbs of dogs whose hind limb circulation was compromised for 12 hours by proximal tourniquet application.[235] Twenty-four hours after tourniquet removal, the hind limbs of four dogs were treated with HVPC for 5 min daily for 14 days, while four control dogs did not receive HVPC treatment. After the 14-day study, period control dogs developed severe gangrene, whereas dogs treated with HVPC walked without limping and had no observable differences between their normal and traumatized limbs. A case report has also reported a positive outcome following HVPC treatment of a patient with an infected wound.[128] However, in the latter study the patient was treated simultaneously with HVPC and antibiotics; therefore, no conclusion can be made regarding

Text continued on page 498

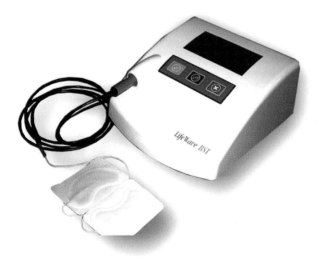

Figure 26•30 *The Lifewave BST LVBPC device used in a clinical study on pressure ulcers (Lifewave Hi-Tech Medical Devices Ltd., Tel Aviv, Israel).[233]*

Table 26•7 Studies of Pressure Ulcers Treated With Conductive Electrical Stimulation (LVMPC and LVBPC)

Author and Reference	Study Design (N)	Wound Diagnosis	Dressing Type, ES Parameters, Protocol	Current Type and Patient Study Groups	Number of Patients or Wounds	% Patients or Wounds Healed/Time (wks)	Other Information Provided by Authors
Gentzkow et al[122]	Double-blind, placebo controlled N = 40	Pressure ulcers stages II–IV	SWC plus ES: PD: 132 μsec PF: 128 pps mA: 35 P: (−) until ulcer débrided then change every 3 days until wound reached stage II, at which time PF was changed to 64 pps WF: rectangular	LVMPC; Wounds tx 30 min BID for 4 wks Control: SWC plus placebo ES Placebo crossover wounds	21 19 15	0/4 0/4 0/4	Healing rate/wk: Active ES: 12.5%/wk to 49.8% of initial size Sham ES: 5.8%/wk to 23.4% of initial size Sham ES: Healed 13.4% of initial size Active ES: Healed 47.9% of initial size
Gentzkow et al[123]	Prospective, baseline-controlled N = 61	Pressure ulcers Stages III, IV	SWC first 4 wks Second 4 wks: SWC plus ES; PD: 1 40 μsec PF: 128 pps mA: 35 P: (−) until wound débrided, then alternated +/− if wound condition worsened WF: rectangular	LVMPC; Wounds tx 3C min BID for 4 wks or longer All patients served as their own controls. Criteria for wound improvement were: Improvement of 2 or more wound characters Improvement of 1 or more wound stages	61	23% closed in a mean of 8.4 wks. (13.2% of stage IV and 34.8% of stage III)	Improvement of 2 or more wound characters: Week 2 = 60.7% Week 4 = 80.4% Last week = 82.0% Improvement of 1 or more wound stages: Week 2 = 27.9% Week 4 = 58.8% Last week = 73.8%
Barczak et al[229]	Double-blind, placebo controlled N = 24	Pressure ulcers, grade 3–5 [Daniel[230]] In patients with SCI	SWC plus ES: PD: 140 PF: 128 pps mA: 38 P: (−) until wound granulated then +/− change every 3 days WF: rectangular	LVMPC; ES group Pacebo group	24/33 10/16 14/17	First 28 days: ↓/day = 1.1% ↓/day = 2.0% Median healing 73% faster for ES group (P = 0.028).	Plastic surgery after 28 days: 86/12 wks 69/12 wks

Author	Study type	Subjects	Intervention	Group	N	Healed	Outcome
Wood et al[119]	Double-blind RCT N = 74	Pressure ulcers stage II, III	SWC (assumed) plus 3, 1-min ES tx/wk of 300 μA at 0.5 pps and 3, 3-min tx of 600 μA at 0.5 pps for 8 weeks to wound edge. P: Not reported. WF: Not reported.	LVMPC; ES group Placebo group	74 43 31	58/8 3/8	Decrease wound size >80%: 73% 13%
Karba et al[111]	Case series	Pressure ulcers	Dressing not reported ES 60 min/day PD: 250 μsec PF: 40 mA: 15-20 W: symmetrical	LVBPC	14		100% of PUs healed in 5.5 wks.
Stefanovska et al[114]	Case series	7 SCI with 9 pressure ulcers	Dressing not reported. ES 20 min BID to wound edge PD: 250 μsec PF: 40 pps mA: <50 WF: Not reported	LVBPC	9	8/9 healed in mean of 14.4 wks	Mean healing rate = 0.07 cm²/day.
Baker et al[130]	RCT	80 SCI patients with 185 pressure ulcers	SWC plus ES: 30 min TID to wound edge 1. WF = asymmetrical PD: 100 μsec PF: 50 pps mA: Submotor On/off = 7.7 sec 2. WF: symmetrical PD: 300 μsec PF: 50 pps mA: Submotor 3. Microcurrent PD: 10 μsec PF: 1 pps mA: 4, Submotor On/off: 7.7 4. Controls	LVBPC 1. 2. 3. 4. Controls	35 32 18 19	Not reported.	Mean wound area % decrease/wk ↓ 63.7 50.6 38.5 29.2
Frantz[231]	Double-blind RCT	Pressure ulcers	SWC plus ES: (parameters not reported). ES for 30 min TID for 8 wks. Controls tx with SWC	LVBPC (TENS) (ES active) Control	19 15	42/8 20/8	All ulcers in ES group healed by 20 wks.

Continued

Table 26•7 Studies of Pressure Ulcers Treated With Conductive Electrical Stimulation—cont'd

Author and Reference	Study Design (N)	Wound Diagnosis	Dressing Type, ES Parameters, Protocol	Current Type and Patient Study Groups	Number of Patients or Wounds	% Patients or Wounds Healed/Time (wks)	Other Information Provided by Authors
Adunsky et al[233]	Double-blind RCT	Pressure ulcers	SWC plus ES: (parameters not reported) 20 min TID for 2 wks then BID Controls received placebo ES plus standard moist care. 8-wk study with 12-wk follow-up	LVBPC (ES active) Control	35 28	Not reported	Ulcer area decrease and rate of healing better in active ES than control group through day 45. Between days 46 and 57 there were no differences between groups. Time needed for wound closure 52% longer for control group.
Griffin et al[127]	RCT N = 17	Pressure ulcers in SCI men	SWC plus ES 60 min/day/20 days PD: 20–60 μsec PF: 100 pps V: 200 P: (–) Dosage: 500 μC/sec	HVPC active Control (placebo ES)	8 9	On days 5, 15, 20, ES active group had significantly greater wound size reductions than placebo group.	20% reduction in wound size/wk for 4 wks

BID, twice daily; ES, electrical stimulation; HVPC, high-voltage pulsed current; LVBPC, low-voltage biphasic pulsed current; LVMPC, low-voltage monophasic pulsed current; P, polarity; PD, pulse duration; PF, pulse frequency; PU, pressure ulcer; RCT, random controlled trial; SCI, spinal cord injury; SWC, standard wound care; TID, three times daily; tx, treatment; WF, waveform.

Table 26•8 Clinical Wound Healing Studies With High-Voltage, Monophasic Pulsed Current (HVPC)

Author and Reference	Study Design (N)	Wound Diagnosis	Dressing Type, ES Parameters, Protocol	Current Type and Patient Study Groups	Number of Patients or Wounds	% Patients or Wounds Healed/Time (wks)	Other Information Provided by Authors
Kloth et al[234]	RCT Single blind N = 16	Mixed	SWC plus ES 45 min/day PD: 20–60 μsec PF:105 pps V: Submotor Dosage: 342 μC/sec P: (+) initially then (−/+) alternate daily	HVMPC active 5 days/wk Control (placebo crossover)	9 7	100/7.3 wks 0/17 wks	Healing rate/wk 45% 11.6% larger 38%/wk in 8.3 wks
Griffin et al[127]	RCT N = 17	Pressure ulcers in SCI men	SWC plus ES 60 min/day/ 20 day PD: 20–60 μsec PF: 100 pps V: 200 P: (−) Dosage: 500 μC/sec	HVPC active Control (placebo ES)	8 9	On days 5, 15, 20, ES active group had significantly greater wound size reductions than placebo group.	20% reduction in wound size/wk for 4 weeks
Franek et al[237]	RCT N = 79	Venous leg ulcers	SWC, compression plus ES PD: 20 μsec PF: 100 pps V:100 50 min, 6 days/wk, 7 wks P: (−) 3 wks until wound clean, then (+) 4 wks	HVPC Topical medications Unna's boot	33 32 14	41/7 65/6 76/5.5	Rate of wound area change greater in group tx with HVPC but no statistical significant difference between groups. Rate of slough clearance and the degree of GT development after 2 wks were significantly greater for wounds tx with HVPC (P <0.003).
Polak et al[238]	RCT N = 42	Venous leg ulcers	SWC plus ES PD: 100 μsec PF: 100 pps V: 100 50 min, 6 days/wk, 7 wks P: (−) until wound clean, then (+) to 7 wks	HVPC Topical medications 6 wks	22 20	73.4/7 47/7	1.4 cm² per week = rate of surface area reduction 1.0 cm² per week = rate of surface area reduction

Continued

Table 26-8 Clinical Wound Healing Studies With High-Voltage, Monophasic Pulsed Current (HVPC)—cont'd

Author and Reference	Study Design (N)	Wound Diagnosis	Dressing Type, ES Parameters, Protocol	Current Type and Patient Study Groups	Number of Patients or Wounds	% Patients or Wounds Healed/Time (wks)	Other Information Provided by Authors
Franek et al[239]	RCT N = 110	Venous leg ulcers	SWC plus ES, medication, compression, surgery. PD: 100 μsec PF: 100 pps P: Not reported V: 100 50 min/day, 6 days/ wk, 7 wks	Four groups A. tx with HVPC, medication, compression B. tx with compression, medication C. tx with HVPC, surgery, compression, medication D. tx with surgery, compression, medication	28 27 28 27	Main outcome measure: Number of completely healed wounds (see next column for statistical significance between groups)	A, B $P = 0.03$ B, C $P = 0.03$ B, D $P = 0.03$ in favor of groups A, C, D Conclusion: HVPC efficient tx for healing VLU not treated with previous surgery
Houghton et al[240]	RCT double blind N = 27	Diabetic, venous, arterial	SWC plus active ES: PD: 100 μsec PF: 100 pps V: 150 P: (−) 45 min, 3 × wk for 4 wks; Placebo ES plus SWC	HVPC Active Placebo	20 22	0/4 0/4	% decrease in wound size: 44.3%/4 wks 16%/4 wks
Peters et al[241]	RCT double-blind N = 40	Diabetic foot ulcers	SWC plus active ES: PD: Not reported PF: 80 pps V: 50 P: (−) for 10 min followed by 8 min of 8 pps repeated for 8 hr at night for 12 wks via Dacron mesh sock. Placebo ES and offloading	HVPC Active ES and offloading Placebo and offloading	18 17	65/12 35/12 $P = 0.058$	After stratification by compliance, significantly more compliant patients in both groups healed than non-compliant patients

Study	Design	Wound type	ES parameters	Group	N	Outcome	Results
Goldman et al[242]	Case series; historical controls N = 6	Diabetic ischemic foot ulcers	SWC plus ES: PD: Not reported; PF: 80–100 pps; P: Not reported; V: 80–330 to sensory threshold, 1 hr/day, 7 day/wk for 1–9 mo	HVPC	6	4/7.2 mo, 2 had amputation	Mean $TcPO_2$ before HVPC was 2 mm Hg; after ES began was 33 mm Hg, indicating ↑ perfusion
Goldman et al[243]	Single case	Diabetic, expanding right calf gangrene: $TcPO_2$ <20 mm Hg	SWC plus ES: PD: Not reported; PF:100 pps; V: 150; P: (–); 1 hr × 4 or more days/wk for 250 days	HVPC		Wound healed after 250 days of ES at home	$TcPO_2$ ↑ from 20 mm Hg to 50 mm Hg, indicating ↑ perfusion
Goldman et al[244]	5-yr retrospective, observational study N = 22	Inframalleolar ischemic wounds	SWC plus ES: PD: Not reported; PF: 100 pps; V: 100; P: Not reported. 1 hr/day or SWC	HVPC / Controls	11 / 11	90/12 / 29/12	ES group $TcPO_2$ ↑ 6–26 mm Hg ($P < 0.05$) suggests that HVPC enhances microcirculation
Goldman et al[245]	Prospective pilot N = 8	Infrapopliteal ischemic wounds	SWC plus active or placebo ES at home: PD: Not reported; PF: 100 pps; V: 360 or sensory threshold; P: (–) 1 hr/day for 7 days for 14 wks	HVPC / Active ES plus SWC / Placebo ES plus SWC	4 / 4	After 4 wks area of wounds ↓ significantly ($P < 0.05$); After 4 wks area of wounds ↑ 50%	Measured by laser Doppler, $TcPO_2$ ↑ significantly at wks 8 ($P < 0.01$) and 12 ($P < 0.05$)
Burdge et al[246]	Retrospective study, historic controls N = 30	Diabetic lower extremity wounds	SWC plus ES: parameters not reported	HVPC; Mean number of ES tx = 22.3	45	35/45 (77.8%) healed in mean of 14.2 wks.	At mean follow-up of 39.8 wks, 31 (68.9%) wounds remained closed.

ES, electrical stimulation; HVPC, high-voltage pulsed current; P, polarity; PD, pulse duration; PF, pulse frequency; RCT, random controlled trial; SCI, spinal cord injury; SWC, standard wound care; tx, treatment; WF, waveform.

Table 26•9 Clinical Wound Healing Studies on Lower Extremity Vascular and Diabetic Wounds With Direct Current and Pulsed Currents

Author and Reference	Study Design (N)	Wound Diagnosis	Dressing Type, ES Parameters, Protocol	Current Type and Patient Study Groups	Number of Patients or Wounds	% Patients or Wounds Healed/Time (wks)	Other Information Provided by Authors
Wolcott et al[116]	Historic controls N=75 Embedded RCT N=16	Venous and arterial	SWC plus ES: µA: 200–800 P: Switched (–), (+), (–) 6 hr/day, 0.8–15.4 wks	DC Active DC control	75 Bilateral wounds 8 8	40/9.6 95/15.4 32/15.4	Healing rate/wk: 53 paraplegics = 9.3%; 5 venous disease = 14.4%; 15 arterial disease = 14.0% Healing rate/wk: 13.4% 5.0%
Assimacopoulos[115]	Case series N=8	Venous	SWC plus ES: µA = 50–100 Polarity (–)	DC	8	100/30	Biopsy 1 yr after healed: dense hyalinized collagen
Junger et al[124]	Case series N=15	Venous Previous tx of compression therapy failed to show clinical progress over a mean of 6.5 years.	SWC plus ES: ES parameters; PD: 140 µsec PF: 128 pps µA: 630 WF: rectangular P: (–) until wound granulated then (+), µA = 315 and 64 pps during epithelialization	LVMPC Wounds tx 30 min/day for 38 days	15	After 38 days, mean ulcer area ↓ 63% ($P < 0.01$) from 16 cm² to 6 cm²	Capillary density ↑ from 8.05 capillaries/mm² to 11.55 capillaries/mm² ($P < 0.039$)
Lundberg et al[112]	RCT double-blind N=64	Diabetic ulcers	SWC 2 groups: Active ES PD = 1 ms PF = 80 pps mA = Tingling paresthesia 20 min BID Placebo ES	LVBPC Active Placebo controls	32 32	42/12 15/12	% ulcers healed: 2 wks = 0% ES vs 4% placebo; 4 wks = 12% ES vs 7% placebo 8 wks = 25% ES vs 11% placebo 12 wks = 42% ES vs 15% placebo
Karba et al[111]	Historic controls N=82	Vascular	Dressing not reported. ES 60 min/day PD = 250 µsec PF = 40 mA = 15–20 WF: symmetrical	LVBPC	82	73/82	90% of vascular ulcers healed in 10 wks

Study	Design & N	Population	Treatment parameters	Groups	N	Outcome	Healing rates (%) / Results
Baker et al[131]	RCT N = 92	Diabetic ulcers	SWC plus 3 ES groups, 30 min, TID to wound edge plus controls: A. Asymmetrical biphasic PC; PD: 100 μsec PF: 50 mA: Submotor B. Symmetrical biphasic PC; PD: 300 μsec PF: 50 pps mA: Submotor C. Microcurrent PD: 10 μsec PF: 1 pps mA: 4 D. Controls	IVBPC Group A Group B Group C Group D	29 24 20 19	Not reported	Healing rates (%) 27 24 20 19 ES with group A protocol significantly ↑ the healing rate by nearly 60% over both groups C and D that received no ES.
Debrecini et al[132]	Prospective, historic controls N = 18	24 ischemic LEs, 10 were diabetic	SWC plus vascular drugs and ES: PD: Not reported PF: 1–2 pps mA: 15–30 P: Not reported 20 min/day for 1 yr.	IVBPC	12 ischemic ulcers; 6 LE gangrene	After 1 yr, 20/24 reported ↓ ischemic pain; halted progress of gangrene or healed ulcers	For 5–6 yr prior, all patients treated with pentoxifylline and vasodilator or antiplatelet drugs, none of which had positive effects
Alon et al[236]	Historic controls N = 12	Diabetic neuropathic ulcers	SWC plus ES: PD: 20–60 μsec PF: Not reported V: Not reported P: Anode	HVPC	12	80/2.6 mo	None reported
Franek et al[237]	RCT N = 79	Venous leg ulcers	SWC, compression plus ES. PD: 20 μsec PF: 100 pps V :100 50 min, 6 days/wk, 7 wks. P: (–) 3 wks until wound clean then (+) 4 wks	HVPC Topical medications Unna's boot	33 32 14	41/7 65/6 76/5.5	Rate of wound area change greater in group treated with HVPC but no statistically significant difference between groups Rate of slough clearance and the degree of GT development after 2 wks were significantly greater for wounds treated with HVPC (P < 0.003)

Continued

Table 26•9 Clinical Wound Healing Studies on Lower Extremity Vascular and Diabetic Wounds With Direct Current and Pulsed Currents—cont'd

Author and Reference	Study Design (N)	Wound Diagnosis	Dressing Type, ES Parameters, Protocol	Current Type and Patient Study Groups	Number of Patients or Wounds	% Patients or Wounds Healed/Time (wks)	Other Information Provided by Authors
Polak et al[238]	RCT N = 42	Venous leg ulcers	SWC plus ES PD: 100 μsec PF: 100 pps V: 100 50 min, 6 days/wk, 7 wks P: (−) until wound clean, then (+) to 7 wks	HVPC Topical medications 6 wks	22 20	73.4/7 47/7	1.4 cm² per week = rate of surface area reduction 1.0 cm² per week = rate of surface area reduction
Franek et al[239]	RCT N = 110	Venous leg ulcers	SWC plus ES, medication, compression, surgery. PD: 100 μsec PF: 100 pps V: 100 50 min/day, 6 days/wk, 7 wks	Four groups A. tx with HVPC, medication, compression B. tx with compression, medication C. tx with HVPC, surgery, compression, medication D. tx with surgery, compression, medication	28 27 28 27	1° outcome measure: Number of completely healed wounds (see next column for statistical significance between groups)	A, B P = 0.03 B, C P = 0.03 B, D P = 0.03 in favor of groups A, C, D Conclusion: HVPC efficient tx for healing VLU not treated with previous surgery
Houghton et al[240]	RCT double-blind N = 27	Diabetic, venous, arterial	SWC plus Active ES: PD: 100 μsec PF: 100 pps V: 150 P: (−) 45 min, 3 ×/wk for 4 wks; Placebo ES plus SWC	HVPC Active Placebo	20 22	0/4 0/4	% decrease in wound size: 44.3%/4 wks 16%/4 wk
Peters et al[241]	RCT double-blind N = 40	Diabetic foot ulcers	SWC plus Active ES: PD: Not reported PF: 80 pps V: 50 P: (−) for 10 min followed by 8 min of 8 pps repeated for	HVPC Active ES and offloading Placebo and offloading	18 17	65/12 35/12 P = 0.058	After stratification by compliance, significantly more compliant patients in both groups healed than noncompliant patients

Study	Design	Wound type	Parameters	Group	N	Outcome	Results
Goldman et al[242]	Case series; historical controls N = 6	Diabetic ischemic foot ulcers	SWC plus ES: PD: Not reported PF: 80–100 pps P: Not reported V: 80–330 to sensory threshold, 1 hr/day, 7 days/wk for 1–9 mo 8 hr at night for 12 wks via Dacron mesh sock. Placebo ES and offloading	HVPC	6	4/7.2 mo, 2 had amputation	Mean TcPO$_2$ before HVPC was 2 mm Hg; after ES began rose to 33 mm Hg, indicating ↑ perfusion
Goldman et al[243]	Single case	Diabetic, expanding right calf gangrene: TcPO$_2$ <20 mm Hg	SWC plus ES: PD: Not reported PF: 100 pps V: 150 P: (–) 1 hr for 4 or more days/wk for 250 days	HVPC	1	Wound healed after 250 days of ES at home	TcPO$_2$ ↑ from 20 mm Hg to 50 mm Hg indicating ↑ perfusion
Goldman et al[244]	5-yr Retrospective, observational study N = 22	Inframalleolar ischemic wounds	SWC plus ES: PD: Not reported PF: 100 pps V: 100 P: Not reported. 1 hr/day or SWC	HVPC Controls	11 11	90/12 29/12	ES group TcPO$_2$ ↑ 6–26 mm Hg ($P < 0.05$) suggests that HVPC enhances microcirculation
Goldman et al[245]	Prospective pilot N = 8	Infrapopliteal ischemic wounds	SWC plus active or placebo ES at home: PD: Not reported PF: 100 pps V: 360 or sensory threshold P: (–) 1 hr/day for 14 wks for 7 days	HVPC Active ES plus SWC Placebo ES plus SWC	4	After 4 wks area of wounds ↓ significantly at ($P <0.05$) After 4 wks, area of wounds ↑ 50%	Measured by laser Doppler, TcPO$_2$ ↑ significantly at wks 8 ($P < 0.01$) and 12 ($P < 0.05$)
Burdge et al[246]	Retrospective study, historic controls N = 30	Diabetic lower extremity wounds	SWC plus ES: Parameters not reported	HVPC Mean number of ES tx = 22.3	45	35/45 (77.8%) healed in mean of 14.2 wks.	At mean follow-up of 39.8 wks, 31 (68.9%) wounds remained closed.

BID, two times daily; ES, electrical stimulation; GT, granulation tissue; HVPC, high-voltage pulsed current; P, polarity; PD, pulse duration; PF, pulse frequency; RCT, random controlled trial; SWC, standard wound care; TID, three times daily; tx, treatment; VLU, venous leg ulcers; WF, waveform.

a treatment effect from HVPC. A study by Akers and Gabrielson reports the results of a noncontrolled comparative trial in which 14 patients had their pressure ulcers treated with one of three treatment regimens.[125] The three treatment groups were those treated with whirlpool once daily, whirlpool plus HVPC twice daily, and HVPC alone twice daily. The investigators did not identify the numbers of patients in the three groups, the number or duration of treatments, or the ES parameters. Moreover, patients in the three groups were not comparable in that those who received ES alone had sensory loss while those in the other groups had some sensory perception. Based on a comparison of wound pretreatment size with weekly wound surface area measurements, patients treated with ES alone showed the greatest change in wound surface area, followed by the combined ES and whirlpool group and the group treated with whirlpool alone. Owing to the small sample size and the broad variability within the groups, there were no statistical differences between the three groups.

Twelve clinical studies, all of which are randomized controlled trials, have investigated the effects of HVPC on chronic wound healing.[126,127,236-246] In two of the studies, the authors mentioned that the charge quantities delivered to the wound tissues were 342 and 500 µQ/sec.[126,127] These charge values or dosages of electrical current coincide with the range of charge values previously reported in the five low-voltage PC studies.[57,121-124] In a controlled study, Kloth and Feedar randomly assigned 16 patients with dermal ulcers of mixed etiologies to either an active ES or placebo ES group.[126] Wounds of both groups received standard moist wound care 24 hours a day. In addition, the nine wounds of the active ES group received 45 min of directly applied HVPC 5 days a week at 105 pps, with the voltage set to the submotor level. Initially, the anode was placed over the wound, but in four patients whose wounds were treated with active ES, the wound electrode polarity was alternated daily when there was no change in measurable progress toward wound closure. Seven patients in the control group received 45 min of placebo ES plus standard care to the ulcer 5 days per week. The wounds of patients in the treatment group healed completely in a mean of 7.3 weeks at a rate of 45% per week. Patients in the control group experienced a mean increase in wound size of 29% during a mean period of 7.4 weeks. The wounds of three patients assigned to a control subgroup treated with standard wound care increased in area by 1.2% over 8.7 weeks. However, when these three patients were reassigned to a treatment crossover group, their wounds healed at an average rate of 38% a week, with complete healing occurring in an average of 8.3 weeks.

In a single-blind RCT, Griffin et al assessed the efficacy of HVPC for healing stage II, III, or IV pressure ulcers in men with spinal cord injury.[127] Of 17 patients with pressure ulcers in the pelvic region, eight were randomly assigned to the active ES group and nine to the placebo ES group. All wounds were treated daily with standard moist wound care. In addition, wounds in the active ES group received 60 min of ES treatment on 20 consecutive days with the cathode applied to deliver current directly to the wound. The stimulator was set to deliver 100 pps and 200 V, which produced 500 µQ/sec at the treatment electrode. Ulcer surface area was measured before and after ES treatment on days 5, 10,

15, and 20. Percentage of change from pretreatment ulcer size was calculated for each measurement interval. On days 5, 15, and 20, ulcers in the HVPC group had significantly greater mean wound area reductions compared to their pretreatment size than ulcers in the placebo group.

Polish investigators have reported that ES with HVPC also enhances healing of chronic leg ulcers. Franek et al enrolled 79 patients in a study that compared the effects of HVPC, topically applied medications, and Unna's boot on healing of chronic venous leg ulcers.[237] In addition to being treated with one of these interventions, wounds of all patients were treated with dressings and compression bandaging. They randomized 65 patients to have their ulcers treated either with HVPC ($N = 33$) or topical medications ($N = 32$). A subset of 14 patients who served as controls had their ulcers treated with Unna's boot. At the outset of the study, all groups were identical with respect to patient and wound characteristics. The HVPC was delivered directly to wounds through saline-moist gauze for 50 min, 6 days per week, for an average of 7 weeks. To clear the wound of slough and pus, polarity of the treatment electrode was negative (1–3 weeks), after which the polarity was switched to the anode. All groups showed a significant decrease in wound size compared to baseline measurements ($P < 0.001$). The rate of wound area change was greatest for the group treated with HVPC, but there were no statistically significant differences between the groups. The rate of slough clearance and the degree of granulation tissue development after 2 weeks were significantly greater for wounds treated with HVPC ($P < 0.003$). The authors concluded that HVPC was an efficient treatment for enhancement of venous leg ulcer healing.

In a second clinical study from Poland, Polak et al further evaluated the effect of HVPC on venous leg ulcers.[238] In this 7-week study, they randomly allocated 22 patients to a HVPC treatment group and 20 patients to a control group whose ulcers were treated with topical medications. Patients in the control group had their wounds treated daily with fresh medications for an average of 6 weeks. Patients in the ES group had their wounds treated for 50 min, 6 days per week, for an average of 7 weeks. Wounds were treated with the cathode until clean, followed by anode polarity for the remaining study period. ES treatment parameters were pulse duration, 100 µsec; frequency, 100 pps; and 100 V. The investigators reported that ulcers treated with ES were reduced in area by 73.4% compared to a 47% area reduction for control wounds and that the rate of surface area reduction for ES-treated wounds (1.4 cm² per week) exceeded that of controls (1.0 cm² per week). In addition, the wound volume of ES-treated wounds decreased 91.3% versus 68% for controls, and weekly healing rate expressed as volume reduction was 1.0 cm³ for ES-treated ulcers compared to 0.6 cm³ for controls.

A recent additional clinical study from the Polish research group compared the effect of HVPC on healing of surgically and conservatively treated patients with venous leg ulcers.[239] In this RCT investigators randomized 110 patients with venous leg ulcers to four study groups. Group A ($N = 28$) wounds were treated with HVPC, compression, and medication. Group B ($N = 27$) wounds were treated with compression and medication. Group C ($N = 28$) wounds were treated with surgery, HVPC, compression, and medication, and group D ($N = 27$) wounds were treated with surgery, compression, and medication. Groups A and C received the ES part of their treatment regime for 50 min daily, six times a week, for 7 weeks. ES parameters were pulse duration, 100 μsec; frequency, 100 pps; and 100 V. The four groups were homogenous in terms of patients and wound characteristics. The primary outcome measure (number of completely healed wounds) showed a statistically significant difference between groups A and B ($P = 0.03$), B and C ($P = 0.03$), and B and D ($P = 0.03$) in favor of groups A, C, and D. The authors concluded that HVPC is an efficient conservative method to enhance healing of chronic venous leg ulcers that were not subjected to previous surgical intervention.

In another study designed as a randomized, double-blind, prospective clinical trial, Houghton et al divided 27 subjects with 42 chronic leg ulcers (wound age longer than 3 months) into subgroups according to primary etiology of the wound (diabetic, venous insufficiency, arterial insufficiency).[240] They then randomly assigned them to wound treatments with active HVPC (150 V, 100 pps, 100 μsec pulse duration) or placebo HVPC for 45 min, three times daily for 4 weeks. Negative polarity of the active electrode placed on saline-moist gauze over the wound was maintained throughout the 4-week treatment period. During the days when wounds were not treated with ES and when ES was not applied to the wounds, they were treated with standard moist wound care based on wound etiology. The results for all wounds demonstrated that active HVPC applied over the 4-week period reduced wound surface area to nearly one half of initial size, which was over two times greater than that which occurred in wounds treated with placebo ES ($P < 0.05$). Following the 4-week protocol, in seven patients with bilateral venous ulcers there was also a statistically significant difference in wound size between ulcers treated with active ES and placebo ES ($P < 0.05$). Using the Pressure Sore Status Tool (PSST), the investigators also compared wound appearance between pretreatment, posttreatment, and a 1-month follow-up evaluation. They found that active ES produced a statistically significant improvement in wound appearance compared with placebo-treated wounds ($P < 0.05$).

In another randomized, double-blind, placebo-controlled, 12-week trial, investigators assessed the effect of HVPC as an adjunct to healing diabetic foot ulcers.[241] Forty patients with diabetic foot ulcers and loss of sensation due to neuropathy were randomized to active HVPC and placebo HVPC. At the outset of the study, there were no significant differences between active and placebo ES groups in patient characteristics and clinical variables. Active (subsensory) ES was delivered to the ipsilateral lower extremity at 50 V, 80 pps, and pulse duration of 100 msec via a Dacron-mesh silver nylon stocking nightly for 8 hours. Compliance was divided into compliant patients who used the ES device for 20 hours or more a week on average and noncompliant patients who used the ES device less than 20 hours per week. Following 12 weeks of the research protocol, 65% of the wounds in the active ES group closed compared with 35% of wounds in the placebo ES group ($P = 0.058$). Regarding compliance, significant differences were found among patients in the active ES group (71% closed) compared with 50% closed among noncompliant patients in

the same group. In the placebo ES group, 39% of compliant patient wounds closed compared with 29% of noncompliant patient wounds ($P = 0.038$). The authors concluded that ES using HVPC enhances healing of diabetic foot ulcers when used adjunctively with weight off-loading and local wound care.

Since 2002, Goldman et al have published findings from four small but intriguing studies related to salvaging the ischemic lower extremities with HVPC stimulation.[242-245] In a case series, they taught six adult patients to use HVPC at home to treat their critically ischemic (defined as $TcPO_2$ <10 mm Hg), nonsurgical, malleolar, or inframalleolar wounds that had a mean $TcPO_2$ of 2 plus or minus 2 mm Hg at the wound edge. After ES commenced, periwound $TcPO_2$ increased exponentially until it exceeded 20 mm Hg, about 40 days into the protocol, and the rate of healing changed to positive. The investigators suggested that the improved periwound cutaneous microcirculation resulted from a statistically significant increase in mean $TcPO_2$ of periwound skin to 33 plus or minus 18 mm Hg. Wounds of four patients healed after 207 days of ES, and two patients underwent amputation.[242] In another report, they used HVPC to reverse a rapidly expanding ischemic, cutaneous gangrene on the left posterior calf of a patient with end-stage renal disease.[243] Hypoxia was verified by $TcPO_2$ less than or equal to 20 mm Hg with calf periwound $TcPO_2$ of 20 mm Hg and 12 mm Hg at the heel. To the patient's calf wound, necrotic heel, and fourth toe, home caregivers applied cathodal HVPC 1 hour daily, 5 to 7 days per week, at 150 V and 100 pps. While not receiving ES, the wounds were treated with standard care for ischemic wounds. Both the left calf and heel lesions closed 250 and 234 days, respectively, after beginning ES therapy. During the extended treatment period, the transition to positive healing rate occurred concurrent with an increase in periwound $TcPO_2$ from 20 to 50 mm Hg (calf) and 15 to 50 mm Hg (heel). In a 5-year retrospective observational study, Goldman et al continued their clinical studies to determine if HVPC augments ischemic wound healing and increases periwound perfusion.[244]

The study was carried out on successive patients with ischemic lower extremity wounds who were poor candidates for revascularization. One group of 11 patients had HVPC applied directly to their wounds at more than 100 V, 100 pps, 1 hour daily, in addition to 23 hours of standard wound care. A second group of 11 patients with ischemic wounds had their lesions treated with standard care alone. Outcome measures included planimetry of wound areas, digital wound appearance, and $TcPO_2$ monitoring of microcirculation. The group treated with HVPC plus standard care had smaller wound areas from weeks 20 through 52 after the start of treatment compared with the group that received standard care alone ($P < 0.05$). One year after initiating treatment, 90% of HVPC-treated wounds had closed, compared with 29% of the wounds that were treated with standard care alone. For the HVPC group, maximum $TcPO_2$ improved from 6 plus or minus 8 mm Hg at baseline to 26 plus or minus 20 mm Hg ($P < 0.05$). These results suggest that HVPC facilitates microcirculation and the healing of ischemic wounds.

Continuing their clinical research to determine if HVPC augments ischemic wound healing and increases periwound microcirculation, Goldman et al conducted a prospective, randomized, single-blinded, sham-controlled clinical pilot study on a homogenous subset of patients with infrapopliteal ischemic wounds.[245] For the purpose of their study, they defined ischemia as periwound $TcPO_2$ less than 20 mm Hg, which they deemed the threshold below which healing is not favorable. Eight patients were enrolled with ischemic wounds at or below the knee, periwound $TcPO_2$ less than 20 mm Hg, with wounds open for at least 4 weeks before enrollment in the study, and arteriosclerotic disease was confirmed by magnetic resonance angiography, pulse volume recording, or angiogram. Patients were randomized to have their wounds treated with active or placebo HVPC. Active HVPC or placebo HVPC was applied at home 1 hour per day, 7 days per week, for 14 weeks. Wounds were monitored at regular intervals for wound area, wound appearance, and microcirculation, the latter of which was measured by $TcPO_2$ and laser Doppler flow. After 4 weeks, wounds treated with placebo HVPC increased in area by 50%, which was expected since ischemic wounds tend to increase in size. During the same period, wounds treated with active HVPC underwent a significant decrease in size ($P < 0.05$). After week 4, wounds in both groups demonstrated positive healing rates, but the healing rate in the control group continued to lag behind the healing rate of the active HVPC-treated wounds during the remainder of the 14-week period.

Most recently, Burdge et al reported positive limb salvage outcomes following HVPC adjunctive treatment of 40 full-thickness diabetic wounds on the lower extremities of 30 patients.[246] The wounds had a mean age of 25 weeks and a mean surface area of 7.8 cm^2. Comorbid conditions that contributed to the complexity of these wounds included neuropathy (83.3%), peripheral vascular disease (76.7%), cardiac disease (36.7%), infection (33.3%), osteomyelitis (16.7%), and morbid obesity (10.0%). ES was added to the conservative management of these wounds after they had failed to improve, despite previous interventions that included vascular evaluation, surgical treatment as indicated, aggressive off-loading, infection control, and débridement. The mean number of ES treatments was 22.3. During a mean time of 14.2 weeks, 35 (77.8%) wounds healed, and during a mean follow-up of 39.8 weeks, 31 (68.9%) wounds remained closed. Of the four wounds (8.9%) that recurred, additional ES treatments healed two wounds, one required below knee (BK) amputation, and treatment options were being considered for the fourth wound. Ten (22.2%) wounds failed to heal, resulting in a transmetatarsal amputation for one patient (one wound) and BK amputations for five patients (six wounds).

High-Voltage, Biphasic Multimodulated Current

Recently, investigators have reported use of a conductive electrical stimulation device called Aptiva™ Move (Lorenz Neurovasc, Mississauga, Ontario, Canada), which has a biphasic, asymmetrical charge-balanced waveform with an adjustable negative phase amplitude between 0 and 300 V, a variable pulse frequency between 0 and 1 pps, and a pulse duration that varies between 10 and 100 μsec. (Fig. 26.31) During therapy with this device, electrical stimulation is described as sequences of negative phase signals with multiple modulations of pulse amplitude, frequency, and duration. The combination of these modulations is termed Frequency Rhythmic Electrical Modulation System or FREMS™. Although no studies on the effects of FREMS on wound healing were found, two studies describe its effects on painful diabetic neuropathy and on the induced expression of vascular endothelial growth factor (VEGF) in patients with diabetic polyneuropathy. In a study by Bosi et al, 31 patients with painful diabetic neuropathy who had decreased nerve conduction velocity (< 40 m/sec) and increased vibration perception threshold (> 25 V) were enrolled in a randomized, double-blind, crossover study designed to compare the effects of active and placebo FREMS.[247] Each patient received two series of 10 treatments of either FREMS or placebo in random sequence, with each series lasting no more than 3 weeks. The investigators found that patients treated with active FREMS had a significant decrease in daytime and nighttime VAS pain scores (both $P < 0.02$). In addition, these patients also demonstrated a significant increase in sensory tactile perception as assessed by monofilament, a decrease in foot vibration perception threshold as measured by a bioesthesiometer, and an increase in motor nerve conduction velocity (all $P < 0.01$). No significant changes were observed in patients who received placebo FREMS. The same measurements taken at a 4-month follow-up and compared with baseline measurements showed that a significant carryover benefit had persisted for all measures that had shown improvement at the end of the study. No carryover effect was apparent within the crossover analysis. The authors concluded that FREMS is a safe and effective treatment of diabetic neuropathic pain

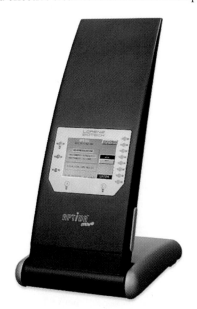

Figure 26•31 *The Aptiva Move HVBPC device used in clinical studies on neuropathic pain and expression of VEGF (Lorenz Neurovasc, Mississauga, Ontario, Canada).[246,247]*

and is able to modify some parameters of peripheral nerve function.

In the second study, Bevilacqua et al assessed the effects of the FREMS signal versus a standard TENS signal on the expression of VEGF in 10 subjects (four males and six females) with type 2 diabetic polyneuropathy and 10 nondiabetic subjects (five males and five females).[248] Subjects received TENS for 10 min followed by 30 min without ES, followed by FREMS for 10 min over the forearm volar surface. Blood samples for VEGF assay were obtained from the contralateral arm every 2 min during TENS/FREMS applications and every 10 min during the 30-min intervals. Laboratory analysis revealed a significant increase in plasma VEGF during FREMS in both nondiabetic and diabetic subjects (maximum response 89.4 ± 80.3 pg/mL and 48.5 ± 18.3 pg/mL, respectively; $P < 0.01$ versus baseline), with a lower but still significant response in diabetic subjects. No changes in VEGF were observed during TENS stimulation. The authors hypothesized that VEGF expression during FREMS stimulation may help explain the positive effects on nerve conduction velocity in diabetic polyneuropathy, possibly mediated by favorable effects on vasa nervorum microangiopathy. The findings from these two studies may have implications for the treatment of pain associated with diabetic polyneuropathy and for enhancing wound healing, but additional research is needed to support these assumptions.

Strength of Evidence for Electrical Stimulation as a Wound Healing Intervention

For the healing of chronic wounds by ES, the strength of evidence based on clinical trials is substantial. In 2000 the Paralyzed Veterans of America provided administrative and financial support to develop and publish a clinical practice pressure ulcer treatment guideline in which ES was assigned a stand-alone recommendation (number 17) based on a strong strength-of-evidence rating from three RCTs.[249] The recommendation reads, "Use electrical stimulation to promote closure of stage III or IV pressure ulcers combined with standard wound care interventions."

Meta-Analyses of Electrical Stimulation Wound Healing Research Studies

Perhaps the most compelling evidence of the efficacy of ES for enhancing the rate of wound healing is supported by two meta-analyses. For their meta-analysis, Gardner et al selected 15 ES studies on chronic wound healing that included placebo-controlled, randomized trials ($N = 8$); nonrandomized trials ($N = 5$); a nonrandomized, placebo-controlled trial ($N = 1$); and one study with a descriptive design.[250] Data analyzed from these studies included 24 ES samples (591 wounds) and 15 control samples (212 wounds) and included ulcers caused by pressure, venous and arterial insufficiency, and diabetic neuropathy. They calculated the mean percentage of healing per week for the ES and control samples and found that the percentage of healing per week

was 22% for the ES samples versus 9% for control samples. The net effect of ES on chronic wounds was reported to be a mean percentage of healing per week of 13.5%, which represented a 144% increase in healing of ES-treated wounds over control wounds. Based on 95% confidence intervals for ES and control samples, the studies revealed a 90% probability that the net healing effect of ES is 3.7% per week or more, which conservatively represents an increase of 40% or more over the control rate. These findings were similar for both placebo-controlled studies and for all the studies reviewed, including non-placebo-controlled trials.

More recently, Houghton and Woodbury performed a meta-analysis that assessed the effect of ES on promoting chronic wound closure.[251] They searched electronic databases and bibliographies to find articles published before October 2006. To qualify for inclusion in the meta-analysis, studies had to meet inclusion criteria that included (1) controlled clinical trials that had a between-group statistical comparison, (2) a population of adult humans with chronic skin ulcers who had undergone ES treatment using surface electrodes, and (3) wound size that was assessed objectively before and after treatment. In addition, consensus between four independent reviewers was required to reject articles. Of 2265 articles reviewed, 19 studies were selected for the review that involved a total subject number of 888 (ES group = 522; control group = 366). Of the 19 studies selected, 12 had data to support the ES accelerated wound healing whereas seven studies reported no differences between ES and control groups. Data were pooled from five studies that assessed the proportion of completely healed wounds. The overall effect size in favor of ES treatment was 3.93 ($P < 0.0006$). Studies that tended to show better responses to ES were those that used randomization, large sample sizes ($N = 25$), had similar subject characteristics at baseline, pressure ulcers, or used ES parameters, including a monophasic PC, negative or alternating polarity, and a relatively high pulse frequency (64 pps). The evidence from this meta-analysis provides strong support that ES can significantly improve the proportion of chronic wounds healed.

Most recently, the European Pressure Ulcer Advisory Panel and the USA National Pressure Ulcer Advisory Panel jointly developed the International Pressure Ulcer Treatment Guide, which states: "Consider the use of direct contact (capacitive) electrical stimulation (ES) in the management of recalcitrant Category/Stage III and IV pressure ulcers to facilitate wound healing. (Strength of Evidence = A, based on data from Sackett Level 1 studies)."[252]

Considerations for Wound Treatment with Conductive Electrical Stimulation

The clinical studies cited in the previous sections have confirmed that ES combined with standard wound care accelerates the rate of wound healing faster than standard care alone, despite the fact that clinical researchers in these studies used a variety of ES devices and waveforms (DC, LVMPC, LVBPC, HVPC) and stimulation parameters. Irrespective of the positive outcomes reported, reviewers of ES clinical research related to wound healing have frequently argued that the evidence supporting the intervention is compromised by the lack of consistency in the type of current and stimulation parameters reported in the literature. What has been overlooked by most evaluators of the ES literature is that there is the common denominator of electrical charge "dosage" delivered into the wound tissues as has been reported in several of the RCTs that used either LVMPC or HVMPC with different paramenters.[121-124,126,127,238] By mathematical calculation, we have found that the dosage falls within a narrow range of 250 to 500 µC/sec. The formulas for calculating electrical charge dosages that are used clinically to enhance the rate of wound healing with low- and high-voltage PC are shown in Figures 26.25 and 26.26, respectively. However, it must be emphasized here that because of variables such as periwound skin and subcutaneous tissue resistance, conductivity of electrodes, and other factors, it is not known whether exogenous currents applied to recalcitrant wound tissues mimic the physiological currents that are involved in tissue repair.

Measuring the Wound Edge Electric Field

As previously indicated, the epidermis generates a transepithelial potential (TEP) of 20 to 50 mV across itself, inside (dermis) positive and outside (dermis) negative.[27] Any wound of the epidermis creates a low-resistance pathway, and the TEP at the wound site is 0 mV. However, the TEP of the intact epidermis around the wound is still present, resulting in a lateral voltage gradient or electric field along the edge of skin surrounding the wound. There is evidence that this lateral electric field stimulates keratinocytes in the area to migrate toward the wound, with the optimal response occurring at an endogenous field strength of 100 mV/mm. If there was a way to measure and determine the magnitude of the lateral electric field at the wound edge, it may be possible to deliver an exogenous "healing" current into the wound tissues that more closely mimics the physiological wound current. Intriguingly, Reid et al and Nuccitelli and colleagues have developed a bioelectric field imager that can determine the electric field strength along the wound edge.[25,253] The instrument (Dermacorder®, BioElectroMed Corporation, Burlingame, CA) vibrates a small sensor perpendicular to the skin about 100 µm above the surface and uses the oscillating capacitance signal to determine the surface potential of the epidermis just beneath the stratum corneum. By measuring the surface potential in many positions along the wound edge, a spatial map of the surrounding electric field can be generated. (Fig 26.32) On the arms and legs of 40 adults, Nuccitelli et al inflicted lancet wounds and measured the lateral surface wound field between the stratum corneum and epidermis near the wounds.[254] Ten males and ten females in the 18- to 29-year-old age group demonstrated a mean electric field of 163 plus or minus 59 mV/mm, whereas 10 males and 10 females in the

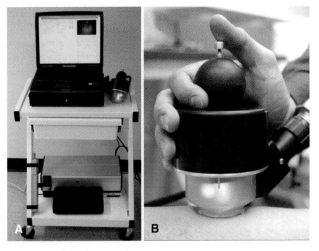

Figure 26•32 (A and B) The Dermacorder is a bioelectric field imager that can determine the endogenous electric field strength along the wound edge (BioElectroMed Corp., Burlingame, CA).[25,250]

65- to 80-year-old age group exhibited a mean electric field of 78 plus or minus 15 mV/mm. These findings for the groups evaluated demonstrate that the mean electric field for an acute wound in the older individuals was half that of the younger group. The investigators suggested that since the surface field for the acute wound is larger than the field within the epidermis, increasing the epidermal field to the optimal 100 mV/mm in older individuals might increase the rate of wound healing. They plan on repeating the measurements on chronic wounds.

Other Factors to Consider When Selecting Conductive Electrical Stimulation for Enhancement of Wound Healing
Type of Current and Waveform

As mentioned earlier in the chapter, the two types of current that are primarily used to enhance wound healing are DC and PC. Although the effects of both currents have been studied in vitro and in animal studies, clinical trials with PC (LVMPC and HVMPC combined) far outnumber those for DC. Although the LVMPC waveform from Dermapulse has not been available in the United States for over a decade, the same signal may become available if the woundEL™ receives FDA clearance for marketing in the United States. (Fig. 26.28) HVMPC is the current that is supported by strong evidence from clinical studies and is presently the most widely used for wound healing in the United States. The monophasic waveform represented by this current is twin-peaked, and the pulse duration varies from 20 to 200 µsec, as shown in Figure 26.18. The HVMPC stimulators also provide choices for polarity and pulse frequency, which influence cell motility and electric field dosage, respectively, delivered to the wound. (See Box 26.1)

active electrode was positioned directly over the wound, which was protected from the electrode by a conductive hydrogel wafer. The second carbon rubber 4 × 4 cm² active electrode on a conductive hydrogel wafer was placed over the plantar longitudinal arch. The latter two electrodes were held in place with Velcro straps (FASTENation™, Clifton, NJ).

Polarity: Negative for active electrodes.

Pulse Frequency: 100 pps.

Voltage: If patient perceives the stimulation, increase and stop at sensory threshold (100–300 V). However, because patient has neuropathy, stop advancing the voltage if the motor threshold is reached (observed as muscle fasciculations) before sensory threshold is reached, then decrease the voltage very slightly until fasciculations disappear (this will correspond to sensory level stimulation). In Mr. P's case, muscle fasciculations were observed at 155 V before he perceived sensory threshold. The muscle fasciculations disappeared by decreasing V to 150, which is the voltage his wife was instructed to deliver to the extremity daily.

Treatment Duration/Frequency: ES treatment is given 1 hour, 7 days a week, for 6 weeks. Standard wound care as described above is provided during remaining 23 hours each day.

Treatment Outcomes

After 6 weeks of the treatment protocol described above, the weekly measurements were compared with baseline data as follows.

Integument: Wound bed changed from 100% to 75% yellow fibrin.

Sensory Perception and Reflexes: Loss of protective sensation persists, and reflexes are diminished.

Pain: No change in ambulatory calf pain, but nocturnal RLE pain is improved from VAS 7/10 to 6/10.

MMT and ROM of RLE: No changes.

Vascular: TcPO₂ proximal to toes increased from 10 to 14 mm Hg and above lateral malleolus increased from 14 to 19 mm Hg. Periwound dermal perfusion improved from 25 to 32 laser Doppler units.

Psychological: Mr. P states that having less pain at night allows him to sleep better, which has given a boost to his daily energy level.

Continued Treatment

Being especially encouraged by the small gains made in TcPO₂ and periwound dermal perfusion, Mr. P's vascular surgeon extended the ES and SOC protocol another 12 weeks. After 18 weeks of this treatment, the following changes occurred.

Integument: Wound bed changed from 75% to 40% yellow fibrin.

Sensory Perception and Reflexes: Mr. P states that occasionally during the ES treatment he feels slight tingling in his lower leg, but not in his foot.

Pain: Mr. P states that he can walk about 8 min before cramping and pain begins and that the night pain in his RLE improved to 5/10.

MMT and ROM of RLE: There are no changes.

Vascular: TcPO₂ proximal to toes increased from 14 mm Hg to 18 mm Hg and above the lateral malleolus increased from 19 mm Hg to 24 mm Hg. Periwound dermal perfusion improved from 32 to 40 laser Doppler units.

Psychological: Mr. P states that he continues having less pain at night, allowing him to sleep. He and his wife indicate they are very encouraged with the improvement made thus far. The vascular surgeon recommended continuation of the treatment protocol indefinitely.

Final Outcome After 14 Months of ES and SOC Protocol

Mr. P continued to make measurable improvements monthly, and after 9 additional months (14 months total) his wound had closed. He indicated that he could feel steady tingling in his RLE during ES treatment, and he is able to perceive 10 grams of monofilament pressure in his leg above the lateral and medial malleoli, but not the plantar surface of his foot. His TcPO₂ increased from 18 mm Hg to 25 mm Hg proximal to his toes and from 24 mm Hg to 35 mm Hg above the lateral malleolus. Periwound dermal perfusion improved from 40 to 62 laser Doppler units.

Mr. P and his wife are very encouraged by the steady progress made which has improved his quality of life and has allowed him to avoid amputation.

References

1. Piccolino, M: Animal electricity and the birth of electrophysiology: The legacy of Luigi Galvani. Brain Res Bull 1998; 46:381–407.
2. Piccolino, M: Luigi Galvani's path to animal electricity. C R Biol 2006; 329:303–318.
3. Becker, RO, Marino, AA: Electromagnetism and Life. Albany, NY, State University of New York Press, 1982.
4. Moruzzi, G: The electrophysiological work of Carlo Matteucci: 1964. Brain Res Bull 1996; 40:69–91.
5. Volta, A: On the electricity excited by the mere contact of conducting substances of different kinds. Philos Trans R Soc Lond A 1800; 90:403–431.
6. Bernstein, J: Elektrobiologie. Die Lehre von den elektrischen Vorgangen im Organismus auf moderner Grundlage dargestellt. Braunschweig, Germany, Vieweg und Sohn, 1912.
7. Hodgkin, AL, Huxley, AF: Movement of sodium and potassium ions during nervous activity. Cold Spring Harb Symp Quant Biol 1952; 17:43–57.

8. Borgens, RB, Jaffe, LF, Cohen, MJ: Large and persistent electrical currents enter the transected lamprey spinal cord. Proc Natl Acad Sci U S A 1980; 77:1209–1213.

9. Borgens, RB: Voltage gradients and ionic currents in injured and regenerating axons. Adv Neurol 1988; 47:51–66.

10. Du Bois-Reymond, E: Untersuchungen uber thierische Elektricitat, Zweiter Band, Zweite Abtheilung (Erste Lieferung). Berlin, Georg Reimer, 1860, pp 1–387.

11. Du Bois-Reymond, E: Vorläufiger Abriss einer Untersuchung uber den sogenannten Froschstrom und die electomotorischen Fische. Ann Phy U Chem 1843; 58:1–30.

12. Piccolino, M: Luigi Galvani and animal electricity: Two centuries after the foundation of electrophysiology. Trends Neurosci 1997; 20:443–448.

13. Piccolino, M: The bicentennial of the Voltaic battery (1800–2000): The artificial electric organ. Trends Neurosci 2000; 23:147–151.

14. McCaig, CD, Rajnicek, AM, Song, B, et al: Controlling cell behavior electrically: Current views and future potential. Physiol Rev 2005; 85:943–978.

15. Robinson, KR, Messerli, MA: Left/right, up/down: The role of endogenous electrical fields as directional signals in development, repair, and invasion. Bioessays 2003; 25:759–766.

16. Nuccitelli, R: Endogenous electric fields in embryos during development, regeneration, and wound healing. Radiat Prot Dosimetry 2003; 106:375–383.

17. Borgens, RB, Vanable, JW Jr, Jaffe, LF: Bioelectricity and regeneration. I. Initiation of frog limb regeneration by minute currents. J Exp Zool 1977; 200:403–416.

18. Borgens, RB, Vanable, JW Jr, Jaffe LF: Bioelectricity and regeneration: Large currents leave the stumps of regenerating newt limbs. Proc Natl Acad Sci U S A 1977; 74:4528–4532.

19. Borgens, RB, Vanable, JW Jr, Jaffe, LF: Role of subdermal current shunts in the failure of frogs to regenerate. J Exp Zool 1979; 209:49–56.

20. Illingworth, CM, Barker, AT: Measurement of electrical currents emerging during the regeneration of amputated fingertips in children. Clin Phys Physiol Meas 1980; 1:87.

21. Chiang, M, Robinson, KR, Vanable, JW Jr: Electrical fields in the vicinity of epithelial wounds in the isolated bovine eye. Exp Eye Res 1992; 54:999–1003.

22. Reid, B, Song, B, McCaig, CD, et al: Wound healing in rat cornea: The role of electric currents. FASEB J 2005; 19:379–386.

23. Wang, E, Reid, B, Lois, N, et al: Electrical inhibition of lens epithelial cell proliferation: An additional factor in secondary cataract? FASEB J 2005; 19:842–844.

24. Zhao, M, Song, B, Pu, J, et al: Electrical signals control wound healing through phosphatidylinositol-3-OH kinase-gamma and PTEN. Nature 2006; 442:457–460.

25. Reid, B, Nuccitelli, R, Zhao, M: Non-invasive measurement of bioelectric currents with a vibrating probe. Nat Protoc 2007; 2:661–669.

26. Barker, AT, Jaffe, LF, Vanable, JW Jr: The glabrous epidermis of cavies contains a powerful battery. Am J Physiol 1982; 242:R358–366.

27. Foulds, IS, Barker, AT: Human skin battery potentials and their possible role in wound healing. Br J Dermatol 1983; 109:515–522.

28. Borgens, RB: Endogenous ionic currents traverse intact and damaged bone. Science 1984; 225:478–482.

29. McCaig, CD, Zhao, M: Physiological electrical fields modify cell behaviour. Bioessays 1997; 19:819–826.

30. Shi, R, Borgens, RB: Three-dimensional gradients of voltage during development of the nervous system as invisible coordinates for the establishment of embryonic pattern. Dev Dyn 1995; 202:101–114.

31. Levin, M: Large-scale biophysics: Ion flows and regeneration. Trends Cell Biol 2007; 17:261–270.

32. Candia, OA: Electrolyte and fluid transport across corneal, conjunctival, and lens epithelia. Exp Eye Res 2004; 78:527–535.

33. Levin, MH, Kim, JK, Hu, J, et al: Potential difference measurements of ocular surface Na+ absorption analyzed using an electrokinetic model. Invest Ophthalmol Vis Sci 2006; 47:306–316.

34. Klyce, SD: Electrical profiles in the corneal epithelium. J Physiol 1972; 226:407–429.

35. Klyce, SD, Beuerman, RW, Crosson, CE: Alteration of corneal epithelial ion transport by sympathectomy. Invest Ophthalmol Vis Sci 1985; 26:434–442.

36A. Klyce, SD, Crosson, CE: Transport processes across the rabbit corneal epithelium: A review. Curr Eye Res 1985; 4:323–331.

36B. Vanable, JW Jr: Integumentary potentials and wound healing. In: Borgens, RB, Robinson, KR, Vanable, JW, et al (eds): Electric Fields in Vertebrate Repair. New York, Alan R. Liss, 1989.

37. Jaffe, LF, Vanable, JW Jr: Electric fields and wound healing. Clinics in dermatology 1984; 2:34–44.

38. Cheng, K, Davis, SC, Oliveira-Gandia, M, et al: Confirmation of the electrical potential induced by occlusive dressings. Abstract 28. Presented at: Eighth Annual Symposium on Advanced Wound Care, San Diego. Wayne, PA, Health Management Publications, 1995.

39. Alvarez, OM, Mertz, PM, Smerbeck, RV, et al: The healing of superficial skin wounds is stimulated by external electrical current. J Invest Dermatol 1983; 81:144–148.

40. Winter, G: Movement of epidermal cells over the wound surface. New York, Pergamon Press, 1964, pp 113.

41. McGinnis, ME, Vanable, JW Jr: Wound epithelium controls stump currents. Dev Biol 1986; 116:174–183.

42. Gupta, B, Arora, P, Singh, VS, et al: Topical amiloride ointment accelerates healing of mechanical skin ulcers in albino rabbits and patients. Methods Find Exp Clin Pharmacol 2006; 28:101–107.

43. Sta Iglesia, DD, Vanable, JW Jr: Endogenous lateral electric fields around bovine corneal lesions are necessary for and can enhance normal rates of wound healing. Wound Repair Regen 1998; 6:531–542.

44. Vanhaesebroeck, B: Charging the batteries to heal wounds through PI3K. Nat Chem Biol 2006; 2:453–455.

45. Huttenlocher, A, Horwitz, AR: Wound healing with electric potential. N Engl J Med 2007; 356:303–304.

46. Ojingwa, JC, Isseroff, RR: Electrical stimulation of wound healing. J Invest Dermatol 2003; 121:1–12.

48. Cooper, MS, Schliwa, M: Motility of cultured fish epidermal cells in the presence and absence of direct current electric fields. J Cell Biol 1986; 102:1384–1399.

47. Bourguignon, GJ, Jy, W, Bourguignon, LY: Electric stimulation of human fibroblasts causes an increase in Ca2+ influx and the exposure of additional insulin receptors. J Cell Physiol 1989; 140:379–385.

49. Dineur, E: Note sur la sensibilies des leukocytes a l'electricité. Bull Seances Soc Belge Microscopic (Bruxelles) 1891; 18:113.

50. Erickson, CA, Nuccitelli, R: Embryonic fibroblast motility and orientation can be influenced by physiological electric fields. J Cell Biol 1984; 98:296–307.

51. Fukushima, Gruler, KH: Studies of galvanotaxis of leukocytes. Med J Osaka Univ 1953; 4:195.

52. Lee, RC, Canaday, DJ, Doong, H: A review of the biophysical basis for the clinical application of electric fields in soft-tissue repair. J Burn Care Rehabil 1993; 14:319–335.

53. Monguio, J: Uber die polare wirkung des galvanischen stromes auf leukozyten. Z Biol 1933; 93:553–556.

54. Orida, N, Feldman, JD: Directional protrusive pseudopodial activity and motility in macrophages induced by extracellular electric fields. Cell Motil 1982; 2:243–255.

55. Rapp, B, de Boisfleury-Chevance, A, Gruler, H: Galvanotaxis of human granulocytes. Dose-response curve. Eur Biophys J 1988; 16:313–319.

56. Stromberg, BV: Effects of electrical currents on wound contraction. Ann Plast Surg 1988; 21:121–123.

57. Weiss, DS, Eaglstein, WH, Falanga, V: Exogenous electric current can reduce the formation of hypertrophic scars. J Dermatol Surg Oncol 1989; 15:1272–1275.

58. Yang, WP, Onuma, EK, Hui, SW: Response of C3H/10T1/2 fibroblasts to an external steady electric field stimulation. Reorientation, shape change, ConA receptor, and intramembranous particle distribution and cytoskeleton reorganization. Exp Cell Res 1984; 155:92–104.

59. Fang, KS, Farboud, B, Nuccitelli, R, et al: Migration of human keratinocytes in electric fields requires growth factors and extracellular calcium. J Invest Dermatol 1998; 111:751–756.

60. Sivamani, R, Garcia, MS, Isseroff, RR: Wound re-epithelialization: Modulating kerationcyte migration in wound healing. Front Biosci 2007; 12:2849–2868.

61. Sheridan, DM, Isseroff, RR, Nuccitelli, R: Imposition of a physiologic DC electric field alters the migratory response of human keratinocytes on extracellular matrix molecules. J Invest Dermatol 1996; 106:642–646.

62. Nishimura, KY, Isseroff, RR, Nuccitelli, R: Human keratinocytes migrate to the negative pole in direct current electric fields comparable to those measured in mammalian wounds. J Cell Sci 1996; 109(Pt 1):199–207.

63. Ferrier, J, Ward, A, Kanehisa, J, et al: Electrophysiological responses of osteoclasts to hormones. J Cell Physiol 1986; 128:23–26.

64. Soong, HK, Parkinson, WC, Bafna, S, et al: Movements of cultured corneal epithelial cells and stromal fibroblasts in electric fields. Invest Ophthalmol Vis Sci 1990; 31:2278–2282.

65. Grahn, JC, Reilly, DA, Nuccitelli, RL, et al: Melanocytes do not migrate directionally in physiological DC electric fields. Wound Repair Regen 2003; 11:64–70.

66. Sillman, AL, Quang, DM, Farboud, B, et al: Human dermal fibroblasts do not exhibit directional migration on collagen I in direct-current electric fields of physiological strength. Exp Dermatol 2003; 12:396–402.

67. Dieckgraefe, BK, Weems, DM, Santoro, SA, et al: ERK and p38 MAP kinase pathways are mediators of intestinal epithelial wound-induced signal transduction. Biochem Biophys Res Commun 1997; 233:389–394.

68. Sammak, PJ, Hinman, LE, Tran, PO, et al: How do injured cells communicate with the surviving cell monolayer? J Cell Sci 1997; 110(Pt 4):465–475.

69. Tran, PO, Hinman, LE, Unger, GM, et al: A wound-induced [Ca2+]i increase and its transcriptional activation of immediate early genes is important in the regulation of motility. Exp Cell Res 1999; 246:319–326.

70. Dieckgraefe, BK, Weems, DM: Epithelial injury induces egr-1 and fos expression by a pathway involving protein kinase C and ERK. Am J Physiol 1999; 276:G322–330.

71. Song, B, Zhao, M, Forrester, JV, et al: Electrical cues regulate the orientation and frequency of cell division and the rate of wound healing in vivo. Proc Natl Acad Sci U S A 2002; 99:13577–13582.

72. Zhao, M, Forrester, JV, McCaig, CD: A small, physiological electric field orients cell division. Proc Natl Acad Sci U S A 1999; 96:4942–4946.

73. Song, B, Zhao, M, Forrester, J, et al: Nerve regeneration and wound healing are stimulated and directed by an endogenous electrical field in vivo. J Cell Sci 2004; 117:4681–4690.

74. Zhao, M, Bai, H, Wang, E, et al: Electrical stimulation directly induces pre-angiogenic responses in vascular endothelial cells by signaling through VEGF receptors. J Cell Sci 2004; 117:397–405.

75. Zhao, M: Electric stimulation and angiogenesis: Electrical signals have direct effects on endothelial cells. In: Janigro, D (ed): The Cell Cycle in the Central Nervous System. Totowa, NJ, Humana Press, 2006, pp 495–509.

76. Bai, H, McCaig, CD, Forrester, JV, et al: DC electric fields induce distinct preangiogenic responses in microvascular and macrovascular cells. Arterioscler Thromb Vasc Biol 2004; 24:1234–1239.

77. Eberhardt, A, Szczypiorski, P, Korytowski, G: Effect of transcutaneous electrostimulation on the cell composition of skin exudate. Acta Physiol Pol 1986; 37:41–46.

78. Mertz, P, Davis, S, Cazzaniga, A, et al: Electrical stimulation: Acceleration of soft tissue repair by varying the polarity. Wounds 1993; 5:153.

79. Zhao, M, Jin, T, McCaig, CD, et al: Genetic analysis of the role of G protein-coupled receptor signaling in electrotaxis. J Cell Biol 2002; 157:921–927.

80. Jaffe, LF: Electrophoresis along cell membranes. Nature 1977; 265:600–602.

81. Poo, M, Robinson, KR: Electrophoresis of concanavalin A receptors along embryonic muscle cell membrane. Nature 1977; 265:602–605.

82. Fang, KS, Ionides, E, Oster, G, et al: Epidermal growth factor receptor relocalization and kinase activity are necessary for directional migration of keratinocytes in DC electric fields. J Cell Sci 1999; 112(Pt 12):1967–1978.

83. Zhao, M, Pu, J, Forrester, JV, et al: Membrane lipids, EGF receptors, and intracellular signals co-localize and are polarized in epithelial cells moving directionally in a physiological electric field. FASEB J 2002; 16:857–859.

84. Zhao, M, Dick, A, Forrester, JV, et al: Electric field-directed cell motility involves up-regulated expression and asymmetric redistribution of the epidermal growth factor receptors and is enhanced by fibronectin and laminin. Mol Biol Cell 1999; 10:1259–1276.

85. Mycielska, ME, Djamgoz, MB: Cellular mechanisms of direct-current electric field effects: Galvanotaxis and metastatic disease. J Cell Sci 2004; 117:1631–1639.

86. Robinson, KR. The responses of cells to electrical fields: A review. J Cell Biol 1985; 101:2023–2027.

87. Brown, MJ, Loew, LM: Electric field-directed fibroblast locomotion involves cell surface molecular reorganization and is calcium independent. J Cell Biol 1994; 127:117–128.

88. Erskine, L, Stewart, R, McCaig, CD: Electric field-directed growth and branching of cultured frog nerves: Effects of aminoglycosides and polycations. J Neurobiol 1995; 26:523–536.

89. Stewart, R, Erskine, L, McCaig, CD: Calcium channel subtypes and intracellular calcium stores modulate electric field-stimulated and -oriented nerve growth. Dev Biol 1995; 171:340–351.

90. Palmer, AM, Messerli, MA, Robinson, KR: Neuronal galvanotropism is independent of external Ca(2+) entry or internal Ca(2+) gradients. J Neurobiol 2000; 45:30–38.

91. Trollinger, DR, Isseroff, RR, Nuccitelli, R: Calcium channel blockers inhibit galvanotaxis in human keratinocytes. J Cell Physiol 2002; 193:1–9.

92. Onuma, EK, Hui, SW: A calcium requirement for electric field-induced cell shape changes and preferential orientation. Cell Calcium 1985; 6:281–292.

93. Onuma, EK, Hui, SW: The effects of calcium on electric field-induced cell shape changes and preferential orientation. Prog Clin Biol Res 1986; 210:319–327.

94. Onuma, EK, Hui, SW: Electric field-directed cell shape changes, displacement, and cytoskeletal reorganization are calcium dependent. J Cell Biol 1988; 106:2067–2075.

95. Pullar, CE, Isseroff, RR, Nuccitelli, R: Cyclic AMP-dependent protein kinase A plays a role in the directed migration of human keratinocytes in a DC electric field. Cell Motil Cytoskeleton 2001; 50:207–217.

96. Nuccitelli, R, Smart, T, Ferguson, J: Protein kinases are required for embryonic neural crest cell galvanotaxis. Cell Motil Cytoskeleton 1993; 24:54–66.

97. Pullar, CE, Isseroff, RR: Cyclic AMP mediates keratinocyte directional migration in an electric field. J Cell Sci 2005; 118:2023–2034.

98. Pu, J, Zhao, M: Golgi polarization in a strong electric field. J Cell Sci 2005; 118:1117–1128.

99. Finkelstein, E, Chang, W, Chao, PH, et al: Roles of microtubules, cell polarity, and adhesion in electric-field-mediated motility of 3T3 fibroblasts. J Cell Sci 2004; 117:1533–1545.

100. American Physical Therapy Association. Electrotherapeutic Terminology in Physical Therapy: Section on Clinical Electrophysiology. American Physical Therapy Association, Alexandria, VA, 2001.

101. Conductive Coupling. Available at: http://en.wikipedia.org/wiki/Conductive_coupling. Accessed March 17, 2009.

102. Inductive Coupling. Available at: http://en wikipedia.org/wiki/Inductive_coupling. Accessed March 17, 2009.

103. Gerleman, DG, Barr, JO: Instrumentation and product safety. In: Nelson, RM, Hayes, KW, Currier, DP (eds): Clinical Electrophysiology, ed. 3. Stamford, CT, Appleton & Lange, 1999, p 35.

104. Beard, RB, Hung, BN, Schmukler, R: Biocompatibility considerations at stimulating electrode interfaces. Ann Biomed Eng 1992; 20:395–410.

105. Procacci, P, Corte, D, Zoppi, M, et al: Pain threshold measurements in man. In: Bonica, JJ (ed): Recent Advances in Pain Therapy. Springfield, IL, Charles C Thomas, 1974, pp 36, 109.

106. Mueller, EE, Loeffel, R, Mead, S: Skin impedance in relation to pain threshold testing by electrical means. J Appl Physiol 1952; 5:746–752.

107. Ojingwa, JC, Isseroff, RR: Electrical stimulation of wound healing. J Invest Dermatol 2003; 121(1):1–12.

108. Westerhof ,W, Bos, JD: Trigeminal trophic syndrome: A successful treatment with transcutaneous electrical stimulation. Br J Dermatol 1983; 10:601–604.

109. Kaada, B: Promoted healing of chronic ulceration by transcutaneous nerve stimulation (TNS). Vasa 1983; 12:262–269.

110. Kaada, B, Emru, M: Promoted healing of leprous ulcers by transcutaneous nerve stimulation. Acupunct Electrother Res 1988; 13:165–176.

111. Karba, B, Vodovnik, L: Promoted healing of chronic wounds due to electrical stimulation. Wounds 1991; 3:16–23.

112. Lundeberg, TC, Eriksson, SV, Malm, M: Electrical nerve stimulation improves healing of diabetic ulcers. Ann Plast Surg 1992; 29:328–331.

113. Barron, JJ, Jacobson, WE, Tidd, G: Treatment of decubitus ulcers. A new approach. Minnesota Med 1985; 68:103–106.

114. Stefanovska, A, Vodovnik, L, Benko, H, et al: Treatment of chronic wounds by means of electric and electromagnetic fields. Value of FES parameters for pressure sore treatment. Med Biol Eng Comput 1993; 31(Pt 2):213–220.

115. Assimacopoulos, D: Low intensity negative electric current in treatment of ulcers of leg due to chronic venous insufficiency: Preliminary report of three cases. Am J Surg 1968; 115:683–687.

116. Wolcott, LF, Wheeler, PC, Hardwicke, HM, et al: Accelerated healing of skin ulcers by electrotherapy: Preliminary clinical results. South Med J 1969; 62:795–801.

117. Gault, WR, Gatens, PF: Use of low intensity direct current in management of ischemic skin ulcers. Phys Ther 1976; 56:265–269.

118. Carley, PJ, Wainapel, SF: Electrotherapy for acceleration of wound healing: Low intensity direct current. Arch Phys Med Rehabil 1985; 66:443–446.

119. Wood, JM, Evans, PE, Schallreuter, KU, et al: A multi-center study on the use of pulsed low intensity direct current for healing chronic stage II and III decubitus ulcers. Arch Dermatol 1993; 129:999–1009.

120. Canaday, DJ, Lee, RC: Scientific basis for clinical application of electric fields in soft tissue repair. In: Brighton, CT, Pollack, SR (eds): Electromagnetics in Biology and Medicine. San Francisco, San Francisco Press, 1991.

121. Feedar, JA, Kloth, LC, Gentzkow, GD: Chronic dermal ulcer healing enhanced with monophasic pulsed electrical stimulation. Phys Ther 1991; 71:639–649.

122. Gentzkow, GD, Pollack, SV, Kloth, LC, et al: Improved healing of pressure ulcers using Dermapulse, a new electrical stimulation device. Wounds 1991; 3:158–170.

123. Gentzkow, GD, Alon, G, Taler, GA, et al: Healing of refractory stage III and IV pressure ulcers by a new electrical stimulation device. Wounds 1993; 5:160–172.

124. Junger, M, Zuder, D, Steins, A, et al: Treatment of venous ulcers with low frequency pulsed current (Dermapulse): Effects on cutaneous microcirculation. Der Hautartz 1997; 18:879–903.

125. Akers, TK, Gabrielson, AL: The effect of high voltage galvanic stimulation on the rate of healing of decubitus ulcers. Biomed Sci Instrum 1984; 20:99–100.

126. Kloth, LC, Feedar, JA: Acceleration of wound healing with high voltage, monophasic, pulsed current. Phys Ther 1988; 71:503–508.

127. Griffin, JW, Tooms, RE, Mendlus, RA, et al: Efficacy of high voltage pulsed current for healing of pressure ulcers in patients with spinal cord injury. Phys Ther 1991; 71:433–442.

128. Fitzgerald, GK, Newsome, D: Treatment of a large infected thoracic spine wound using high voltage pulsed monophasic current. Phys Ther 1993; 73:355–360.

129. Newton, RA, Karselis, TC: Skin pH following high voltage pulsed galvanic stimulation. Phys Ther 1983; 63:1593–1596.

130. Baker, LL, Rubayi, S, Villar F, et al: Effect of electrical stimulation waveform on healing of ulcers in human beings with spinal cord injury. Wound Rep Reg 1996; 4:72–79.

131. Baker, LL, Chambers, R, DeMuth, SK, et al: Effects of electrical stimulation on wound healing in patients with diabetic ulcers. Diabetes Care 1997; 20:405–412.

132. Debreceni, L, Gyulai, M, Debreceni, A, et al: Results of transcutaneous electrical stimulation (TES) in cure of lower extremity arterial disease. Angiology 1995; 46:613–618.

133. Bourguignon, GJ, Bourguignon, LYW: Electric stimulation of protein and DNA synthesis in human fibroblasts. FASEB J 1987; 1:398–402.

134. Bourguignon, GJ, Bergouignan, M, Khorshed, A, et al. Effect of high voltage pulsed galvanic stimulation on human fibroblasts in cell culture. J Cell Biol 1986; 103:344a.

135. Falanga, V, Bourguignon, GY, Bourguignon, LYW: Electrical stimulation increases the expression of fibroblast receptors for transforming growth factor-beta. J Invest Dermatol 1987; 88:488–492.

136. Cheng, N, Van Hoof, H, Bockx, E, et al: The effects of electric currents on ATP generation, protein synthesis, and membrane transport in rat skin. Clin Orthop 1982; 171:264–272.

137. Cheng, K, Goldman, R: Electric fields and proliferation in a dermal wound model: Cell cycle kinetics. Bioelectromagnetics 1998; 19:68–74.

138. Rowley, B: Electrical current effects on E coli growth rates. Proc Soc Exp Biol Med 1972; 139:929–934.

139. Wolcott, L, Wheeler, P, Hardwicke, H, et al: Accelerated healing of skin ulcers by electrotherapy: Preliminary clinical results. South Med J 1969; 62:795–801.

140. Rowley, B, McKenna, J, Chase, G, et al: The influence of electrical current on an infecting microorganism in wounds. Ann NY Acad Sci 1974; 238:543–551.

141. Barranco, S, Spadero, J, Berger, T, et al: In vitro effect of weak direct current on *Staphylococcus aureus*. Clin Orthop 1974; 100:250–255.

142. Chu, CS, McManus, AT, Pruitt, BA, et al: Therapeutic effects of silver nylon dressings with weak direct current on *Pseudomonas aeruginosa* infected burn wounds. J Trauma 1988; 28:1490–1493.

143. Deitch, E, Marino, A, Malakanok, V, et al: Electrical augmentation of the antibacterial activity of silver nylon. Presented at: Proceedings of the 3rd Annual BRAG, San Francisco, CA, October, 1983.

144. Deitch, E, Marino, A, Gillespie, T, et al: Silver nylon: A new antimicrobial agent. Antimicrob Agents Chemother 1983; 23:356–359.

145. Marino, A, Deitch, E, Albright, J: Electric silver antisepsis. IEEE Trans Biomed Eng 1985; 32:336–337.

146. Colmano, G, Edwards, S, Barranco, S: Activation of antibacterial silver coatings on surgical implants by direct current: Preliminary studies in rabbits. Am J Vet Res 1980; 41:964–966.

147. Thibodeau, E, Handelman, S, Marquis, R: Inhibition and killing of oral bacteria by silver ions generated with low intensity direct current. J Dent Res 1978; 57:922–926.

148. Alvarez, O, Mertz, P, Smerbeck, R, et al: The healing of superficial skin wounds is stimulated by external electrical current. J Invest Dermatol 1983; 81:144–148.

149. Falcone, A, Spadero, J: Inhibitory effects of electrically activated silver material on cutaneous wound bacteria. Plast Reconstr Surg 1986; 77:445–458.

150. Becker, R, Spadero, J: Treatment of orthopedic infections with electrically generated silver ions. J Bone Joint Surg Am 1978; 60:871–881.

151. Ong, P, Laatsch, L, Kloth, L: Antibacterial effects of a silver electrode carrying microamperage direct current in vitro. J Clin Electrophysiol 1994; 6:14–18.

152. Laatsch, L, Ong, P, Kloth, L: In vitro effects of two silver electrodes on select wound pathogens. J Clin Electrophysiol 1995; 7:10–15.

153. Guffey, J, Asmussen, M: In vitro bactericidal effects of high voltage pulsed current versus direct current against *Staphylococcus aureus.* J Clin Electrophysiol 1989; 1:5–9.

154. Kincaid, C, Lavoie, K: Inhibition of bacterial growth in vitro following stimulation with high voltage, monophasic pulsed current. Phys Ther 1989; 69:651–655.

155. Szuminsky, N, Albers, A, Unger, P, et al: Effect of narrow, pulsed high voltages on bacterial viability. Phys Ther 1994; 74:660–667.

156. Merriman, HL, Hegyi, CA, Albright-Overton, CR, et al: A comparison of four electrical stimulation types on *Staphylococcus aureus* growth in vitro. J Rehabil Res Develop 2004; 41(2):139–146.

157. Daeschlein, G, Assadian, O, Kloth, LC, et al: Antibacterial activity of positive and negative polarity low-voltage pulsed current (LVPC) on six typical Gram-positive and Gram-negative bacterial pathogens of chronic wounds. Wound Rep Regen 2007; 15:399–409.

158. Perez, R, Rivas, Y, Gil, J, et al: Assessment of the effects on wound healing and gene expression of a bio-electric dressing (CMB) using a porcine wound model and a real time RT-PCR. Presented at: Abstracts of the World Union of Wound Healing Societies Symposium, Toronto, Ontario, Canada, June, 2008.

159. Costerton, B, Ellis, K, Lam, K, et al: Antibiotic effectiveness is increased in the presence of even a weak, intermittent electrical field. Antimicrob Agents Chemother 1994; 38:2803–2809.

160. McLeod, B, Dirckx, P: The combination of electricity plus antibiotic is more effective against biofilm cells than either is alone. The Center for Biofilm Engineering, Montana State University, Bozeman, MT. Available at: http//www.erc.montana.edu. Accessed 01/13/05.

161. Janigro, D, Perju, C, Fazio, V, et al: Alternating current electrical stimulation enhanced chemotherapy: A novel strategy to bypass multidrug resistance in tumor cells. Biomedical Central Cancer 2006; 17(6):72 Abstract. Available at: http://www.biomedcentral.com/1471-2407/6/72/abstract. Accessed 11/29/07.

162. Assimacopoulos, D: Wound healing promotion by the use of negative electric current. Am Surg 1968; 34:423–431.

163. Bigelow, J: Effect of electrical stimulation on canine skin and percutaneous device: Skin interface healing. In: Brighton, CT, Black, J, Pollack, SR (eds): Skin Interface Healing and Electrical Properties of Bone and Cartilage. New York, Grune and Stratton, 1979, p 289.

164. Carey, L, Lepley, D: Effect of continuous direct electric current on healing wounds. Surg Forum 1962;13:33–35.

165. Castillo, E, Sumano, H, Fortoul, T, et al: The influence of pulsed electrical stimulation on the wound healing of burned rat skin. Arch Med Res 1995; 26:185–189.

166. Konikoff, JJ: Electrical promotion of soft tissue repairs. Biomed Eng 1976; 4:1–5.

167. Smith, J, Romansky, N, Vomero, J, et al: The effect of electrical stimulation on wound healing in diabetic mice. J Am Podiatr Assoc 1984; 74:71–75.

168. Cruz, N, Bayron, F, Suarez, A: Accelerated healing of full-thickness burns by the use of high voltage pulsed galvanic stimulation in the pig. Ann Plast Surg 1989; 23:49–55.

169. Taskan, I, Ozyazgan, I, Tercan, M, et al: A comparative study of the effect of ultrasound and electrostimulation on wound healing in rats. Plast Reconstr Surg 1997; 100:966–972.

170. Dunn, M, Doillon, C, Berg, R, et al: Wound healing using a collagen matrix: Effect of DC electrical stimulation. J Biomed Mater Res 1988; 22(suppl):191–206.

171. Bach, S, Bilgrav, K, Gottrup, F, et al: The effect of electrical current on healing skin incision. Eur J Surg 1991; 157:171–174.

172. Mertz, P, Davis, S, Cazzaniga, A, et al: Electrical stimulation: Acceleration of soft tissue repair by varying the polarity. Wounds 1993; 5:153–159.

173. Brown, M, Gogia, P: Effects of high voltage stimulation on cutaneous wound healing in rabbits. Phys Ther 1987; 67:662–667.

174. Brown, M, McDonnell, M, Menton, D: Electrical stimulation effects on cutaneous wound healing in rabbits. Phys Ther 1988; 68:955–960.

175. Reed, BV: Effect of high voltage pulsed electrical stimulation on microvascular permeability to plasma proteins: a possible mechanism in minimizing edema. Phys Ther 1988; 68:491–495.

176. Taylor, K, Mendel, F, Fish, D, et al: Effect of high voltage pulsed current and alternating current on macromolecular leakage in hamster cheek pouch microcirculation. Phys Ther 1997; 77:1729–1740.

177. Thornton, R, Mendel, F, Fish, D: Effects of electrical stimulation on edema formation in different strains of rats. Phys Ther 1998; 78:386–394.

178. Matylevich, NP, Chu, CS, McManus, AT, et al: Direct current reduces plasma protein extravasation after partial–thickness burn injury in rats. J Trauma 1996; 4:424–429.

179. Chu, CS, Matylevich, NP, McManus, AT, et al: Direct current reduces wound edema after full-thickness burn injury in rats. J Trauma 1996; 40:738–742.

180. Chu, CS, McManus, AT, Mason, AD Jr, et al: Multiple graft harvestings from deep partial-thickness scald wounds healed under the influence of weak direct current. J Trauma 1990; 30:1044–1049.

181. Politis, MJ, Zanakis, MF, Miller, JE: Enhanced survival of full-thickness skin grafts following the application of DC electrical fields. Plast Reconst Surg 1989; 84:267–272.

182. Im, JM, Lee, WPA, Hoopes, JE: Effect of electrical stimulation on survival of skin flaps in pigs. Phys Ther 1990; 70:37–40.

183. Kjartansson, J, Lundeberg, T, Samuelson, U: Transcutaneous electrical nerve stimulation (TENS) increases survival of ischaemic musculocutaneous flaps. Acta Physiol Scand 1988; 134:95–99.

184. Greenberg, J, Hanly, AJ, Davis, SC, et al: The effect of electrical stimulation (RPES) on wound healing and angiogenesis in second degree burns. Presented at: 13th Annual Symposium on Advanced Wound Care, Dallas, TX, April 1–4, 2000.

185. Mohr, T, Akers, T, Wessman, HC: Effect of high voltage stimulation on blood flow in the rat hind limb. Phys Ther 1987; 67:528–533.

186. Mehri, M, Helme, R, Khalil, A: Age related changes in sympathetic modulation of sensory nerve activity in rat skin. Infamm Res 1998; 47:239–244.

187. Kanno, S, Oda, N, Abe, M, et al: Establishment of a simple and practical procedure applicable to therapeutic angiogenesis. Circulation 1999; 99:2682–2687.

188. Patterson, C, Runge, MS: Therapeutic angiogenesis: The new electrophysiology? Circulation. 1999; 99:2614–2616.

189. Kaada, B: Vasodilation induced by transcutaneous nerve stimulation in peripheral ischemia (Raynaud's phenomenon and diabetic polyneuropathy). Eur Heart J 1982; 3:303–308.

190. Kaada, B, Eielson, O: In search of the mediators of skin vasodilation induced by transcutaneous nerve stimulation: I. Failure to block the response by antagonists of endogenous vasodilators. Gen Pharmacol 1983; 4:623–625.

191. Kaada, B, Ensen, O: In search of the mediators of skin vasodilation induced by transcutaneous nerve stimulation: II. Serotonin implicated. Gen Pharmacol 1983; 14:635–639.

192. Kaada, B, Helle, KB: In search of the mediators of skin vasodilation induced by transcutaneous nerve stimulation: IV. In vitro bioassay of the vaso-inhibitory activity of sera from patients suffering from peripheral ischemia. Gen Pharmacol 1984; 15:115–121.

193. Kaada, B, Hegland, O, Oktedalen, O, et al: Failure to influence the VIP level in the cerebrospinal fluid by transcutaneous stimulation in humans. Gen Pharmacol 1984; 15:563–568.

194. Dooley, DM, Kasprak, M: Modification of blood flow to the extremities by electrical stimulation of the nervous system. South Med J 1976; 69:1309–1312.

195. Owens, S, Atkinson, ER, Lees, DE: Thermographic evidence of reduced sympathetic tone with transcutaneous nerve stimulation. Anesthesiology 1979; 50:62–65.

196. Wong, RA, Jette, PV: Changes in sympathetic tone associated with different forms of transcutaneous electrical nerve stimulation in healthy subjects. Phys Ther 1984; 64:478.

197. Ernst, M, Lee, M: Sympathetic vasomotor changes induced by manual and electrical acupuncture of the hoku point visualized by thermography. Pain 1985; 21:25–29.

198. Ebersold, MI, Laws, ER, Jr, Albers, JW, et al: Measurements of autonomic function before, during, and after transcutaneous stimulation in patients with chronic pain and in control subjects. Mayo Clin Proc 1977; 52:228–231.

199. Skudds, RJ, Helewa, A, Skudds, RA: The effects of transcutaneous electrical nerve stimulation on skin temperature in asymptotic subjects. Phys Ther 1995; 75:621–626.

200. Currier, DP, Petrilli, CR, Threlkeld, AJ: Effect of medium frequency electrical stimulation on local blood circulation to healthy muscle. Phys Ther 1986; 66:937–940.

201. Tracy, JE, Currier, DP, Threlkeld, AJ: Comparison of selected pulse frequencies from two different electrical stimulators on blood flow in healthy subjects. Phys Ther 1988; 68:1526–1530.

202. Hecker, B, Carron, H, Schwartz, DP: Pulsed galvanic stimulation: Effects of current frequency and polarity on blood flow in healthy subjects. Arch Phys Med Rehabil 1985; 66:369–373.

203. Cramp, A, Gilsensan, C, Lowe, A, et al: The effect of high and low frequency transcutaneous electrical nerve stimulation upon cutaneous blood flow and skin temperature in healthy subjects. Clin Physiol 2000; 20:150–157.

204. Petrofsky, J, Schwab, E, Lo, T, et al: Effects of electrical stimulation on skin blood flow in controls and around stage III and IV wounds in hairy and non-hairy skin. Med Sci Monitor 2005; 11:CR309–316.

205. Petrofsky, J, Schwab, E, Lo, T, et al: The thermal effect on the blood flow response to electrical stimulation. Med Sci Monitor 2007; 13:CR 498–504.

206. Lawson, D, Petrofsky, J: A randomized control study on the effect of biphasic electrical stimulation in a warm room on skin blood flow and healing rates in chronic wounds of patients with and without diabetes. Med Sci Monitor 2007; 13:CR 258–263.

207. Wikstrom, S, Svedman, P, Svensson, H, et al: Effect of transcutaneous nerve stimulation on microcirculation in intact skin and blister wounds in healthy volunteers. Scand J Plastic Surg Hand Surg 1999; 33:195–201.

208. Cosmo, P, Svensson, H, Bornmyr, S, et al: Effect of transcutaneous nerve stimulation on the microcirculation in chronic leg ulcers. Scan J Plast Reconstr Surg Hand Surg 2000; 34:61–64.

209. Young, KC, Railton, R, Harrower, ADB, et al: Transcutaneous oxygen tension measurements as a method of assessing peripheral vascular disease. Clin Phys Physiol Meas 1981; 2:147–151.

210. Sheffield, C, Sessler, D, Hopf, H, et al: Centrally and locally mediated thermoregulatory responses alter subcutaneous oxygen tension. Wound Repair Regen 1996; 4:339–345.

211. Gagnier, K, Manix, N, Baker, L, et al: The effects of electrical stimulation on cutaneous oxygen supply in paraplegics. Phys Ther 1988; 68:835–839.

212. Dodgen, P, Johnson, B, Baker, L, et al: The effects of electrical stimulation on cutaneous oxygen supply in diabetic older adults (abstr). Phys Ther 1987; 67:793.

213. Peters, E, Armstrong, D, Wunderlich, R, et al: The benefit of electrical stimulation to enhance perfusion in persons with diabetes mellitus. J Foot Ankle Surg 1998; 37:396–400.

214. Rodriguez, G, Claus-Walker, J, Kent, M, et al: Adrenergic receptors in insensitive skin of spinal cord injury patients. Arch Phys Med Rehabil 1986; 67:177–113.

215. Bogie, K, Nuseibeh, I, Bader, D: Transcutaneous gas tension in the sacrum during the acute phase of spinal cord injury. Proceedings of the Institute of Mechanical Engineers, Part H. J Engr Med 1992; 206:1–6.

216. Mawson, A, Siddiqui, F, Connolly, B, et al: Sacral transcutaneous oxygen tension levels in the spinal cord injured: Risk factors for pressure ulcers? Arch Phys Med Rehabil 1993; 74:745–751.

217. Patterson, R, Cranmer, H, Fisher, S, et al: The impaired response of spinal cord injured individuals to repeated surface pressure loads. Arch Phys Med Rehabil 1993; 74:947–953.

218. Mawson, A, Siddiqui, F, Connolly, B, et al: Effect of high voltage pulsed galvanic stimulation on sacral transcutaneous oxygen tension levels in the spinal cord injured. Paraplegia 1993; 31:311–319.

219. Bolton, L, Foleno, B, Means, B, et al: Direct current bactericidal effect on intact skin. Antimicrob Agents Chemother 1980; 18:137–144.

220. Cukjati, D, Robnik-Sikonja, M, Rebersek, S, et al: Prognostic factors in the prediction of chronic wound healing by electrical stimulation. Med Biol Eng Comput 2001; 39:542–550.

221. Katelaris, PM, Fletcher, JP, Little, JM, et al: Electrical stimulation in the treatment of chronic venous ulceration. Aust N Z J Surg 1987; 57: 605–607.

222. Feldman, DS, Andino, RV, Jennings, JA: Clinical evaluation of an electrical stimulation bandage (POSIFECT dressing). Poster presentation at: ETRS/EWMA/DFGW Conference, Stuttgart, Germany, 2005.

223. Hampton, S, Collins, F: Treating a pressure ulcer with bio-electric stimulation therapy. Br J Nurs 2006; 15:S14–18.

224. Hampton, S, King, L: Healing an intractable wound using bio-electric stimulation therapy. Br J Nurs 2005; 14:30–32.

225. White, R, Cutting, K, Bhatti, JZ, et al: Electrical stimulation (E-Stim) in the healing of chronic wounds compromised by bacterial biofilm. Poster presentation at: Tissue Viability Society Annual Conference, Birmingham, UK, April 26–27, 2006.

226. Hampton, S, Kerr, A, Ling, L: Bio-electrical stimulation of chronic wounds: POSiFECT bio-electric wound care dressing. Poster presentation at: Wounds UK Conference, Harrogate, England, November 14–16, 2005.

227. Blenkinsopp, SA, Khouri, AE, Costerton, JW: Electrical enhancement of biocide efficacy against *Pseudomonas aeruginosa* biofilms. App Environ Microbiol 1992; 58:3770–3773.

228. Khoury, AE, Lam, K, Ellis, BD, et al: Prevention and control of bacterial infections associated with medical devices. Am Soc Artific Intern Org J 1992; 38:M174–M178.

229. Barczak, M, Kluger, P, Kluger, J, et al: Therapeutic effectiveness of electric stimulation in paraplegic patients with pressure sores [dissertation of M. Barczak]. Medical School of the University of Ulm, Germany, 2001.

230. Daniel, RK, Kerrigan, CL: Principles and physiology of skin flap surgery. In: McCarthy, J (ed): Plastic Surgery. Philadelphia, WB Saunders, 1990, pp 275–328.

231. Frantz, RA: The effectiveness of transcutaneous electrical nerve stimulation (TENS) on decubitus ulcer healing in adult patients. In: Funk, SG, Tornquist, EM, Champagne, et al (eds): Key Aspects of Recovery: Improving Nutrition, Rest, and Mobility. New York, Springer, 1990, pp 197–205.

232. Sumano, H, Mateos, G: The use of acupuncture-like electrical stimulation for wound healing of lesions unresponsive to conventional treatment. Am J Acupuncture 1999; 27:5–14.

233. Adunsky, A, Ohry, A: Decubitus direct current treatment (DDCT) of pressure ulcers: Results of a randomized double-blinded placebo controlled study. Arch Gerontol Geriatr 2005; 41:261–269.

234. Kloth, LC: Electrical stimulation for wound healing: A review of evidence from in vitro studies, animal experiments, and clinical trials. Lower Extrem Wounds 2005; 4:23–44.

235. Young, GH: Electric impulse therapy aids wound healing. Mod Vet Prac 1996; 47:60–64.

236. Alon, G, Azaria, M, Stein, H: Diabetic ulcer healing using hugh voltage TENS. (Abstracted) Phys Ther 1986; 66:775.

237. Franek, A, Polak, A, Kucharzewski, M: Modern application of high voltage stimulation for enhanced healing of venous crural ulceration. Med Eng Phys 2000; 22:647–655.

238. Polak, A, Franek, A, Hunka-Zurawinska, H, et al: High voltage electrostimulation in treatment of venous crural ulceration. Wiadomosci Lekarskie 2000; LIII:7–8.

239. Franek, A, Taradaj, J, Polak, A, et al: Efficacy of high voltage stimulation for healing of venous leg ulcers in surgically and conservatively treated patients. Phlebologie 2006; 35:1–7.

240. Houghton, PE, Kincaid, CB, Lovell, M, et al: Effect of electrical stimulation on leg ulcer size and appearance. Phys Ther 2003; 83:17–28.

241. Peters, EJG, Lavery, LA, Armstrong, DG, et al: Electrical stimulation as an adjunct to heal diabetic foot ulcers: a randomized clinical trial. Arch Phys Med Rehabil 2001; 82:721–724.

242. Goldman, R, Brewley, B, Golden, M: Electrotherapy reoxygenates inframalleolar ischemic wounds on diabetic patients. Adv Skin Wound Care 2002; 15:112–120.

243. Goldman, R, Brewley, B, Cohen, R, et al: Use of electrotherapy to reverse expanding cutaneous gangrene in end-stage renal disease. Adv Skin Wound Care 2003; 16:363–366.

244. Goldman, R, Brewley, B, Zhou, L, et al: Electrotherapy reverses inframalleolar ischemia: A retrospective, observational study. Adv Skin Wound Care 2003; 16:79–89.

245. Goldman, R, Rosen, M, Brewley, B, et al: Electrotherapy promotes healing and microcirculation of infrapopliteal wounds: A prospective pilot study. Adv Skin Wound Care 2004; 17:284–290, 290–294.

246. Burdge, JL, Hartman, JF, Wright, ML: The role of high voltage, pulsed electrical stimulation in limb salvage for diabetic patients. Abstract (Oral presentation) 38.4. 2008 Symposium on Advanced Wound Care and the Wound Healing Society, S 144. San Diego, CA.

247. Bosi, E, Conti, M, Vermigli, C, et al: Effectiveness of frequency-modulated electromagnetic neural stimulation in the treatment of painful diabetic neuropathy. Diabetologia 2005; 48:817–823.

248. Bevilacqua, M, Dominquez, LJ, Barrella, M, et al: Induction of vascular endothelial growth factor release by transcutaneous frequency modulated neural stimulation in diabetic polyneuropathy. J Endocrinol Invest 2007; 30:944–947.

249. Clinical Practice Guideline: Pressure Ulcer Prevention and Treatment Following Spinal Cord Injury. Paralyzed Veterans of America, Washington, DC, 2000.

250. Gardner, SE, Frantz, RA, Schmidt, FL: Effect of electrical stimulation on chronic wound healing: A meta-analysis. Wound Rep Regen 1999; 7:495–503.

251. Houghton, PE, Woodbury, MG: Electrical stimulation therapy to promote wound closure: A meta-analysis. Wounds 2007; 19:A27.

252. European Pressure Ulcer Advisory Panel and National Pressure Ulcer Advisory Panel. Treatment of pressure ulcers: Quick Reference Quide. Washington DC: National Pressure Ulcer Advisory Panel; 2009.

253. Nuccitelli, R, Nuccitelli, P, Ramlatchan, S, et al: Imaging the electric field associated with mouse and human skin wounds. Wound Repair Regen 2008; 16:432–441.

254. Nuccitelli, R, Nuccitelli, P, Li, C, et al: The electric field at human skin wounds declines sharply with age. Poster presentation at: 21st Symposium on Advanced Wound Care & Wound Healing Society meeting, San Diego, CA, April, 2008.

chapter 27

Electromagnetic Stimulation for Wound Repair

Luther C. Kloth, MS, PT, CWS, FACCWS, FAPTA
Arthur A. Pilla, PhD

Principles of Electromagnetic Radiation

In this chapter we will cover the use of exogenously applied, time-varying electromagnetic (EM) fields from the nonionizing radio frequency (RF) part of the EM spectrum, which, when placed near open or closed wounded soft and hard tissues, will induce a healing electric field inside those tissues that is proportional to the rate of change of the magnetic field. In this context we will present the evidence for the use of nonthermal pulsed electromagnetic fields (PEMF), pulsed radio frequency energy (PRF), and low-level thermal PRF, which may also be referred to as pulsed shortwave diathermy (PSWD), as adjunctive treatments for patients with chronic wounds. Please note that continuous shortwave diathermy (CSWD) is also derived from the 27.12-MHz frequency, but because it is capable of generating vigorous tissue heating if tissues are in well vascularized tissues, it is generally not used for wound healing applications. Table 27.1 lists devices and their acronyms.

> ▶ **PEARL 27•1** It is important to emphasize here that all of these alternative wound healing interventions are derived from a primary continuous RF sinusoidal wave (27.12 MHz) called a "carrier," which can be modulated to produce nonthermal PEMF and PRF and mild thermal PSWD, each of which will be described later.

What Is Electromagnetic Radiation?

EM radiation is a type of energy that is created when electric charges are accelerated. When electric charges move, they produce waves of electric and magnetic energy in space. A familiar example is electric charges that move back and forth as alternating current emitted from a radio station tower (antenna) and that travel (broadcast) at the speed of light through space as RF radiation. These waves have a distinctive frequency and wavelength and can be reflected, refracted, and absorbed when they interact with matter.

What Is Frequency and How Does It Affect Tissues?

The frequency of EM radiation corresponds to the number of waves per second that cross a fixed point in space. EM waves are typically sine waves that cover a vast range of frequencies and corresponding wavelengths. Lower energy levels represented by the spectrum are produced by lower-frequency sine waves (eg, 60 Hz for electric power), whereas very high frequencies (10^{19} Hz) produce high-energy level gamma rays. RF radiation is the area or band of the EM spectrum in which most radio communication takes place and consists of propagating sine waves typically between 10 kilohertz (kHz) and 300 gigahertz (GHz) (1 kHz = 1×10^3 Hz; 1 GHz = 1×10^9 Hz.)[1] (Fig. 27.1) The electromagnetic spectrum also includes the familiar waves of visible light, infrared, and ultraviolet. Unlike the lower pulsed current frequencies used to excite nerve and muscle cell membranes,

Table 27•1	List of Devices and Their Acronyms
Acronym	**Device/EM Energy**
PEMF	Pulsed electromagnetic field
PRF	Pulsed radio frequency
PSWD	Pulsed shortwave diathermy
CSWD	Continuous shortwave diathermy

the higher RFs are not capable of depolarizing motor nerves or eliciting contractions from skeletal muscle because the duration of each cycle of alternating current in this frequency range is too short to cause migration of ions through cell membranes of nerve or muscle.[2] Another advantage of EM energy in the RF range is that, unlike photons produced by x-rays and sufficiently high frequencies (ionizing radiation) that have enough energy to eject electrons (ionize) from atoms or molecules, RF signals do not. When a cell's contents are ionized, very reactive compounds called *free radicals* are formed that can damage vital parts of the cell. Cells are equipped to deal with some free radicals, which can be produced by normal metabolism, but excessive ionizing radiation can overpower a cell's ability to control and repair the free radical damage and thus disrupt normal function. The damage from ionizing radiation that cannot be repaired accumulates over time in the cell, hindering or preventing mitosis and causing permanent tissue damage. Ionizing radiation may also directly damage DNA and RNA.[3] The ultraviolet wavelength of 100 nm and frequency 3×10^{15} Hz,

is conventionally taken as the dividing line between ionizing and nonionizing radiation.[3] Energy from the RF part of the spectrum may or may not penetrate the skin. Regardless, RF energy is only a fraction of that required to produce ionization in tissue. Therefore, with RF energy, no mutations are induced nor does DNA single-strand uncoupling occur, such as that which results from ionizing x-ray radiation therapy used in cancer treatment.[3] However, as shown in Figure 27.1, RF waves that have appropriate dosage parameters are capable of producing thermal energy that may be used to therapeutically heat body tissues such as occurs with mild thermal level PSWD. Recall that all frequencies in the EM spectrum travel through a vacuum at the speed of light and that they consist of two components, an electric field and a magnetic field that transmit electric and magnetic energy (electromagnetic waves) through space. The magnetic component of the EM signal has a negligible physiological effect on the tissue target. The induced electric field can interact with electric charges, for example, ions, to produce the desired effect. It is fundamental that, for EM waves to have an effect on target tissues within the body, they must be absorbed by those tissues that contain cells and molecules. This fact is upheld by the law of Grotthus-Draper, which states that only radiation that is absorbed can produce chemical change. However, absorbed radiation does not necessarily cause a chemical reaction. Absorbed radiation may simply be converted into heat, or it may be reemitted as light of a different wavelength, which is the phenomenon called *fluorescence*. Thus, while waves from one part of the spectrum may be absorbed when they encounter an object, waves from other parts of the spectrum may either be reflected or pass through the object. Nonionizing RF waves delivered to the body for therapeutic purposes cause atoms and molecules to vibrate and rotate without ionization.

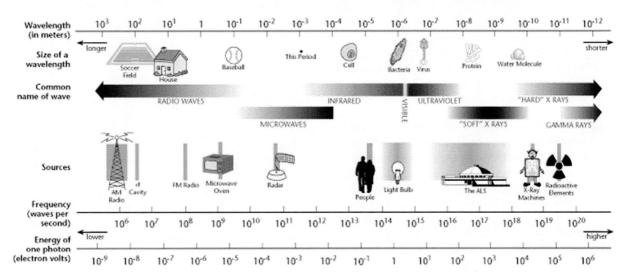

Figure 27•1 *Electromagnetic radiations showing the radio frequency part of the spectrum.* www.lbl.gov/MicroWorlds/ALSTool/EMSpec/EMSpec2.html

Energy from the RF field is transferred to tissue by increasing the vibrational and rotational energy of dipoles (primarily water) in the tissue.

▶ **PEARL 27•2** At the carrier frequency of interest (27.12 MHz), and in the near field, that is, with the tissue target placed next to the transmitting antenna (patient treatment coil applicator), the primary component of the EM signal is the electric field that produces the desired physiological thermal effect of heat or nonthermal cellular signaling.

▶ **PEARL 27•3** Thus, RF effects on cells and molecules are generally limited to nonthermal (PEMF and PRF) and low-level thermal (PSWD) through changes that occur secondary to increased kinetic activity rather than the direct breaking of chemical bonds.[3]

Because of the high demands for the use of various frequencies for communication, the Federal Communications Commission (FCC) has very carefully regulated what frequencies can be used in television and radio transmission, radar, and medical applications. In the past the FCC allowed the use of three different RF frequencies in the medical applications of PEMF, PRF, and PSWD. However, for practical electronic reasons, only the 27.12-MHz frequency is used in these devices in the United States.

What Is Wavelength?

The time that elapses between successive peaks of a propagating RF sine wave is called the *period* of the wave. The distance traveled by EM waves in one period is the wavelength. (Fig. 27.2) EM wavelengths are inversely related to frequency and can range from one-billionth of a meter up to miles. All of these wavelengths do not pass through the body with equal ease, however; there is no simple relationship between wavelength and the ability of these EM waves to travel through the body almost unimpeded. This explains why you can listen to a radio when a person or a wall is between you and a broadcasting radio. Wavelengths of RF described above used for tissue healing and therapy lie between 3×10^5 and 3×10^{-3} meters. It is within this range that the wavelengths are found for devices used to deliver the PEMF, PRF, and PSWD signals previously mentioned.

▶ **PEARL 27•4** The wavelength that corresponds to the FCC-approved frequency of 27.12 MHz is 11 meters. This wavelength readily penetrates human skin and produces electric fields at a depth that is sufficient for most therapeutic uses.

Modulation of the Radio Frequency Carrier Wave

As previously mentioned, the RF carrier wave (27.12 MHz) is used to produce PEMF, PRF, and PSWD treatment signals. RF waves may be delivered to the body either as continuous oscillations or by periodically interrupting the

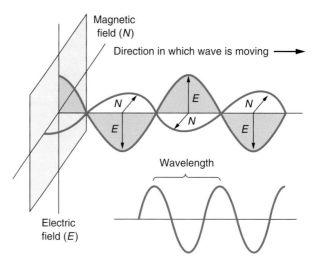

Field and wavelength relationships in an electromagnetic wave

Figure 27•2 *Magnetic and electric field components at right angles to each other and wavelength of an electromagnetic wave. (From: Yost MG: Nonionizing radiation questions and answers. In: Clemmensen J: Nonionizing Radiation: A Case for Federal Standards? San Francisco, San Francisco Press, 1993, p.2, with permission)*

continuous waves at regular intervals to produce pulses or bursts of RF energy. Continuous waves of RF are associated with increasing tissue temperature, first observed by Nagelschmidt in 1906.[4] RF devices that deliver continuous waves used for therapeutic heating are called continuous shortwave diathermy (CSWD) machines, and they are capable of producing high to moderate tissue heating effects (*diathermy* means to heat through) for adjunctive treatment of a variety of musculoskeletal conditions. (Table 27.2) RF devices that deliver pulses of RF waves are referred to as pulsed radio-frequency (PRF) and pulsed shortwave diathermy (PSWD) devices. PRF devices that have low average power output produce nonthermal effects on absorbing tissues, whereas PRF devices with high average power produce pulsed shortwave diathermy (PSWD), which has low heating effects. The pulsed version created from RF was originally reported to elicit a nonthermal biological effect by Ginsberg.[5] In contrast to PRF and PSWD devices, PEMF devices operate with a different modulated waveform frequency. Figure 27.3 shows waveforms for PRF and PSWD (bottom) and PEMF (top). Several differences in the characteristics of the two signals are evident. The most visible difference is pulse shape. The PRF signal is characterized by sequences of sine waves contained within rectangular burst envelopes that typically have a duration of 65 µsec. Each pulse or burst envelope contains 1760 sine waves of the 27.12 MHz carrier RF. The frequency of this pulsed signal varies between 80 and 600 pulses per second, and the duty cycle is less than 4%. The PEMF pulse duration and the pulse frequency may vary between 1 and 100 msec and 1 and 100 pulses per second, respectively. Each of the three signals that have been briefly described will be addressed in greater detail below, in the order of PEMF, PRF, and PSWD.

Table 27•2 **Characteristics and Effects of Radio Frequency Devices**

Device	Signal/Frequency	Pulse Duration	Induced Voltage	Effects on Tissues/Cells
PEMF	Sinusoidal; 27.12 MHz; 1–100 pps	1–100 msec	mV/cm	Nonthermal and cellular; no nerve/muscle excitation
PRF	Sinusoidal; 27.12 MHz, 80–600 pps	42 and 65 μsec	V/cm	Nonthermal, cellular, and circulatory; no nerve/muscle excitation
PSWD	Sinusoidal; 27.12 MHz; 3.9% duty cycle	95 μsec	V/cm	Mild heating, circulatory; no nerve/muscle excitation
CSWD	Sinusoidal; 27.12 MHz	Continuous	V/cm	Moderate to high heating; enhances collagen extensibility; no nerve/muscle excitation

PEMF, pulsed electromagnetic field; PRF, pulsed radio frequency; PSWD, pulsed shortwave diathermy; CSWD, continuous shortwave diathermy.
Modified with permission from Sussman, C: Induced electrical stimulation: Pulsed radio frequency and pulsed electromagnetic fields. In: Sussman C, Bates-Jensen B (eds): Wound Care: A Collaborative Practice Manual for Health Professionals, ed. 3. Philadelphia, Lippincott Williams & Wilkins, 2007, p 557.

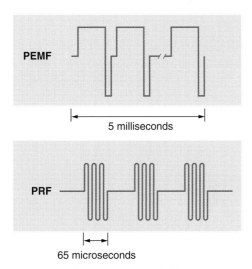

5 milliseconds

65 microseconds

Figure 27•3 *Pulsed electromagnetic field (PEMF) signal was designed for bone growth stimulation, while the pulsed radiofrequency (PRF) signal is used primarily for treatment of soft tissue closed and open wounds. Note that the PEMF signal is asymmetrical with a 5-ms duration, while the PRF signal consists of 65-μsec rectangular pulse bursts. (From Markov MS, Pilla AA: Electromagnetic field stimulation of soft tissues: Pulsed radio frequency treatment of post-operative pain and edema. Wounds 1995; 7:144, with permission)*

▶ **PEARL 27•5** Depending on the average power delivered to the body by these pulses of RF energy, tissue temperature may or may not increase. Thus, PRF may have either thermal or nonthermal effects on tissues.

▶ **PEARL 27•6** Another main difference between the two signals is the magnitude of the induced voltage, which is in the V/cm range for PRF and mV/cm for PEMF.[6]

Pulsed Electromagnetic Fields for Bone Tissue Repair

The number of people who have received substantial clinical benefit from the exogenous application of pulsed electromagnetic fields (PEMF) is likely in the millions worldwide and increasing rapidly as new clinical indications emerge. PEMF and PRF therapies present as alternatives to many pharmacological treatments with no pharmacokinetic limitations and no known toxicity or side effects. This chapter reviews the scientific and clinical evidence that shows that PEMF and PRF can modulate molecular, cellular, and tissue function in a physiologically significant manner. In Chapter 26, enhanced soft tissue healing was reported to be augmented by the use of capacitively (conductively) coupled electric stimulators that have electrodes in direct contact with wound and periwound skin. Such technologies deliver waveforms similar to those produced by pulsed current devices currently cleared by the FDA for relief of acute and chronic pain.[6,7] Unlike the direct contact (conductive coupling) method described in Chapter 26, here emphasis will be on PEMF and PRF technologies that inductively couple the signal to the tissue target and have been reported to be clinically effective for healing bone fractures and soft tissue repair, respectively.

▶ **PEARL 27•7** PEMF devices produce physiologically effective voltage and current in tissue without the necessity of skin or wound tissue contact.[6,8] In addition, the Center for Medicare Services (CMS) determined in 2004 that PRF research had produced sufficient positive clinical outcomes to permit reimbursement for its off-label use in the treatment of chronic wounds, such as pressure ulcers, diabetic leg and foot ulcers, as well as chronic wounds caused by arterial and venous insufficiency.[9]

Background—Pulsed Electromagnetic Field–Induced Osteogenesis

The development of modern PEMF therapeutics was stimulated by the clinical problems associated with nonunion and delayed union bone fractures. It started with an attempt to answer the fundamental orthopedic question of how bone adaptively and structurally responds to mechanical stresses by suggesting that an electric signal may be involved in the transduction of the mechanical (weight loading) signal to cellular activity. This led to the suggestion that superimposing an exogenous PEMF upon the endogenous bioelectric fields that occur following bone fracture may help in the treatment of difficult-to-heal fractures. The first animal studies employed microampere level direct currents (DC) delivered via implanted electrodes. Remarkably, this resulted in new bone formation, particularly around the cathode.[10] As these studies progressed, it became clear that the new bone growth resulted from the chemical changes around the electrodes caused by electrolysis.[11] The first therapeutic devices were based on these early animal studies and used implanted and semiinvasive electrodes that delivered DC to the fracture site.[12,13] This was followed by the development of clinically preferable, externally applied electromagnetic field technologies.[14-17] Subsequent studies concentrated on the direct effects of electromagnetic fields, leading to devices that provided a noninvasive, noncontact means of applying an electric signal to a cell or tissue target. Therapeutic uses of these technologies in orthopedic practice have led to clinical applications, approved by regulatory bodies worldwide, for treatment of recalcitrant fractures and spine fusion and recently for osteoarthritis of the knee.[18-27] Additional clinical indications for PEMF have been reported in double-blind studies for the treatment of avascular necrosis and tendinitis.[28-30]

At present, the clinical PEMF technologies in use for bone repair consist of DC electrodes implanted directly into the repair site or noninvasive capacitive or inductive coupling. *Direct current* is applied via one electrode (cathode) placed in the tissue target at the fracture site and the anode placed in soft tissue. DC currents of 5 to 100 µA are sufficient to stimulate osteogenesis.[18] The *capacitive or conductive coupling* (CC) technique uses external skin contact electrodes placed over a cast on opposite sides of the fracture site.[31] This requires openings in the cast or orthosis to allow skin access. Sinusoidal waves of 20 to 200 kHz are typically employed to induce 1 to 100 mV/cm electric fields in the repair site.[32] The *inductive coupling* (PEMF) technique induces a time-varying electric field at the recalcitrant fracture site by applying a time-varying magnetic field via one or two non-skin contact electric coils. (Fig. 27.4) The induced electric field parameters are determined by frequency characteristics of the applied magnetic field and the electrical properties of the tissue target.[15,16,33,34] Several waveform configurations have been shown to be physiologically effective. Peak time-varying magnetic fields of 0.1 to 20 gauss (G) that induce 1 to 150 mV/cm peak electric fields in a 3-cm diameter tissue target have been used.[15,35] The relationship between inductively coupled waveform characteristics and their ability to produce physiologically significant bioeffects will be considered below.

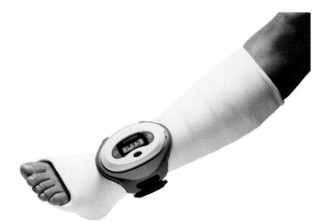

Figure 27•4 *PEMF induction of an electric field into a fracture site to promote healing. A non-surgical option for long bone and small bone nonunion and delayed union fractures, the device may be worn over a cast, orthopedic device, of clothing without lessening its effectiveness. (Physiostim™ Model 3202, permission of Orthofix Inc., McKinney, TX)*

Cellular Studies/Bone Repair

Cellular studies have addressed effects of PEMF on signal transduction pathways and growth factor synthesis. The clinical benefit to bone repair is enhanced production of growth factors upregulated as a result of the fracture trauma. The induced electric field thus acts as a signal that modulates the normal process of molecular regulation of bone and soft tissue repair mediated by growth factors.

> ▶ **PEARL 27•8** The important overall result from these studies is that PEMF signals can stimulate the secretion of growth factors (eg, insulin-like growth factor II) following a short-duration trigger stimulus.

Studies underlying this working model have shown effects on calcium ion transport,[36] a 28% increase in cell proliferation,[37] a fivefold increase in IGF-II release,[38] and increased IGF-II receptor expression in osteoblasts.[39] Increases of 53% and 93% on IGF-I and II, respectively, have also been demonstrated in rat fracture callus.[40] Additionally, PEMF stimulation of TGF-β and mRNA by threefold in a bone induction model in the rat has been reported.[41] The latter study also suggests that the increase in growth factor production by PEMF may be related to the induction of cartilage differentiation.[42] Moreover, it also suggests that the responsive cell population is most likely mesenchymal cells,[43] which are recruited early during PEMF treatment to enhance cartilage formation. Upregulation of TGF-β mRNA by 100%, as well as collagen and osteocalcin synthesis by PEMF has been reported in the human osteoblast-like cell line MG-63.[44,45] PEMF stimulated a 130% increase in TGF-β1 in bone nonunion cells.[46] That the upregulation of growth factor production in bone may be a common denominator in the soft tissue level mechanisms underlying electromagnetic stimulation is supported by several key studies.[47-50]

Use of specific inhibitors suggests PEMF acts through a calmodulin-dependent (CaM-dependent) pathway.[48] This follows reports that specific PEMF and PRF signals, as well as weak static magnetic fields, modulate Ca^{2+} binding to CaM by a twofold acceleration in Ca^{+2} binding kinetics in a cell-free enzyme preparation.[51-57]

> **PEARL 27•9** PEMF has been reported to increase angiogenesis by threefold in an endothelial cell culture.[58] A recent study confirms this and suggests PEMF increases in vitro and in vivo angiogenesis through a sevenfold increase in endothelial release of FGF-2.[59]

PRF signals configured on the basis of a transduction mechanism that involves Ca^{2+} binding to CaM are discussed below, along with several basic and clinical examples. It is useful to consider that PRF signals are configured to act as a first messenger for a second messenger, which in turn modulates biochemical cascades related to tissue growth and repair. The likely second messenger is Ca^{2+} binding to CaM, which activates epithelial or neuronal nitric oxide synthase (eNOS or nNOS) to produce nitric oxide (NO). The result is that PRF can act to reduce the inflammatory phase of tissue repair and then accelerate the remaining phases of repair by directly modulating the appropriate growth factor release at the appropriate time and with the correct kinetics. A scheme for PEMF/PRF acceleration of tissue healing based upon this model is shown in Figure 27.5.

Animal Studies—Bone Repair

PEMF signals have been reported to accelerate bone repair in a wide variety of conditions, including osteotomies,[60,61] osseus

PEMF/PRF Mechanism for Tissue Repair

PEMF
Ca^{2+} + CaM ⟶ Ca/CaM
PEMF accelerates Ca^{2+} binding to CaM (milliseconds)

Ca/CaM + eNOS ⟶ NO
Ca/CaM activates eNOS, catalyzes NO release (seconds)

Anti-inflammatory:
downregulates iNOS & IL-1?
increases Blood & Lymph Flow
Pain/Edema Decrease (seconds/minutes)

(seconds/minutes)
NO ⟶ cGMP ⟶ Growth Factors (mins/hours)

FGF-2 (VEGF) Angiogenesis (hours/days)
TNF-? Collagen/Granulation (days)
TGF-? Remodeling (days/weeks)

Figure 27•5 *A schematic showing a proposed mechanism for PEMF/PRF-modulated tissue repair. The RF signal induces sufficient voltage and current to accelerate Ca^{2+} binding to CaM. This accelerates the production of NO from endothelial NOS, which acts rapidly as an anti-inflammatory. There follows accelerated production of cGMP, which starts the growth factor cascades. (From A. Pilla with permission)*

defects,[62,63] osteopenia,[64-67] and a bone disuse model.[68] Experimental models of bone repair show enhanced cell activity, proliferation, calcification, and increased mechanical strength with DC currents in spinal arthrodeses,[69-73] fusion,[74] and other experimental bone repair conditions.[75-79] The mechanical strength of late-phase osteotomy gap healing in the dog was 35% stronger in PEMF-treated limbs,[75] and PEMF increased bone ingrowth into hydroxyapatite implants in cancellous bone by 50%.[76]

Clinical Studies—Bone Healing

PEMF technologies have been used clinically to treat fresh fractures, osteotomies, spine fusions, and delayed and nonunion fractures. The efficacy of PEMF stimulation on bone repair has been studied in a formal meta-analysis.[8] Twenty RCTs were identified. Fifteen trials supported electromagnetic field (EMF) effectiveness, and five failed to show effectiveness. Most studies used PEMF. In all cases, the primary outcome measure was bone healing assessed by radiographs and clinical stability test. Results from pooled trials of 765 cases supported the effectiveness of PEMF stimulation of bone repair. However, because of the inability to pool data from all studies, conclusions regarding PEMF efficacy in bone repair were only suggestive. PEMF significantly accelerated union of femoral and tibial osteotomies in randomized, placebo-controlled studies by approximately 50%.[80-82]

Bone Healing–Spinal Fusions

PEMF has been used to promote healing of spinal fusions for the treatment of chronic back pain from worn or damaged intervertebral discs. This is measured by the increase in successful fusions from 50% to approximately 80% using PEMF as adjunctive treatment. This application has also been subjected to meta-analysis.[83] Five RCTs and five nonrandomized case controlled studies showed positive results for the enhancement (by 60%) of spine fusion by electrical and electromagnetic stimulation. There are many studies and reviews that show electrical and electromagnetic stimulation is effective in promoting spinal arthrodesis.[84-88]

Bone Healing—Recalcitrant Extremity Fractures

The effectiveness of PEMF in promoting healing of recalcitrant fractures has been reviewed.[89] Twenty-eight studies of nonunited tibial fractures treated with PEMF were compared with 14 studies of similar fractures treated with bone graft with or without internal fixation. The overall success rate for the surgical treatment of 569 nonunited tibial fractures was 82%, while that for PEMF treatment of 1718 nonunited tibial fractures was 81%, suggesting it is significantly more advantageous for the patient to use PEMF than to submit to invasive surgery for the first bone graft. There are several observational studies suggesting the efficacy of PEMF techniques in stimulating healing of delayed unions and nonunions.[90-98] Studies comparing PEMF with bone graft show their equivalence in promoting union of delayed union or nonunion fractures.[89,99-101] Finally, there is a promising study on the effects of PEMF on distraction osteogenesis for the correction of bone length discrepancies.[102]

▶ **PEARL 27•10** PEMF technologies now constitute the standard armamentarium of orthopedic clinical practice. Since the success rate for these interventions has been reported to be equivalent to that for the first bone graft, a huge advantage to the patient ensues because PEMF therapy is noninvasive and is performed on an out-patient basis.

PEMF therapy also provides significant reductions in the cost of health care since no operative procedures or hospital stays are involved. This also applies for the increased success rate of spinal fusions with PEMF. Thus, the clinical effects of PEMF on hard tissue repair are physiologically significant and often constitute the method of choice when standard of care has failed to produce adequate clinical results. It is interesting to note that PEMF may be the best modulator of the release of the growth factors specific to each stage of bone repair, certainly more so than the exogenous application of the same growth factors.

Biophysical Considerations of Pulsed Electromagnetic Field Therapeutics

The biophysical mechanism(s) of interaction of weak electric and magnetic fields on biological tissues as well as the biological transductive mechanism(s) have been vigorously studied. At present, the most generally accepted biophysical transduction step is ion/ligand binding at cell surfaces and junctions that modulate a cascade of biochemical processes resulting in the observed physiological effect.[103-106] A unifying biophysical mechanism that could explain the vast range of reported results and allow predictions of which EMF signals and exposures are likely to induce a clinically meaningful physiological effect has been proposed.[107-109]

Electromagnetic bioeffects from relatively weak signals (below heating and excitation thresholds) can be produced with a time-varying electric field, $E(t)$, induced from an applied time-varying magnetic field, $B(t)$. The PEMF clinical devices in present use for bone repair and PRF devices for wound repair induce 1 to 100 mV/cm peak E at the treatment site.[8,35,83] Determination of the amplitude and spatial dosimetry of the induced EMF within the tissue target site has been rigorously studied for the laboratory dish with coils oriented vertically or horizontally.[110-112] Models have been created for the distribution of induced voltage and current in human limbs and joints.[113,114] Three-dimensional visualizations of clinical PEMF signals have been reported.[115] Thus, the distribution of current in a given tissue target from a coil placed in proximity to that target is relatively well understood, and adequate dosage should present no problem in clinical applications of PRF for wound repair.

Inductively Coupled Clinical Pulsed Electromagnetic Field Waveforms

The electric field induced via a time-varying magnetic field waveform is directly related to the electrical characteristics of the coil employed and the current waveform applied to the coil. Induced electromotive force (emf) is proportional to the rate of

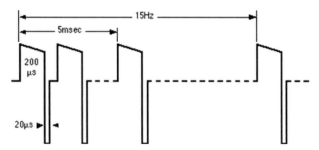

Figure 27•6 *Induced electrical field in tissue from the time-varying magnetic fields used in PEMF devices for clinical applications to bone repair. The waveform consists of bursts of asymmetrical pulses. Peak E is 1–10 mV/cm in a 2-cm cell/tissue target. Positive clinical and biological effects have been reported for this signal. (From A. Pilla with permission.)*

change of current in the coil (dI_{coil}/dt), which produces the shape of the induced electric field. A pulse-type induced electric field waveform in common clinical use for bone repair is shown in Figure 27.6. Note that this is the in situ waveform, that is, the PEMF stimulus at the cell/tissue level. The rationale behind the configuration of this waveform was based on the assumption that the induced electric field (and associated induced current density) is the primary stimulus. In other words, the magnetic component was considered to be the carrier or coupler, not significantly contributing to the biological effect.

The waveform shown in Figure 27.6 represents the time variation of the electric field signal induced in a cell/tissue target (eg, fracture site). The distribution of current flow depends upon the geometry of coil and target. The basic rule is that the voltage induced will be defined by the distribution of magnetic flux within the tissue and the electrical properties of the target. The induced E field will be greater when the magnetic field intercepts a greater cross-sectional area of the sample, that is, maximum E field in the target depends upon target size. Peak E field and associated current density, J, at a radius of 2 cm is often used for dosimetry comparisons. It is also convenient to use dB/dt (rate of change of the magnetic field with time) as a measure of the peak induced electric field, assuming identical target size, for a given PEMF signal. For example, a common clinical bone repair signal produces a 20-G peak magnetic field in 20 μsec. Thus, $dB/dt = 10^6$ G/sec for which peak $E_\phi(t) = 1$ V/m = 10 mV/cm at a radius of 2 cm in the target, a typical dose metric for PEMF bone-growth stimulators.

The Pulsed Electromagnetic Field Transduction Mechanism

For a living cell or tissue to respond functionally to an exogenous electric field, it is necessary that it reach and be detected at the appropriate molecular, cellular, or tissue site. An important step, therefore, is the characterization of the electrical properties of cells and tissues. It has been proposed that a complete description of the electrical properties of cells and tissues should include the electrical equivalents of the electrochemical processes that could be involved in the signal transduction pathway.[15] The electrical equivalents of electrochemical processes at cell surfaces and junctions and their relevance to EMF therapeutics have been described.[15,33,108,116,117] Thus, induced current can affect cell surfaces and junctions via a complex, but readily discernible set of electrochemical steps that are representative of the cell's real-time response to perturbations in its charged environment for any given functional state.

The electrochemical pathways involved in the transduction of an exogenous EMF signal into a physiologically significant endpoint appear to be operationally similar to the initial gating process involved in the production of the action potential via membrane depolarization.[118] It is therefore appropriate to consider the configuration of EMF waveforms in terms of an informational approach, or signaling in contrast to one designed to supply energy to drive the biochemical cascade. Examples of the latter would be the use of direct currents large enough to cause cells to move along the electric field in wound repair applications and electroporation, wherein short voltage pulses are applied with sufficient electric field to temporarily cause the cell membrane to become permeable to macromolecules such as DNA or chemotherapeutic agents.

The Electrochemical Information Transfer Model

It was proposed by Pilla in 1972 that nonthermal, subthreshold electromagnetic fields may directly affect ion binding and/or transport and possibly alter the cascade of biological processes related to tissue growth and repair.[116] This electrochemical information transfer (EIT) hypothesis postulated the cell membrane as the site of interaction of low-level electromagnetic fields through modulation of the rate of binding of, for example, calcium ion to receptor sites as a first step in a biochemical cascade relevant to the desired clinical outcome.

Equivalent electrical circuit models representing electrochemical processes at cell surfaces and junctions have been derived.[15,33,109,117] Typically, most calculations consider a membrane model that consists of a capacitance, C_d, in parallel with an ionic leak pathway, R_M (see Fig. 27.3). While all membranes exhibit these properties, this simple model does not completely describe the dielectric properties of a functioning membrane, particularly with respect to the EMF transduction pathway. Impedance measurements on isolated cells have revealed the existence of relaxation processes that appear to reflect the kinetics of ion or ligand binding, as well as follow-up biochemical reactions.[118-122] Thus, a more general description of membrane dielectric properties, which takes into account electrochemical processes relevant to EMF sensitivity, considers an ion-binding step that precedes and possibly triggers a subsequent chemical reaction at the membrane surface.

The EIT model strongly guided the creation of the first clinically effective PEMF signal for recalcitrant fracture repair.[16,17] According to the EIT model, the requirements for an effective waveform could be met if it contained frequency components of sufficient amplitude within the time constant of the proposed target pathway.[15] Transmembrane ion transport, for which kinetics is in the millisecond range, was chosen as the target pathway for bone repair.[118] This, coupled with practical restrictions on the size of the coil

for patient use, led to the pulse burst waveform shown in Figure 27.6. It was supposed that the cell would ignore the short opposite polarity pulse and respond only to the envelope of the burst that had a duration of 5 msec, enough to induce sufficient amplitude in the kilohertz frequency range. Although the reasoning behind the asymmetric pulse in this waveform was erroneous because the EIT model was not yet complete and required further knowledge of the transduction mechanism, this signal is nonetheless effective for bone repair. It continues to be part of the standard armamentarium of the orthopedist for the nonsurgical noninvasive treatment of recalcitrant bone fractures.

Dosimetry for Pulsed Electromagnetic Field Signals

Classical biophysical lore suggests that, unless the amplitude and frequencies of an applied electric field are sufficient to trigger an excitable membrane (eg, heart pacemaker), to produce tissue heating, or to move an ion along a field gradient, there could be no effect. This was a formidable obstacle in the quest for therapeutic applications of weak EMF signals. However, the classical biophysics position had to be changed as the evidence for weak (nonthermal) EMF bioeffects became overwhelming. The clinical evidence offered by many double-blind clinical studies, coupled with the database of hundreds of thousands of successful treatments of delayed and nonunion bone fractures registered with the FDA, simply could no longer be ignored. Noninvasive PEMF treatment is actually as successful as the first bone graft, to the huge benefit of the patient. The task was to provide solid testable models for the biophysical mechanism of weak electric field bioeffects.

> **PEARL 27•11** The underlying problem for any model that claims to describe the biophysical mechanism of weak EMF bioeffects relates to whether the induced signal can be detected at the molecular/cellular/tissue target in the presence of thermal noise, that is, signal-to-thermal noise ratio (SNR). SNR compares the amplitude of a desired signal (eg, the noise produced by an induced electric field) to the amount of undesirable background noise (eg, thermal or cell membrane noise) that has mixed with it. The higher the ratio, the less obtrusive is the background noise.

Considering the cell membrane as the target, the burden of proof is to show that the induced voltage is not buried in thermal and other voltage noise, that is, that the applied signal is detectable. Without resorting to signal processing or metabolic amplification, it is still necessary to attempt to understand the remarkable sensitivity of biological systems to weak electric fields. In terms of target geometry, certainly the spherical cell model is oversimplified and cannot represent the geometric complexity of cellular and tissue EMF targets. For example, the successful outcome of a healing fracture, wherein bone tissue differentiates both functionally and spatially, is a clinically relevant illustration of cell-cell communication.[123] This suggests the target for the PEMF signals used to affect nonunions and delayed unions of bone is a highly organized ensemble of cells. In fact, all organized tissue is developed and maintained by an ensemble of complex geometry cells that have coordinated activity.[124] The most prevalent cell shape in living system tissue is elliptical and flattened, with processes extending in at least two directions. Gap junctions provide pathways for ionic and molecular intercellular communication.[125] They are present in all tissues, including bone.

The presence of gap junctions in the cells of an organized or organizing (repairing) tissue cause the induced transmembrane voltage (V_M) to be substantially higher than that for the same cell in isolation for the same applied EMF. The frequency range in which increased V_M occurs versus that for a single isolated cell is shifted toward a substantially lower range. This places different frequency requirements on the induced electric field waveform dependent upon whether the target is a macromolecule, single cell, or tissue. As array length increases beyond 1 mm, the rate of increase in V_M diminishes because of the dissipation of intracellular current via transmembrane resistance (R_M). In the case of myelinated nerve axons, R_M is substantially higher, and array lengths above 1 cm can provide further significant increases in V_M.[126]

Assuming Ca^{2+} binding to CaM, signal-to-thermal noise ratio (SNR) may be evaluated for molecular, cellular, or tissue targets. An interesting example is wound repair. A common model is the full-thickness linear incision performed through the skin down to the fascia on the dorsum of adult Sprague-Dawley rats.[127] Acceleration of wound repair is assessed by tensile strength measurements at 21 postoperative days. At this time point, untreated (control) strength is approximately one third that of the fully healed wound. One study used the PEMF signal commonly employed for bone repair and reported no effect.[128] (Fig. 27.7) A second, more recent study

used a PRF signal, having a carrier frequency of 27.12 MHz specifically configured to enhance Ca^{2+} binding to CaM with the specific goal of enhancing growth factor release. A 59% increase in tensile strength versus controls at 21 days ($P < 0.001$) was reported.[129] SNR analysis for the signals used in these studies is shown in Figure 27.8. It is clear that the induced electric field produced by the PEMF bone repair signal consisting of a 5-msec burst of bipolar pulses (200/20 μsec asymmetrical duration), repeating at 15/sec and inducing a gross peak electric field of 1 mV/cm ($dB/dt = 10^6$ G/sec), produced very low induced voltage across the Ca/CaM pathway. The resultant SNR was below the detection threshold. In contrast, the PRF signal that consisted of a 2-msec burst of 27.12-MHz sinusoidal waves repeating at 1/sec, $dB/dt = 10^7$ G/sec, produced a significantly larger induced voltage with a larger effect on Ca^{2+} binding.

A recent study compared the effects of the PEMF bone repair signal used in the example above ($dB/dt = 10^6$ G/sec) with a 65-μsec burst of rectangular pulses of 4-μsec and 12-μsec duration per polarity repeating at 1.5 bursts/sec ($dB/dt = 10^4$ G/sec) on bone repair in a rat osteotomy model.[79] In this study the standard clinical bone repair PEMF signal produced a twofold increase in new woven bone and callus stiffness, whereas the 4/12-μsec signal was ineffective. SNR, assuming a Ca/CaM target pathway, reveals peak SNR greater than 1 for the clinical PEMF signal and peak SNR less than 1 for the 4/12-μsec signal. Note that modulation of the Ca/CaM pathway for bone repair requires frequency components of sufficient amplitude in the 10^2 to 10^4 Hz range, and neither of these signals was configured accordingly.

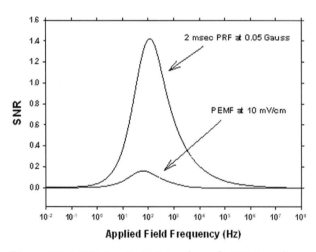

Figure **27•7** *SNR in a Ca/CaM pathway for PEMF and PRF waveforms used in a rat cutaneous wound model. The PEMF asymmetrical repetitive pulse bone repair signal produced low (below detection threshold) SNR and had no effect on wound repair. The 27.12-MHz PRF repetitive sinusoidal burst produced sufficient SNR for detection in the Ca/CaM pathway and enhanced tensile strength by 59% at 21 days. (From: Strauch, B, et al (129) with permission.)*

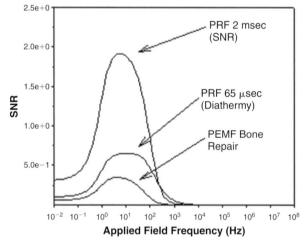

Figure **27•8** *SNR for PRF signals consisting of a 2000-μsec burst of 27.12-MHz sinusoidal waves repeating at 5/sec (configured a priori for the Ca/CaM pathway), a 65-μsec burst at 600/sec (a diathermy-based signal in clinical use for soft tissue repair), and the original PEMF bone healing signal consisting of a 5-msec burst of 200/20-μsec pulses repeating at 5/sec. Both PRF signals were predicted effective, the 65-μsec signal significantly less so since it was not matched to the bandpass of Ca^{2+} binding. The PEMF bone repair signal was predicted ineffective. (From Pilla (139) with permission.)*

Pulsed Electromagnetic Field Stimulation for Chronic Wound Healing (Lower Extremity Venous and Arterial Insufficiency Leg Ulcers)

In a double-blind trial to determine the effect of nonthermal PEMF on venous leg ulcers, Ieran and colleagues randomly assigned 44 patients to a treatment group (*N* = 22, active PEMF device) and to a control group (*N* = 22, inactive PEMF device).[130] Patients in both groups were treated 4 hours a day for 90 days. The active device delivered PEMF from a noncontact coil at 75 Hz and 2.8 mT intensity for the amount of time just stated. Because of patient noncompliance with the protocol or other reasons for patient exclusion, the data analysis was done on 18 patients in the treatment group and on 19 patients in the control group. At day 90, 6 patients (31.5%) were healed in the control group compared with 12 patients (66.6%) in the treatment group (*P* < 0.02). Within 1 year from the start of the study, 8 patients (42.1%) had healed among the control group, and 16 patients (88.8%) had healed among the treatment group (*P* < 0.005). No ulcers worsened in the treatment group, while four ulcers worsened in the control group. After healing, the rate of recurrence of ulcers was greater in the control group (50%) than in the treatment group (25%). In a before-and-after study, Duran et al reportedly used PEMF to treat 18 venous leg ulcers 10 times for 15 minutes each session.[131] They reported that reepithelialization resulted in a significant decrease in mean surface area of 33% after 10 treatment days. In another study labeled a double-blind randomized, controlled trial, Todd et al treated 19 patients with venous leg ulcers twice weekly with PEMF over a 5-week period.[132] Their device reportedly delivered a field strength of 60 units (not identified) at 5 Hz for 15 minutes by placing noncontact coils on opposite sides of the wound over the dressings. Outcome measures included ulcer size, pain level, lower leg girth, and presence of infections. After removing data from one patient from the active treatment group who had a very large ulcer that slanted the mean pretreatment and posttreatment wound areas, they reported a trend toward a positive healing effect but no statistical difference between the active and inactive treatment groups.

In a prospective, randomized, double-blind, placebo-controlled, multicenter study, Stiller et al assessed the efficiency of PEMF treatment on the healing of intractable venous leg ulcers.[133] Patients were instructed to treat themselves 3 hours daily at home for 8 weeks with a portable PEMF device. PEMF parameters derived from bone healing research were 3.5-msec pulse duration, a biphasic delta B waveform, and an intensity of about 22 G. At week 8 the active group had a 47.7% reduction in wound surface area, compared to a 43.3% increase for the placebo group (*P* < 0.0002). Additional evaluations by the investigators revealed that 50% of the wounds in the active group closed or distinctly improved versus 0% in the placebo group, and 0% of the active group worsened compared with 54% of the placebo group (*P* < 0.001). Significant reductions in wound depth and pain (both *P* < 0.04) occurred for the active

group. From in vitro research, Canedo-Dorantes et al found that extremely low-frequency (ELF) PEMF interacts with peripheral blood mononuclear cells (PBMCs) via Ca^2 channels, activating signal transduction cascades, which in turn promote cytokine synthesis, changing cell-proliferation patterns.[134] They then configured ELF frequencies to interact in vitro with the proliferation patterns of PBMC obtained from normal human subjects. Since, as mentioned above, ELF interacts with peripheral blood mononuclear cells, they applied the ELF peripherally (to the arms rather than directly to the wounds) as the sole treatment to 26 patients with 42 chronic venous or arterial leg ulcers that had not responded to previous medical and/or surgical treatments in a before-and-after design. The purpose of PEMF application approach was to ascertain whether the ELF could alter systemic effects by interaction with action potentials at the peripheral (lower extremity) wound site. They theorized that ELF frequencies previously tested on normal human volunteers could increase proliferation of PBMCs in the bodies of patients with chronic leg ulcers. The treatment involved placing an arm into a chamber containing a magnetic field for 2 to 3 hours, three times a week, for a 4-month period. The strength of the ELF inside the chamber was 36.36 G. Based on before-and-after wound surface area measurements and photographs, the investigators divided patient's data into "responders" (closed wounds or wounds reduced greater than 50%) and "nonresponders," who had at least one wound that decreased in size less than 50% or increased in size. Twenty-nine wounds that earlier were unresponsive to medical-surgical treatment responded to ELF and began to heal by week 2. By the end of study, 15 arterial and 14 venous wounds were in the responder groups while 2 arterial and 11 venous ulcers were in the nonresponder groups. After ELF treatment over the 4-month study period, 69% of all wounds were either closed or had healed more than 50%. Defective wound healing was observed in ulcers associated with arterial occlusion, hypertension, severe lipodermatosclerosis, nonpitting edema and obesity.

> ▶ **PEARL 27•12** The positive outcomes seen in this study could be attributed to the greater overall electrical energy dosage accumulated over the 8-week study period compared with the previously cited studies that introduced considerably less electrical energy into the wounds.[131,132]

Although the five small studies on venous leg ulcers described above and summarized in Table 24.4 have reported positive chronic wound healing effects with PEMF signals that are configured for treatment of nonunion and delayed union fractures, more research is needed to establish the efficacy of these signals in being able to significantly enhance healing of chronic wounds.

Summaries Regarding PEMF

As shown in Figure 27.6, PEMF signals may be very specifically configured to modulate Ca^{2+} binding to calmodulin, which in turn can affect a variety of biochemical cascades, starting with a very rapid anti-inflammatory component and ending with the modulation of growth factors important to tissue repair.

Nonthermal Pulsed Radio Frequency for Soft Tissue Wound Repair
Animal Studies (Induced Wounds)

A recent study showed the PEMF signal used for bone repair accelerated wound closure in diabetic and normal mice.[135] Cell proliferation and CD31 density were significantly increased in the PEMF-treated groups. Cultured medium from human umbilical vein endothelial cells exposed to PEMF exhibited a threefold increase in FGF-2, which facilitated healing when applied to wounds.[136] Skin on diabetic mice exposed to nonthermal PRF did not exhibit tissue necrosis and demonstrated oxygen tensions and vascularity comparable to those in normal animals.[135] PRF signals produced a statistically significant several-fold increase in neovascularization in an arterial loop model, suggesting an important clinical application for the angiogenesis that is so critical to wound repair.[137,138] PRF signals, configured a priori assuming a Ca/CaM transduction pathway, accelerated wound repair in a rat cutaneous wound model by approximately 60% as measured by tensile strength.[129] A similar 70% increase in tensile strength in an Achilles tendon model in the rat has been reported.[139] In another study investigators reported that acute wounds induced in rabbits treated with nonthermal PRF had lower contraction but higher epithelialization rates than control wounds.[140]

Design of Pulsed Radio Frequency Signals for Clinical Wound Repair

Having established the rationale for the a priori configuration of PEMF and PRF signals to obtain a predicted bioeffect, the following cases demonstrate specific applications to clinical wound repair.

▸ **PEARL 27•13** For all of the clinical results presented in Figures 27.14 through 27.17, the a priori SNR analysis was applied to a nonthermal PRF signal. This signal had the standard 27.12 MHz sinusoidal carrier, for which pulse modulation (burst duration and repetition rate) was configured according to an assumed Ca/CaM transduction pathway.

Signal configuration is proceeded by evaluation of SNR in a two-step pathway involving Ca^{2+} binding to CaM, followed by Ca^{2+}/CaM binding to epithelial or neuronal nitric oxide synthase (eNOS and nNOS, respectively), which mediates nitric oxide (NO) release. Assuming this pathway, Figure 27.8 shows SNR for PRF signals consisting of a 2000-μsec burst of 27.12-MHz sinusoidal waves repeating at 5/sec (configured a priori for the Ca/CaM pathway), or a 65-μsec burst at 600/sec (a diathermy-based signal in clinical use for soft tissue repair), and the original PEMF bone healing signal consisting of a 5-msec burst of 200/20-μsec pulses repeating at 5/sec. Both

PRF signals were predicted to be effective, the 65-μsec signal significantly less so since it was not matched to the bandpass of Ca^{2+} binding. The PEMF bone repair signal was predicted to be ineffective. The validity of this approach was reported on Achilles tendon repair in the rat.[139] The significance of results such as these was to permit the design of cost-effective clinical PRF units that are simple, portable, and even disposable. The PRF signal configured a priori for the Ca/CaM transduction pathway was employed in all of the devices for which the clinical results are reported below.

Pulsed Radio Frequency Nonthermal Devices

Nonthermal PRF is created by modulating the primary 27.12-MHz RF carrier by using a timing mechanism in the device to interrupt the carrier frequency waves so the output is turned on and off at preset intervals, allowing bursts of pulse trains to be emitted from the treatment coil. Hence, within each burst or pulse train is a series of high-frequency sine wave oscillations. The pulse train duration, or "on time," is usually separated by a longer lasting "off time." (Fig. 27.3 bottom)

▸ **PEARL 27•14** The biophysics community defines a nonthermal PRF device as one that raises the temperature of the target tissue less than 1°C after exposure for 1 hour.[174]

Some nonthermal PRF devices allow the clinician a few choices of pulse burst durations, while others provide a fixed burst duration, which typically is 65 μsec. The pulse train frequency within bursts can be varied and determines the duration of the off time between bursts. At 27.12 MHz, there are 27.12×10^6 cycles in 1 sec and 27.12 cycles in 1 μsec. Therefore, for FDA class III nonthermal PRF devices with fixed 65-μsec pulse durations, such as the Diapulse® (Diapulse Corporation of America, Great Neck, NY) and the former solid-state MRT 911® (Electropharmacology Inc., Pompano Beach, FL), each burst contains 1762.8 oscillations. (Fig. 27.9) At a maximum frequency choice of 600 pulses per second (pps), each complete period lasts 1666.66 μsec (1.7 ms), and the interval between successive pulses is 1601.66 μsec. At a frequency choice of 400 pps, each period lasts 2500 μsec (2.5 ms) and the interval between successive pulses is 2435 μsec.[141] At 600 pps, the duty cycle is 65/1666 = 0.039, or less than 4%, while at 400 pps, the duty cycle is 65/2500 = 0.026, or less than 2.6%. Thus, with nonthermal PRF devices such as the Diapulse and the former MRT 911 that have fixed 65-μsec pulse durations, when the peak pulse power is preset by a clinician, a manual increase in the pulse frequency from a minimum of 80 pps toward the maximum of 600 pps will increase the mean power accordingly. With nonthermal PRF devices, as with thermal PRF devices, the power driving the patient treatment coil does not represent the level of absorbed power in the tissues. The power driving the treatment coil can be measured either as peak pulse power, which, for Diapulse and the former MRT 911, ranges from 185 to 975 W, or as mean power, which (for both devices) is much lower, ranging from 7.5 to 38 W.

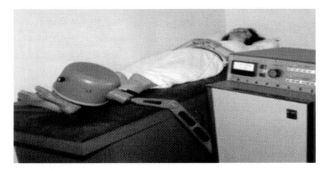

Figure 27•9 *Diapulse™ nonthermal PRF device. (Courtesy of Diapulse Corp., Great Neck, NY.)*

These values are determined by the settings of peak power and pulse frequency. Another nonthermal PRF device, the Provant CPI® (Regenesis Biomedical, Scottsdale, AZ), has a fixed 42-μsec burst duration. (Fig. 27.10) Since the MRT 911, the Diapulse, and Provant CPI® devices are described and categorized by the FDA as class III, none of the three devices (according to the FDA class III definition) are supposed to induce any significant tissue-heating effect, even at the highest peak power and pulse frequency settings.[141] Of the three devices, the MRT 911 is no longer on the market; however, a newer version, the disposable SoftPulse Torino II (Ivivi Health Sciences, San Francisco, CA) has a burst duration that varies from 2 to 5 msec, with frequencies between 1 and 5 pps and maximum power < 1 watt. (Fig 27.11) The most recent version of this SofPulse technology (Fig. 27.12) requires less than 10 watts of peak input power to induce a magnetic field in tissue that is 50-fold less intensity (0.05 G) compared to the 2 G intensity delivered by the other three nonthermal PRF devices using >400 W peak input power. Nonthermal PRF signals were originally used for the treatment of infections in the preantibiotic era and are now widely employed for the reduction of posttraumatic and postoperative pain and edema.[142]

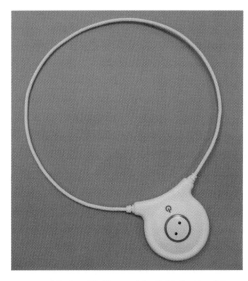

Figure 27•11 *Torino II disposable PRF device (Courtesy of Ivivi Health Sciences, San Francisco, CA)*

> ▶ **PEARL 27•15** Since 38 W or more of mean power is used as a measure of the heating effect for thermal PRFD, less than 38 W mean power driving the treatment coil is used as an indicator of minimal or no heating effect for nonthermal PRF.

> ▶ **PEARL 27•16** If transient, imperceptible tissue heating with these devices does occur with each burst, there should be no accumulative heating effect as long as perfusing blood dissipates the thermal energy.

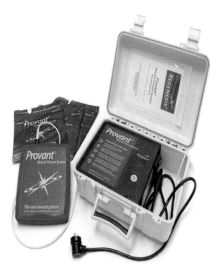

Figure 27•10 *Provant CPI™ nonthermal PRF device. (Courtesy of Regenesis Biomedical Inc., Scottsdale, AZ.)*

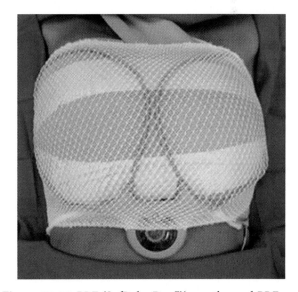

Figure 27•12 *PRF (SofPulse Duo™, nonthermal PRF device (Courtesy of Ivivi Health Sciences, San Francisco, CA) in use to control postoperative pain following breast augmentation surgery. (From Heden P, Pilla A (143) with permission.)*

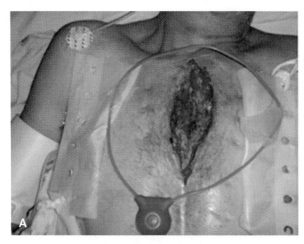
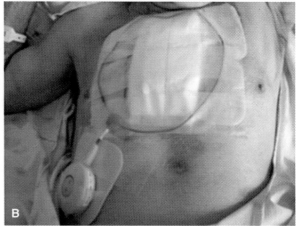

Figure 27•13 *Case 1: (A) PRF treatment started in hospital with Ivivi Roma clinic device. Note coil is positioned above wound that is within coil perimeter. (B) Patient is discharged after 1 week with disposable PRF device. Coil is incorporated in dressing. (Courtesy B. Strauch, MD, Albert Einstein School of Medicine, New York, NY.)*

Nonthermal Pulse Radio Frequency in Postsurgical Wound Pain Suppression

A PRF signal configured a priori for the Ca/CaM pathway was tested clinically in a randomized double-blind pilot study on 30 patients for its effect on pain reduction immediately after breast augmentation.[143] The PRF signal used in this study was configured a priori, assuming a Ca/CaM transduction pathway, and consisted of a 2-msec burst of 27.12-MHz sinusoidal waves repeating at 2 bursts/sec and at 0.05-G peak amplitude (SofPulse; Ivivi Health Sciences, San Francisco, CA). (Fig. 27.12) The PRF signal is inductively coupled and can thus be applied through clothing or dressings, requiring no contact with the skin. PRF was delivered from a small (2.5-cm diameter, 1-cm thick) battery-powered generator to a single-turn 15-cm diameter electrical coil. A portable and disposable PRF device (Torino II, Ivivi Technologies Inc., Northvale, NJ) was placed on the patient as part of normal postsurgical procedure, and the signal was activated before the patient left the operating room. (Fig. 27.13) Once active, the PRF device automatically provided a 30-minute treatment according to a regimen as follows: every 4 hours for the first 3 postoperative days; then every 8 hours for the next 3 days; and every 12 hours until the follow-up visit, normally at postoperative day (POD) 7. Pain was assessed twice daily using a validated Visual Analogue Scale (VAS).

The results are shown in Figure 27.14. Bars represent the mean postoperative VAS pain score for all breasts and at POD 7 for both the active and sham groups. Mean (± SD) VAS score was 54 plus or minus 9 mm for all groups postoperatively. Mean VAS decreased to 17 plus or minus 4.4 mm in the treated group (218%, $P < 0.001$ vs postoperative mean VAS) and to 31 plus or minus 5.6 mm in the sham group (74%, $P < 0.001$- vs postoperative mean VAS). The difference in mean pain between the active and sham cohorts was also statistically significant ($P < 0.001$), suggesting postsurgical use of PRF therapy could produce a clinically meaningful reduction in pain by nearly a factor of 3. A 2-fold increased

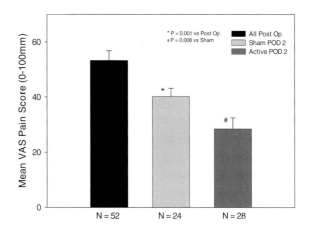

Figure 27•14 *Effect of PRF therapy on postsurgical pain from breast augmentation. Bars represent the mean VAS pain score at POD 2 vs initial postsurgical VAS score. Mean VAS score was 54 ± 9 mm for all groups postoperatively. Mean VAS decreased to 28 ± 4.3 mm in the treated group (87%, P < 0.001 vs postoperative) and to 40 ± 3.5 mm in the sham group (32%, P < 0.001 vs postoperative), representing a clinically meaningful reduction in pain by approximately 2.7-fold. (From Heden P, Pilla A (126) with permission.)*

reduction in pain by PEMF was already observed by POD 2. Active patients also had a concomitant decrease in pain medication by a factor of 2.9 by POD 7.[143]

A second randomized double-blind clinical study using the same PRF signal configured to target the anti-inflammatory cascade involving the CaM/NO/cGMP signaling pathway reported postoperative pain decreased by 300% by 5 hrs postsurgery, accompanied by a 275% decrease in IL-1β in the wound bed at the same postoperative time.[143A] Twenty-four healthy women, who were candidates for breast reduction for medical reasons, were admitted to this double-blind, placebo-controlled randomized study. Breast reduction was performed by the same surgeon using the standard Wise or vertical incision techniques with superomedial pedicles. Patients were equally divided into active and sham groups. A disposable dual coil radio frequency PEMF device (Ivivi Health Sciences, UB, San Francisco, CA), placed in the post surgical support bra normally used for all patients, was activated on transfer of the patient to the recovery stretcher. The PEMF signal, configured, *a priori*, to modulate Ca^{2+} binding to CaM, consisted of a 2 msec burst of 27.12 MHz sinusoidal waves repeating at 2 bursts/sec. Peak magnetic field was 0.05G which induced an average electric field of 32 ± 6 mV/cm in a 9 cm^3 target in each breast. An active PEMF device automatically provided a 20 minute treatment every 4 hours for the observation period of 24–48 hours post-surgery. Sham devices were activated in exactly the same manner as the active devices, but produced no RF signal in tissue. The primary outcome measure was the effect of non-thermal RF on the rate of post surgical pain reduction, using a Visual Analog Scale (VAS) which patients self-recorded throughout the overnight hospital stay. Postoperative pain medication was monitored for each patient. Wound exudates were analyzed for IL-1β, TNF-α, VEGF, and FGF-2.

Mean VAS scores showed this RF signal produced a 57% decrease in mean pain scores at 1 hour (P < 0.01), and a 300% decrease at 5 hours post-op (P < 0.001), persisting to 48 hours post-surgery in the active, versus no significant change in the control group. There was a concomitant 2.2-fold reduction in narcotic use in active patients over the first 24 hours postsurgery (P = 0.002). Mean IL-1β concentration in the wound exudates of treated patients was 275% lower at 5 hours postsurgery (P < 0.001) vs the sham group. There were no significant differences found for TNF-α, VEGF, and FGF-2 concentrations in the first 18 hours post-op.

These randomized placebo-controlled double-blind pilot studies confirm that non-thermal radio frequency PEMF therapy significantly reduced post-operative pain and narcotic use in the immediate post-operative period. It was also shown that PRF produced a significant reduction of IL-1β in the wound bed within the same post-op time frame. This non-thermal RF signal can provide its effect independent of pharmacokinetic limitations since the time-varying magnetic field appears instantaneously in all compartments of the target tissue. This could explain the rapidity of the PRF effect. It is intriguing to consider that the known effects of PEMF on NO release via effects on Ca^{2+} binding to CaM which, in turn, activates the constitutive nitric oxide synthases (cNOS) may be applicable here. NO from cNOS is known to downregulate inducible NO synthase (iNOS, not CaM-dependent) and IL-1β.

These studies provides further evidence that pulsed electromagnetic field therapy (PEMF) can rapidly reduce pain levels and pain medication requirements in the immediate post-operative period. The concomitant reduction of IL-1β in the wound bed, possibly via NO/cGMP signaling, suggests that PEMF could have a profound effect upon wound repair outcomes. The current availability of both economical and disposable PEMF devices could easily translate to many, if not most, post-surgical situations, leading to lower morbidity, shorter hospital stays, increased productivity, and a reduction in the cost of health care.

> **PEARL 27•17** The postoperative use of PRF using disposable economical devices could help decrease post-surgical patient morbidity in many surgical procedures. The technique is clinically simple to use and may also contribute to reduced costs for health care, particularly for more complex surgical procedures.

Nonthermal Pulsed Radio Frequency Clinical Studies—Effects on Pain, Edema, and Function Associated with Acute Soft Tissue Trauma (Closed Wounds)

In the soft tissue closed-wound area, nonthermal PRF signals are now employed for the reduction of acute posttraumatic and postoperative pain and edema. In a study designed to evaluate the effects of nonthermal PRF (Diapulse) on pain, edema, and disability associated with inversion ankle sprains, Wilson demonstrated that PRF reduced pain and disability in several acute ankle sprains significantly better than did thermal shortwave diathermy (SWD) treatment.[144,145] In one study, Wilson compared the nonthermal effects of PRF with the placebo effects of PRF.[144] He assigned patients with recent inversion ankle sprains to two match-paired groups of 20. The treatment group received a 1-hour treatment of PRF daily for 3 days. For these treatments, a PRF device with a frequency of 27.12 MHz was set to provide a peak pulse power of 975 W for each 65-msec pulse. The off time interval between successive pulses was approximately 1600 msec. The control group received a 1-hour PRF placebo treatment daily for 3 days. Wilson reported that, statistically, symptoms of pain and disability were relieved more rapidly in the treatment than in the control group; however, there was no significant difference between the two groups regarding improvement in swelling. To assess the possibility that the beneficial effects observed in the treatment group might have resulted from an increase in blood flow owing to some small, transient degree of heating (which is the mode of action attributed to thermal SWD), a second clinical study was conducted to compare the effects of nonthermal PRF with thermal SWD.[145] The same number of patients with recent inversion ankle injuries were assigned in matched pairs to two groups and, depending on the group, received either a 1-hour treatment of PRF or two 15-minute treatments within 1 hour of inductive thermal SWD daily for 3 days. Analysis of the data revealed statistically significant differences—at the 1.0% level of confidence in reduction of swelling and at the 0.1% level in reduction of pain and disability—by PRF compared with SWD. In comparing total energy delivered to patients in the two groups, it was found that those treated with SWD received approximately 22.5 watt-hours compared to 15 watt-hours received by patients treated with PRF. The fact that better clinical responses were produced with less energy was interpreted by Wilson as support for the idea that beneficial results occurred because of specific nonthermal effects.[144] It is widely accepted, however, that heat applied in the early stages following soft-tissue trauma may exacerbate the inflammatory response to injury. Thus, it is possible that patients in this study who were treated with heat either did not improve or got worse, whereas those who received PRF would have improved spontaneously without any treatment. This question could have been resolved if the design of the study had included a control group.

In a prospective, randomized, double-blind study, Pennington et al also evaluated the effects of nonthermal PRF (Diapulse) on pain and edema in 50 military personnel with grade I and II ankle sprains when PRF was applied between 1 and 24 hours, 25 and 48 hours, and 49 to 72 hours after the injury.[146] They found a statistically significant ($P < 0.01$) decrease in edema in ankles treated with an active PRF signal (4.7%) versus control ankles treated with an inactive PRF signal (0.95%). They also reported that pain was reduced by 64% and 33% in ankles treated with active and inactive PRF signals, respectively, and that the favorable outcomes resulted in a significant decrease in time loss from military training.

Additionally, double-blind clinical studies have been reported for acute ankle sprains, wherein PRF edema reduction was sevenfold versus the control group, and acute whiplash injuries, in which pain decreased by 50% and range of motion increased by 75% in the treated versus control patients.[147-149] In contrast to outcomes reported in the above-mentioned studies, Barker et al reported no significant differences between two groups of patients following nonthermal PRF treatment or placebo applications to acute ankle sprains with respect to range of motion, gait, pain, or swelling.[150]

Nonthermal PRF has also produced positive outcomes in the treatment of hand injuries and the accompanying inflammatory symptoms of pain, edema, and compromised function. Barclay et al evaluated 60 matched pairs of patients with hand injuries that had occurred within 36 hours of enrollment into his research study.[151] In the PRF-treated group, by the third day all but two of the patients had complete resolution of edema compared with the control group, whose swelling increased compared to baseline measurements. By the third day, 17 patients in the treatment group were symptom free, and by the seventh day only 1 patient in the treatment group had slight loss of function while the other 30 patients had been discharged. In comparison, of the 30 patients in the control group, 3 had been discharged, while the other 27 were still symptomatic with pain, edema, and loss of function.

In a study on burn wounds treated with PRF, Ionescu et al observed that pain and edema formation were prevented and related local symptoms were reduced.[152] When the investigators compared samples of some proteins and enzymes found in normal and burned tissues before and after PRF therapy, they found that the enzymatic activities of skin decrease when the skin is traumatized or burned. Interestingly, they found that the enzymatic activity of the burned skin significantly improved after PRF treatment and that the sooner the treatment is administered after being burned, the sooner the normal enzyme activity is restored.

▶ **PEARL 27•18** With respect to the pain and swelling that accompanies trauma and burns and the associated loss of function, the three studies mentioned—Pennington,[146] Barclay,[155] and Ionescu[152]—have shown that early intervention with PRF during the inflammatory phase resulted in successful outcomes in terms of reduced pain, swelling, and earlier return to functional activities.

A meta-analysis was performed on randomized clinical trials that used PEMF and PRF signals on injuries involving soft tissues and joints.[8] The results showed that both PEMF and PRF were effective in accelerating repair of soft tissue (closed wound) injuries,[146-149,153] as well as providing symptomatic relief in patients with osteoarthritis and other joint conditions.[25-27]

Nonthermal Pulsed Radio Frequency Chronic Open Wound Case Studies

The PRF signal configured a priori for the Ca/CaM pathway has been used with success for hundreds of chronic wounds, typically in long-term acute care facilities. The following series of case studies is typical of the results obtained with either clinic-only (SoftPulse Roma[3], Ivivi Health Sciences, San Francisco, CA) or portable/disposable (SoftPulse Torino II, Ivivi Health Sciences, San Francisco, CA) devices. The hospital treatment regimen was typically two times daily manually and after discharge in a home setting automatically every 4 hours for the first 3 days, every 8 hours the next 3 days, and two times daily thereafter for the life of the disposable unit (7–10 days), which is usually replaced at 6 to 7 days.

Nonthermal Pulsed Radio Frequency for Chronic Wound Healing—Clinical Research Reports
(Pressure Ulcers)

Duma-Drzewinska and Buczyski used a nonthermal PRF device at a mean power of 38 W for 20 minutes to treat 27 pressure ulcers, followed by a 15-minute application at a mean power of 15.2 W to the suprarenal and liver areas once or twice daily until complete wound healing was documented by photography.[154] Eleven of 12 superficial ulcers healed 100% in 4 weeks and 4 of 15 deep ulcers healed 100%. However, a much longer period of time was required to close the deep ulcers, but this time was not reported.

Studies have been reported in which PRF-treated pressure ulcers closed by 84% versus 40% closure in untreated wounds in one study and 60% closure versus no closure in the control group in another study.[155-156] In a double-blind study, Salzberg et al randomized 30 male spinal cord–injured patients with stage II and III pressure ulcers to receive two 30-minute treatments from either an active or a placebo nonthermal PRF device (Diapulse) for 12 weeks or until healed.[155] Ten patients with stage II ulcers were randomized to an active device and 10 others to a placebo device. The 10 patients with stage III ulcers were also evenly distributed to active and placebo devices. The 10 patients with stage II ulcers who were treated with the active device had a significantly shorter median time to complete healing of the ulcer (13.0 days) compared to that of the placebo group (31.5 days; $P = 0.002$). The stage III ulcers treated with an active device also healed faster than ulcers treated with the placebo device, but the small sample size precluded statistical analysis. Itoh et al reported the results from a case series study in which nonthermal PRF with Diapulse was used at 600 pps, a peak pulse power setting of 6 (38 W mean power) for 30 minutes two times daily, plus standard wound care to treat 9 stage II and 13 stage III pressure ulcers over a period of 9 months.[157] They reported that all 9 stage II ulcers healed in a mean of 2.3 weeks, after standard wound care had failed to heal them over a mean of 8 weeks. The 13 stage III ulcers that failed to heal over a mean of 35 weeks with standard wound care closed over a mean of almost 9 weeks.

Wilson reported on the results of an uncontrolled study in which 32 patients, ages 77 to 88 years, with 25 stage II, 11 stage III, and 14 stage IV refractory pressure ulcers were treated with PRF (Diapulse) for which no treatment parameters were mentioned.[158] Patients served as their own controls since all received standard wound care for several weeks up to 2 years prior to inclusion in the study. Clinically significant healing was observed for most wounds between 3 and 7 days. Although wound exudation increased in most wounds during the first 2 days of PRF treatment, it was minimal in all wounds by the third day of treatment. All except one wound closed, but that ulcer improved considerably before the patient died from other causes.

In a study involving 20 nonambulatory patients with pressure ulcers of the trochanter and sacrum, Seaborne et al randomized them into four groups of five for treatment with what they referred to as PSWD.[159] Each group was treated over a period of 7 days with one of four interventions, which included an electrostatic field at either 20 or 110 pps and PEMF (likely PRF) nonthermal at 20 and 119 pps. The number and duration of patient treatments was not reported. Using an ABAB multifactorial analysis, the investigators reported a highly significant decrease in wound surface area for each treatment group, without significant differences between the groups.

In a randomized, double-blind, placebo-controlled study, Ritz et al evaluated the wound healing effects of a PRF device (Provant® Wound-Closure System, Regenesis Biomedical Inc., Scottsdale, AZ) on 34 patients with chronic pressure ulcers, of which 60% were more than 6 months old.[160] Inclusion criteria were stage II and III pressure ulcers in patients who were 18 years of age or older. Exclusion criteria were changed in Norton Risk Assessment score greater than or equal to 7 within 30 days; osteomyelitis; immune dysfunction or repeated systemic infection; cancer; concurrent treatment with other wound healing devices (eg, hyperbaric oxygen (HBO), electrical stimulation). Patients with stage II and stage III wounds were separately randomized to groups that received 30-minute twice-daily active PRF plus SWC or placebo PRF plus SWC. Patients and caregivers were blinded to group

assignments. Patients were followed for 12 weeks, until wound closure, or until they were discharged. ANOVA, chi-square, and *t* tests were used as appropriate to determine alpha levels, set a priori at 0.05. PRF induced significantly more wound closures than did placebo. At 6 weeks, 100% of stage II active PRF wounds were closed compared to 36% of placebo-treated wounds, ($P \leq 0.005$). By 12 weeks, 64% of placebo wounds had closed. Stage II active PRF wounds healed 60% faster (26 days) than stage II placebo wounds (66 days, $P \leq 0.005$). At 12 weeks, 59% of stage III active PRF wounds were closed, compared to 14% for placebo wounds ($P \leq 0.01$). Active PRF wounds had an average 87% decrease in surface area compared to a 56% reduction for placebo wounds ($P \leq 0.05$). The results from this study suggest that PRF delivered by the Provant Wound Closure System accelerates closure of stage II and III pressure ulcers. (See Fig. 27.10) (The pressure ulcer studies described above are summarized in Table 27.3.)

Venous Leg Ulcers

Kenkre et al described the device they used on venous leg ulcers (VLU) as an "electromagnetic therapy" machine (Elmedistrall, United Kingdom) that generated perpendicular electric and magnetic fields delivered via a pulse generator capable of creating frequencies of 100, 600, or 800 Hz.[161] The pulsed current generated a magnetic field strength of 25 microteslas (μT), which was delivered to the patient through a pair of electrodes positioned on the patient's involved lower extremities by means of an elastic bandage. The parameters mentioned seem to classify this device as a PRF apparatus. The aim was to establish the potential efficacy, tolerability, and side effect profile of electromagnetic therapy as an adjunct to conventional dressings in the treatment of VLUs. Nineteen patients who demonstrated unsatisfactory healing for at least the previous 4 weeks were randomized to active or placebo PRF treatment. All patients received a 30-minute treatment on weekdays for a total of 30 days, after which patients were followed during a 4-week observation period, with dressing changes only, and final assessment on day 50. Of the 19 patients recruited, 9 were treated with the placebo device, one group of 5 was treated with active 600 Hz, and a second group of 5 received active 800 Hz. Sixty-eight percent of patients treated with active PRF devices achieved improvements in ulcer size, and 21% closed completely. At day 50 patients treated with electromagnetic therapy at 800 Hz were found to have significantly greater healing ($P < 0.05$) and pain control ($P < 0.05$) than placebo therapy or treatment with 600 Hz. All patients reported improved mobility at the end of the study. The electromagnetic therapy was well tolerated by patients, with no differences between groups in reporting adverse events. This study is summarized in Table 27.4.

Diabetic Foot Ulcers

A recent case study by Larsen and Overstreet was found in which two patients with complex diabetic ankle and/or foot ulcers were treated with electromagnetic energy from a PRF device (Provant Wound Therapy System).[162] (Fig. 27-9) One case, a 59-year-old male with a 24-month history of a refractory wound over his left Achilles tendon had a 14-year history of poorly controlled type I diabetes mellitus, anemia, and hypertension. Over the previous 2 years of treatment, consisting

Table 27•3 Pressure Ulcer Clinical Trials with Nonthermal Pulsed Radio Frequency

Investigator	Salzberg et al[155]	Itoh et al[157]	Wilson[158]	Seaborne, Quirion-DeGirardi, and Rousseau[159]	Ritz et al[160]
Study design	DB-RCT	Uncontrolled Unblinded	Uncontrolled	Blinded RCT	Prospective, DB, RCT, placebo controlled
Type of device	PRF (Diapulse)	PRF (Diapulse)	PRF (Diapulse)	ES vs PRF	PRF (Provant)
Frequency	600 pps 65 μsec	600 pps 65 μsec	Not reported	20 pps ES 110 pps ES 20 Hz PRF 110 Hz PRF	Not reported
Amplitude	Peak power	Peak power	Not reported	Not reported	Not reported
Treatment duration	30 min twice daily for 12 wks	30 min twice daily	Not reported	Not reported	30 min twice daily for 12 wks
Treatment effect	Stage II Exp group: 84% closed at 1 wk Median no. days to complete closure = 13 Placebo group: 40% closed at 1 wk Median no. days to closure = 31.5 Stage III ulcer area Exp group: Wounds decreased in size mean of 70.6% Placebo group: Wounds decreased in size 20.7%	All wounds closed. Stage II mean size = 5.56 cm². Closed mean of 2.33 wks Stage III mean size = 8.78 cm² Mean healing/wk: Stage II 57% Stage III 8.9%	Initial increase in wound exudates 1–2 days. All wounds closed except 1.	All groups demonstrated highly significant decrease in wound surface area. No statistical difference between groups.	Stage II Exp group: At 6 wks 100% closed vs 36% for placebo. Stage III Exp group: At 12 wks 50% closed vs 14% for placebo.
Method of measurement	Wound area	Wound area	Observational	Wound area	Wound area
Wound etiology and number	Pressure ulcers/SCI N = 10 stage II N = 10 stage III	Pressure ulcers N = 9 stage II N = 13 stage III	Pressure ulcers N = 25 stage II, N = 11 stage III, N = 14 stage IV	Pressure ulcers N = 20 (4 groups of 5)	Pressure ulcers N = 19 stage II 15 stage III

Modified with permission from Kloth, L, Ziskin, M: Diathermy and pulsed radiofrequency radiation. In: Michlovitz, S (ed): Thermal Agents in Rehabilitation, ed. 3. Philadelphia, F.A. Davis, 1996, p 188.
DB-RCT = double blind randomized controlled trial; RCT = randomized controlled trial

Table 27•4 Effects of PEMF on Venous Leg Ulcers

Investigator	Ieran, Zaffuto, Bagnacani[130]	Duran et al[131]	Todd et al[132]	Stiller et al[133]	Canedo-Dorantes et al[134]	Kenkre et al[161]
Study design	DB-CT	Observational	DB-RCT	DB-RCT	Before-after	DB-RCT
Type of device	PEMF	PEMF	PEMF	PEMF	PEMF (ELF)	PRF
Frequency	75 Hz	Not reported	5 Hz	25% duty cycle	Not reported	600 Hz 800 Hz
Amplitude	2.8 mT	Not reported	Field strength 60 (units not reported)	0.06 mV/cm 22 G	Field strength 36.36 G	25 µT
Treatment duration	4 hr/day for 90 consecutive days	15 min for 10 treatments	15 min 2/wk for 5 wks	3 hrs/day for 8 weeks	2–3 hrs, 3/wk for 4 mo	30 min 5/wk for 30 days
Treatment effect	Wounds closed: 66% exp 31% control	33% decrease in mean surface area	Mean decrease of ulcer size was 7% for both exp and controls. Girth of ulcerated leg: Exp: decrease 2.8% Control: increase 1.2%	*Wound surface area:* Exp 47.1% decrease Control 48.7% decrease *Wound depth decrease:* Exp 46% Control 3.8% *Granulation quality and quantity:* Exp 14.1% decrease in un-healthy granulation Control 0% decrease *Clinical assessment based on 8-point scale:* Exp 50% closed Control 54% worse	After 4 mo, 69% of all wounds either closed or had decreased in size >50%.	*Wound surface area:* Placebo Group: ↓14.2% 20 days ↓21.8% 30 days 600-Hz Group: ↑28.2% 20 days ↑76% 30 days 800-Hz group: ↓24.7% 20 days ↓38% 30 days
Posttreatment effect	Wounds closed: 89% exp 42% controls					Day 50 800-Hz group had significantly greater healing (63%) than placebo group (34%).
Method of measurement	Wound closure	Decrease in wound surface area	Decrease in wound surface area	Wound characteristics	Decrease in wound surface area	Decrease in wound surface area
Wound etiology and number	Venous ulcers N = 44	Venous ulcers N = 18	Venous ulcers N = 19	Venous ulcers N = 31	Venous and arterial ulcers N = 42	Venous leg ulcers N = 19

Modified with permission from Sussman, C: Induced electrical stimulation: Pulsed radio frequency and pulsed electromagnetic fields. In: Sussman, C, Bates-Jensen, B (eds): Wound Care: A Collaborative Practice Manual for Health Professionals, ed. 3. Philadelphia, Lippincott Williams & Wilkins, 2007, p 570. .

DB-CT = double blind controlled trial; DB-RCT = double blind randomized controlled trial

Table 27•5 Postsurgical Clinical Trials with Nonthermal Pulsed Radiofrequency Stimulation

Investigator	Goldin et al[166]	Cameron[167]	Kaplan and Weinstock[168]	Aronofsky[169]	Comorosan, Paslaru, and Popovici[170]
Study design	DB-RCT	Study 1: DB controlled Study 2: Uncontrolled	DB-RCT	CT (nonrandomized, unblinded)	CT
Type of device	PRF (Diapulse)	PRF (Diapulse)	PRF (Diapulse)	PRF (Diapulse)	PRF (Diapulse)
Frequency	400 pps/600 pps 65 µsec	400 pps 65 µsec	400 pps/600 pps 65 µsec	600 pps 65 µsec	400 pps/600 pps 65 µsec
Amplitude	25.3 W/38 W	Med power (4)	Peak power (6) Med power (4)	Peak power	Peak power (6) Med power (4)
Treatment duration	10 min hepatic 20 min wound every 6 hrs for 7 days	Study 1: 20 min hepatic 20 min wound Twice a day for 4 days Study 2: Same as in study 1	30 min postsurgery and 4 hrs later	Gr 1: 15 min 24 hrs preoperative and 10 min preoperative Postoperative: 24, 48, 72 hrs Gr 2: 10 min postoperative Postoperative: 24, 48, 72 hrs Gr 3: no PRF	10 min hepatic 15 min wound
Treatment effect	90% or more healing for 59% of treatment group 29% healing for placebo group (NS)	Study 1: Treatment group little improvement for abdominal incision re suture removal; all others had sutures removed on fifth postoperative day. Study 2: Shorter hospital stay for treatment group	Postoperative day 3: Severe/moderate edema Exp: 80% ↓ edema Placebo: 58% ↓ edema	Inflammation 72 hrs post operative: Gr 1: None 75% Mod 20% High 30% Gr 3: None 2% Mod 57% High: 37% Pain 72 hrs postoperative: Gr 1: None 63% Mod 30% High 6.7% Gr 3: None 7% Mod 57% High 37% Healing group 1: 3–5 days postoperative Group 2: 5–7 days postoperative Group 3: 10–12 days postoperative	Plasma: fibronectin concentration ↑ on postoperative day 7 in treatment group; lower than baseline in control group
Method of measurement	Degree of pain	Retrospective review of medical records Subjective measurements	Likert-like scale grading for edema, erythema, pain	Not reported	Observation of inflammation/infection processes, scar formation, and laboratory measurements
Wound etiology and number	Split-thickness skin graft donor sites N= 29 Exp N= 38 placebo	Heterogeneous surgical wounds N study 1 = 100 N study 2 = 81	Postsurgical podiatric patients	Oral surgery N= 90 (30/group)	Heterogeneous surgical wounds N = 15 Exp N = 10 Control

Modified with permission from Sussman, C: Induced electrical stimulation: Pulsed radio frequency and pulsed elecromagnetic fields. In: Sussman, C, Bates-Jensen, B (eds): Wound Care: A Collaborative Practice Manual for Health Professionals, ed. 3. Philadelphia, Lippincott Williams & Wilkins, 2007, p 561.
DB-RCT = double blind randomized controlled trial; CT = controlled trial

of débridement, serial custom orthotics, silver-impregnated dressings, and platelet-derived growth factor (Regranex, Ortho McNeil Pharmaceuticals, Sommerville, NJ), the wound size increased with the development of a second adjacent wound. Adjunctive PRF treatment of 30 minutes twice a day was initiated when the patient's glycosylated hemoglobin levels (HbA$_{1c}$) was 12.9% and the combined surface area of his two Achilles tendon wounds was 1.75 cm^2. Other interventions included off-loading, sharp débridement, and silver-based and petrolatum gauze dressings. After the first 10 weeks of therapy, the wound decreased in surface area by 54.3%. In spite of poor glucose control (HbA$_{1c}$ varied from 8.0% to 10.3%), the wound closed in 16 weeks at a healing rate of 1.56 mm^2/day and remained closed at a 9-month follow-up.

A second case involved a 79-year-old male with a right transmetatarsal (2-5) amputation that was performed for a draining, conspicuously infected, second toe, with underlying osteomyelitis. The patient presented 3 days postoperatively with a wide dehiscence of the surgical site that measured 7 cm^2 in surface area and was noticeably inflamed. Collectively, he had several other conditions that could be considered impediments to healing, including obesity, hypertension, type II diabetes mellitus, a history of peripheral neuropathy, posttraumatic stress disorder, chronic obstructive pulmonary disease, and colon cancer. His HbA$_{1c}$ was within normal limits at 6.2%. Treatment of his wound consisted of débridement, off-loading, silver-based dressings, and PRF 30 minutes twice a day. The wound closed within 16.7 weeks at a healing rate of 6.0 mm^2/day and remained closed at a 7-month follow-up. In these two cases, patients received comprehensive standard wound care without alteration, other than the addition of PRF therapy. Although these reports are anecdotal, the results suggest that PRF treatment may have prevented amputation, possibly by enhancing blood perfusion.

Nonthermal Pulsed Radio Frequency—Blood Perfusion Studies

Regarding PRF and blood perfusion, Mayrovitz and Larsen conducted a study on the effects of nonthermal PRF (MRT SofPulse) on microvascular perfusion in healthy individuals by exposing the right forearms of nine men and women to PRF having a pulse duration of 65 μsec, a pulse frequency of 600 pps, and a duty cycle of 0.039 for 45 minutes.[163] After 40 minutes with laser Doppler instrumentation, they recorded a 29% increase in cutaneous blood perfusion compared with no change in perfusion in the left (control) forearms. In a second study, the same investigators evaluated the effects of PRF (MRT SofPulse) on perfusion in periwound skin of 15 subjects who had had diabetes for at least 5 years and each of whom had an ulcer on the foot or toe of one lower extremity for a minimum of 8 weeks.[164] The intact contralateral lower limb served as the control. Noninvasive vascular testing revealed that 9 subjects had peripheral arterial disease in the ulcer-bearing limb; however, these limbs had pretreatment perfusion and volume much greater than the control limb. With PRF parameters of 65 μsec, 600 pps at peak power, and the induction coil 1.5 cm above the ulcer surface, and a single 45-minute treatment at the periulcer site, an increase in laser

Doppler perfusion occurred due mainly to an increase in blood volume. There was no change in any laser Doppler parameter at the contralateral control site nor was there an increase in skin temperature at either site. These findings suggest that if resting perfusion is marginally insufficient to allow timely ulcer healing, an increase in perfusion secondary to PRF stimulation may enhance perfusion enough to allow ulcer healing.

Unlike the previous study by Mayrovitz and Larsen who applied PRF directly over periwound skin,[164] Erdman used the consensual or indirect approach by applying nonthermal PRF from the inductive coil of Diapulse over the epigastrium to see if blood flow changes occurred to the feet of 20 healthy young adults.[165] Using cutaneous thermometry he measured an increase in foot temperature of 2.0°C and an average blood volume increase of 1.75-fold at the maximum power output settings. There were no changes in rectal temperatures or pulse rates. The foot-warming effect continued for a short time after the treatment was terminated. These findings suggest that PRF may be applied remotely over the epigastrium to elicit enhanced perfusion to the distal lower extremities.

Nonthermal Pulsed Radio Frequency—Postsurgical Wounds

Goldin et al conducted a controlled, double-blind clinical study that compared donor sites of medium-thickness split-skin grafts treated with an active nonthermal PRF device ($N = 29$) with control donor sites treated with a placebo PRF device ($N = 38$).[166] Patients in both groups received a 30-minute treatment before receiving medication prior to surgery and then received a 1-hour treatment daily for 7 days after surgery. The active PRF treatment group received a peak output of 975 W at a frequency of 400 pps and a pulse duration of 65 μsec. The mean power output was 25.3 W. Wounds were evaluated daily by medical staff unaware of the patients' grouping. On the seventh postoperative day, dressings were removed and the percentage of wound area healed was determined. In the active treatment group, 17 of 29 patients had wounds that were healed 90% or more, compared with only 11 of 38 patients in the placebo group. Data analysis revealed that this difference was statistically significant.

Cameron reported favorable results in postsurgical wound healing from a "double-blind" study using Diapulse in which 100 patients were assigned to an active PRF group or a placebo PRF group.[167] The credibility of the reported findings from this study is uncertain because many results were based on observational subjectivity, and other interventions were used along with PRF, making it difficult to evaluate the effects of PRF.

In a study of 100 patients who received a variety of podiatric surgical procedures (fewer than five), Kaplan and Weinstock randomly applied placebo or active nonthermal PRF postsurgically with Diapulse.[168] They delivered PRF to the epigastrium with the signal frequency set at 400 pps and to the surgical site with the frequency set at 600 pps. The power levels and treatment durations for the two treatment sites were 4 for 15 minutes and 6 for 15 minutes, respectively. A modified Likert scale was used to grade the tissues for pain, edema, and erythema. A drawback to this study is that they descriptively reported significant reductions in severe to moderate edema for the active PRF group on the third postoperative day (80%) versus the placebo group (58%), but reported nothing regarding the effects of PRF on pain or erythema.

The use of nonthermal PRF (Diapulse) to reduce pain and edema and improve the rate of soft-tissue healing has also been reported following dental surgical procedures. In a nonrandomized controlled trial, Aronofsky divided 90 patients who had had dental surgery into three groups of 30.[169] One group was treated with active PRF for 72 hours, both preoperatively and postoperatively; a second group was treated with active PRF 72 hours only postoperatively, and a third group that served as controls received placebo PRF. PRF pulse frequency was set at 600 pps and peak power output. Patients in both active PRF groups reportedly exhibited substantially less time for their wounds to heal compared to wounds of patients in the control group, and inflammation and pain were absent at 72 hours for the preoperative/postoperative and postoperative treatment groups.

In a double-blind clinical trial, Bentall and Eckstein used both the indirect and direct application methods of transmitting PRF (Diapulse) to the epigastrium and scrotum of 50 pairs of boys who had undergone orchidopexy.[153] One boy in each pair served as the control. The objective was to assess the effects of PRF on postsurgical bruising and edema. Repeated circumferential measurements and pictures of the scrotum were recorded before and after surgery. PRF pulse frequency was set at 500 pps with the intensity at

level 5 for 20 minutes over the scrotum and at 500 pps and intensity at 4 over the epigastrium for 10 minutes. The treatment protocol was performed three times daily for the first 4 postoperative days. The investigators reported a trend toward reduced edema buildup and significantly enhanced reduction of posttraumatic bruising.

One other noncontrolled study by Comorosan et al also used the indirect and direct methods of transmitting nonthermal PRF (Diapulse) over the epigastrium and the postsurgical trauma site.[170] They selected 15 patients to be treated with PRF and 10 others who served as controls. They initiated treatment on the second postoperative day and continued for 5 successive days. PRF was transmitted to the postsurgical site at 600 pps and maximum power output for 20 minutes, followed by epigastric application at 400 pps at a power level of 4 for 10 minutes. The criteria used to evaluate the effects of PRF included disappearance of edema, hematoma, and parietal seroma; lack of inflammation and infection; presence or absence of keloid scaring; and the level of postoperative site sensitivity. Subjectively, the investigators reported that after 5 days, all of these characteristics were noticeably improved. The credibility of the reported findings from this study is uncertain because results were based on observational subjectivity. A summary of these studies is presented in Table 27.4.

Summary Regarding Pulsed Radio Frequencies

The technology of pulsed radio frequencies has certainly advanced due to a greater understanding of the mechanism of action of EMF therapeutic signals. The clinician has at hand a powerful armamentarium of PRF tools that allow

▶ **Case Study 27•1** | **60-Year-Old Male; Episternal After Post Cardiac Surgery**

(See Figs. 27.15 and 27.16)

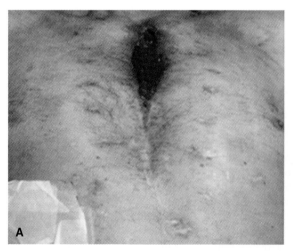
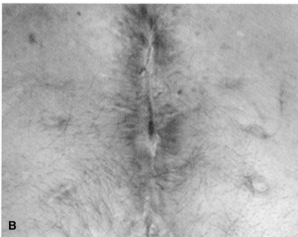

Figure 27•15 *Case 1: (A) Progress at 4 weeks after discharge using disposable PRF unit. (B) Wound resolved at 8 weeks. Therapy regimen was as described for Figure 27.13. (Courtesy B. Strauch, MD, Albert Einstein School of Medicine, New York, NY)*

▶ **Case Study 27•2** 79-Year-Old Female with Large Open Wound Secondary to Right Mastectomy for Papillary Carcinoma

NPWT in place at admission; discontinued due to pain. (Fig 27.16)

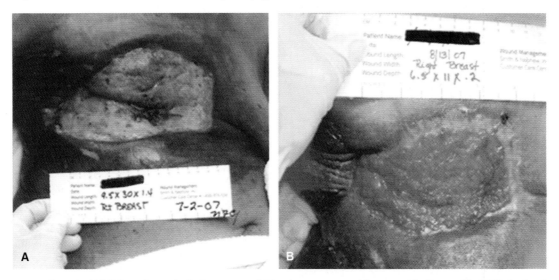

Figure 27•16 *Case 2: (A) Wound at admission; treated 30 minutes every 4 hours with disposable PRF device (see Figure 27.13B). (B) Wound after 41 days of treatment; wound volume had decreased by 96%; patient deferred graft and was discharged. (Courtesy NF Cher, RN, MSA, CWOCN, Regency Hospital, Macon, GA.)*

▶ **Case Study 27•3** A Patient Admitted with Open Venous Insufficiency Wounds

Standard treatment started 11/06; wounds nonhealing despite conservative therapy. (Fig. 27.17)

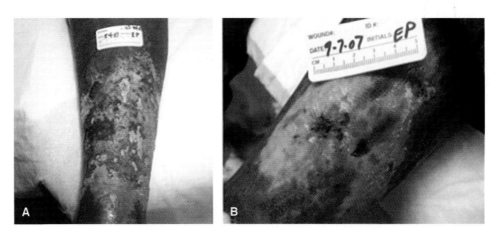

Figure 27•17 *Case 3: (A) Wound after 10 months conservative treatment; PRF with disposable unit is started (B) Healed at 12 weeks with no recurrence as of spring 2008. (Courtesy P. Justice RN, CWS, FACCWS, Indian Health Service, Skiatook, OK.)*

greater treatment flexibility and use with a wider array of patients, at the same time reducing the cost of health care. The clinical wound healing results presented here strongly suggest that PRF therapy has considerably advanced. Portable, even disposable, economical devices are now available for all aspects of wound repair. Although FDA regulatory clearance restricts PRF indications to postoperative pain and edema reduction, it is clear that all stages of wound repair appear to be modulated by specifically configured PRF signals.

Pulsed Shortwave Diathermy— Mild Thermal Effects on Wound Healing

At the beginning of the chapter, we addressed modulation of the RF carrier wave (27.12 MHz) that is used to produce nonthermal PEMF, PRF, and pulsed shortwave diathermy (PSWD) treatment signals. We said that depending on the average power delivered to the body by these pulses of RF energy, tissue temperature may or may not increase. Some of the effects of PRF and PSWD on wound healing are shown in Table 27.5.

▸ **PEARL 27•19** As we have seen prior to this section, both PEMF and PRF devices produce mean power outputs less than 38 watts that classify them as being nonthermal and therefore capable of having nonthermal effects on tissues. On the other hand, RF devices that have higher average power outputs between 38 and 80 watts (PSWD) are capable of elevating tissue temperature to produce mild thermal effects (38°–40°C) in superficial to deep absorbing wound tissues that are vascularized sufficiently to dissipate the mild heat.[171]

Continuous Shortwave Diathermy Versus Pulsed Shortwave Diathermy

Both continuous shortwave diathermy (CSWD) and pulsed shortwave diathermy (PSWD) use the 27.12-MHz RF carrier frequency. CSWD may be used safely on individuals who are sensate and can respond to painful stimuli and who have blood perfusion that is sufficient to dissipate local and regional heating through blood flow. In patients with arterial insufficiency of the extremities (peripheral arterial disease), heating is contraindicated because of poor heat dissipation, which places them at higher risk for burns.[174] PSWD has frequency rates between 1 and 7000 pps, and the pulse duration varies between 65 and 400 μsec. The combination of longer pulse durations and higher frequencies provide more energy to the tissues, which results in a greater thermal effect. The clinical use of the thermal effects of CSWD and thermal/nonthermal effects of PRF may be divided into two categories: (1) functional restoration and analgesia and (2) facilitation of healing of acutely injured soft tissue and chronic dermal ulcerations.

▸ **PEARL 27•20** When the RF carrier is not interrupted into pulses or bursts of energy, it is called CSWD, which generally has a power output range between 55 and 500 watts,[172] and is capable of raising the temperature of deep, well-vascularized soft tissues to between 38°C and 45°C for enhancing the resiliency of structures that have a high collagen content.[173]

Rationale for Treating Wounds with Mild Thermal Energy (Pulsed Shortwave Diathermy)

The beneficial effects of heat on tissue healing have been recognized for centuries. The literature on the history of medicine has long made reference to the use of a variety of heat methods to treat wounds. Early civilizations used various heat applications to promote drainage and healing of boils, provide analgesia, and limit the spread of infection. Hippocrates himself once said, "Wounds love warmth; naturally, because they exist under shelter; and naturally they suffer from the opposite."[175]

▸ **PEARL 27•21** Increasing wound and periwound tissue temperature increases oxygen delivery, and oxygen uptake increases subsequent to an increase in blood perfusion.[176-180]

These findings are especially important with respect to tissue healing because, in addition to subcutaneous oxygen tension being correlated with tissue perfusion, it is also correlated with an increased resistance to infection and acceleration of wound healing.[176-188] Moreover, through its effect on fibroblasts, tissue oxygen tension impacts collagen deposition and scar tensile strength and, through oxidative killing, is an important defense against pathogens that colonize wounds.[189-192] In an experimental study on rats, Ninnikoski et al found that when the temperature of the wound area in ischemic wounds was intermittently elevated by infrared heat,[193] a statistically significant increase in healing rate was observed. They proposed that the increased rate of healing in response to heat was due to increased blood perfusion and oxygen delivery to the wound tissues.

Bello et al measured the temperature of wound tissue and periwound skin and found that compared to body core temperature, average wound and periwound skin temperatures were 5.6°F and 4.5°F cooler, respectively, than core temperature.[194] They proposed that because of the relatively low temperature of wound and periwound tissues, a controlled level of heat applied to these tissues could be beneficial to wound healing. In fact, Kloth et al and others have reported positive wound healing outcomes from mild thermal effects produced by an infrared device that maintained the wound temperature at 38°C.[195-197]

Suggested Protocols for Pulsed Shortwave Diathermy Treatment of Wounds

Based on the earlier definitions of mild and vigorous tissue heating by Lehman and deLateur,[173] Kloth and Ziskin proposed a protocol for the adjunctive use of PSWD for wound healing in the acute, subacute, and chronic inflammatory phases of healing.[198] They divided PSWD power output into four dosage levels that corresponded to percentages of maximum output: level 1 (lowest, subthermal); level 2 (low, mild heat sensation); level 3 (medium, moderate, comfortable heat sensation); and level 4 (high, vigorous heating, well tolerated, decrease to just below maximum tolerance). Table 27.6 shows the lowest- and low-thermal dosage levels of PSWD that may be use at the discretion of the clinician to enhance healing of well-vascularized wounds.

Pulsed Shortwave Diathermy Blood Flow Studies on Healthy Subjects

Some PSWD devices allow selection of parameters that provide mild heating of tissues. Examples of such devices are the Magnatherm SSP® (International Medical Electronics, Kansas City, MO) and the Megapulse® II (Accelerated Care Plus, Reno, NV) (Figs. 27.18 and 27.19), respectively. The Magnatherm SSP device has two treatment applicators designed to allow each to be set at the same or different thermal dosages. Heating effects are produced at high pulse frequencies and long pulse durations, whereas nonthermal effects are produced at low pulse frequencies and short pulse durations. The Megapulse II device also provides several pulse-frequency and pulse-duration options for producing thermal and nonthermal effects in soft tissues.

In reviewing the literature related to the use of PSWD to enhance blood flow, only three studies were found. Silverman

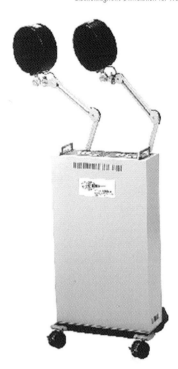

Figure 27•18 *Magnatherm SSP diathermy device that has the capability for mild tissue heating (PSWD) and vigorous tissue heating (CSWD). (Courtesy of International Medical Electronics Ltd., Kansas City, MO.)*

and Pendleton compared the effects of CSWD and PSWD on lower-extremity perfusion in healthy young adults.[199] They used plethysmography to measure blood flow changes to the calf and foot and also measured skin temperature before and after indirect applications of PSWD or CSWD to the

Table 27•6 Dosage Guide for Shortwave Diathermy							
Condition Treated	Heat Dosage Level	Duration of Treatment	Frequency of Treatment	Heat Sensation Reported by Patient	Output of Energy from Device (%)	Rate of Tissue Temperature Rise (°C/min)	Tissue Temperature Increase Goal (°C)
Acute inflammation	1. Lowest	1–3 min	Daily 1–2 wks	None; dose is just below sensation of heat.	1/4 maximum output	0.4–0.8	37.5–38.5
Subacute inflammation	2. Low	3–5 min	Daily 1–2 wks	Barely felt	1/2 maximum output	0.8–1.2	38.5–40.0
Repair phase	3. Medium	5–7 min	Daily 1–2 wks	Distinct but pleasant heat sensation	3/4 maximum output	1.2–2.0	40.0–42.0
Chronic conditions	4. High	5–7 min	Daily or 2/wk for 1 wk to 1 mo	Definite heat sensation, well within tolerance	3/4 maximum output	2.0–2.7	42.0–44.0

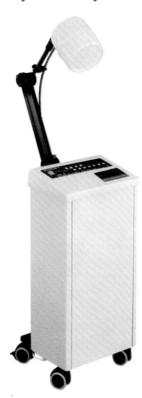

Figure 27•19 *Magnapulse II diathermy device that has the capability for nonthermal PRF, mild thermal PSWD, and vigorous heating (CSWD). (Courtesy of Accelerated Care Plus, Reno, NV.)*

abdominal area. Following 20 minutes of both CSWD and PSWD independently set at a high mean power setting of 65W and 2400 pps or low mean power of 15 W and 600 pps, they recorded mean increases in foot circulation of 165% with PSWD and 195% with CSWD, both at the high mean power settings. No circulatory changes occurred with either device at the low power setting. The mean skin temperature increase was 5.3°C with CSWD and 5.8°C with PSWD. The foot temperature increased 1.9°C and 2.2°C, respectively. The skin of the abdomen of subjects who received low power increased 3.1°C and 3.4°C, respectively, for CSWD and PSWD. These changes in temperature and blood flow are statistically significant, which verifies the thermal capability of PSWD. However, the differences between the CSWD and PSWD devices were not statistically significant,

In another study that evaluated the effects of diathermy on lower-extremity perfusion, Santoro et al applied thermal PSWD to the legs of 10 patients diagnosed with moderate to severe peripheral arterial disease.[200] They delivered PSWD via two coil applicators to the plantar surface of the foot and the ipsilateral midanterior thigh simultaneously for 30 minutes, 5 days a week, for 20 days over 1 month. For patients with both limbs affected, both coil applicators were placed over the plantar surfaces of both feet. During the first 20 minutes of the protocol, the PSWD device was set at 100% of its maximum power output (95 μsec pulse duration and 7000 pps). During the remaining 10 minutes, the power output was reduced to 10% of maximum (95 μsec pulse duration and 700 pps), which was described as a "cooling phase." In five patients they measured skin temperature, TcPO$_2$, and segmental Doppler blood pressure and superficial blood flow with a laser Doppler flowmeter. In these five patients, the percentage of change between the pre-TcPO$_2$ and post-TcPO$_2$ measurements was insignificant in the treated limb, but significant in the untreated limb ($P < 0.0001$). They suggested that the untreated limb could have experienced reflex vasodilation owing to circulation of warmed blood and sympathetic nerve activity. Subjectively, 60% of the patients felt the treatments helped them to walk farther, especially following treatment. However, no long-term vasodilation effects were detected over the 1-month of treatment.

In a randomized study, Santiesteban and Grant used PSWD at a dosage of 700 pps and a power setting of 12 (approximately 120 W) to treat 25 patients, either immediately after or 4 hours after foot surgery.[201] Two coil applicators were used, with one placed over the plantar surface of the postoperative foot and the other over the ipsilateral inguinal area. If foot surgery was bilateral, the coil applicators were placed over the plantar surfaces of both feet. They reported that patients who received the treatment had hospital stays that averaged 8 hours shorter and required lower dosages of analgesic medications than did 25 patients in the control group. Although these investigators did not measure blood flow, it is possible that enhanced perfusion secondary to heating led to improvement of patients who were discharged earlier.

▸ **Box 27•1 Similarities between Thermal PSWD and Non-thermal PRF**

- PSWD and PRF provide comparative dosimetry and uniformity of the induced magnetic field in wound and periwound tissues.
- PSWD and PRF provide postoperative reduction of pain and edema.
- PSWD and PRF enhance tissue perfusion, either directly or consensually, and secondarily increase tissue oxygen saturation.
- PSWD and PRF can be applied without making contact with wound or periwound tissues, thus obviating pain and avoiding wound contamination.
- PSWD elevates tissue temperatures.
- PSWD can mildly increase temperature within deep wounds, tunnels, and abscessed areas.
- PRF excites cellular activity and cell membrane transduction mechanisms.
- PRF can be transmitted through clothing, wound dressings, compression bandages, casting materials, and splints.

Modified with permission from Sussman, C: Induced electrical stimulation: Pulsed radio frequency and pulsed electromagnetic fields. In: Sussman, C, Bates-Jensen, B (eds): Wound Care: A Collaborative Practice Manual for Health Professionals, ed. 3. Philadelphia, Lippincott Williams & Wilkins, 2007, p 573.

Safety Concerns

Pulsed Radio Frequency

Because PRF signals can interfere with electronic devices, for example, hearing aids and watches, ask patients to remove such devices before treating them with PRF. Also, avoid applying PRF over metal objects on the patients or in their clothing, because the signal will reflect the energy away from the intended tissue target.

Pulsed Shortwave Diathermy

In addition to the safety concerns mentioned for PRF, the presence of metal in the patient (eg, orthopedic hardware, shrapnel) or in contact with the patient (jewelry, zippers, bra fasteners and underwires, metal bed parts) should not be in the PSWD field because they can be selectively heated and cause burns. PSWD can also melt or ignite synthetic materials such as some types of patient clothing. Because of the potential for excessively heating a moist dressing in the wound, which could cause wound tissue burning, prior to performing the PSWD treatment of a wound the clinician should replace any moist dressings with a dry sterile gauze dressing. If the wound is likely to produce significant exudates that will moisten the dry gauze during the PSWD treatment, stop the treatment as often as needed and replace the moist dressing with a dry one.

Clinician Safety

Some older PRF and PSWD devices may not have adequate shielding around device applicators and cables, allowing some energy to be dissipated into the immediate area close to the equipment. Normally, clinicians in close proximity to the equipment will absorb a small amount of EMF energy when they are within 0.5 m from the cables and 0.2 m from the inductive coil treatment applicators. When clinicians are at least 1.0 m from the applicator and 0.5 m from the cables during operation of the device, there is little danger of absorbing harmful energy.[202] Table 27.7 lists FDA contraindications, warnings, and cautions for PRF and PSWD.

Table 27•7 FDA Contraindications, Warnings, and Cautions for Pulsed Radio Frequency and Pulsed Shortwave Diathermy	
PSWD	**PRF**
Do not treat over ischemic tissue with inadequate blood flow.	Do not use as a substitute for treatment of internal organs.
Do not treat over metallic implants.	Do not use on patients who have any implanted metallic lead or wire, or any implanted system that may contain a metallic lead including devices such as pacemakers. This device and related diathermy devices may have adverse effects on electronic pacemakers or implanted defibrillators in cardiac patients, and on nerve stimulators.
Do not use on patients with cardiac pacemakers.	Do not use on patients who are pregnant.
Do not treat in any region where the presence of primary or metastatic growth is known or suspected.	Do not treat over immature bone.
Do not treat over immature bone.	
Do not treat over acute osteomyelitis without adequate drainage or before adequate drainage has been established.	
Do not treat patients who have a tendency to hemorrhage (including menses).	
Do not treat over pelvic or abdominal region or lower back during pregnancy.	
Do not treat transcerebrally.	
Do not use over anesthetized areas.	
Avoid situations that could concentrate the field, including moist dressings, perspiration, adhesives.	
Use caution when treating patients with heat sensitivity.	
Use caution when treating patients with inflammatory processes.	

Data from International Medical Electronics, Magnatherm® Model 1000 Instruction Manual (International Medical Electronics, Kansas City, MO) and Electropharmacology, MRT® sofPulse™ User's Manual (MRT, Boca Raton, FL).

Summary

Both nonthermal PEMF and thermal/nonthermal PRF technologies have important clinical applications to pain suppression and facilitation of tissue healing. The biophysical effects of these electromagnetic energies is a function of the time varying parameters of the signals that are transmitted to the target tissues. Various conditions for which PEMF and continuous and pulsed PRF are beneficial have been discussed.

References

1. Erwin, DN: An overview of the biological effects of radiofrequency radiation. Mil Med 1983; 148:113–117.
2. Kloth, LC, Ziskin, MC: Diathermy and pulsed radiofrequency radiation. In: Michlovitz, SL (ed): Thermal Agents in Rehabilitation, ed. 3. Philadelphia, FA Davis, 1996, pp 231–254.
3. Yost, MG: Nonionizing radiation questions and answers. In: Clemmensen, J: Nonionizing Radiation: A Case for Federal Standards? San Francisco, San Francisco Press, 1993, p 8.
4. Nagelschmidt, CF: Lehrbuch der Diathermie fur Srzye und Studierende, von Franz Nagelschmidt. Berlin, Germany, J Springer, 1913.
5. Ginsberg, AJ: Ultrashort radio waves as a therapeutic agent. Med Record 1934; 140:651–653.
6. Markov, MS, Pilla, AA: Electromagnetic field stimulation of soft tissues: Pulsed radio frequency treatment of post-operative pain and edema. Wounds 1995; 7:143–151.
7. American Physical Therapy Association: Electrotherapeutic Terminology in Physical Therapy: Section on Clinical Electrophysiology. American Physical Therapy Association, Alexandria, VA, 2001.
8. Akai, M, Hayashi, K: Effect of electrical stimulation on musculoskelctal systems: A meta-analysis of controlled clinical trials. Bioelectromagnetics 2002; 23:132–143.
9. Centers for Medicare and Medicaid Services. Decision memo for electrostimulation for wounds (CAG-00068R), 2003. http://www.cms.hhs.gov/transmittals/downloads/R7NCD.pdf
10. Spadaro, JA: Electrically stimulated bone growth in animals and man. Clin Ortho 1977; 122:325–329.
11. Black, J: Electrical Stimulation: Its Role in Growth, Repair, and Remodeling of the Musculoskeletal System. New York, Praeger, 1987.
12. Brighton, CT: The treatment of non-unions with electricity. J Bone Joint Surg 1981; 63A:8–12.
13. Friedenberg, ZB, Harlow, MC, Brighton, CT: Healing of non-union of the medial malleolus by means of direct current. J Trauma 1971; 11:8831–8834.
14. Pilla, AA: Electrochemical events in tissue growth and repair. In: Miller, I, Salkind, A, Silverman, H (eds): Electrochemical Bioscience and Bioengineering. Princeton, Electrochemical Society, 1973, pp 1–17. Electrochemical Society Symposium Series.
15. Pilla, AA: Mechanisms of electrochemical phenomena in tissue growth and repair. Bioelectrochem Bioenergetics 1974; 1:227–243.
16. Bassett, CAL, Pawluk, RJ, Pilla, AA: Acceleration of fracture repair by electromagnetic fields. Ann NY Acad Sci 1974; 238:242–262.
17. Basset, CAL, Pilla, AA, Pawluk, R: A non-surgical salvage of surgically-resistant pseudoarthroses and non-unions by pulsing electromagnetic fields. Clin Orthop 1977; 124:117–131.
18. Bassett, C, Mitchell, S, Gaston, S: Treatment of ununited tibial diaphyseal fractures with pulsing electromagnetic fields. J Bone Joint Surg 1981; 63A:511–523.
19. Bassett, C, Mitchell, S, Schink, M: Treatment of therapeutically resistant nonunions with bone grafts and pulsing electromagnetic fields. J Bone Joint Surg 1982; 64A:1214–1224.
20. Bassett, C, Valdes, M, Hernandez, E: Modification of fracture repair with selected pulsing electromagnetic fields. J Bone Joint Surg 1982; 64A:888–895.
21. Mooney, V: A randomized double blind prospective study of the efficacy of pulsed electromagnetic fields for interbody lumbar fusions. Spine 1990; 15:708–715.
22. Goodwin, CB, Brighton, CT, Guyer, RD, et al: A double blind study of capacitively coupled electrical stimulation as an adjunct to lumbar spinal fusions. Spine 1999; 24:1349–1357.
23. Zdeblick, TD: A prospective, randomized study of lumbar fusion: Preliminary results. Spine 1993; 18:983–991.
24. Linovitz, RJ, Ryaby, JT, Magee, FP, et al: Combined magnetic fields accelerate primary spine fusion: A double-blind, randomized, placebo controlled study. J Am Acad Orthop Surg 2000; 67:376.
25. Nicolakis, P, Kollmitzer, J, Crevenna1, R, et al: Pulsed magnetic field therapy for osteoarthritis of the knee–A double-blind sham-controlled trial. Wien Klin Wochenschr 2002; 16:678–684.
26. Zizic, T, Hoffman, P, Holt, D, et al: The treatment of osteoarthritis of the knee with pulsed electrical stimulation. J Rheumatol 1995; 22:1757–1761.
27. Mont, MA, Hungerford, DS, Caldwell, JR, et al: The use of pulsed electrical stimulation to defer total knee arthroplasty in patients with osteoarthritis of the knee. Orthopedics 2006; 29 (10): 887–892.
28. Aaron, RK, Lennox, D, Bunce, GE, et al: The conservative treatment of osteonecrosis of the femoral head. A comparison of core decompression and pulsing electromagnetic fields. Clin Orthop 1989; 249:209–218.
29. Steinberg, ME, Brighton, CT, Corces, A, et al: Osteonecrosis of the femoral head. Results of core decompression and grafting with and without electrical stimulation. Clin Orthop 1989; 249:199–208.
30. Binder, A, Parr, G, Hazelman, B, et al: Pulsed electromagnetic field therapy of persistent rotator cuff tendinitis: A double blind controlled assessment. Lancet 1984; 1:695–697.
31. Brighton, C, Pollack, S: Treatment of recalcitrant non-unions with a capacitively coupled electrical field. J Bone Joint Surg 1985; 67A:577–585.
32. Brighton, CT, Hozack, WJ, Brager, MD, et al: Fracture healing in the rabbit fibula when subjected to various capacitively coupled electrical fields. J Orthop Res 1985; 3:331–340.
33. Pilla, AA: Electrochemical information transfer at living cell membranes. Ann N Y Acad Sci 1974; 238:149–170.
34. Pilla, AA: Weaktime-varying and static magnetic fields: From mechanisms to therapeutic applications. In: Stavroulakis, P (ed): Biological Effects of Electromagnetic Fields. New York, Springer Verlag, 2003, pp 34–75.
35. Aaron, RK, Ciombor, DM, Simon, BJ: Treatment of nonunions with electric and electromagnetic fields. Clin Orthop 2004; 419:21–29.
36. Fitzsimmons, RJ, Ryaby, JT, Magee, FP, et al: Combined magnetic fields increase net calcium flux in bone cells. Calcif Tissue Int 1994; 55:376–380.
37. Fitzsimmons, RJ, Baylink, DJ, Ryaby, JT, et al: EMF-stimulated bone cell proliferation. In: Blank, MJ (ed): Electricity and Magnetism in Biology and Medicine. San Francisco, San Francisco Press, 1993, pp 899–902.
38. Fitzsimmons, RJ, Ryaby, JT, Mohan, S, et al: Combined magnetic fields increase IGF-II in TE-85 human bone cell cultures. Endocrinology 1995; 136:3100–3106.
39. Fitzsimmons, RJ, Ryaby, JT, Magee, FP, et al: IGF II receptor number is increased in TE 85 cells by low amplitude, low frequency combined magnetic field (CMF) exposure. J Bone Min Res 1995; 10:812–819.
40. Ryaby, JT, Fitzsimmons, RJ, Khin, NA, et al: The role of insulin-like growth factor in magnetic field regulation of bone formation. Bioelectrochem Bioenergetics 1994; 35:87–91.

41. Aaron, RK, Ciombor, DM, Jones, AR: Bone induction by decalcified bone matrix and mRNA of TGFb and IGF-1 are increased by ELF field stimulation. Trans Orthop Res Soc 1997; 22:548.

42. Ciombor, DM, Lester, G, Aaron, RK, et al: Low frequency EMF regulates chondrocyte differentiation and expression of matrix proteins. J Orthop Res 2002; 20:40–50.

43. Aaron, RK, Ciombor, DM: Acceleration of experimental endochondral ossification by biophysical stimulation of the progenitor cell pool. J Orthop Res 1996; 14:582–589.

44. Aaron, RK, Ciombor, DM, Jolly G: Stimulation of experimental endochondral ossification by low-energy pulsing electromagnetic fields. J Bone Min Res 1989; 4:227–233.

45. Lohmann, CH, Schwartz, Z, Liu, Y, et al: Pulsed electromagnetic field stimulation of MG63 osteoblast-like cells affects differentiation and local factor production. J Orthop Res 2000; 18:637–646.

46. Guerkov, HH, Lohmann, CH, Liu, Y, et al: Pulsed electromagnetic fields increase growth factor release by nonunion cells. Clin Orthop 2001; 384:265–279.

47. Zhuang, H, Wang, W, Seldes, RM, et al: Electrical stimulation induces the level of TGF-beta1 mRNA in osteoblastic cells by a mechanism involving calcium/calmodulin pathway. Biochem Biophys Res Commun 1997; 237:225–229.

48. Brighton, CT, Wang, W, Seldes, R, et al: Signal transduction in electrically stimulated bone cells. J Bone Joint Surg 2001; 83:1514–1523.

49. Bodamyali, T, Bhatt, B, Hughes, FJ, et al: Pulsed electromagnetic fields simultaneously induce osteogenesis and upregulate transcription of bone morphogenetic proteins 2 and 4 in rat osteoblasts in vitro. Biochem Biophys Res Commun 1998; 250:458–461.

50. Aaron, RK, Boyan, BD, Ciombor, DM, et al: Stimulation of growth factor synthesis by electric and electromagnetic fields. Clin Orthop 2004; 419:30–37.

51. Markov, MS, Ryaby, JT, Kaufman, JJ, et al: Extremely weak AC and DC magnetic field significantly affect myosin phosphorylation. In: Allen, MJ, Cleary, SF, Sowers, AE, et al (eds): Charge and Field Effects in Biosystems, ed. 3. Boston, Birkhauser, 1992, pp 225–230.

52. Markov, MS, Wang, S, Pilla, AA: Effects of weak low frequency sinusoidal and DC magnetic fields on myosin phosphorylation in a cell-free preparation. Bioelectrochem Bioenerg 1993; 30:119–125

53. Markov, MS, Pilla, AA: Ambient range sinusoidal and DC magnetic fields affect myosin phosphorylation in a cell-free preparation. In: Blank, M (ed): Electricity and Magnetism in Biology and Medicine, San Francisco, San Francisco Press, 1993, pp 323–327.

54. Markov, MS, Pilla, AA: Static magnetic field modulation of myosin phosphorylation: Calcium dependence in two enzyme preparations. Bioelectrochem Bioenerg 1994; 35:57–61.

55. Markov, MS, Pilla, AA: Modulation of cell-free myosin light chain phosphorylation with weak low frequency and static magnetic fields. In: Fry, AH (ed): On the Nature of Electromagnetic Field Interactions with Biological System. Austin, TX, RG Landes, 1994, pp 127–141.

56. Markov, MS, Muehsam, DJ, Pilla, AA: Modulation of cell-free myosin phosphorylation with pulsed radio frequency electromagnetic fields. In: Allen, MJ, Cleary, SF, Sowers, AE (eds): Charge and Field Effects in Biosystems, ed. 4. World Scientific, Hackensack, NJ, 1994, pp 274–288.

57. Markov, MS, Pilla, AA: Weak static magnetic field modulation of myosin phosphorylation in a cell-free preparation: Calcium dependence. Bioelectrochem Bioenerg 1997 43:235–240.

58. Yen-Patton, GP, Patton, WF, Beer, DM, et al: Endothelial cell response to pulsed electromagnetic fields: Stimulation of growth rate and angiogenesis in vitro. J Cell Physiol 1988; 134:37–39.

59. Tepper, OM, Callaghan, MJ, Chang, EI, et al: Electromagnetic fields increase in vitro and in vivo angiogenesis through endothelial release of FGF-2. J FASEB 2004; 18:1231–1233.

60. Bassett, CAL, Pawluk, RJ, Pilla, AA: Acceleration of fracture repair by electromagnetic fields. Ann N Y Acad Sci 1974; 238:242–262.

61. Bassett, CAL, Pawluk, RJ, Pilla, AA: Augmentation of bone repair by inductively coupled electromagnetic fields. Science 1974; 184:575–578.

62. Cane, V, Botti, P, Farnetti, P, et al: Electromagnetic stimulation of bone repair: A histomorphometric study. J Orthop Res 1991; 9:908–917.

63. Cane, V, Botti, P, Soana, S: Pulsed magnetic fields improve osteoblast activity during the repair of an experimental osseous defect. J Orthop Res 1993; 11:664–670.

64. Brighton, CT, Katz, MJ, Goll, SR, et al: Prevention and treatment of sciatic denervation disuse osteoporosis in the rat tibia with capacitively coupled electrical stimulation. Bone 1985; 6:87–97.

65. Brighton, CT, Luessenhop, CP, Pollack, SR, et al: Treatment of castration induced osteoporosis by a capacitively coupled electrical signal in rat vertebrae. J Bone Joint Surg 1989; 71A:228–236.

66. Skerry, TM, Pead, MJ, Lanyon, LE: Modulation of bone loss during disuse by pulsed electromagnetic fields. J Orthop Res 1991; 9:600–608.

67. Ryaby, JT, Haupt, DL, Kinney, JH: Reversal of osteopenia in ovariectomized rats with combined magnetic fields as assessed by x-ray tomographic microscopy. J Bone Min Res 1996; 11:S231.

68. McLeod, KJ, Rubin, CT: The effect of low-frequency electrical fields on osteogenesis. J Bone Joint Surg 1992; 74A:920–929.

69. Connolly, J, Ortiz, J, Price, R, et al: The effect of electrical stimulation on the biophysical properties of fracture healing. Ann N Y Acad Sci 1974; 238:519–529.

70. Petersson, C, Holmar, N, Johnell, O: Electrical stimulation of osteogenesis: Studies of the cathode effect on rat femur. Acta Orthop Scand 1982; 53:727–732.

71. France, JC, Norman, TL, Santrock, RD, et al: The efficacy of direct current stimulation for lumbar intertransverse process fusions in an animal model. Spine 2001; 26:1002–1008.

72. Nerubay, J, Marganit, B, Bubis, JJ, et al: Stimulation of bone formation by electrical current on spinal fusion. Spine 1986; 11:167–169.

73. Toth, JM, Seim, HB, Schwardt, JD, et al: Direct current electrical stimulation increases the fusion rate of spinal fusion cages. Spine 2000; 25:2580–2587.

74. Dejardin, LM, Kahanovitz, N, Arnoczky, SP, et al: The effect of varied electrical current densities on lumbar spinal fusions in dogs. Spine 2001; 1:341–347.

75. Inoue, N, Ohnishi, I, Chen, D, et al: Effect of pulsed electromagnetic fields (PEMF) on late-phase osteotomy gap healing in a canine tibial model. J Orthop Res 2002; 20:1106–1114.

76. Fini, M, Cadossi, R, Cane, V, et al: The effect of pulsed electromagnetic fields on the osteointegration of hydroxyapatite implants in cancellous bone: A morphologic and microstructural in vivo study. J Orthop Res 2002; 20:756–763.

77. Smith, TL, Wong-Gibbons, D, Maultsby, J: Microcirculatory effects of pulsed electromagnetic fields. J Orthop Res 2004; 22:80–84.

78. Ibiwoyea, MO, Powella, KA, Grabinera, MD, et al: Bone mass is preserved in a critical-sized osteotomy by low energy pulsed electromagnetic fields as quantitated by in vivo micro-computed tomography. J Orthop Res 2004; 22:1086–1093.

79. Midura, RJ, Ibiwoye, MO, Powell, et al: Pulsed electromagnetic field treatments enhance the healing of fibular osteotomies. J Orthop Res 2005; 23:1035–1046.

80. Borsalino, G, Bagnacani, M, Bettati, E, et al: Electrical stimulation of human femoral intertrochanteric osteotomies. Clin Orthop 1988; 237:256–263.

81. Mammi, GI, Rocchi, R, Cadossi, R, et al: The electrical stimulation of tibial osteotomies: A double-blind study. Clin Orthop 1993; 288:246–253.

82. Traina, G, Sollazzo, V, Massari, L: Electrical stimulation of tibial osteotomies: A double blind study. In: Bersani, F (ed): Electricity and Magnetism in Biology and Medicine. New York, Plenum Press, 1999, pp 137–138.

83. Akai, M, Kawashima, N, Kimura, T, et al: Electrical stimulation as an adjunct to spinal fusion: A meta-analysis of controlled clinical trials. Bioelectromagnetics 2002; 23:496–504.

84. Kahanovitz, N: Electrical stimulation of spinal fusion: A scientific and clinical update. Spine 2002; 2:145–150.

85. Oishi, M, Onesti, S: Electrical bone graft stimulation for spinal fusion: A review. Neurosurgery 2000; 47:1041–1056.

86. Rogozinski, A, Rogozinski, C: Efficacy of implanted bone growth stimulation in instrumented lumbosacral spinal fusion. Spine 1996; 21:2479–2483.

87. Meril, AJ: Direct current stimulation of allograft in anterior and posterior lumbar interbody fusions. Spine 1994; 19:2393–2398.

88. Goodwin, CB, Brighton, CT, Guyer, RD, et al: A double-blind study of capacitively coupled electrical stimulation as an adjunct to lumbar spinal fusions. Spine 1999; 24:1349–1356.

89. Gossling, HR, Bernstein, RA, Abbott, J: Treatment of ununited tibial fractures: A comparison of surgery and pulsed electromagnetic fields (PEMF). Orthopedics 1992; 15:711–719.

90. Paterson, D, Lewis, G, Cass, C: Treatment of delayed union and nonunion with an implanted direct current stimulator. Clin Orthop 1980; 148:117–128.

91. Brighton, C, Black, J, Friedenberg, Z: A multicenter study of the treatment of non-union with constant direct current. J Bone Joint Surg 1981; 63A:2–13.

92. Bassett, C, Mitchell, S, Gaston, S: Treatment of ununited tibial diaphyseal fractures with pulsing electromagnetic fields. J Bone Joint Surg 1981; 63A:511–523.

93. Heckman, J, Ingram, A, Loyd, R: Nonunion treatment with pulsed electromagnetic fields. Clin Orthop 1981; 161:58–66.

94. Bassett, C, Mitchell, S, Schink, M: Treatment of therapeutically resistant nonunions with bone grafts and pulsing electromagnetic fields. J Bone Joint Surg 1982; 64A:1214–1224.

95. Brighton, C, Pollack, S: Treatment of recalcitrant non-unions with a capacitively coupled electrical field. J Bone Joint Surg 1985; 67A:577–585.

96. Sedel, L, Christel, P, Duriez, J, et al: Acceleration of repair of non-unions by electromagnetic fields. Rev Chir Orthop Reparatrice Appar Mot 1981; 67:11–23.

97. DeHaas, W, Watson, J, Morrison, D: Noninvasive treatment of ununited fractures of the tibia using electrical stimulation. J Bone Joint Surg 1980; 62B:465–470.

98. Dunn, AW, Rush, GA: Electrical stimulation in treatment of delayed union and nonunion of fractures and osteotomies. South Med J 1984; 77:1530–1534.

99. Sharrard, W: A double blind trial of pulsed electromagnetic fields for delayed union of tibial fractures. J Bone Joint Surg 1990; 72B:347–355.

100. Scott, G, King, J: A prospective double blind trial of electrical capacitive coupling in the treatment of non-union of long bones. J Bone Joint Surg 1994; 76A:820–826.

101. Brighton, C, Shaman, P, Heppenstall, R: Tibial nonunion treated with direct current, capacitive coupling, or bone graft. Clin Orthop 1995; 321:223–234.

102. Fredericks, DC, Piehl, DJ, Baker, JT, et al: Effects of pulsed electromagnetic field stimulation on distraction osteogenesis in the rabbit tibial leg lengthening model. J Pediatr Orthop 2003; 23:478–483.

103. Brighton, CT, Wang, W, Seldes, R, et al: Signal transduction in electrically stimulated bone cells. J Bone Joint Surg 2001; 83A:1514–1523.

104. Aaron, RK, Boyan, BD, Ciombor, DM, et al: Stimulation of growth factor synthesis by electric and electromagnetic fields. Clin Orthop 2004; 419:30–37.

105. Seegers, JC, Engelbrecht, CA, van Papendorp, DH: Activation of signal-transduction mechanisms may underlie the therapeutic effects of an applied electric field. Med Hypotheses 2001; 57:224–230.

106. Nelson, FR, Brighton, CT, Ryaby, J, et al: Use of physical forces in bone healing. J Am Acad Orthop Surg 2003; 11:344–354.

107. Pilla, AA, Muehsam, DJ, Markov, MS, et al: EMF signals and ion/ligand binding kinetics: Prediction of bioeffective waveform parameters. Bioelectrochem Bioenerg1999; 48(1):27–34.

108. Pilla, AA: Weak time-varying and static magnetic fields: From mechanisms to therapeutic applications. In: Stavroulakis, P (ed): Biological Effects of Electromagnetic Fields, Springer Verlag, 2003, pp 34–75.

109. Pilla, AA: Mechanisms and therapeutic applications of time varying and static magnetic fields. In: Barnes, F, Greenebaum, B (eds): Biological and Medical Aspects of Electromagnetic Fields. Boca Raton, FL, CRC Press, 2006, pp 351–411.

110. Pilla, AA, Sechaud, P, McLeod, BR: Electrochemical and electric current aspects of low frequency electromagnetic current induction in biological systems. J Biol Phys 1983; 11:51–57.

111. McLeod, BR, Pilla, AA, Sampsel, MW: Electromagnetic fields induced by Helmholtz aiding coils inside saline-filled boundaries. Bioelectromagnetics 1983; 4:357–370.

112. Hart, FX: Cell culture dosimetry for low-frequency magnetic fields. Bioelectromagnetics 1996; 17:48–57.

113. van Amelsfort, AMJ: An analytical algorithm for solving inhomogeneous electromagnetic boundary-value problems for a set of coaxial circular cylinders. [dissertation] Eindhoven University, The Netherlands, 1991.

114. Buechler, DN, Christensen, DA, Durney, CH, et al: Calculation of electric fields induced in the human knee by a coil applicator. Bioelectromagnetics 2001; 22:224–231.

115. Zborowski, M, Midura, RJ, Wolfman, A, et al: Magnetic field visualization in applications to pulsed electromagnetic field stimulation of tissues. Ann Biomed Eng 2003; 31:195–206.

116. Pilla, AA: Electrochemical information and energy transfer in vivo. In: Proceedings of the 7th IECEC, Washington, DC, American Chemical Society, 1972, pp 761–764.

117. Pilla, AA: Electrochemical information transfer at cell surfaces and junctions: Application to the study and manipulation of cell regulation. In: Keyser, H, Gutman, F, (eds): Bioelectrochemistry. New York, Plenum Press, 1980, pp 353–396.

118. Plonsey, R, Fleming, DG: Bioelectric Phenomena. New York, McGraw-Hill, 1969.

119. Pilla, AA, Margules, G: Dynamic interfacial electrochemical phenomena at living cell membranes: Application to the toad urinary bladder membrane system. J Electrochem Soc 1977; 124:1697–1706.

120. Pilla, AA: Membrane impedance as a probe for interfacial electrochemical control of living cell function. In Blank, M (ed): Adv Chem Ser. Washington DC. American Chemical Society, 1980; 188:339–359.

121. Margules, G, Doty, SB, Pilla, AA: Impedance of living cell membranes in the presence of chemical tissue fixative. In Blank, M (ed): Adv Chem Ser. Washington, DC, American Chemical Society, 1980, 188:461–484.

122. Schmukler, RE, Kaufman, JJ, Maccaro, et al: Transient impedance measurements on biological membranes: Application to red blood cells and melanoma cells. In: Blank, M, (ed): Electrical Double Layers in Biology, New York, Plenum Press, 1986, pp 201–210.

123. Doty, SB: Morphological evidence of gap junctions between bone cells. Calcif Tissue Int 1981; 33:509.

124. Loewenstein, WR: Junctional intracellular communications: The cell-to-cell membrane channel. Physiol Rev 1981; 61:829–841.

125. Sheridan, JD, Atkinson, MM: Cell membranes: Physiological roles of permeable junctions: Some possibilities. Ann Rev Physiol 1985; 47:337–353.

126. King, RW: Nerves in a human body exposed to low-frequency electromagnetic fields. IEEE Trans Biomed Eng 1999; 46:1426–1431.

127. Paul, RG, Tarlton, JF, Purslow, PP, et al: Biomechanical and biochemical study of a standardized wound healing model. Int J Biochem Cell Biol 1997; 29:211–220.

128. Glassman, LS, McGrath, MH, Bassett, CA: Effect of external pulsing electromagnetic fields on the healing of soft tissue. Ann Plastic Surg 1986; 16:287–295.

129. Strauch, B, Patel, MK, Navarro, A, et al: Pulsed magnetic fields accelerate wound repair in a cutaneous wound model in the rat. Plast Reconstr Surg 2007; 120:425–430.

130. Ieran, M, Zaffuto, S, Bagnacani, M, et al: Effect of low frequency electromagnetic fields on skin ulcers of venous origin in humans: A double blind study. J Orthop Res 1990; 8:276–282.

131. Duran, V, Zamurovic, A, Stojanovk, S, et al: Therapy of venous ulcers using pulsating electromagnetic fields—Personal results. Med Pregl 1991; 44:485–488.

132. Todd, D, Heylings, D, Allen, G, et al: Treatment of chronic vari-cose ulcers with pulsed electromagnetic fields: A controlled pilot study. Ir Med J 1991; 84:54–55.

133. Stiller, MJ, Pak, GH, Shupack, JL, et al: A portable pulsed elec-tromagnetic field (PEMF) device to enhance healing of recalci-trant venous ulcers: A double-blind, placebo-controlled clinical trial. Br J Dermatol 1992; 127:147–154.

134. Canedo-Dorantes, L, Garcia-Cantu, R, Barrera, R, et al: Healing of chronic arterial and venous leg ulcers with systemic electromag-netic fields. Arch Med Res 2002; 33:281–289.

135. Callaghan, MJ, Chang, EI, Seiser, N, et al: Pulsed electromag-netic fields accelerate normal and diabetic wound healing by in-creasing endogenous FGF-2 release. Plast Reconstr Surg 2008; 121:130–41.

136. Goodman, E, Greenebaum, B, Frederiksen, J: Effect of pulsed magnetic fields on human umbilical endothelial vein cells. Bioelectrochem Bioenerg 1993; 32:125–132.

137. Roland, D, Ferder, M, Kothuru, R, et al: Effects of pulsed magnetic energy on a microsurgically transferred vessel. Plast Reconstr Surg 2000; 105:1371–1374.

138. Weber, RV, Navarro, A, Wu, JK, et al: Pulsed magnetic fields applied to a transferred arterial loop support the rat groin com-posite flap. Plast Reconstr Surg 2004; 114:1185–1189.

139. Strauch, B, Patel, MK, Rosen, DJ, et al: Pulsed magnetic field therapy increases tensile strength in a rat Achilles' tendon repair model. J Hand Surg 2006; 31A:1131–1135.

140. Kelpke, S, Feldman, D: Alterations in PEMF: The effect on wound healing. Wound Repair Regen 1994; 2:81–85.

141. Kloth, LC, Ziskin, MC: Diathermy and pulsed radio frequency radiation. In: Michlovitz, SL (ed): Thermal Agents in Rehabilita-tion, ed. 3. FA Davis, Philadelphia, 1996, pp 231–254.

142. Ginsberg, AJ: Ultrashort radiowaves as a therapeutic agent. Med Record 1934; 140:651–653.

143. Heden, P, Pilla, AA: Effects of pulsed electromagnetic fields on post operative pain: A double-blind randomized pilot study in breast augmentation patients. Aesth Plast Surg 2008: 32(4):660–666.

143A. Rohde C, Chiang A, Adipoju O, Casper D, Pilla AA. Effects of Pulsed Electromagnetic Fields on IL-1β and Post Operative Pain: A Double-Blind, Placebo-Controlled Pilot Study in Breast Reduction Patients. Plast Reconstr Surg. 2009 Nov 17. [Epub ahead of print].

144. Wilson, DH: Treatment of soft tissue injuries by pulsed electrical energy. Brit Med J 1972; 2:269–270.

145. Wilson, DH: Comparison of short wave diathermy and pulsed electromagnetic energy in treatment of soft tissue injuries. Physiotherapy (Br) 1974; 60(10):309–310.

146. Pennington, GM, Danley, DL, Sumko, MH, et al: Pulsed, non-thermal, high frequency electromagnetic energy (Diapulse) in the treatment of grade I and grade II ankle sprains. Mil Med 1993;158:101–104.

147. Pilla, AA, Martin, DE, Schuett, AM, et al: Effect of pulsed radiofre-quency therapy on edema from grades I and II ankle sprains: A placebo controlled, randomized, multi-site, double-blind clinical study. J Athl Train 1996; S31:53.

148. Foley-Nolan, D, Barry, C, Coughlan, RJ, et al: Pulsed high frequency (27 MHz) electromagnetic therapy for persistent neck pain: A double-blind placebo-controlled study of 20 patients. Orthopedics 1990; 13:445–451.

149. Foley-Nolan, D, Moore, K, Codd, M, et al: Low energy high frequency pulsed electromagnetic therapy for acute whiplash injuries: A double blind randomized controlled study. Scan J Rehab Med 1992; 24:51–59.

150. Barker, AT, Barlow, OS, Porter, J, et al: A double-blind clinical trial of lower power pulsed shortwave therapy in the treatment of a soft tissue injury. Physiotherapy 1985; 71:500–504.

151. Barclay, V, Collier, R, Jones A: Treatment of various hand injuries by pulsed electromagnetic energy (Diapulse). Physiotherapy 1983; 69:186–188.

152. Ionescu, A, Ionescu, D, et al. Study of efficicacy of Diapulse therapy on the dynamics of enzymes in burned wound. Presented at: Sixth International Congress on Burns. San Francisco, CA, August 1982.

153. Bentall, RHC, Eckstein, HB: A trial involving the use of pulsed electromagnetic therapy on children undergoing orchidopexy. Z Kinderchirurgie 1975; 17(4):380–385.

154. Duma-Drzewinska, A, Buczyski, AZ: Pulsed high frequency currents (Diapulse) applied in treatment of bed sores. Pol Tyg Lek 1978; 33:885–888.

155. Salzberg, CA, Cooper, SA, Perez, P, et al: The effects of non-thermal pulsed electromagnetic energy on wound healing of pressure ulcers in spinal cord-injured patients: A randomized, double-blind study. Ostomy Wound Manage 1995; 41:42–51.

156. Kloth, LC, Berman, JE, Sutton, CH, et al: Effect of pulsed radio fre-quency stimulation on wound healing: A double-blind pilot clinical study. In Bersani, F (ed): Electricity and Magnetism in Biology and Medicine. New York, Plenum Press, 1999, pp 875–878.

157. Itoh, M, Montemayor, JS Jr, Matsumoto, E, et al: Accelerated wound healing of pressure ulcers by pulsed high peak power electromag-netic energy (Diapulse). Decubitus 1991; 4:24–25, 29–34.

158. Wilson, CM: Clinical effects of Diapulse technology in treatment of recalcitrant pressure ulcers. Poster presentation at the Seventh Annual Clinical Symposium on Pressure Ulcer and Wound Management. Orlando, FL, Sept. 15–17, 1992.

159. Seaborne, D, Quirion-DeGirardi, C, Rousseau, M: The treatment of pressure sores using pulsed electromagnetic energy (PEME). Physiother Can 1996; 48:131–137.

160. Ritz, MC, Gallegos, R, Canham, MB, et al: PROVANT® wound-closure system accelerates closure of pressure wounds in a randomized, double-blind, placebo-controlled trial. Ann N Y Acad Sci 2002; 961:356-359.

161. Kenkre, J, Hobbs, F, Carter, Y, et al: A randomized controlled trial of electromagnetic therapy in the primary care management of venous leg ulceration. Fam Pract 1996; 13:236–240.

162. Larsen, JA, Overstreet, J: Pulsed radio frequency energy in the treatment of complex diabetic foot wounds: Two cases. J Wound Ostomy Continence Nurs 2008; 35:523–527.

163. Mayrovitz, HN, Larsen, PB: Effects of pulsed magnetic fields on skin microvascular blood perfusion. Wounds: A Compendium of Clinical Research and Practice 1992; 4:192–202.

164. Mayrovitz, HN, Larsen, PB: A preliminary study to evaluate the effect of pulsed radio frequency field treatment on lower extremity peri-ulcer skin microcirculation of diabetic patients. Wounds: A Compendium of Clinical Research and Practice 1995; 7:90–93.

165. Erdman, W: Peripheral blood flow measurements during application of pulsed high frequency currents. Orthopedics 1960; 2:196–197.

166. Goldin, JH, Broadbent, NRG, Nancarrow, JD, et al: The effects of Diapulse on the healing of wounds: A double-blind randomized controlled trial in man. Br J Plast Surg 1981; 34:267–270.

167. Cameron, BM: A three phase evaluation of pulsed high frequency radio short waves (Diapulse): 646 patients. Am J Orthop 1964; 6:72–78.

168. Kaplan, EG, Weinstock, RE: Clinical evaluation of Diapulse as adjunctive therapy following foot surgery. J Am Podiat Assoc 1968; 58:218–221.

169. Aronofsky, DH: Reduction of dental postsurgical symptoms using non-thermal, high peak power electromagnetic energy. Oral Surg Oral Med Oral Pathol 1971; 32:688–696.

170. Comorosan, S, Paslaru, L, Popovici, Z: The stimulation of wound healing processes by pulsed electromagnetic energy. Wounds 1992; 4:31–32.

171. van den Bouwhuijsen, F, Maassen, V, Meijer, M, et al. A Manual of Pulsed and Continuous Shortwave Diathermy, ed. 2. Delft, Holland, Enraf-Nonius, 1990, Publication No. 1419.762.

172. Diathermy units: Microwave and shortwave units. In: Product Comparison System. Plymouth Meeting, PA, ECRI, 1988, pp 1–10.

173. Lehman, J, deLateur, B: Therapeutic heat. In: Lehman, J (ed): Therapeutic Heat and Cold, ed. 4. Baltimore, Lippincott Williams & Wilkins, 1990.

174. Brown, G: Diathermy: A renewed interest in a proven therapy. Phys Ther Today 1993; Spring:78–80.

175. Majno, F: The Healing Hand: Man and Wound in the Ancient World. Cambridge, Harvard University Press, 1975, p 181.

176. Abramson, DI: Changes in blood flow, oxygen uptake and tissue temperatures produced by the topical application of wet heat. Arch Phys Med Rehabil 1961; 42:305–311.

177. Rabkin, J, Hunt, T: Local heat increases blood flow and oxygen tension in wounds. Arch Surg 1987; 122:221–229.

178. Randall, BF, Imig, CJ, Hines, HM: Effects of some physical therapies on blood flow. Arch Phy Med Rehabil 1952; 33:73–76.

179. Wessman, HS, Kottke, FJ: The effect of indirect heating on peripheral blood flow, pulse rate, blood pressure, and temperature. Arch Phys Med Rehabil 1967; 48:567–571.

180. Stoner, HB, Barker, P, Riding, GSG, et al: Relationships between skin temperature and perfusion in the arm and leg. Clin Physiol 1991; 11:27–30.

181. Sheffield, CW, Sessler, GL, Hopf, HW, et al: Centrally and locally mediated thermoregulatory responses after subcutaneous oxygen tension. Wound Repair Regen 1996; 4:339–344.

182. Gottrup, F, Firmin, R, Rabkin, J, et al: Directly measured tissue oxygen tension and arterial tension assess tissue perfusion. Crit Care Med 1987; 15:1030–1035.

183. Jonsson, K, Jensen, JA, Goodson, WH, et al: Assessment of perfusion in postoperative patients using tissue oxygen measurements. Br J Surg 1987; 74:263–266.

184. Jonsson, K, Hunt, TK, Mathes, SJ: Oxygen as an isolated variable influences resistance to infection. Ann Surg 1988; 208:783–787.

185. Hohn, DC, Mackay, RD, Halliday, B, et al: Effect of O2 tension on microbicidal function of leukocytes in wounds and in vitro. Surg Forum 1976; 27:18–21.

186. Jonsson, K, Jensen, JA, Goodson, WH, et al: Tissue oxygenation anemia and perfusion in relation to wound healing in surgical patients. Ann Surg 1991; 214:605–609.

187. Pai, MP, Hunt, TK: Effect of varying oxygen tension on healing of open wounds. Surg Gynecol Obstet 1972; 135:756–759.

188. Niinikoski, J: Cellular and nutritional interaction in healing wounds. Med Biol 1980; 58.303–305.

189. Hunt, TK: The effect of varying ambient oxygen tensions on wound metabolism and collagen synthesis. Surg Gynecol Obstet 1972; 135:561–565.

190. Shandall, A, Lowndes, R, Young, HL: Colonic anastomotic healing and oxygen tension. Br J Surg 1984; 72:606–609.

191. Babior, BM: Oxygen-dependant microbial killing by phagocytes. N Eng J Med 1978; 298:659–661.

192. Bemheim, P, Hunt, TK: Natural resistance to infection: Leukocyte functions. J Burn Care Rehabil 1992; 13:287–290.

193. Niinikoski, J, Rajamaki, A, Kulonen, E: Healing of open wounds: Effects of oxygen, distributed blood supply, and hyperemia by infrared radiation. Acta Chir Scand 1971; 137:399–403.

194. Bello, YM, Lopez, AP, Philips, TJ: Wound temperature is lower than core temperature. Abstract presentation at: 11th Annual Symposium on Advanced Wound Care, Miami Beach, FL. April 18–22, 1998.

195. Kloth, LC, Berman, JE, Dumit-Minkel, S, et al: Effects of a normothermic dressing on pressure ulcer healing. Adv Skin Wound Care 2000; 13:68–74.

196. Kloth, LC, Berman, JE, Nett, M, et al: A randomized controlled clinical trial to evaluate the effects of a noncontact normothermic wound therapy on chronic full-thickness pressure ulcers. Adv Skin Wound Care. 2002; 15:270–276.

197. Whitney, JD, Salvadalena, G, Higa, L, et al: Treatment of pressure ulcers with noncontact normothermic wound therapy: Healing and warming effects. J Wound Ostomy Continence Nurs 2001; 28:244–252.

198. Kloth, LC, Ziskin, MC: Diathermy and pulsed radio frequency radiation. In: Michlovitz, SL (ed): Thermal Agents in Rehabilitation, Philadelphia, FA Davis, p 231, 1996.

199. Silverman, D, Pendleton, L: A comparison of the effects of continuous and pulsed short-wave diathermy on peripheral circulation. Arch Phys Med Rehabil 1968; 49:429–436.

200. Santoro, D, Ostranderl, L, Lee, BY, Cagir, B: Inductive 27.12 MHz diathermy in arterial peripheral vascular disease. Proceedings of the 16th International IEEE/EMBS Conference, Baltimore, MD. Publication date: Nov. 3–6, 1994, vol 2, pages 777–778. IEEE Press.

201. Santiesteban, J, Grant, C: Post-surgical effect of pulsed short-wave therapy. J Am Podiatr Med Assoc 1979; 75:306–309.

202. Ourllet-Helstrom, SR: Miscarriages among female physical therapists who report using radio and microwave frequency electromagnetic radiation. Am J Epidemiol 1993; 138:775–786.

Ultrasound for Wound Débridement and Healing

Luther C. Kloth, MS, PT, CWS, FACCWS, FAPTA

Jeffrey A. Niezgoda, MD, FACHM, FAPWCA, FACEP

Introduction

Ultrasound (US) has been used by various health-care specialists for over 60 years. Biological effects in tissues exposed to US were first reported by Wood and Loomis in 1927.[1] They demonstrated lysis of red blood cells and hindrance of mobility in mice following exposure to high-frequency (300 kHz), high-intensity sound waves. The application of US for medical treatment was introduced in Germany in the late 1930s, and in the United States in the late 1940s.[2,3] The purpose of this chapter is to describe the physical properties and biological effects of ultrasound and how they can be used to enhance wound healing.

Physics and Generation of Ultrasound—Piezoelectric Effect

Ultrasound is produced by vibration of piezoelectric transducer disks that are located in the treatment handpiece behind a metal plate or probe that serves to transmit the acoustic energy to the patient's tissues. The ceramic disks are crystals such as barium titanate or lead zirconate titanate that are capable of transducing electrical energy into sound energy or vice versa. There are two types of piezoelectric effect: direct and indirect (also called reverse).[4] (Fig. 28.1) The direct piezoelectric effect generates an electric voltage across the disk when it is mechanically compressed. If the

crystal is expanded instead of compressed, a voltage of opposite polarity is generated. If acoustic energy from a sound wave at a given frequency impinges upon a crystal, it will expand and contract at the same frequency and will cause an oscillating voltage to be generated across the crystal face. The direct piezoelectric effect is used to convert US into an electrical signal that duplicates the sound pattern.

The reverse piezoelectric effect is the contraction or expansion of a crystal when an alternating current voltage is applied across its surface. A change in the polarity of the applied voltage causes a contracted crystal to expand and vice versa. Thus, a piezoelectric crystal can be used to generate US at any desired lower (eg, 20–40 kHz) or higher (1–3 MHz) sound wave frequency.

> **PEARL 28•1** Ultrasound is generated when an alternating voltage at any frequency makes the crystal vibrate (repetitively expand and contract) at the frequency of the electrical oscillation.

Ultrasound Frequency

US is nonionizing radiation and therefore does not impose the hazards attributed to ionizing radiation, such as cancer production and chromosome breakage.[4] Because sound waves are produced by vibration of piezoelectric disks, the resulting mechanical energy that is transferred to tissues causes molecules to oscillate. The number of oscillations a molecule undergoes in 1 sec defines the frequency of a sound wave and

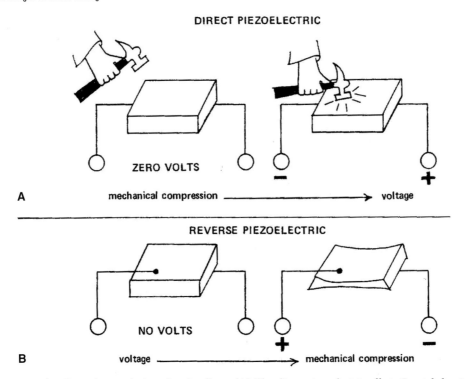

DIRECT PIEZOELECTRIC

ZERO VOLTS

A   mechanical compression ⟶ voltage

REVERSE PIEZOELECTRIC

NO VOLTS

B   voltage ⟶ mechanical compression

Figure 28•1 *Direct and indirect (reverse) piezoelectric effects. (A) The direct piezoelectric effect. Crystals having piezoelectric properties produce positive and negative electrical charges when they are mechanically compressed or expanded. (B) The reverse (indirect) piezoelectric effect. These same crystals expand and contract or vibrate at the same frequency as that of an alternating voltage that is applied to them. (Used by permission of: Starky C: Ultrasound. In: Starky C (ed): Therapeutic Modalities, ed. 2. Philadelphia, F.A. Davis, 1993, p 272.)*

is expressed in units of hertz (Hz); that is, 1 Hz = 1 cycle per second (cps), 1 kHz = 1000 cps, and 1 MHz = 1 million cps. The human ear is sensitive only to sound frequencies between 16 Hz and 20 kHz. US is acoustic energy having frequencies greater than 20 kHz, which are inaudible to the human ear. While audible sound spreads out in all directions, US beams are well collimated, similar to a light beam leaving a flashlight. (Fig. 28.2) For a given source of sound, the higher the frequency, the less the beam diverges from its direction of propagation and the greater the absorption of energy in tissue per unit of distance traveled.

▶ **PEARL 28•2** The more recent lower kilohertz frequencies are used clinically for open wound treatment applications, whereas the higher megahertz frequencies are primarily used for treating closed wound inflammatory soft tissue conditions, as well as for Doppler vascular assessment and for fetal imaging.

Wavelength

US is a mechanical form of energy that causes molecules in tissues to oscillate or vibrate above the upper limit of human hearing. US is transmitted in the form of compression waves, like ripples on a pool of water.[5] In tissues the repeating sonic pressure waves create regions in which molecules are alternately compressed into areas of high (compression) and low

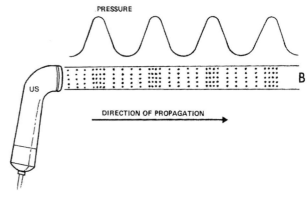

PRESSURE

US

DIRECTION OF PROPAGATION

B

Figure 28•2 *A collimated US beam (B) emitted from an US applicator. The acoustic pressure wave is illustrated as areas of high molecular concentration corresponding to the peaks of the pressure wave, whereas areas of low molecular concentration correspond to the valleys of the pressure wave. Thus, molecular concentration is proportional to acoustic pressure and varies sinusoidally along the direction of wave propagation. (Used by permission of: McDiarmid, T, Ziskin, MC, Michlovitz, SL: Therapeutic ultrasound. In: Michlovitx, SL (ed): Thermal Agents in Rehabilitation, ed. 3. Philadelphia, FA Davis, 1996, p 170.)*

(rarefaction) molecular densities. The molecular concentration is proportional to acoustic pressure and varies sinusoidally along the direction of wave propagation, with peak pressure occurring at the areas of high molecular density as shown in Figure 28.2. The wavelength is the distance between two successive peaks on the waveform in a specified medium (eg, soft tissues) and is inversely related to frequency. The wavelength (λ) is related to the frequency (f) and velocity (c) of the wave by the equation $\lambda = c/f$. The velocity of US in water, blood, and soft tissue is 1540 meters per second. Thus, at a frequency of 1 MHZ the wavelength is $1540/10^6$, or 1.5 mm, and the wavelength at 25 kHz is 61.6 mm.

Attenuation of Ultrasound Energy

When US at a given frequency passes through tissues, molecules vibrate back and forth at that frequency, and with increasing depth of penetration, the energy progressively decreases due to scattering and absorption. Scattering is deflection of sound away from the direction of propagation when it strikes a higher density reflecting surface such as bone or tendon. Absorption is transfer of US energy to tissues and occurs in part because of the internal friction in tissue that needs to be overcome in the passage of sound. The higher the frequency, the more rapidly the molecules are forced to move against this friction. Note in Figure 28.3 that as the US beam penetrates farther into the tissues, a greater proportion of the energy will have been absorbed, and therefore there is less energy available to achieve therapeutic effects. Also note in Figure 28.3 that at the higher frequency (3 MHz) more energy is absorbed in the first centimeter of tissue than occurs at the lower frequency of 1 MHz. Ultrasound imparts its effects on tissues through thermal and nonthermal mechanisms. Both low (kilohertz)

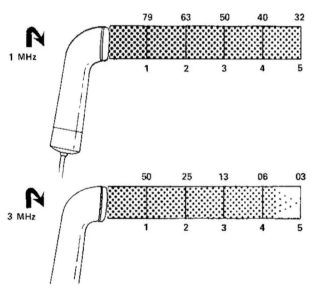

Figure 28•3 *Attenuation of US energy in soft tissue at 1 and 3 MHz assuming that uniform attenuation is approximately 1 dB/cm/MHz. (Used by permission of: McDiarmid, T, Ziskin, MC, Michlovitz, SL: Therapeutic ultrasound. In: Michlovitx, SL (ed): Thermal Agents in Rehabilitation, ed. 3. Philadelphia, FA Davis, 1996, p 171.)*

and high (megahertz) US frequencies simultaneously produce thermal and nonthermal effects in tissues. The thermal effect and absorption increase with higher frequencies (1 and 3 MHz), whereas nonthermal effects are predominant with lower frequencies (20–40 kHz) and when US is pulsed. The thermal and nonthermal effects of US will be presented later.

> ▶ **PEARL 28•3** The predominant thermal effects of 1 and 3 MHz are commonly used to enhance blood flow and to elevate the temperature of periwound tissues and musculoskeletal conditions that limit joint range of motion. The predominant nonthermal effects of US frequencies between 20 and 40 kHz are employed for débridement, bactericidal effect, and healing of acute and chronic wounds.

Continuous and Pulsed Ultrasound Treatment Modes

In the continuous treatment mode, the sound waves and intensity remain constant during the treatment period. In this mode, regardless of frequency, given a constant intensity and treatment duration, the amount of acoustic energy delivered to the tissues will be greater than that in the pulsed mode. If 1 or 3 MHz US is being used primarily to heat tissues, then the continuous mode of application is appropriate. In the pulsed treatment mode, the continuous US waves are intermittently interrupted. The pulse feature is like an intermittent windshield wiper accessory on your car. The output will be on for a short time and off for a short time. The term duty cycle is used to specify what fraction of time the US is on during one pulse period and may be calculated using the following equation:

$$\text{Duty cycle} = \frac{\text{duration of pulse on time}}{\text{pulse period (time on + time off)}}$$

Generally, the choice of duty cycles range from 0.05 (5%) to 0.5 (50%) for megahertz US devices and between 0.5 (50%) and 0.9 (90%) for kilohertz devices. If the frequencies between 20 and 40 kHz are being used for wound débridement purposes, the continuous mode will have a greater fibrolytic effect than the pulsed mode because more energy per unit of time is delivered to the tissues in the continuous mode. Pulsing US reduces the total amount of energy transmitted, and thus for megahertz US, it may be used to guard against excessive heating, while for the kilohertz frequencies it can be used to reduce discomfort that may be experienced during treatment with the continuous mode. Although using the pulsed mode decreases the intensity level for both the megahertz and kilohertz US frequencies, there is still sufficient energy during each pulse to produce the predominately nonthermal effects, which are known to stimulate the wound healing process.[6] Figure 28.4 illustrates both US modes of application.

Intensity

Intensity is the characteristic most often used by practitioners in selecting the desired dosage of an ultrasonic treatment. Intensity reflects the strength of the acoustic vibrations at a given location in the tissues being treated. It is the amount of power per unit area and is expressed as watts per square

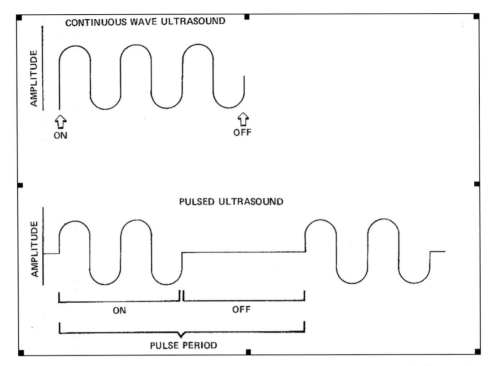

Figure 28•4 *Continuous wave and pulsed wave ultrasound. The duty cycle of the pulsed mode illustrated is 2 msec ÷ 4 msec = 0.5 = 50%. (Used by permission of: McDiarmid, T, Ziskin, MC, Michlovitz, SL: Therapeutic ultrasound. In: Michlovitz, SL (ed): Thermal Agents in Rehabilitation, ed. 3. Philadelphia, FA Davis, 1996, p 173.)*

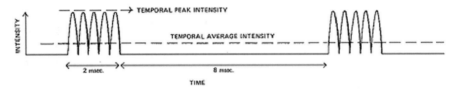

Figure 28•5 *A typical pulsed pattern. The total pulse period is 10 msec. The pulse duration is 2 msec. The duty cycle is 0.20 (20%). (Used by permission of: McDiarmid, T, Ziskin, MC, Michlovitz, SL: Therapeutic ultrasound. In: Michlovitz, SL (ed): Thermal Agents in Rehabilitation, ed. 3. Philadelphia, FA Davis, 1996, p 175.)*

centimeter (W/cm^2). For 1- and 3-MHz therapeutic US devices operating in the continuous mode, the radiating area of the applicator (sound head) determines the average US intensity for a given power setting. The applicator spatial average intensity (SAI) can be calculated by dividing the ultrasonic power (W/cm^2) by the effective radiating area of the applicator. For example, if a 10 cm^2 applicator radiates 20 W of US power, the SAI is 2 W/cm^2. When the pulsed mode is used with the megahertz and kilohertz frequencies, the US intensity will be zero when the sound is off and at its maximum when the pulse is on. (Fig. 28.5) The maximum intensity is called the temporal peak intensity (TPI). The temporal average intensity (TAI) is determined by averaging the intensity over both the on and off periods. For example, at the megahertz frequencies, pulsing US with a duty cycle of 0.5 (50%) and a TPI of 2.0 W/cm^2 would have a TAI of 1.0 W/cm^2; if the duty cycle is 0.25 (25%), the TAI would be 0.5 W/cm^2. With pulsed US at the megahertz frequencies, the TAI is reduced proportionately to the amount of time

the sound is off. Therefore, if 1-MHz or 3-MHz pulsed US is applied to periwound tissues, less tissue heating will occur, even though the TPI is unchanged; nevertheless, the nonthermal effects of pulsed US will be transmitted to the periwound tissues. The most commonly used duty cycle for megahertz US application to periwound tissues seems to be 20%.[4] The values for SAI, TPI, and TAI have not been determined for the kilohertz US devices that are used for wound débridement and healing applications. Information related to intensity of kilohertz US devices will be provided later in this chapter.

Transmitting Ultrasound to the Patient—Coupling Mediums

Unlike radio waves and audible sound waves, which travel through space, megahertz US must be transmitted from the treatment applicator to the patient by a medium or coupling agent. A good medium is characterized by the ability to transmit a significant percentage of the US; therefore, it should be nonreflective. The optimal medium for transmission is distilled water, which reflects only 0.2% of the US energy.[7] The US applicator is placed in contact with the coupling medium, which is placed on the surface of the skin. Low-frequency kilohertz US is generally transmitted by water (saline) coupling through contact with wound tissues; however, one kilohertz device (Celleration MIST®, Celleration Inc. Eden Prairie, MN) uses saline vapor as the coupling medium. In this instance, the applicator does not make contact with the wound tissues.

Aqueous Coupling Mediums

Tap water is an excellent medium for transmitting megahertz US to the patient. (Fig. 28.6) However, since tap water contains air bubbles that prevent US transmission, it is best to let the water stand in the treatment container undisturbed for up to 24 hours to allow the gaseous bubbles to settle out before using it with megahertz US noncontact immersion treatments. If tap water is used without removal of gas bubbles, the intensity of US may be increased by approximately 0.5 W/cm² to account for attenuation caused by air.

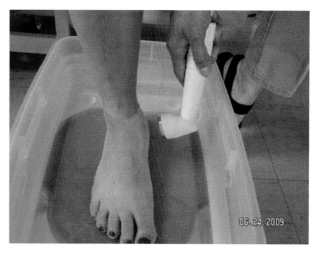

Figure 28•6 *Megahertz US being administered by the noncontact immersion method using water as the coupling medium to transmit the acoustic energy. While moving the US applicator in a circular or linear overlapping pattern, it is maintained at approximately 1 cm away from the patient's skin.*

> **PEARL 28•4** Water may be selected as the coupling agent when treating wounds with megahertz US on smaller and more irregular body parts, such as the hand, wrist, foot, or ankle. When megahertz US is used, the applicator and the part of the body to be treated are immersed in water held in a clean container, and the applicator (transducer) metal surface need not make contact (1 cm away) with the periwound skin. (Fig. 28.6) This noncontact method is also employed by the kilohertz MIST® device.

> **PEARL 28•5** When using kilohertz US devices that require necrotic tissue contact for débridement, other aqueous wound irrigation mediums may be used, such as standard physiological saline (0.9% NaCl) and nonstandard irrigant antiseptic solutions, for example, 0.125 Dakin's solution and hypochlorous acid.

Aqueous Gel as a Coupling Medium

Amorphous aqueous gel or a hydrogel sheet containing 96% water may be used to transmit megahertz US to the tissues. Both types are applied to the periwound skin. Ultrasound is transmitted into the tissue by placing the applicator in contact with the amorphous gel and moving it slowly (4–5 cm/sec) in overlapping circular or parallel strokes. Prior to placing the US applicator on a hydrogel sheet, it is best to apply a thin film of aqueous gel to the surface of the hydrogel sheet, which enhances ease of movement of the applicator over the surface of the sheet without compromising US transmission.

Biophysical Effects of Ultrasound That Pertain to Wound Healing

The biophysical effects produced by the interaction of US with tissues can be classified in two ways.

1. *Thermal.* Effects produced by the ability of US to increase tissue temperature
2. *Nonthermal.* Effects that are attributed to mechanisms other than elevation of tissue temperature

The mechanisms of some of the biological changes caused by megahertz US may be thermal or nonthermal or a combination of both, whereas biological changes caused by kilohertz US are primarily attributed to nonthermal effects.

Thermal Effects of Megahertz Ultrasound

If the wound healing practitioner believes that warming of wound and periwound tissues will enhance healing processes, the thermal effects of megahertz US may be used to raise tissue temperature at a depth of 5 cm. Low-frequency kilohertz US is used primarily for its nonthermal effects. Although some thermal energy is generated with kilohertz US devices that are used for wound débridement, this energy is virtually negated by the cooling action of the saline coupling medium. Recall that US energy absorption and the subsequent tissue temperature elevation are frequency dependent, so the higher the frequency, the greater the attenuation of energy in superficial tissues. At 3 MHz most of the energy is absorbed within a depth of 1 to 2 cm. (Fig. 28.3) At 1 MHz there is less attenuation in superficial tissues, allowing more energy to be available for absorption in deeper tissues. In general a 3-MHz frequency should be used in warming tissues up to 1 to 2 cm from the skin surface, and a 1-MHz frequency should be used in warming tissues deeper than 1 to 2 cm from the skin surface.

Effects of Tissue Warming on Perfusion and Oxygen Saturation

The primary response of human skin to locally applied external heat is an increase in capillary perfusion.[8] This occurs together with enhanced transport of oxygen and anabolic substrates via the arterioles and with removal of catabolic waste products via the venules.[9] Rabkin and Hunt first reported the beneficial effect of local heat application from a source other than US to open wounds in hospitalized patients.[10] They found that local heat application was associated with a threefold increase in capillary flow and a mean increase in subcutaneous oxygen tension of 39.5 mm Hg. Other investigators have shown that subcutaneous oxygen is correlated not only with an increase in perfusion, but with resistance to infection, secondary to oxidative killing by neutrophils of pathogens that colonize wounds.[11,12] Increasing tissue oxygen tension secondary to tissue warming has also been reported to enhance wound healing by effecting collagen deposition and scar tensile strength.[13,14] Using therapeutic heat from other sources, other studies have demonstrated that elevating tissue temperature increases local blood flow.[15-17] Numerous other studies have shown that 10 to 20 min of US at intensities greater than 2 W/cm², 1 MHz, continuous mode, increased skeletal muscle temperature

and muscle blood flow.[18-20] Elevating the local temperature to between 40° and 45°C is generally acceptable for well-vascularized tissues, but temperatures above this cause thermal necrosis and must be avoided. Figure 28.7 shows an ultrasound device that provides continuous and pulsed modes and frequencies of 1 and 3 MHz that may be used for warming wound and periwound tissues and for wound pain suppression. The nonthermal effects of kilohertz US, which are considered to have a greater impact on tissue and wound healing, are addressed later in this chapter.

▶ **PEARL 28•6** Because heat is normally dissipated by circulating blood, if the local circulation is compromised or has been obstructed, levels of US that would be suitable for well-perfused tissues could cause thermal damage.

Pain Suppression by Megahertz Ultrasound (Possible Treatment for Wound-Related Pain)

Following treatment with megahertz US, pain threshold is usually increased. Although the mechanism by which US reduces pain is unclear, tissue heating could activate large-diameter pain fibers or alter the response to stimulation of pain receptors (free nerve endings). Lehmann et al found that pain threshold was elevated after US application to the arm at 1.5 W/cm² for 2 min.[21] Because they found similar changes with infrared and diathermy, they attributed elevation of the threshold for activation of free nerve endings to

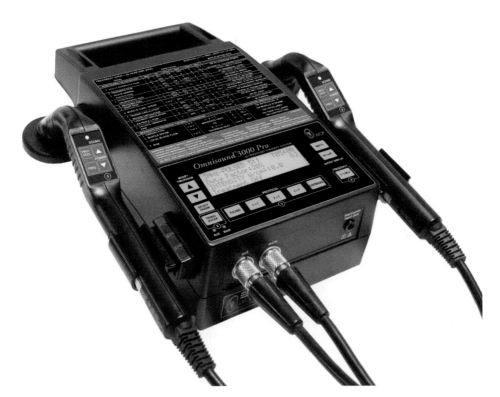

Figure **28•7** *An ultrasound device that offers continuous and pulsed modes at 1- and 3-MHz frequencies that may be used for enhancing wound blood flow and healing secondary to warming wound and periwound tissues and for suppressing wound related pain. (Used by permission of Accelerated Care Plus, Reno, NV.)*

thermal effects. Thus, in patients who experience wound-related pain, megahertz US applied to the periwound skin for enhancing blood flow may also provide temporary relief of pain.

Nonthermal Effects of Ultrasound

Both high-frequency (1 and 3 MHz) and low-frequency US (20–40 kHz) in the continuous and pulsed modes produce the nonthermal effects of cavitation and acoustic streaming that can cause physiological changes that affect tissue-healing processes.[22]

Cavitation

Unlike heating, which occurs more readily at higher US frequencies, cavitation is more prominent at lower frequencies. Cavitation strength is inversely proportional to frequency, thus its effect is significantly more pronounced at long-wavelength kilohertz frequencies than at short wavelength megahertz frequencies. Cavitation is the vibrational effect of US on microsized gas bubbles that form due to the accumulation of dissolved gas in the path of the US beam. Under appropriate conditions, changes in local pressure produced by US can cause the formation of these microsized gas bubbles or cavities in biological fluids such as blood, lymph, wound exudates, and tissue fluids and in US coupling media such as water and physiological saline. Periods of high and low pressure in the US field can cause the bubbles to increase and decrease in size, respectively. *Stable cavitation* occurs in a low-intensity field where the gaseous bubbles maintain their integrity and vibrate in response to the cyclic acoustic pressure changes but do not significantly increase and decrease in size while compressed during the high-pressure peaks and low-pressure valleys of the US wave. Stable cavitation acts to enhance the acoustic streaming phenomena. *Unstable* or *transient cavitation* occurs in a high-intensity field where the microbubbles significantly increase in size and violently implode during the low-pressure part of the US wave cycle. On implosion the bubbles release a large amount of energy, which can be detrimental to healthy cells and tissues.[22,23] (Fig. 28.8) There is no evidence to suggest that this phenomenon occurs with high-frequency (megahertz) US as long as movement of the sound applicator is not delayed during treatment.[23] Recent studies have shown that kilohertz US can remove nonviable tissue in a localized, controlled manner and that enhanced acoustic backscatter is highly correlated with the erosion process.[24,25]

> ▶ **PEARL 28•7** However, in unstable cavitation with kilohertz US, desirable tiny shock waves produced by bubble implosions cause preferential and rapid liquefaction and fragmentation (débridement) of adherent necrotic fibrin, loose slough, and microorganisms on wound surfaces.[7]

Acoustic Microstreaming

Acoustic microstreaming is described as a small-scale eddying of fluids near a vibrating structure such as cell membranes and the surface of stable cavitation gas bubbles.[6,26] In essence it

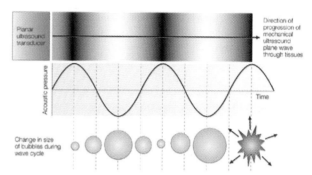

Figure 28•8 *Unstable cavitation occurs in a high-intensity field where micron-size gas bubbles significantly increase in size and violently implode during the low-pressure part of the US wave cycle. Tiny shock waves produced by bubble implosions cause preferential and rapid emulsification of necrotic fibrin and slough and fragmentation of bacteria and biofilms on wound surfaces. (www.nature.com/nrc/ journal/v5/n4/fig_tab/nrc1591_F2html. Kennedy, JE: High intensity focused ultrasound in the treatment of solid tumors. Courtesy of Nature Reviews/Cancer. 5, 321–337, April, 2005. Accessed on April 17, 2009.)*

refers to high-velocity fluid gradients along the boundaries between cell membranes, bubbles, and tissue fibers as a result of the US pressure wave and is augmented by stable cavitation. Figure 28.9 shows a schematic for possible US enhancement of membrane permeability leading to calcium influx into a fibroblast cell, which in turn leads to increased collagen synthesis and fibroblast proliferation. Another clinically important change in membrane function due to acoustic streaming is serotonin release from platelets.[27,28] In addition to serotonin, platelets contain chemotactic factors that promote the migration of cells necessary for repair to the injury site.[29] Also, low-frequency US (27 kHz) has been shown to increase endothelial

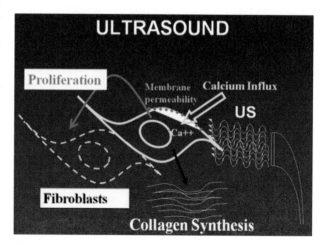

Figure 28•9 *Illustration showing conceptual US triggering of enhanced fibroblast cell membrane permeability, leading to Ca influx, collagen synthesis, and fibroblast proliferation. (Courtesy of Pamela Houghton, BSPT, PhD, University of Western Ontario, London, ON, Canada.)*

cell nitric oxide synthase activity and nitric oxide synthesis in vitro,[30] and investigators have further shown that 40-kHz US at intensities from 0.25 to 0.75 W/cm² improved perfusion and reversed acidosis in acutely ischemic skeletal muscle through a nitric oxide–dependent mechanism.[31] The end result of the combined effects of stable cavitation and acoustic streaming is that the cell membrane and organelles become "excited" (upregulated), thereby increasing the activity levels of the entire cell.[32]

> **PEARL 28•8** Acoustic microstreaming has been shown to alter cell membrane permeability and second messenger activity, which in turn may result in increased protein synthesis, degranulation of mast cells, and increased production of growth factors by macrophages.[28-33]

Frequency Resonance Hypothesis

The primary basis of the frequency resonance hypothesis is that the mechanical energy within the US wave is absorbed by proteins, theoretically altering the structural conformation of an individual protein or the function of a multimolecular complex. In addition, the sonic wave may induce resonant activity in the protein, modulating the molecule's or multimolecular complex's effect or function.[32] Signal transduction pathways may also be stimulated from mechanical energy generated by US. Such stimulation may produce a wide range of cellular effects that influence wound healing. Examples of US-induced cellular effects include increases in nitric oxide levels, fibrinolysis, macrophage responsiveness, leukocyte adhesion, collagen production, growth factor production, and angiogenesis.[30,33—44]

Low-Frequency (Kilohertz) Ultrasound Devices—Features and Specifications

This section will describe, according to increasing frequency, the four kilohertz US devices that are commercially available. The four frequencies are 22.5, 25, 35, and 40 kHz. All four of the devices transmit acoustic energy, which has the physical properties of cavitation and microstreaming described earlier. Recall that cavitation intensity is inversely proportional to frequency, and because lower frequencies have longer wavelengths, at higher power output levels more acoustic energy is transmitted to tissues per unit of time. Ultrasound dose or power is measured in watts per square centimeter (W/cm²) of the treatment probe tip or applicator. Thus, the combination of lower frequency and higher power create stronger doses of US. To further explain, when a blunt US treatment tip vibrating at ultrasonic frequencies is placed onto a liquid medium such as moist necrotic fibrin, the back-and-forth motion of the tip will cause sudden compression and then decompression of microbubbles in the surrounding saline coupling medium. Consequently, increasing and decreasing pressure waves are generated, and cavitation bubbles fill voids created by the pressure differentials. The bubbles grow with each excursion of the vibrating probe tip, and if the amplitude of vibration of the probe tip is high enough, the bubbles will implode and release forces strong enough to fragment and disintegrate necrotic tissue. Figure 28.10 shows the relationship between the US wave and the distal displacement of the vibrating US probe tip or transducer applicator. Ultrasonic wound therapy is emerging as an alternative method to surgical-sharp débridement for wound care. While US débridement produces results that are nearly as rapid and complete as the sharp technique, it is typically better tolerated as being less painful, both during the actual procedure as well as after débridement. Patients are typically débrided once or twice per week. Most wounds show decreased bioburden and improved appearance after three or four débridements. The procedure is suspended once these objectives have been attained. The typical débridement is 3 to 5 min for a wound less than the size of the patient's palm.

> **PEARL 28•9** Using cavitation as a mechanism for tissue fragmentation and emulsification offers a significant benefit in that cavitation is tissue selective as long as the clinician directs the moving contact treatment probe at nonviable tissue.

SonicOne®

SonicOne® (Misonix, Farmingdale, NY), the contact, low-thermal US device shown in Figure 28.11, operates at a frequency of 22.5 kHz in the continuous or pulsed mode. Pulsed mode settings range from 50% down to 90%. Thus, at a setting of 90%, if the pulse repetition rate is 1 sec, the US would be on for 0.9 sec and off for 0.1 sec. The pulsed mode allows the vibrating tissue at the probe tip to relax for a few microseconds during the pulse off time. During pulse on times, tissue vibrations are accelerated, and hydrodynamic forces at the probe tip are maximized to fragment and emulsify nonviable fibrin and slough and destroy bacteria and biofilms on the wound surface. As mentioned earlier, because the pulsed mode reduces the total acoustic energy per unit of time going to the tissue, it may be used to improve patient comfort. To ensure that patients are comfortable during the débridement procedure, they can be premedicated with topical 4% lidocaine (Xylocaine) applied to the wound and periwound area 10 to 20 min prior to the procedure. The US output level is not given as a readout in watts of power; rather, the readout is shown as numbers between 0 and 5, which represent a relative indication of the

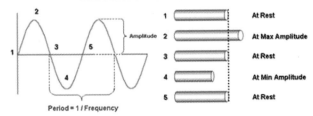

Wave Motion to Probe Movement

1	At Rest
2	At Max Amplitude
3	At Rest
4	At Min Amplitude
5	At Rest

Period = 1 / Frequency

Figure 28•10 *The relationship between the US wave and the distal displacement of the vibrating US probe tip or applicator. (www.nature.com/nrc/journal/v5/n4/fig_tab/ nrc1591_F2.html. Accessed on April 17, 2009.)*

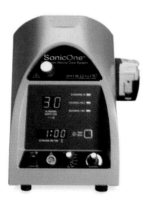

Figure 28•11 *The SonicOne®. This US device operates at 22.5 kHz and offers continuous and pulsed modes. Through light tissue contact, strong cavitation expeditiously and selectively fragments microorganisms and biofilms and emulsifies nonviable adherent fibrin and loose slough, creating a clean wound bed that provides a favorable environment for wound healing to advance. (Courtesy of Misonix Inc. Farmingdale, NY.)*

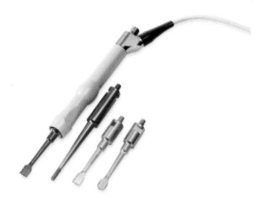

Figure 28•12 *The SonicOne® handpiece and detachable treatment probes with different configurations to accommodate wound topographical surfaces. Handpiece and probes can be sterilized in an autoclave. (Courtesy of Misonix Inc., Farmingdale, NY.)*

percentage of output amplitude (amplitude of vibration) or the clinician-controlled back-and-forth excursion of the treatment probe tip across the necrotic tissue. This device uses 0.9% saline as the coupling and irrigation medium, which is delivered to the metal treatment probe tip by special disposable tubing and a volumetric pump shown on the side of the device in Figure 28.11. The US atomizes the saline, creating a vapor of microbubbles that transmit the US to the wound surface via treatment probe contact. The treatment handpiece

and several treatment probes having different configurations to accommodate wound topographical surfaces are shown in Figure 28.12. See Table 28.1 for a summary and comparison of specifications and features of the four kilohertz US devices used for wound healing applications.

▶ **PEARL 28•10** The SonicOne will keep the frequency, amplitude, and treatment probe tip vibration displacement relatively constant while delivering more or less energy, depending upon tissue type and force applied by the clinician against the tissue with the probe.

Table 28•1	Summary and Comparison of Specifications and Features of the Four Kilohertz Ultrasound Devices Used for Wound Healing Applications			
	Low-Frequency Ultrasound			
Features	**Misonix Inc. SonicOne™ 22.5 kHz**	**Soring Inc. Sonoca 180™ 25 kHz**	**Arobella Medical Qoustic Wound Therapy System™ 35 kHz**	**Celleration, Inc. MIST Therapy System™ 40 kHz**
Intensity (Watts)	Auto gain control (45–50 W)	Variable 40%–100% (up to 60 W)	Variable 10%–100% (<50 W)	Preset based on wound size (0.1–0.5 w/cm²)
Distal tip displacement	Up to 180 μm	Up to 150 μm	50–70 μm	60–70 μm
Mode	Continuous or pulsed	Continuous	Continuous or pulsed	Continuous
Coupling	Sterile saline vapor	Sterile saline vapor	Sterile saline vapor	Sterile saline vapor
Treatment time	Usually 2–5 min	Usually 2–5 min	Usually 2–5 min	Wound size dependent 3–20 cm
Wound contact with applicator	Yes; autoclavable metal probes	Yes; autoclavable metal probes	Yes; autoclavable curette shaped	No; 1.5–2.5 cm from wound; disposable applicator

Sonoca 180®

The Sonoca 180® (Soring Inc., North Richland Hills, TX) contact/noncontact, low-thermal US device, shown in Figure 28.13, operates at a frequency of 25 kHz in the continuous mode. It can deliver an acoustic power of up to 60 W, creating a vibration displacement of approximately 150 μm at a 15-mm² treatment probe tip. Like the previous device, the US output is not given as a readout in watts of power; rather, the readout shows a percentage of maximum output ranging between 40% and 100%. Generally, the output range for most patients is between 60% and 80%, which will provide output amplitude (amplitude of vibration) that will create appropriate back-and-forth vibration excursion of the treatment probe tip to débride by fragmentation and emulsification of necrotic fibrin and slough and destroy bacteria and biofilms. To ensure that patients are comfortable during the débridement procedure, they can be premedicated with topical 4% lidocaine (Xylocaine) applied to the wound and periwound area 10 to 20 min prior to the procedure. This device also uses 0.9% saline as the coupling and irrigation medium, which is delivered to the treatment probe tip by gravity feed through IV tubing down the canula of the handpiece to the metal treatment probe tip, where it emerges as an atomized vapor of microbubbles that are delivered to the nonviable tissue by probe contact. The treatment handpiece and several treatment probes having different configurations to accommodate wound topographical surfaces are shown in Figure 28.14A and B, respectively. See Table 28.1 for a summary and comparison of specifications and features of the four kilohertz US devices used for wound healing applications.

> **PEARL 28•11** In addition to the direct contact mode, this device may be used for noncontact US, in which the probe tip is held 5 to 10 mm away from the wound surface for extra irrigation and for transmitting the nonthermal microstreaming effect to tissues and cells.

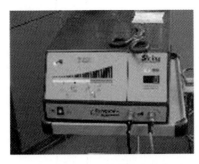

Figure 28•13 *The Sonoca 180®. This US device operates at 25 kHz and offers the continuous mode. Through tissue contact, strong cavitation expeditiously and selectively fragments microorganisms and biofilms and emulsifies nonviable adherent fibrin and loose slough, creating a clean wound bed that provides a favorable environment for wound healing to advance. (Courtesy of Soring Inc., North Richland Hills, TX.)*

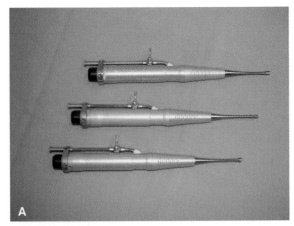

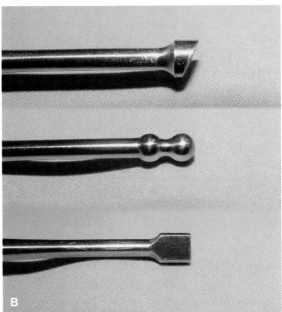

Figure 28•14 *(A and B) The Sonoca 180® handpiece (A) and treatment probes (B) with different configurations to accommodate wound topographical surfaces. Handpiece and probes can be sterilized in an autoclave. (Courtesy of Soring Inc., North Richland Hills, TX.)*

Qoustic Wound Therapy System™

The Qoustic Wound Therapy System™ (Arobella Medical LLC, Minnetonka, MN), a contact/noncontact low-thermal US device shown in Figure 28.15A, operates at a frequency of 35 kHz in the continuous and pulsed modes. Like the two previous devices, the US output is not given as a readout in watts of power; rather, the readout shows a percentage of maximum output ranging between 10% and 100%, with adjustable increments of 5%. The Qoustic Wound Therapy System tip will deliver a derived power (per international standard IEC 61847) of 732.42 mW/cm² at a generator setting of 100%. Because the generator scaling is 1 to 1 (ie, 100% generator output equates to 100% tip power output, and 10% tip output equates to 10% handpiece power output), the theoretical tip power output will scale to 659.18 mW/cm² at 90% and

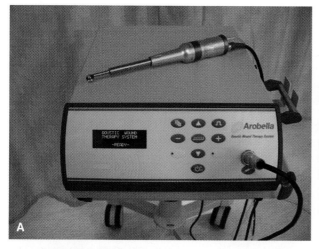

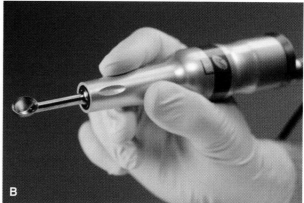

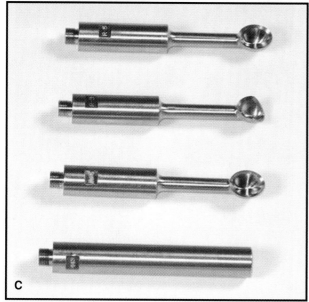

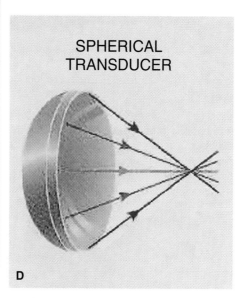

SPHERICAL
TRANSDUCER

Figure 28•15 *(A) The Qoustic Wound Therapy System™. This US device operates at 35 kHz and offers continuous and pulsed modes. Through contact with the tissue, strong cavitation expeditiously and selectively fragments microorganisms and biofilms and emulsifies nonviable adherent fibrin and lose slough, creating a clean wound bed that provides a favorable environment for wound healing to advance. In addition, through noncontact with healthy tissue, wound healing is stimulated by the combined effects of less-intense cavitation and microstreaming. (Courtesy of Arobella Medical LLC, Minnetonka, MN.) (B) The Qoustic Wound Therapy System™ handpiece and (C) different configurations of the curette-shaped treatment probe to accommodate wound topographical surfaces. (Courtesy of Arobella Medical LLC, Minnetonka, MN.) (D) Spherical (curette-shaped) transducer. Ultrasound beams may be focused by curving the piezoelectric plate. Focusing allows fast and focused delivery of acoustic energy for enhanced antibacterial and débridement effects. (Used by permission of Science and Medicine Inc., Hynynen, K: Focused ultrasound surgery guided by MRI. Science & Medicine 1996; 3. Available at: http://www.advanced-surgical.com/Documents/Science_and_Medicine/index.htm. Accessed May 14, 2009.)*

73.24 mW/cm² at 10%. When the device is set on "pulse," the pulse mode applies a duty cycle to the handpiece. The pulse mode is an 80% duty cycle of the percentage of the power setting; that is, approximately 80% of that percentage of power setting is delivered. The duty cycle is currently set to 80% over a 1-sec period, meaning the handpiece will be on (sonating) for 800 msec and off (no sonation) for 200 msec. The effect of the pulse mode, though nonlinear, creates approximately an 80% reduction in cavitation and microstreaming,

which in turn reduces some of the thermal effects from a given power setting percentage and also reduces discomfort the patient may be experiencing during treatment.

Generally, for débridement purposes, the output range for most patients is between 80% and 100%, which will provide an effective back-and-forth vibration displacement of the treatment probe tip. Also for this device, to ensure that patients are comfortable during the débridement procedure, they can be premedicated with topical 4% lidocaine (Xylocaine) applied to the wound and periwound area 10 to 20 minutes prior to the procedure. This device also uses 0.9% saline as the coupling and irrigation medium, which is delivered to the treatment probe tip by gravity feed through IV tubing down the canula of the handpiece to the metal treatment probe tip, where it emerges as an atomized vapor of microbubbles that impact the nonviable tissue by probe contact. The metallic probe configuration is uniquely shaped like a curette with a blunt edge. (Fig. 28.15B) For general débridement purposes, the curettelike applicator can be placed with its concave "cup" inverted over the nonviable tissue so the tiny shock waves produced by microcavitations, fragment the nonviable tissue and microorganisms. Using the inverted method of the applicator, reduces aerosolization and contamination.[45] In addition, this method also focuses and concentrates the US waves, thereby enhancing the débridement effectiveness. Other variations of the curettelike applicator are shown in Figure 28.15C.

> ▸ **PEARL 28•12** This unique curette design enhances wound débridement via the delivery of highly focused US energy directly to the wound surface with the additional benefit of reducing aerosolization and the volume of coupling solution.[46]

In addition to the direct contact mode, this device may be used without contact, whereby the probe tip is held 5 to 10 mm away from the wound surface for extra irrigation and for transmitting the nonthermal microstreaming effect to tissues and cells. The curette probe may also be navigated across the nonviable tissue by placing it on its side to take advantage of combining cavitation with the curette edge.

> ▸ **PEARL 28•13** However, the combined effects of a weaker cavitation effect and microstreaming may account for the positive wound healing outcomes reported from several clinical studies to be discussed later. An advantage of the noncontact method of transmitting US to the wound is that there is no pain associated with the procedure.

MIST Therapy® System

The MIST Therapy® System (Celleration Inc., Eden Prairie, MN), the noncontact, nonthermal US device shown in Figure 28.16A, operates at a frequency of 40 kHz in the continuous mode. The clinician's handpiece is configured with a spiked recess that punctures the bottom of an inserted container of saline, which allows the saline to be delivered to the US transducer where it is atomized into a fine mist. (Fig. 28.16B) The vapor, or mist, complements the transmission of the 40-kHz US to wound tissues, just as water has been used for decades by physical therapists as a noncontact coupling medium for transmitting 1- and 3-MHz US to tissues. At a therapeutic intensity of 0.2 to 0.8 W/cm² and a distance of 5 to 15 mm from the plastic applicator leading edge, a nominal transducer displacement of 65 µm is created. Because the metal transducer makes no contact with the wound tissue, there is no tissue heating, and more of the acoustic pressure is absorbed by the tissues. At power settings

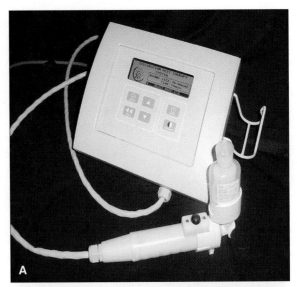

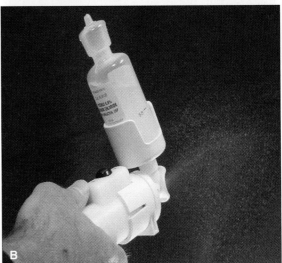

Figure **28•16** *(A and B) MIST Therapy® System. This US device operates at 40 kHz and offers the continuous mode. Without contacting the tissue, moderate cavitation expeditiously destroys microorganisms and biofilms and with successive treatments emulsifies nonviable adherent fibrin and loose slough, creating a clean wound bed that provides a favorable environment for wound healing to advance. In addition, through noncontact with healthy tissue, wound healing is stimulated by the combined effects of less-intense cavitation and microstreaming. (Courtesy of Celleration Inc. Eden Prairie, MN.)*

between 0.2 and 0.8 W/cm² and at an applicator distance of 0.5 to 1.5 cm from the wound surface, the acoustic pressure will vary between 1300 and 2200 pascals. (Personal communication with Michael Peterson of Celleration, Inc.) (Fig. 28.17A and B) The effects these acoustic pressures may have on cells will be discussed later. Wound treatment with the MIST therapy device is performed by the clinician, keeping the US applicator 0.5 to 1.5 cm from the wound and performing slow, even strokes of the treatment head vertically across the wound using multiple

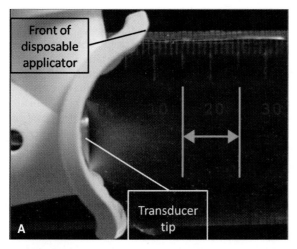

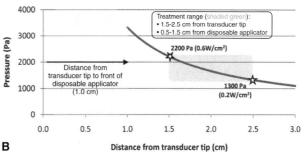

Figure 28•17 *(A) Noncontact treatment range from reference points relating to the transducer tip (energy source) and the disposable applicator (point closest to patient and used as clinical treatment reference). (B) Acoustic pressure levels associated with the MIST Therapy® System. The prescribed noncontact treatment range from the leading edge of the disposable applicator is 0.5 to 1.5 cm. (Courtesy of Celleration Inc., Eden Prairie, MN.)*

Table 28•2 The Four Kilohertz US Devices Available in the United States, Their FDA-Cleared Indications, and Clinical Features					
Devices FDA 510k	Selective Débridement	Fibrinolysis	Antibacterial	Pain	Aerosolization
SonicOne™ Misonix, Inc. Wound débridement, surgical fragmentation, and aspiration of soft and hard tissues	Yes	Yes	Yes	Yes	Yes
Sonoca 180™ Soring, Inc. Selective dissection and fragmentation of tissue at the operation site	Yes	Yes	Yes	Yes	Yes
Qoustic Wound Therapy System™ Arobella Medical, LLC Selective dissection and fragmentation of tissues, wound débridement, and cleansing of the site for removal of debris, exudates, fragments, and other matter through the use of ultrasonic energy and/or fluid irrigation	Yes	Yes	Yes	No	Yes
MIST Therapy™ Celleration, Inc. Promotes wound healing through cleansing and maintenance débridement by removal of slough fibrin, tissue exudates, and bacteria	No	Yes	Yes	No	Yes

passes, followed by movement of the treatment head horizontally across the wound using multiple passes. Although this device has the acoustic properties of microstreaming and cavitation, the lower intensity and shorter wavelength, compared with the previous three devices, renders a less-prominent cavitation effect, making débridement less aggressive. Table 28.2 lists the four kilohertz US devices that presently are commercially available in the United States and their FDA-cleared indications, which govern what the manufacturers can say about their devices in their marketing materials.

Experimental Effects of Kilohertz Ultrasound on Wound Healing
Fibrinolytic Effects

Several investigators have used US frequencies of 1 and 3 MHz and reported enhanced enzymatic fibrinolysis in vitro and in animal models.[46-53] Unfortunately, a drawback of using high-frequency US on humans for fibrinolytic denaturation of necrotic tissue is that, as the intensity is increased, tissue heating may become excessive and cause thermal necrosis of viable cells. Moreover, at megahertz frequencies tissue absorption and penetration of US are less than that which occurs at kilohertz frequencies.[54] On the other hand, low-frequency US (20–60 KHz) has been reported to have several positive treatment effects in animals and humans. McDonald and Nichter found that 50- to 60-kHz US abolished particulate debris and bacteria from the surface of induced wounds in rats.[55] Suchkova et al have shown that low-frequency (40 kHz), low-intensity (0.25 W/cm^2) US significantly increased enzymatic fibrinolysis in vitro compared with no US ($P < 0.0001$) and that acceleration of fibrinolysis increased with power output ($P < 0.001$).[56] Other investigators have found that both continuous and pulsed mode US at low US frequencies of 27, 40, and 100 kHz significantly accelerated fibrinolysis of radio-labeled fibrin, with the greatest effect observed at 27 kHz, continuous mode.[57] Bessette et al treated full-thickness experimentally infected burns in rats with US and showed by electron microscopy that fibroblasts increased lysosomal activity and enhanced collagen synthesis without detrimental effects.[58]

Antimicrobial Effects

Numerous cell culture and animal studies have reported that kilohertz US not only has direct antimicrobial effects, but it also works in synergy with antibiotics and antiseptic agents to enhance killing of planktonic bacteria and bacteria in biofilms.

Schoenbach and Song found that in experimentally infected rat burns, daily US treatments significantly reduced bacterial counts and improved survival over controls.[59] Scherba et al evaluated the germicidal efficacy of 26-kHz US on aqueous suspensions of *Eschericia coli, Staphylococcus aureus, Bacillus subtilis,* and *Pseudomonas aeruginosa* bacteria and on fungus (*Trichophyton mentagrophytes*) and viruses (feline herpes virus type 1 and feline calicivirus).[60] For all bacteria except *E. coli* they found that the percentage killed increased with exposure time and increased intensity. A significant reduction in fungal growth occurred compared with controls, with a reduction in growth increasing with intensity. Growth of feline herpes virus declined significantly with intensity, but there was no effect on feline calicivirus. The authors attributed the antimicrobial effect to unstable cavitation. In 44 Sprague-Dawley rats with uniform paravertebral incisions, Nichter et al compared the efficacy of various wound débridement methods used to avert infection following primary closure of contaminated rat wounds.[61] Each wound was inoculated with a standard number of *S. aureus* (2×10^7 to 7×10^7 bacteria per 0.1 mL) and treated before closure by one of four débridement methods: (1) surgical scrubbing, (2) high-pressure (8 psi) irrigation, (3) 50-kHz ultrasound, or (4) soaking. Control wounds were closed without débridement. After 7 days, each animal was evaluated for the presence of gross infection. US-treated wounds had a 25% incidence of gross infection, compared with irrigation (75%), scrubbing (82%), and soaking (89%). All of the control wounds developed flagrant infection. Other reports have described US-enhanced germicidal effects of antibiotic and antiseptic agents on bacteria and biofilms.[62-66] Additionally, investigators found lower-frequency US significantly more effective than higher frequency in decreasing bacterial viability

within a biofilm.[67] Schulze designed an in vitro model to evaluate the antibacterial effectiveness of 25-kHz US on four planktonic bacterial species commonly found in chronic wounds. (Personal communication) They used an immersion prototype with bacteria cultured in a test tube to simulate a cavity wound containing serous exudates and physiological saline. This model allowed the US treatment probe to be immersed in the culture fluid that served as the US coupling medium. Bacteria were sonated at different US power outputs and exposure times. Schulze found that bacterial killing was most effective with 100% US power output delivered for 120 sec. (Fig. 28.18A and B) Pearson et al have reported that direct contact of 27-kHz US to *Acineobacter baumannii* cells had a significant antibacterial effect on these highly antibiotic-resistant isolates that were recovered from soldiers returning from Iraq.[68] Using a previously described protocol for an in vitro model, the bacterial suspension was set to a 0.5 McFarland standard and then serially diluted to approximately 100,000 CFU/mL. Initial colony counts were taken prior to sonation. Test solutions were treated with the Sonoca 180 at 60% output in 10-sec bursts, followed by 50-sec cool down periods, until a total of 129 sec of sonation was achieved. Aliquots were taken and plated after each 20 sec of sonation. Bacterial death was measured both by colony counts after 24 hours of growth and acridine orange staining using a standard protocol. After US treatment, a significant log decrease in bacterial load was noted, with less than 5% viable bacteria identified after the 120-sec treatment. In contrast to the previous study, Wagner et al used 40-kHz US delivered noncontact via a saline vapor for 2.5 min to destroy *S. aureus* growing in vitro.[69] (Fig. 28.19A–D) Niezgoda has also observed clinically that direct-contact kilohertz US is capable of reducing methicillin-resistant *Staphylococcus aureus* (MRSA), vancomycin-resistant enterococci (VRE), and other pathogens.[70] The findings from these in vitro studies suggest that US is capable of killing bacteria, at least in a laboratory setting. However, clinically effective antimicrobial treatments should decrease more than surface bacteria; they should also penetrate to greater depths below the wound surface to kill pathogens that contribute to infection. More clinical research is warranted to determine the germicidal effects of kilohertz US.

> **PEARL 28•14** Several other studies have reported that kilohertz frequency US enhances the action of antibiotics and antiseptic drugs.[63-65] Researchers also found that US works in synergy with gentamicin and vancomycin to sterilize biofilms of *Escherichia coli and Staphylococcus epidermidis*, respectively, and to kill a greater number of bacteria in biofilms of *Pseudomonas aeruginosa*.[66-68]

Recently, Serena et al conducted a four-part study to assess the effect of 40-KHz noncontact US (NCUS) on bacterial counts in experimental and chronic wounds.[71] In the first part of the study, they determined the tissue depth at which NCUS could have a physiological effect, based on the assumption that there are differences in wound bioburden penetration for intact skin versus wounded skin. They used a pig model to measure the transfer of a lipophilic dye into intact and

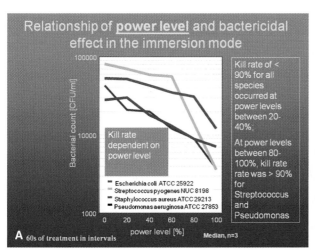

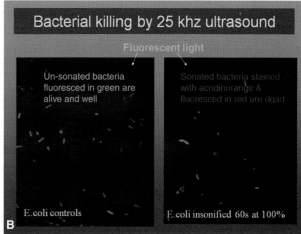

Figure 28•18 *(A) In vitro antibacterial effect. Schulze et al reported that 25-kHz US (Sonoca 180®) applied in vitro (aqueous immersion method) at power levels between 20% and 40% for 2 min produced a kill rate of less than 90% for four bacterial species.[69] At power levels between 80% and 100%, the kill rate was greater than 90% for S. pyogenes and P. aeruginosa. (B) From Schulze's work, the left picture shows unsonated, intact E. coli; the right picture shows E. coli cell fragments after being sonated at 100% power for 60 sec. (From Schulze CH, Oesser S, Seifert J. Investigations into the antibacterial effect of low frequency ultrasound applied by using the spherical Soring Sonoca probe tip Sonotrode. Endotoxin Laboratory for Surgical Research, Christian-Albrechts-Universitat, Michaelisstrase 5, D-24105, Kiel, Germany. Personal communication, 2004.)*

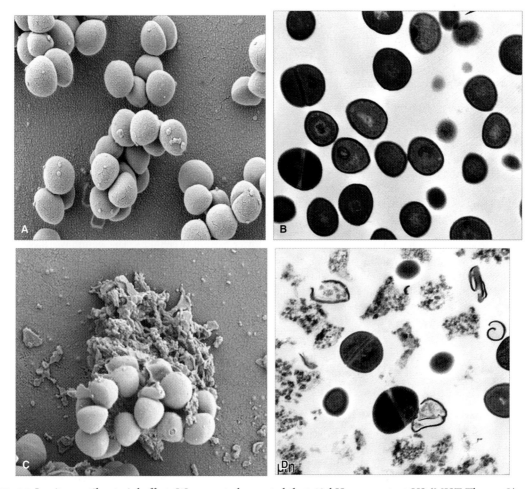

Figure 28•19 *In vitro antibacterial effect. Wagner et al reported that 40-kHz noncontact US (MIST Therapy®) applied in vitro for 2.5 min destroyed S. aureus.[71] (A and B) Intact S. aureus cells following exposure to saline for 2.5 min as viewed by scanning electron microscopy (SEM). (C and D) Damaged cells after exposure to 2.5 min of 40-kHz, noncontact ultrasound as viewed by transmission electron microscopy (TEM).*

wounded skin treated with NCUS or placebo US. Using in vitro assessment, they found that compared to placebo, NCUS penetrated farther into both wounded (3.0 mm to 3.5 mm vs 0.35 mm to 0.50 mm) and intact (2.0 mm to 2.5 mm vs 0.05 mm to 0.07 mm, respectively) pig skin. In the second part of the study, they used an in vitro model to stain and count live versus dead bacteria and found that 0% of placebo-treated, 33% of *P. aeruginosa,* 40% of *E. coli,* and 27% of *Enterococcus faecalis* bacteria were dead after one 5-min exposure. In the third part of the study, the investigators inoculated bacteria into induced pig wounds on the right and left sides of four animals. All four animals received four 4-min NCUS treatments to wounds on their left sides. On the right side, wounds of pigs 1 and 2 were treated with a silver antimicrobial dressing, pig 3 received placebo NCUS, and pig 4 wounds were treated with a moist gauze dressing. Bacteria were collected from wounds on days 1, 3, 5, and 7. After four treatments with NCUS over a 7-day period, overall bacterial quantity was reduced with US from 7.2 to 6.7 CFU/g of tissue and from 7.2 to 5.7 CFU/g with the silver dressing. For wounds treated with the NCUS placebo and moist gauze dressing, bacterial growth increased from 7.2 to 8.6 CFU/g of tissue. In the fourth part of the study, 11 patients with stage III pressure ulcers containing bacterial counts greater than 10^5 CFU/g of tissue received NCUS three times per week to their wounds for 2 weeks. Treatment durations were based on wound surface area. In this small clinical study, the quantities of seven bacteria were reduced from a mean baseline bacterial count of 4×10^7 to a mean count of 2×10^7 after 2 weeks of NCUS treatment. The authors concluded that taken together, these four studies indicate that NCUS can be used to reduce bacterial quantity.

Cell Viability and Morphology

In an in vitro study, Conner-Kerr et al assessed the effects of 35-kHz US delivered via the Qoustic Wound Therapy System (QWTS) on neuroblastoma (SHSY-5Y) viability and morphology.[72] They found that while this US frequency did not decrease cell viability, there was a trend toward increased viability compared to control cells at 24 hours after treatment. In addition, US-treated cells exhibited enhanced metabolic response, increased cell attachment to the medium, increased cell body size and axon elongation, and increased layering of cells in a three-dimensional structure. They concluded that their results suggest a putative mechanism for 35-kHz US modulation of persistent wound pain through a direct effect on neuronal function and possible facilitation of neuronal proliferation that may have implications for neuronal regeneration.

Clinical Research Findings for Contact Kilohertz Ultrasound
Effect on Wound Débridement

Ultrasonic wound débridement is best achieved with the 22.5-kHz, 25-kHz, or 35-kHz frequencies applied through contact with the wound surface. This débridement method is considered to reside between surgical-sharp and mechanical on the spectrum of débridement techniques. Ultrasonic débridement results in removal of necrotic tissue and slough via fibrinolysis, whereby necrotic proteins are denatured and are mechanically flushed from the wound base by the impact of the coupling solution without damaging viable underlying tissue. As previously mentioned, the tissue microcavitations produced by low-frequency US have also been shown to achieve a highly effective bactericidal effect.

▸ **PEARL 28•15** The results of this form of débridement are as immediate as sharp or surgical débridement, more aggressive and complete than mechanical débridement, and better tolerated due to pain than surgical-sharp débridement.

Low-frequency or kilohertz US that is transmitted through light contact with the wound is primarily used to ablate nonviable fibrinous tissue from the wound surface and to destroy microorganisms and biofilms as previously mentioned.[61-68] Débridement of necrotic or devitalized tissue and destruction of pathogens from the wound surface is a vital component of wound bed preparation that enhances clinical management efforts. Necrotic tissue on the wound can alter the normal healing cascade, thereby contributing to chronicity. Steed et al demonstrated that aggressive, ongoing surgical débridement converts a chronic nonhealing ulcer into an acute healing wound.[73] Breuing et al used 25-kHz US to débride wounds of varying etiologies on 17 patients over a period of 8 months.[74] They reported that nine of the wounds (53%) closed primarily or with the aid of a skin graft, six wounds (35%) decreased in size by 50% or more, and the remaining wounds of two patients (12%), one with sickle cell anemia and one with a venous leg ulcer, reduced in surface area by 20% and 30%, respectively. Ultrasound at a frequency of 25 kHz is reported by Stanisic et al to have produced rapid and thorough débridement of adherent fibrin from two patients with venous leg ulcers and one patient with a sacral pressure ulcer.[75] Figure 28.20A and B show wound images taken before (Fig. 28.20A) and after US débridement (Fig. 28.20B) of a venous ulcer located on the right anterior edematous leg of a 46-year-old male with a history of morbid obesity, sleep apnea, lymphedema, and lower-extremity cellulitis. The wound was 95% covered with adherent fibrin after 1 week of attempted débridement with collagenous enzyme. Although the patient did not complain of wound-related pain (Visual Analogue Scale [VAS] = 0), as a precautionary measure prior to performing US débridement 4% Xylocaine (lidocaine) was applied to the wound bed and periwound border for 10 to 20 min to make him comfortable during the procedure. In addition, the US intensity was adjusted as necessary so the patient experienced no pain. In one 6-min session, the wound was débrided with Sonoca 180 without any harmful macroscopic effects, which resulted in the clean wound shown in Figure 28.20B. Had the selective sharp method been used to débride the wound, the amount of time required for complete removal of the fibrinous tissue wound have been increased significantly. Clinically, the same débridement outcome has been achieved with 25-kHz US, which rapidly and selectively emulsifies adherent fibrin without harmful macroscopic changes in granulation tissue.[76]

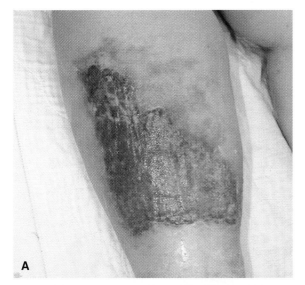

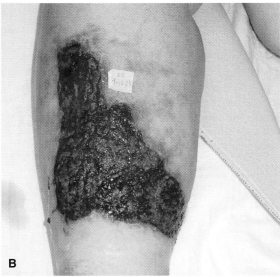

Figure 28•20 *(A and B) Wound images taken before (A) and after 25-kHz US débridement (B) of a venous leg ulcer following 1 week of attempted débridement with collagenous enzyme. Prior to the procedure, the patient's wound was pre-medicated for 10 to 20 min with topical 4% Xylocaine (lido-caine) applied to the wound bed and periwound. Complete débridment required 6 min without any harmful macroscopic effects observed. (From Stanisic MM, Provo BJ, Larson DL, et al: Wound débridement with 25 kHz ultrasound. Adv Skin Wound Care 2005; 18:484–490. Used by permission of Lippincott Williams and Wilkins Inc., Hagarstown, MD.)*

In a pilot study Tan et al evaluated the use of 25-kHz US (Sonoca 180) on débridement of venous leg ulcers as an adjunct to compression bandage therapy.[77] They recruited 19 patients with leg ulcerations of at least 6 months duration. Over repeated intervals of 2 to 3 weeks, each leg received an average of 5.7 US débridement treatments, each of which ranged from 5 to 20 min depending on ulcer size. Compression bandages were reapplied after each US débridement

treatment. They reported that symptomatic relief of pain and odor was achieved in six patients, whereas seven patients achieved complete wound closure, while no response was observed in the remaining eight patients. They concluded that kilohertz US débridement may heal some chronic ulcers when standard compression therapy has failed. More controlled clinical studies to evaluate the effect of kilohertz contact ultra-sound on wound-related pain are necessary.

Thorough coverage of the negative effects necrotic tissue has on wounds, as well as all of the débridement methods (except ultrasonic débridement), are presented in Chapter 11.

Effect on Blood Flow

In a recent clinical case series, Suzuki et al evaluated the effect of 35-kHz US (Qoustic Wound Therapy System) on perfusion in the periwound skin of 17 patients with lower-extremity wounds.[78] They nonrandomly assigned the patients to an ultrasound débridement group ($N = 9$) and a sharp débride-ment control group ($N = 7$). The US group received one 5-min, 35-kHz wound débridement followed by room-temperature saline irrigation, whereas the control group received one sharp wound débridement with scalpel fol-lowed by room-temperature saline irrigation. Using a skin perfusion pressure (SPP) monitor, they measured SPP at the same periwound skin areas before and after the US and sharp débridement procedures. They found that the nine patients in the US group had a significant increase in SPP values (mean = 9.11 mm Hg, SD = 4.34) while the eight pa-tients in the control group showed a negligible increase in SPP values (mean = 1.2 mm Hg, SD = 0.84). They concluded that 35-kHz US produces a vasodilatation effect and in-creased perfusion in the periwound skin of lower-extremity wounds as verified by a statistically significant increase in SPP values after US wound treatment ($P < 0.001$). More controlled clinical studies to evaluate the effect of kilohertz contact ultrasound on wound blood flow are essential.

Effect on Wound-Related Pain

Niezgoda conducted a study to measure the levels of pain experienced by patients during débridement with three kilohertz US devices.[79] A series of 25 patients were asked to score their pain following wound débridement with either the 22.5-kHz SonicOne or the 25-kHz Sonoca 180 devices. At a subsequent visit, the patients underwent wound débridement with the 35-kHz Qoustic Wound Therapy Sys-tem, and pain scores were again recorded. Pain was rated using an analog pain scale of 0 to 10, with 0 as no pain and 10 as severe pain. All patients had débridement of their wound using the same predébridement preparation and procedure. Ninety-six percent (24/25) of patients reported less pain during débridement with use of the Qoustic Curette™. The average pain score for débridement with the other US débridement devices was 7.1 compared to 3.2 with the Qoustic Qurette. In addition to the report of less pain during the débridement procedure in the wound clinic, several patients reported decreased need for oral narcotic pain medications later that day, hours after the débridement with the Qoustic Qurette. The investigator attributed the outcome of less pain to lower tissue shear forces occurring with the more highly focused 35-kHz device. Controlled clinical studies to evaluate the effect of kilohertz contact ultrasound on wound-related pain are required.

Practical Considerations for Wound Débridement With Kilohertz Ultrasound Contact Devices

Power and Pulse Settings

The design of the system, handpiece, and probes allows for variation in the amount of ultrasonic energy applied to the wound bed and adjacent tissues. As described earlier, a variety of control parameters and probes can be used, depending on the amount of devitalized tissue, fibrin, or necrotic tissue requiring removal and the sensation or pain level experienced by the patient. Current commercial devices deliver ultrasound at frequencies that are preset by the manufacturer (eg, 22.5, 25, and 35 kHz). However, all allow for the amplitude (power output) to be adjusted for the level of débridement aggressiveness required. Some systems can also operate in "pulse mode," in which the delivery of ultrasound is intermittent. This has been found to further decrease the patient's pain.

Aerosolization

Some of the contact kilohertz débridement devices have splash guard attachments; however, there still may be some splash, splatter, or aerosolization of the coupling solution during the procedure. Therefore, most manufacturers recommend the use of personal protective equipment (gown, mask, gloves). To comply with infection control policy some clinics have adopted the practice of removing nonessential equipment from exam rooms prior to US wound procedures as well as draping for protection of fixed equipment, including the US unit. Some manufacturers of kilohertz US devices have reduced the risk of contamination by developing unique probe designs that focus, direct, and control the ultrasonic energy.[45]

Sterilization Procedure

Cleaning of the contact US device can be divided into disinfection of the unit and sterilization of the probe tips. Following a débridement, the device should be cleaned by wiping all surfaces using a facility-approved disinfection solution. Cleaning should include the US unit, all power and control cables, foot pedal, and cart. All probe tips should be sterilized per facility policy. The handpieces and probe tips are treated per individual manufacturer's recommendation. Some clinics use central sterilization, while others have small autoclave units available to them within the clinic.

Clinical Setting

The treatment setting for use of kilohertz US devices is dependent upon availability of the equipment and trained personnel. These devices are marketed with a rolling cart for portability, which allows use in the clinic, at the bedside, or in the operating room or surgical suite. The hospital outpatient wound clinic is often the primary treatment location. The high cost of individual ultrasound units and attachments generally precludes having units in multiple hospital departments for delivery of therapy in other outpatient or subacute environments.

Utilization Protocol

The Table 28.3 describes general procedural steps for performing contact US débridement. The information is provided as a guideline and is not intended to supersede manufacturer's recommendations or facility policy.

Table 28•3 **General Procedural Steps for Performing Contact Ultrasound Débridement***	
Procedural Steps	**Comments**
1. Assess patient and patient's comfort, current pain level, history of pain with débridement, and current analgesic regimen.	• Assess patients pain, consider topical anesthesia (4% lidocaine) or oral/parenteral narcotics. • Reassess pain frequently during treatment.
2. Assess wound to determine wound treatment regimen, including treatment location, intensity, duration, irrigation solution, and frequency of subsequent treatments.	• RNs, PTs and physician extenders require a written order for procedure.
3. Set up the US device in accordance with the manufacturer's manual. Select irrigation solution and prime IV tubing. Select probe tip. Assemble handpiece (attach ultrasound cable to unit and tubing and tip to probe).	• Standard irrigant: sterile 0.9% NaCl. • Nonstandard irrigant: antibiotic solution, 0.125 Dakin's, hypochlorous acid.
4. Wash hands and apply personal protective equipment: gloves, mask, fluid-resistant gown, eye protection, and shoe covers. Apply equipment protective covering. Protect patient with absorbent pads (Chux).	• Standard precautions include personal protective equipment for splash and aerosolization of fluids. • Follow infection control procedures if patient is in contact isolation.

Table 28•3	General Procedural Steps for Performing Contact Ultrasound Débridement*—cont'd

Procedural Steps	Comments
5. Power up device. Select intensity (power) setting. Select pulse mode on/off.	• Do not operate device without irrigation fluid.
6. Prime ultrasound handpiece with irrigant and set drip rate to wet surface of the wound.	• Excess fluid will add to splash and aerosolization.
7. Place probe in contact with wound bed/irrigant. Activate ultrasound by depressing foot pedal.	• In order for ultrasound energy to be transmitted, the probe tip must be in contact with fluid or moist wound bed.
8. With probe in contact with fluid or wound bed, pass the probe head with a slow continuous motion across the entire wound surface. DO NOT STOP IN ONE SPOT for an extended period of time; sweep over and return for repeated treatment.	• The thermal effects of ultrasound are multiplied if the sound waves are allowed to reflect back up to the stationary probe tip, creating a standing wave.
9. Continue the débridement using sweeping motion until treatment is complete or patient no longer tolerates procedure.	• Monitor and record elapsed time of procedure as well as intensity used.
10. Turn off machine.	• Discontinues ultrasound production.
11. Gently wipe dry periwound tissue and reassess the patient and the wound.	• Measure and photograph as indicated.
12. Apply appropriate dressing to wound as ordered.	
13. Remove equipment protection covering prior to moving unit from area of use. Wipe connector lines with facility-approved disinfectant. Disassemble handpiece and device and perform sterile process. Remove personal protection equipment and dispose of properly. Have treatment room cleaned prior to next client use.	• Sterilization process per manufacturer's recommendation in accordance with facility policy.

*This information is provided as a guideline and is not intended to supersede manufacturer's recommendations or facility policy.

Contact Kilohertz Ultrasound Treatment Indications, Precautions, Expected Clinical Outcomes

Indications:
• Locally infected wounds
• Wounds with impaired circulation
• Wounds with the need for débridement, irrigation, and topical treatment
• Pressure ulcers, diabetic foot ulcers, arterial ulcers, venous ulcers, surgical wounds

Precautions:
• Untreated advancing cellulitis with signs of systemic response
• Wounds with metal components, such as joint replacements, plates, and screws
• Wounds associated with implanted electronic devices
• Uncontrolled pain

Expected Clinical Outcomes:
• Wound débridement
• Decreased pain
• Reduced bioburden
• Reduction of systemic and topical antibiotic usage
• Decreased time to closure

Clinical Effects of Noncontact 40-Kilohertz Ultrasound
Effect on Wound-Related Pain

In a retrospective chart review, Gehling and Samies reported that 15 consecutive patients with painful, recalcitrant lower-extremity wounds treated for 2 to 4 weeks with 40-kHz noncontact ultrasound MIST Therapy (NCUS) had mean pretreatment VAS pain scores of 8.07 that decreased to a mean of 1.76 after treatment.[80] None of the patients reported worsening pain after the treatment started. In another retrospective study with the same 40-KHz NCUS device, Bell and Cavorsi found that in paired analyses of 26 participants for whom numeric pain ratings were available at the start and the end of US treatment, the mean pain rating was reduced by 1.8 points ($P = 0.0010$).[81] In a small case series, Waldrop and Serfass evaluated the analgesic effect of 40-kHz NCUS on six nonrandomly selected patients with seven partial to full-thickness thermal burns.[82] They administered NCUS treatment of 3 to 20 min (depending on wound size) up to five times weekly for 1 to 6 weeks. Patients reported no pain with removal of fibrin, slough, and eschar. Exudate was reduced to minimal amounts of serous fluid in 1 to 3 weeks, and wound areas decreased to a mean of 76% in 3 weeks. All patients reported complete pain reduction, and reepithelialization was complete in 1 to 6 weeks. More controlled clinical studies to evaluate the effect of NCUS on wound-related pain are warranted.

Effect on Wound Débridement

Ramundo and Gray systematically reviewed the literature to determine whether 40-kHz NCUS effectively removes necrotic debris from the bed of chronic wounds and promotes wound healing.[83] They reviewed MEDLINE and CINAHL databases from January 1996 to February 2008 using the following key words: *therapeutic ultrasound, ultrasonic,* and *ultrasonic mist.* They also included prospective studies that compared NCUS to a sham device, to another débridement method, or to alternative treatment for wound healing. They concluded that there is insufficient evidence to determine whether NCUS effectively débrides necrotic tissue in chronic wound beds. On the other hand, they noted that there was limited evidence for wound healing (see the next section), which suggests that NCUS promotes wound healing when used in conjunction with standard wound care.

Effect on Wound Healing— Retrospective Studies

Several clinical studies of various designs have reported that 40-kHz NCUS enhances wound healing. Haan and Lucich performed a retrospective analysis of the effects of NCUS on the healing progression of chronic wounds.[84] Outcome measures included amount of devitalized tissue, amount and type of wound drainage, and surface area following treatment with NCUS. They performed a chart review of 48 consecutive patients treated with NCUS at a single center between January 2006 and October 2007. Data from paired comparisons of baseline versus posttreatment values for wound area, tissue characteristics, drainage, and pain were analyzed. Treatment frequency and duration were also recorded. Following a mean of 2.1 NCUS treatments per week for 4.1 min per session over 5.5 weeks, they found that the median wound area decreased by 92% from baseline (6.2 cm² to 0.2 cm², $P < 0.0001$). Additionally, the proportion of wounds with greater than 75% granulation tissue increased from 37% to 89% ($P < 0.0001$) and the proportion of wounds without fibrin slough or eschar increased from 31% to 75% ($P < 0.0001$) and from 72% to 94% ($P = 0.02$), respectively. Realizing the study limitations of a retrospective design, lack of a control group, and small sample, the authors concluded that as an adjunct to standard wound care (SWC), NCUS seems to improve characteristics associated with wound healing, including decreased necrotic tissue, increased granulation tissue and decreased wound area.

In another previously mentioned retrospective review of 76 patient charts, investigators set the primary effective study endpoint as the percentage of change in area of nonhealing wounds from the beginning to the end of treatment with NCUS.[80] In addition to SWC, patients received 40-kHz NCUS a mean of 5.1 min per session for a mean of 2.3 times per week over a median period of 4.3 weeks. They reported that the median wound area decreased by 79% from the start to the end of NCUS treatments (from 2.5 to 0.6 cm²). Furthermore, the proportion of patients with greater than 75% granulation tissue increased from 32% before NCUS to 46% after 40-kHz NCUS treatment.

In a third retrospective, observational study at a single site, Kavros et al evaluated the effect of 40-kHz NCUS in the treatment of chronic lower extremity wounds.[85] Wounds of 163 patients were treated with NCUS plus SWC, while wounds of 47 control patients received SWC alone. All wounds in both groups received SWC and were followed for 6 months. NCUS treatments were given three times per week for 90 days or until closed. They reported that a greater percentage of wounds treated with NCUS plus SWC closed compared with wounds treated with SWC alone (53% vs 32%, $P = 0.009$). In addition, the slope of the regression line in the NCUS arm (1.4) was steeper than the slope in the control arm (0.22, $P + 0.002$), indicating a faster rate of healing in the NCUS arm. They concluded that the rate of healing and complete wound closure improved significantly when NCUS was combined with SWC.

Effect on Wound Healing with 30- and 40-Kilohertz Ultrasound—Prospective Studies

In 1997 two groups of investigators at separate health-care facilities in Germany performed RCTs to evaluate the effects of 30-kHz US on wound healing using an experimental device. In studies by Weichenthal et al and Peschen et al, 38 patients and 24 patients, respectively, with chronic venous leg ulcers were randomized to have their wounds treated with SWC alone (controls) or with SWC plus 30-kHz US (treatment).[86,87] In both studies the US treatment was administered by having patients immerse their leg or ankle ulcer into a container of water that contained a fixed stainless steel US transducer. The wound was positioned approximately 5 cm from the transducer, and the US power was set to deliver 100 mW/cm² for 10 min, three times a week, using water as the coupling agent. In the Weichenthal et al study, wound size was recorded after 3 and 8 weeks. They found that after 3 weeks of treatment (and to a greater extent after 8 weeks of treatment) the US group showed a markedly improved response compared with the control group. In the control group, the mean wound area decreased by 11%, whereas in the US group the mean ulcer area decreased 41% ($P < 0.05$). In the Peschen et al study, wound size was recorded after 12 weeks of treatment. They found that after 12 weeks of treatment the control ulcers showed a mean decrease of 16.5% in wound area, while the mean area of the US-treated wounds decreased by 55.4 % ($P < 0.007$). Investigators of both groups concluded that 30-kHz US is a helpful treatment for venous leg ulcers, particularly when SWC has failed.

In a randomized, controlled, single-center trial, Kavros et al systematically assigned 35 patients with chronic, ischemic leg and foot ulcers to receive 40-kHz NCUS plus SWC (treatment group) and 35 other patients with the same wound etiology to receive SWC alone (control group) for 12 weeks or until wound closure.[88] Wounds of patients in the treatment group received NCUS three times per week for 5 min per treatment. The investigators reported that a significantly higher percentage of patients treated with NCUS plus SWC achieved greater than 50% wound healing at 12 weeks than those treated with SWC alone (63% vs 29%, P <0.001). They concluded that the rate of healing chronic, ischemic leg and foot ulcers improved significantly when 40-kHz NCUS was combined with SWC.

In a noncomparative clinical outcomes study, completed over an 8-month period, Ennis et al used 40-kHz NCUS to treat wounds of 23 patients with 29 lower-extremity lesions of various etiologies.[89] During the 2 weeks prior to treating the wounds with NCUS, patients received SWC. After patients were treated with SWC for 2 weeks, if their wound had failed to achieve an area reduction greater than 15%, they were deemed qualified to receive NCUS plus SWC. The investigators reported that 69% of the wounds treated with 40-kHz NCUS plus SWC healed and that the healing response was evident within 4 weeks of treatment. Ennis et al also reported positive wound healing outcomes from a randomized, double-blind, controlled, multicenter trial that evaluated healing effects of 40-kHz NCUS.[90] In this study 55 patients with non-healing diabetic foot ulcers received SWC and either active NCUS (N = 27) or sham NCUS (N = 28). After 12 weeks of care, the proportion of wounds healed (defined as complete epithelialization without drainage) in the active NCUS group was significantly higher than that in the sham control group (40.7% vs 13.3%, P = 0.0366).

Effect on Wound Healing—Clinical Case Studies

In an open label, nonrandomized, baseline controlled case series of 51 patients with chronic foot and leg ulcerations of various etiologies, Kavros and Schenck reported that the mean SWC treatment time was 9.8 plus or minus 5.5 weeks versus 5.5 plus or minus 2.8 weeks of treatment with 40-kHz NCUS (P = 0.0001).[91] Following these treatment periods, the mean percentage of wound volume reduction achieved was 37.3% plus or minus 18.6% for the SWC group versus 94.9% plus or minus 9.8% for the NCUS group. They concluded that NCUS improved the healing rate and closure of refractory lower-extremity wounds.

Other case studies have also reported favorable wound healing outcomes following wound treatment with NCUS.[92]

Effects of High-Frequency (Megahertz) Ultrasound on Wound Healing—Overview

These frequencies (often referred to as "therapeutic US") also transmit acoustic energy, which has the physical properties of stable cavitation and microstreaming described earlier. However, with megahertz US, stable cavitation and microstreaming are less intense than the unstable cavitation associated with kilohertz US. This is because intensity is inversely proportional to frequency, and since higher frequencies have shorter wavelengths, at the power (wattage) levels used for megahertz US, less acoustic energy is transmitted to tissues per unit time. Recall that the more prominent unstable cavitation produced by 22.5, 25 and 35 kilohertz US frequencies is a major contributing source of energy by which contact US débrides via fragmentation and emulsification of nonviable, adherent fibrin, and slough. The combination of stable cavitation and microstreaming that are characteristic of megahertz US do not generate the destructive energy levels that are associated with kilohertz US frequencies. Owing to the lower-level nonthermal effects that 1- and 3-MHz acoustic energy has on tissues and cells, these frequencies are also used to treat open wounds by applying the US to the periwound skin with either aqueous gel or water immersion as the coupling medium. Using this approach rather than direct insonation into the wound bed avoids the risk of wound contamination. Bear in mind that megahertz US is also capable of generating thermal energy in soft tissues. This was addressed earlier in the section titled "Thermal Effects of Megahertz Ultrasound." Although mild heating of closed and open wounds may be desirable when the objective is to enhance blood flow, generally the nonthermal effects of US on wound healing are considered more desirable and are supported by more research evidence. Therefore, the focus of this section is to review how the combined effects of stable cavitation and acoustic streaming excite or upregulate the cell membrane, thereby increasing the activity levels of the entire cell. Essentially, the US energy acts as a trigger for this process, but it is the increased cellular activity that is actually responsible for the therapeutic benefits of the acoustic energy.[93-97] The combined effects of stable cavitation and microstreaming associated with 1- and 3-MHz US that may impact wound healing include a temporary increase in uptake of calcium ions by fibroblasts.[98,99] In addition, with the ultrasound pulsed at a 20% duty cycle and a frequency of 1 MHz, intensity levels as low as 0.5 W/cm² have been shown to increase collagen synthesis by fibroblasts.[31] This effect is highly significant for cell membrane permeability changes. In particular, the important second messenger, calcium, could act as an intracellular signal for some of the events that lead to ultrasound-induced stimulation of tissue repair.[100] Other plausible examples include increased collagen synthesis (release of growth factors from mast cells and macrophages) and stimulation of angiogenesis.[35-38,41,42] Another clinically significant change in membrane function resulting from acoustic streaming is serotonin release from platelets.[27,28] In addition to serotonin, platelets contain chemotactic factors that promote migration of cells essential for successful repair to the wound site.[29] If streaming can stimulate serotonin release, it may also stimulate the release of these factors, thus stimulating wound healing.

> ▶ **PEARL 28•16** Megahertz frequency US is a physical technology that has been used for decades by physical therapists to facilitate healing of musculoskeletal tissues (eg, muscle, fascia, tendon, ligament, joint capsule) that are wounded or inflamed, but not exposed because the skin remains intact following many accidents or sports injuries. The two high-frequency devices (1 and 3 MHz) that are used to treat these "closed wounds" are available in commercial devices (Fig. 28.7).

Using the biophysical effects just described as background, the demonstrated effects of nonthermal megahertz US on the three phases of wound healing are discussed next.

Inflammatory Phase

Immediately after connective tissue is injured, platelets and mast cells are activated, releasing pharmacologically active agents that initiate acute inflammation. Inflammation, which is accompanied by pain, erythema, and swelling, is often considered to be an adverse condition. Frequently, anti-inflammatory medications are prescribed to reduce swelling and relieve pain, an appropriate course of action for chronic inflammatory conditions. Acute inflammation, however, unlike chronic inflammation, is not a disease, but the normal response of tissues to injury. It is part of the healing process and as such should be accelerated rather than suppressed. Ultrasonic therapy administered in the pulsed mode applied shortly after injury can accelerate the inflammatory phase of repair and in doing so can accelerate wound healing.[101, 102]

A single treatment of therapeutic US applied during the early inflammatory phase can stimulate the release of histamine from mast cell degranulation.[37,102] In addition to histamine, mast cells contain a wide range of chemical mediators, including chemotactic agents that attract neutrophils and monocytes to the wound site.[103] Many of these agents are preformed and stored in granules. If their release is enhanced by ultrasound, this would help to explain why clinicians find ultrasonic therapy particularly valuable if applied after bleeding has stopped but during the first 24 hours after injury, while the tissues are still in the early part of the acute inflammatory phase of repair. In a randomized controlled trial (RCT) on induced wounds in rats, Leung et al evaluated the effect of megahertz pulsed (1:4) US on acute inflammation of soft tissue injuries by measuring levels of prostaglandin E_2 (PGE_2) and leukotriene B_4 (LTB_4) before and after exposure to four different US intensities (0, 0.5, 1.5, 2.3 w/cm^2) for a 5-min treatment on postinjury days 1, 5, or 10.[98] They found that levels of PGE_2 and LTB_4 were higher in all intensity subgroups that received the highest intensity (2.3 w/cm^2) on postinjury day 2. On postinjury day 11, LTB_4 was significantly decreased, but PGE_2 was significantly increased. They concluded that pulsed US may stimulate inflammation of acute ligament injury.

Mast cell degranulation is generally triggered by membrane changes involving increased transport of calcium ions into the cell.[103] Possibly, membrane perturbation induced by US therapy can increase calcium ion transport into mast cells, as it does in fibroblasts.[98,99]

On arriving at the wound site, monocytes leave the blood vessels and are transformed into macrophages. Together with the neutrophils, they remove dead cells, debris, and microorganisms from the wound. Provided the wound is not colonized, the number of neutrophils in the wound begins to decrease after a few days, marking the end of the early part of the inflammatory phase of repair. The late part of the inflammatory phase is characterized by a continued increase in the number of macrophages, with a decrease in the number of neutrophils. The granules of neutrophils and macrophages, especially the latter, contain chemotactic agents and growth factors that are necessary for the development of new connective tissue at the site of injury.[104] On their release, these agents

and growth factors stimulate pericytes (undifferentiated mesenchymal cells), fibroblasts, and endothelial cells to produce granulation tissue at the wound site. Treatment of U937 cells (an unstimulated form of macrophage that can be maintained in vitro) with therapeutic levels of US has resulted in the release of growth factors that stimulate fibroblast proliferation.[105] Treatment in the late part (24–48 hours) of the acute inflammatory phase, when macrophages containing these factors are gathering at the wound site, is therefore recommended, for early release of these factors could accelerate the onset of the proliferative phase of repair.

Although therapeutic US can accelerate the early inflammatory phase of repair, it is not an anti-inflammatory agent.[106] Clinical research on the resolution of postoperative edema revealed that an apparent anti-inflammatory response following low-intensity US therapy was mainly a placebo effect.[106] Furthermore, the same study showed that pulsed US average intensities of 0.5 W/cm^2 and above were proinflammatory in that they stimulated mast cell activity. However, this response was masked by its anti-inflammatory, placebo-induced effects.

Proliferative Phase

This phase overlaps with, and is initiated by, the late part of the inflammatory phase of repair, generally beginning about 3 days after injury. During the proliferative phase, a highly vascularized, collagen-rich granulation tissue develops at the site of injury. In the case of excised lesions of the skin, granulation tissue becomes covered superficially by epidermal cells. Granulation tissue, a temporary reparative tissue, is gradually replaced by scar tissue during the subsequent remodeling phase. This tissue is very cellular, containing macrophages (which secrete chemotactic and growth factors, thereby controlling its development), pericytes, endothelial cells, and fibroblasts, which synthesize collagen to form the extracellular matrix. The matrix is rich in fibronectin (the substrate over which cells contributing to the granulation tissue migrate), type III collagen, and hyaluronic acid.[107] Initially, the growth factors secreted by the macrophages are essential, because they attract the other cells of the granulation tissue to the wound area and stimulate their proliferation. Later in the proliferative phase, however, the need for them appears to be reduced. The number of macrophages falls, while the number of fibroblasts and endothelial cells increases. The fibroblasts, very important in repair, mainly provide the connective tissue matrix and are also the chief contractile cells of the wound. As myofibroblasts, they help to reduce the size of the tissue defect (responsible for wound contraction).[107] Clearly, endothelial cells are vital, being essential for angiogenesis, forming the new blood capillaries that transport metabolites to and from the reparative tissue. Evidence exists that both fibroblast activity and angiogenesis can be affected by therapeutic ultrasound in a manner conducive to the acceleration of tissue repair.

The exposure of fibroblasts in vitro to megahertz US has been shown to stimulate additional secretion of collagen, the fibrous protein that increases the tensile strength of connective tissues.[35] This increase may be triggered by a temporary US-induced increase in their calcium ion content following reversible alterations in membrane permeability.[98,99] Shear stresses associated with acoustic streaming and possibly also with stable cavitation have been implicated in the production of these effects in vitro.[98,99] Nonthermal levels of US can stimulate fibroblast activity in vivo, but whether cavitation is involved remains to be determined.[108]

> **PEARL 28•17** Treatment with US during the inflammatory and early proliferative phases of repair can accelerate wound contraction, presumably directly by its effects on fibroblasts and indirectly by growth factors released from macrophages.[111]

Wound contraction, the reduction of a skin defect by the centripetal movement of the surrounding intact skin, reduces the need for scar-tissue production. During wound contraction, fibroblasts develop temporarily into myofibroblasts, specialized contractile and secretory cells, that become linked together and aligned in such a way that when they contract, the edges of the wound are pulled together.[107,109] They resemble smooth muscle cells, and since the latter can be induced to contract by therapeutic levels of US, possibly myofibroblast contraction may be affected in a similar manner. Although wound contraction can be accelerated by US, no evidence exists that the total amount of contraction is affected.[109,110]

Quantitative data are available to support the hypothesis that treatment of injured skin with therapeutic US during the inflammatory and early proliferative phases of repair can accelerate healing of the dermis.[105,111] The method used is based on the observation that, during repair, different types of cells arrive at and then leave the wound site in a characteristic sequence. The first to arrive, during the inflammatory phase, are neutrophils and macrophages. Provided that the wound is not contaminated, the neutrophils decrease significantly within a few days, marking the end of the early part of the inflammatory process. However, macrophages continue to increase in number. During the proliferative phase, the number of fibroblasts and endothelial cells increases, while the number of macrophages gradually falls. Because each group of cells reaches a maximum and then decreases, the rate of repair progress can be quantified by assessing the relative numbers of each cell type at different times after wounding.[111] By 5 days after injury, there are fewer macrophages, but significantly more fibroblasts in wounds treated with US at either 1 or 3 MHz (0.5 W/cm², pulsed 2 msec on/8 msec off for 5 min daily) compared with sham-insonated controls.[111] This suggests that wounds treated with ultrasound in this manner leave the inflammatory phase and enter the proliferative phase of repair more rapidly than the controls. Thus, treatment with US can be shown to accelerate dermal repair.

> **PEARL 28•18** In addition to affecting mast cells, macrophages, and fibroblasts, treatment with therapeutic US can also stimulate endothelial cell activity. In chronically ischemic muscle, treatment with US resulted in development of new capillaries, and blood flow was restored at an accelerated rate.[115] Treatment with US during the first 4 days after injury has been shown to result in a statistically significant increase in the rate at which blood capillaries and other vessels develop within the granulation tissue.[116]

Since angiogenic factors are present in the granules of mast cells and macrophages, the stimulation observed may be due, at least to some extent, to an accelerated liberation of their release.[112-114]

Remodeling Phase

During this phase, which overlaps with the preceding proliferative phase, the initial, apparently random deposition of collagen fibers is changed. Collagen fibers are removed from some locations and newly synthesized fibers are deposited in others. This results in a more regular pattern thought to be correlated with the mechanical forces to which the tissue is subjected during normal activity. Additionally, some of the type III collagen is replaced by type I collagen. Ideally, remodeling should continue until the scar tissue, which replaces granulation tissue at the site of injury, becomes both structurally and functionally identical to preinjury tissue. In the case of injured dermis and deeper soft tissues, this ideal state is never reached. The scar tissue remains weaker and less elastic than uninjured dermis indefinitely.

Exposure to therapeutic levels of US during remodeling has been used in attempts to improve the mechanical properties of mature scar tissue, with limited success.[115,116] An alternative approach is to begin treatment immediately after injury, a technique that has been shown to have more dramatic effects on the mechanical properties of the scar tissue. Full-thickness skin wounds treated with therapeutic levels of US (0.5 W/cm², 3 MHz, pulsed 2 msec on/8 msec off for 5 min, three times weekly for 2 weeks) developed significantly stronger and yet more elastic scar tissue than control, sham-sonated wounds. However, the scar tissue remained mechanically less satisfactory than uninjured skin.[108,117] The increased strength of the treated scar tissue is believed to be due to its increased collagen content, while the increased elasticity could be related to a change in collagen fiber pattern. Scanning electron microscopy has shown that the pattern in ultrasonically treated scar tissue is that of a three-dimensional lattice, similar to the uninjured dermis, whereas in sham-treated controls the fiber arrangement is less regular. Change in fiber angle in the lattice arrangement in response to the application of a tensile force to the tissue would permit a limited amount of elongation, followed by recoil when the force was reduced and the fibers returned to their original position. It could also increase the amount of energy the scar tissue can absorb before breaking.[118]

Several investigators have studied the effects of US on acute induced wounds in animals. Dyson et al found that low dosages of pulsed US increased granulation tissue growth in full-thickness wounds in rabbits, whereas high dosages produced no change.[119] Drastichova et al reported that US applied to incisional wounds in guinea pigs increased wound breaking strength, but another study failed to demonstrate any change.[120,121] In a controlled study on induced wounds in Yucatan pigs, Byl et al found that low-dose US (pulsed mode, 20% duty cycle, 1 MHz, 0.5 W/cm² for 3 days and 1.5 W/cm² for 2 days) increased collagen deposition, wound breaking strength, and wound closure.[122] In a second study on Yucatan pigs, Byl et al found that both wound breaking strength and hydroxyproline (an indicator of collagen deposition) were significantly higher in a low-dose US group compared to the results of a high-dose US group after 10 days of treatment.[123]

Based on the evidence provided from basic science research, the clinician may consider using US to produce desirable cellular ultrastructural changes during each of the three phases of wound healing. In doing so, one should pay close attention to the treatment parameters reported to be effective in the studies just described.

Clinical Research—Effects of Megahertz Ultrasound on Venous Leg Ulcers

Eleven clinical trials related to determining the effects of US on wound healing have been published. Of these studies, seven evaluated the effects of US on venous ulcer healing and four evaluated the effects on pressure ulcer healing. The seven venous ulcer studies will be reviewed first in chronological order.

In a 4-week controlled blind trial involving venous ulcers having durations between 6 and 360 months, Dyson et al randomized 25 patients into two groups.[124] One group of 13 patients had 3-MHz pulsed US applied to their periwound skin at a 20% duty cycle, 1 W/cm², for 5 to 10 min, three times a week for 4 weeks. To 12 control ulcers they applied sham US in a double-blind manner to the periwound skin. The authors did not indicate whether the mean baseline wound size was the same for the two groups or if there was a significant difference between them. After the 4-week protocol, wounds that had been treated with active US were significantly smaller than the control wounds (active US = 66.4 ± 8.8% of baseline size vs sham US = 91.6 ± 8.9% of baseline size). Given that small wounds heal faster than large wounds, the results of this study may be confounded if the mean wound size of the experimental group was smaller than the control group at the beginning of the study.

In an 8-week study by Roche and West, patients with 26 venous ulcers being treated with standard wound care were randomized to active ($N = 13$) and sham ($N = 13$) US groups, but the randomization resulted in the mean ulcer size being larger in the active US group.[125] While the sham group received only standard wound care for 8 weeks, the active group received standard care plus 3-MHz pulsed US at a 20% duty cycle and 1 W/Cm², three times a week for 8 weeks. Despite the mean size of wounds in the active group being larger at the outset of the study, the authors reported that at the end of 8 weeks, there was a greater reduction in mean wound size for the active US group than for the sham group ($P < 0.01$). The results of this study indicate that the larger wounds treated with US plus standard care healed faster than the small wounds ($P < 0.001$) that received standard care alone.

Callam et al used the Roach and West research design in a study in which they randomized 108 patients with leg ulcers (87% venous) to a treatment group ($N = 52$) that received US plus standard care to their wounds and a control group ($N = 56$) that received standard care alone.[126,125] In addition to standard care, the treatment group also received 1-MHz pulsed US (duty cycle not stated) at 0.5 W/cm² once weekly for 12 weeks. At the end of 12 weeks (excluding 11 patients who withdrew from the treatment group and 15 patients who withdrew from the control group), the proportion of ulcers healed was 20% greater in the US group than in the control group. This 20% difference between the two groups was significant ($P < 0.05$). However, following Callam's report, Lundeberg et al and Eriksson et al used pulsed and continuous mode US, respectively, but failed to show significant differences in the proportion of healed venous leg ulcers or ulcer area for wounds that received active US versus sham US.[127,128]

The results of these five studies demonstrate equivocal findings, making it difficult to draw any conclusions regarding the efficacy of MHz US in facilitating the healing of venous ulcers. Interestingly, the results from a 1998 meta-analysis by Johannsen et al that pooled data from the US studies just cited, report a nonstatistically "beneficial effect" between ultrasound and placebo ultrasound in the treatment of chronic leg ulcers.[129] Their analysis also suggested that US has the best effect when delivered in low doses to the periwound skin. The studies Johannsen et al used for their meta-analysis are presented in Table 28.4.[129]

A study published in 2002 by Swist-Chmielewska et al evaluated the effects of 1-MHz US on venous ulcer healing.[130] Patients were randomized to groups that received 1 W/cm² (group A), 0.5 W/cm² (group B), and standard wound care (group C). They found the rate of wound area and wound volume changes were greatest for group B, but were only statistically significant in comparison with group A. Although they did not report a statistically significant difference between groups B and C, they concluded that faster ulcer healing occurred in wounds treated with US at 0.5 W/cm².

A recent RCT (2008) was found that evaluated the effects of 1-MHz US on venous ulcer healing after all patients in the study had received vascular surgery consisting of the following options: crossectomy, partial stripping of the greater or lesser saphenous vein, local phlebectomy and ligation of insufficient perforators. The US treatments commenced 5 days after the surgical intervention. In this study Dolibog et al assigned 70 patients to groups A and B.[131] Ulcers of the A group were treated with water immersion pulsed US at a 20% duty cycle and 0.5 W/cm², plus a moist wound dressing, compression stockings, and drug therapy. The US energy was applied directly to the ulcers; the duration of treatment was based on wound size; and treatments were repeated daily, 6 days a week for 7 weeks. The dressing and compression stockings were changed daily, and daily drug therapy consisted of vitamin supplements. Group B control ulcers were treated with moist dressings, compression stockings, and vitamin supplements daily. They found there were no statistically significant differences between groups for wound surface area, length, width, or volume and concluded from their findings that there are no indications that US promotes healing of venous leg ulcers after they undergo surgical intervention.

Clinical Research—Effects of Megahertz Ultrasound on Pressure Ulcers

Four studies were found that investigated the effect of US on healing of pressure ulcers. In a noncontrolled case series, Paul et al reported that, of 23 patients with pressure ulcers, 13 wounds healed.[132] Wounds were treated with an US dosage

Table 28•4 Modus Operandi and Outcomes of Clinical Trials Used by Johannsen et al in Their Meta-Analysis of Megahertz Ultrasound Effects on Chronic Leg Ulcers

Study Variables		Peschen et al[89]	Dyson et al[127]	Roche and West[128]	Callam et al[129]	Lundeberg et al[130]	Eriksson et al[131]
Ulcer etiology		Venous	Venous	Venous	Venous primarily (94/108)	Venous	Venous
Method of randomization		Alternately	Alternately	Random distribution	Permuted blocks	Permuted blocks	Alternately
Number of subjects	Control	12	12	13	41 (15 dropouts)	15	13
	US	12	13	13	41 (11 dropouts)	17	12
Area treated		Wound surface and periwound	Periwound	Periwound	Periwound	Wound surface	Wound surface
Frequency of treatment		3/week	3/week	3/week	1/week	3/week	2/week
US frequency		30 kHz	3 MHz	3 MHz	1 MHz	1 MHz	1 MHz
US intensity		100 mW/cm²	1 W/cm²	1 W/cm²	0.5 W/cm²	0.5 W/cm²	1 W/cm²
Continuous or pulsed/duty cycle		Continuous	1:5	1:4	Pulsed	1:9	Not reported
Treatment duration		10 min	5–10 min	5–10 min	1 min/area of transducer	10 min	10 min max
% Healing results							
4 weeks	Control	↓8%; SD 20	↓7.4%; SD 8.9	↓28%; SD 27.3	↓30%; SD 61.6 5 closed	↓19; SD 9 1 closed	↓27; SD 12 1 closed
	US	↓27%; SD 24	↓34% SD 8.8	↓35%; SD 21.9	↓48%; SD 49.8 6 closed	↓24; SD 12 2 closed	↓35; SD 14 2 closed
	No. ulcers closed	Not reported	Not reported	Not reported			
8 weeks	Control	↓20%; SD 24	Not reported	↓7%; SD 36.7	↓60%; SD 41.9 6 closed	↓47; SD 10 3 closed	↓5.2; SD 13 4 closed
	US	↓40%; SD 23	Not reported	↓35.3%; SD 30.1	↓80%; SD 24.6 14 closed	↓53; SD 8 5 closed	↓68; SD 9 5 closed
	No. ulcers closed	Not reported	Not reported	Not reported			

Modified with permission from Johannsen, F, Gam, AN, Karlsmark, T.: Ultrasound therapy in chronic leg ulceration: A meta-analysis: Wound Repair Regen 1998; 6: 121–126.

of between 0.5 and 1 W/cm^2 (frequency and mode not mentioned). In addition to the 13 wounds healed, 5 demonstrated definite improvement, and 5 showed equivocal responses. Unfortunately, very little can be concluded from the results of this study.

In a double-blind study by McDiarmid et al, patients with partial-thickness (stage II) pressure ulcers were enrolled and randomized into two groups.[133] The wounds of one group were treated three times weekly with 3-MHz US, pulsed at a 20% duty cycle, and at an intensity of 0.8 W/cm^2 for 5 to 10 min. Wounds of the second group received sham US for 5 min, three times weekly. Over the course of the study, 7 patients were discharged from the institution, 6 died, and 9 withdrew. This left 10 patients in the US active group and 8 in the US sham group. Taking clean versus infected wounds into consideration, the authors indicated that US therapy appeared to improve the healing rate of infected ulcers but not clean ulcers. Because of the weak cavitation effect from megahertz US, it is doubtful that the apparent increased healing rate of infected wounds occurred because the bacterial burden was reduced by US fragmentation of bacteria.

Two other studies examined the effect of US on pressure ulcer healing. The design of one study and the results of the other make it very difficult to draw firm conclusions from either study.[134,135] Nussbaum and coworkers, compared nursing care alone, nursing care plus laser, and nursing care alternated with ultrasound or ultraviolet C (UVC) on pressure ulcer healing in 16 spinal cord injury patients with 18 wounds.[134] Although they reported that US/UVC treatment had a greater effect on wound healing than did nursing care either alone or combined with laser, the underlying question remains: Would the same treatment effect have occurred with either US alone or UVC alone? This is an important question with regard to wound healing interventions because Medicare and private insurance companies want to know whether a particular treatment is more efficacious than standard care alone, even though standard care may be based on expert opinion. If clinical research demonstrates that a particular intervention facilitates wound healing faster than standard care, then clinicians will gradually substitute the new treatment for standard care. One other randomized study failed to demonstrate a significant treatment effect by US on pressure ulcers.[135]

Megahertz Ultrasound Protocol for Treatment of Chronic Wounds

1. Evaluate the wound to determine its phase of healing.
2. For all three wound healing phases, select pulsed mode US at a 20% duty cycle, (virtually all clinical wound studies that report positive treatment effects used a 20% duty cycle).
3. Measure the depth of the wound to help determine whether 1 or 3 MHz will be used.
4. Cleanse the periwound skin with mild soap and water, followed by rinsing.
5. For full-thickness (cavity) wounds, apply US transmission gel to the intact periwound skin that will be insonated.
6. For partial-thickness wounds, apply a sterile sheet hydrogel (96% H$_2$O) directly over the wound. The hydrogel should be large enough to cover the entire wound as well as 4 to 6 cm of periwound skin, so that at the therapist's discretion, US may be delivered to both the wound and the periwound skin (Fig. 28.21A).

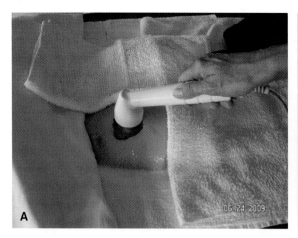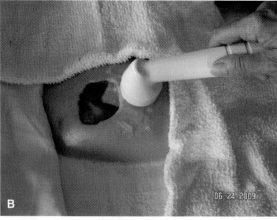

Figure 28•21 *(A) Megahertz US may be delivered to partial-thickness wounds by using a hydrogel sheet for coupling. The hydrogel sheet should be large enough to cover the wound and extend onto the periwound skin far enough so that, at the discretion of the clinician, the US energy can be delivered to wound and periwound skin. The US applicator should be moved 4 to 5 cm/sec in overlapping parallel or circular strokes. (B) For full-thickness wounds, US can be delivered only to the periwound skin by using a hydrogel sheet or sterile amorphous US gel as optional coupling agents.*

7. Cleanse the US applicator with an antibacterial approved agent to avoid cross-contamination of the wound.

8. Ask the patient to inform you if he or she experiences any discomfort during the treatment (eg, periosteal pain).

9. Select the following intensities (W/cm²) for the following wound phases[122]:
   • inflammatory: 0.3
   • reparative: 0.5
   • early remodeling: 0.5 to 1

10. For full-thickness wounds, or if the wound is in the inflammatory or proliferative phase, apply sterile amorphous US gel to the intact periwound skin and treat each periwound skin surface area that is approximately two times the surface area of the US applicator for 5 min daily (for larger wounds select a larger US applicator). If the wound is in the remodeling phase, treat three times a week for 2 weeks to increase the scar tensile strength. (Fig. 28.21B)

Precautions for Ultrasound

US must be used cautiously in patients with the following conditions:

1. *Wound inflammation.* Use only nonthermal US to avoid severe exacerbation of acute inflammation.

2. *Fractures.* Avoid lingering over a fracture site to avoid inducing pain in the site.

To ensure cautious use, the following are important:

1. Use the lowest intensity that produces the required effect, since higher intensities may be damaging.

2. Move the applicator constantly at about 4 cm/sec throughout treatment to avoid the painful and/or damaging effects of standing waves.

3. If the patient feels any additional pain during treatment, either reduce the intensity to a pain-free level or abandon the treatment.

4. Use properly calibrated and maintained equipment. If there is any doubt, do not proceed with treatment.

Contraindications to Ultrasound

US should not be used in patients with a cancerous growth in the wound or periwound skin or over the following areas:

• Pregnant uterus
• Central nervous system tissue
• Joint cement
• Plastic joint components
• Pacemaker (or near it)
• Thrombophlebitis
• Reproductive organs and the eyes

▶ **Case Study 28•1** | **Effect of 25-kHz Ultrasound Débridement on a Stage III Infected Sacral Pressure Ulcer**

History

CK is a 53-year-old female with a 30-year history of multiple sclerosis. She has significant disability, with motor and cognitive deficits and diffuse lower-extremity weakness and spasm. She has been confined to a wheelchair for several years. During an acute care hospitalization, she developed an iatrogenic stage III right sacral pressure ulcer. The wound was deteriorating despite pressure relief efforts, including a pressure relief mattress and wheelchair cushion. Local wound care was performed by a home nursing agency and consisted of wet-to-dry dressings.

Date 11/21: Patient was seen in initial wound care consultation. Appearance of the wound showed minimal pale granulation with an adherent area of fibrin slough. (Fig. 28.22A)

Wound measurements were 7 cm × 5 cm × 1.9 cm. Sharp débridement was performed, and cultures were obtained. Wound care regimen was changed to include an enzymatic débriding agent. Recommendations were made for continued aggressive pressure relief and nutritional support.

Date 12/06: Patient returned for wound clinic follow-up. Wound appearance showed persistent fibrin slough. (Fig. 28.22B)

Wound measurements were 6 cm × 3.5 cm × 2.2 cm. Wound culture from initial visit was positive for vancomycin-resistant enterococci and resistant *Pseudomonas aeruginosa.* Treatment with 25-kHz US was initiated. Fig. 28.22C shows improved appearance of the wound after US débridement. A quantitative wound culture was obtained after débridement. An enzymatic agent was continued, with aggressive pressure relief and nutritional support.

Date 12/13: Patient returned to wound care follow-up and repeat US therapy per protocol. Appearance showed increased quantity and quality of granulation tissue. (Fig. 28.22D) Wound measurements were 5.8 cm × 3.4 cm × 1.6 cm. The previous week's culture was negative for VRE or *Pseudomonas*. The wound was again treated with US. Before and after US quantitative wound culture was obtained. Wound care regimen is unchanged.

Date 01/17: Patient returned for wound care follow up. Appearance now shows complete granulation of wound base. (Fig. 28.22E) Wound measurements were 4.3 cm × 2.7 cm × 1.1 cm. Wound cultures remain negative for VRE and *Pseudomonas*.

Date 3/28: Wound closed. (Fig. 28.22 F)

Continued

▶ **Case Study 28•1** **Effect of 25-kHz Ultrasound Débridement on a Stage III Infected Sacral Pressure Ulcer—cont'd**

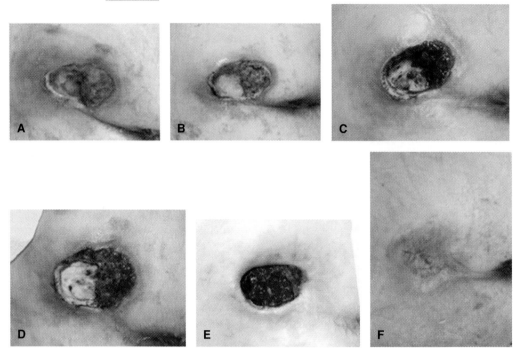

Figure 28•22 *Positive changes in a stage III infected sacral pressure ulcer after adding 25-kHz ultrasound débridement to the standard wound care regimen.*

References

1. Wood, RW, Loomis, AL: The physical and biological effects of high frequency waves of great intensity. Philosophical Magazine and Journal of Science 1927; 4:417–420.
2. Buchtala, V: The present state of ultrasonic therapy. Br J Phys Med 1952; 15:3–6.
3. Kuitert, JH, Harr, ET: Introduction to clinical application of ultrasound. Phys Ther Rev 1955; 35:19–22.
4. McDiarmid, T, Ziskin, MC, Michlovitz, SL: Therapeutic ultrasound. In: Michlovitx, SL (ed): Thermal Agents in Rehabilitation, ed. 3. Philadelphia, FA Davis, 1996, pp 168–212.
5. Ter Haar, GR: Basic physics of therapeutic ultrasound. Physiotherapy 1987; 73:110–114.
6. Dyson, M: Mechanisms involved in therapeutic ultrasound. Physiotherapy 1987; 73:116–120.
7. Williams, R: Production and transmission of ultrasound. Physiotherapy 1987; 73:113–116.
8. Stoner, HB, Barker, P, Riding, GS, et al: Relationship between skin temperature and perfusion in the arm and leg. Clin Physiol 1991; 11:27–40.
9. Sheffield, CW, Sessler, DI, Hopf, HW, et al: Centrally and locally mediated thermoregulatory responses alter subcutaneous oxygen responses. Wound Repair Regen 1996; 4:339–445.
10. Rabkin, JM, Hunt, TK: Local heat increases blood flow and oxygen tension in wounds. Arch Surg 1987; 122:221–225.
11. Babior, BM: Oxygen-dependent microbial killing by phagocytes. N Eng J Med 1978; 298:659–668.
12. Jonsson, K, Hunt, TK, Mathes, SJ: Oxygen as an isolated variable influences resistance to infection. Ann Surg 1988; 208:783–787.
13. Hunt, TK: The effect of varying ambient oxygen tensions on wound metabolism and collagen synthesis. Surg Gynecol Obstet 1972; 135:561–567.
14. Shandall, A, Lowndes, R, Young, HL: Colonic anastomic healing and oxygen tension. Br J Surg 1985; 72:606–609.
15. Baker, RJ, Bell, GW: The effect of therapeutic modalities on blood flow in the human calf. J Orthop Sports Phys Ther 1991; 13:23–27.
16. Borrell, RM, Parker, R, Henley, EJ, et al: Comparison of in vivo temperatures produced by hydrotherapy, paraffin wax treatment, and fluidotherapy. Phys Ther 1980; 60:1273–1276.
17. Abrahamson, DI, Mitchell, RE, Tuck, S Jr, et al: Changes in blood flow, oxygen uptake, and tissue temperatures produced by the topical application of wet heat. Arch Phys Med Rehabil 1969; 42:305–318.
18. Paul, ED, Imig, CJ: Temperature and blood flow studies after ultrasonic irradiation. Am J Phys Med 1955; 34:370–376.
19. Abrahamson, DI, Burnett, C, Bell, Y, et al: Changes in blood flow, oxygen uptake, and tissue temperature produced by therapeutic physical agents. I. Effect of ultrasound. Am J Phys Med 1960; 39:51–62.
20. Bickford, RH, Duff, RS: Influence of ultrasonic irradiation on temperature and blood flow in human skeletal muscle. Circ Res 1953; 1:534–538.
21. Lehmann, JF, Bruner, GD, Stow, RW: Pain threshold measurements after therapeutic application of ultrasound, microwaves, and infrared. Arch Phys Med Rehabil 1958; 39:560–565.
22. Young, S: Ultrasound therapy. In: Kitchen, S (ed): Electrotherapy: Evidence-Based Practice, ed. 11. New York, Churchill Livingstone, 2002, pp 211–230.
23. Watson, T: Available at: Ultrasound: The Basics, http//www.electrotherapy.org/electro/modalities/ultrasound%20basics.htm. Accessed on 04/08/09.
24. Xu, Z, Ludomirsky, A, Eun, LY, et al: Controlled ultrasound tissue erosion. IEEE Trans Ultrason Ferroelectr Freq Control 2004; 51:726–736.

25. Xu, Z, Fowlkes, JB, Rothman, ED, et al: Controlled ultrasound tissue erosion: The role of dynamic interaction between insonation and microbubble activity. J Acoust Soc Am 2005; 117:424–435.

26. Dyson, M, Suckling, J: Stimulation of tissue repair by ultrasound: A survey of the mechanisms involved. Physiotherapy 1978; 64:105–108.

27. Williams, AR: Release of serotonin from platelets by acoustic streaming. J Acoust Soc Am 1974; 56:1640–1649.

28. Williams, AR, Sykes, SM, O'Brien, WD: Ultrasonic exposure modifies platelet morphology and function in vitro. Ultrasound Med Biol 1977; 2:311–317.

29. Ginsberg, M: Role of platelets in inflammation and rheumatic disease. Adv Inflamm Res 1981; 2:53–58.

30. Altland, OD, Dalecki, D, Suchkova, VN, et al: Low intensity ultrasound increases endothelial cell nitric oxide synthase activity and nitric oxide synthesis. J Thromb Haemost 2004; 2:637–643.

31. Suchkova, VN, Baggs, RB, Sahni, SK, et al: Ultrasound improves tissue perfusion in ischemic tissue through a nitric oxide dependent mechanism. Thromb Haemost 2002; 88:865–870.

32. Johns, LD: Nonthermal effects of therapeutic ultrasound: The frequency resonance hypothesis. J Athletic Training 2002; 37:293–299.

33. Dyson, M: Non-thermal cellular effects of ultrasound. Brit J Cancer 1982; 45(suppl):165–171.

34. Dyson, M: Therapeutic applications of ultrasound. In: Nyborg, WL, Ziskin, MC (eds): Biological Effects of Ultrasound. Clinics in Diagnostic Ultrasound. New York, Churchill Livingstone, 1985, pp 121–133.

35. Harvey, W, Dyson, M, Pond, JB, et al: The stimulation of protein synthesis in human fibroblasts by therapeutic ultrasound. Rheumatol Rehabil 1975; 14:237–241.

36. Webster, DF, Pond, JB, Dyson, M, et al: The role of cavitation in the in vitro stimulation of protein synthesis in human fibroblasts by ultrasound. Ultrasound Med Biol 1988; 4:343–351.

37. Fyfe, MC, Chahl, LA: Mast cell degranulation: A possible mechanism of action of therapeutic ultrasound. Ultrasound Med Biol 8(suppl):62–65.

38. Young, SR, Dyson, M: Macrophage responsiveness to therapeutic ultrasound. Ultrasound Med Biol 16:809–816.

39. Maxwell, L, Collecutt, T, Gledhill, M, et al: The augmentation of leukocyte adhesion to endothelium by therapeutic ultrasound. Ultrasound Med Biol 1994; 20:383–390.

40. Ito, M, Azuma, Y, Ohta T, et al: Effects of ultrasound and 1,25-dihydroxyvitamin D3 on growth factor secretion in co-cultures of osteoblasts and endothelial cells. Ultrasound Med Biol 2000; 26:161–166.

41. Doan, N, Reher, P, Meghji, S, et al: In vitro effects of therapeutic ultrasound on cell proliferation, protein synthesis, and cytokine production by human fibroblasts, osteoblasts, and monocytes. J Oral Maxillofac Surg 1999; 57:409–419.

42. Young, SR, Dyson, M: The effect of therapeutic ultrasound on angiogenesis. Ultrasound Med Biol 1990; 16:261–269.

43. Francis, CW: Ultrasound enhanced thrombolysis. Echocardiography 2001; 18:239–246.

44. Reher, P, Harris, M, Whiteman, M, et al: Ultrasound stimulates nitric oxide and prostaglandin E2 production by human osteoblasts. Bone 2002; 31:236–241.

45. Niezgoda, JA: Reducing aerosolization and contamination: The next generation of ultrasound assisted wound therapy (abstract). Presented at: 22nd Annual Clinical Symposium on Advances in Skin & Wound Care, Nashville, TN, October 11–14, 2007.

46. Lauer, CG, Burge, R, Tang, DB, et al: Effect of ultrasound on tissue-type plasminogen activator-induced thrombolysis. Circulation 1992; 86:1257–1264.

47. Francis, CW, Onundarson, PT, Carstensen, EL, et al: Enhancement of fibrinolysis in vitro by ultrasound. J Clin Invest 1992; 90:2063–2068.

48. Blinc, A, Francis, CW, Trudnowski, JL, et al: Characterization of ultrasound-potentiated fibrinolysis in vitro. Blood 1993; 81:2636–2643.

49. Tachibana, K: Enhancement of fibrinolysis with ultrasound energy. J Vasc Interv Radiol 1992; 3:299–303.

50. Kudo, S: Thrombolysis with ultrasound effect. Jikeikai Med J 1989; 104:1005–1012.

51. Hamano, K: Thrombolysis enhanced by transcutaneous ultrasonic irradiation. Jikeikai Med J 1991; 106:533–542.

52. Kornowski, R, Meltzer, RS, Chernine, A, et al: Does external ultrasound accelerate thrombolysis? Results from a rabbit model. Circulation 1994; 89:339–344.

53. Riggs, PN, Francis, CW, Bartos, SR, et al: Ultrasound enhancement of rabbit femoral artery thrombolysis. Cardiovasc Surg 1997; 5:201–207.

54. Suchkova, V, Carstensen, EL, Francis, CW: Ultrasound enhancement of fibrinolysis at frequencies of 27 to 100 kHz. Ultrasound Med Biol 2002; 28:377–382.

55. McDonald, WS, Nichter, LS: Debridement of bacterial and particulate-contaminated wounds. Ann Plast Surg 1994; 33:142–147.

56. Suchkova, V, Siddiqi, FN, Carstensen, EL, et al: Enhancement of fibrinolysis with 40 kHz ultrasound. Circulation 1998; 98:1030–1035.

57. Suchkova, V, Carstensen, EL, Francis, CW: Ultrasound enhancement of fibrinolysis at frequencies of 27 to 100 kHz. Ultrasound Med Biol 2002; 28:377–382.

58. Bassett, RW, Cusenz, B, Meenaghan, MA, et al: Comparison of ultrasonic wound debridement to whirlpool and Silvadene® therapy in infected burn wounds. Anat Rec 1982; 202:164–170.

59. Schoenbach, SF, Song, IC: Ultrasonic debridement: A new approach in the treatment of burn wounds. Plast Reconstr Surg 1980; 66:34–37.

60. Scherba, G, Weigel, RM, O'Brien, WD: Quantitative assessment of the germicidal efficacy of ultrasonic energy. Appl Environ Microbiol 1991; 57:2079–2084.

61. Nichter, LS, McDonald, S, Gabriel, K, et al: Efficacy of debridement and primary closure of contaminated wounds: A comparison of methods. Ann Plast Surg 1989; 23:224–230.

62. Ukhov, AI, Petrus, VS, Shvaidetslaia, GV, et al: Potentiation of the action of antibiotics by ultrasound. Antibiot Med Biotekhnol 1985; 30:684–687.

63. Pitt, WG, McBride, MO, Lunceford, JK, et al: Ultrasonic enhancement of antibiotic action on gram negative bacteria. Antimicrob Agents Chemother 1994; 38:2577–2582.

64. Niezgoda, JA: The combined use of ultrasound assisted wound therapy and cadexomer iodine in the management of an abdominal wound complicated by tunneling and resistant organisms (abstract). Presented at: 22nd Annual Clinical Symposium on Advances in Skin & Wound Care, Nashville, TN, October 11–14, 2007.

65. Johnson, LL, Peterson, RV, Pitt, WG: Treatment of bacterial biofilms on polymeric biomaterials using antibiotics and ultrasound. J Biomaterials Science, Polymer Edition 1998; 9:1177–1185.

66. Carmen, JJ, Roeder, BL, Nelson, JL, et al: Ultrasonically enhanced vancomycin activity against *Staphylococcus epidermidis* biofilms in vivo. J Biomater Appl 2004; 18:237–245.

67. Qian, Z, Sagers, RD, Pitt, WG: The effect of ultrasonic frequency upon enhanced killing of *P. aeruginosa* biofilms. Ann Biomed Eng 1997; 25:69–76.

68. Pierson, T, Niezgoda, JA, Learmonth, S, et al: Abstracts of the 18th Annual Symposium on Advanced Wound Care, HMP Communications, San Diego, CA, April 23, 2005. Abstract 323.

69. Wagner, SA, Kavros, SJ, Vetter, EA, et al: The effect of mist ultrasound transport technology on common bacterial wound pathogens (abstract). Presented at: Symposium on Advanced Wound Care, Las Vegas, NV, April 30–May 3, 2001.

70. Niezoda, JA: Ultrasonic-assisted wound treatment vs MRSA, VRE, and other pathogens (abstract supplement). Presented at: 17th Annual Symposium on Advance Wound Care & Medical Research Forum on Wound Repair, Orlando, FL, May 2–5, 2004.

71. Serena, T, Lee, SK, Lam, K, et al: The impact of non-contact, non-thermal, low frequency ultrasound on bacterial counts in experimental and chronic wounds. Ostomy Wound Manage 2009; 55:22–30.

72. Conner-Kerr, T, Fox, H, Garland, E, et al: Effects of low frequency ultrasound delivered via the Qoustic Wound Therapy System™ on neuroblastoma (SHSY-5Y) viability and morphology (abstract). Symposium on Advanced Wound Care and Wound Healing Society, Dallas, TX, April, 26–29, 2009. Abstract LB-042.

73. Steed, DL, Donohoe, D, Webster, MW, et al: Effect of extensive debridement and treatment on the healing of diabetic foot ulcers. Diabetic Ulcer Study Group. J Am Coll Surg 1996; 183:61–64.

74. Breuing, KH, Bayer, L, Neuwalder, K, et al: Early experience using low frequency ultrasound in chronic wounds. Ann Plast Surg 2005; 55:183–187.

75. Stanisic, MM, Provo, BJ, Larson, DL, et al: Wound debridement with 25 kHz ultrasound. Adv Skin Wound Care 2005; 18:484–490.

76. Nelson, KM, Verhage, M, Niezgoda, JA, et al: Ultrasonic assisted wound treatment: A novel technique for wound debridement. Poster presented at: Clinical Symposium on Advances in Skin and Wound Care, October, 16–19, 2003, Chicago, IL. Abstract 36.

77. Tan, J, Abisi, S, Smith, A, et al: A painless method of ultrasonically assisted debridement of chronic leg ulcers: A pilot study. Eur J Vasc Endovasc Surg 2007; 33:234–238.

78. Suzuki, K, Cowan, L, Aronowitz, J, et al: Low frequency ultrasound therapy of lower extremity wounds significantly increases the peri-wound skin perfusion pressure (abstract). Presented at: the Diabetic Foot Global Conference. Los Angeles, CA, 2009.

79. Niezgoda, JA: Reducing painful debridement: Ultrasound assisted wound therapy (abstract supplement). Presented at: 22nd Annual Clinical Symposium on Advances in Skin and Wound Care, Nashville, TN, October, 11–14, 2007.

80. Gehling, ML, Samies, JH: The effect of noncontact, low intensity, low frequency therapeutic ultrasound on lower extremity chronic wound pain: A retrospective chart review. Ostomy Wound Manage 2007; 53:44–50.

81. Bell, AL, Cavorsi, J: Noncontact ultrasound therapy for adjunctive treatment of nonhealing wounds: Retrospective analysis. Phys Ther 2008; 88:1517–1528.

82. Waldrop, K, Serfass, A: Clinical effectiveness of non-contact, low frequency, non-thermal ultrasound in burn care. Ostomy Wound Manage 2008; 54:66–69.

83. Ramundo, J, Gray, M: Is ultrasonic mist therapy effective for debriding chronic wounds? J Wound Ostomy Continence Nurs 2008; 35:579–583.

84. Haan, J, Lucich, S: A retrospective analysis of acoustic pressure wound therapy: Effects on the healing progression of chronic wounds. J Am Coll Cert Wound Spec 2009; 1:28–34.

85. Kavros, SK, Liedl, DA, Boon, AJ, et al: Expedited wound healing with noncontact, low frequency ultrasound therapy in chronic wounds: A retrospective analysis. Adv Skin Wound Care 2008; 21:416–423.

86. Weichenthal, M, Mohr, P, Stegmann, W: Low-frequency ultrasound treatment of chronic venous ulcers. Wound Repair Regen 1997; 5:18–22.

87. Peschen, M, Weichenthal, M, Schopf, E, et al: Low frequency ultrasound treatment of chronic venous leg ulcers in an outpatient therapy. Acta Derm Venereol 1997; 77:311–314.

88. Kavros, SK, Miller, JL, Hanna, SW: Treatment of ischemic wounds with noncontact, low frequency ultrasound: The Mayo Clinic experience, 2004–2006. Adv Skin Wound Care 2007; 20:221–226.

89. Ennis, WJ, Valdes, W, Gainer, M, et al: Evaluation of clinical effectiveness of MIST ultrasound therapy for the healing of chronic wounds. Adv Skin Wound Care 2006; 19:437–460.

90. Ennis, WJ, Formann, P, Mozen, N, et al: Ultrasound therapy for recalcitrant diabetic foot ulcers: Results of a randomized, double-blind, controlled, multi-center study. Ostomy Wound Manage 2005; 51:24–39.

91. Kavros, SJ, Schenck, EC: Use of non-contact low frequency ultrasound in the treatment of chronic foot and leg ulcerations: A 51 patient analysis. J Am Podiatr Med Assoc 2007; 97:95–101.

92. Serena, T: Wound closure and gradual involution of an infantile hemangioma using a noncontact, low frequency ultrasound therapy. Ostomy Wound Manage 2008; 54:68–71.

93. Watson, T: Masterclass. The role of electrotherapy in contemporary physiotherapy practice. Man Ther 2000; 5:132–141.

94. Watson, T, Young, S: Therapeutic ultrasound. In: Watson, T: Electrotherapy: Evidence Based Practice. Edinburgh, Churchill Livingstone/Elsevier, 2008.

95. Watson, T: Ultrasound in contemporary physiotherapy practice. Ultrasonics 2008; 48:321–329.

96. Dinno, MA, Dyson, M, Young, SR, et al: The significance of membrane changes in the safe and effective use of therapeutic and diagnostic ultrasound. Phys Med Biol 1989; 34:1543–1552.

97. Leung, MC, Ng, GY, Yip, KK, et al: Effect of ultrasound on acute inflammation of transected medial collateral ligaments. Arch Phys Med Rehabil 2004; 85:963–966.

98. Mummery, CL: The effect of ultrasound on fibroblasts in vitro [dissertation]. University of London, 1978.

99. Mortimer, AJ, Dyson, M: The effect of therapeutic ultrasound on calcium uptake in fibroblasts. Ultrasound Med Biol 1988; 14:499–506.

100. Rasmussen, H, Weismann, DM: Modulation of cell function in the calcium messenger system. Rev Physiol Biochem Pharmacol, 1983; 95:111–148.

101. Dyson, M: Mechanisms involved in therapeutic ultrasound. Physiother J Chartered Soc Physiother 1987; 73(3):8–12.

102. Hashish, LL: The effects of ultrasound therapy on post-operative inflammation [dissertation]. University of London, 1986.

103. Yurt, RW: Role of the mast cell in trauma. In: Dineen, P, Hildick-Smith, G, (eds): The Surgical Wound. Philadelphia, Lea and Febiger, 1987, p 37.

104. Clark, RAF: Cutaneous tissue repair: Basic biologic considerations. J Am Inst Dermatol 1985; 13:701–707.

105. Dyson, M, Young, SR: Acceleration of tissue repair by low intensity applied during the inflammatory phase. American and Canadian Physical Therapy Association Joint Congress, 1988. Abstract RP-PL 97.

106. Goddard, N: Ultrasound has no anti-inflammatory effect. Ann Rheum Dis 1983; 42:582–586.

107. Gabbini, G, Ryan, GB, Majno, G: Presence of modified fibroblasts in granulation tissue and their possible role in wound contraction. Experientia 1971; 27:549–554.

108. Webster, DF: The effect of ultrasound on wound healing [dissertation]. University of London, 1980.

109. Dyson, M, Small, D: Effects of ultrasound on wound contraction. In: Millner, R, Corbet, U, (eds): Ultrasound Interactions in Biology and Medicine. New York, Plenum, 1983, pp 151–162.

110. ter Haar, GR, Dyson, M, Talbert, D: Ultrasonically induced contraction of mouse uterine smooth muscle in vivo. Ultrasonics 1978; 16:175–182.

111. Young, S: The effect of therapeutic ultrasound on the biological mechanisms involved in dermal repair [dissertation]. University of London, 1988.

112. Hogan, RD, Burke, KM, Franklin, TD: The effect of ultrasound on microvascular hemodynamics in skeletal muscle: Effects during ischemia. Microvasc Res 1982; 23:370–376.

113. Hosseinpour, AR: The effects of ultrasound on angiogenesis and wound healing [dissertation]. University of London, 1988.

114. Martin, BM, Gimbrone, MA Jr, Unanue, ER, et al: Stimulation of non-lymphoid mesenchymal cell proliferation by a macrophage-derived growth factor. J Immunol 1981; 126:1510–1515.

115. Bierman, W: Ultrasound in the treatment of scars. Arch Phys Med Rehabil 1954; 35:209–214.

116. Markham, DE, Wood, MR: Ultrasound for Dupuytren's contracture. Physiotherapy 1980; 66:55–58.

117. Dyson, M: The effect of ultrasound on the rate of wound healing and the quality of scar tissue. In: Mortimer, A, Lee, N (eds): Proceedings of the International Symposium on Therapeutic Ultrasound. Manitoba, Canadian Physiotherapy Association, Winnipeg, 1981, p 110.

118. Forester, JC: Mechanical, biomechanical, and architectural features of surgical repair. Adv Biol Med Phys 1973; 14:1–5.

119. Dyson, M, Pond, JB, Joseph, J, et al: The stimulation of tissue regeneration by means of ultrasound. Clin Sci 1968; 35:273–280.

120. Drastichova, V, Samohyl, J, Slavetinska, A: Strengthening of sutured skin wound with ultrasound in experiments on animals. Acta Chir Plast 1973; 15:114.

121. Shamberger, RC, Talbot, TL, Tipton, HW, et al: The effect of ultrasonic and thermal treatment on wounds. Plast Reconstr Surg 1981; 68:860.
122. Byl, NN, McKenzie, AL, West, JM, et al: Low-dose ultrasound effects on wound healing: A controlled study on Yucatan pigs. Arch Phys Med Rehabil 1992; 73:656.
123. Byl, NN, McKenzie, A, Wong, T, et al: Incisional wound healing: A controlled study of low and high dose ultrasound. J Orthop Sports Phys Ther 1993; 18:619.
124. Dyson, M, Franks, C, Suckling, J: Stimulation of healing of varicose ulcers by ultrasound. Ultrasonics 1976; 14:232–236.
125. Roche, C, West, J: A controlled trial investigating the effect of ultrasound on venous ulcers referred from general practitioners. Physiotherapy 1984; 70:475–482.
126. Callam, MJ, Harper, DR, Dale, JJ, et al: A controlled trial of weekly ultrasound therapy in chronic leg ulceration. Lancet 1987; 8:204–206.
127. Lundeberg, T, Nordström, F, Brodda-Jansen, G, et al: Pulsed ultrasound does not improve healing of venous ulcers. Scand J Rehab Med 1990; 22:195–197.
128. Eriksson, SV, Lundeberg, T, Malm, M: A placebo controlled trial of ultrasound therapy in leg ulceration. Scand J Rehab Med 1991; 23:211–213.

129. Johannsen, F, Gam, AN, Karlsmark, T: Ultrasound therapy in chronic leg ulceration: A meta-analysis. Wound Repair Regen 1998; 6:121–126.
130. Swist-Chmielewska, D, Franek, A, Brzezinska-Wcislo, L, et al: Experimental selection of best physical and application parameters of ultrasound in the treatment of venous crural ulceration. Pol Merkur Lekarski 2002; 12:500–505.
131. Dolibog, P, Franek, A, Taradaj, J, et al: Efficiency of therapeutic ultrasound for healing venous leg ulcers in surgically-treated patients. Wounds 2008; 20:334–340.
132. Paul, BJ, Lafratta, CW, Dawson, AR, et al: Use of ultrasound in the treatment of pressure sores in patients with spinal cord injury. Arch Phys Med Rehabil 1960; 41:438–449.
133. McDiarmid, T, Burns, PN, Lewith, GT, et al: Ultrasound and the treatment of pressure sores. Physiotherapy 1985; 71:66–70.
134. Nussbaum, EL, Biemann, I, Mustard, B: Comparison of ultrasound/ultraviolet-C and laser for treatment of pressure ulcers in patients with spinal cord injury. Phys Ther 1994; 74:812–823.
135. ter Riet, G, Kessels, AGH, Knipschild, P: A randomized clinical trial of ultrasound in the treatment of pressure ulcers. Phys Ther 1996; 76;1301–1311.

Light Therapies

Teresa Conner-Kerr, PT, PhD, CWS

Humans have always sought the rays of the sun to treat a plethora of ailments. The therapeutic use of sunlight is known as *heliotherapy*. Heliotherapy involves controlled exposure of the skin to sunlight, with graduated increases in exposure time to avoid burning. Due to differences in the types of light rays that are present during the day and during the different seasons, it is recommended that individuals expose their skin to the sun in the morning during the summer and at noon during the winter.[1] While many remain skeptical regarding the benefits of sunlight exposure, an evolving science is demonstrating the positive attributes of select wavelengths of light on human health. New technologies are being developed to deliver specific wavelengths of light to treat both physical and psychological ailments. The science behind these photo or light therapies, along with their potential benefits, will be discussed in this chapter.

Heliotherapy and Chromotherapy

To find evidence of the central importance of the sun in human history, one has only to look at the deities that humans have worshipped through the ages. Sun gods can be traced to every continent, and most take a male form. We find sun deities in mythology from Africa, China, Europe, Indonesia, and Japan.[2-4]

In the early cultures, Egypt was perhaps the civilization most influenced by the sun.[2-4] In Egyptian history, there were at least seven deities associated with the sun, including Ra, and many others followed. The ancient Egyptians recognized the curative powers of the sun and used sunlight to treat skin disorders and wounds. It is thought that early Egyptians constructed temples with rooms specifically designed to radiate particular colors of light. Individuals were placed in these rooms according to their illness. The Egyptians also used gemstones to produce colored light that was focused on sick individuals. This is probably the origin of color therapy, or *chromotherapy*. The Chinese also have a rich history of using color therapy to treat illness. This practice dates to the second millennium BC.

Like the Egyptians before them, the Greeks used color therapy in the treatment of illness. Sunlight was prescribed for a variety of ailments, including epilepsy, paralysis, asthma, and malnutrition. The Greeks built temples specifically designed to break up sunlight into its component colors of light.[1] Each color was used to treat a particular disorder. This practice was named *heliotherapy*, after Heliopolis, the Greek city of the sun. The term heliotherapy is used to refer to the treatment of human illness with sunlight. Traditionally, heliotherapy involved sunbathing. Sunbathing or sunlight exposure is still prescribed for certain illnesses today, especially seasonal affective disorder (SAD), or as it is commonly known, the winter blues. Most of the time, however, light treatment, or phototherapy, as it is commonly known in the medical field, involves exposure to specific wavelengths of light delivered via a variety of medical devices. We will discuss these devices in this chapter.

History of Heliotherapy

The first person to systematically record and describe the use of sunlight (heliotherapy) for medicinal purposes was Herodotus.[3,4] Through his travel and observations, Herodotus surmised a relationship between sun exposure and biological responses. In his writings he described the difference in degree of calcification between the skull bones of Egyptian and Persian soldiers. He ascribed the increased thickness of Egyptian soldiers' skulls to heightened sun exposure as a result of the cultural practice of shaving the scalp. Observations made by

Herodotus and others lead to the acceptance and widespread use of heliotherapy. This use persisted until the advent of Christianity. However, nothing more was written regarding heliotherapy until the 18th century.

In 1796 significant attention was refocused on the use of sunlight for the treatment of human maladies.[3,4] Scientists began to consider whether sunlight was beneficial to healing. Ebemaier, a student at the University of Gottingen, became the first person to propose a relationship between the lack of sun exposure and the development of rickets. Some years later, Niels Finsen wrote a paper on the influence of light on skin. He demonstrated the ability of sunlight to induce a delayed erythema in unprotected skin. It is also interesting to note that at about this same time the psychological effects of sun deprivation were also recorded. Liberman,[1] a recognized pioneer and expert on light in medicine, refers to the writings of Hufeland in 1796. Hufeland writes of the impact of light on the human psychological condition in his book, *Macrobiotics*. He states, "Even the human being becomes pale, flabby, and apathetic as a result of being deprived of light, finally losing his vital energy."

Shortly thereafter, Niels Finsen discovered the germicidal properties of sunlight. These properties were first demonstrated in 1877 using an unboiled Pasteur's solution.[3,4] Soon, Downes and Blunt demonstrated the growth-inhibiting effect of sunlight on bacteria. Downes and Blunt would later demonstrate that violet-colored light near the ultraviolet portion of the electromagnetic spectrum had the greatest bactericidal properties. However, it was not until later, when Duclaux (1885) and Ward (1892) demonstrated the bactericidal effects of sunlight in the absence of heat production, that the bactericidal properties of sunlight were accepted.

Bernhard and Morgan were the first to demonstrate that particular wavelengths of light were bactericidal.[3,4] They showed that ultraviolet (UV) radiation below 329 nm was bactericidal. In the years between 1890 and 1909, UV energy was shown to be bactericidal to many bacteria, including, *Mycobacterium tuberculosis, Staphylococcus, Streptococcus, Bacillus,* and *Shigella dysenteriae.* As a result of these findings, UV radiation became a common treatment for tuberculosis of the skin in this preantibiotic era.

The importance of this treatment in the early 1900s was reflected in the awarding of the Nobel Prize for Medicine and Science 1903 to Finsen for his work on the treatment of tuberculosis-induced skin lesions.[3,4] Since the early 1900s, research has focused on the use of UV radiation to control or prevent surgical wound infection, facilitate wound healing, and to treat acne. Interest in UV continues today, with researchers investigating its potential use for equipment and facility disinfection as well as treatment for skin wounds infected with antibiotic-resistant bacteria.

Similarly, there has also been interest in the potential health benefits of other wavelengths of light during the past two centuries.[1] In 1917, Einstein opened a new era in light therapy with his theoretical proposal regarding "stimulated emission of radiation."[5-7] This theoretical concept later gave rise to the groundbreaking work by Arthur Schawlow and Charles Townes in 1958 on the maser (microwave amplification by stimulation emission of radiation), the early forerunner of the laser (light amplification by stimulated emission of radiation). The maser, like the

laser, excites or adds energy to atoms or molecules, which leads to a biological response in animal and human tissue. With the creation of the first laser by physicist Theodore Maiman in 1960, interest grew quickly in the potential medical applications for this device. In 1971, the first study in an English-based journal demonstrating a positive effect of the laser on wound healing was published by Mester.[7] Interest in the applications of laser and other devices that use infrared technology has continued to grow since the 1970s, with a number of new technologies introduced to the wound-care market.

Electromagnetic Radiation— Terms and Definitions

Electromagnetic waves are generated as a result of the motion of electrically charged particles. Electromagnetic waves are also referred to as electromagnetic radiation because they radiate from electrically charged particles.[8] According to the electromagnetic wave theory, energy is transmitted by oscillatory motion. This oscillatory motion is described by the following terms:

1. *Wavelength* is the distance between identical points of a propagating wave of a given frequency. It is denoted by the lambda (λ) symbol and is measured in nanometers, centimeters, or meters.
2. *Peak* is the crest of the wave or point of maximal upward displacement.
3. *Trough* is the point of maximum downward displacement.
4. *Frequency* is the number of peaks that pass by a given point per second. It is denoted by the (f) symbol and measured in hertz (Hz) or 1 wave crest/second.

The following equation demonstrates the relationship of wavelength to frequency, where C = wave speed:

$$f = C/\lambda$$

As can be seen from the equation, wavelength is inversely proportional to frequency. Higher frequency electromagnetic waves have shorter wavelengths, whereas lower frequency electromagnetic waves have longer wavelengths. This concept is clearly illustrated in Figure 29.1.

The wavelength of radiant energy is important to consider when selecting a form of electromagnetic energy for patient treatment. Wavelength determines the depth of penetration by electromagnetic radiation.[8] Longer wavelengths penetrate deeper into tissue than do shorter ones. For example, a wavelength of 850 nm penetrates to 40 mm, an 800-nm wavelength penetrates to 30 mm, and a 660-nm wavelength penetrates to approximately 10 mm. It is also important to distinguish between depth of penetration and depth of effect, as the biological cascade of events set in motion by electromagnetic energy treatment can extend beyond the treatment depth.

Tissue pigmentation also influences absorption of electromagnetic energy, particularly in the ultraviolet band. Tissues with less pigmentation are more sensitive to the effects of ultraviolet energy due to decreased amounts of melanin available to protect the nucleus of keratinocytes. Tissues with greater melanin content provide increased protection from

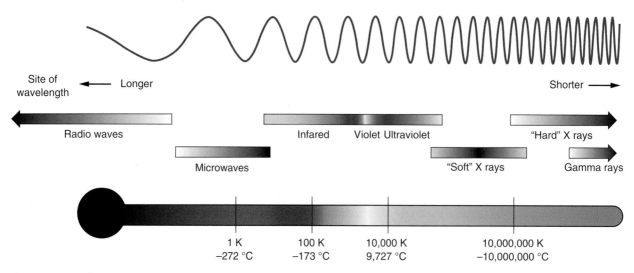

Figure 29•1 *Electromagnetic spectrum.*

ultraviolet radiation. As a result of this absorption, less energy is available to deeper tissues.

There are other factors that influence the treatment parameters of electromagnetic radiation for open wounds. Electromagnetic radiation travels through empty space as well as through air and other substances.[8] However, the velocity with which electromagnetic radiation travels decreases as the density of the intervening medium increases. Therefore, the density of tissues targeted for treatment with electromagnetic radiation must be taken into account when determining treatment intensities. High protein content in human tissues typically attenuates electromagnetic energy transmission, and the intensity of treatment must be adjusted.

Delivery of electromagnetic radiation to a target tissue is influenced by the medium in four different ways.[8] It is

1. reflected by the medium,
2. absorbed by the medium,
3. refracted by the medium, and
4. transmitted through the medium.

Electromagnetic energy reflected by the medium is lost to the target tissue, while electromagnetic energy refracted (bent on transmission) by the medium may not reach the intended tissue. Electromagnetic radiation that traverses a medium may be attenuated to some degree by absorption. However, the energy that leaves the tissue is lost to treatment. Only electromagnetic radiation that is absorbed by target tissues produces a treatment effect. Treatment parameters must be optimized to produce the intended effect on tissues.

Four separate laws govern treatment of human tissues, including open wounds, with electromagnetic energy.[8] They are Grotthuss-Draper law, inverse square law, cosine law, and Bunsen Roscoe law of reciprocity. According to the Grotthuss-Draper law, different wavelengths of electromagnetic energy induce different responses in human tissues, and the effect produced by these wavelengths is dependent on the degree of tissue absorption.

The inverse square law describes the relationship between the distance from the source of electromagnetic radiation to the target tissue.[8] This law states that the intensity of the treatment varies inversely with the square of the distance between the source and treatment target. As the treatment source is removed from the target tissue, the intensity decreases due to divergence of the electromagnetic energy waves. Therefore, the treatment source must be appropriately placed in relationship to the patient in order for an effective dose to be delivered.

The third law governing treatment with electromagnetic energy is the cosine law. This law states that the greatest absorption of energy occurs when the source is placed at right angles to the tissue.[8] This law speaks to the importance of treatment setup.

The final law, the Bunsen Roscoe law of reciprocity, states that intensity and duration of the treatment dose are inversely proportional.[8] This equation also demonstrates that the same energy dosage may be delivered while using different treatment times or intensities. This allows the clinician flexibility in designing treatment protocols while preserving the total energy delivery required to produce a biological response.

> **PEARL 29•1** When treating a patient with a phototherapy device,
>
> - select the wavelength required to induce the desired biological effect,
> - adjust intensity of energy delivered to tissues according to treatment distance,
> - place the device so that the light is delivered at a right angle to the treatment area, and
> - adjust the intensity of the treatment with changes in treatment times to ensure adequate delivery of energy and to prevent harm to tissues.

Electromagnetic Spectrum

The electromagnetic spectrum (EMS) is a range of radiant energy forms that vary in wavelength and travel in a self-propagating wave through space or matter. The EMS denotes the full range of electromagnetic radiations that have been documented. Electromagnetic radiation (EMR) includes, from lowest to highest frequency, radio waves, microwaves, infrared radiation, visible light, ultraviolet radiation, X-rays, and gamma rays. EMR is classified according to the frequency of the wave, with the highest frequency waves having the shortest wavelengths (see Fig. 29.1). Radio waves are the lowest-frequency waves, with wavelengths of thousands of meters (10^3 m) or as tall as a skyscraper, whereas the shortest waves are the gamma rays, which are as small as atomic nuclei. If measuring the various wavelengths of EMR in inches, the wavelengths of the EMR from shortest to longest range from 0.0000000000003937 of an inch to 21,456.69 inches. (Fig. 29.1)

EMR sources for phototherapy devices are found near the center of the EMS. Energy from the infrared, visible, and ultraviolet regions of the spectrum is used in photo or light therapy devices to treat open wounds. These three energy bands are present in sunlight. Sunlight radiation is a broad, continuous spectrum, with peak intensities in the blue-green spectrum. The importance of the blue-green spectrum of light to human health is becoming more apparent as our knowledge is increased in regard to chromophores.[1]

Infrared Radiation

The wavelength for infrared radiation (IR) is slightly longer than that for visible light.[8] IR is divided into two energy bands, a short or near band and a long or far infrared band. The short or near IR band is 800 to 1500 nm in length, and the long or far infrared band is 1500 to 15,000 nm in length. The frequency of these waves is lower than that for visible light.

Visible Light

Humans can detect visually only a small portion of the EMS (~1%).[8] Visible light falls in the 400- to 800-nm wavelength range of the EMS.

Ultraviolet Radiation

Ultraviolet radiation (UVR) has a slightly higher frequency and shorter wavelength than visible light. UVR wavelengths are between 180 and 400 nm.[9] UVR is typically separated into three energy bands based on their wavelengths and associated biological effects. These bands include ultraviolet-A (UVA), ultraviolet-B (UVB), and ultraviolet-C (UVC).[9-11]

Depending on the source referenced, the wavelength range for the three bands of UVR may vary slightly. The International Commission on Illumination (CIE) divided the bands into the following wavelength ranges: UVA (400–315 nm), UVB (315–280 nm), and UVC (280–100 nm).[10] On the other hand, the World Health Organization (WHO) defines the bands somewhat differently. According to the WHO, the UVA wavelengths range from 400 to 320 nm, UVB from 320 to 280 nm, and UVC from 280 to 200 nm.

Some sources also subdivide UVA into two distinct bands, UVA1 and UVA2.[9] UVA2 wavelengths are thought to induce biological effects more similar to those of UVB, the sunburn band. UVA1 wavelengths range from 340 to 400 nm and UVA2 wavelengths are 320 to 340 nm in length.

UVA, or long-wave, UV radiation is referred to as near UV and is the closest to the visible light component of the EMS. UVB is the middle component of the UVR spectrum of radiation and is known as the sunburn band. It is thought to be the most harmful of the two bands and is linked to photoaging and skin cancer.[12-16] UVC is the shortest wavelength of UVR. It does not penetrate the ozone layer and plays no role in inducing skin cancer due to excessive sun exposure. UVC is bactericidal in nature and has been used since the 1900s for its germicidal effects.

Biological Effects of the Spectral Components of Sunlight

Visible light can be broken up into its component wavelengths when shone through a prism (see Table 29.1). This process demonstrates the different colors of light found in visible light. These single wavelengths produce pure, spectral, or monochromatic colors. The order of color that is found when visible light is split into its components is wavelength dependent, with colors arranged from longest to shortest in the spectrum. The longest wavelength gives rise to the color red and the

Table 29•1 Component Colors of Visible Light and Their Wavelengths

Spectral Light Colors	Wavelength (nm)
Red	620–750
Orange	590–620
Yellow	570–590
Green	495–570
Blue	450–495
Violet	380–450

shortest to the color violet. The order of the wavelengths from longest to shortest can be remembered with the pneumonic "Roy G. Biv" (R, red; O, orange; Y, yellow; G, green; B, blue; I, indigo; V, violet). Wavelengths for individual colors are listed in Table 29.1.

Plants and Humans as Photocells

A photocell is a type of photodetector or light detector that is energized when energy strikes it. Plant cells are well-known photocells and use sunlight to generate the cellular energy source, adenosine triphosphate (ATP), from simple and complex carbohydrates through the process of photosynthesis. In this process, electromagnetic energy from the sun is converted to chemical energy by the green pigment chlorophyll. When electromagnetic radiation strikes a pigment and is absorbed, one of the three following events occurs: energy is dissipated as heat, energy is emitted as a longer wavelength (fluorescence), or radiation may trigger a chemical reaction, such as photosynthesis.

Work conducted by John Ott also demonstrated an effect of light on chloroplast behavior in the cells of the Elodea grass.[17] In his research, he found that chloroplasts followed an organized streaming pattern of movement inside the cells when exposed to full natural sunlight. However, filtering of ultraviolet light produced a clumping effect on chloroplast streaming. The chloroplasts would slow and form a clump at the end of the cell. When ultraviolet light was added back to the paradigm, the chloroplasts returned to their original organized streaming pattern. Changes in the composition of shorter and longer wavelengths of light through the use of filters produced similar reactions, with slowing and clumping of chloroplasts.

It is also interesting to note that Halobacteria, microbes that grow in high-salt environments, contain a purple pigment similar to that found in human retinas. This pigment known as bacteriorhodopsin generates ATP from sunlight in much the same way as chlorophyll.[17] The findings of the above studies suggest that the ability to harness energy from the sun by both plant and bacterial cells may be universal. Studies performed by Ott using epithelial cells from rabbit retinas further support a role for mammalian cells as photocells. Ott showed that filtering certain wavelengths of sunlight also produced changes in cell function. A blue-light filter induced changes in cell morphology, and filtering red light produced weakening of the cell wall.

Other studies examining the effect of different types of light on human physiology and behavior have provided evidence that human physiology can be influenced by sunlight and artificial light. Work by Hollwich in 1980 comparing the effects of artificial cool-white light versus full-spectrum sunlight demonstrated a differential effect on the production of adrenocorticotropic hormone (ACTH) and cortisol.[18] ACTH and cortisol levels were increased to stresslike levels in individuals exposed to the artificial cool-white light, whereas no changes were detected in individuals exposed to full-spectrum sunlight. Similarly, Gerard in 1958 demonstrated that red light increased normal subjects' blood pressure, respiratory rate, and eye-blink frequency when viewed on a screen.[1,19] These same physiological responses decreased in the presence of white or blue light.

Phototherapy Treatment Devices

Modern approaches to phototherapy began with the use of ultraviolet light boxes and infrared lamps and continue today with new light-emitting devices. Infrared heat lamps and Birtcher cold quartz lamps were routinely used by physical therapists in the past century. These devices gave way to halogen lamps, infrared bandages, lasers, and, more recently, light-emitting diodes and cluster probes.

Laser, the technology central to recent advancements in light delivery systems, entered the health-care arena in the 1960s. Lasers, which produce a uniform and coherent monochromatic beam of light, are used today at high intensities in surgical dissection and at low intensities to stimulate tissue healing, relieve pain, and reduce wound bioburden.

When lasers were originally introduced, they were used at high intensities to coagulate body proteins. Because of the high intensities used and their associated thermal effects, the term *hot laser* evolved. Subsequently, the terms *low-level,* or *cold, laser,* were developed to describe low-intensity laser treatments that did not produce significant elevation of tissue temperatures. These low-level, or cold, lasers were adopted for applications in wound and tissue healing and pain control due to their photo biomodulation effects. Therapists have been slow to adopt low-level or cold laser in the United States. Cold lasers are routinely used in Europe, China, and Canada for wound healing.

Current phototherapeutic devices employ a number of new technologies, including clusters of light-emitting diodes (LEDs), laser diodes (LDs), and superluminescent diodes (SLDs), cluster probes that use a mixture of the aforementioned light sources.[20,21] Lasers and laser diodes produce electromagnetic or light energy through the process of stimulated emission of photons of light. On the other hand, LEDs or SLDs produce light through a spontaneous emission of photons of light.

Lasers produce light that is coherent (beam stays together), collimated (directional), and monochromatic (one wavelength/color). In contrast, light produced by LEDs and SLDs is polychromatic in nature with a narrow range of wavelengths.[20] Since LEDs and SLDs are not collimated or coherent, they produce a wider beam of energy as compared to a true laser. The importance of this lack of coherence or collimation by LEDs and SLDs is not known since light that enters tissue is routinely refracted or bent by proteins in the tissues, particularly collagen. As a result, divergence of laser light occurs in tissue to some extent. Therefore, the effects of LEDs and SLDs may be comparable to those of lasers. However, this remains a topic of interest and research.

Light-Emitting Diodes

LEDs emit a form of radiant or light energy in the visible or infrared range of the electromagnetic spectrum. LEDs are not lasers.[20] They spontaneously release a narrow range of wavelengths from closely related color spectra that are minimally divergent.

Laser Diodes

LDs are true lasers that derive light from an LED source and as such produce a single wavelength of light.[20]

Superluminescent Diodes

SLDs use high-intensity, narrow-frequency, light-emitting diodes to deliver a focused treatment.[20] SLDs do not use laser technology but rather produce an amplified spontaneous emission with a narrow frequency range and beam angle that is wider than a LD but between that of an LED and LD.

Cluster Probes

Cluster probes combine the above-described technologies to produce a device that capitalizes on the benefits of each of the aforementioned devices.[20] Cluster probes contain multiple individual light sources that allow different wavelengths of electromagnetic energy to be mixed. The cluster probe design also allows a larger treatment area to be covered in a single treatment session.

Ultraviolet Radiation
Biological Effects

As discussed previously, wavelength determines the depth of penetration by electromagnetic radiation.[8,9] Longer wavelengths penetrate deeper into tissue than do shorter ones. Since ultraviolet radiation from the UVA band has the longest wavelength, this band of wavelengths penetrates the farthest into human skin. UVA penetrates to the level of the papillary layer of the dermis. This layer is located directly beneath the epidermis and constitutes the most superficial layer of the dermis.

UVB rays are intermediate in length between those of the UVA and UVC bands.[9] However, these somewhat shorter rays do completely penetrate the epidermis. UVB rays reach only as far as the stratum basale of the epidermis in intact skin while UVC radiation reaches just to the level of the upper layers of the epidermis. (Fig. 29.2)

Specific biological effects are also associated with particular wavelengths (see Table 29.1).[9] The shortest wavelengths of ultraviolet radiation are known for their bactericidal effects. Peak bactericidal effects are achieved with ultraviolet radiation from the 250 to 270 nm range in the C band. Shorter wavelengths also induce the greatest degree of erythema and tanning. These effects are seen at 254 nm and 297 nm for erythema and 254 nm and 299 nm for tanning. Interestingly, these peak effects on erythema induction and tanning occur with wavelengths from both the UVC and UVB bands. (Table 29.2)

Table 29•2	Comparison of the Peak Biological Effects of Ultraviolet-B Versus Ultraviolet-C	
Peak Biological Effects	**UVB**	**UVC**
Bactericidal	–	+
Erythema induction	+	+
Tanning	+	+

Under normal conditions, ultraviolet energy, primarily in the UVB band, causes acute, late, and chronic skin reactions.[10,14,22] Acute reactions are known as early cutaneous effects that occur during the first 60 hours of exposure. These acute effects include induction of immediate hyperpigmentation, epidermal hyperplasia, and acute inflammatory changes. Late changes occur after 60 to 336 hours of exposure and include secondary hyperpigmentation, hyperplasia, and fibrosis. Late changes include elastosis and carcinoma after chronic exposure for more than 336 total hours of exposure.

▶ **PEARL 29•2** For peak biological effectiveness, select a UVC lamp to treat wound infections.

Acute or Early Cutaneous Effects

As discussed above, erythema is a well-known effect of UV exposure. Erythema results from the acute inflammatory response of the skin to UV exposure. Erythema occurs due to a vasodilation of blood vessels in the papillary dermis secondary to the release of inflammatory mediators. Peak erythematous effects occur with exposure to 297-nm and 254-nm UV wavelengths.[9] These wavelengths cross both the UVC and UVB spectrum. However, it is important to note that under normal conditions human skin is not exposed to UVC as it does not penetrate the ozone layer.

Erythema produced by exposure to longer wavelengths has a greater latency and lasts for a longer period of time than that produced by shorter wavelengths.[9,11] Shorter wavelengths of UV appear to be more potent. UV-induced erythema is associated with a latent period of 2 to 3 hours. However, the exact mechanism that underlies this latent appearance of erythema is unknown. A number of theories have been offered to explain the latent induction of erythema. It is thought that this response is due to the synthesis of some diffusible biological mediator from damaged epidermal cells.[14] The time between exposure and synthesis of a mediator would explain the delay in response.

Once this mediator is produced, it is thought to diffuse to the dermis where it enhances blood vessel permeability. This mediator has yet to be identified. However, there are several likely candidates, including histamine, bradykinin, and prostaglandins.[14,35] In the past, prostaglandins were thought to be the most likely candidate for this role as a diffusible mediator, although work by Hensby using prostaglandin antagonists has produced inconclusive results.[23] Thus, the

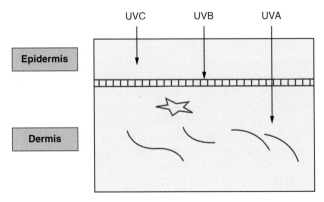

Figure **29•2** *Depth of penetration of ultraviolet radiation.*

role that prostaglandins play in mediating erythema is unclear.

Work by Brauchle has demonstrated a significant increase in vascular endothelial growth factor (VEGF) after ultraviolet radiation exposure.[24] VEGF expression in cultured keratinocytes after irradiation with sublethal levels of UVB increased. Irradiation of quiescent keratinocytes also produced an increase in mRNA levels as well as elevated levels of VEGF in culture media. Since VEGF is known to enhance vascular permeability, it is a likely candidate for mediating the induction of erythema after UV treatment.

Holtz has further defined the sequence of events that accompany the induction of erythema in the skin.[25] He showed that UV-induced erythema is accompanied by an intercellular edema in stratum spinosum or the prickle cell layer of the epidermis. The detection of this intercellular edema in stratum spinosum is also consistent with the separation of the upper and lower epidermal layers that occurs upon exposure to high-intensity UV radiation. The induction of this separation by the accumulation of intercellular fluid may account for the ability of UV radiation to stimulate débridement.

Holtz also demonstrated an accumulation of white cells in local blood vessels.[25] These phagocytic white blood cells may contribute through autolysis to the localized débriding effect observed by Conner-Kerr when rats were exposed to UVC treatment.[26] Increased lysosomal activity and leakage of lysosomal enzymes has been detected and may also contribute to this débridement effect.

An additional acute or immediate effect of UV exposure is skin thickening or hyperplasia.[14,27] UV is used clinically to stimulate reepithelialization. In a rat model, Conner-Kerr demonstrated decreased epibole and a more organized progression of epithelial cells across the wound base with brief exposure of the wound bed to UVC.[26] UV rays appear to increase epithelial hyperplasia. Research indicates that DNA changes are seen within 4 to 7 hours after irradiation of the epidermis.[10,14,22] Epidermal cells in stratum basale have been shown to accumulate glycogen at 12 hours and to increase RNA levels by 24 hours. These changes are seen in both the basal and prickle cell layer. These increased levels of RNA are thought to reflect ultimately an increased rate of protein synthesis to support repair mechanisms.

Work by Kaiser et al has directly demonstrated that UVB facilitates wound epithelialization.[28] This finding is further supported by the increased production of interleukin-1 (IL-1) by epithelial cells treated with UV radiation. Interleukin-1 is known to play a role in enhancing wound epithelialization, thus providing support for the current treatment approach of using UV to enhance epithelialization of wound bed. This treatment approach may be particularly useful when combined with sharp débridement for indolent wounds with fibrotic edges.

Late Cutaneous Effects

Late effects of long-term ultraviolet treatment include elastosis, loss of skin elasticity, and carcinoma.[22,29,34] Elastosis has been observed traditionally in the skin of individuals who have had significant lifetime exposure to ultraviolet B rays. Elastosis is characterized by the degeneration of the connective tissue fibers, collagen and elastin, in the dermis.

With histological evaluation of the skin, elastosis presents with basophilic degeneration of connective tissue fibers. These changes are not seen in adjacent areas that have been protected from prolonged exposure to ultraviolet B radiation from the sun.

Lifetime exposure to UVB radiation is well accepted as a causative factor in certain types of skin cancers.[10] Long-term exposure to UVB is known to cause the following:

1. Increased number of skin cancers at chronically exposed sites
2. Increased incidence of skin cancer in light-skinned people who work outdoors
3. Increased incidence of skin cancer in light-skinned people who live near the equator
4. Increased incidence of skin cancer in experimental animal models with prolonged exposure (hours)

Bactericidal Effects

Ultraviolet energy is bactericidal across all three bands. In vitro testing has demonstrated the effectiveness of UVA, UVB, and UVC radiation in killing microbes. However, longer treatment times are required to produce a decrease in bacterial numbers when a light source that produces all three bands of UV light is used as compared to a pure UVC source.[31] This contention is supported by work performed by High and High.[31] They demonstrated that UV radiation delivered by the Kromayer lamp (model 10), which produces wavelengths from all three UV bands, was effective in eliminating a wide range of wound pathogens in vitro. Treatment times were based on induction of skin erythema. Classically, UV treatment times have been determined based on the condition to be treated and the level of erythema desired (see Table 29.3). Doses delivered at a second degree erythemal dose (E_2) and greater were effective in killing common wound pathogens. However, complete eradication of microorganisms was obtained only with a fourth degree or E_4 dose which resulted in severe damage to the skin.

In contrast, UVC light treatment in vitro has been shown to effectively eliminate a number of different wound pathogens, including those expressing antibiotic resistance with treatment times as short as 3 seconds.[32,33] These short treatment times are well below those required to induce even an E_1 response.

UVC light treatment delivered with the V-254 lamp, which selectively emits UVC energy, produced a 99.99% kill rate for many common wound pathogens.[32,33] In vitro testing under optimal growth conditions for microbes demonstrated the effectiveness of UVC irradiation in eradicating both prokaryotic organisms such as bacteria and eukaryotic organisms such as yeast or multicellular fungi at short exposure times. Furthermore, UVC was shown to be effective in killing multicellular eukaryotic wound pathogens at treatment times shorter than those currently advocated for prokaryotic (bacterial) organisms. However, research findings indicated that multicellular eukaryotic organisms require 10 times the exposure time (30 seconds) for a 99.9% kill rate as compared with the most susceptible eukaryotic organism (3 seconds).

Research also indicates that short UVC exposure times can produce a 99.99% kill rate for common antibiotic-resistant

Table 29•3 Erythemal Dosing

Dose	Time to Response	Time to Resolution	Skin Reaction
Suberythemal (SED)	Not detectable visually	NA	None observed
Minimal erythemal (MED)	4–6 hours	Within 24 hours	Slight reddening
First degree erythemal (E_1)	4–6 hours	48 hours	Mild reddening
Second degree erythemal (E_2)	4–6 hours	3–4 days	Mild sunburn with exfoliation and pigmentation of the skin
Third degree erythemal (E_3)	2 hours	Several days	Severe sunburn with significant erythema, blistering, exfoliation, and pigmentation
Fourth degree erythemal (E_4)	2 hours	Several days	Same as E_3 but with significant tissue swelling and exudate

bacterial pathogens in vivo as well as in vitro (see Table 29.4).[32] Using an optimal growth model in vitro, 99.99% of methicillin-resistant *Staphylococcus aureus* (MRSA) can be killed with only 5 seconds of UVC irradiation. Similar results were obtained for vancomycin-resistant enterococci (VRE). Additionally, a 100% reduction of MRSA was found in rats with acute surgical wounds that were inoculated with 10^6 MRSA and then exposed to once-daily UVC treatment for 30 seconds for 5 days.[26] Interestingly, rat acute surgical wounds treated with a UV light source that produced all three UV light bands (UVA, UVB, UVC) did not produce a difference in posttreatment bacterial levels. UVC is known to be the most effective band for killing microorganisms, with peak bactericidal effects in the 250 to 270 nm range. Therefore, the mixed light source may not have produced a high enough percentage of UVC to be effective in killing microorganisms.

Effects of Ultraviolet Irradiation on Wound Healing in Animal Models

A number of different animal models have been used to study the effects of UVA, UVB, and UVC irradiation on wound healing (see Table 29.5). These models include the rat, hairless guinea pig, rabbit, and pig.[34-38] UVB had positive effects on wound healing in both the rat and rabbit, but not the hairless guinea pig. UVA and UVB treatment of rat acute surgical wounds resulted in a significantly increased rate of wound closure between day 4 and day 15 of treatment compared with untreated controls on the contralateral side of the animal. No decrement in wound tensile strength was detected over this time frame. Results from this study also suggest that the effects of UVA and UVB are localized and not systemic, since healing of the contralateral wounds was not enhanced.

Similarly, UVA and UVB modestly increased the rate of tissue regeneration in acute full-thickness wounds of the pinna of rabbit ears.[34] The UVA- and UVB-treated wounds healed more rapidly than untreated controls. Positive findings were also documented using histopathological analysis. Significant increases in epithelialization rates and collagen deposition were detected as compared with untreated control tissue.

In contrast, the opposite effects were detected using the hairless guinea pig model. Acute surgical wounds induced in hairless guinea pigs pretreated with UVA or UVB radiation every other day for 16 weeks did not exhibit enhanced wound closure rates.[36,37] Wound tensile strength was significantly less in both the UVA- and UVB-treated animals, and marked endothelial swelling and eosinophilic infiltration was detected in

Table 29•4 Ultraviolet-C Treatment Time (sec) Required to Produce 99.99% Kill

	MRSA	VRE	*Pseudomonas*
In vitro			
3 sec			*
5 sec	*	*	
In vivo			
30 sec	*		

MRSA, methicillin-resistant *S. aureus*; VRE, vancomycin-resistant enterococci.

Table 29•5 Effects of Ultraviolet-A, -B, and -C on Wound Healing in Animal Models

	UVA	UVB	UVC
Rats	+	+	+
Hairless guinea pig	–	–	ND
Rabbit	+	+	ND
Pig	ND	ND	0

+, positive effect; –, negative effect; 0, no observed effect; ND, no data.

the irradiated group. Pure UVA irradiation of wounds in hairless guinea pigs also produced decreased wound tensile strength. However, the relevance of these studies remains unclear as the unusually long duration of treatment (16 weeks in the first study and 21 weeks in the second study) and the use of a pretreatment UV paradigm are incongruent with current clinical practice.

In comparison, no deleterious effects of UVC on wound healing rates have been demonstrated using a porcine or rodent model. Research using the porcine model did not demonstrate any significant effect of UVC irradiation on wound tensile strength.[38] However, studies using an acute surgical wound model in rodents demonstrated that a 30-second UVC treatment once daily for 5 days produced a cleaner and smoother transition area between the periwound and the wound bed with no tissue curling.[39] The pattern of wound contraction was also altered as compared to the infected, untreated control. These findings are consistent with those of Morykwas et al.[40] Morykwas et al demonstrated increased secretion of fibronectin into the culture medium of fibroblasts after UVC irradiation.[40] Fibronectin is an extracellular matrix protein that appears to play a role in wound contraction. It provides a point of contact for fibroblast migration and contraction of the wound bed by myofibroblasts. Enhanced fibronectin secretion may account for the positive effects observed after UVC treatment of rat acute surgical wounds. (Table 29.5)

Effects of Ultraviolet Irradiation on Human Tissue

Experimental data exist to suggest a positive role for UV irradiation in enhancing wound healing; however, very few well-controlled clinical studies have been done. The majority of studies that have been conducted, dating to 1945, have found positive effects of UVA and UVB on wound healing.[41] An article detailing the increased rate of wound healing and reduction of wound infection in two soldiers, one with a traumatic wound and the other with a pressure wound, was published by Stein and Shorey.[41] Both wounds were chronic and had not progressed toward healing until UV treatment was instituted. Both ulcers healed after the initiation of UV therapy. The traumatic wound healed within 10 days of initiating UV therapy, and the pressure ulcer healed in less than 2 months.

A randomized, controlled trial involving elderly individuals with superficial pressure ulcers demonstrated enhanced healing rates.[42] UV-treated pressure ulcers closed in approximately 6 weeks compared with an average of 10 weeks for control ulcers. A clinical study conducted by Crous and Malherbe found similar results in individuals with ulcers due to venous insufficiency.[43] However, closure was not achieved. UVA and UVB treatment parameters were based on erythemal dosing as described previously. An E_1 dose was used for periwound skin and granulation tissue and an E_4 dose for necrotic tissue.

Nussbaum et al also examined the effects of UV irradiation on pressure ulcer healing.[44] She used a mixed protocol of UVC and ultrasound compared to cold laser or moist wound healing. While the combination of UVC and ultrasound treatment was found to enhance healing of pressure ulcers over that of cold laser or moist wound healing, it is difficult to determine the exact effect of UVC since it was delivered in combination with the ultrasound treatments. Therefore, it is not clear as to what effect either of the modalities had individually.

The effects of UVC on skin infections have also been studied. The effectiveness of UVC on skin infections was studied by Taylor in 56 individuals.[45] These individuals had skin lesions due to the following infections: tinea pedis, tinea capitis, sporotrichosis, and tinea corporis. Treatment times between 2 and 5 minutes were delivered over a 5- to 7-day period, with individuals receiving an average of 3.2 treatments. A positive effect was demonstrated in 50 patients, with most showing significant clearing of the infection within 1 week.

Taylor et al also demonstrated the effectiveness of UVC irradiation on reducing bacterial numbers in individuals undergoing total joint arthroplasty.[46,47] UVC energy was delivered through an overhead light source for 10 minutes after the surgical procedure was initiated. Study results indicated that the UVC treatment was effective in significantly reducing bacterial levels in both the surgical theatre air and surgical wounds, with the effectiveness of treatment increasing with higher doses. UVC treatment delivered at 100 $\mu W/cm^2$ (study group $N = 18$) produced an 87% decrease in bacterial levels compared to a 92% decrease with 300 $\mu W/cm^2$ (study group $N = 13$).

Work by Moggio et al demonstrated similar results with significantly lower numbers of airborne bacteria detected over the surgical site after UV irradiation.[48] Only 0.15% of 1322 individuals undergoing surgery experienced a surgical site infection following UV irradiation of the air above the surgical site. Berg et al also demonstrated similar findings in operating rooms when a blue light application was compared to UV treatment.[49] The UV-treated room produced operating room air quality that was similar to air quality produced by ultraclean air filtering. Additionally, no adverse effect of UVC exposure was detected on operating room personnel by either Berg or Taylor.[46,49]

Recent research has also examined the effectiveness of UVC in decreasing bacterial numbers in chronic wounds.[50] The following bacteria, *Pseudomonas aeruginosa*, *S. aureus*, and MRSA were reduced with a single UVC treatment for 180 seconds. Consistent with in vitro testing, *P. aeruginosa* was most sensitive to the UVC treatment.[33] UVC was not as effective against MRSA as compared to the other bacteria. Only a one-level reduction in MRSA numbers was detected after the standard 180-second treatment time.[11] Data from this small study indicate that multiple treatments of 180 seconds may be required to completely eradicate MRSA from chronic wounds.

Ultraviolet-C Treatment Paradigm

The paradigm presented for ultraviolet treatment is based on a comprehensive review of the literature and expert opinion. Evolving evidence supports a role for ultraviolet from the C band in the treatment of wounds with detrimental levels of wound pathogens. In the past, wound infection has been defined as 10^5 microorganisms per gram of tissue harvested from a wound bed. However, this definition has been reconsidered in recent years. Currently, wound infection is defined in relation to a number of factors, including patient (host) response, virulence of the offending microorganism, and number of microorganisms present in a gram of wound tissue.

In the past, erythemal dosing was used to determine the treatment times for an infected wound. Increasing degrees of erythema and ultimately "burning" were induced in the patient's skin. The degree of erythema prescribed for treatment was dependent on the state of the wound and the response of the individual's skin to ultraviolet radiation. Slow-healing wounds with high numbers of bacteria were treated with either a first-degree (E_1) or second-degree (E_2) erythemal dose. An E_1 dose induces a slight reddening of the skin that resolves in 48 hours, and an E_2 dose is similar to a mild sunburn. All doses are calculated based on individual skin response. Treatment times must be determined with test exposures to ensure particular skin responses.

The erythemal dosing regimen may prove beneficial when applied at lower erythemal doses since it induces an acute inflammatory response by the individual's skin. This acute inflammatory response may assist with clearing offending microorganisms and stimulating healing through the activation of the immune system, recruitment of white cells, and release of endogenous growth factors.

However, it is the contention of the author and colleagues that treatment times based on minimal lethal dose for individual organisms may be more effective and may minimize or prevent damage to treated tissues.[26,32,33] Strong erythemal doses produce direct tissue damage through inducing a burn. In vitro and in vivo studies in the author's laboratory indicate that periods of time as little as 5 seconds long are required to eliminate most bacteria in vitro and 30 seconds in vivo. In a small case series, 180-second exposure was required to more effectively eliminate antibiotic-resistant bacteria in humans.[50] However, extensive studies examining reduced times with multiple exposures versus longer treatment times over fewer exposures has yet to be performed. Optimum parameters with the total energy required to eliminate individual wound pathogens have not been established. The treatment paradigm proposed in Figure 29.3 is based on the best available evidence.

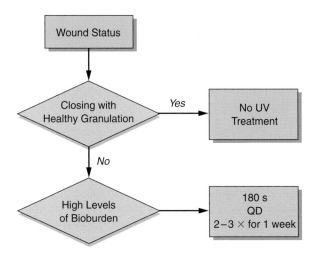

Figure 29•3 *UVC treatment paradigm for wounds with high levels of bioburden.*

Ultraviolet Equipment Selection for Stimulating Wound Healing

UVA and UVB have been studied to the greatest extent in relation to wound healing in both animal and human studies. Research indicates that UVB in particular stimulates wound healing through the promotion of increased epithelialization and dermal vascularity. Molecular studies suggest a role for UVB radiation in facilitating wound healing through the stimulation of cytokines such as IL-1 or VEGF.[51,52] However, skin damage and skin cancer is also associated with long-term exposure to this band of UV radiation. For this reason, short exposure times for a very limited number of total exposures should be considered, with protection in place for the surrounding epidermis.

Very limited data are available to support the use of UVC to stimulate wound healing in humans or animals. A study by Nussbaum et al demonstrated increased rates of pressure ulcer healing in individuals treated with UVC and ultrasound combined.[44] The observed rates of healing were greater than those observed in a randomized controlled clinical trial using UVB radiation. However, no definitive conclusion can be drawn since Nussbaum employed a combined ultrasound/UVC treatment group without a separate ultrasound or UVC treatment group for comparison.

Ultraviolet-A and Ultraviolet-B Equipment Selection

UVA and UVB lamps may be used to stimulate wound healing. A number of UVA/UVB lamps are available for purchase. Many of these lamps also have an infrared generator. Because of their design, these lamps may be prone to tilting or turning over, and the clinician is encouraged to select a high-quality model with a stable base.

Ultraviolet-C Equipment Selection

UVC lamps may be used to stimulate wound healing but are most often used for their bactericidal effects. The peak germicidal wavelengths range from 250 to 270 nm in length. Peak effects are often associated with the 254-nm wavelength. A number of different types of UVC generators are available that selectively produce UVC at the 254-nm wavelength. Most of today's UVC generators are halogen lamps, and they are readily available. When selecting a lamp, the clinician must be careful to choose one that emits a nearly pure UVC spectrum with peak production of the 254-nm wavelength in order to obtain the greatest effect. The clinician is also advised to select a halogen lamp with the largest faceplate so that larger wounds can be treated more efficiently.

Periwound Preparation

The periwound should be protected from UV exposure due to the possible risk for skin damage and resulting carcinoma, particularly with the UVB lamps. Protection of the skin can be easily accomplished with draping materials or application of petrolatum jelly.

▶ **PEARL 29•3** Cover the periwound area with petrolatum jelly or draping material to prevent any unwanted skin exposure.

Wound Bed Preparation

UV energy will not penetrate most dressings, including transparent film dressings. All dressings should be removed from the wound bed and the wound bed débrided. UV energy is not deeply penetrating, and necrotic tissue should be removed to enhance wound bed exposure. The wound should also be cleansed to remove necrotic tissue and loose debris. This can be accomplished by a variety of mechanisms, including pulsatile lavage with suction or through the use of ultrasonic débridement. Wounds covered with minimal necrotic tissue may be flushed with saline using a syringe or pressurized canister. One research study has demonstrated an added benefit to decreasing microorganism numbers in an in vitro wound model when coadministering jet lavage and UV radiation.[53]

> **PEARL 29•4** Remove all dressing material and cleanse the wound bed in order to provide maximum exposure of the target tissues to the ultraviolet light. UVC will not penetrate most dressing materials.

Determining Treatment Distance

UVC lamps are placed 1 inch or 2.54 cm from the wound surface. Many lamps have 1-inch spacers attached to their undersurface that will allow the lamp to be placed on the patient's skin over the top of the wounds. If spacers are not available, then they can be easily constructed from sterile tongue depressor tips and affixed to the lamp. They should be replaced at each treatment session.

UVA and UVB lamps should be placed approximately 30 inches from the wound bed. However, treatment distances may vary depending on selected treatment intensities. The following laws should be observed during patient treatments when using either a UVA/UVB lamp or a UVC lamp: (1) Grotthuss-Draper law, (2) inverse square law, (3) cosine law and (4) Bunsen Roscoe law of reciprocity.

Indications for Ultraviolet Treatment

UV treatment is indicated for the following wounds:

1. Recalcitrant wounds
2. Necrotic wounds
3. Infected acute or chronic wounds

Contraindications for Ultraviolet Treatment

UV treatment is contraindicated for the patient with the following conditions:

1. Pulmonary tuberculosis
2. Hyperthyroidism
3. Systemic lupus erythematous
4. Cardiac, renal, and hepatic disease
5. Acute eczema or psoriasis
6. Herpes simplex

Adverse Reactions

Adverse reactions may occur with UV treatment. These reactions include severe pain due to itching or burning. If the patient experiences these reactions, then UV therapy should be discontinued. Application of a hydrogel dressing may provide skin cooling and pain relief.

Administration of Ultraviolet Therapy

UV therapy should be delivered by a skilled individual licensed in the application of biophysical energy technologies.

Documentation

The following should be documented in the patient record:

- Treatment duration
- Treatment frequency
- Type of UV lamp
- UV lamp output (intensity and dosage)
- Patient position
- Wound location
- Preparation and protection of the periwound
- Preparation of the wound bed
- Patient response to treatment

Visible and Infrared Light (Lasers, Light-Emitting Diodes, and Superluminescent Diodes)

Biological Effects of Lasers

The low-level or cold laser produces a variety of effects in biological tissues.[54,55] These effects are described as photobiomodulation. Laser has been shown to both stimulate (photobiostimulation) and inhibit (photobioinhibition) biological processes in both animals and humans. These effects result from the interaction of chromophores (naturally occurring pigments in the body) with the light energy provided by the laser.

Both plants and animals have cells that contain chromophores. These chromophores are involved in day-to-day biochemical processes necessary for life, including photosynthesis for plants and cellular respiration in animals. Laser light derived from the infrared or visible light (600–1200 nm) sections of the electromagnetic spectrum is absorbed by biological pigments or chromophores in plants and animals.[1,2]

The energy provided by a laser light source powers cellular processes. This energy can penetrate the dermis and interact with a number of human chromophores.[1,2,54-56] Mammalian chromophores include respiratory chain enzymes, melanin, hemoglobin, and myoglobin. Longer wavelength of light such as those derived from the infrared spectrum influence a greater number of cellular chromophores as compared to the shorter wavelengths of the visible light spectrum. Visible light energy is absorbed by melanin, hemoglobin, and myoglobin.

Research indicates that cells from damaged tissues are more sensitive to the effects of laser light as compared to normally functioning cells.[57] Inflamed, edematous, and ischemic tissues have been shown to benefit from low-level laser energy. Cells in these tissues have a lower threshold for excitation or energy transfer and thus benefit from exposure to light energy.

▶ Case Study 29•1 | UVC for the Treatment of an Infected Pressure Ulcer

Medical History

R.J. was a 72-year-old nonambulatory male resident of a long-term care facility with a trochanteric pressure ulcer. His medical diagnoses included cancer, hypertension, and diabetes. He required maximum assistance for bed mobility. He had previously developed a pressure ulcer in his sacral area.

Reason for Referral

Client was referred to physical therapy due to impaired bed mobility and the presence of a clinically infected stage III trochanteric pressure ulcer.

Wound Examination

The wound was a stage III trochanteric pressure ulcer with copious drainage and a foul odor. A hardened black eschar had recently been removed. The wound margin was indurated, and the periwound was erythematous. Semiquantitative swab

cultures of this wound indicated that it contained high numbers of methicillin-resistant *S. aureus* (MRSA).

Treatment Plan and Outcome

Beginning on April 4, the wound was further débrided and cleansed. A single application of UVC was applied to the wound bed for 180 seconds at 1 inch from the wound bed surface at a dose of 15 mW. To determine if one application of UVC for 180 seconds was effective, the wound was cultured and the culture submitted for analysis by the semi-quantitative swab method. The periwound skin was protected with a sterile drape. Results from the clinical laboratory tests indicated that the wound had very low numbers of microorganisms after 180 seconds of UVC treatment. This case study demonstrates the rapid treatment effects of UVC therapy in reducing the number of bacteria on the surface of the wound bed.

Much of the beneficial effects of lasers are mediated by light energy from the 600 to 900 nm range of the electromagnetic spectrum.[54,56] Wavelengths in this range produce the following biological effects: increased cellular proliferation and differentiation, increased mitochondrial production of ATP, increased RNA synthesis, and increased release of chemotactic factors from mast cells.[54,58] (Table 29.6) Other positive biological effects of laser light generated from these wavelengths that may facilitate wound healing include enhanced leukocyte infiltration, increased macrophage activity, increased fibroblast proliferation, increased growth factor release, enhanced epithelialization rates, and improved tissue tensile strength (see Table 29.6).

> ▶ **PEARL 29•5** Consider phototherapy devices delivering wavelengths of energy between 600 and 900 nm to promote wound healing.

Table 29•6 | Biological Effects of Laser Light

Biological Effects

- Increased cellular proliferation
- Increased cellular differentiation
- Increased mitochondrial ATP production
- Increased RNA synthesis
- Increased release of chemotactic factors
- Increased leukocyte infiltration
- Increased macrophage activity
- Increased fibroblast proliferation
- Increased growth factor release
- Increased epithelialization rates
- Increased tissue tensile strength

Effects of Laser Therapy on Specific Wound Healing Processes

Laser light therapy stimulates many of the cells involved in the wound healing process (see Table 29.7). The processes listed below are enhanced by laser therapy.

Fibroplasia/Fibroblast Proliferation

Low-level laser light enhances fibroplasia through the stimulation of macrophages. Enhanced synthesis and release of chemical mediators by macrophages that play an important role in directing fibroblastic proliferation have been detected after exposure to the 660-, 820-, and 870-nm wavelengths.[59,60] Fibroblast proliferation in cell culture has also been shown to increase when cocultured with macrophage-like cells receiving laser treatment at the pulsing frequencies of 2.28, 18.24, and 292.30 Hz.[58,61]

Collagen Synthesis

Low-level laser exposure has been shown to stimulate collagen production in a number of in vitro studies.[60-62] Human skin fibroblast irradiation with a helium-neon laser increased collagen production up to four times that of controls when a treatment paradigm of four consecutive exposures at 24-hour intervals was used.[60] In another study, human skin fibroblasts exposed to helium-neon and gallium arsenide lasers demonstrated an enhanced proliferation rate of fibroblasts and procollagen synthesis.[61]

Muscle Cell Proliferation

Research has also demonstrated a positive effect of low-level laser on muscle cell proliferation. Cultured muscle satellite/precursor cells and isolated muscle fibers exposed to low-level laser have been shown to increase their proliferation rate.[63] Low-level laser also increased the pool of satellite cells available for differentiation into muscle cells.

Table 29•7 Effects of Specific Wavelengths of Laser Light on Wound Healing Processes		
Wound Healing Processes	**Wavelengths**	**Type of Laser**
Stimulation of macrophage activity	660, 820, 870	Semiconductor
Collagen synthesis	633	Helium-neon
ATP synthesis	633	Helium-neon
Immune system stimulation (T-cell and B-cell activity)	488, 541, 633	Argon, helium-neon
Bacterial binding by lymphocytes	633	Helium-neon

ATP Synthesis

A positive effect of low-level lasers on adenosine triphosphate (ATP) production by mitochondria has also been demonstrated in vitro.[65,67] Cultured mitochondria isolated from Wistar rat livers were treated with low-level laser irradiation by a helium-neon laser using 5 J/cm^2. ATP synthesis was increased by 70% as compared to untreated controls. This effect appeared to be mediated by an enhanced rate of electron transport in the inner membrane of mitochondria, as the effect could be quenched with an electron transport inhibitor.

Immune System Stimulation

Energy emitted by low-level lasers has also been shown to stimulate the activity of white cells harvested from individuals with breast cancer. T- and B-lymphocyte activity increased in vitro after treatment of cells with either a helium-neon (633 nm) or an argon (488 or 541 nm) laser at an energy density of 30 W/cm^2.[65] Both the argon and helium-neon laser stimulated T- and B-lymphocyte activity, which is important for fighting bacterial invaders. Longer-duration time periods resulted in more active T cells, with the maximum increase in percentage of active T cells detected at 10 minutes of irradiation time. Argon laser treatment at 488 nm produced the largest increase in B cells as compared to controls.

Additionally, low-level laser irradiation has also been found to increase the ability of lymphocytes to bind microorganisms.[65,66] Lymphocytes from human peripheral blood exposed to a helium-neon laser at an energy density of 5 J/cm^2 demonstrated an increased affinity for salmonella. Increased binding sites for salmonella and an increased ability of lymphocytes to bind salmonella were found after treatment with the helium-neon laser.

Oxygen Transfer

A study by Asimov et al indicates that laser may enhance tissue healing by increasing the effectiveness of oxygen transfer by oxyhemoglobin from red blood cells in blood vessels of the skin.[56] Absorption of photons of light causes the dissociation of oxygen from the hemoglobin molecule so that it is available for transfer to tissues. The increased effectiveness with which oxygen is transferred to the tissues may relieve hypoxic states that are often associated with chronic wounds. It may also provide relief to ischemic tissues. In determining dosage and wavelength selection (laser choice), the absorption of laser light by melanin and scattering caused by collagen must be taken into account. Wavelengths of 585 nm appear to be more effective in promoting molecular oxygen dissociation and thus availability to tissues. However, more research is needed to confirm the optimal wavelengths for enhancing oxygen availability. (Table 29.7)

Biological Effects of Light-Emitting Diodes

Infrared energy from LED lights has also been shown to stimulate cellular proliferation of a variety of cell types and to penetrate 23 mm into tissue.[67] LED-treated cells have demonstrated cellular proliferation rates of 150% to 200% of untreated cells. Cultured human muscle cells grew seven times faster than their untreated counterparts, whereas skin cells grew five times faster.[68]

Effects of Laser and Light-Emitting Diodes on Wound Healing in Animal Models

Beneficial effects of low-level laser treatment on wound healing were demonstrated in a variety of animal models.[54] Enhanced healing of experimentally induced wounds in cows, pigs, dogs, rabbits, rats, and mice were detected after irradiation with low-level laser. However, the most pronounced effect on wound healing was found in cow skin followed by rat skin. Pig skin was less responsive compared to the skin of cows and rats.

This research indicates that the effect of low-level laser irradiation is more pronounced in loose-skinned animals such as the cow and rat.[54,69,70] Similar to humans, pigs have a more tightly anchored skin that is less mobile. This may explain the outcome of a recent meta-analysis of the literature that found that low-level laser treatment has a more positive effect on wound healing in animals than humans. However, this effect may also have been due to the greater power associated with larger subject numbers in the animal studies.

A number of different effects of low-level laser have been found in animal models. These include more rapid healing and closure of wounds, enhanced formation of granulation tissue, improved alignment of collagen in tendons, increased tensile strength of tendons, and accelerated healing of fractures.[54] These effects were associated with helium-neon and gallium arsenide laser treatments. Doses between 4 to 10 J/cm^2 were required to produce positive effects.

Low-level laser treatment has also been shown to increase prostaglandin production and mast cell activation and degranulation in animals. This effect may stimulate wound healing because prostaglandins play an important role in the early inflammatory process by increasing vascular permeability. Mast cells serve as a source of chemical mediators, which are important to the wound healing process.

In 1985, Mester et al investigated the effects of the helium-neon laser at an energy density of 1 J/cm^2 on E- and F-type prostaglandin production in dorsal rat wounds.[62] Both types of prostaglandins significantly increased at 4 posttreatment days in the laser-treated wounds compared to control wounds. Mast cell degranulation has also been demonstrated in vitro using a low-power laser set to different pulsing frequencies.[71] Mast cell degranulation occurred with exposure to 20 and 292 Hz.

Enhanced wound healing in animals has also been measured after treatment with LEDs. An increased rate of wound healing in diabetic mice treated with infrared LEDS developed by NASA was demonstrated by Whelan et al.[72]

Effects of Laser and Light-Emitting Diodes on Wound Healing in Humans

The effects of the lower-level laser on wound healing in humans was first studied by Andre Mester.[55,73] He studied the effects of low-power laser on healing in various types of chronic wounds. He claimed to have attained a 90% rate of healing in more than 1000 patients using low doses of laser light energy (4 J/cm^2 or less). A number of other researchers have demonstrated positive treatment effects of laser on a variety of wound types, including surgical wounds, cutaneous fissures, and venous ulcerations, among others.[54]

In a comprehensive review of the literature, Belanger identified 14 studies of varying quality that demonstrated a positive effect of low-level laser therapy on wound and ulcer healing in humans.[55] Belanger ranked 12 of these 14 studies at the highest levels of evidence (level I and II). Only three studies with an evidence ranking of I or II found no benefit to low-level laser therapy. A meta-analysis by Barham et al in 2004 produced similar results. Aggregate analysis of the available data provided from both human and animal studies demonstrated a large overall positive effect of low-level laser treatment on wound healing.[54]

Barham also calculated the effect size for time to healing using nine studies that met the inclusion criteria for the meta-analysis.[54] Only one study had a negative effect size. This study was fraught with experimental design flaws, including differences in standard of care for the treated versus nontreated group. In this study, wounds treated with occlusive dressings healed more quickly than control or laser-treated wounds. The other studies examined in this meta-analysis exhibited a positive effect size ranging from +0.06 to +9.10.

The meta-analysis of the literature performed by Barham also indicated that low-level laser treatment is more effective when delivered early in the phases of wound healing.[54] Wounds treated at or around day three after injury resulted in the greatest acceleration of wound healing. This finding is congruent with research, which has demonstrated that low-level laser accelerates the inflammatory and proliferative phases of wound healing.

Findings by Barham also provide information as to which type of laser is most effective in stimulating wound healing.[54] Research data involving eight different types of laser were examined. A positive-effect size was detected for each of the different laser types, with the krypton laser demonstrating the greatest effect on wound healing. However, caution must be used in interpreting this finding as the krypton laser was represented in only one study. High calculated effects of approximately the same size, +3.23, +3.05, and +3.02, were found for the argon, helium-neon, and galium arsenide lasers, respectively.

Evidence to support the use of LEDs in treating nonhealing or slow-healing human wounds is evolving. Work by Whelan et al has demonstrated that LEDs have the ability to rescue epithelial cells in children undergoing radiation and chemotherapy.[74] Infrared LEDs prevented the development of oral mucositis and acute mouth ulcers in these children. LEDs used to deliver monochromatic infrared energy at 890 nm have also been shown to enhance wound healing in recalcitrant ulcers.[75-77] Individuals treated with this technology demonstrated a significant enhancement of healing rates. This LED has also been shown to increase sensation in individuals diagnosed with diabetic peripheral neuropathy and loss of protective sensation. Similar results have been reported in both small uncontrolled and controlled clinical trials.[77-81] The mechanism of action is unknown, but it is thought that the LED light stimulates nitric oxide production and an associated vasodilation and/or enhances oxygen dissociation from hemoglobin and its transfer to surrounding tissues. However, clinicians must exercise care with this treatment device as reports of superficial burns have been reported.

Laser Treatment Paradigm

Dose

A diversity of parameters has been used in laser studies conducted to date. Animal studies have demonstrated a positive effect of helium-neon and gallium arsenide laser treatment on wound healing when delivered at doses between 4 and 10 J/cm^2.[54] Similarly, Mester et al purported a 90% rate of healing in more than 1000 patients using a dose of laser light energy at 4 J/cm^2 or less.[55,73] Current laser treatment regimens use this dose as a benchmark for treatment. Low-power lasers do not produce heat, so there should be no appreciable tissue heating. These lasers should deliver less than 500 mW of energy during a treatment cycle.

▶ **PEARL 29•6** Consider a dose of between 4 and 10 J/cm^2 when using a helium-neon or gallium arsenide laser to promote wound healing.

Treatment Time

Treatment time depends on the intensity at which the laser light energy is delivered. Less time is needed to treat an area when high intensities are used. For example, a 10-mW laser would take 100 seconds to deliver the same energy as a

50-mW laser would in 20 seconds. Most laser devices have a programmed activation cycle with a preset time of exposure in seconds. Dosage is determined by the output of the laser in milliwatts, the time of exposure in seconds, and the beam surface area of the laser in square centimeters. A rotation of the laser at several intervals to ensure thorough treatment of the target area is recommended by some manufacturers. High-intensity treatments (dose delivered at greater than 500 mW) or extended treatment times can be detrimental to healing since the total energy applied to the tissue exceeds safe exposure levels.

Treatment Distance

The laser is typically placed in direct contact with an interface material covering the wound, such as a thin film dressing to prevent contamination of the device. The laser may be stationary during treatment of selected tissue areas or it may be moved from one treatment area to another continuously in a stroking pattern. However, it must be moved slowly to allow optimal dosing. The periwound area may also be treated with the laser.

Equipment Selection

Laser Classes

At this time, four classes of lasers exist based on their potential to modulate biological processes to induce tissue damage and their power level.[54,82] These classes include the lasers listed in Table 29.8. Class 3B lasers are used by clinicians trained in physical energy technologies to modulate the inflammatory response and to stimulate wound healing, to provide pain relief, and to encourage peripheral nerve regeneration.

▸ **PEARL 29•7** Select a class 3B laser to modulate inflammatory responses and to promote wound healing.

Laser Type and Characteristics

Several types of low-level lasers are available to the wound care clinician. The helium-neon laser produces a red-colored light from the visible light spectrum, whereas the galium arsenide and the galium aluminum arsenide lasers use infrared light. Infrared lasers penetrate the body more deeply than do the helium-neon laser. The depth of penetration of laser light is dependent on its wavelength.[8,56,83] Absorption of laser light

by melanin in the basal layers of the epidermis and scattering by collagen in the dermis limits the amount of laser energy available to interact with chromophores in the skin. The helium-neon laser penetrates only superficially (2–5 mm), whereas the infrared-based lasers, gallium arsenide (1–2 cm) lasers, and the gallium aluminum arsenide (3–5 cm) lasers, penetrate the body more deeply.

The power range of lasers used for stimulating wound healing is 10^{-3} to 10^{-1} W, with wavelengths between 300 and 10,600 nanometers.[84] Common lasing mediums include helium and neon (632.8 nm), ruby (694 nm), and argon (488 nm).[56] Others include newer laser technology that employs semiconductor laser diodes, such as gallium arsenide (904 nm) and gallium aluminum arsenide (830 nm).

Results of a meta-analysis of the literature by Barham indicate that the krypton laser is most effective for stimulating wound healing.[54] However, there is limited evidence to support this finding. Further research is needed to establish the optimal laser type for use in stimulating wound healing.

▸ **PEARL 29•8** Select an infrared-based laser such as the gallium arsenide (1–2 cm) or the gallium aluminum arsenide (3–5 cm) for penetration into soft tissue.

Wound and Periwound Preparation

Prior to application of the laser, dressing should be removed and the wound and periwound tissue should be thoroughly cleansed to remove wound drainage, coagulated blood, and necrotic tissue. Presence of exudates diminishes laser penetration, as does necrotic tissue. However, a transparent film dressing should be placed over the wound to avoid contamination of the laser device.

▸ **PEARL 29•9** Remove all dressing material and cleanse the wound bed in order to provide maximum exposure of the target tissues to laser treatment.

Indications for Laser Treatment

Laser treatment is indicated as follows:

1. Recalcitrant wounds
2. Necrotic wounds
3. Infected acute or chronic wounds

Table 29•8 Classification of Lasers

Class of Laser	Power Density	Potential to Cause Harm	Clinical Use
1	<0.5 mW	None to very minimal	Subclinical
2	<1 mW	Minimal	Subclinical
3A	<5 mW	Minimal	Subclinical
3B	<500 mW	Potential to damage eyes; caution with long treatment times or extended use	Photobiomodulation used for wound care, pain relief, and nerve regeneration
4	>500 mW	Damaging to eyes and skin; use extreme caution	Photothermal effects used in surgery

Contraindications for Laser Treatment

Laser treatment is contraindicated as follows:

1. Do not use over cancerous growths.
2. Avoid direct exposure to the eyes due to possible retinal burns. Use appropriate eye protection for the clinician and patient.
3. As a general precaution, do not use during the first trimester of pregnancy.
4. Do not treat over the thyroid gland.

Adverse Reactions

No adverse reactions have been documented in the literature.

Administration of Laser or Light-Emitting Diode Therapy

Low-level laser or LED therapy should be performed by a skilled individual licensed in the application of physical energy technologies. To prevent overexposure or inappropriate exposure of other areas, laser should not be administered by the patient or care giver.

Documentation

The following should be documented in the patient record:

- Treatment parameters (wavelength, mode: pulsed vs continuous, energy density, frequency, total irradiation time)
- Treatment duration
- Treatment frequency
- Type of treatment device
- Patient position
- Wound location
- Preparation and protection of the periwound
- Preparation of the wound bed
- Patient response to treatment

Summary

Phototherapy has been used since time began for the treatment of human ailments. Perhaps it is because of this history or the ubiquity of the energy form that we often overlook the benefits of this therapy for chronic wound management. Both basic and clinical science provides a foundation for the use of phototherapy in the treatment of wounds. Evidence supports the use of Ultraviolet C for reducing wound bioburden, especially in the presence of antibiotic resistant bacteria such as MRSA. LASER and related modalities have evolving evidence indicating that IR energy modulates many biological processes and can be used to facilitate healing. It is imperative in this era of evidence-based practice that we familiarize ourselves with the levels and types of evidence required to fully understand the biophysical technologies available to us. As we see the adoption of many traditional and new forms of biophysical energies by medicine, nursing and others, it behooves all professions to seek out the full evidence that supports the use of these energies in wound healing.

▶ **Case Study 29•2** **Laser Therapy for the Management of an Arterial Ulcer**

Medical History

M.G. was a 65-year-old ambulatory female who lives with her sister in a two-story townhouse. She has smoked for the last 48 years and has type 2 diabetes. She has a nonhealing, arterial wound over the right lateral malleolus. Her medical diagnoses additionally include hypertension, congestive heart failure, and chronic obstructive pulmonary disease. She has very low endurance and mild claudication pain. She uses a wheelchair for long-distance travel.

Reason for Referral

She was referred to physical therapy due to a nonhealing arterial ulcer on right lateral malleolus and decreased endurance.

Wound Examination

The ulcer was dry with a light-pink granulation bed. The ulcer was 5 cm in length and 2 cm in width at the widest point. The depth of the wound was less than 3 to 4 mm. The Achilles tendon was visible in distal edge of the wound. The periwound was dry and hair loss was apparent below the knees on both extremities. Posterior tibial and dorsalis pedis pulses could be detected in both feet upon palpation.

Treatment Plan and Outcome

The ulcer was treated three times per week for 8 weeks with a helium-neon laser and with a transparent film dressing. The laser treatment was delivered with a stroking method to produce a crosshatch effect. A total treatment dose of 60 J/cm² was used at each treatment session. The wound closed at the end of the ninth week.

▶ **PEARL 29•10** Biophysical technologies, including phototherapy devices, should only be applied by skilled clinicians with a license to provide such treatments and to determine appropriate treatment paradigms.

References

1. Liberman, J: Light and Medicine of the Future. Rochester, VT, Bear & Company, 1991, pp 119–138.
2. Samina, T, Yousuf, A, Mohsin Raza, S: A critical analysis of chromotherapy and its scientific evolution. Evid Based Complement Alternat Med 2005; 2:481–488.
3. Licht, S: History of ultraviolet light therapy. In: Licht, S (ed): Therapeutic Electricity and Ultraviolet Radiation, ed. 2. New Haven, CT, Elizabeth Licht Publishing, 1967, pp 191–212.
4. Licht, S: History of ultraviolet therapy. In: Stillwell, GK (ed): Therapeutic Electricity and Ultraviolet Radiation, ed. 3. Baltimore, Lippincott Williams & Wilkins, 1983, pp 228–261.
5. What is a Maser? Available at: http://einstein.stanford.edu/content/faqs/maser.html. Accessed 02/06.
6. Singer, JR: Masers. New York, John Wiley, 1959.
7. Charles Townes: The Maser. Available at: http://web.mit.edu/invent/iow/townes.html Accessed 02/06.
8. Weisberg, J: Electromagnetic spectrum. In: Hecox, B, Mehreteab, TA, Weisberg, J (eds): Physical Agents: A Comprehensive Text for Physical Therapists. Norwalk, CT, Appleton & Lange, 1994, pp 50.
9. Weisberg, J: Ultraviolet irradiation. In: Hecox, B, Mehreteab, TA, Weisberg, J (eds): Physical Agents: A Comprehensive Text for Physical Therapists. Norwalk, CT, Appleton & Lange, 1994, pp 377–378.
10. Moseley, H: Sources of ultraviolet radiation. In: Moseley, H (ed): Non-Ionising Radiation: Microwaves, Ultraviolet and Laser Radiation. Philadelphia, IOP Publishing, 1988, p 110.
11. Hayes, KW: Ultraviolet radiation. In: Hayes, KW (ed): Manual for Physical Agents, ed. 5. Norwalk, CT, Appleton & Lange, 1999.
12. Schwarz, T, Urbanski, A, Luger, TA: Ultraviolet light and epidermal cell-derived cytokines. In: Luger, TA, Schwarz, T (eds): Epidermal Growth Factors and Cytokines. New York, Marcel Dekker, 1994, p 303.
13. Scott, BO: Clinical uses of ultraviolet radiation. In: Stillwell, GK (ed): Therapeutic Electricity and Ultraviolet Radiation, ed. 3. Baltimore, Lippincott Williams & Wilkins, 1983, pp 228–261.
14. Stenback, F: Health hazards from ultraviolet radiation. Public Health Rev 1982; 10:229.
15. Daniels, F: Ultraviolet light and dermatology. In: Stillwell, GK (ed): Therapeutic Electricity and Ultraviolet Radiation, ed. 3. Baltimore, Lippincott Williams & Wilkins, 1983, pp 263–303.
16. van der Leun, JC: On the action spectrum of ultraviolet erythema. Res Prog Org Biol Med Chem 1972; 3:711–736.
17. Ott, JN: Health and Light. Columbus, OH, Ariel Press, 1973.
18. Hollwich, F, Dieckhues, B: The effect of natural and artificial light via the eye on the hormonal and metabolic balance of animal and man. Ophthalmologica 1980; 180:188–197.
19. Gerard, RM: Differential effects of colored lights on psychophysiological functions [dissertation]. UCLA, 1958.
20. Cameron, MH: A shining light. Adv Dir Rehabil 2005; 14:39–42.
21. Conner-Kerr, T: Wound technology: The future is now. Extended Care Product News 2005; 104:34–39.
22. Harm, W: UV carcinogenesis. In: Harm, W (ed): Biological Effects of Ultraviolet Radiation. New York, Cambridge University Press, 1980, p 191.
23. Hensby, CN, Plummer, NA, Black, AK, et al: Time course of arachidonic acid, prostaglandins E2 and F2 alpha production in human abdominal skin following irradiation with ultraviolet wavelengths (290–320 nm). Adv Prostaglandin Thromboxane Res 1980; 7:857–860.
24. Brauchle, M, Funk, JO, Kind, P, et al: Ultraviolet B and H_2O_2 are potent inducers of vascular endothelial growth factor expression in cultured keratinocytes. J Biol Chem 1996; 271:93–97.
25. Holtz, F: Pharmacology of ultraviolet radiation. Br J Phys Med 1952; 5:201.
26. Conner-Kerr, TA, Sullivan, PK, Keegan, A, et al: UVC reduces antibiotic resistant bacterial numbers in living tissue. Ostomy Wound Manage 1999; 45:84.
27. Scott, BO: Clinical uses of ultraviolet radiation. In: Stillwell, GK (ed): Therapeutic Electricity and Ultraviolet Radiation, ed. 3. Baltimore, Lippincott Williams & Wilkins, 1983, pp 228–261.
28. Kaiser, MR, Davis, SC, Mertz, PM: The effect of ultraviolet irradiation-induced inflammation on epidermal wound healing. Wound Repair Regen 1995; 3:311–315.
29. Schwarz, T, Urbanski, A, Luger, TA: Ultraviolet light and epidermal cell-derived cytokines. In: Luger, TA, Schwarz, T (eds): Epidermal Growth Factors and Cytokines. New York, Marcel Dekker, 1994, p 303.
30. Daniels, F: Ultraviolet light and dermatology. In: Stillwell, GK (ed): Therapeutic Electricity and Ultraviolet Radiation, ed. 3. Baltimore, Lippincott Williams & Wilkins 1983, pp 263–303.
31. High, AS, High, JP: Treatment of infected skin wounds using ultraviolet radiation: An in vitro study. Physiotherapy 1983; 69:359–360.
32. Conner-Kerr, TA, Sullivan, PK, Gaillard, J, et al: The effects of ultraviolet radiation on antibiotic-resistant bacteria in vitro. Ostomy Wound Manage 1998; 44:50–56.
33. Sullivan, PK, Conner-Kerr, T: A comparative study of the effects of UVC irradiation on select procaryotic and eucaryotic wound pathogens. OstomyWound Manage 2000; 46:44–50.
34. El-Batouty, MF, El-Gindy, M, El-Shawaf, I, et al: Comparative evaluation of the effects of ultrasonic and ultraviolet irradiation on tissue regeneration. Scand J Rheumatol 1986; 15:381–386.
35. Das, SK, Brantley, SK, Davidson, SF: Wound tensile strength in the hairless guinea pig following irradiation with pure ultraviolet-A light. Br J Plast Surg 1991; 44:509–513.
36. Davidson, SF, Brantley, SK, Das, SK: The effects of ultraviolet radiation on wound healing. Br J Plast Surg 1991; 44:210–214.
37. Davidson, SF, Brantley, SK, Das, SK: The reversibility of UV-altered wound tensile strength in the hairless guinea pig following a 90-day recovery period. Br J Plast Surg 1992; 45:109–112.
38. Basford, JR, Hallman, HO, Sheffield, CG, et al: Comparison of cold quartz ultraviolet, low-energy laser, and occlusion in wound healing in a swine model. Arch Phys Med Rehabil 1986; 67:151.
39. Sullivan, PK, Conner-Kerr, TA, Dixon, S, et al: The effect of UVC irradiation on wound closure. Presented at: 2000 Symposium on Advanced Wound Care & Medical Research Forum on Wound Repair, Dallas, TX, April 2000.
40. Morykwas, MJ, Mark, MW: Effects of ultraviolet light on fibroblast fibronectin production and lattice contraction. Wounds 1998; 10:111–117.
41. Stein, I, Shorey, MM: Ultraviolet radiation in the treatment of indolent, soft-tissue ulcerations. Physiother Rev 1945;25(6):272–274.
42. Willis, EE, Anderson, TW, Beattie, BL, et al: A randomized placebo controlled trial of ultraviolet light in the treatment of superficial pressure sores. J Am Geriatr Soc 1983; 31:131.
43. Crous, L, Malherbe, C: Laser and ultraviolet light irradiation in the treatment of chronic ulcers. Physiotherapy 1988; 44:73.
44. Nussbaum, EL, Biemann, I, Mustard B: Comparison of ultrasound/ultraviolet-C and laser for treatment of pressure ulcers in patients with spinal cord injury. Phys Ther 1994; 74:812–825.
45. Taylor, R: Clinical study of ultraviolet in various skin conditions. Phys Ther 1972; 52:279–282.
46. Taylor, GJ, Chandler, L: Ultraviolet light in the orthopaedic operating theatre. Br J Theatre Nurs 1997; 6:10–14.
47. Taylor, GJS, Bannister, GC, Leeming, JP: Wound disinfection with ultraviolet radiation. J Hospital Infection 1995; 30:85–93.
48. Moggio, M, Goldner, JL, McCollum, DE, et al: Wound infections in patients undergoing total hip arthroplasty. Ultraviolet light for the control of airborne bacteria. Arch Surg 1979; 114:815–823.
49. Berg, M, Bergman, BR, Hoborn, J: Shortwave ultraviolet radiation in operating rooms. J Bone Joint Surg 1989; 71:483–485.
50. Thai, TP, Keast, DH, Campbell, KE, et al: Effect of ultraviolet light C on bacterial colonization in chronic wounds. Ostomy Wound Manage 2005; 51:32–45.

51. Mertz, PM, Davis, SC, Oliveira-Gandia, M, et al: The wound environment: Implications from research studies for healing and infection. Wounds 1996; 8:1–8.

52. Mertz, PM: Interleukin-1 enhances epidermal wound healing. Lymphokine Res 1990; 9:465–473.

53. Taylor, GJ, Leeming, JP, Bannister, GC: Effects of antiseptics, ultraviolet light, and lavage on airborne bacteria in a model wound. J Bone Joint Surg Br 1993; 75:724–730.

54. Barham, CD, Bounkeo, JM, Brannon, WM, et al: The effect of laser therapy in the treatment of wounds: A meta-analysis of the literature [masters thesis]. Graduate Program of Physical Therapy, North Georgia College and State University, Dahloneg, GA, 2003.

55. Belanger, AY: LASER. In: Belanger, AY (ed): Evidence-Based Guide to Therapeutic Physical Agents. Philadelphia, Lippincott Williams & Wilkins, 2003, pp 191–221.

56. Asimov, MM, Asimov, RM, Rubinov, AN: Spectrum of the effect of laser radiation on hemoglobin of the blood vessels of skin. J Appl Spect 1998; 65:919–922.

57. Martin, R: LASER-accelerated inflammation/pain reduction and healing. Practical Pain Management Nov/Dec 2003; 3(6):20–25.

58. Abergel, RP, Lyons, RF, Castel, JC, et al: Biostimulation of wound healing by lasers: Experimental approaches in animal models and in fibroblast cultures. J Derm Surg Oncol 1987; 13:127–133.

59. Young, S, Bolton, P, Dyson, M, et al: Macrophage responsiveness to light therapy. Laser Surg Med 1989; 9:497–505.

60. Rajaratnam, S, Bolton, P, Dyson, M: Macrophage responsiveness to laser therapy with varying pulsing frequencies. Laser Ther 1994; 6:107–111.

61. Abergel, RP, Lam, TS, Meeker, CA, et al: Biostimulation of procollagen production by low energy lasers in human skin fibroblast cultures. Clin Res 1984; 32:567A.

62. Mester, E, Mester, AF, Mester, A: The biomedical effects of laser application. Laser Surg Med 1985; 5:31–39.

63. Shefer, G, Partridge, TA, Heslop, L, et al: Low energy laser irradiation promotes the survival and cell cycle entry of skeletal muscle satellite cells. J Cell Sci 2002; 115(Pt 7):1461–1469.

64. Passarella, S, Casamassima, E, Molinari, S, et al: Increase of proton electrochemical and ATP synthesis in rat liver mitochondria irradiated in vitro by HeNe. FEBS Lett 1984; 175:95–99.

65. Kupin, VI, Bykov, VS, Ivanov, AV, et al: Potentiating effects of laser radiation on some immunological traits. Neoplasma 1982; 29:403–406.

66. Passarella, S, Casamassima, E, Quagliariello, E, et al: Quantitative analysis of lymphocyte-salmonella interaction and effect of lymphocyte irradiation by helium-neon laser. Biochem Biophys Res Comm 1985; 130:546–552.

67. Marovino, T: Cold LASERS in pain management. Pract Pain Manage Sept/Oct 2004; 4(6):37–42.

68. Whelan, HT, Smits, RL, Buchman, EV, et al: Effect of NASA light-emitting diode irradiation on wound healing. J Clin Lasers Med Surg 2001; 19:305–314.

69. Lee, P, Kim, K, Kim, K: Effects of low incident energy levels of infrared laser irradiation on healing of infected open skin wounds in rats. Laser Ther 1993; 5:59–64.

70. Graham, DJ, Alexander, JJ: The effects of argon laser on bovine aortic endothelial and smooth muscle cell proliferation and collagen production. Curr Surg 1990; 47:27–30.

71. El Sayed, SO, Dyson, M: Comparison of the effect of multiwavelength light produced by a cluster of semiconductor diodes and of each individual diode on mast cell number and degranulation in intact and injured skin. Laser Surg Med 1990; 10:559–568.

72. Whelan, HT, Buchmann, EV, Dhokalia, A, et al: Effect of NASA light-emitting diode irradiation on molecular changes for wound healing in diabetic mice. J Clin Laser Med Surg 2003; 21:67–74.

73. Mester, E, Spiry, T, Szende, B, et al: Effect of laser rays on wound healing. Am J Surg 1971; 122:532–535.

74. Whelan, HT, Connelly, JF, Hodgson, BD, et al: NASA light-emitting diodes for the prevention of oral mucositis in pediatric bone marrow transplant patients. J Clin Laser Med Surg 2002; 20:319–324.

75. Horwitz, LR, Burke, TJ, Carnegie, D: Augmentation of wound healing using nonochromatic infrared energy. Exploration of a new technology for wound management. Adv Wound Care 1999; 12:35–40.

76. Horwitz, LR, Burke, TJ: Effect of monochromatic infrared energy on venous stasis ulcers. Wound Care Institute Newsletter 1999 Jan–Feb; 4(1):

77. Kochman, A: Restoration of sensation, improved balance, and gait reduction in falls in elderly patients with use of monochromatic infrared photo energy and physical therapy. J Geriatr Phys Ther 2004; 27:16–19.

78. Kochman, AB, Carnegie, DH, Burke, TJ: Symptomatic reversal of peripheral neuropathy in patients with diabetes. J Am Podiatr Med Assoc 2002; 92:125–130.

79. Leonard, DR, Farooqi, MH, Myers, S: Restoration of sensation, reduced pain, and improved balance in subjects with diabetic peripheral neuropathy: A double-blind, randomized, placebo-controlled study with monochromatic near infrared treatment. Diabetes Care 2004; 27:168–172.

80. Powell, MW, Carnegie, DE, Burke, TJ: Reversal of diabetic neuropathy and new wound incidence: The role of MIRE. Adv Skin Wound Care 2004; 17:295–300.

81. Prendergast, JJ, Miranda, G, Sanchez, M: Improvement of sensory impairment in patients with peripheral neuropathy. Endocrine Pract 2004; 10:24–30.

82. Cameron, M: Laser and light. Seminar presentation. January 2005, Torrance, CA.

83. Mendez, T, Pinheiro, A, Pacheco, M, et al: Dose and wavelength of laser light have influence on the repair of cutaneous wounds. J Clin Laser Med Surg 2004; 22:19–25.

84. Posten, W, Wrone, DA, Dover, JS, et al: Low-level laser therapy for wound healing: Mechanism and efficacy. Dermatol Surg 2005; 31:334–340.

chapter 30

Compression Therapy

Joseph M. McCulloch, PhD, PT, CWS, FACCWS, FAPTA

Fluid accumulates in extravascular tissues in response to changes in various forces normally controlling vessel permeability. Local factors include hydrostatic pressure changes and blockage of lymphatic channels, whereas on a systemic level, protein imbalance can result in generalized swelling. While most swelling is referred to as "edema," the general use of this term can lead to misunderstanding of the underlying pathology and, subsequently, inappropriate treatment. Critical distinctions exist between normal tissue edema and lymphedema, which is due to a dysfunctional lymphatic system. The reader is referred to Chapter 18 for a detailed discussion of this condition.

As is known from the Starling equation (Box 30.1), under normal conditions a state of near equilibrium exists at the capillary membranes. The amount of fluid filtering out from the capillaries almost equals absorption. The disequilibrium that exists favors accumulation in the interstitial tissues, and this is effectively handled by the lymphatic system under normal conditions.[1,2] The Starling equation suggests that effectively applied local pressure can facilitate reabsorption of fluid by veins and lymphatics.

> **Box 30•1** **Starling Equation**
>
> $$F = c(P_c - P_t) - (\Pi_c - \Pi_t)$$
> F = Net filtration
> c = Filtration coefficient
> P_c = Capillary blood pressure
> P_t = Tissue pressure
> Π_c = Capillary oncotic pressure
> Π_t = Tissue oncotic pressure

> **PEARL 30•1** A disequilibrium exists between filtration and absorption in the vascular system that favors accumulation of fluid in the interstitial tissues.

Accumulation of fluid in the interstitium can greatly impede wound healing, yet it is seldom addressed as treatment plans are developed for management of wounds. While surgeons are quick to recognize and correct limb-threatening ischemia associated with a compartment syndrome, little attention is directed to handling low-level continuous swelling that occurs in chronic states of inflammation and gravity-dependent conditions. This is despite the fact that swelling has been demonstrated to be a significant deterrent in wound healing.[3-5]

Fortunately for patients, a significant number of options exist to treat local swelling, improve tissue oxygenation, alleviate venous hypertension, and promote an environment conducive to wound healing. This chapter presents a variety of such options from short-stretch bandages to dynamic compression pumps that can be tailored to meet the needs of individual patients. When appropriately applied, compression can facilitate the healing of venous leg ulcers and other wounds. To the contrary, however, compression that is inappropriately applied can result in delayed healing and tissue necrosis.

Bandaging

Of the broad variety of compression bandages available for clinical use, each comes with its merits and concerns. Before selecting any bandage device, clinicians should be mindful of four principles addressed by Clark.[6]

1. What are the elastic properties of the bandage and how is it constructed?
2. What is the size and shape of the extremity?

3. How skilled is the clinician, patient, or caregiver at bandage application?
4. What will be the level of physical activity the patient will undertake?

Regardless of how superior a bandage is alleged to be, improper application or use can render the device ineffective, if not dangerous. Clinicians must always be alert to the fact that proper bandaging is not only an art, but also a science. Laplace's law (Box 30.2) tells us that the pressure exerted by a bandage is directly proportional to bandage tension and the number of layers applied, while inversely proportional to the radius of curvature of the limb.[7,8] This means, therefore, that attention should be paid not only to the elastic tension of the selected wrap but also to the number of layers applied and the size of the extremity. Much greater pressure is exerted over areas of small circumference due to the small radius of curvature. This is a special concern over such bony areas as the ankle.

▸ **PEARL 30•2** Laplace's law dictates that sub-bandage pressure will be proportional to tension and number of layers applied while inversely proportional to limb circumference.

Short-Stretch Bandages

Bandages are typically classified according to elasticity and layers of application (single versus multilayer). Short-stretched bandages are named for their relative anti-elasticity. While some short-stretch wraps may be slightly elastic, their extensibility is negligible when compared to the traditional elastic wraps. Short-stretch bandages are generally crepe-type products manufactured from cotton or combinations of cotton and viscose. They have limited extensibility and elasticity, allowing them to be applied firmly over a joint without causing significant pressure.[9] Many short-stretch bandages also are stiff, which helps the bandage remain rigid and resist geometric changes in the extremity during exercise.[10] Such wraps are highly effective in managing swelling associated with lymphedema. Short-stretch bandages are noted for their lower resting pressure but high working pressure, making them excellent for decreasing edema and improving venous hemodynamics.[11] They can achieve resting pressures of around 30 to 60 mm Hg, though this pressure tends to decrease over a 24-hour period as the individual moves around and swelling begins to subside.[12] Short-stretch bandages are quite popular in the management of lymphedema.[13-16] This is discussed in greater detail in Chapter 18. One example of a short-stretch bandage in common use is Comprilan® (Beiersdorf Medical, Charlotte, NC). (Fig. 30.1)

Another bandage in common use that qualifies as a short-stretch wrap is Unna's boot (Tyco Healthcare/Kendall, Mansfield, MA). Unna's boot consists of a gauze bandage impregnated with various substances, including zinc oxide, calamine, and gelatin. The consistency of the additives constitutes a paste that helps the gauze wrap mold to the extremity and form a semirigid support. (Fig. 30.2) While originally designed as a means of providing support and delivering zinc to aid wound healing, the latter effect has not been documented as effective. To the contrary, it has been shown that applying an Unna'a boot directly over an open wound serves to produce an environment similar to a wet-to-dry dressing. Wounds have been demonstrated to heal at a more rapid rate when first covered with a synthetic dressing.[17] Lippman and Briere found that the high working pressure of Unna's boot worked to improve calf pump function and reduce ambulatory venous hypertension.[18,19]

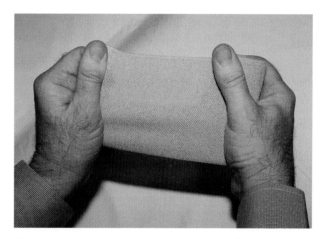

Figure 30•1 *Example of a short-stretch bandage.*

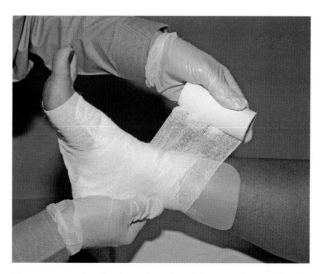

Figure 30•2 *Application of an Unna's boot with a synthetic dressing.*

▸ **Box 30•2** | **Laplace's Law**

$$P \propto T/R$$
P = Sub-bandage pressure
T = Tension of application (a measure of the degree of elastic stretch of the bandage)
R = Radius of curvature of the limb
$\propto$ = Proportional to

▶ **PEARL 30•3** Applying an Unna's boot directly over a wound will make it function as a wet-to-dry dressing. An appropriate dressing should first be applied to promote moist wound healing. The true benefit of an Unna's boot is from its semirigid support.

Long-Stretch Bandages

Long-stretch bandages are so named because of their extensibility and elastic recoil. These bandages contain elastomeric fibers that permit the bandage to stretch and then cause it to return almost to its original shape. As noted by Laplace's law, the tension exerted by such wraps has the potential to significantly increase sub-bandage pressure. Long-stretch bandages have a high working pressure as well as a high resting pressure, making them potentially dangerous for patients with arterial occlusive disease.[11] There is some evidence to suggest, however, that because of their ability to sustain pressure, elastic bandages may be more effective than inelastic ones for immobile patients or those with a fixed ankle, as long as circulatory perfusion is not compromised.[10,20]

It is generally recommended that long-stretch bandages be applied in a spiral fashion, with 50% overlap and 50% elastic extension. This is a difficult task indeed when no guided system exists and patients are trying to apply wraps to their own extremities. Some controlled tension wraps have been developed to address this problem. The dressing Setopress® (ConvaTec, Bristol-Myers Squibb Co., Skillman, NJ) has a series of green and brown rectangles imprinted on the bandage. When the bandage is properly elongated, the appropriate rectangle becomes a square to indicate desired pressure for that size limb. Another compression bandage, Surepress® (ConvaTec, Bristol-Meyers Squibb Co.) has, in addition to a series of rectangles, a center line to serve as a guide to provide 50% overlap of successive layers. (Fig. 30.3)

▶ **PEARL 30•4** For proper use of a long-stretch bandage, it should be applied at 50% stretch with 50% overlap of layers.

Although compression bandaging has proven highly effective in promoting venous ulcer healing, its effect on transcutaneous oxygen tension ($TcPO_2$) is worthy of consideration. Gaylarde and colleagues discovered that arteriolar vasoconstriction was a common finding in patients with venous distention.[21] Vasoconstriction was triggered by the sympathetic venoarterial reflex. The result of the increased arterial resistance was skin hypoxia. External compression was affective in decreasing venous distention and restoring blood flow to the skin. The reversal of hypoxia by compression was pressure dependent. Compression of 40 to 50 mm Hg was effective in restoring skin $TcPO_2$ to recumbent levels. The authors gave a word of caution, however, because pressures at 40 to 50 mm Hg while the patient was supine resulted in a fall in $TcPO_2$. They suggested that calf external pressure should not exceed 10 mm Hg in the supine position.

Multicomponent Compression

Various manufacturers have developed bandage systems with a variety of components designed to improve fit and

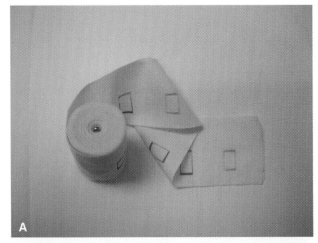
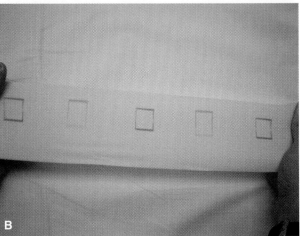

Figure 30•3 *(A) Setopress compression wrap. (B) Demonstration of lengthening of compression wrap converting rectangle to square.*

speed healing. In the past, the terminology associated with these systems referred to them being "multilayer." As noted in the consensus document published by the World Union of Wound Healing Societies, use of the term *layer* can be problematic, as there is no such thing as a single-layer bandage because there will always be some overlap of material during application.[10] We should instead be speaking of the components used in the systems (eg, cotton padding, short- or long-stretch bandages).

Some multicomponent bandage systems consist simply of a cotton or foam contact layer with a compression wrap, whereas others incorporate multiple components for absorption and long- and short-stretch characteristics. Most multicomponent bandage systems are designed to deliver a gradient pressure of 40 mm Hg at the ankle, decreasing to around 17 mm Hg at the proximal calf.[11]

One multicomponent system is Coban™ 2 (3M, Saint Paul, MN), which consists of an absorbent foam contact wrap covered with a short- to medium-stretch cohesive bandage. A four-component system, Profore (Smith & Nephew, Largo, FL), combines both short- and long-stretch bandages with an absorbent padding and an outer cohesive wrap. This compression system has been demonstrated to provide sustained compression for up to 1 week. Four-component bandage systems have been proven to increase the percentage of ulcers healed at 24 and 12 weeks in two trials when compared to single-component compression.[22-25] Several smaller studies did not find any significant differences between four-component bandaging and two inelastic compression devices (Unna's boot and short-stretch bandage). However, both four-component and short-stretch bandages healed venous ulcers more quickly than did paste bandages alone.[22,25]

Considerations Prior to Use of Compression Bandaging

As stated at the outset of this chapter, bandaging is both an art and a science. Effective bandaging requires that the wraps be applied consistently, with care being taken to apply proper pressure while taking into consideration the geometry of the body part. Prior to wrapping an extremity, an assessment must be made of the arterial supply. This may be as simple as performing an assessment of peripheral pulses or may require that an ankle-brachial index be performed. This is discussed in greater detail in Chapter 7. Individuals who have critical limb ischemia or ischemic pain should have a thorough vascular evaluation before ever considering compression bandaging. Critical limb ischemia has been defined as meeting either of the following criteria:

1. Persistently recurring ischemic rest pain that requires the regular use of analgesia for greater than 2 weeks, with an ankle systolic pressure less than or equal to 50 mm Hg or a toe systolic pressure less than or equal to 30 mm Hg
2. Ulceration or gangrene involving the toes or foot, with an ankle systolic pressure less than or equal to 50 mm Hg or a toe systolic pressure less than or equal to 30 mm Hg[10,26]

The presence of comorbidities such as diabetes should also be considered because compression could cause delayed healing if applied at too great a pressure. Risk factors associated with delayed healing include such factors as mixed arteriovenous disease, venous ligation, history of hip-knee replacement, popliteal reflux, recurring ulcers, impaired mobility, ulcers greater than 5 cm² or longer than 6 months in duration, and fibrin present over more than 50% of the wound.[10,27-29]

Alternative Compression Systems

Several appliances exist that are designed to effect the calf muscle pump and improve venous function, yet do not fall into the category of a compression wrap or bandage. The first is the Circaid (Coloplast Corp., Marietta, GA), which is an inelastic device consisting of a mesh stocking with multiple adjustable Velcro® (Velcro USA Inc., Manchester, MA) straps around the leg from the ankle to the upper calf. (Fig. 30.4) The Velcro closure helps to provide a sustained compression while making the device easily removable for frequent dressing changes.[30-32] Spence and Cahall evaluated the effect of Circaid and 30- to 40-mm Hg compression stockings on venous hemodynamics.[33] They found that Circaid performed significantly better than compression stockings in decreasing venous reflux and improving calf muscle function.

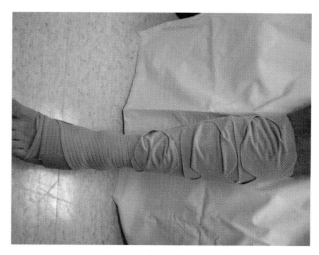

Figure 30•4 *The Circaid compression system.*

Intermittent Compression Therapy

Intermittent compression therapy (ICT) is demonstrated to be effective in promoting healing and preventing recurrence of venous ulcers.[34-36] ICT is provided when the patient is positioned supine and the lower extremities are elevated slightly. Pressure levels are generally set to about 50 mm Hg but are never greater than diastolic blood pressure. Box 30.3 provides guidelines for ICT. (Fig. 30.5)

ICT should not be used in individuals with acute deep venous thrombophlebitis or severe ischemic disease. Congestive heart failure is not an absolute contraindication to ICT, but patients with this disease should be monitored closely for signs of respiratory distress. Additionally, individuals with significant lymphedema may not respond effectively to ICT because lymphatic fluid is high protein in nature and hard to move from the extremities. Lymphedema is best handled by complete

> **Box 30•3 Guidelines for Intermittent Compression Therapy***

1. Gently cleanse the wound (avoid whirlpool and the dependent position).
2. Place the extremity into a plastic bag and then into the compression sleeve.
3. Elevate the extremity slightly.
4. Allow pumping for 30 minutes to an hour at a pressure less than diastolic.
5. Use a compression/relaxation ratio of 90:30 seconds.
6. Apply a semirigid or short-stretch dressing to the extremity after pumping if the patient is going to be ambulatory. If the individual will be fairly inactive, a long-stretch bandage may be indicated.
7. Treat one to two times per week as an outpatient or daily if home ICT is available.

*See Figure 30.5.

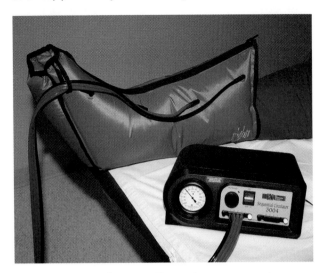

Figure 30•5 *Application of intermittent pneumatic compression.*

decongestive therapy which involves specialized massage techniques combined with compression bandaging.[37] ICT may be useful as an adjunct in certain conditions. The reader is referred to Chapter 18 for more information.

Although it appears evident that ICT is effective in reducing edema and assisting the dysfunctional calf muscle pump in removing venous blood from the extremities, additional benefits also may be realized. In a study of 19 subjects with symptoms of chronic venous insufficiency, Kessler and associates found that when patients were treated with 13-week cycles of ICT during 2-hour sessions twice weekly, symptoms improved in 16 of the 19 subjects (84%).[38] Additionally, enhanced fibrinolytic activity was noted in 6% of the subjects. The increased fibrinolytic potential was attributed to increased urokinase plasminogen activator, probably released from perturbed endothelial cells.

Smith and colleagues undertook a randomized controlled study to evaluate two regimens for treatment of venous ulcers.[36] Both treatment programs involved débridement, nonadherent dressings, and graduated compression stockings. One group of 21 patients additionally received 4 hours of sequential intermittent pneumatic compression daily. Ten of these patients healed completely compared to only 1 of 24 patients in the control group. The median rate of healing for the intermittent compression group was a 19.8% area compared to a 2.1% area for controls.

Kolari et al and Falanga et al also reported the successful use of ICT in the management of venous leg ulcers in hospitalized patients.[39,40] The greatest utility of pump therapy, however, appears to be in long-term outpatient and home use.

Graduated Compression Stockings

Another method used to control edema and promote wound healing in persons with venous insufficiency is support stockings. Support stockings, such as Jobst garments (Beirsdorf-Jobst Inc., Charlotte, NC), can be custom fitted; others, such as Medi stockings (Medi USA, Arlington Heights, IL) and Juzo stockings (Juzo Inc., Cuyahoga Falls, OH), can be semi-custom fit by selecting the garment that best accommodates the individual's ankle and calf girth and extremity length. (Fig. 30.6) Although a true custom-fitted stocking would fit an individual best, and theoretically provide the best compression, many people, especially elderly persons, find them difficult to don and doff because they are too tight when the leg swells. Because these garments work only if they are used, clinicians should use good judgment and involve patients in stocking selection. In individuals with mobility impairment, a donning device often helps the patient don stockings. (Fig. 30.7)

Compression stockings generally come in four classes. Class I stockings provide 20 to 30 mm Hg pressure and are designed for management of simple varicosities or mild swelling. Class II stockings deliver 30 to 40 mm Hg pressure and are indicated for moderate swelling, severe varicosities,

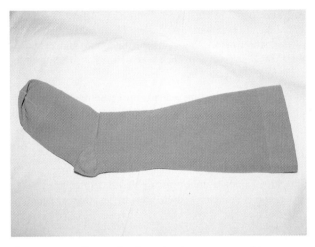

Figure 30•6 *Example of an elastic support stocking.*

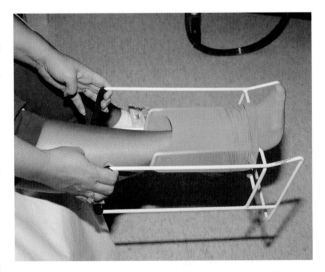

Figure 30•7 *Patient using a donning device to apply compression hosiery.*

and chronic venous insufficiency. Class III (40 to 50 mm Hg) and IV (60 plus mm Hg) stockings are typically used for severe edema, postthrombotic lymphatic edema, and elephantiasis.[30] Most patients with healed venous insufficiency ulcers use class II or III stockings.

Patients with chronic venous insufficiency are at high risk for reulceration, and for this reason compression stockings must be worn consistently.[11] Samson and Showalter noted that 78% of patients with ulcer recurrence had failed to consistently wear their stockings.[41] Mayberry et al found that 100% of their patients who did not wear stockings reulcerated.[5] This was compared to only a 16% reulceration rate when stockings were worn.

One mistake often made by clinicians is to fit patients for custom stockings before the extremity is effectively reduced to a desirable size. The only thing accomplished by fitting an edematous limb with a custom garment is to keep the limb at that size. Effective use of complex decongestive therapy, pneumatic compression therapy, and bandaging can effectively reduce limb size prior to fitting the patient for custom garments.

> ▸ **PEARL 30•5** Patients should be fit for custom compression garments only after the extremity has been reduced to the desired size by serial wrapping and/or intermittent compression therapy.

Implications of Treatment

Cullum et al, in an extensive literature review on the treatment of venous insufficiency, found 22 articles supporting compression therapy.[42] The data from the studies lead to the conclusion that high compression (35–45 mm Hg) was better than low compression (15–25 mm Hg), and multicomponent systems (short or long stretch) were more effective than single-component compression. Based on these findings, The International Leg Ulcer Advisory Board made the following recommendations[43]:

- *For mobile patients.* Either elastic or inelastic (long or short stretch) multicomponent compression is recommended.
- *For immobile patients.* Elastic (long stretch) multicomponent compression is recommended.

Compression with short-stretch bandages was not recommended in an immobile patient since these bandages depend upon calf muscle pump function to work effectively.

With regard to intermittent compression therapy, it is advocated for reduction of edema, facilitating the healing of venous ulcers, and in prophylaxis. ICT is a good adjunct to other therapy techniques designed to reduce limb volume and prepare the patient for custom stockings.

Summary

As stated at the outset of this chapter, numerous factors influence the development of edema and lymphedema. Effective treatment of any swollen extremity will likely incorporate some aspect of compression therapy. This is especially the case when managing patients with venous insufficiency and ulceration. Great care should be taken by clinicians to select appropriate compression modalities and reinforce with patients the need for appropriate use.

▸ **Case Study 30•1** **Management of a Recalcitrant Venous Insufficiency Ulcer**

History/Subjective

The patient is a 65-year-old African American female who presented to our clinic with a diagnosis of a chronic venous insufficiency ulceration of the right lower extremity that had been present for greater than 1 year. The patient related that she had been receiving wound care that consisted of various dressings and compression wraps. The wound had shown some signs of improvement, but then began to enlarge. Her medical history is significant for hypertension, hyperlipidemia, and varicose veins. Present medications are aspirin (325 mg by mouth daily), atenolol (25 mg daily), Lipitor® (20 mg daily), and furosemide (20 mg twice a day). Her social history is negative for alcohol, tobacco, or drug abuse. She is a widow and is retired and tends to her own house and yard work.

Physical Examination

On examination, the patient is noted to be a well-developed, well-nourished female in no acute distress. Examination of all systems was unremarkable, with the exception of the integumentary system. She was noted to have a 5.8 × 8 cm full-thickness ulceration over the right medial ankle just proximal to the medial malleolus. (Fig. 30.8) The wound had a good, rich granulation base, but there was minimal evidence of epithelialization. A mild pedal edema was also present. Peripheral pulses were good, with no signs of ischemia noted.

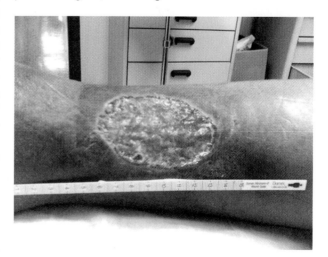

Figure 30•8 *Appearance of wound on admission to wound center.*

Continued

▸ **Case Study 30•1** | **Management of a Recalcitrant Venous Insufficiency Ulcer — cont'd**

Treatment

The patient was begun on intermittent compression therapy (ICT) at 50 mm Hg for 30 minutes. Following ICT the wound was dressed with a calcium alginate dressing that was covered by a thin adhesive foam dressing. The extremity was then wrapped with an Unna's boot, which would be changed two times per week in the clinic. The patient was given no restrictions and was encouraged to ambulate and to elevate the extremity when not active.

Within the first few weeks of treatment, the lower-extremity edema began to subside, and there was a 25% reduction in wound surface area. (Fig. 30.9) This slowly began to change, however, and the wound surface area began to again increase. The patient was sent for further vascular workup, at which time an ultrasound was performed on the veins of the right lower extremity from the level of the iliac down to the distal tibial veins. There was normal vessel compression, a phasic response, and color filling, with distal augmentation at all appropriate levels. Of note, however, was a +3 reflux involving the superficial femoral, popliteal, lesser saphenous, and below-knee greater saphenous veins. There were also numerous midcalf varicosities noted.

It was determined by the vascular surgeon that surgical intervention was necessary. The patient was taken to the vascular laboratory so that her saphenous vein could be marked. She was then taken to the operating room where she underwent stripping of the vein. Following surgery, the extremity was compressed with a long-stretch elastic bandage with a cotton padding. Patient did well postoperatively and was discharged from the hospital with instructions to return to the wound care center for follow-up management.

On return to the wound care center, the patient's ulcer was noted to be granular and clean and measured 5.5 × 7.5 cm in surface area. (Fig. 30.10) She was again started on ICT, and a home compression unit was prescribed so that daily treatments could be performed. The wound was dressed with alginate and a thin foam and compressed with a four-component dressing system that was changed weekly until the home compression system arrived. Once home compression was begun, the patient was supplied with a controlled-tension long-stretch bandage, and this was reapplied daily after ICT. The wound continued to reduce in size, and the lower-extremity girth stabilized. At this time, the patient was fitted with custom support hosiery, and the wound went on to completely resolve. (Fig. 30.11) At present, the patient remains healed, performs prophylactic ICT several times per week, and wears support hosiery daily.

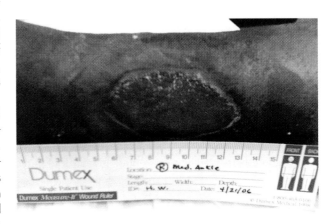

Figure 30•10 *Appearance of wound following saphenous vein stripping.*

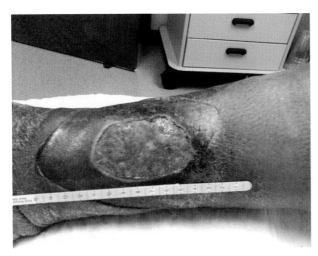

Figure 30•9 *Appearance of wound after several weeks of intermittent compression therapy and wound care.*

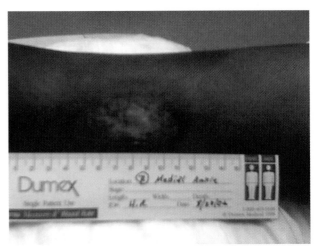

Figure 30•11 *Appearance of extremity at discharge.*

References

1. Partsch, H: Understanding the pathophysiological effects of compression. In: Calne, S (ed) EWMA Position Document: Understanding Compression Therapy. London, Medical Education Partnership, 2003, p 17.

2. Guyton, A: Textbook of Medical Physiology. Philadelphia, WB Saunders, 1991.

3. Armstrong, DG, Nguyen, HC: Improvement in healing with aggressive edema reduction after debridement of foot infection in persons with diabetes. Arch Surg 2000; 135:1405–1409.

4. Miller, S: Compression therapy for foot wounds: Overview and case reports. Wounds 2005; 17:278–281.

5. Mayberry, J, Moneta, GL, Taylor, LM Jr, et al: Fifteen-year results of ambulatory compression therapy for chronic venous ulcers. Surgery 1991; 109:575–581.

6. Clark, M: Compression bandages: Principles and definitions. In: Calne, S (ed) EWMA Position Document: Understanding Compression Therapy. London, Medical Education Partnership, 2003, p 17.

7. Reichardt, L: Venous ulceration: Compression as the mainstay of therapy. J Wound Ostomy Continence Nurs 1999; 26:39–47.

8. Blair, S, Wright, D, Backhouse, CM, et al: Sustained compression and healing of chronic venous ulcers. Br Med J 1988; 297:1159–1161.

9. Thomas, S: Compression bandaging in the treatment of venous leg ulcers. World Wide Wounds, 1998. Available at: http://www.worldwidewounds.com/1997/september/Thomas-Bandaging/bandage-paper.html. Accessed Dec. 30, 2009.

10. World Union of Wound Healing Societies (WUWHS): Principles of best practice: Compression in venous leg ulcers. A consensus document. London, Medical Education Partnership, 2008.

11. Trent, J, Falabella, A, Eaglstein, W, et al: Venous ulcers: Pathophysiology and treatment options. OstomyWound Manage 2005; 51:38–53.

12. Partsch, H: The use of pressure change on standing as a surrogate measure of the stiffness of a compression bandage. Eur J Vasc Endovasc Surg 2005; 30:415–421.

13. Szubs, A: Lymphedema: Classification, diagnosis, and therapy. Vasc Med 1998; 3:145–156.

14. Foldi, M: Treatment of lymphedema [editorial]. Lymphology 1994; 27:1–5.

15. Foldi, E, Foldi, M, Weissleder, H: Conservative treatment of lymphedema of the limbs. Angiology 1985; 36:171–180.

16. Boris, M, Weindorf, S, Lasinski, B, et al: Lymphedema reduction by noninvasive complex lymphedema therapy. Oncology 1994; 8:95–106, 109–110.

17. Davis, L, McCulloch, J, Neal, B, et al: The effectiveness of Unna boot and semipermeable film vs Unna boot alone in the healing of venous ulcers. OstomyWound Manage 1992; 38:19–21.

18. Lippmann, H, Briere, J: Physical basis of external supports in chronic venous insufficiency. Arch Phys Med 1971; 52:555–559.

19. Lippman, H, Fishman, L, Farrar, RH, et al: Edema control in the management of disabling chronic venous insufficiency. Arch Phys Med Rehabil 1994; 75:436–471.

20. European Wound Management Association (EWMA): EWMA Position Document: Understanding Compression Therapy. London, Medical Education Partnership, 2003.

21. Gaylarde, P, Sarkany, I, Dodd, HJ: The effect of compression on venous stasis. Br J Dermatol 1993; 128:255–258.

22. Fletcher, A, Cullum, N, Sheldon, T: A systematic review of compression treatment for venous leg ulcers. Br Med J 1997; 315:576–580.

23. Hafner, J, Botonakis, I, Burg, G: A comparison of multilayer bandage systems during rest, exercise, and over 2 days of wear time. Arch Dermatol 2000; 136:857–863.

24. Scriven, J, Taylor, L, Wood, A, et al: A prospective randomised trial of four-layer versus short stretch compression bandages for the treatment of venous leg ulcers. Ann R Coll Surg Engl 1998; 80:215–220.

25. Thompson, B, Hooper, P, Powell, R, et al: Four-layer bandaging and healing rates of venous leg ulcers. J Wound Care 1996; 5:213–216.

26. Second European consensus document on chronic critical leg ischaemia. Eur J Vasc Surg 1992; 6(suppl A):1–32.

27. Margolis, D, Berlin, J, Strom, B: Risk factors associated with the failure of a venous leg ulcer to heal. Arch Dermatol 1999; 135:920–926.

28. Margolis, D, Berlin, J, Strom, B: Which venous leg ulcers will heal with limb compression bandages? Am J Med 2000; 109:15–19.

29. Chaby, G, Viseux, V, Ramelet, A, et al: Refractory venous leg ulcers: A study of risk factors. Dermatol Surg 2006; 32:512–19.

30. Choucair, M, Phillips, T: Compression therapy. Dermatol Surg 1998; 24:141–148.

31. Blecken, S, Villavicencio, J, Kao, T: Comparison of elastic versus nonelastic compression in bilateral venous ulcers: A randomized trial. J Vasc Surg 2005; 42:1150–1155.

32. Bergan, J, Sparks, S: Non-elastic compression: An alternative in management of chronic venous insufficiency. J Wound Ostomy Continence Nurs 2000; 27:83–89.

33. Spence, R, Cahall, E: Inelastic versus elastic leg compression in chronic venous insufficiency: A comparison of limb size and venous hemodynamics. J Vasc Surg 1996; 24:783–787.

34. McCulloch, J: Intermittent compression for the treatment of a chronic stasis ulcer. Phys Ther 1981; 91:1452.

35. McCulloch, J, Marler, K, Neal, M, et al: Intermittent pneumatic compression improves venous ulcer healing. AdvWound Care 1994; 7:22–26.

36. Smith, PC, Sarin, S, Hasty, J, et al: Sequential gradient pneumatic compression enhances venous ulcer healing: A randomized trial. Surgery 1990; 108:871–875.

37. Weissleder, H, Schuchhardt, C: Lymphedema Diagnosis and Therapy, ed. 2. Bonn, Kagerer Kommunikation, 1997, p 270.

38. Kessler, C, Hirsch, D, Jacobs, H, et al: Intermittent pneumatic compression in chronic venous insufficiency favorably affects fibrinolytic potential and platelet activation. Blood Coagul Fibrinolysis 1996; 7:437–446.

39. Kolari, P, Pekanmaki, K: Intermittent pneumatic compression in healing venous ulcers. Lancet 1986; 2:1108.

40. Falanga, V, Eaglstein, W: A therapeutic approach to venous ulcers. J Am Acad Dermatol 1986; 14:777–784.

41. Samson, H, Showalter, D: Stockings and the prevention of recurrent venous ulcers. Dermatol Surg 1996; 22:373–376.

42. Cullum, N, Nelson, E, Fletcher, AW: Systematic reviews of wound care management: (5) beds; (6) compression; (7) laser therapy, therapeutic ultrasound, electrotherapy, and electromagnetic therapy. Health Technol Assess 2001; 5:1–221.

43. Marston, W, Vowden, K: Compression therapy: A guide to safe practice In: Calne, S (ed) EWMA Position Document: Understanding Compression Therapy. London, Medical Education Partnership, 2003, p 17.

chapter 31

Negative-Pressure Wound Therapy

Stanley Keith McCallon, MPT, DPT, CWS, FACCWS

Introduction

The use of negative-pressure wound therapy (NPWT) has increased dramatically in recent years in the United States and Europe, due in part to case studies and controlled trials demonstrating the effectiveness of the therapy. The process of applying negative pressure to wounds has been referred to by many names in the literature, including vacuum-assisted closure (V.A.C.®), topical negative pressure (TNP), vacuum-sealing technique (VST), subatmospheric pressure dressing (SPD), and sealed surface wound suction (SSS). The current NPWT nomenclature generally describes the controlled application of subatmospheric pressure to a wound using an electrical pump to intermittently or continuously convey pressure through connecting tubing to a specialized wound dressing to promote healing.

History

Subatmospheric pressure has been used in wound care for centuries through the use of drains from body cavities. However, the use of suction drainage was practiced more routinely beginning in the middle of the 20th century for the postsurgical removal of blood, bile, and other exudates.[1] Early studies reported the use of closed wound suction for prophylactic drainage, which appeared to greatly improve wound healing, minimize postoperative complications, and reduce the duration of hospitalization following surgery.[1]

Fleck and Frizzell reported that by the early 1980s, the principle of applying constant suction to promote healing gained renewed interest with surgeons. It was thought that a key factor in facilitating wound healing was the ability to contain, control, and remove excess fluid, air, or material that may disrupt the healing process.[2]

Several studies can be found in the Russian medical literature that analyze the benefits of vacuum treatment for purulent wounds following surgical débridement.[3-7] Kostiuchenok et al reported that the use of vacuum treatment in combination with surgical débridement significantly reduced the bacterial burden in the subject wounds and improved healing.[3] Davydov et al similarly found that the use of vacuum treatment in conjunction with surgical treatment in patients with purulent lactation mastitis reduced the bacterial load in the wound and reduced wound healing time as well as boosted immune system function.[4] In 1987 Usopov and Yeplifanov used a rabbit model to study the effects of vacuum treatment in the clinical setting in an effort to evaluate beneficial settings for negative pressure and duration of treatment.[5] Davydov et al published another study in 1988 evaluating the bacteriological and cytological properties of purulent wounds following vacuum treatment.[6] Over 200 patients had perforated drains placed in the depths of their purulent wounds following surgical incision and drainage. The drains were connected to a hemispherical chamber to cover the wound and connected to a vacuum source 1 hour a day for 6 days. A comparative group received the surgical intervention alone. Subsequently, tissues were obtained for biopsy from both groups. The authors concluded that vacuum treatment and surgical débridement in conjunction shortened the inflammatory process and reduced the local bacterial counts more effectively than did débridement alone.[6]

Back in North America, research into the benefits of negative pressure was beginning to take shape. Chariker et al discussed the benefits of closed suction wound drainage in 1989 for the management of incisional and cutaneous fistulas.[8] Evaluating a small number of fistulas over the course of 3 years, the authors placed moistened gauze in the wound base and then placed a Jackson-Pratt Mini Snyder flat drain over the gauze. The entire wound was then draped with an occlusive dressing to create an airtight seal. The drain was then connected to continuous suction at a pressure of –60 to –80 mm Hg and left in place for 3 to 5 days. The dressing protocol has been subsequently referred to as the Chariker-Jeter system or approach. The average closing time for the fistulas treated was 16 days, with a reported cost savings versus conventional dressings of the time.[8] In 1991 Nakayama and Soeda reported using adhesive drapes and suction drains to create "vacuum packages" on free skin grafts on hands.[9] Brock et al later described the technique of providing temporary closure of abdominal surgical wounds when conditions prevented immediate closure.[10] The group described a multiple-layer technique in which a polyethylene sheet was placed in contact with the wound, followed by a moist sterile surgical towel, then covered with a polyester sheet backed with acrylic adhesive. A silicone drain was placed between the second and third layers and connected to 100- to 150-mm Hg continuous suction.[10]

Perhaps the most comprehensive and broad-reaching research to that time was published in the *Annals of Plastic Surgery* in 1997. Drs. Morykwas and Argenta from the Bowman Gray School of Medicine in Winston-Salem, North Carolina, published a pair of studies that established foundational scientific mechanisms of action as well as treatment parameters for subatmospheric pressure therapy.[11-12] Morykwas elucidated a technique to expedite wound healing, which entailed placing a cut-to-fit open-cell polyurethane ether foam into contact with the wound bed. The foam was connected to a noncollapsible evacuation tube, and the entire wound was covered with an adhesive drape to create an airtight seal. The tubing was then connected to a vacuum unit creating 125 mm Hg of negative pressure to the wound site. The technique was labeled "vacuum-assisted closure" and abbreviated V.A.C.® (Kinetic Concepts Inc., San Antonio, TX) as a trademark of the company that owned the license and patent rights. Using a porcine model, the authors studied the effects of subatmospheric pressure on wound tissue by measuring blood flow to the wound and adjacent tissue using a laser Doppler. They also infected subject wounds with injections of 1 mL of saline containing 10^8 *Staphylococcus aureus* and *Staphylococcus epidermis* organisms. The results demonstrated an increase in local functional blood perfusion, accelerated rates of granulation tissue formation, a decrease in tissue bacterial levels, and an increase in nutrient blood flow as determined by survival of random pattern flaps.[11] Argenta and Morykwas also reported use of vacuum-assisted closure for treatment of difficult wounds of varying etiologies. The authors used the same technique as described in the aforementioned Morykwas study to treat acute, subacute, and chronic wounds as an alternative to previously used treatment such as serial saline-moistened gauze dressings. Of the 300 wounds evaluated for the study, 175 (of which 141 were pressure related) were classified as chronic wounds, 94 as subacute, and 31 as acute in etiology. All wounds were treated at a –125 mm Hg continuous setting for the first 48 hours and then switched to an intermittent setting (5 minutes on/2 minutes off) at –125 mm Hg. All dressings were changed at 48-hour intervals. All patients were treated with negative pressure until the wounds were completely healed, progressed to the point where they could be closed by a surgical procedure (skin graft or muscle flap), or until the patient refused further treatment or died. Using these endpoints, 296 of the 300 wounds had a positive response to NPWT.[12]

Mechanisms of Action

The effects of NPWT are thought to promote wound healing through multiple actions, including the removal of exudate from the wounds to help establish fluid balance, provision of a moist wound environment, removal of slough, a potential decrease in wound bacterial burden, a reduction in edema and third-space fluids, an increase in the blood flow to the wound, an increase in growth factors, and the promotion of white cells and fibroblasts within the wound.[13] Negative-pressure wound therapy also brings tissues together, promoting contraction, which allows the tissues to stick together through natural tissue adherence thereby increasing rates of healing.[13] These proposed mechanisms of action will be explored in greater detail within this chapter; however, several have not been fully elucidated within the scientific literature.

Moist Wound Environment

Wet-to-dry or wet-to-moist saline gauze dressings have been used for years due to their relative ease of application and low cost. The disadvantages of traditional gauze dressings include risk of wound desiccation, increased exposure to biological contaminants, wound bed disruption from frequency of dressing changes (2–4 times per day or more), and increased pain associated with tissue adherence and desiccation.[14] Ovington, in her often-cited work on the benefits of moist wound healing, noted that "traditional" dressings such as wet-to-dry or wet-to-moist gauze dressings may cause pain, wound reinjury, and delayed wound healing.[14] The practice of wet-to-dry saline gauze dressings was designed to serve as a form of mechanical débridement.[15] This method has been criticized for removing viable tissue as well as nonviable tissue and being traumatic to granulation tissue and to new epithelial cells.[16] One of the distinct characteristics of the closed airtight system used in NPWT is the promotion of moist wound healing through the creation of a normothermic, humid wound environment optimal for cell growth and the reduction of passive loss of moisture vapor from the wound.[17] Pain management has become a focal point in treatment of all patients, including those with wounds. Pain may be reduced through use of NPWT compared to many other dressing options for management of large and/or complex wounds. Krasner has helped quantify and illuminate pain experienced by patients with wounds through the chronic wound pain experience model.[18] Cyclic acute wound pain is described by Krasner as nociceptive pain occurring at regular time cycles, such as dressing changes and turning or repositioning.[18] The frequency with which NPWT dressings are changed (most protocols call for dressing changes every 48–72 hours) may help reduce cyclic acute pain experiences for the patient compared to other dressing options. Additionally, maintenance of a moist wound environment helps reduce pain. Krasner provided suggestions on ways of managing wound-related pain during use of negative pressure wound therapy, including soaking.[19] For more clinical suggestions for pain management in patients receiving NPWT, refer to Box 31.1.

Increased Blood Flow

In 1997 Morykwas et al used laser Doppler velocimetry to measure effects of NPWT on blood flow of wound tissue in porcine models.[11] Two circular defects, 2.5 cm in diameter, were excised down to the deep fascia of the muscles over the spine. Laser Doppler needle probes were then inserted into the subcutaneous tissue and deep back muscles adjacent to the defect. A foam dressing was then placed into the anterior wound and subatmospheric pressure applied in 25-mm Hg increments from 0 to 400 mm Hg for 15-minute intervals as blood flow was evaluated. Blood flow was recorded in a similar fashion on the posterior wound, but subatmospheric pressure was applied in an intermittent mode. Their study demonstrated a fourfold increase in microvascular blood flow over baseline with use of negative pressure at 125 mm Hg while blood flow was inhibited at pressures at or above –400 mm Hg. Interestingly, the increases in blood flow of the anterior wound declined after 5 to 7 minutes of continuous application of subatmospheric pressure, whereas the posterior wound treated with intermittent therapy demonstrated increased flow with each successive "on" cycle of treatment and returned to baseline during the "off" cycle.[11] (Fig. 31.1) Chen et al also observed an increase in blood flow to wounds experimentally created in the ears of white rabbits and treated with NPWT. Microscopic examination and image pattern analysis revealed that increased blood flow was the result of increased vascular diameter, blood flow velocity, and blood volume, as well as increased angiogenesis and endothelial proliferation.[20]

Wackenfors et al used a porcine model to further study the impact of NPWT (ranging from –50 to –200 mm Hg) on blood flow in the immediate and adjacent vicinity of an acute wound.[21-22] Among findings of the studies was the observation that NPWT decreased blood flow (hypoperfusion) in the immediate proximity of treated wounds but increased blood flow (hyperperfusion) in areas 1.5 to 3.0 cm away from the wound.

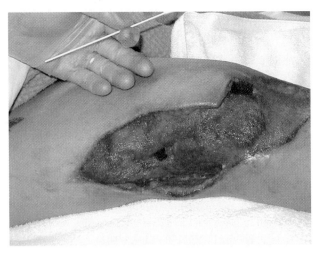

Figure 31•1 *Photo of patient with right lower-extremity traumatic wound. Beefy red granulation tissue response often seen with NPWT indicative of increased blood flow to wound tissue (Black foam NPWT dressing pieces are seen in photo).*

The authors found an increase in blood flow to the hypoperfused areas during "off" cycles, suggesting the presence of a reactive hyperemia. Due in part to the contrasting regional effects on blood flow, investigators in this study relate the beneficial effects of negative pressure more to its ability to reduce edema and to tamponade superficial bleeding than to its ability to increase blood flow.[21-22]

Swedish researchers used negative pressure on normal and ischemic myocardium to demonstrate stimulation of blood flow.[23] Lindstedt et al employed a porcine model and laser Doppler velocimetry to measure blood flow in the myocardium before, during, and after application of negative pressure. Doppler probes were sewn into the heart muscle and the heart exposed through a 5-cm-diameter hole for direct application of negative pressure via polyurethane foam. The study found that application of –50 mm Hg pressure induced a near twofold increase in microvascular blood flow in normal, ischemic, and reperfused myocardium.[23] The investigators' selection of 50 mm Hg of negative pressure was premised on earlier studies by Wackenfors et al suggesting that negative pressures of 75 to 125 mm Hg stimulate blood flow to a depth of 25 mm in skeletal tissue, whereas lower pressures stimulate skeletal muscle at more superficial depths.[22]

▶ **Box 31•1** **Pain Management During Negative-Pressure Wound Therapy**

- Educate patient and caregivers about NPWT purpose, benefits, and possible discomfort.
- Saturate dressings with normal saline prior to removal.
- Monitor patient's perceived pain level and provide appropriate analgesics if necessary to alleviate any discomfort; premedicate patient an appropriate amount

of time (dependent on analgesic administration route) before dressing change.
- Ramp negative pressure incrementally to target pressure if patient experiences discomfort adjusting to therapy; adjust target pressure to patient tolerance if required.
- Reassess patient frequently after pain-relief measures are initiated and document accurately.

Edema Reduction

The ongoing inflammatory response around a wound results in local tissue edema, a condition that adversely affects diffusion of needed nutrients and oxygen from the vascular bed to the wound.[24] All types of wounds are known to contain cytotoxic compounds, including proteases, cytokines, metalloproteases, and oxygen-free radicals, all of which are produced largely by neutrophils.[25-28] These compounds break down the extracellular matrix and granulation tissue found in wounds, and it has been suggested that they inhibit migration of needed repair cells (cytokines) into the wound, thus delaying wound closure.[26,28] These compounds have been found in the effluent obtained from human wounds treated with NPWT, suggesting that removal of cytotoxic compounds might be a viable mechanism by which NPWT enhances wound healing.[27] Morris et al noted that negative pressure may directly stimulate wound healing by simply creating a pressure gradient that "pulls" materials or cells from the wound bed or from surrounding tissues into the wound bed and then into the dressing of the NPWT device for removal.[29]

Healing in acute and chronic wounds is impaired by the presence of excessive fluid in the periwound spaces (eg, interstitium). Excessive fluid creates a myriad of problems, including impaired blood flow, tissue hypoxia, ischemia, and thrombosis.[30-32] Localized peripheral edema compresses the microvasculature and lymphatic system.[33-34] Morykwas et al postulated that the application of subatmospheric pressure resulted in an increase in localized blood flow due to active removal of the excess interstitial fluid from tissues immediately surrounding the wound, decompressing small blood vessels and restoring blood flow.[11] Recent burn literature has also demonstrated the benefits of edema reduction through use of NPWT with the vacuum-assisted closure device. Kamolz et al found that use of the V.A.C. on acute partial thickness hand burns resulted in hyperperfusion and prevention of burn progression.[35] The authors noted that the burn pathophysiology model includes impairment of blood flow within the zone of stasis created by active edema formation surrounding the burn. This zone of stasis may result in burn progression (eg, partial-thickness burn progressing to full-thickness injury) within a very short time. Morykwas et al also demonstrated in the porcine model that application of subatmospheric pressure is capable of preventing progression of partial-thickness burns.[11]

Lambert et al suggested that the pressure gradient may act by simply pulling or drawing greater numbers of keratinocytes into and across the wound, thereby increasing the population of cells necessary for wound healing.[36] Negative-pressure gradients also may favor approximation of soft tissue and reduce the likelihood of soft tissue retraction.[37] Similarly, the simple action of bringing and holding the wound edges closer together would promote wound healing.[29] (Figs. 31.2 and 31.3)

Mechanical Deformation

Despite the benefits of edema reduction, some wounds have shown positive responses to NPWT in the absence of appreciable fluid extraction. This response has been attributed to a

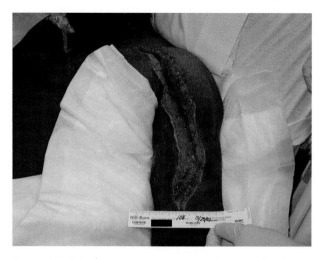

Figure 31•2 *Left anterior upper-extremity wound status after surgical removal of infected vascular shunt (NPWT day #0).*

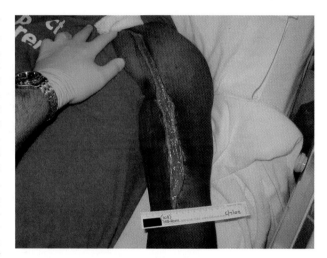

Figure 31•3 *Left anterior upper-extremity wound seen in Fig. 31.2 following 13 days of NPWT treatment.*

cellular level action described as mechanical deformation or microdeformation.[38] Mechanically stretching isolated cells from several organs is known to stimulate cell mitosis, cell proliferation, and angiogenesis.[39,40] Several in vivo studies support the mechanical stress theory as a mechanism for increasing cellular proliferation and angiogenesis.[41-44] Specific signaling molecules and genes that lead to cellular changes in response to this type of cell deformation have been identified.[39,40] It has been suggested that the application of negative pressure disrupts the balance between the extracellular matrix and the intracellular cytoskeleton, resulting in release of various intracellular second messengers, including some that upregulate cell growth.[38] (Fig. 31.4) Using the V.A.C. foam as a contact medium with wound tissue, Saxena et al demonstrated through computer modeling based on histological studies that the pressures used with the V.A.C. create tissue strain sufficient to deform cells by as much as 20%, a change known to induce cell proliferation in vitro.[38] (Fig. 31.5) It is very likely that

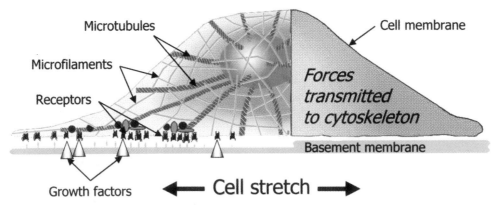

Figure 31•4 *Schematic view of a cell (with cytoskeleton elements) showing the cell can extend by attachment to the extracellular matrix and/or by application of external force. (Reproduced with permission from: Saxena, V, Hwang, C-W, Huang, S, et al: Vacuum assisted closure: Microdeformations of wounds and cell proliferation. Plast Reconstr Surg 2004; 114(5):1086–1096.)*

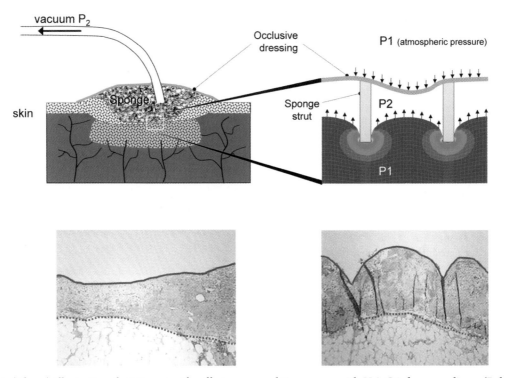

Figure 31•5 *(Above) Illustration depicting specific effect on wound tissue seen with V.A.C.® foam medium. (Below, left) Histological section of wound biopsy specimen at 7 days without application of the V.A.C. foam sponge. (Below, right) Different area of same wound tissue after 7 days of V.A.C. (Reproduced with permission from: Saxena, V, Hwang, C-W, Huang, S, et al: Vacuum assisted closure: Microdeformations of wounds and cell proliferation. Plast Reconstr Surg 2004; 114(5):1086–1096.114(5):1086–1096.)*

negative pressures also can create such changes in a human wound.[38,45] Numerous studies have suggested that intermittent negative pressure is more effective than continuous negative pressure for proliferative growth of granulation tissue because continuous pressure causes less cell deformation and intermittent application of pressure causes repeated stimulation of cellular level second messengers.[11,45]

The role of matrix metalloproteinases (MMPs) in wounds has been evaluated at great length in the scientific literature.

MMPs, a family of zinc-dependent endopeptidases, degrade the extracellular matrix and promote endothelial migration and growth factor production.[46] Elevated levels of MMPs, such as MMP-9 and MMP-2, frequently seen in chronic wounds, can also inhibit angiogenesis by generating inhibitors such as angiostatin and endostatin.[47-51] (Fig. 31.6) Greene et al recently studied the effects of NPWT using V.A.C. foam as a contact medium with the wound tissue and demonstrated significant reductions in MMP levels of treated

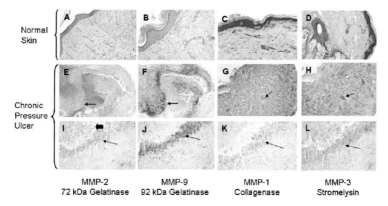

Figure 31•6 *Immunohistochemical localization of matrix metalloproteinases (MMP-2, MMP-9, MMP-1, and MMP-3) in biopsies of normal skin (top row) and biopsies from chronic pressure ulcers. The arrows in panels E, F, I, J, K, and L indicate regions of inflammatory cells. Arrows in panels G and H indicate vessels. Magnification in panels A to H is 40× and in panels I to L is 100×. Note the absence or low levels of MMPs in normal skin compared with the intense immunostaining for MMPs in the sections of chronic pressure ulcers. In addition, the intense immunostaining of MMP-2 and MMP-9 are strongly associated with regions that contain high numbers of polymorphonuclear inflammatory cells. (Reproduced with permission from: Schultz, GS, Ladwig, G, Wysocki, A: Extracellular matrix: Review of its roles in acute and chronic wounds. World Wide Wounds 2005; August. Available from: http://www.worldwidewounds.com/2005/august/Schultz/Extrace-Matric-Acute-Chronic-Wounds.html.)*

chronic wounds.[52] The authors found that MMP-2 (active and latent) and MMP-9 levels decreased between 15% and 76% during the first and second weeks of NPWT treatment in areas of V.A.C. foam contact and also found a corresponding twofold to threefold increase in microvessel density, suggesting increased angiogenesis.[52] Interestingly, areas without foam contact but underneath the occlusive negative-pressure drape showed overall increases in MMP-2 and MMP-9 levels compared to the levels taken before NPWT treatment, at which time patients were receiving wet-to-dry saline gauze dressing changes.[52] The gelatinases MMP-9 and MMP-2 are found at significantly higher levels in nonhealing wounds but will return to normal levels as wound healing progresses to closure.[47-51,53-54] The complete role of NPWT in converting chronic wounds back to an acute stage of wound healing remains under clinical investigation.

Bioburden Reduction

An open wound becomes contaminated with bacteria from the surrounding skin within 48 hours, and correspondingly, most acute wounds and all chronic wounds have measurable bacterial counts.[55] In the absence of cellulitis, it is often not possible to distinguish normal colonization from excessive bacteria or critical colonization. Indeed, a recent article by White and Cutting examined the need for clinicians to conclude that delayed healing is more likely than not to be microbiological in origin.[56] Significant impairments to wound healing occur in the presence of infection, clinically defined as that point of critical colonization of microorganisms measuring 10^5 colony-forming units per square centimeter of wound surface or gram of tissue.[57-58] Wound infection is particularly problematic in patients with compromised immune defenses. In critically ill patients, it is crucial to ensure the optimization of the patient's nutritional status in order to meet the demands of tissue repair and immune function.[59]

The presence of excessive bacteria in a wound will inevitably delay the healing process. Kostiuchenok et al found that suction treatment of a purulent wound after surgical débridement significantly reduced the microbe count in the wound tissues.[3] Similar findings were published by Morykwas et al in 1997 where it was reported that tissue bacterial counts decreased significantly after 4 days of NPWT treatment.[11] In the Morykwas study, five swine models with two circular surgically created defects measuring 2.5 cm were injected with 1 mL of saline containing 10^8 organisms, including *Staphylococcus aureus* and a pig isolate of *Staphylococcus epidermis*. Foam dressings were applied to both the experimental and control wounds and secured with adhesive drape. Negative pressure at 125 mm Hg was applied to the experimental defect. Serial 3-mm punch biopsy tissues from both wounds were obtained over the following 2 weeks. Biopsy results indicated that the number of organisms per gram of tissue decreased significantly between treatment days 4 and 5 in the wounds treated with NPWT, whereas levels in control wounds took an average of 11 days to decrease below 10^5 organisms per gram of tissue.[11] However, a study by Moues and associates in 2004 demonstrated conflicting results for human subjects.[60] In that study, patients with full-thickness wounds that could not be closed due to infection, contamination, or chronic character were randomized into two groups: NPWT or conventional moist gauze treatment. Investigators were allowed to choose between normal saline, nitrofuralam solution, acetic acid solution, or sodium hypochlorite as moistening agents for the control group, whereas a standard NPWT dressing was applied every 48 hours to the experimental wounds. The study results indicated a significant reduction in the wound surface area for NPWT-treated wounds but no difference in bacterial load reduction for either group. During NPWT, a clear shift in bacterial species was noted, with a decrease in the number of nonfermentative negative rods and an increase seen in the number of *S. aureus*. The authors concluded that NPWT had a similar effect on bacterial load as conventional treatment but had a statistically significant impact on wound size reduction.[60]

Some NPWT devices use antimicrobial gauze as the contact medium. The gauze is impregnated with 0.02% polyhexamethylene biguanide (PHMB), a powerful antiseptic that has the ability to suppress microbial growth on fiber when contamination is present. It has a broad range of effectiveness against gram-positive and gram-negative microorganisms, including some multi-drug-resistant strains such as methicillin-resistant *Staphylococcus aureus* (MRSA).[61] The Kinetic Concepts Inc. (KCI) product line offers silver-impregnated foam to use on highly contaminated or infected wounds. V.A.C. Granufoam® Silver (Kinetic Concepts Inc.) is an open-celled reticulated foam that is microbonded with metallic silver that, upon exposure to wound fluid, oxidates to ionic silver.[62] Ionic silver has become increasingly popular as an anti-infective agent for wound care due to its large spectrum of antimicrobial coverage and minimal side effects.[63] A recent modification of the NPWT system—NPWT with instillation—allows for intermittent instillation of solutions into the wound (V.A.C. Instill™ from Kinetic Concepts Inc. is one example). Instead of the traditional single tubing, the NPWT with instillation uses two sets of tubing. (Fig. 31.7) The instillation fluid drips by gravity through the first tubing to saturate the sponge and bathe the wound. The irrigation tubing is then occluded. Fluid is allowed to sit in the wound for a predetermined period of time (from 1 second to 1 hour), after which vacuum is applied to the suction tubing, thereby removing the irrigation fluid and wound exudate and collapsing the sponge. Suction is continuously maintained until the entire cycle is repeated according to the amount of time programmed into the unit (1 minute to 12 hours). Typical instillation solutions include normal saline, antibiotics, antifungals, antiseptics, and local anesthetics.[64] It is important to note that clinically infected wounds should be monitored very closely and may require more frequent dressing changes than noninfected wounds. If there are signs of the onset of systemic infection or advancing infection at the wound site, the physician should be contacted to determine if the NPWT should be discontinued.[62]

Clinical Applications

Negative-pressure wound therapy has been demonstrated to deliver positive outcomes in all patient care settings across a broad spectrum of wound types. Indications for use include chronic, acute, traumatic, subacute, and dehisced wounds, partial-thickness burns, ulcers (eg, diabetic and pressure), as well as flaps and grafts.[62] (Box 31.2)

NPWT is currently a widely accepted treatment for wounds of multiple etiologies and has been adapted and used by surgeons in the thoracic, general, trauma, burn, orthopedic, urologic, and plastic/reconstructive specialties.[65-73] It is important to remember that no one modality or treatment is a panacea for all wounds. Many factors should be considered before initiating NPWT, including the patient's general ability

> **Box 31•2** **Negative-Pressure Wound Therapy Indications**

- Pressure ulcers (stage III and IV)
- Orthopedic trauma wounds
- Diabetic ulcers
- Postoperative flaps
- Autologous meshed grafts
- Bioengineered tissue grafts
- Open abdominal wounds
- Surgical dehisced wounds
- Partial-thickness burns

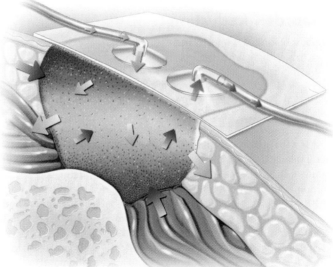

Figure 31•7 *Illustration depicting two-way system in V.A.C. Instill™ product. Yellow arrows indicate instillation of fluid through foam, and blue arrows indicate return flow of fluids under negative pressure. (Courtesy of KCI Licensing Inc., 2007.)*

Courtesy KCI Licensing, Inc., San Antonio, TX 11/2007

to heal, nutritional and circulatory status, bioburden, and presence of necrotic tissue.[74] (Box 31.3)

The patient should be determined to have adequate ability to heal or stimulate angiogenesis. Consideration should be given to overall health issues, including systemic respiratory function, use of anti-inflammatory/corticosteroid medications, and history of radionecrosis or hypoxia. As detailed in Chapter 4, adequate nutrition is absolutely essential to wound healing. Baseline and ongoing nutritional assessments should be performed to determine the patient's nutritional status.[74] (Box 31.4)

Adequate circulation to the wound site is also essential for wound healing as it allows for transport of oxygen, cytokines, and other growth factors. While NPWT is helpful to increase local perfusion of wound tissue, it will not be effective if the patient has macrocirculatory deficiencies such as proximal arterial occlusion. Bioburden should be considered before initiating NPWT. Appropriate measures should be taken in the event that heavy microbial colonization will limit wound healing.[75] Deeper soft tissue or bone infection will require more aggressive treatment prior to NPWT initiation. Surgical débridement and targeted antibiotic coverage is considered

the gold standard for treatment of chronic osteomyelitis.[76] Proper wound bed preparation including débridement of eschar and devitalized tissue is essential to ensure success with any treatment modality, including NPWT. NPWT may be initiated in the presence of a small amount of soft necrotic slough, but in general the wound bed should be devoid of most necrotic tissue.[77] Due to the potential for exudate and fluid removal with NPWT, care should be taken to assess the patient's hydration status before and during NPWT. Extrinsic factors that affect wound healing must be addressed, including pressure off-loading (for horizontal, recumbent, and ambulatory positions), moisture control, and reduction of shear and friction.[74-75] (Box 31.5)

Pain control should be considered for all patients, including those receiving NPWT. Frequent assessments should be performed to ensure adequate pain control measures are in place during and between treatments. (See Box 31.1) Measures can also be taken to ensure the periwound skin is protected during NPWT. These measures include the use of skin protection preparations and absorptive dressings such as hydrofibers and hydrocolloids when appropriate to protect the periwound from excessive moisture or adhesion problems.[78] (Figs. 31.8 through 31.10) Pressure relief should also be provided to ensure that collection tubes and plastic ports do not cause tissue damage.[77] (Fig. 31.11) In deeper wounds, it is imperative to accurately identify the number and kind of materials placed in the cavity to ensure all foreign objects are removed at subsequent dressing changes.

▸ **Box 31•3** | **Negative-Pressure Wound Therapy Contraindications**

- Malignancy in wound
- Untreated osteomyelitis (débridement of necrotic tissue/ bone and appropriate antibiotic therapy recommended before initiating NPWT)
- Wound with exposed blood vessels, anastomotic sites, organs, or nerves
- Necrotic tissue with eschar and/or hardened slough
- Nonenteric or unexplored fistula
- Patients with bleeding disorder or inadequate wound hemostasis

---

▸ **Box 31•4** | **Before Initiating Negative-Pressure Wound Therapy**

- Débride eschar and hardened slough
- Reduce bioburden through cleansing with appropriate solutions, cleansers, or topical antimicrobial dressings
- Assess for adequate blood supply
- Identify and correct intrinsic factors that affect healing (eg, protein deficiency, heavy bioburden, hyperglycemia)
- Identify and correct extrinsic factors that affect healing (eg, excessive pressure, friction, shear, and excessive moisture from incontinence)
- Ensure proper training of staff/caregivers who will be responsible for changing dressing, monitoring the treatment, and troubleshooting problems

---

▸ **Box 31•5** | **During Negative-Pressure Wound Therapy**

- Provide adequate pain control to patient, if needed, during dressing-change procedures and/or NPWT treatment. (Box 31.1).
- Prepare periwound skin with alcohol-free skin preparation for protection and help with adhesion of drape. (Fig. 31.9)
- Address periwound maceration, if present, with use of absorptive, protective materials (eg, hydrofiber or hydrocolloid). (Fig. 31.10)
- Frequently check seal to ensure airtight status.
- Count number of pieces of foam or other dressing material and record on drape with indelible ink to notify others during subsequent dressing change.
- Ensure removal of all pieces of foam or other contact materials with each dressing change.
- Monitor fluid status on patients receiving NPWT (especially pediatric and geriatric patients).
- Cover any exposed structures with nonadherent sterile dressings prior to initiation of NPWT.
- Do *not* take NPWT pumps into magnetic resonance imaging (MRI), hyperbaric oxygen therapy (HBOT) environments, or into the presence of flammable anesthetics.

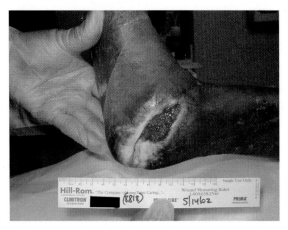

Figure **31•8** *Photo of patient with left medial ankle wound receiving NPWT. White-colored periwound tissue represents area of tissue maceration from excessive hydration.*

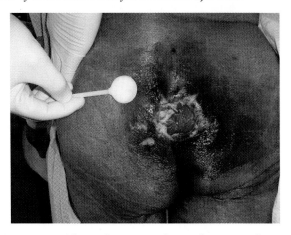

Figure **31•9** *Photo of patient with sacral pressure ulcer. Note the application of alcohol-free skin preparation film via a sterile applicator. The use of skin preparations serves to protect the periwound skin and remove oils from skin to allow better adhesion of NPWT film drapes.*

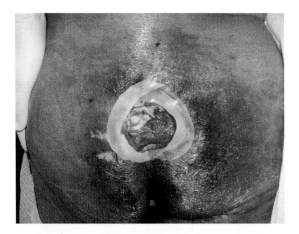

Figure **31•10** *Photo of patient with sacral pressure ulcer. Note periwound region has been dressed with a thin hydrocolloid cut to fit in order to protect periwound skin from excess moisture.*

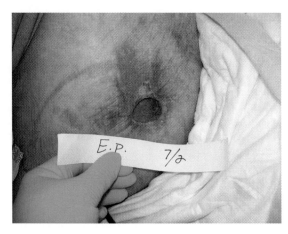

Figure **31•11** *Photo of patient with sacral pressure ulcer that has been treated with NPWT. Note areas of redness and periwound skin breakdown related to excessive pressure from NPWT tubing and inappropriate contact with dressing.*

Efficacy

Hundreds of patient case series, case studies, and anecdotal accounts can be found in the medical literature regarding NPWT, most involving evaluation of the V.A.C. product. The treatment has been used on wounds of all etiologies with positive outcome data reported. Case studies and series are valuable but provide no clinically objective, comparative information to allow the clinician to deduce if a certain treatment is more or less effective than another. As a result of multiple confounding factors when evaluating human wounds, single-arm trials that lack a control group are insufficient to determine if improvement is related only to the intervention being tested.[79] Therefore, properly conducted randomized controlled trials (RCTs), which contain an experimental and concurrent control group, permit the evaluator to measure the treatment effect above that related to optimization of standard treatment. Randomized assignment to treatment group and an independent, blinded outcomes measurement are also essential in removing bias and distributing confounding factors.[79] Early literature on NPWT was based on results of experimentation on the animal model, but there have been several randomized controlled trials on humans in the intervening years. However, some have criticized the relative small number of RCTs in the literature as insufficient support of the hypothesis that NPWT is more effective than current standard care in reducing wound healing times, costs, and overall wound healing outcomes.[29,79-80] A Cochrane review conducted by Evans and Land in 2001 found only two appropriate RCTs on a total of 34 patients were available at that time and determined that those studies contained methodological and statistical weaknesses that provided weak evidence that NPWT was more effective than saline gauze dressings in healing chronic human wounds.[80] In 2004 Samson et al conducted an evidence report and technology assessment for the Agency of Healthcare Research and Quality (AHRQ) on low-level laser and NPWT (vacuum-assisted closure).[79] The report provided an overview of clinical and methodological issues relevant to evaluating evidence on NPWT for acute and chronic wound healing and determined that only well-controlled, randomized trials could be used to reach conclusions on treatment efficacy. The authors identified only six trials (out of 467 studies) that met the inclusion criteria for the review and determined those trials were of small size and poor quality.[15,60,67,81-83] Samson et al suggested that future research demonstrating the efficacy of NPWT should address how to improve the delivery of care, quality of care, cost effectiveness, and outcomes of wound treatments in various care settings.[79] More recently, Armstrong and Lavery published a large, multicenter RCT on the use of NPWT following partial diabetic foot amputation.[74] In that study a total of 162 patients were randomly assigned to the NPWT ($N = 77$) group receiving dressing changes with the V.A.C. system or were assigned to the control ($N = 85$) group receiving standard moist wound care (alginates, hydrocolloids, foams, or hydrogels in accordance with a standardized guideline). Inclusion criteria included patients aged 18 or older with diabetic foot amputations to the transmetatarsal level of the foot, adequate glucose control, and evidence of adequate perfusion. Wounds were treated until closed or until completion of a 112-day assessment period, with dressing changes every 48 hours for NPWT group and every 24 hours or at discretion of attending clinician for the control group.[74] Measures were taken to ensure proper off-weighting therapy and nutritional assessment and intervention if needed. Outcomes indicated that NPWT yielded a higher proportion of healed wounds, faster time to wound closure, a more rapid and robust granulation tissue response, and a potential trend toward reduced risk for a second amputation as compared to the control group.[74] The authors self-identified some potential weaknesses of the study, such as performance bias, and there were some external criticisms including confusion over actual endpoints, low power, and poor descriptions of adverse events.[84-86] A subsequent resource utilization and economic cost evaluation of the treatments provided in the Armstrong and Lavery trial was recently presented.[87] Resource utilization and costs for inpatient hospital care, surgical procedures, reamputations, postbaseline débridements, antibiotics, outpatient treatment visits, dressing changes, and dressing materials were calculated and analyzed in a post hoc retrospective study. The results of the cost analysis revealed no difference in the number of admissions or length of stay between the NPWT and control groups. However, more surgical procedures, additional dressing changes, and more necessitated outpatient treatment visits for the control moist wound healing group led to increased cost versus the NPWT group. On average, the direct cost per patient treated 8 weeks or longer, independent of clinical outcome, was $27,270 for the NPWT group and $36,096 for the control group.[87] Several more randomized controlled trials have appeared in the literature recently, including studies on posttraumatic hematomas and surgical incisions and chronic leg ulcers.[66,69] While there is growing evidence that NPWT treatment is clinically beneficial, additional large, well-designed randomized trials are needed to demonstrate the efficacy and cost effectiveness of negative-pressure therapy.[29,79-80]

Commercially Available Negative-Pressure Wound Therapy Products

Several NPWT products are available on the United States commercial market. Here, each available product is generally described and illustrations and photographs are provided for identification purposes. Additional information can be obtained by using the provided manufacturer contact information. The clinician and end user are responsible for discerning the benefits and efficacy of any particular product or system.

Boehringer Wound Systems LLC Products

Boehringer Wound Systems LLC is a subsidiary of Boehringer Laboratories, which has over 30 years of experience in hospital suction systems, anesthesia instrumentation, and sterile consumables. The Engenex™ Advanced Negative Pressure Wound Therapy System (Boehringer Wound Systems LLC, Norristown, PA) uses a wound contact layer with Bio-Dome™ dressing technology. The Bio-Dome dressing is multilayered in a corrugated fashion and features multiple dimples on the contact surface through which the negative pressure is delivered, allowing granulation tissue growth. (Fig. 31.12) The dressing should be cut slightly smaller than the wound and placed with the Bio-Dome surface side in contact with the wound tissue. The dressing is also available with the EasyRelease™ contact layer, which is designed to minimize wound tissue adherence and reduce the risk of pain with dressing removal.

The Engenex Wound Flo™ suction pump operates within a 30- to 75-mm Hg vacuum range that can be adjusted by the clinician. A color-coded indicator system provides a visual indication of the system operation, and an internal hour meter tracks the hours of satisfactory vacuum delivery. An alarm will sound if a leak is detected in the system, and a rechargeable battery is incorporated in the pump unit. The Engenex Wound Flo suction pump is connected to the Bio-Dome dressing via a single lumen, noncollapsible tubing and an Opti-Flo™ tube attachment device (T.A.D.) that is thermally welded to adherent element covering the Bio-Dome. A 500-mL collection canister features an integrated shut-off filter that stops suction when the canister is full. (Fig. 31.13)

In addition to general NPWT contraindications, the Engenex system is contraindicated for emergency airway aspiration, pleural/mediastinal/chest tube drainage, surgical suction, or application over exposed blood vessels, organs, or nerves. For complete details on this product, see the website for "Instructions for Use" at www.boehringerwound.com.

Medela Inc. Products

Medela Inc., headquartered in Switzerland, operates a global medical technology and breastfeeding supply organization. The Medela Healthcare Division offers medical suction devices for use in multiple practice settings, with application for plastic surgery, cardiothoracic drainage, endoscopy, airway suction, and wound care. The Invia® Healing System (Medela Inc. USA, McHenry, IL) is a NPWT system introduced in the United States in the acute care setting in April of 2007, with

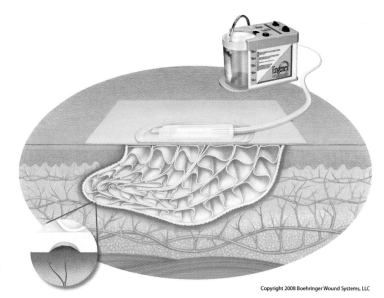

Figure 31•12 *Illustration showing cross-section of the Bio-Dome™ dressing in contact with the wound tissue. Inset shows magnified depiction of dressing interaction with wound tissue. (Used with permission of Boehringer Wound Systems LLC.)*

Copyright 2008 Boehringer Wound Systems, LLC

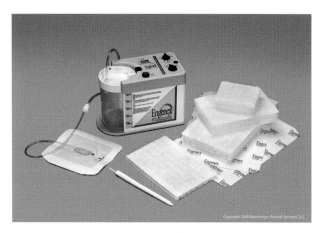

Figure 31•13 *Engenex™ product line. (Used with permission of Boehringer Wound Systems LLC).*

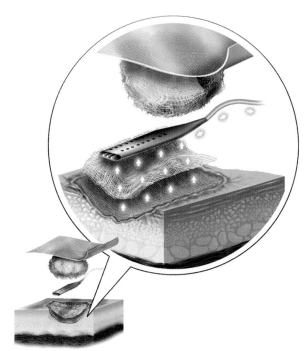

Figure 31•14 *Illustration depicting the Chariker-Jeter dressing sequence. (Used with permission from Medela Inc.)*

plans for subsequent introduction to long-term care, extended care, and home care.

The Invia Healing System uses an antimicrobial gauze dressing and nonadherent wound contact layer. The antimicrobial gauze is impregnated with 0.02% polyhexamethylene biguanide (PHMB), a broad-spectrum antiseptic. The wound dressing kit uses the Chariker-Jeter design with a gauze layer and flat suction drain. (Fig. 31.14) Routine dressing changes are recommended every 48 hours, unless the wound is infected, for which the manufacturer recommends dressing changes every 12 to 24 hours.

The suction for the system is supplied by the Medela-manufactured Vario 18 AC/DC c/i aspirator pump. (Fig. 31.15) Dressing supply kits come in a variety of sizes and sterile disposables for use. (Fig. 31.16) In addition to the general contraindications for NPWT, Medela Healthcare suggests exercising precautions in patients with unexplored fistulas, tunnels, or sinus tracts and patients at risk for bleeding. A full list of recommendations and instructions for use can be found on the company's website at www.inviahealingsystem.com.

Kinetic Concepts Inc. Products

Kinetic Concepts Inc (KCI USA Inc.), a global medical technology company, designs, manufactures, and markets a family of NPWT products known collectively as the Vacuum Assisted Closure (V.A.C.®) therapy system (Kinetic Concepts Inc., San Antonio, TX). (Fig. 31.17) The V.A.C. devices are cleared by the FDA for use in all care settings, including the home setting.

The V.A.C. system uses Granufoam®, an open-cell, reticulated, hydrophobic polyurethane foam that serves as the contact medium with the wound tissue. The dressing can be cut to conform to the geometry of the wound and consists of

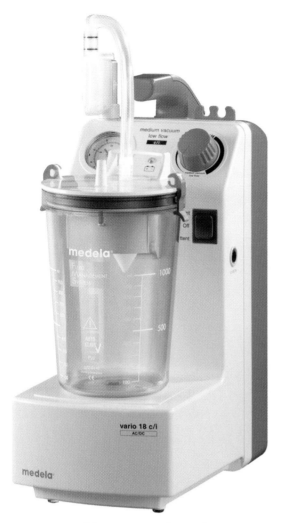

Figure 31•15 *Medela® Vario18 AC/DC c/i aspirator pump. (Used with permission from Medela Inc.)*

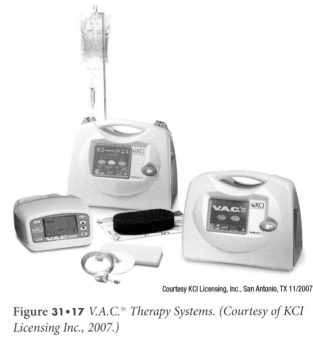

Courtesy KCI Licensing, Inc., San Antonio, TX 11/2007

Figure 31•17 *V.A.C.® Therapy Systems. (Courtesy of KCI Licensing Inc., 2007.)*

thousands of micropores that collect and move fluid under suction. (Fig. 31.18) The Granufoam dressings, with pore sizes in the 400- to 600-micron size, come in regular black and silver-impregnated varieties and are available in many different sizes and configurations. A white foam dressing is also available and has a smaller pore size for use in sensitive areas or in cases in which granulation tissue in-growth needs to be avoided. Most of the V.A.C. systems use a single-tube evacuation system that connects to the disposable foam dressing via the SensaT.R.A.C.® pad. (Fig. 31.19) In general, the dressings are changed every 48 hours for patients receiving continuous or intermittent NPWT. More frequent dressing changes are recommended for infected wounds. The V.A.C. Instill™ system has a two-way system, with one tube to allow instillation of

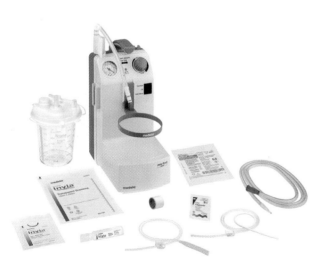

Figure 31•16 *Invia® Healing System product line. (Used with permission from Medela Inc.)*

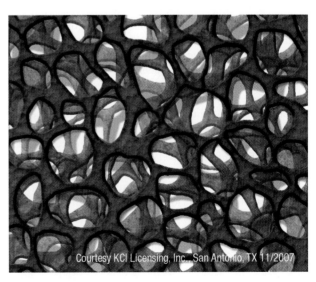

Courtesy KCI Licensing, Inc., San Antonio, TX 11/2007

Figure 31•18 *V.A.C.® Granufoam® dressing and artist rendition close-up. (Courtesy of KCI Licensing Inc., 2007.)*

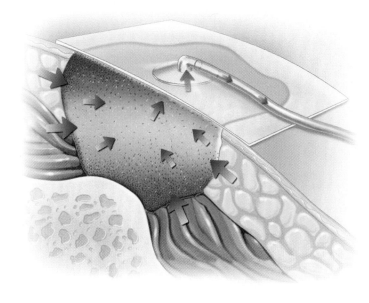

Figure 31•19 *Illustration of SensaT.R.A.C.® pad in contact with V.A.C.® foam. (Courtesy of KCI Licensing Inc., 2007.)*

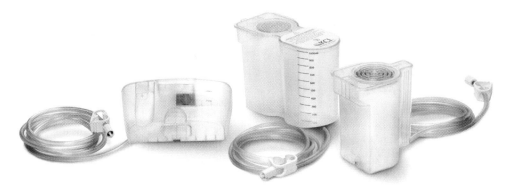

Figure 31•20 *V.A.C.® Canisters. (Courtesy of KCI Licensing Inc., 2007.)*

solution and another to allow removal of fluid. (Fig. 31.7) The Instill system can be used with a range of solutions, including topical cleansers, topical antibiotics, topical antifungals, topical antiseptics, and topical anesthetics.[62]

Suction for the V.A.C. system is provided by a self-contained pump unit that features a LED display, and pressures are provided in 25-mm Hg increments up to 200 mm Hg. The pump unit accommodates a disposable canister (either 500 mL or 1000 mL size, depending on unit) that contains an agent that solidifies and decontaminates the exudate and a valve that prevents backflow. (Fig. 31.20) The pump system has an alarm in the event that the desired target negative pressure is not met due to leak in the system or in the event that the canister is full. It has a long-life rechargeable battery incorporated into the pump casing.

V.A.C. dressings come in a variety of shapes, sizes, and configurations. (Fig. 31.21) In addition, the clinician can create a bridge to allow negative-pressure suction but relocate the tubing and SensaT.R.A.C. pad away from bony prominences. (Fig. 31.22) For a complete list of available dressings, systems, and instructions for use, see the website for KCI USA Inc. at www.woundvac.com or www.kci1.com.

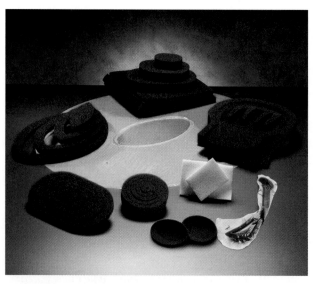

Figure 31•21 *V.A.C.® Dressings. (Courtesy of KCI Licensing Inc., 2007.)*

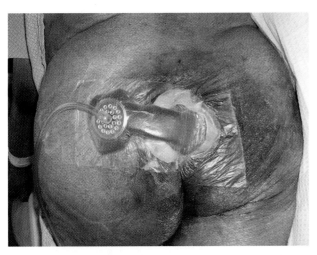

Figure 31•22 *Photo of patient with sacral pressure ulcer demonstrating the bridging technique of reducing pressure from bony prominence.*

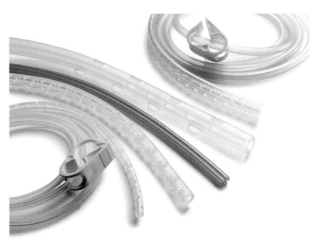

Figure 31•23 *Smith & Nephew NPWT tubes and drains. (Used with permission of Smith & Nephew.)*

Smith & Nephew Products

In May 2007 Smith and Nephew, a global medical technology business, announced the acquisition of BlueSky Medical Group Inc. and BlueSky's NPWT products. Smith & Nephew operates in 31 countries and offers a large number of wound-related products and devices through its Advanced Wound Management division.

The Smith & Nephew NPWT products use an oil-emulsified nonadherent layer as the primary wound contact layer followed by a moistened antimicrobial gauze to fill the wound base. A flexible silicone drain, available in different sizes and applications, is then placed in the wound base on top of the gauze, using the previously described Chariker-Jeter approach.[8] (Fig. 31.23) The remainder of the wound is filled with the moistened antimicrobial gauze and covered with a transparent adhesive film dressing to create an airtight seal. (Fig. 31.24)

The Versatile 1™ EZ Care (Smith & Nephew, Largo, FL) pump comes in a tabletop design and is capable of delivering negative pressure in the range of 40 mm Hg to 200 mm Hg in either continuous or intermittent settings. (Fig. 31.25) The unit has a 40-hour battery life and alarms for low battery and low pressure. The pump also comes in a portable version called the V1STA™ portable system. (Fig. 31.26) The unit weighs just over 4 pounds, can operate for 4 hours on battery power, and has several alarm conditions, including low battery, low vacuum, and high vacuum. The manufacturer recommends negative-pressure therapy in the 40 to 80 mm Hg range with use of both the Versatile 1 EZ Care pump and the V1STA portable system.

A number of dressing kits are available, depending on the wound size, location, and amount or type of exudate. (Fig. 31.27) The Wooding-Scott™ kits include an irrigation/aspiration drain that allows the clinician to deliver saline and/or medication to the wound site and remove it via suction without changing the dressing each time. For more information on the product offerings and instructions for use, see the company's website at www.smith-nephew.com.

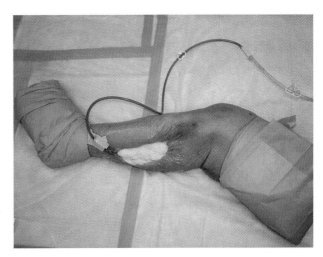

Figure 31•24 *Photo of patient with left lateral leg wound receiving NPWT using Smith & Nephew system. (Used with permission of Smith & Nephew.)*

Kalypto Medical Products

The NPD 1000 Negative Pressure Wound Therapy System is a small, portable system comprising a battery-operated electromechanical pump with an accessory wound dressing. (Fig. 31.28) The system uses a small device mated with a closed dressing. In lieu of a separate collection canister, the wound dressing is designed to absorb and contain wound exudate.

The NPD 1000 pump provides negative pressure in two modes, intermittent and continuous, in pressure ranges from –40 mm Hg to –125 mm Hg. In continuous mode, the pump holds the dressing at the prescribed pressure continuously between dressing changes. In intermittent mode, the pump cycles between the prescribed pressure and atmospheric pressure by venting the bandage with a solenoid valve. The dressing is held at the therapeutic negative pressure for 5 minutes and vented to atmospheric pressure for 2 minutes. Polyvinyl chloride (PVC) tubing connects the dressing to the pump via a pressure port fitting. The dressing has three windows near

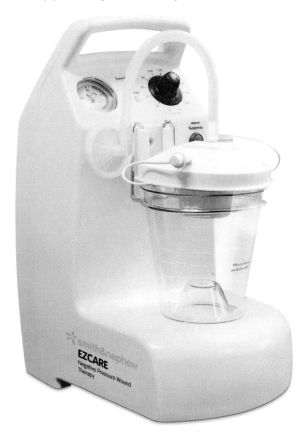

Figure 31•25 *Smith & Nephew EZ CARE Versatile 1™ NPWT pump. (Used with permission of Smith & Nephew.)*

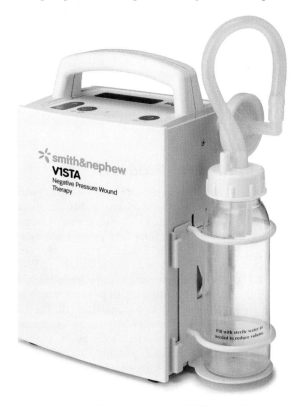

Figure 31•26 *Smith & Nephew VISTA™ NPWT pump. (Used with permission of Smith & Nephew.)*

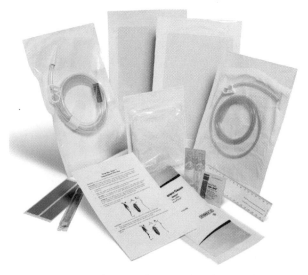

Figure 31•27 *Smith & Nephew NPWT dressing kits. (Used with permission of Smith & Nephew.)*

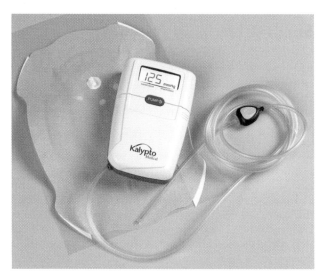

Figure 31•28 *The NPD 1000 Negative Pressure Wound Therapy System. (Used with permission of Kalypto Medical.)*

the pressure port to monitor when the dressing is nearing its exudate capacity.

The NPD 1000 dressing is composed of the following:

• Semiocclusive outer layer that maintains the negative pressure
• Pressure port with an in-line hydrophobic, antibacterial, 0.2-μm filter and fitting to which the NPD pump system is attached via PVC tubing
• Hydrogel gasket to seal the wound area
• Superabsorbent nonwoven polymer matrix to absorb exudates
• Nonstick Silverlon® wound contact layer

The Kalypto control unit is a fully portable, battery-powered device. The NPD 1000 dressing serves as the wound contact layer and wound effluent collection site. (Fig. 31.28) A full list of instructions for use can be found at the company's website, www.kalyptomedical.com.

▶ Case Study 31•1 | Orthopedic Trauma Case

History

Mr. B is a 25-year-old male motorcycle driver involved in a head-on collision with an oncoming motor vehicle resulting in significant trauma to left upper extremity. His left arm went through the windshield of the oncoming vehicle and pulled Mr. B off his motorcycle. He was then thrown from the vehicle, resulting in a near traumatic amputation of his left upper extremity at the shoulder. The previous medical history is unremarkable.

Mr. B was taken to a Level 1 trauma center for multiple surgeries to include orthopedic repair of his humerus and a neurovascular repair of the brachial plexus. He was later transferred to a long-term acute care facility for intensive wound management and rehabilitation. He is alert and oriented, and he cared for his wife and infant son prior to the accident. Past treatment at the trauma center consisted of saline-moistened gauze dressing changes up to four times daily and general passive range of motion exercises.

Systems Review

Integument: Patient has a large soft tissue defect to left anterior, superior, and posterior shoulder related to trauma. Heavy serosanguinous exudate is present, with no odor or purulence noted. There are multiple cuts and abrasions to soft tissue of left biceps, triceps, and forearm. Multiple glass and rock fragments are imbedded in soft tissue.

Anthropometric Characteristics: The left upper extremity is approximately 3 to 4 cm larger than right upper extremity at corresponding points. Patient's height is 5'10"; weight is 165 lbs.

Joint Integrity, Manual Muscle Testing (MMT), Range of Motion, Posture: Mr. B has significant loss of fine and gross motor control in left upper extremity. There is poor strength in all major muscle groups, and range of motion is passively within normal limits at elbow, hand, and fingers. There are significant limitations at the left shoulder with postoperative restrictions of 45 degrees abduction and flexion imposed by surgeon.

Pain: Patient reports excruciating pain with gauze-dressing removal; pain at wound site is reported at 9 out of 10 on a visual analog scale with every dressing change. Current pain management includes oral medication.

Ventilation, Respiration, Circulation: Patient has normal breath sounds, with 16 breaths per minute. His resting heart rate is 68 beats per minute (increased to 100 beats per minute during dressing changes), and blood pressure is within normal limits. Patient is negative for venous or arterial disease, and biphasic Doppler signal is present at left radial artery (triphasic on right radial artery).

Laboratory Results: Laboratory test results are as follows: white blood cells: 10,500/μL; red blood cells: 3.8 million/μL; prealbumin: 10 mg/dL; hemoglobin: 12.2 gm/dL; hematocrit: 38%. A quantitative swab culture and sensitivity of wound tissue revealed multiple bacterial organisms, including methicillin-sensitive *Staphylococcus aureus* and *Pseudomonas Aeruginosa*.

Sensory and Reflex Integrity: Mr. B has loss of proprioception, and biceps reflex is diminished.

Motor Function, Gait, Balance: Patient requires minimal assistance with bed mobility and transfers, with contact guard assistance for ambulation of 150 feet. His balance is fair plus in sitting and standing.

Orthotic, Prosthetic, Supportive, Assistive, and Adaptive Devices: Patient has an orthopedic brace to left shoulder and a straight cane on the right side for balance with ambulation.

Aerobic Capacity and Endurance: Abilities are diminished compared to age group and premorbid level.

Self-Care: Mr. B requires maximum assistance with dressing and is independent with feeding and oral care. He requires minimum assistance for bed mobility and transfers.

Work and Community: Mr. B is employed as general laborer in a plumbing supply warehouse.

Test and Measures:

1. Girth measurements
2. Pain assessment
3. Range of motion with goniometer
4. Handheld Doppler
5. Blood chemistry including albumin

Recommended Interventions

Wound Management: Discontinue gauze-dressing changes. Initiate negative-pressure wound therapy at −125 mm Hg continuous setting, with dressing changes three times weekly. Consider use of silver-impregnated primary dressing due to the high risk of infection and heavy bioburden. Prepare periwound area by shaving hair in axilla to assist with adherence of NPWT drape. Monitor wound drainage output and document accordingly. (Figs. 31.29 through 31.32)

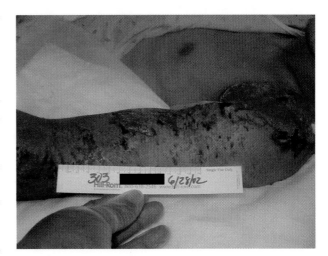

Figure 31•29 *Photo of patient with left upper-extremity/shoulder traumatic wound on presentation to therapist.*

Continued

▶ **Case Study 31•1** | **Orthopedic Trauma Case—cont'd**

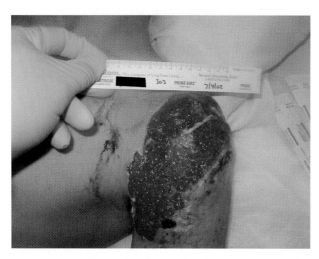

Figure 31•30 *Photo of patient with left upper-extremity/ shoulder traumatic wound following 6 days of NPWT.*

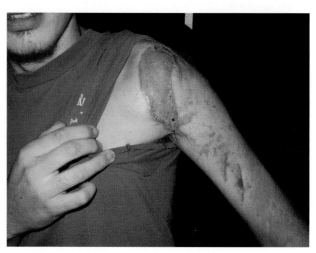

Figure 31•32 *Photo of patient in previous photos 14 days status after application of split-thickness skin graft to cover soft tissue defect.*

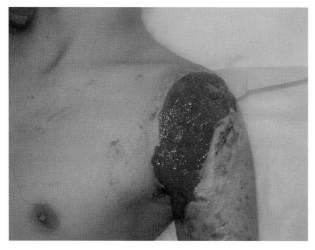

Figure 31•31 *Photo of patient with left upper-extremity/ shoulder traumatic wound following 15 days of NPWT.*

Pain Management: Work with physician and patient to formulate effective pain management plan; administer pain medication before NPWT dressing changes and allow for sufficient time to optimize analgesia. Assess pain level before, during, and after dressing change, and reformulate plan as needed.

Exercise and Rehabilitation: Provide extensive rehabilitation program of range of motion and strengthening, activities of daily living retraining, gait training, and consultation with dietician/ nutritionist for dietary supplementation to address nutritional deficits.

Educational Considerations: Education should be provided in the following areas: wound care, NPWT-related education (troubleshooting tips, importance of airtight seal, etc.), self-care issues, coping with trauma.

Other Considerations: Provide periodic removal of imbedded foreign objects (small glass fragments and rock particles) as they are pushed to skin surface; monitor fluid balance carefully (input and output on regular intervals); positioning of the upper extremity in an elevated position and mild compressive wrap to decrease edema to left upper extremity. Provide social services consultation to address the need for a support group and communication with employer.

References

1. Fox, J, Golden, G: The use of drains in subcutaneous surgical procedures. Am J Surg 1978; 132:573–574.
2. Fleck, CA, Frizzell, LD: When negative is positive: A review of negative pressure wound therapy. Extended Care Product News 2004; 92:20–25.
3. Kostiuchenok, II, Kolker, VA, Karlov, VA: The vacuum effect in the surgical treatment of purulent wounds. Vestnik Khirurgii 1986; 9:18–21.
4. Davydov, YA, Malafeeva, AP, Smirnov, AP: Vacuum therapy in the treatment of purulent lactation mastitis. Vestnik Khirurgii 1986; 9:66–70.
5. Usupov, YN, Yepifanov, MV: Active wound drainage. Vestnik Khirugii 1987; 4:42–45.
6. Davydov, YA, Larichev, KG, Abramov, AY, et al: The bacteriological and cytological assessment of vacuum therapy of purulent wound. Vestnik Khirugii 1988; 10:48–52.
7. Davydov, YA, Larichev, KG, Abramov, AY: Concepts for clinical biological management of the wound process in the treatment of purulent wounds using vacuum therapy. Vestnik Khirugii 1991; 2:132–135.
8. Chariker, ME, Jeter, KF, Tintle, TE, et al: Effective management of incisional and cutaneous fistulae with closed suction wound drainage. Contemp Surg 1989; 34:59–63.

9. Nakayama, Y, Soeda, S: A new dressing method for free skin grafting in hands. Ann Plast Surg 1991; 26:499–502.

10. Brock, W, Barker, D, Burns, R: Temporary closure of open abdominal wounds: The vacuum pack. Am Surg 1995; 61:30–35.

11. Morykwas, MJ, Argenta, LC, Shelton-Brown, EI, et al: Vacuum-assisted closure: A new method for wound control and treatment: Animal studies and basic foundation. Ann Plast Surg 1997; 38:553–562.

12. Argenta, L, Morykwas, M: Vacuum-assisted closure: A new method for wound control and treatment: Animal studies and basic foundation. Ann Plast Surg 1997; 38: 563–576.

13. Miller, MS, Lowery, CA: Negative pressure wound therapy: A rose by any other name. Ostomy Wound Manage 2005; 51:44–49.

14. Ovington, LG: Hanging wet-to-dry dressings out to dry. Home Healthc Nurse 2001; 19:477–483.

15. Joseph, E, Hamori, CA, Bergman, S, et al: A prospective randomized trial of vacuum-assisted closure versus standard therapy of chronic nonhealing wounds. Wounds 2000; 12:60–67.

16. Alverez, OM, Mertz, PM, Eaglestein, WH: The effectiveness of occlusive dressings on collagen synthesis and re-epithelization in superficial. J Surg Res 1983; 35:142–148.

17. Xia, Z, Sato, A, Hughes, MA, et al: Stimulation of fibroblast growth by intermittent radiant heat. Wound Rep Reg 2000; 8:138–144.

18. Krasner, DL: Caring for the person experiencing chronic wound pain. In: Krasner, DL, Rodeheaver, GT, Sibbald, RG (eds): Chronic Wound Care: A Clinical Source Book for Healthcare Professionals, ed. 3. Wayne, PA, HMP Communications, 2001, pp 79–89.

19. Krasner, DL: Managing wound pain in patients with vacuum-assisted closure devices. Ostomy Wound Manage 2002; 48:38–43.

20. Chen, SZ, Li, J, Li, XY, et al: Effects of vacuum-assisted closure on wound microcirculation: An experimental study. Asian J Surg 2005; 28:211–217.

21. Wackenfors, A, Sjogren, J, Gustafsson, R, et al: Effects of vacuum-assisted closure therapy on inguinal wound edge microvascular blood flow. Wound Rep Regen 2004; 12:600–606.

22. Wackenfors, A, Gustafsson, R, Sjogren, J, et al: Blood flow responses in the peristernal thoracic wall during vacuum-assisted closure therapy. Ann Thorac Surg 2005; 79:1724–1730.

23. Lindstedt, S, Malmsjo, M, Ingemansson, R: Blood flow changes in normal and ischemic myocardium during topically applied negative pressure. Ann Thorac Surg 2007; 84:568–573.

24. Venturi, ML, Attinger, CE, Mesbahi, AN, et al: Mechanisms and clinical applications of the vacuum-assisted closure (VAC) device. Am J Clin Dermatol 2005; 6:185–194.

25. Yager, DR, Nwomeh, BC: The proteolytic environment of chronic wounds. Wound Repair Regen 1999; 7:433–441.

26. Mustoe, T: Understanding chronic wounds: A unifying hypothesis on their pathogenesis and implications for therapy. Am J Surg 2004; 187:65S–70S.

27. Yager Dorne, R, Zhang, LY, Liang, HX, et al: Wound fluids from human pressure ulcers contain elevated matrix metalloproteinase levels and activity compared to surgical wound fluids. J Invest Derm 1996; 107:743–748.

28. Henry, G, Garner, WL: Inflammatory mediators in wound healing. Surg Clin North Am 2003; 83:483–507.

29. Morris, GS, Brueilly, KE, Hanzelka, H: Negative pressure wound therapy achieved by vacuum-assisted closure: Evaluating the assumptions. Ostomy Wound Manage 2007; 53:52–57.

30. Sevitt, S: Local blood flow changes in experimental burns. J Pathol Bacteriol 1949; 61:427–442.

31. Noble, HGS, Robson, MC, Krizek, TJ: Dermal ischemia in the burn wound. J Surg Res 1977; 23:117–125.

32. Lund, T, Wug, H, Reed, RK: Acute post burn edema: Role of strongly negative interstitial fluid pressure. Am J Physiol 1986; 255:1069–1074.

33. Reuler, JB, Cooney, TG: The pressure sore: Pathophysiology and principles of management. Ann Intern Med 1981; 94:661–665.

34. Witkowski, JA, Parish, LC: Histopathology of the decubitus ulcer. J Am Acad Dematol 1982; 6:1014–1021.

35. Kamolz, LP, Andel, H, Haslik, W, et al: Use of subatmospheric pressure therapy to prevent burn wound progression in human: First experiences. Burns 2004; 30:253–258.

36. Lambert, K, Hayes, P, McCarthy, M: Vacuum assisted closure: A review of development and current applications. Eur J Vasc Endovasc Surg 2005; 29:219–226.

37. Fenn, CH, Butler, PE: Abdominoplasty wound-healing complications: Assisted closure using foam suction dressing. Br J Plast Surg 2001; 54:348–351.

38. Saxena, V, Hwang, CW, Huang, S, et al: Vacuum assisted closure: Microdeformations of wounds and cell proliferation. Plast Reconstr Surg 2004; 114:1086–1096.

39. Iwasaki, H, Eguchi, S, Ueno, H, et al: Mechanical stretch stimulates growth of vascular smooth muscle cells via epidermal growth factor receptor. Am J Physiol Heart Circ Physiol 2000; 278:H521–H529.

40. Sanchez-Esteban, J, Wang, Y, Gruppuso, PA, et al: Mechanical stretch induces fetal type II cell differentiation via an epidermal growth factor receptor-extracellular-regulated protein kinase signaling pathway. Am J Respir Cell Mol Biol 2004; 30:76–83.

41. Ryan, TJ, Barnhill, RL: Physical factors and angiogenesis. In: Nurgent, J, O'Connor, M (eds): Development of the vascular system. Ciba Foundation Symposium 100. London, Pittman Books, 1983, pp 80–84.

42. Urschel, JD, Scott, PG, Williams, HTG: The effect of mechanical stress on soft and hard tissue repair: A review. Br J Plast Surg 1988; 41:182–186.

43. Cherry, GW, Austad, E, Pasyk, K, et al: Increased survival and vascularity of random-pattern skin flaps elevated in controlled, expanded tissue. Plast Reconstr Surg 1983; 72:680–687.

44. Olenius, M, Dalsgaard, C, Wickman, M: Mitotic activity in expanded human skin. Plast Reconstr Surg 1993; 91:213–216.

45. Venturi, ML, Attinger, CE, Mesbahi, AN, et al: Mechanisms and clinical applications of the vacuum-assisted closure (VAC) device. Am J Clin Dermatol 2005; 6:185–194.

46. Rundhaug, JE: Matrix metalloproteinases, angiogenesis, and cancer. Clin Cancer Res 2003; 9:551–554.

47. Tarlton, JF, Vickery, CJ, Leaper, DJ, et al: Postsurgical wound progression monitored by temporal changes in the expression of matrix metalloproteinase-9. Br J Dermatol 1997; 137:506–516.

48. Chen, C, Schultz, GS, Bloch, M, et al: Molecular and mechanistic validation of delayed healing rat wounds as a model for human chronic wounds. Wound Repair Regen 1999; 7:486–494.

49. Wysocki, AB, Staiano-Coico, L, Grinnell, F: Wound fluid from chronic leg ulcers contains elevated levels of metalloproteinases MMP-2 and MMP-9. J Invest Dermatol 1993; 101:64–68.

50. Ladwig, GP, Robson, MC, Liu, R, et al: Ratios of activate matrix metalloproteinase-9 to tissue inhibitor of matrix metalloproteinase-1 in wound fluids are inversely correlated with healing of pressure ulcers. Wound Repair Regen 2002; 10:26–37.

51. Lerman, OZ, Galiano, RD, Armour, M, et al: Cellular dysfunction in the diabetic fibroblast: Impairment in migration, vascular endothelial growth factor production, and response to hypoxia. Am J Pathol 2003; 162:303–312.

52. Greene, AK, Puder, M, Roopali, R, et al: Microdeformation wound therapy: Effects on angiogenesis and matrix metalloproteinases in chronic wounds of 3 debilitated patients. Ann Plast Surg 2006; 56:418–422.

53. Moses, MA, Marikovsky, M, Harper, JW, et al: Temporal study of the activity of matrix metalloproteinases and their endogenous inhibitors during wound healing. J Cell Biochem 1996; 60:379–386.

54. Greene, AK, Puder, M, Roy, R, et al: Urinary matrix metalloproteinases and their endogenous inhibitors predict hepatic regeneration after murine partial hepatectomy. Transplantation 2004; 78:1139–1144.

55. Bowler, PG: Wound pathophysiology, infection, and therapeutic options. Ann Med 2002; 34:419.

56. White, RJ, Cutting, KF: Critical colonization—The concept under scrutiny. Ostomy Wound Manage 2006; 52:50–56.

57. Raahave, D, Friis-Moller, A, Bjerre-Jepsen, K, et al: The infective dose of aerobic and anerobic bacteria in postoperative wound sepsis. Arch Surg 1986; 121:924.

58. Robson, MC, Shaw, RC, Heggers, JP: The reclosure of postoperative incisional abscesses based on bacterial quantification of the wound. Ann Surg 1970; 171:279.

59. Arnold, M, Barbul, A: Nutrition and wound healing. Plast Reconstr Surg 2006; 117:42S–58S.

60. Moues, CM, Vos, MC, Van Den Bernd, GJCM, et al: Bacterial load in relation to vacuum-assisted closure wound therapy: A prospective randomized trial. Wound Repair Regen 2004; 12:11–17.

61. Mulder, GD, Cavorsi, JP, Lee, DK: Polyhexamethylene Biguanide (PHMB): An addendum to current topical antimicrobials. Wounds 2007; 19:173–182.

62. VAC Physician and Caregiver Reference Manual. San Antonio, TX, Kinetic Concepts, 2007.

63. Ip, M, Lui, SL, Poon, VKM, et al: Antimicrobial activities of silver dressings: An in vitro comparison. J Med Microbiol 2006; 55:59–63.

64. Wolvos, T: Wound instillation—The next step in negative pressure wound therapy. Lessons learned from initial experiences. Ostomy Wound Manage 2004; 50:56–66.

65. Argenta, LC, Morykwas, MJ, Marks, MW, et al: Vacuum-assisted closure: State of clinical art. Plast Reconstr Surg 2006; 117:127S–142S.

66. Stannard, JP, Robinson, JT, Ratcliffe-Anderson, E, et al: Negative pressure wound therapy to treat hematomas and surgical incisions following high-energy trauma. J Trauma 2006; 60:1301–1306.

67. Eginton, MT, Brown, KR, Seabrook, GR, et al: A prospective randomized evaluation of negative-pressure wound dressings for diabetic foot wounds. Ann Vasc Surg 2003; 17:645–649.

68. Carson, SN, Overall, K, Lee-Jahshan, S, et al: Vacuum assisted closure used for healing chronic wounds and skin grafts in the lower extremities. Ostomy Wound Manage 2004; 50:52–58.

69. Vuerstaek, JDD, Vainas, T, Wuite, J, et al: State of the art treatment of chronic leg ulcers: A randomized controlled trial comparing vacuum assisted closure with modern wound dressings. J Vasc Surg 2006; 44:1029–1037.

70. Oczenski, W, Waldenberger, F, Nehrer, G, et al: Vacuum assisted closure for the treatment of cervical and mediastinal necrotizing fasciitis. J Cardiothor Vasc Anesth 2004; 18:33–338.

71. Phelps, JR, Fagan, R, Pirela-Cruz, M: A case study of negative pressure wound therapy to manage acute necrotizing fasciitis. Ostomy Wound Manage 2006; 52:54–59.

72. Moisidis, E, Heath, T, Boorer, C, et al: A prospective, blinded, randomized, controlled clinical trial of topical negative pressure use in skin grafting. Plast Reconstr Surg 2004; 114:917–922.

73. Parrett, BM, Matros, E, Pribaz, JJ, et al: Lower extremity trauma: Trends in the management of soft tissue reconstruction of open tibia-fibula fractures. Plast Reconstr Surg 2006; 117:1315–1322.

74. Armstrong, DG, Lavery, LA: Negative pressure wound therapy after partial diabetic foot amputation: A multicentre, randomised controlled trial. Lancet 2005; 366:1704–1710.

75. de Leon, J: Negative pressure wound therapy in pressure ulcer management. Ostomy Wound Manage 2005; 51(suppl):3S–8S.

76. Carek, PJ, Dickerson, LM, Sack, JL: Diagnosis and management of osteomyelitis. Am Fam Physician 2001; 63:2413–2420.

77. Niezgoda, JA: Incorporating negative pressure therapy into the management strategy for pressure ulcers. Ostomy Wound Manage 2004; 50(suppl):26–29.

78. Short, B, Claxton, M, Armstrong, DG: How to use VAC therapy on chronic wounds. Podiatry Today 2002; 15:48–54.

79. Samson, DJ, Lefevre, F, Aronson, N: Wound-Healing Technologies: Low-Level Laser and Vacuum-Assisted Closure. Evidence Report/Technology Assessment No. 111. No. 05-E005-2. Rockville, MD, Agency for Healthcare Research and Quality, 2004.

80. Evans, D, Land, L: Topical negative pressure for treating chronic wounds. Brit J Plast Surg 2001; 54:238–242.

81. Ford, CN, Reinhard, ER, Yeh, D, et al: Interim analysis of a prospective, randomized trial of vacuum-assisted closure versus the health-point system in the management of pressure ulcers. Ann Plast Surg 2002; 49:55–61.

82. McCallon, SK, Knight, CA, Valiulus, JP, et al: Vacuum-assisted closure versus saline-moistened gauze in the healing of postoperative diabetic foot wounds. Ostomy Wound Manage 2000; 46:28–32, 34.

83. Wanner, MB, Schwarzl, F, Strub, B, et al: Vacuum-assisted wound closure for cheaper and more comfortable healing of pressure sores: A prospective study. Scand J Plast Reconstr Surg Hand Surg 2003; 37:28–33.

84. Chantelav, E: Negative pressure therapy in diabetic foot wounds. Lancet 2006; 367:726–727.

85. Maegele, M, Gregor, S, Peinemann, F, et al: Negative pressure therapy in diabetic foot wounds. Lancet 2006; 367:725–726.

86. Williams, DT: Negative pressure therapy in diabetic foot wounds. Lancet 2006; 367:725.

87. Apeqvist, J, Armstrong, DG, Lavery, LA, Boulton, AJ: Diabetic foot ulcer and VAC resource utilization and economic cost based on a randomized trial. Presented at 20th Annual Symposium on Advanced Wound Care and the Wound Healing Society Meeting, April 28–May 1, 2007, Tampa, FL.

chapter 32

Oxygen Therapy—Management of the Hypoxic Wound

Jeffrey A. Niezgoda, MD, FACHM, FAPWCA, FACEP

Eric P. Kindwall, MD

Introduction

A chronic wound is defined as a wound that has failed to progress through the stages of healing in an orderly fashion to produce anatomic tissue integrity and restored functional capability.[1] Many factors are recognized as contributing to wound chronicity, but impaired tissue perfusion that results in poor tissue oxygenation and tissue hypoxia is often at the top of the list. This chapter will discuss the importance of oxygen in wound healing and the role of adjunctive technologies such as hyperbaric oxygen therapy (HBOT) in the management of the hypoxic wound.

Biochemistry of Oxygen

Oxygen is the third most common element in the universe. In fact, approximately 21% of the air we breathe is composed of oxygen, and most of this exists in a biatomic form as O_2 molecules. This is the form that living organisms can best use. The remaining composition of air consists of about 79% nitrogen and less than 1% inert gases such as argon, carbon dioxide, neon, helium, and hydrogen. Air enters the alveoli, diffuses into the pneumatocytes, and then moves into the bloodstream. Given an atmospheric pressure of about 760 mm Hg at sea level, the partial pressure of oxygen (PaO_2) in the air is around 150 mm Hg. But when losses due to vapor pressure and pulmonary diffusion gradients are considered, the partial pressure of oxygen actually reaching the bloodstream is less than 100 mm Hg.[2]

Once in the blood, oxygen is preferentially bound to the hemoglobin molecules on the red blood cells, and at sea level the average person has essentially 100% saturation of the hemoglobin molecules. However, the plasma can also carry dissolved oxygen, and, in fact, this system provides a great reserve in oxygen-carrying capacity.

> ▶ **PEARL 32•1** Under normal atmospheric pressure, the average person has about 0.3 volume percent of dissolved oxygen in his or her plasma. However the oxygen-carrying capacity of the plasma is immense, and this reserve capacity is exactly the target of the supraphysiological oxygen levels provided by HBOT.[2,3]

Oxygenated blood flows to distal tissues, and under normal physiological conditions the oxygen is off-loaded to provide the energy substrates to fuel tissue metabolism. Oxygen delivery can be negatively impacted by conditions that inhibit uncoupling of oxyhemoglobin (such as tissue acidosis) or, as mentioned previously, conditions that prevent adequate tissue perfusion (ie, peripheral arterial disease, edema, and conditions causing vessel sludging or trauma). With regard to wound healing, normal tissue oxygenation is critical to collagen synthesis, epithelialization, angiogenesis, and bacterial killing.[4-7]

Definition of the Hypoxia Wound and Chronic Ulcer

Wounds that have failed to progress through the normal stages of the wound healing process are considered to be chronic, non-healing wounds, especially if they have persisted longer than 4 to 6 weeks. The four phases of normal wound healing and their durations are the hemostasis phase (0–3 hours), the inflammatory phase (0–3 days), the proliferative phase (3–21 days), and the maturation phase (21 days–1.5 years). Although the process may go awry anywhere along the pathway, chronic wounds are generally considered to be stagnant within either the inflammatory or the proliferative stages of the normal healing cascade. Therefore, the treatment of these nonhealing wounds and ulcers generally involves exploration, discovery, and correction of the factors that prevent normal healing from proceeding in an orderly fashion. Although poor tissue perfusion is a common cause of wound healing compromise, other factors can also pose a significant impediment to normal wound healing. These factors include infection, tissue edema, tissue trauma, unrelieved pressure, or underlying medical conditions that unfortunately too often remain undiagnosed (such as diabetes, collagen vascular disease, renal insufficiency, protein energy malnutrition) and can challenge the restoration of normal healing. Any or all of these conditions can arrest wound healing and, in fact, can occur simultaneously. Thus, recognition and correction of the underlying conditions responsible for the delay in wound healing is not always straightforward.

Generally speaking, living tissue needs oxygen and nutrients to thrive, and in the case of wound healing, to regenerate. In normal wound healing, both hypoxia and normal amounts of oxygen are necessary for progression of the phases of the healing. Hypoxia stimulates macrophages to release mitogens, which in turn stimulate fibroblast replication and the release of angiogenic factors.[7] Oxygen is also essential for collagen synthesis by fibroblasts. Intermittent tissue hyperoxygenation allows for periods of hypoxia. During the hypoxic periods, angiogenic factors are released, initiating neoangiogenesis and propagation of the healing cascade. New capillaries, however, cannot advance unless they are surrounded by a supportive collagen matrix. The role of oxygen in wound healing has become increasingly more apparent. The maturation of collagen, development of new endothelium, and obliteration of dead space by healthy granulation tissue are all oxygen-dependent processes. With the development of a healthy collagen matrix, capillary buds invade rapidly, and new capillary arcades are formed in the advancing vascular system. Referred to as granulation tissue formation, granulation obliterates dead space, allowing wound healing to proceed.[8-10]

Although white cells can phagocytize bacteria at relatively low oxygen tensions, they are unable to kill bacteria unless they are in an environment of at least 30 mm Hg partial pressure of oxygen. In patients with ischemic wounds, such as diabetic foot ulcers, oxygen tensions in peripheral soft tissue and bone are often much lower than 30 mm Hg. Under these circumstances, infections quickly become fulminant. Edema, frequently associated with infection, potentiates the tissue ischemia and creates a vicious circle of ischemia, more edema, and increasing tissue injury.[11]

⏵ **PEARL 32•2** It is clear that in the setting of tissue hypoxia (less than 30 mm Hg) healing will be impaired. Likewise, correction of tissue ischemia and improved oxygen delivery has been clearly shown to improve wound healing. In patients with large vessel stenosis, this is accomplished by vascular bypass or by endovascular intervention, but for those causes in which smaller vessels are damaged, such as in radiation injury or diabetes, improved oxygen-carrying capacity, increased oxygen diffusion, and correction of localized ischemia at a cellular level may allow neovascularization and healing to occur in tissues that were previously unresponsive.

While the obvious solution to this problem seems to be the restoration of normal blood flow, in reality it is often much more complicated than this because the patient's underlying medical condition(s) often prevents the complete reversal of the hypoxic process. In these cases, it is often advantageous to consider the use of supplemental oxygen to augment the normal healing process. In fact, this is one of the main reasons to use hyperbaric oxygen in the treatment of such patients.

Definition of Hyperbaric Oxygen Therapy

Hyperbaric oxygen therapy (HBOT), defined as treatment during which a patient inhales 100% oxygen at pressures exceeding 1.4 atmospheres absolute (ATA), has been used worldwide for more than 50 years in the treatment of many chronic nonhealing wounds and ulcers.[12] Treatments are given in an airtight chamber occupied by either several patients simultaneously (multiplace chamber; Fig. 32.1) or in smaller chambers containing only one patient at any one time (monoplace chamber). (Fig. 32.2) While multiplace chambers traditionally tend to be quite large and expensive in design, construction, and operation, technological advances over the past

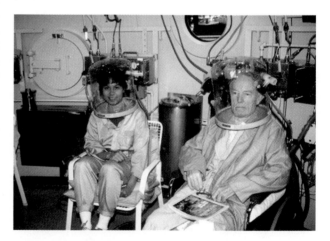

Figure 32•1 *Multiplace hyperbaric chamber. Patients breathing 100% oxygen via hood tent.*

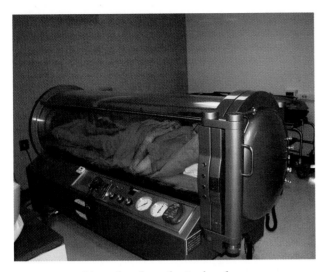

Figure 32•2 *Monoplace hyperbaric chamber.*

15 to 20 years have led to an increase in the number of monoplace chambers in use today. In multiplace chambers, several patients are treated simultaneously in an environment of pressured air while breathing pure oxygen delivered via mask or hood tent that is pressurized to correspond to the chamber pressure. In a monoplace chamber, a single patient is placed in an environment of pure oxygen under the desired treatment pressure. For routine conditions, hyperbaric oxygen therapy (HBOT) is typically administered between 2.0 and 2.5 ATA, with 90 minutes of oxygen breathing interrupted briefly by an "air break" (5–10 minutes of air breathing). The safety record of HBOT in this country is excellent, and the technology has become a vital part of the growth of comprehensive wound care programs across the nation.[13,14]

History of Hyperbaric Oxygen Therapy

The first nondiving use of hyperbaric oxygenation (HBO) was for cardiac surgery by the Dutch surgeon Ite Boerema in 1956. Before the heart-lung machine was available, Boerema was able to extend circulatory arrest time for several minutes by compressing both the patient and the surgical team in the hyperbaric chamber. While under pressure, the patient breathed 100% O_2 in order to "drench" the tissues with oxygen, as Boerema termed it. Soon, the investigators in Amsterdam also discovered its dramatic effect in treating gas gangrene. Other surgeons began building chambers in England and the United States. Smith and Sharp in Glasgow were the first to treat carbon monoxide poisoning in 1960.[12]

These early advances were followed by a lull in hyperbaric development as researchers, chiefly surgeons, were exploring the possible effects of HBO on other maladies. The treatment of completed stroke was tried without success, and a preliminary study of its salutary effects on senility was eventually not substantiated. Hyperbaric quackery became common, with oxygenation being touted for everything from increasing sexual vigor to breast firming and enlargement and the removal of skin wrinkles. As the use of the heart-lung machine in the late 1960s became commonplace, the need for hyperbaric surgery became vanishingly small, surgeons who had been the principle researchers began to leave the field, and many large and expensive surgical chambers closed.[15]

In 1976 there were only 37 clinical chambers operating in the United States. To stem the tide of quackery and to provide insurers with guidance as to what was legitimate to treat with hyperbaric oxygen, the Undersea and Hyperbaric Medical Society (then known simply as the Undersea Medical Society) established the Committee on Hyperbaric Oxygen. The committee surveyed the field and published a short list of disorders treated with HBOT that had a scientific basis and had been clinically demonstrated to have merit. These were deemed reimbursable by the committee, and Blue Cross/Blue Shield adopted it as their source document.[16] With a scientific basis established, the number of chamber facilities began to grow. By 1983 there were approximately 110 chambers in operation in the United States, and today there are over 700. Typically, new hyperbaric facilities are established as an integral component of wound care clinics, and few are listed purely as hyperbaric facilities.

Mechanism of Action of Hyperbaric Oxygen Therapy

An uncompromised patient, breathing air at sea level, will typically have an arterial PaO_2 of 100 mm Hg. The majority of this oxygen will be carried bound to hemoglobin, with only a small percentage of oxygen physically dissolved in the plasma. In this setting, the normal diffusion radius for an oxygen molecule is 64 microns at the end arteriole and about 36 microns from the venous system, where the PaO_2 might be as low as 34 mm Hg. (Fig. 32.3) However, this same patient breathing 100% oxygen at 3 ATA will have an enormous increase in the amount of oxygen physically dissolved in the plasma

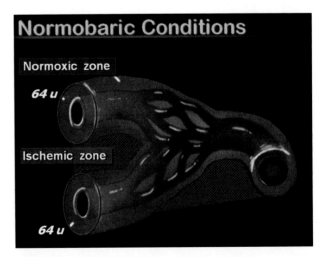

Figure 32•3 *Oxygen diffusion normobaric air. (Courtesy Bob Bartlett MD.)*

(6.9 volume percent) compared to the volume of oxygen dissolved at 1 ATA (0.3 volume percent). The brain only uses 6.1 volume percent per pass, so the brain is fully oxygenated from oxygen dissolved in the plasma. In fact, plasma PaO_2 values well in excess of 1500 to 1800 mm Hg are routinely achieved in hyperbaric patients. In this setting the hemoglobin never desaturates, and thus hemoglobin plays a minimal role in the transport of oxygen. Tissue oxygen partial pressures can reach 250 to 300 mm Hg, far above the normal 30 to 40 mm Hg when breathing air at 1 atmosphere. This 18- to 20-fold rise in dissolved oxygen establishes a tremendous gradient between the plasma and the peripheral tissues. It is this steep oxygen gradient that stimulates and initiates neoangiogenesis. In addition to this supraphysiological oxygen gradient, there is a significant increase in oxygen diffusion distance from the tissue capillary beds (247 microns).[17] (Fig. 32.4)

Given that the intercapillary distance in living tissue is less than 247 microns, it should be apparent that the fourfold increase in the oxygen diffusion radius provided by HBOT is an effective countermeasure against any tissue hypoxia that may be present. In addition, the supraphysiological oxygen levels seen in hyperbaric patients can also reduce tissue edema through a compensatory vasoconstriction effect caused by an autoregulatory mechanism inherent in the vasculature. Thus, hyperbaric oxygen has a multifactorial mode of action: increased oxygen levels in the plasma available to diffuse farther into hypoxic tissues while reducing tissue edema through compensatory vasoconstriction.[12]

It is well documented that HBOT can induce angiogenesis and neovascularization in hypoxic tissues. Lee et al demonstrated that hyperbaric oxygen induces expression of vascular endothelial growth factor (VEGF) in human umbilical vein endothelial cells (HUVECs), both through transcription and translation within the cells.[18] They also showed that pure oxygen given at normobaric pressures (1 ATA) had no similar effect and therefore concluded that the benefits of pure oxygen seem to be unrealized unless the pressure at which it is given is significantly increased. Shiekh et al showed that VEGF levels in hypoxic wounds rose by approximately 40% within 5 days of starting HBOT, but then

dropped to control levels within 3 days of stopping the treatment.[19] They concluded that the angiogenic effect of HBOT was due to an increase in VEGF levels induced by hyperbaric oxygen and that hypoxia was not necessarily the only requirement for wound VEGF production. Ahmad and colleagues also demonstrated via laser Doppler imaging that, in addition to an increase in angiogenesis, there was a 20% increase in wound bed perfusion following 10 days of HBOT.[20] Marx et al showed that normobaric oxygen had no angiogenic properties above those associated with normal revascularization in rabbit mandibles irradiated with 60 Gy of gamma radiation.[21] They observed that hyperbaric oxygen demonstrated an eightfold to ninefold increase in vascular density over both normobaric oxygen and air-breathing controls. Therefore, the angiogenic benefits of HBOT in hypoxic, hypovascular tissue seem to be quite significant, and indeed, the authors' clinical experience supports this observation.

Molecular oxygen is universally considered to be simply a consumable substrate to support our metabolism. At the time Boerema conducted his initial surgical experiments, this was considered to be its only property or function. But as research has delved deeper into the mechanisms of why HBOT produces the results seen clinically, oxygen was found to have other properties. Under increased pressure, it becomes a pharmacological agent having the properties of a drug, but in excess it can also be toxic to the body.

In only a limited number of circumstances is a great surfeit of oxygen necessary or even desirable. But in treating some disorders, we make use of the druglike attributes of HBO alluded to above. For example, HBO acts as a potent vasoconstrictive agent that can reduce intracranial pressure by one half. However, it does not cause vasoconstriction in postischemic muscle, sustaining blood flow to damaged tissues. It preserves adenosine triphosphate in cell membranes and dramatically reduces edema, allowing cells to control their own osmolarity. It prevents reperfusion injury in posthypoxic tissue [22-24]

HBOT has been demonstrated to have a positive impact on limiting the deleterious effects of reperfusion injury. It blocks guanylate cyclase, the trigger molecule for beta-2 integrin, which forms the leukocyte adhesion molecule. Thus, following ischemia or sepsis, leukocytes do not stick to the capillary walls to block circulation when the patient is treated early with HBOT. Every leukocyte in the body is rendered "nonsticky" for about 8 hours following a single HBO exposure. It also blocks the action of the intracellular adhesion molecule (the ICAM mechanism) that causes any leukocytes that become adherent to the capillary wall to bore through to the tissues surrounding the vessel, releasing the super oxide anion, proteinases, and elastase that liquefy tissue following crush injury and other forms of ischemia.[24,25]

Many nonhealing wounds do not heal because they are chronically infected or hypoxic. Because oxygen levels below 40 mm Hg do not allow leukocytes to kill bacteria, raising the tissue levels much higher than normal improves white cell bactericidal function. At oxygen partial pressures of 150 mm Hg, white cell killing ability is doubled or tripled beyond that found in even normally oxygenated leukocytes.[11]

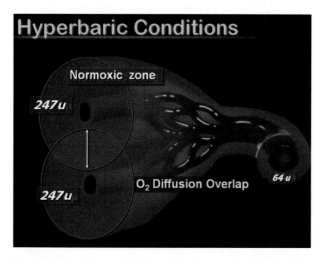

Figure 32•4 *Oxygen diffusion hyperbaric oxygen. (Courtesy Bob Bartlett MD.)*

▶ **PEARL 32•3** It is important to note that oxygen levels remain high for a prolonged period following HBOT. After a 90-minute treatment at 2 ATA, the arterial levels fall to normal within a couple of minutes of treatment cessation, but oxygen levels in muscle tissue remain significantly elevated for up to 3 hours, and in subcutaneous tissues for 4 hours, from the start of treatment. (Fig. 32.5)

This phenomenon allows the use of HBOT sessions twice or three times a day to enhance tissue oxygenation for extending periods of time, rather than only when the patient is actually in the chamber.

For all the above reasons, wound healing centers have eagerly adopted HBOT as its mechanisms have been clarified.

Indications for Hyperbaric Oxygen Therapy

The Centers for Medicare and Medicaid Services (CMS) has evaluated the use of HBOT in this country and has issued a National Coverage Determination (NCD) to define its policy regarding the reimbursement for hyperbaric services. While they are not obligated to follow the CMS guidelines, most insurance providers in this country do indeed follow the NCD when considering reimbursement for these services. A list of both approved diagnoses as well as other conditions (eg, stroke, cerebral palsy) that are not considered to be reimbursable conditions can be found on the CMS website.[26] There are free-standing hyperbaric centers that offer treatment to patients with a noncovered diagnosis, typically on a cash basis. Indeed, there have been both published and anecdotal reports that HBOT may be efficacious in the treatment of certain of these conditions. Definitive randomized trials are clearly needed to investigate these claims.

Of the diagnoses listed as covered by CMS, some of the most common conditions treated with HBOT include the diabetic foot ulcer (DFU), chronic refractory osteomyelitis (CROM), and both osteoradionecrosis (ORN) and soft tissue radionecrosis (STRN). Less common (but equally important) indications for HBOT include necrotizing soft tissue infections, decompression sickness (DCS), and carbon monoxide (CO) poisoning. HBOT is the treatment of choice for DCS and CO poisoning, and the timely treatment of both of these conditions can prevent many of the long-term neurological sequelae often seen in patients not receiving hyperbaric oxygen.[13,27]

While it is beyond the scope of this chapter to discuss the nuances of the treatment plans for each of these conditions, some generalizations can be made. For most patients, hyperbaric oxygen therapy is administered on a daily basis. Although more serious conditions such as necrotizing soft tissue infections, DCS, and CO poisoning often require the use of HBOT on a more frequent basis, twice or three times daily (BID or TID), most chronic conditions can be treated using daily treatments. The patient is placed within the hyperbaric chamber for 90 to 120 minutes for a total of 20 to 35 treatments, with ongoing wound care on a regular basis. Often, the use of HBOT is in conjunction with both medical and surgical treatment interventions aimed at correction of the underlying cause(s) of the nonhealing wound. In fact this point cannot be overstated as HBOT should always be used as part of a multidisciplinary treatment plan and not simply as standalone therapy. While there certainly may be exceptions to this rule (DCS and CO poisoning), this important point should not be forgotten. Thus, if a clinician is considering the use of HBOT for a patient, a general evaluation by a wound specialist who will look for other causes of the nonhealing wound is advised.

Hyperbaric Oxygen Therapy Contraindications

As with any drug, there is a proper therapeutic range for HBOT and overdoses are toxic. HBOT is never given at pressures greater than 3 ATA as higher pressures will evoke grand mal seizures (Paul Bert effect). Even at 3 ATA, exposure longer than 3 hours will cause nearly everyone to have a seizure. For this reason, clinical protocols limit the maximum exposure time at 3 ATA to 90 minutes. In the clinical practice of treating wounds, the longest protocol typically used is 2 hours at 2 ATA.

Likewise, there may be significant contraindications in some patients. An absolute contraindication to HBOT, particularly in the monoplace chamber, is untreated pneumothorax. The danger is that this could develop into an expanding tension pneumothorax during treatment. Significant expansion of extrapleural air during decompression could severely compromise the patient's respirations and even block blood return to the heart. This problem can be circumvented in patients with a pneumothorax by inserting a chest tube on the affected side prior to treatment.

Other contraindications are the concomitant administration of doxorubicin (Adriamycin®) and bleomycin with HBOT. Both are cancer chemotherapeutic drugs, and doxorubicin in animals has caused 70% mortality when combined with HBOT, presumably due to cardiac toxicity. Bleomycin is known to cause "bleomycin lung," and it is made fulminant by the addition of oxygen. It has been reported that therapeutic levels of 1 ATA oxygen given years after bleomycin therapy was complete could

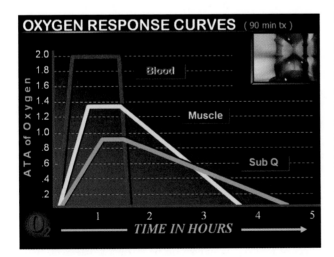

Figure 32•5 *Hyperbaric oxygen response curves. (Courtesy Bob Bartlett MD.)*

re-evoke bleomycin lung. However, recent reports show that patients with a previous history of bleomycin therapy have been treated successfully with HBOT. It is probably safe to use HBOT if the bleomycin was discontinued more than 6 months previous to treatment. Nevertheless, pulmonary function should be closely monitored in these patients.[14,28]

Risks and Side Effects of Hyperbaric Oxygen Treatment

As mentioned above, the use of HBOT is widely considered to be quite safe; however, there are certain conditions that might make a patient an unsuitable candidate for the hyperbaric chamber. Ear squeeze or failure to equalize the middle ear during compression is the most frequent side effect of HBOT. Equalizing the pressure in the middle ear during compression is a learned technique, but may be made difficult by excess mucus from allergies or upper respiratory infections. Thus, a relative contraindication to HBOT includes upper respiratory infections that make ear equalization difficult or impossible. As patients are very carefully pressurized during their initial treatment, tympanic membrane rupture should not occur because pressurization is halted when the patient indicates distress. Oral decongestants such as Sudafed® or other over-the-counter drugs can be used to advantage. Nasal sprays can be used, but they are less effective, even if given 15 or 20 minutes prior to treatment, and they are not used routinely as dependence can develop quickly.

If the patient sustains a significant ear squeeze, there will usually be so much resulting edema that the patient will not be compressible for several days. For this reason, the first HBOT treatment should be initiated very carefully. However, should the patient feel unable to tolerate additional hyperbaric treatment sessions, this is usually resolved by having an ear, nose, and throat (ENT) specialist place tympanostomy tubes in both ear drums. Indeed, this procedure can often be performed quite comfortably in the specialist's office between hyperbaric sessions. Another practice employed to minimize the risks of barotrauma is that of gentle compression and decompression rates, and indeed this technique is quite effective in minimizing the risk of both pulmonary and tympanic membrane injury. Serous otitis or fluid retention in the ear secondary to oxygen breathing may rarely occur and can also be managed with decongestants.

Sinus squeeze is much less common, and the only remedy is to use decongestants. If the problem persists, the services of an ENT specialist should be enlisted. Frontal sinus squeeze is the most painful, and a patient who experiences it must not be forced to continue except in an absolute emergency as the pain can be unbearably severe.

Alternobaric vertigo is the only problem that will sometimes appear during decompression. Air escapes easily from the eustachian tube during decompression, sometimes making crackling sounds but not causing pain. However, some patients may suddenly develop true vertigo as depressurization begins. It is benign and usually lasts only seconds, but can cause alarm to the patient. It is caused by the slight build up in middle ear pressure as gas expansion begins and before the eustachian tube opens. If one inner ear is damaged, the signal sent by the eighth cranial nerve is asymmetric and the brain interprets it as spinning. The same result occurs if one eustachian tube opens up before the other. The patient need only be given reassurance.

Pulmonary oxygen toxicity does not occur with any of the treatment protocols in use clinically. Oxygen is toxic to the lung if administered for more that 6 continuous hours at 2 ATA. There is a drop in vital capacity as surfactant production ceases, and patchy atelectasis becomes evident on X-ray. Repeated and prolonged exposure to pure oxygen at higher pressures is thought to cause an increased amount of oxygen free-radical production, with subsequent tissue injury to which there is a fibrotic response. Acutely, the appearance of pulmonary edema, increasing alveolar oxygen gradients, and pulmonary hemorrhage eventually results in interstitial fibrosis and type II pneumonocyte production. If exposure continues, microhemorrhages appear, and eventually the result is irreversible fibrosis. This is rarely seen clinically as the longest continuous exposure is only for 2 hours at 2 ATA. Even with repetitive exposures on the same day, the lung recovers well between treatments. Even 5-minute "air breaks" or air breathing periods every 20 minutes will double the time required before toxicity appears.

At pressures greater than 2 ATA, cerebral or central nervous system (CNS) oxygen toxicity can cause problems. A common wound treatment protocol is 2.4 ATA for 90 minutes, with a 5-minute air break midtreatment. Even so, every hyperbaric clinician will eventually encounter a patient who has a lower than normal seizure threshold and who will manifest CNS toxicity as a seizure. There is no way of predicting who will seize, but a patient with a known seizure disorder may be at increased risk. This is probably mediated by an inhibition of the GABA pathways with concomitant loss of GABA-mediated inhibitory neurochemical activity. Oxygen seizures are benign, and management simply consists of lowering the fractional concentration of inspired oxygen (FiO_2). This is done by removing the mask or hood in the multiplace chamber. In the monoplace chamber, the patient is decompressed after the tonic phase of the seizure is completed, usually in short bursts to avoid breath holding and air trapping that could cause a gas embolism.

Pneumothorax occurring in the chamber is a potential risk, but fortunately it is extremely rare. By definition, treatment in a hyperbaric chamber occurs at pressures in excess of 1.4 atmospheres, thus the possibility exists that excess pressure can accumulate in inadequately ventilated portions of the lung, predisposing those areas to rupture under pressure. Therefore, any patients with a history of an air-trapping condition such as asthma, emphysema, or COPD must have a thorough evaluation. Consultation with a pulmonologist should be considered if there are any concerns noted. Pneumothorax occurring in the monoplace chamber poses a particular problem because there is no way to insert a chest tube prior to decompression. If it occurs, the side where it is located must be determined. A thoracentesis tray is made ready, the patient is rapidly decompressed and the physician quickly inserts a chest tube to relieve the intrathoracic pressure. In the multiplace chamber, a chest tube is inserted prior to decompression, and this obviates the problem.

Visual changes in the form of lens refraction can be a side effect of HBOT. Distant vision or myopia worsens in many patients after 20 to 30 treatments, particularly if they are over the age of 40. On the other hand, presbyopia is improved, and some patients say they can read again without reading glasses. These changes are usually temporary and revert to the pretreatment state within 6 weeks of the cessation of HBOT. Patients with early cataracts may not completely regain their pretreatment status, however, and may require a new prescription for glasses.

In the past, there was concern that a history of optic neuritis (with the possibility of HBOT causing blindness), a history of thoracic surgery (fear of air trapping), and pregnancy (retinitis of the newborn and premature closure of the patent ductus) were contraindications to HBOT. None of the above has been proven to be a serious threat in practice. Glaucoma is not a contraindication to HBOT as the eye consists of solids, gels, and liquids that are incompressible and do not deform. Only gas-containing spaces in the body or in hardware accompanying the patient can cause problems secondary to pressure changes. Confinement anxiety may occasionally occur. It is best managed by reassurance and sedatives.[14,28]

Safety Considerations

Although there has never been an explosion or fire in a hospital based hyperbaric chamber in the United States, disastrous chamber fires have been reported abroad. Considerable attention to safety is paramount for hyperbaric operations due to the risk of fire. While pure oxygen is not flammable, it vigorously supports combustion, and therefore this concern is valid. However, this risk can be managed very effectively through the use of environmental controls. In both the monoplace and multiplace environments, patients are treated in an uncontaminated environment. Strict contraband monitoring and precautions against potential sources of combustion are vigorously enforced. Patients should not wear lipstick or alcohol-based perfumes or hairspray. Volatile flammable liquids such as alcohol should not be allowed in the chamber because static electricity has ignited liquids in pure oxygen in laboratory tests. It is essential that patients never be treated in their street clothes: There have been serious, fatal chamber fires (outside the United States) because patients have brought lighters and hand warmers into the chamber in their pockets. Hospital cotton clothing is routinely employed to minimize this concern and decrease the risk of static discharge. In the monoplace chamber, patients are also grounded with a wrist strap and grounding wire. The multiplace chamber patient is compressed in air (rather than 100% oxygen) and breathes 100% oxygen via a mask, thus the issue of static discharge is not as pronounced as in the monoplace environment. Nonetheless, every effort is made to ensure that all potential sources of combustion are eliminated from the hyperbaric chamber environment.

The many "foreign objects" or items of hardware that are attached to or accompany patients in the chamber have often caused worry. Internal cardiac pacemakers and even internally implanted defibrillators are completely safe at therapeutic pressures. Insulin pumps should be emptied prior to treatment as there can be a precipitous fall in blood sugar levels in diabetic patients while they receive HBOT. External metal fixators for fractures as well as fiberglass

casts are safe. In the oxygen-filled monoplace chamber, remove electronic hearing aids and watches. Glasses and contact lenses are permitted, but glasses with titanium frames should be removed as breakage of titanium wire can occasionally cause fire. Petrolatum or Vaseline® dressings have been safely used for over 40 years, even in the monoplace chamber, as there is no ignition source. They are simply covered with gauze during treatment.

Given all of the aforementioned safety precautions, patients treated with HBOT in the United States routinely complete 40 to 60 hyperbaric treatments without any untoward side effects during the course of their treatment.[14,28]

Rationale for Use of Hyperbaric Oxygen Therapy in the Hypoxic Wound

HBOT is appropriate and indicated for the management of several classifications of compromised wound types. The majority of these wounds have similar pathergy in that they all manifest wound healing compromise due to varying degrees of tissue hypoxia. It is well established that local-tissue hypoxia and infection are two of the primary defects underlying compromised healing in the diabetic foot ulcer (DFU). Hyperbaric oxygen therapy specifically treats both of these underlying factors. Thus, a short discussion of the use of hyperbaric oxygen as an adjunct in the management of the DFU is presented as an example of the benefit of HBOT in the generic "hypoxic wound." The use of HBOT in the care of the patient with a DFU is based on a rational physiological basis, favorable in vitro studies, and animal research that has elucidated mechanisms of action in aerobic and anaerobic infections and wound healing.[29-32] These effects are corroborated by extensive clinical experience.[33-35]

> **PEARL 32•4** Hyperbaric oxygen therapy provides a significant increase in tissue oxygenation in the hypoperfused, infected wound. This elevation in oxygen tension in the hypoxic wound induces powerful positive changes in the wound-repair process. Hyperbaric oxygen therapy promotes wound healing by directly enhancing fibroblast replication, collagen synthesis, and the process of neovascularization in ischemic tissue. By providing molecular oxygen at the cellular level, it also significantly increases leukocyte bactericidal activity.

The increase in tissue oxygenation, which leads to the increased formation of oxygen radicals within the leukocyte, is bactericidal or bacteriostatic to anaerobic organisms, and it may be as effective as specific antibiotic therapy, providing an added effect.

The Centers for Medicare and Medicaid Services (CMS) recently approved the use of HBOT for the management of the diabetic foot ulcer. Strict criteria have been established. The patient must have diabetes (type 1 or type 2) and a lower-extremity wound (Wagner grade 3–5) due to diabetic disease. The wound must have failed standard wound care as demonstrated by no measurable signs of healing for 30 days (decrease in volume or size, decrease in exudate, or decrease in necrotic tissue). Standard therapy must include assessment of vascular status, optimization of nutrition/glucose control, débridement, moist dressings, off-loading, and treatment of infection. Once these criteria have been satisfied and HBOT initiated, the wound must be reevaluated every 30 days during the HBOT course. Continued HBOT will not be covered if there are no measurable signs of healing during the 30-day period.

Clinical Literature

Although there is extensive literature describing the surgical management of the diabetic foot, it is difficult to adequately compare different approaches to therapy. The principal obstacles to interpretation of most studies are the influence of the bias introduced by "clinical judgment" and the lack of objective documentation of the severity of complicating local and systemic factors. Recently, a protocol for the management of diabetic foot wounds has been tested in a prospective, randomized fashion.[36]

In 1982 a retrospective report of 70 patients with nonhealing wounds treated with adjuvant hyperbaric oxygen therapy suggested beneficial effects for this modality.[37] This report included diabetic patients with soft tissue infection, underlying osteomyelitis, failed skin grafts, and nonhealing amputation sites. In this series, 60% of the patients healed or showed significant improvement despite the presence of ischemia, infection, or neuropathic changes.

In a prospective controlled study, Baroni et al studied the effect of HBOT on the management of grade 3 and 4 diabetic foot lesions.[38] The groups were matched for lesion size, subfascial involvement, and duration and severity of diabetes. All patients were hospitalized, underwent daily débridement, and were maintained under strict metabolic control. The study (hyperbaric oxygen, or HBO) group consisted of 18 patients, of whom 16 healed and 2 underwent amputation. In the control group ($N = 10$), 1 patient healed, 5 showed no change, and 4 underwent amputations ($P = 0.001$). A retrospective review in the same center revealed an amputation rate of 40% between 1979 and 1981. Once HBO therapy became available, the amputation rate dropped dramatically to 11%. Baroni concluded that HBOT was effective in the treatment of grade 3 and 4 diabetic foot lesions as evidenced by a higher healing rate and a drastic decrease in amputation rate.

In a large clinical series of 168 patients with grade 3 and 4 diabetic foot lesions, Davis reported a 70% success rate with a combined management protocol consisting of daily débridement, specific antibiotic therapy, aggressive wound care, metabolic control, and daily HBOT for 30 to 60 days.[39] Most treatment failures were seen in older patients with significant occlusive vascular disease and absent pedal pulses. Oriani and colleagues reported on the effect of HBO for the treatment of grade 4 diabetic foot lesions. In this series, the HBO group consisted of 62 patients, and the matched control group had 18.[40] There was no significant difference in age, severity, or duration of diabetes, or its complications. All patients were hospitalized and underwent daily débridement, strict metabolic control, and specific antibiotic therapy. In the HBO group, 96% of the patients healed, while 4% underwent amputation. In the control group, 66% achieved primary healing, and 33% required amputation ($P < 0.001$).

In addition, Wattel et al evaluated the role of transcutaneous oximetry in predicting outcome in a prospective series of 59 consecutive patients with diabetic foot lesions treated with HBO therapy.[41] In this study, the patients received an average of 29 plus or minus 19 treatment sessions at 2.5 ATA, 100% O_2 for 90 minutes, twice daily. The benefit of HBO therapy was shown in this study with a healing rate of 87% and an amputation rate of 13%. More importantly, the outcome was predicted by transcutaneous oxygen ($TcPo_2$) measurements in the hyperbaric chamber. The healed group attained a chamber $TcPo_2$ of 786 plus or minus 258 mm Hg as compared to 323 plus or minus 214 mm Hg for the amputation group ($P < 0.005$). In this study, a minimum value of 450 mm Hg was shown to correlate with a successful outcome. In another large retrospective series of patients with diabetic foot lesions, Stone et al showed that the HBO-treated group ($N = 87$) had a higher limb salvage rate (73% vs 53%) than the nontreated group ($N = 382$).[42] These studies strongly suggest that HBO therapy should be an integral part of the treatment regimen of the diabetic foot to minimize lower-extremity amputations and that $TcPo_2$ measurements may be of significant value in predicting outcome.

More recently, in a prospective, randomized study, Faglia et al evaluated the effectiveness of HBOT in decreasing major lower-extremity amputations in diabetic patients with Wagner's grade 2, 3, and 4 lesions.[36] All patients were evaluated and treated following a comprehensive protocol, including aggressive surgical débridement, culture-specific antibiotics, appropriate revascularization, strict metabolic control of diabetes, daily wound care, and prevention of mechanical stress. The HBO group consisted of 35 patients with the following Wagner classification lesions: grade 4 ($N = 22$), grade 3 ($N = 9$), and grade 2 ($N = 4$). The control group consisted of 33 patients with grade 4 ($N = 20$), grade 3 ($N = 8$), and grade 2 ($N = 5$). The transcutaneous oxygen measurements on the dorsum of the foot for the HBO group were 23.25 plus or minus 10.6 mm Hg as compared to 21.29 plus or minus 10.7 mm Hg in the control group. There were no significant differences in the clinical characteristics of the groups, including presence of infection, sensory motor neuropathy, or severity of peripheral vascular disease. The treated group underwent an average of 38 plus or minus 8 sessions at 2.5 ATA on 100% O_2 for 90 minutes. The average chamber $TcPo_2$ value was 493 plus or minus 152 mm Hg.

In this trial, a significant difference in major amputation rates was observed between the two groups. The HBO group underwent three major amputations (8.6%, one above knee amputation (AKA), two below knee amputations (BKA)), with 11 (33.3%, four AKA, seven BKA) major amputations in the control group ($P = 0.016$). Furthermore, the foot TcPo$_2$ values were significantly higher in the HBO-treated group (37 ± 16.1 mm Hg) than in the control group (26 ± 13.5 mm Hg) at the time of discharge ($P = 0.0002$). The results obtained in this landmark randomized trial clearly document and define the effectiveness of HBO therapy in addition to a comprehensive protocol in decreasing major amputations in the diabetic with a compromised foot. Moreover, the transcutaneous oximetry data provides objective documentation of improved tissue oxygenation after HBO treatment.

Patient Selection

As previously mentioned, not all patients are good candidates for hyperbaric oxygen therapy. Besides the contraindications mentioned above, not all patients will respond to HBOT, for various reasons. Therefore, in order to predict whether a patient might receive benefit from this treatment modality, especially in the case of a nonhealing lower-extremity wound or ulceration, transcutaneous oximetry is often a very useful tool. Transcutaneous oxygen mapping (TCOM) is the technique in which a specialized instrument is used to simultaneously measure transcutaneous oxygen pressures in several areas of the skin. It is painless, inexpensive, and can usually be performed quite easily at the bedside.

The concept of measuring the oxygen delivery to the cutaneous tissue is fairly straightforward. After a small area of the skin is thoroughly cleaned of any loose debris, a specialized electrode is placed on the skin to warm it to a specified temperature. This warming action induces vasodilation in small vessels within the skin, and the oxygen content is then measured by the same electrode. Tissue oxygen levels of 35 to 40 mm Hg and higher obtained in room air at normobaric pressures are generally considered to be normal; thus, wound healing in these areas is not likely to be compromised due to hypoxia. However values of 30 mm Hg or less indicate impaired wound healing, with impaired immune function and fibroblast proliferation rates being the two most significant impediments to the normal healing process in these patients. It is also important to note that abnormally low transcutaneous oxygen values can be caused by several disease processes, and once an abnormal value has been documented, a further diagnostic work-up is indicated to more fully define the exact cause for the tissue hypoxia.

For example, while patients with either peripheral arterial disease (PAD) or diabetes may have abnormally low transcutaneous oximetry values, the mechanism behind each is vastly different. In the case of the patient with PAD, it is often macrovascular disease that accounts for the diminished distal blood flow, thus these patients will likely benefit from a vascular work-up with referral to the vascular specialist. In contrast is the patient with diabetes, which tends to more dramatically affect the microvasculature. However, as there could certainly be components of both microvascular and macrovascular disease in each of these patients, both deserve further evaluation prior to considering HBOT.

> ▶ **PEARL 32•5** Besides indicating that a basic problem with tissue hypoxia exists, the TCOM study also helps to predict the potential success of HBOT. When normobaric oximetry values are less than 35 to 40 mm Hg, a 100% normobaric oxygen challenge is given via a nonrebreathing face mask. If the abnormally low TCOM values rise to 100 mm Hg or more, the patient will likely benefit from HBOT.

However, this fact does not excuse the patient from a vascular work-up, as many patients have multifactorial components to tissue hypoxia. Thus, the absence of reconstructible arterial disease is a CMS prerequisite for the use of HBOT.[43-45]

Topical Oxygen

A chapter devoted to oxygen therapy would not be complete without a brief discussion of topical oxygen. Topical oxygen therapy is the application of oxygen to the surface of a wound. This is generally accomplished by placing the affected limb in an enclosed acrylic or plastic box and filling it with oxygen. This should not be confused with systemic hyperbaric oxygen therapy, in which the patient breathes 100% oxygen while inside a monoplace or multiplace chamber under greater-than-normal atmospheric pressure. Topical oxygen is frequently (and inappropriately) called "topical hyperbaric oxygen." Use of this term simply adds confusion and is a misapplication of the word *hyperbaric*. Hyperbaric oxygen as defined by the American College of Hyperbaric Medicine is the inhalation of 100% oxygen while the entire patient is enclosed within a chamber at pressures of at least 1.4 ATA or greater. Advocates claim that topical oxygen dissolves in tissue fluids, is bacteriostatic, and stimulates angiogenesis and wound healing.[45] Clinical trials comparing topical oxygen and hyperbaric oxygen have been undertaken in centers in the United States. However, there are only two quantitative studies involving topical oxygen reported in the literature, one controlled and the other using electron microscopy to assess results. Both show an impediment to healing.[4,48]

Summary

Hyperbaric oxygen therapy is an advanced wound care technology that can have a significant positive and powerful effect in the management of patients with compromised wound healing, especially when the primary deficit is tissue hypoxia. When patients are carefully selected and appropriately managed with HBOT as part of a comprehensive wound care strategy, wound healing enhancement can be realized and limb loss avoided.

▶ Case Study 32•1 — Hyperbaric Oxygen Therapy for a Wagner's Stage 3 Diabetic Foot Ulcer

This 52-year-old Hispanic male with a 3-year history of insulin-dependent diabetes and distal neuropathy presented to his podiatrist with a superficial plantar foot ulceration of his right great toe (Wagner 1). Initial management efforts consisted of moist wound care and off-loading with a diabetic pressure-relief shoe. Lack of healing progress prompted a referral to the Center for Comprehensive Wound Care and Hyperbaric Oxygen Therapy. Physical examination revealed 2+ pedal pulses, and transcutaneous oximetry showed normal tissue oxygenation with all values exceeding 40 mm Hg.

Aggressive wound care efforts yielded decreased wound size, but the wound failed to heal. Off-loading was suboptimal due to failure to maintain use of pressure-relief shoes. The patient returned to the Wound Care Clinic and frequently required wound débridement and callus paring.

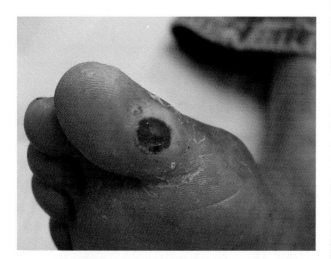

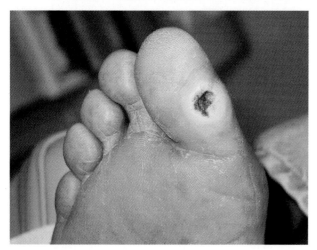

The patient presented on 12/26 with erythema, warmth, and deterioration of the ulcer with purulent drainage. MRI imaging showed bony erosion of the distal phalanx consistent with underlying osteomyelitis.

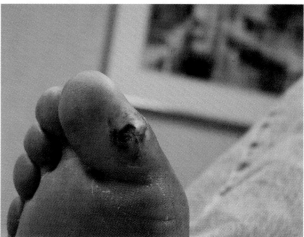

Management included toe amputation and IV antibiotics. Hyperbaric oxygen therapy (HBOT) was initiated as adjunctive therapy for a Wagner's 3 diabetic foot ulcer. The patient was discharged after 3 days' hospitalization for continued outpatient care. HBOT was continued for 15 sessions.

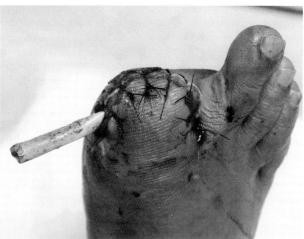

Once the operative incision was healed and the subdermal tissue matured, the patient was fitted with custom diabetic shoes with orthotic inserts. He was advised to perform daily foot monitoring and moisturizing and continue with routine podiatric foot care.

▶ **Case Study 32•1** **Hyperbaric Oxygen Therapy for a Wagner's Stage 3 Diabetic Foot Ulcer—cont'd**

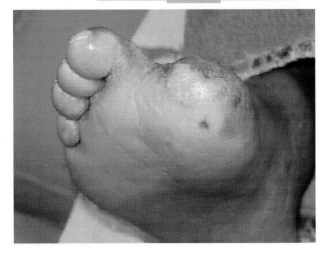
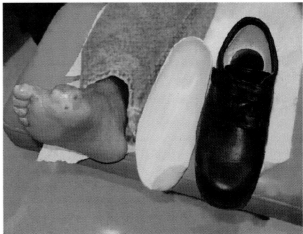

Case Key Points:

- Diabetic patients are at high risk for foot ulceration, which can lead to partial foot or high amputation.
- The risk of developing complicated skin, soft tissue, or bone infection once a diabetic foot ulcer (DFU) is present is significant and efforts to reduce wound bioburden is prudent.

- Appropriate off-loading is paramount in the management of a patient with a DFU.
- HBOT is appropriate as an adjunctive therapy in the management of a patient with a DFU (Wagner 3–5).
- HBOT positively affects angiogenesis, collagen synthesis, and leukocyte function in patients with hypoxic wounds.

References

1. Lawrence, WT: Clinical management of non-healing wounds. In: Cohen, IK, Diegelmann, RF, Lindblad, WJ (eds): Wound Healing. Biochemical and Clinical Aspects. Philadelphia, Saunders, 1992, pp 541–561.
2. Guyton, AC: Physical principles of gaseous exchange. In: Guyton, AC, Hall, JE: Textbook of Medical Physiology. Philadelphia, Saunders, 1981 pp 491–500.
3. Guyton, AC: Transport of oxygen and carbon dioxide in the blood and body tissues. In: Guyton, AC, Hall, JE: Textbook of Medical Physiology. Philadelphia, Saunders, 1981, pp 504–514.
4. Davis, JC, Hunt, TK: Problem Wounds: The Role of Oxygen. New York, Elsevier Science Publishing, 1988.
5. Niinikoski, J: Oxygen and wound healing. Clin Plast Surg 1977; 4:361–374.
6. Niinikoski, J, Rajamaki, A, Kulonene, E: Healing of open wounds: Effects of oxygen, disturbed blood supply, and hyperemia by infrared irradiation. Acta Chir Scand 1971; 137:399–401.
7. Knighton, DR, Hunt, TK, Scheuenstuhl, H, et al: Oxygen tension regulates the expression of angiogenesis factor by macrophages. Science 1983; 221:1283–1285.
8. Stillman, RM: Effects of hypoxia and hyperoxia on progression of intimal healing. Arch Surg 1983; 118:732–737.
9. Hunt, TK, Hopf, H, Hussian, Z: Physiology of wound healing. Adv Skin Wound Care 2000; 13(suppl):6–11.
10. Knighton, DR, Silver, IA, Hunt, TK: Regulation of wound healing angiogenesis-effect of oxygen gradients and inspired oxygen concentration. Surgery 1981; 2:262–270.
11. Hopf, HW, Hunt, TK, West, JM, et al: Wound tissue oxygen tension predicts the risk of wound infection in surgical patients. Arch Surg 1997; 132:997–1004.
12. Hammarlund, C: The physiologic effects of hyperbaric oxygenation. In: Kindwall, EP, Whelan, HT (eds): Hyperbaric Medicine Practice. Flagstaff, AZ, Best Publishing, 2004, pp 37–68.
13. Weaver, LK, Valentine, KJ, Hopkins, RO: Carbon monoxide poisoning: Risk factors for cognitive sequelae and the role of hyperbaric oxygen. Am J Respir Crit Care Med 2007; 176:491–497.
14. Kindwall, EP, Niezgoda, JA (eds): Hyperbaric Medicine Procedures: The Kindwall HBO Handbook. Milwaukee, Aurora Heath Care, 2006.
15. Kindwall, EP: The history of hyperbaric medicine. In: Kindwall, EP, Whelan, HT (eds): Hyperbaric Medicine Practice. Flagstaff, AZ, Best Publishing, 2004, pp 1–20.
16. Kindwall, EP: Report of the Committee on Hyperbaric Oxygenation. Bethesda, MD, Undersea Medical Society, 1977.
17. Krough, A: The number and distribution of capillaries in muscle with calculations of the oxygen pressure head necessary for supplying the tissue. J Physiology 1919; 52:409–415.

18. Lee, CC, Chen, SC, Tsai, SC, et al: Hyperbaric oxygen induces VEGF expression through ERK, JNK and c-Jun/AP-1 activation in human umbilical vein endothelial cells. J Biomed Sci 2006; 13:143–156.

19. Sheikh, AY, Gibson, JJ, Rollins, MD, et al: Effect of hyperoxia on vascular endothelial growth factor levels in a wound model. Arch Surg 2000; 135:1293–1297.

20. Ahmad, Y, Sheikh, MD, Mark, D, et al: Hyperoxia improves microvascular perfusion in a murine wound model. Wound Repair Regen 2005; 13:303–308.

21. Marx, RE, Ehler, WJ, Tayapongsak, P, et al: Relationship of oxygen dose to angiogenesis induction in irradiated tissue. Am J Surg 1990; 160:519–524.

22. Min, L, Yizhang, C, Meiping, D, et al: Involvement of the mitochondrial ATP-sensitive potassium channel in the neuroprotective effect of hyperbaric oxygenation after cerebral ischemia. Brain Res Bull 2006; 69:109–116.

23. Buras, JA, Stahl, GL, Svoboda, KKH, et al: Hyperbaric oxygen down-regulates ICAM-1 expression induced by hypoxia and hypoglycemia: The role of NOS. Am J Physiol Cell Physiol 2000; 278:C292–C302.

24. Nylander, G, Nordström, H, Franzén, L, et al: Effects of hyperbaric oxygen treatment in post-ischemic muscle. A quantitative morphological study. Scand J Plast Reconstr Surg Hand Surg 1988; 22:31–39.

25. Buras, J: Basic mechanisms of hyperbaric oxygen in the treatment of ischemia-reperfusion injury. Int Anesthesiol Clin 2000; 38:91–109.

26. Centers for Medicaid and Medicare Services. Available at: http://www.cms.hhs.gov/transmittals/downloads/R187CP.pdf, May 28th, 2004

27. Weaver, LK, Hopkins, RO, Chan, KJ, et al: Hyperbaric oxygen for acute carbon monoxide poisoning. N Engl J Med 2002; 347:1057–1067.

28. Kindwall, EP, Whelan, HT (eds): Hyperbaric Medicine Practice. Flagstaff, AZ, Best Publishing, 2004.

29. Bassett, BE, Bennett, PB: Introduction to the physical and physiological bases of hyperbaric therapy. In: Davis, JC, Hunt, TK (eds): Bethesda, MD, Undersea Medical Society, 1977, pp 11–24.

30. LaVan, FB, Hunt, TK: Oxygen and wound healing. Clin Plastic Surg 1990; 17:463–472.

31. Mader, JT (ed): Hyperbaric Oxygen Therapy: A Committee Report. Bethesda, MD, Undersea and Hyperbaric Medical Society 1989, pp 37–44.

32. Rabkin, JM, Hunt, TK: Infection and oxygen. In: Davis, J, Hunt, TK (eds): Problem Wounds: The Role of Oxygen. New York, Elsevier, 1988, pp 1–16.

33. Davis, JC: Enhancement of healing. In: Camporesi, E, Barker, AC (eds): Hyperbaric Oxygen Therapy: A Critical Review. Bethesda, MD, Undersea and Hyperbaric Medical Society, 1991, pp 127–140.

34. Davis, JC, Buckley, CJ, Barr, PO: Compromised soft tissue wounds: Correction of wound hypoxia. In: Davis, J, Hunt, TK (eds): Problem Wounds: The Role of Oxygen. New York, Elsevier Science Publishing, 1988, pp 143–152.

35. Perrins, DJ, Davis, JC: Enhancement of healing in soft tissue wounds. In: Camporesi, E, Barker, AC (eds): Hyperbaric Oxygen Therapy: A Critical Review. Bethesda, MD, Undersea and Hyperbaric Medical Society, 1977, pp 229–248.

36. Faglia, E: Adjunctive systemic hyperbaric oxygen therapy in treatment of severe prevalently ischemic diabetic foot ulcer. Diabetes Care 1996; 19:1338–1343.

37. Matos, LA: Preliminary report of the use of hyperbarics as adjunctive therapy in diabetics with chronic non-healing wounds. HBO Review 1983; 4:88–89.

38. Baroni, G, Porro, T, Faglia, E: Hyperbaric oxygen in diabetic gangrene treatment. Diabetes Care 1987; 10:81–86.

39. Davis, JC: The use of adjuvant hyperbaric oxygen in treatment of the diabetic foot. Clin Podiatr Med Surg 1987; 4:429–437.

40. Oriani, G, Meazza, D, Favales, F: Hyperbaric oxygen therapy in diabetic gangrene. J Hyperbaric Med 1990; 5:171–175.

41. Wattel, FE, Mathieu, DM, Fossati, P, et al: Hyperbaric oxygen in the treatment of diabetic foot lesions. J. Hyperbaric Med 1991; 6:263–268.

42. Stone, JA, Scott, R, Brill, LR, et al: The role of hyperbaric oxygen in the treatment of diabetic foot wounds. Diabetes 1995; 44(suppl):71A.

43. Sheffield, PJ, Workman, WT: Transcutaneous tissue oxygen monitoring in patients undergoing hyperbaric oxygen therapy. In: Huch, R, Huch, A (eds): Continuous Transcutaneous Blood Gas Monitoring. New York, Marcel Dekker, 1983, pp 655–660.

44. Fife, CE, Buyukecakir, C, Otto, G, et al: The predictive value of transcutaneous oxygen tension measurement in diabetic lower extremity ulcers treated with hyperbaric oxygen therapy: A retrospective analysis of 1144 patients. Wound Rep Regen 2002; 10:198–207.

45. Ballard, JL, Eke, CC, Bunt, TJ, et al: A prospective evaluation of transcutaneous oxygen measurements in the management of diabetic foot problems. J Vasc Surg 1995; 22:485–492.

46. Heng, MCY: Topical hyperbaric therapy for problem skin wounds. J Dermatol Surg Oncol 1993; 19:784–793.

47. Heng, MCY, Kloss, SG: Endothelial cell toxicity in leg ulcers treated with topical hyperbaric oxygen. Am J Dermatopath 1986; 8:403–410.

48. Leslie, CA, Sapico, FL, Ginunas, VJ, et al: Randomized control trial of topical hyperbaric oxygen for treatment of diabetic foot ulcers. Diabetes Care 1988; 11:111–115.

PART VI | Practice Management

chapter *33*

Documentation for Reimbursement

Pamela G. Unger, PT, CWS, FAPWCA

Wound care clinicians must understand that today's medical record serves as an instrument for demonstrating their ability to plan, coordinate, and evaluate patient care. The patient's chart, which was once used simply to measure patient outcomes, now may end up as evidence in a malpractice claim or used by an insurance company to confirm or challenge the level of service billed.

Documentation in wound care, as in all areas of clinical practice, is critical for reimbursement. The medical record is the primary method of communication between members of the health-care team. Documentation of patient outcomes and responses to treatment are key for evaluating treatment interventions. Demonstrating "the need for skilled/professional intervention" by a wound care professional must be evident in the documentation regardless of the payer source.[1] To ensure payment, a comprehensive individualized plan, indicating the wound problem and goal of treatment, must be in the medical record. While multiple models of documentation exist, one comprehensive source useful in wound care is the *Guide to Physical Therapist Practice.*[2] This American Physical Therapy Association (APTA) publication recommends a five-stage management system—examination, evaluation, diagnosis, prognosis, and intervention—that supports third-party reimbursement.

> ▶ **PEARL 33•1** Accurate and complete patient outcomes must be documented in the medical record.

Treatment of wounds alone does not guarantee payment. Medical complexity, wound chronicity, and collaborative efforts from other members of the wound-care team should be reflected in the medical record. As the health-care industry continues to move toward cost-containment strategies outlined in the Balanced Budget Act of 1997, management of and focus on cost-effective functional outcomes is mandatory.

633

This chapter identifies risk-assessment tools and provides documentation guidelines and examples of history and physical examinations, wound evaluations, and ongoing treatment interventions. General recommendations for billing in different practice settings also are reviewed.

Interdisciplinary Documentation

Pen-and-paper documentation is quickly becoming history. Today's documentation forms include, in addition to the old standby of handwritten notes, telephonic, photographic, and computer-generated correspondence. Regardless of the method of documentation, it is essential that guidelines be developed to assess clinical efficacy and cost effectiveness.

Keeping in mind that the practice setting may vary, wound prevention and treatment are best addressed by a team of experts. Teams may consist of any combination of diabetic educators, dieticians, nurses (Wound Ostomy Continence Nurse), nurse practitioners, occupational therapists, orthotists, pedorthists, physical therapists, physicians, physician assistants, and podiatrists. Physicians of any specialty (dermatology, endocrinology, family practice, infectious disease, orthopedic surgery, plastic-reconstructive surgery, physiatrics, or vascular surgery) may be involved in wound care. The physician with the wound care interest, regardless of specialty, will function as the coordinator of care, using the expertise of other team members to accomplish the wound care goals. Professionals involved in wound care will perform a variety of functions, such as the following:

- *Diabetes educator.* Patient/caregiver education related to diabetes management
- *Dietician.* Nutritional assessments and dietary modifications
- *Nurse.* History and systems review, wound assessment, wound treatments and dressings
- *Occupational therapist.* Functional seating and positioning, functional mobility training related to activities of daily living (ADL), treatment of barriers interfering with function (contractures, edema, motor control, muscle weakness, pain), and wound assessment and treatment of the upper extremity (UE) if the occupational therapist is a certified hand therapist
- *Orthotist/pedorthist.* Fabrication of upper- and lower-extremity orthotics, prostheses, and special footwear
- *Physical therapist.* Wound assessment, wound treatment with therapeutic modalities, débridement and standard wound care, functional seating and positioning, support surfaces, functional mobility training, and treatment barriers interfering with function (contractures, edema, motor control, muscle weakness, and pain)
- *Podiatrist.* Wound assessment, treatment, and reconstructive surgery of the foot and ankle
- *Physician.* Medical management, surgical intervention, and care coordination

The roles and responsibilities of team members may overlap, although each member brings a different viewpoint to the total wound care picture. In many clinical situations, members of the interdisciplinary team will generate a referral to another practitioner, if the referral is supported by appropriate documentation. Often, a well-established wound care team will have the roles and responsibilities of the team members delineated to streamline the evaluation and assessment process. Team members conduct evaluations within their specific scope of clinical practice. In order to provide optimal patient care and reimbursement, a detailed summary of problems within the specific domains of practice, barriers to functional outcomes, treatment interventions, and prognosis must all be addressed and documented. (Box 33.1)

> ▸ **PEARL 33•2** Organize your thoughts before you write them on paper or enter them into the computer.

Comprehensive documentation may be in the form of

- a critical pathway,
- a care plan,
- data and treatment ledgers, and
- interdisciplinary notes.

> ▸ **PEARL 33•3** Develop an accurate and legal abbreviation list.

Examination

Examination of the patient is required before any intervention is performed. The *Guide to Physical Therapist Practice* identifies three components of the initial examination: the patient history, relevant systems review, and tests and measures. According to the Office for Quality Healthcare Research (formerly the Agency for Healthcare Policy and Research [AHCPR]) and the APTA, a complete history and physical examination beyond the wound are critical in creating a comprehensive treatment plan for patients with dermal ulcers, including those caused by pressure, neuropathy, and vascular insufficiency.[3]

All wounds, regardless of etiology, require an assessment of underlying medical conditions that contribute to a delay in wound healing. Information may be obtained from a review of the patient medical record and patient/caregiver interview. The *history review* (Appendix 3) includes general demographics: social history; vocational history; growth and development; living environment; history of current condition; activity level; current medications; laboratory and other diagnostic tests, such as vascular studies and x-rays; past medical history of current condition; past medical/surgical history; family history; health

> ▸ **Box 33•1 General Documentation Guidelines**
>
> 1. Be accurate.
> 2. Be factual.
> 3. Be objective.
> 4. Be thorough.
> 5. Be truthful.
> 6. Avoid late entries.
> 7. Do not assign blame.
> 8. Use appropriate abbreviations.
> 9. Write legibly.

status; and social habits. The wound history and previous treatment interventions are also included.

The *systems review* contains information about the physiological and anatomic status of the cardiopulmonary, integumentary, musculoskeletal, and neuromuscular systems, as well as communication and language skills. The *tests and measures* include anthropometric characteristics, arousal and cognition, assistive and adaptive devises, gait, integumentary integrity, supportive devices, pain, range of motion (ROM), sensory integrity, and circulatory integrity. Treatment of underlying comorbidities may require referrals to other practitioners. For example, evidence of uncontrolled diabetes may require a referral to the primary care physician, endocrinologist, or diabetes educator as part of the comprehensive wound treatment plan.

Risk Assessment

Risk assessments are an efficient means of identifying and documenting patients at low, moderate, or high risk. The interdisciplinary team members working in inpatient settings in hospitals, rehabilitation hospitals, subacute units, skilled nursing facilities (SNFs), and home care programs should identify all at-risk individuals. On admission, or within 24 hours of admission, all patients should receive a systematic skin risk assessment.

The risk assessment can be accomplished by using a validated risk-assessment tool such as the Braden or Norton scales.[4,5] Both scales assess the critical components of risk. The Braden scale (Appendix 1) has been evaluated in diverse sites (medical-surgical units, intensive care units, nursing homes, and home health care), whereas the Norton scale (Appendix 2) has been evaluated only with elderly subjects in hospital settings. The Braden scale appears to be more specific, although there are outliers for each scale. Therefore, patients need to be assessed on an individual basis as it is very important to identify *all* risk factors. (Box 33.2)

The risk assessment tools are only as effective as their correlation to critical pathways, algorithms, and/or treatment interventions. When risk assessment tools are properly correlated, significant cost savings and outcomes for pressure ulcers can be realized.

SNFs and home health settings may use the Minimum Data Set (MDS) and OASIS to establish the patient at risk. With either tool, patients are placed into a resource utilization group (RUG) or home health resource group (HHRG) category

that determines the direction of care, reimbursement, and, ultimately, the most cost-efficient means of providing care.

The Evaluation

The evaluation is performed to establish a diagnosis and prognosis. Interpretation of examination data results in a diagnosis based on a cluster of signs and symptoms. Crucial to evaluation of the wound is establishment of the cause and history. It is also important to identify and classify wound severity by stage, thickness, and/or color. Wounds can be identified as burns, diabetic/neuropathic, arterial/ischemic, pressure, surgical, traumatic, and venous. Pressure ulcers are classified by stages identifying depth of soft tissue damage. This is discussed further in Chapters 6 and 19. Stages for grading pressure ulcers were developed by the National Pressure Ulcer Advisory Panel in 1989 and adopted by the AHCPR in 1994.[6] In 2007, The National Pressure Ulcer Advisory Panel revised the earlier definitions to include *unstageable* and *deep tissue injury* (DTI). The Wagner Ulcer Grade Classification Scale is used to assess neuropathic foot ulcers. (Table 33.1)[7] All other wounds are typically classified as partial thickness or full thickness. (Table 33.2) An additional classification system developed by Marion Laboratories uses a three-color concept (red, yellow, or black) to describe the wound base by percentage. This classification system can be used with any wound type. (Table 33.3) This system addresses the documentation requirement of percentage of necrosis on the wound bed. Once the wound type and classification is identified, the following documentation is required:

- A specific anatomical location
- Size (surface area) or size and depth (volume)
  Wound is easily assessed with a ruler, tape measure caliper (one-dimensional). This is still the most common and reliable method recognized by researchers.[8]
  Planimetry, measurement of the surface area, and the periphery of a plane are figured by tracing its boundaries (two-dimensional).
  Wound assessment systems (VISITRAK, VERG, and MAVIS) use stereophotographic systems to measure wound volume.

> ## Box 33•2 Risk Factors

- Impaired/decreased mobility
- Impaired/decreased functional mobility
- Comorbid conditions such as end-stage renal disease, thyroid disease, diabetes mellitus
- Refusal of some aspects of care or treatment
- Cognitive impairment
- Undernutrition, malnutrition, and hydration deficits
- Healed ulcer (history of a healed ulcer and its stage is important, since these areas are more likely to have recurrent breakdown.)

Table 33•1	Classification by Wagner Scale (Diabetic Foot Ulcer Classifications)
Grade	**Description**
Grade 0	Preulcerous lesion, healed ulcer, bony deformity
Grade 1	Superficial ulcer without subcutaneous tissues involvement
Grade 2	Penetration through the subcutaneous tissue; may expose bone, tendon or ligament, or joint capsule
Grade 3	Osteitis, abscess, or osteomyelitis
Grade 4	Gangrene of digit
Grade 5	Gangrene requiring foot amputation

Table 33•2 Classification of Wound by Thickness

Thickness	Description
Partial thickness	Extends through the first layer of skin (epidermis), but not through the second layer of skin (dermis)
Full thickness	Extends through the epidermis and dermis and may involve subcutaneous tissue, muscle, bone

Table 33•3 Wound Type and Classifications

Type	Classification	Color
Arterial/ischemic	Partial/full thickness[18]	Red, yellow, black[19]
Burns	Partial/full thickness	Red, yellow, black
Diabetic	Wagner scale[20]	Red, yellow, black
Pressure	Stage I–IV, deep tissue injury, unstageable[3]	Red, yellow, black
Surgical	Partial/full thickness	Red, yellow, black
Traumatic	Partial/full thickness	Red, yellow, black
Venous	Partial/full thickness	Red, yellow, black

- Undermining/tunneling
- Stage/thickness
- Wound bed description (color)
- Exudate (color, odor, consistency, quantity)
- Pain
- Periwound condition and appearance

This specific documentation is required for every wound to identify severity and justify reimbursement. These categories are evaluated initially and at least weekly thereafter to monitor progress. Wound care team members will use additional documentation in the form of photographs and tracings to further justify treatment interventions.

Wound care documentation is often found in the form of treatment and objective data ledgers instead of progress notes. This helps to ensure accuracy, consistency, and efficiency of the documentation. Treatment ledger documentation provides an assessment of treatment effectiveness, as well as an easy method of communication to team members and third-party payers.

▶ **PEARL 33•4** Perform a documentation audit to ensure accurate documentation.

Assessment forms may take the form of a flow sheet (Appendix 4) or a single-use form (Appendix 5). Currently, the Pressure Sore Status Tool (PSST) has been validated for content and interrater reliability among enterostomal nurses.[9]

In addition to providing an objective score of the wound status for evaluation and weekly assessments, the PSST provides a complete description of the wound (Appendix 6). A modified version of the tool for evaluation and weekly progress notes (Appendix 7) incorporates additional patient information, references to wound tracing, multiple wound sites, short- and long-term goals, treatment plan, reference to nutritional consultation, and cosignature by the caregiver.

Additional tests and measures with documentation are needed for patients with vascular (arterial and venous) and neuropathic ulcers. Palpation or Doppler ultrasound may be used to assess peripheral pulses (femoral, popliteal, posterior tibial, dorsalis pedis) and to determine the ankle-brachial index when evaluating patients for arterial disease.[10] Evaluation of swelling and a venous Doppler exam may also be used to assess patients for venous disease. In the absence of edema or infection, transcutaneous oxygen measurements ($TcPo_2$) may be used for preliminary assessment of arterial flow and skin oxygen tension. Results of clinical vascular examinations determine the need for follow-up studies in a vascular laboratory. Monofilament testing to determine the presence or absence of protective sensation and light touch is an additional measure used to evaluate neuropathic lower extremities in individuals with diabetes with or without foot ulcers.

Prognosis

The prognosis is the determination of the optimal level of improvement that might be attained in conjunction with the amount of time to reach that level. During the prognostic process, the wound care treatment team develops a plan of care, goals, specific interventions, expected outcomes, frequency of visits, and duration of the episode of care. With patients receiving wound care, it may be necessary to estimate various levels of improvement to be reached at different time intervals throughout the entire episode of care to ensure ongoing reimbursement by third-party payers. Wound chronicity and severity of comorbidities may alter the type, frequency, and length of treatment.

Intervention

The APTA's *Guide to Physical Therapist Practice* defines intervention as "the purposeful and skilled interaction of the physical therapist with the patient/client . . . to produce changes in the condition that are consistent with the diagnosis and prognosis." All patients should receive a coordinated plan of care and have open lines of communication with their caregivers. Certainly, all patients will receive personalized instruction related to their care. Direct interventions may include therapeutic exercise, functional training, manual therapy, assistive devices, support surfaces, therapeutic treatment modalities, mechanical modalities, débridement, and wound management.

Documentation

Beyond evaluation and treatment of the wound, the physical therapy plan of care focuses on restoration of functional loss secondary to the wound problem, as well as the wound-specific treatments. The medical record must include physician orders and evidence of patient/caregiver teaching or training. Efficient documentation is expedited by prepared evaluation forms with standardized functional scales. Documentation of barriers related to restricted functional mobility is also critical. Barrier documentation is best addressed by objective data, such as range of motion (ROM) measurements, manual muscle test grades, and balance or pain scales. A minimum weekly reassessment of function and barriers relative to the short-term goals is essential for documenting progress and justifying continued treatment. A lack of progress does not necessarily indicate the need to stop therapy, but it does indicate the need to reassess the present plan of care. Using a treatment ledger, daily documentation is generally used to identify treatments performed. It is common to chart by exception when recording daily treatment interventions. Charting by exception involves only recording information such as unusual response to treatment, a change in medical status, trial of specific pressure-relieving devices or techniques, or patient/caregiver training and education. Concurrent review of patient evaluations, weekly assessments, and daily documentation are critical for maximizing reimbursement.

Documentation Checklist
- Chief complaint
- History of present illness
- Past medical history, family and social history
- Previous treatments performed
- Review of systems
- Physical assessment
- Risk assessment
- Manual assessments
- Skin and wound assessment
- Procedures performed
- Supplies and tests ordered
- Patient education
- Plan of care
- Discharge plan
- Short- and long-term goals

Electronic Medical Record
When considering the implementation of an electronic medical record (EMR), one must wonder if the added expense will actually help the documentation process. Any EMR that is worth its cost will address the regulatory standards and issues of such groups as the Joint Commission on Accreditation for Healthcare Organizations (JCAHO), Magnet, individual state departments of health, and Centers for Medicare and Medicaid Services. EMRs guarantee that the required documentation for standards compliance is entered into the program.

▶ **PEARL 33•5** Document at the time of the visit and make sure that any sticky notes or scratch paper is discarded.

Using such an EMR reduces the chance of using prohibited abbreviations, facilitates medication reconciliation, and helps demonstrate interdisciplinary communication. It also ensures that the documentation supports charges sent to the billing department, which in turn enhances reimbursement for services. The wound assessment, procedure, and plan of care are all in one place. Diagnoses match the reason for the daily visit and service provided. The EMR is programmed to record the entire patient visit, care planning, and evaluation. Liability exposure is reduced. Built-in measures tie documentation to the person entering it, thereby allowing a quick and easy audit trail. With mandatory or required fields, risk of missing information is significantly reduced. Most evident is the elimination of illegible entries.

▶ **PEARL 33•6** Policies and procedures for skin and wound care should reflect current clinical practice guidelines and be approved by your facility.

The EMR can contribute to improved customer satisfaction for the patient, physician, clinician, and administrator. The patient benefits by the ability of the systems to show pictorial and graphic representations of progress, further assisting in patient participation in care planning. The physician benefits by having ready access to patient care information, the ability to view historical data and trends (with no need to flip through mounds of paper), and progress and/or consultation letters regarding patient care at the touch of a button. Clinicians benefit by the decreased need for narrative notes, easy access to all patient information, a concise and complete chart at the end of a visit, and prompts and mandatory fields to ensure complete documentation. Administration benefits from the elimination of the cost of dictation and transcription, elimination of the cost of record storage, and reassurance that regulatory and legal exposure is being controlled.

Managing quality and performance improvement are essential in the world of pay-for-performance. The EMR is a very effective tool for outcomes and benchmarking. Whether the goal is to compare performance to like programs, set goals for healing, or monitor adherence to clinical practice guidelines, the EMR has revolutionized the way data is collected, collated, and delivered. (Appendix 8)

Billing Recommendations

Currently, reimbursement is contingent on documentation supporting "skilled therapy interventions."[11] All health-care professionals need to carefully examine how patient care is provided and billed. The following guidelines are important considerations to remember when designing a wound care treatment plan:

- benefit to the patient/client
- appropriateness of caregiver
- cost effectiveness of the interventions
- outcome-oriented plans of care

When providing interdisciplinary care, excellent communication between health-care providers and the various care settings is essential.

Billing processes to ensure reimbursement are very systematic. The International Classification of Diseases (ICD-9) is used to identify diagnosis to justify treatment interventions; the ICD-9 codes are updated and published annually.[12] On the Medicare billing form there is space for five diagnostic codes. The diagnoses must include the wound, supporting medical conditions (comorbidities), and those diagnoses that support functional interventions. The ICD-9 codes should be listed in order of importance. All team members involved in billing related to wound care should use the same ICD-9 codes to ensure payment for services provided.

Physicians' Current Procedural Terminology (CPT) refers to codes used to describe predominantly medical services and procedures performed by physician and nonphysician professionals. There are three levels of CPT Codes:

- *Category I.* Codes describing current clinical practice procedure
- *Category II.* Performance measurement codes used as tracking codes to facilitate data collection to decrease the need for record abstraction and chart review, minimizing the administrative burden when entities are seeking to measure the quality of patient care.
  These are services and tests that support nationally established performance measures that have an evidence base contributing to the quality of patient care.
  Codes are optional.
- *Category III.* Emerging technology codes granted by the American Medical Association for the primary purpose of tracking utilization
  No payment is assigned.
  When performing the procedure or service assigned, it is recommended to use the Category III code.

Physical therapists and other health-care providers use CPT codes to describe the services provided. The codes used need to correlate with documentation in the medical record involving the amount of time spent with the patient and the treatment provided. In addition to the CPT code, a system of two-digit modifiers allows the provider to indicate any modifications in the service or procedure. Like the ICD-9 codes, the CPT codes are updated and published annually.[13] (Table 33.4)

In addition to CPT codes, revenue codes are used to identify discipline-specific treatment interventions relative to CPT codes in acute care institutions and hospital-based outpatient wound care programs. Different revenue codes are used by clinicians for the same CPT code intervention, depending on payer type. Physical therapy services are always identified under revenue code 420. Clinical services are often identified under revenue code 510.

The Health Care Financing Administration's Common Procedural Coding System (HCPCS) uses codes to supplement the CPT coding system.[14] The system includes codes for nonphysician services, administration of injectable drugs, durable medical equipment (DME), and office supplies. Wound care clinicians use these codes for durable medical equipment, including wound care supplies and dressings. Selection and use of wound care supplies and dressings depend on the wound size and quantity of product that will be reimbursed on a monthly basis.

Medicare Payment Systems

Reimbursement in SNFs is determined by the Resource Utilization Group (RUG) category. If the SNF resident qualifies for one of the rehabilitation RUG categories (ultra high, high), the therapist must appropriately document the distribution of rehabilitation time in minutes allocated to wound care (eg, treatment, débridement), ADL, positioning, and strengthening. Depending on the resident's RUG category, the medical condition may determine that nursing resources are adequate to care for this patient until the medical condition has stabilized. On medical stabilization, the patient may be moved into a new rehabilitation RUG category. Based on all of the resident's rehabilitation needs, wound care may still be delegated to nursing.

On August 1, 2000, Ambulatory Payment Classifications (APCs) were introduced as a new Medicare Prospective Payment System for hospital outpatient services. Payment for services are predetermined according to the types of services and procedures provided, including supplies for the visit.

Table 33•4	Active Wound Management Codes	
97602	Nonselective débridement	Removal of devitalized tissue from wound(s), nonselective débridement without anesthesia, wet-to-moist dressings, enzymatic, abrasion, includes topical application(s), wound assessments, and instruction(s) for ongoing care May include use of a whirlpool
97597	Selective débridement ≤20 cm²	Removal of devitalized tissue from wound(s), selective débridement without anesthesia, high-pressure water jet with/without suction, sharp selective débridement with scissors, scalpel, and forceps, with or without topical application(s), wound assessments, and instruction(s) for ongoing care May include use of a whirlpool
97598	Selective débridement >20 cm²	
97605	Negative-pressure therapy ≤50 cm²	Negative-pressure wound therapy (eg, vacuum-assisted drainage collection), including topical application(s), wound assessment, and instruction(s) for ongoing care, per session; total wound(s) surface area less than or equal to 50 cm²
97606	Negative-pressure therapy >50 cm²	
0183T	Low-frequency ultrasound	Low-frequency, nonthermal, noncontact ultrasound, including topical application(s) when performed, wound assessment and instruction(s) for ongoing care, per day

American Medical Association: CPT Manual. Chicago, American Medical Association, 2008.

Medicare has the option of providing "pass through" payments of specific supply items for a limited time for items unavailable when APCs were developed. The APC rates are assessed annually. Outpatient hospital-based physical therapy services continue to be reimbursed under the Medicare physician fee schedule.

The Medicare Prospective Payment System for inpatient rehabilitation, inpatient rehabilitation facilities (IRF), was introduced January 1, 2002, for free-standing rehabilitation hospitals and rehabilitation units in acute care hospitals. Patients in these facilities must be able to complete 3 hours of rehabilitation a day. The patient assessment instrument (PAI), updated October 1, 2007, uses information from the patient assessment instrument to classify patients into distinct groups based on clinical characteristics and expected resource needs. The PUSH tool version 3.0 is the assessment tool for wounds.

The Medicare Prospective Payment System for home health, home health reimbursement groups (HHRG), was introduced October 1, 2000. Payments are determined from completion of the OASIS assessment and establishment of a case-mix ratio based on patient acuity. The reimbursement covers a 60-day episode of care and includes all services and nonroutine medical supplies (wound dressings, ostomy and urinary supplies).

In general, accurate assessment and coding of diagnosis, services, and procedures expedites and maximizes reimbursement. Individual insurers may require prior authorizations for evaluation and treatment visits, including specific procedures. Frequently, the insurer requests the ICD-9 and CPT codes before granting authorization. The insurer and/or payer may also request written updates justifying continued treatment intervention. Current documentation from the medical record may be submitted or supplied on a separate form (Appendix 8).

Pay for performance (P4P) has arisen from Centers for Medicare and Medicaid Services (CMS), employers, consumers, providers of all types, and health-care plans taking a closer look at the value provided by our health-care delivery system. There are references that indicate a 50% gap between the care patients require and the care they are rendered. Others indicate that only 40% of patients receive care that is necessary and appropriate. More amazing is that studies have shown that after a major medical advance or practice guideline is released, it takes about 10 years for physicians to change the way they practice.

The CMS hospital reimbursement is based on diagnostic related groups (DRG), regardless of the quality of care delivered. The current evolution in Congress is to revise the Medicare system and base payments on safe, efficient, and effective delivery of care. The solution is *pay for performance*.

In October 2006, CMS announced a new initiative to pay physicians for the quality of the care they provide to seniors and disabled beneficiaries with chronic conditions. The CMS administrator stated, "This is another step toward paying for what we really want: Better care at a lower cost, not simply the amount of care provided." This is presently being tested in four states with 26 quality measures related to the care of patients with diabetes, congestive heart failure, and coronary artery disease. The model will be for all health sectors with payment incentives in which the top 20% of performers for a measure will receive an extra 5% to 6% in reimbursement and the bottom 20% of performers for a measure will lose 5% to 6% in

reimbursement. As the program evolves, this author feels certain that chronic wounds will be included. Hence, it is imperative to develop skin and wound care algorithms that are evidence based and have proven efficacy and cost effectiveness.

The Centers for Medicare and Medicaid Services (CMS) establishes the Medicare program requirements. General provisions of the Social Security Act (SSA) govern Medicare reimbursement for all services.

- Section 1862(a) (1) (A) of the SSA states that no payment may be made for services that "are not reasonable and necessary for the diagnosis or treatment of illness or injury or to improve the functioning of a malformed body member."
- Section 1833 (e) requires that physicians furnish "such information as may be necessary in order to determine the amounts due" to receive Medicare payment.[15]

Over the past 3 years, there has been increasing scrutiny of the use of surgical débridement and active wound management CPT codes. The Office of Inspector General (OIG) report, "Medicare Payments for Surgical Debridements in 2004," has certainly brought the issue of documentation for débridement to the forefront:[16]

- 64% of surgical débridements did not meet the Medicare requirements.
- 39% of surgical débridements were miscoded.
- 29% of surgical débridements were insufficiently documented.
- 1% of surgical débridements were not medically necessary.

The report specifically speaks to the documentation of the depth of débridement. The report indicated that the "physician" used a code that did not accurately reflect the level of tissue, muscle, or bone removed during the débridement. The report went on to clarify that "physicians" frequently coded the level of débridement based on the depth of the wound, not the *extent of tissue removed*. Nurses, physicians, and therapists should include in their documentation

- type, location, and number of wounds,
- wound tissue characteristics,
- the extent of tissue débrided,
- wound measurements,
- indication of regular assessments of the wound, and
- time in/time out.

The OIG report recommended that physicians improve documentation in the medical record to adequately describe procedure(s) actually performed; improve their selection of surgical débridement, selective débridement, and nonselective débridement codes to match the actual work performed; and improve their knowledge of their Medicare contractor's local coverage determinations (LCDs) regarding débridement.

▶ **PEARL 33•7** Review all pertinent Medicare coverage policies and decisions.

Negative-pressure wound therapy is another therapeutic modality that has come under scrutiny of the OIG.[17] This report specifically speaks to the extent to which claims for negative pressure wound therapy devices met Medicare coverage criteria and supplier documentation requirements in 2004.

- Approximately 25% of all negative-pressure wound therapy device claims did not meet Medicare coverage criteria.
- Virtually all claims met supplier documentation requirements.
- For 44% of the claims, the information on the supplier-prepared statement was not fully supported in the medical record.

There was specific emphasis placed on the lack of documentation in the medical record citing type of wound, wound measurements, and treatments prior to negative-pressure wound therapy pump.

The OIG report recommended that CMS ensure claims for the negative-pressure wound therapy device meet Medicare coverage criteria and are paid appropriately. CMS should consider establishing advance coverage determinations of pump claims from suppliers with a high number of claims that have been denied or that have a pattern of overutilization. CMS should consider a face-to-face examination of the patient by the physician, and CMS should consider strengthening the coverage criteria for the pump and increasing prepayment reviews of these claims.

Coverage Decisions

The bulk of wound care treatment interventions do not have national coverage decisions (NCDs), but each payer/carrier has LCDs that clearly state the documentation requirements, such as the following:

- Type, location, and number of wound(s)
- History of wound
- Wound measurements
- Previous treatment regimens
- Indication of regular assessments of the wound
- Wound characteristics indicating healing

Various instructions for the documentation of wound care services can be located under the heading of "wound care." National coverage also clearly outlines documentation requirements. There are five NCDs related to treatment of chronic nonhealing wounds.

1. *Hyperbaric Oxygen Therapy for Hypoxic Wounds and Diabetic Wounds of the Lower Extremities (NCDM 20.29).* The evidence is adequate to conclude that hyperbaric oxygen (HBO) therapy is clinically effective and thus reasonable and necessary in the treatment of certain patients with limb-threatening diabetic wounds of the lower extremity. Medicare has issued a national coverage determination for HBO therapy in the treatment of diabetic wounds of the lower extremities in patients who meet each of the following criteria:
   - Patient has type 1 or 2 diabetes and has a lower-extremity wound that is due to diabetes;
   - Patient has a wound classified as Wagner grade 3 or higher; and
   - Patient has failed an adequate course of standard wound treatment.
2. *Electrostimulation for Wounds (NCDM 270.1.1).* Medicare allows for coverage for the use of electrical and electromagnetic stimulation for chronic stage III and stage IV pressure ulcers, arterial ulcers, diabetic ulcers, and venous ulcers. All other uses of electrical and electromagnetic stimulation for the treatment of wounds are not covered. Electrical stimulation and electromagnetic stimulation for the treatment of wounds will not be covered as an initial primary treatment modality.
3. *Treatment of Decubitus Ulcer (NCDM 270.4).* Hydrotherapy (whirlpool) treatment for decubitus ulcers is a covered service under Medicare for patients when treatment is reasonable and necessary. Some other methods of treating decubitus ulcers, the safety and effectiveness of which have not been established, are not covered under the Medicare program.
4. *Porcine Skin and Gradient Pressure Dressings (NCDM 270.5).* Porcine (pig) skin dressings are covered if reasonable and necessary for the individual patient as an occlusive dressing for burns, donor sites of a homograft, and decubiti and other ulcers.
5. *Pneumatic Compression Devices (NCDM 280.6).* Pneumatic compression devices are covered in the home setting for the treatment of chronic venous insufficiency of the lower extremity only if the patient has one or more venous stasis ulcer(s) that have failed to heal after a 6-month trial of conservative therapy directed by the treating physician. The trial of conservative therapy must include a compression bandage system or compression garment, appropriate dressings for the wound, exercise, and elevation of the limb.

There are two national noncoverage decisions for the treatment of chronic nonhealing wounds.

1. *Autologous Blood-Derived Products for Chronic Non-Healing Wounds (NCDM 270.3).* CMS has determined that the evidence is adequate to conclude that autologous platelet-derived growth factor (PDGF) in a platelet-poor plasma does not improve healing in chronic nonhealing cutaneous wounds and therefore is not reasonable and necessary.
2. *Non-Contact Normothermic Wound Therapy (NNWT) (NCDM 270.3).* There is insufficient scientific or clinical evidence to consider this device as reasonable and necessary for the treatment of wounds.

The NCDs clearly describe the criteria for use, as well as the documentation points required to justify continued treatment. Each and every policy states a decrease in wound size, surface area, or volume; decrease in exudate; and a decrease in necrotic tissue.

▶ **Case Study 33•1** | **Treatment Planning for a Patient with a Diabetic Foot Ulcer**

This 65-year-old man was evaluated by the hospital outpatient-based wound care center following a referral from his primary care physician. He presents with an ulcer on his right plantar-lateral foot, which has been present for the past 12 months. Over the past year, he has had multiple hospitalizations for urinary tract infections and wound infections. He is awaiting a pancreatic transplant, which has been placed on hold due to the open wound.

History Review

Past Medical History: The patient has type 1 diabetes mellitus with peripheral neuropathy, retinopathy, kidney transplant, mild hypertension.

Previous Level of Function: Patient is living alone with support from family and friends. He walks independently and was active in a seniors program at local athletic club.

Current Level of Function: The patient is independent in all ADL, has 100% functional mobility, and wears orthotics in shoes. Primary care physician has recommended complete non-weight-bearing on right lower extremity (LE), using crutches. He is restricted from working his part-time job.

Current Barriers to Function: He has normal ROM in all extremities, excepting bilateral heel cord tightness. Strength at ankle is 3/5 and at plantar flexors 2/5. Pain is 0/10 on the visual analog scale.

Wound Status: Length by width is 3.5 cm × 2.0 cm; depth is 0.2 cm; wound base is 30% yellow fibrin slough, 70% dusky pink; periwound is a 2-cm circumference of callus build-up with 3-cm area of blanchable redness medially; there is no odor; exudate is moderate, cloudy serous.

Diet: Patient has regular diet. Albumin is 3.0 g/dL and HgB A_{1c} 6.7.

Patient Goal

The goal is to return the patient to the active pancreatic transplant list, return to work without restrictions, return to program at the athletic club, and for there to be no need for family and friend support for doctor appointments and dressing changes.

Short-Term Goals (1 month):

1. Safe and independent ambulation with appropriate off-loading shoe or boot, using a single point cane.

2. Decrease the heel cord tightness bilaterally, increase plantar flexor strength to 3/5.
3. Free wound bed of all fibrin slough and decrease wound size by 25%.
4. Provide an exercise program for home without sheer stress on the plantar surface of right foot.

Long-Term Goals (12 weeks):

1. Safe and independent ambulation without assistive device, using orthotic and proper footwear.
2. A 100% closure of wound.
3. Education of foot care, daily examination and routine visits for shoe and orthotic examination.
4. Review appropriate exercise routine on a continuing basis.

Treatment Plan:

1. Moist heat to both calves followed by gentle heel cord stretches
2. Instruct on home exercise program to maintain cardiac exercise and improved dorsiflexion
3. Gait training with single point cane
4. Support boot (or total contact cast) to off-load the right lower extremity
5. Débridement of the callus and fibrin slough
6. Appropriate modalities to promote wound closure (electrical stimulation; low-frequency, noncontact ultrasound)
7. Alginate dressing for fluid absorption (after 2 weeks the wound was dressed with a thin foam dressing)

Outcome

The patient was discharged after 12 weeks with a completely closed wound with maturing scar tissue. He was walking independently, wearing his appropriate footwear at all times. He was back to being first on the pancreatic transplant list.

Functional Maintenance Program

His diabetes mellitus will be monitored monthly by his primary care physician, and he will return to the wound center monthly for foot and orthotic examinations. He has returned to work and the local athletic club as before his wound on the right lower extremity.

(Acknowledgments: Lisa A Barton, MMSc, PT)

Summary

Regardless of the method of documentation, paper or electronic medical record, documentation must be done in a timely manner on admission and at appropriate intervals throughout the treatment regimen. When multiple healthcare professionals are providing care, the documentation must reflect an integrated plan of treatment and must be accurate and consistent. Failure to provide consistent documentation will definitely result in difficulties. Documentation must not only match the service provided to the patient, but also the service billed. Complete and concise documentation facilitates communications between wound care team members and payers, thereby justifying reimbursement. In summary, see Table 33.5 for some dos and don'ts to remember in documentation.

> **PEARL 33•8** All health-care professionals' documentation must be consistent in the medical record in all treatment settings.

Table 33•5 Dos and Don'ts of Documentation

Do	Don't
Date and time all entries	Blame anyone
Use facts and measurements	Use nonstandard abbreviations
Note patient/family education, follow-up, and referral instructions	Obliterate any chart entries
Include all contacts, including phone calls, missed appointments	Make subjective statements about the patient
Limit use of abbreviations	
Note patient refusal, noncompliance with treatment	
Document what is required to demonstrate that the patient was properly cared for	
Correct chart errors appropriately	

References

1. Department of Health and Human Services (DHHS), Centers for Medicare and Medicaid Services (CMS): Outpatient Physical Therapy Manual. Baltimore, DHHS, 2004.
2. Guide to Physical Therapist Practice, 2nd edition, American Physical Therapy Association, Phys Ther. 2001 Jan; 81(1): 9–746.
3. Bergstrom, N, Allman, R, Alvarez, O, et al: Treatment of Pressure Ulcers. Clinical Practice Guideline. No 15. Rockville, MD, Agency for Health Care Policy and Research, 1994.
4. Braden, B, Bergstrom, N: Clinical utility of the Braden scale for predicting pressure sore risk. Decubitus 1989; 2(3):44–46, 50–51.
5. Norton, D, Exton Smith, AN, McLaren, R: An Investigation of Geriatric Nursing Problems in Hospitals. Edinburgh, McClaren Churchill Livingston, 1962.
6. Pressure Ulcer prevalence, cost and risk assessment: consensus development conference statement. Decubitus 1989; May; 2(2):24–28.
7. Wagner, FW: The dysvascular foot: A system for diagnosis and treatment. Foot Ankle 1981; 3:64.
8. Langemo, D, Anderson, J, Hanson. D, et al: Measuring wound length, width, and area: Which technique? Adv Skin Wound Care 2008; 21:42–45.
9. Bates-Jensen, BM, Vredevoe, DL, Brecht, ML: Validity and reliability of the pressure sore status tool. Decubitus 1992; Nov; 5(6):20–28.
10. Burrows, C, Miller, R, Townsend, D, et al: Best practice recommendations for the prevention and treatment of venous leg ulcer: Update 2006. Adv Skin Wound Care 2007; 20:11.
11. Healthcare Financing Administration (HCFA): Outpatient Physical Therapy and Comprehensive Rehabilitation Facility Manual, Sections 270–273. Baltimore, US Department of Health and Human Services, 1998.
12. American Medical Association (AMA): International Classification of Diseases, rev. 9. Clinical Modification, vol 1 and 2. Chicago, AMA, 2007.
13. American Medical Association (AMA): Physician Current Procedural Terminology, CPT 2007. AMA, Chicago, 2007.
14. American Medical Association (AMA): Healthcare Common Procedure Coding System, HCPCS 2007. Chicago, 2007.
15. Medicare law, §§ 42 CRF 411.15 and 424.5 (a) (6), 42 U.S.C. § 1395y (a)(1)(A); 42 U.S.C. § 1395l(e)
16. Levinson, D: Medicare Payments for Surgical Debridement Services in 2004. Washington, DC, Health and Human Services, OEI 02-05-00390, 2005.
17. Levinson, D: Medicare Payments for Negative Pressure Therapy Wound Pumps in 2004. Washington, DC, Health and Human Services, OEI 02-05-00370, 2007.
18. Hess, CT: Clinical Guide: Wound Care, ed. 5. Philadelphia, Lippincott Williams & Wilkins, 2005.
19. McGuckin, M, Stineman, MG, Goin, JE, et al: Venous Leg Ulcer Guideline. King of Prussia, PA, Health Management Publications, 1997.
20. Wagner, FW: The dysvascular foot: A system for diagnosis and treatment. Foot Ankle 1981; 3:64.

chapter 34

Developing a Clinical Wound Care Program

Stephanie Woelfel PT, MPT, CWS, FACCWS

Wound care programs are becoming more prevalent and may exist in a variety of health-care settings. In general, the program will either be inpatient based or outpatient based, thus serving two distinct patient populations, each with its own set of challenges.

In the inpatient setting, there really is no question as to whether to start a program. At the very least, a plan to *prevent* skin breakdown should be in place. In most facilities a formalized wound care program is also a necessity.

Outpatient wound care programs are not quite as clear-cut. Many factors need to be taken into account. These will be explored in more detail later in the chapter.

Inpatient Wound Care Program

Based on the type of inpatient facility, the extent of the wound care program may vary. For example, due to a shorter average length of stay, a short-term acute care program would usually be different from a program in an intensive care unit or a long-term acute care facility in which patients remain longer. The components listed in this chapter will illustrate a very comprehensive wound care program. The reader will need to identify the interventions most appropriate for the specific patient population to be served.

Team Members

Getting the right combination of health-care practitioners is vital to the success of any wound care program. Choose clinicians that have a passion for wound care and who want to be team players. Appointing someone to head a wound care program or to be a member of the wound team rarely works. A significant commitment needs to be made to properly managing patients with wounds as well as staying informed of the rapid changes occurring within this specialty. A clinician without the interest and drive to follow through in these areas can be a detriment to the program as a whole, and patient outcomes will likely suffer.

Likewise, wound management programs are not as successful when there is only one person who ostensibly "holds" the same knowledge as a transdisciplinary team. What happens during times that clinician is not available? No single person can be present 24 hours a day, 365 days a year. There needs to be a team approach so that patient care is consistent and thorough. Only a transdisciplinary team consisting of several practitioners with experience in specific areas of expertise can ensure that patient wound care is optimal.

What should be the makeup of this team of experts? Possible members include therapists (physical and/or occupational), dietitians, nurses, nursing assistants, orthotists/pedorthists, and podiatrists, as well as case managers, social workers, materials managers, and billing and coding specialists. In addition, there are a multitude of physicians that may be a part of the team. These may include infectious disease specialists, plastic surgeons, vascular surgeons, internal medicine physicians, dermatologists, hyperbaric medicine specialists, and physiatrists to name a few. The key is to pull as many of these players together as possible to create a true transdisciplinary team. Each team member will have his or her own focus in treating a patient with a wound. Taken collectively, these contributions will provide a comprehensive view of the issues present and will enhance patient care. (Fig. 34.1)

> ▶ **PEARL 34•1** A true "transdisciplinary" team is necessary for any wound care program to succeed.

Once the team has been assembled, it is important to delineate responsibilities and expectations for the different members. Who are core members of the team and who will be called in as consultants? How is the determination made to get a consultant on board? Who is responsible for the initial evaluation of the patient? These are just some of the questions that need to be answered for the process to flow smoothly and for the program to be a success.

The answers to some of these questions may be influenced by the reimbursement system used by the facility. Physical and occupational therapists working in inpatient facilities are able to bill CPT codes for evaluations and biophysical technologies used for wound care. Medicare patients in inpatient facilities are reimbursed on a diagnosis-related group (DRG) system. Based on the patient's diagnosis and specific comorbidities and complications, the facility is paid a certain amount to care for that patient and is responsible for managing the costs. If a patient is discharged outside the average length of stay for their DRG, they could fall into "short-stay" status (discharged early) or "outlier" status (discharged after their average length of stay). In either of these situations, actual charges billed to the patient become much more important. Thus, it may have been beneficial to have a therapist perform the initial wound evaluation and generate a charge for it.

Certain interventions performed by physicians and other qualified health care providers (ie, excisional débridement) can actually change the patient's DRG and affect reimbursement. For patients in need of débridement, this could be an additional consideration for requesting a surgical consultation.

In skilled nursing facilities where resource utilization group (RUG) categories are used for therapy services, one must be cognizant of the fact that wound care interventions performed by physical or occupational therapists count toward billable minutes. Based on the specific patient situation, this may or may not be desirable.

Reimbursement policies change on a consistent basis and are even more varied when commercial insurance carriers are brought into the mix. It is important to know which fiscal intermediary (FI) or Medicare Administrative Contractor (MAC) issues decisions for your facility and to make sure there is a team member responsible for monitoring this area of practice. This is especially important in light of recent pay for performance and "never events" initiatives. The reader may want to return to Chapter 33 for more detailed information on reimbursement.

Process Standardization

Once the team is in place and roles and responsibilities have been delineated, it is important to standardize the care that patients will be receiving. Standardization in this case does not mean a "cookbook" approach to treating patients with wounds. Clinicians experienced in the field of wound care know that not every stage III pressure ulcer can or *should* be treated in exactly the same way. Rather, the intent is to ensure that all areas affecting the treatment plan have been addressed while individualizing care for each patient.

> ▶ **PEARL 34•2** Standardizing wound program elements such as risk assessments, products, and treatments ensures a comprehensive approach that can be individualized for each patient.

Risk Assessments

The number and types of risk assessment each facility performs will be based largely on the patient population served. There are no specific risk assessment tools for diabetic foot ulcers, arterial insufficiency ulcers, or venous ulcers. Risk *factors* for each of these etiologies are well-defined in the literature, and facilities that deal with a large number of patients with these types of wound should consider creating an internal risk assessment tool to use.

Risk assessment tools for pressure ulcers (Braden scale, Norton scale, etc) are much more prevalent and widely available for use. The vast majority of inpatient wound healing programs will want one of these tools as a cornerstone of their program to help guide preventative measures as well as treatment interventions. Regardless of the tool used, remember that simply assigning a risk category is not enough. Once an at-risk patient is identified, the facility must be able to show what was done to mitigate that risk.[1]

To that end, algorithms can be very helpful. The clinician can follow the "yes/no" format through a series of pathways in order to decide exactly what interventions are the most appropriate for a given patient. The algorithm can delineate products and devices to be used, what team member is responsible for certain interventions, and even give cues for completion of

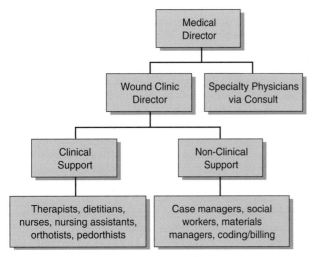

Figure 34•1 *Flow diagram of practitioners. An example of wound team members and their relationship to each other.*

documentation. This step-by-step process reduces the risk of vital information being overlooked. (Fig. 34.2)

Product Formularies and Vendor Selection

There are a plethora of wound care products and devices available on the market, with more being developed every day. At times it can be difficult for even a seasoned wound care clinician to be knowledgeable about all the different options. Developing a comprehensive product formulary is one way to strengthen the wound care team.

There are several benefits to instituting a product formulary:

- *It makes care delivery more consistent.* By limiting the number of products, staff become much more proficient at using what is available, and competence is easier to maintain.
- *It reduces costs.* Standardizing to one specific vendor or product line often results in price breaks or discounts.

When a formulary is promulgated across a corporation, volume discounts may be an added incentive.

- *It allows for easier training.* By choosing one particular vendor for wound or skin care products, one can capitalize on vendor-offered in-service training. Once a great team of clinicians has been assembled, their focus should primarily be evaluating and treating patients, not spending hours training support staff. Many vendors have dedicated staff that will take the time to educate these vital team members at no cost to the facility.

Even though product formularies can be extremely beneficial, one must take great care in deciding on a vendor. Many things must be taken into account, including the primary user of the products, the specific patient mix at the facility, and any group purchasing agreements in effect (especially regarding how much can be purchased "off contract"). A comprehensive product formulary will likely cover about 95% of a facility's needs, but

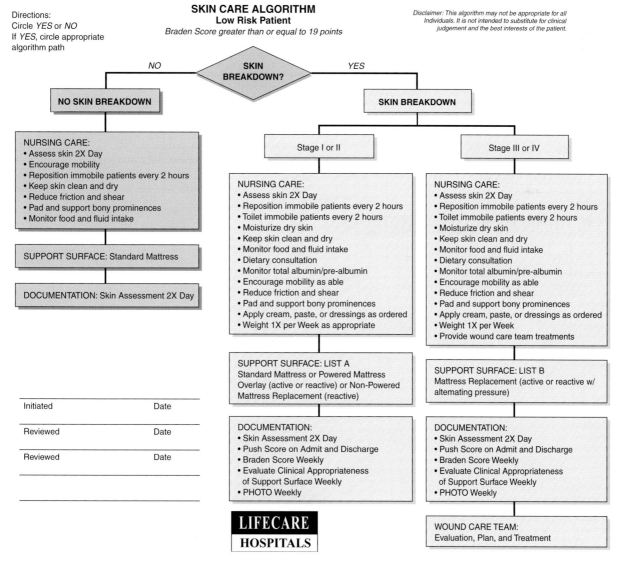

Figure 34•2 *Sample algorithm. Decision-making algorithm for prevention and treatment interventions based on the patient's risk for skin breakdown.*

there should be room to obtain specialty items from another vendor if a specific patient need calls for it. This process should also have its own set of guidelines. A product evaluation team can minimize duplication of products and ensure that there is a clinical need before a new product is added.

Minimally, a formulary should cover the basic dressing categories. These include gauze, impregnated gauze, transparent films, hydrocolloids, hydrogels, foams, alginates (or other absorbent dressing), enzymes, topical antibacterials, and adhesives (tape). Based on the type of patient treated and the different physician specialties involved on the team, different composite dressings, collagen, and biological dressings and skin substitutes may also be appropriate for inclusion.

Another pitfall to avoid in developing a product formulary is any practitioner bias that may exist. Often, team members have developed professional relationships with vendors over time. Formulary decisions should be made as objectively as possible. One way to achieve this goal is by using a quantitative analysis to compare vendors and products. Table 34.1 shows a sample quantitative analysis that may be used to compare two different bed frames.

Each quantitative analysis can be very different. The main stakeholders (typically core members of the wound care team with some administrative input) decide which key characteristics are most important based on what is being evaluated and the type of patients for which it will be used. In addition, they also decide how important each of these characteristics is in the big picture. In the example shown in Table 34.1, "ease of use" was very important (weight value of 20%), while "cost" was less important (weight value of 5%).

Another way to enhance objectivity in the process is to make sure that staff have received equal amounts of in-service training for each product (make sure vendors make themselves available for in-service training on all shifts) and that all products are evaluated for the same amount of time. Once the stakeholders have decided on the product characteristics to be used and their importance, the process is turned over to the end users for evaluation. "End user" does not refer just to other members of the wound care team. An end user is any person who has contact with the product. The bed frame example included end users such as nursing assistants, physicians, housekeeping staff, therapists, and even patients. Patient input can be vital in making some of these decisions, especially where comfort or pain reduction are key characteristics.

Once the end users have had the opportunity to work with the product and complete their evaluations, results can be combined and a decision made. The evaluations are completed by each staff member "scoring" the key characteristics on a 1-to-10 scale. This score is multiplied by the weighted value for that particular characteristic, and these points are then added for the total. Involving all levels of staff in this decision-making process can prove very beneficial. It allows for many different viewpoints regarding the same product and increases staff buy-in when the time comes to implement the new formulary. Since staff were involved in the process from the beginning, they already feel some sense of ownership and understand what was taken into consideration for the final decision. Additionally, some amount of in-service training will have been completed so the learning curve is significantly shorter.

When deciding on formularies, consider all areas of opportunity. Wound care dressings are just the beginning. Think about skin care products, ostomy products, support surfaces, negative pressure, ultrasound, electrical stimulation, Doppler devices, etc. Streamlining each of these areas greatly enhances the effectiveness of the wound program as a whole.

Treatment Algorithms

Just as algorithms were beneficial in standardizing interventions based on risk assessments, they can also be helpful in streamlining wound treatment options. An example of how this may be used in an inpatient setting would be for the wound care team to create treatment algorithms that could be easily implemented by the floor nursing staff. These algorithms can be especially valuable for wound issues that arise when the wound care team is not immediately available. It gives the point-of-care staff an appropriate course of action to initiate while also making sure that the wound care team is notified when the situation warrants. This "trigger" for notification of the wound care team is vital for patients who require more advanced interventions. (Box 34.1) (Fig. 34.3)

Treatment algorithms are appropriate for any type of wound that the facility deals with, from severe pressure ulcers to skin tears to moisture-associated skin damage. In addition to assisting floor staff in making appropriate clinical decisions, treatment algorithms can also help to identify opportunities for improvement. For example, the initial algorithm for stage III pressure ulcers calls for filling the dead space with a gauze dressing. It was noted that all patients with stage III pressure ulcers were having an issue with periwound maceration. One would conclude that a more absorbent dressing was needed, and the treatment algorithm could be changed to reflect this.

Table 34•1 Bed Frame Qualitative Analysis

Key Quality Characteristics	Weight Value	Score (1–10)	Points
Ease of use	20%		
Brake function	15%		
Scale accuracy/ repeatability	15%		
Hoyer lift fits easily under bed	5%		
Ease of patient positioning	10%		
Ease in maneuvering bed	5%		
Fail safety	5%		
Bed exit system	10%		
Cost	5%		
Warranty	10%		
Total			

▶ **Box 34•1** | **Sample Wound Care Algorithm for Stage III Pressure Ulcers**

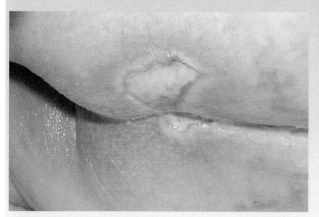

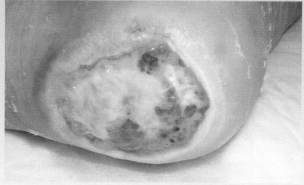

Definition:

The wound shows full-thickness tissue loss. Subcutaneous fat may be visible, but bone, tendon, or muscle is not exposed. Slough may be present but does not obscure the depth of tissue loss. The pressure ulcer may include undermining and tunneling. The depth of a stage III pressure ulcer varies by anatomical location.

- *No* use of hydrogen peroxide or Betadine® in open areas
- Inform attending physician of assessment findings and plan of care
- Hydrogel per formulary = Saf-Gel®
- Appropriate "absorbent dressings" per formulary = Aquacel® or Kaltostat®

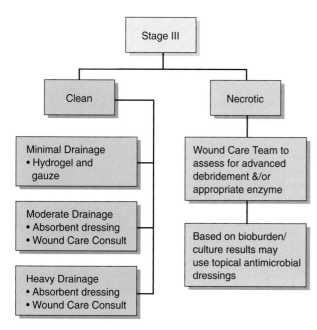

Figure **34•3** *Example of a wound care algorithm for stage III pressure ulcers.*

Another instance in which the consistency of treatment algorithms is beneficial is in the case of a patient with an uncommon wound issue. If a proven treatment algorithm is in place and a patient's wound is not healing as expected, it leads the clinician to explore other variables that might be playing a role. Is there a bioburden issue that needs to be addressed? Did the initial evaluation properly identify wound etiology? Should a biopsy be performed?

As long as a strong product formulary is in place, it is acceptable to have a treatment algorithm that is fairly generic (ie, makes use of dressing categories rather than brand names). This allows the treatment algorithm to remain functional even if product lines or dressing names change. It also prevents the treatment algorithm from becoming too prescriptive. The algorithms are meant to guide patient care, not substitute for good clinical judgment. There will be certain patient scenarios that will deviate from what is standard, and the treatment algorithm should be flexible enough to allow for those cases. It is important that treatment algorithms be reviewed on a regular basis (most facilities will require an annual review by the medical executive committee). This helps to ensure that the current practice of the facility is reflected in the treatment algorithms and allows for regular updates based on new literature and research.

Remember to explore a broader view when thinking about how to use treatment algorithms. In the field of wound care, algorithms for dressings are a clear option, but what about other aspects of care for the patient with wounds? A good example of this would be therapy implications for patients with wounds. Algorithms could easily be created for biophysical technologies to be used with certain wound types, positioning interventions, compensatory and strengthening strategies based on the muscle(s) impacted in a stage IV wound, and lower-extremity therapeutic exercise for patients with arterial or venous insufficiency wounds.[2,3] Although these interventions do not always address the wound bed itself, they positively impact the healing process. This approach capitalizes on the strengths of the different team members and looks at the entire patient, not just the wound itself.

Evaluation and Assessments

Depending on the members of the wound care team, the person primarily in charge of wound evaluation and assessment may change. The reimbursement topics related to this have already been discussed in Chapter 33. The type of wound being assessed may also play a part in deciding which team member is primarily responsible. A patient who presents with denuded and excoriated skin surrounding a stoma site may be best assessed by a wound ostomy continence nurse (WOCN). The patient with a stage IV ischial ulcer and noted contractures may be more appropriate for a physical therapist, certified wound specialist (CWS) to evaluate. The patient who enters the facility emergently with suspected necrotizing fasciitis would be best evaluated by a surgeon.

The same facility may have different disciplines acting as the primary wound team member based on the unit a patient is on or the type of wound the patient presents. Regardless, it is important to clearly define responsibilities and the time frame in which evaluation is to occur. It is also essential to define when reassessments are to occur and who is the responsible party. A strong wound care team is one that is proactive in managing patients and identifying changes in their condition. State and federal guidelines often drive these timelines.

Support Surfaces

Another core piece of a good wound care program is appropriate use of support surfaces. Similar to wound dressings, the world of support surfaces can be difficult to navigate. The National Pressure Ulcer Advisory Panel (NPUAP) has made some significant strides in making this an easier task for clinicians with their Support Surface Initiative.[4] As described in Chapter 19, all major vendors have adopted a common vocabulary related to support surfaces. It makes it much easier to compare products from different vendors and understand the features offered by various surfaces.

Support surfaces have come a long way in the past few years and now offer many options to enhance patient care. Despite this, there is still a key point for all wound team members to recall at all times: no surface replaces the need for patient repositioning! Moving the immobile patient still needs to be a core component of any successful wound care program, and it is one that relies most heavily on support staff, not necessarily the wound care team itself.

It is important to have a continuum of support surfaces available to patients. This is another area in which individualizing the care for each patient is very important. Two patients with almost identical wounds may present very differently. Where an alternating pressure surface may be appropriate for one, the other may benefit more from an air-fluidized surface. Developing a formulary and usage algorithm related to support surfaces can improve patient outcomes as well as significantly reduce costs.[5]

This is also an area for which reassessment time frames should be defined. As a patient's wound(s) heal, he or she may no longer need the air-fluidized bed that makes movement and transfers very difficult. Perhaps after the first week in the facility the patient could be transitioned to a low-air-loss surface, which enables him or her to move more independently in bed and work more easily with the physical therapist. Just as the wound itself is assessed on a regular basis, the support surface should be addressed to see that all the patient's needs are being optimally met.

Patient Safety

All health-care providers integrate safety measures into their daily interactions with patients. The array of devices and biophysical technologies used in the treatment of patients with wounds requires a more formalized approach to patient safety. Using spreadsheets or tables to track necessary interventions increases the likelihood that they will be performed in a timely manner.

Devices that are rented or leased may have preventative maintenance performed by the vendor, but it is important to clarify this from the beginning. The safety of any owned electrical equipment must be checked by biomedical services at least annually and more often if there is a concern with how the piece of equipment is functioning. Equipment such as sterilizers for débridement instruments typically have daily, weekly, biannual, and annual safety checks that must be performed. These will be specified by the manufacturer. Refrigerators that house skin substitutes or medications must have the temperature checked daily. Records of this monitoring and any interventions performed should be maintained in an easily accessible location. State and federal surveyors will often ask to see these documents.

In addition to device safety, there should also be a formal plan in place for safety associated with dressings and treatment algorithms. A policy should be in place to define how new products will be introduced or selected. This ensures that the proper clinicians are involved in evaluating products before they are used with patients. Treatment algorithms should be reviewed by the medical staff annually at a minimum to make sure they still reflect current best practice.

Wound Care Team Meetings

The strengths of a transdisciplinary team are easy to recognize, but these strengths can quickly become weaknesses if there is no regular communication between team members. The surgeon needs to know what supplements the dietitian recommends to elevate the patient's protein stores prior to surgery. The physical therapist needs to know what activities the surgeon wants to limit so that the flap incision heals properly. The links between wound care team members are almost endless and with strong communication are almost seamless. All team members work toward the same goal(s) for the patient but often use very different methods to get there.

Most wound team members see each other in passing throughout the day and discuss different patients as the need arises. However, there is still a place for a more formalized exchange of ideas between members. Perhaps one team member has picked up on a change the others haven't observed, or someone has just attended a conference and has a new intervention to share with the group. A scheduled meeting, whether weekly or monthly, helps facilitate open conversation about patients and also fosters a culture of communication that carries over into the daily routine.

These team meetings are also an excellent place to discuss trends that have arisen and what, if any, action needs to be taken in response. A *root cause analysis* is an excellent way to formally assess trends and identify the details. If there was a positive trend in healing of moisture-associated skin damage this month versus last month, was anything done differently? Was there a new support surface purchased or a new barrier cream used? If a specific cause can be pinpointed, is there any way to expand that good outcome to more patients? On the other hand, if there was a negative trend in increased nosocomial pressure ulcers compared to the previous month, the underlying cause must be identified. Did staffing levels change during that time? Was there an additional trend in the location of these pressure ulcers? Is a new pressure off-loading boot needed to protect patient's heels? Were any of these wounds potentially present earlier as stage I or deep tissue injury but overlooked? This in-depth inspection and discussion about both positive and negative outcomes is essential to the continued growth of any wound care program and will be especially important as reimbursement for performance initiatives expand.

Wound team meetings may also bring forward ideas for new research. The focus throughout health care is on evidence-based practice, and wound care is an area in need of additional data. Trends that are noticed in one facility may pertain to a more global patient population, and sharing these ideas can impact quality of care as well as reimbursement.

Patients and Caregivers as Team Members

The roles and responsibilities of the clinical and professional team members have been discussed at length, but what about patients and their caregivers? They are team members with an important role to play as well. They need to understand what is happening to them medically and physiologically, and it is the responsibility of the wound care team to see that this happens.

▶ **PEARL 34•3** Patients and caregivers are integral members of the wound care team.

Each patient and caregiver will have a different comfort level as it relates to information about wounds. There will also be differences in the way people learn best about their situation. The wound team members need to be sensitive to these individual preferences and adjust the information delivery accordingly. The important thing is that the patient and caregiver is involved in the patient's care and that they understand their responsibilities. Perhaps this responsibility is allowing the staff to help the caregiver turn the patient every 2 hours even though it feels disruptive or following through on elevating the legs when the patient is sitting up in a chair. In some situations the responsibilities are even more involved as patients or caregivers may need to perform actual dressing changes in order for a patient to return home.

Implementing the Inpatient Wound Care Program

Once the wound care team members have been selected and the framework for the program has been solidified, there is still the task of fully implementing the program and making it functional. This is often the most difficult task of all and one that needs to be approached with a significant amount of patience. At times it may be helpful to phase in certain parts of the program one aspect at a time. Perhaps a facility deals mostly with pressure ulcers, and that portion of the program is implemented first. National agencies have resources to help facilities introduce new programs like this piece by piece.[6]

At this phase in the process, the wound care team members themselves need to be the champions of the new program and help the support staff understand their very important roles in the success of the program. Cooperation of the facility administration is paramount at this time because there is a need for significant time and energy to be spent in educating staff about their new responsibilities. There also needs to be a substantial amount of time dedicated to auditing and re-education as the program continues to roll out. Often when programs fail, it is because there were not enough resources set aside for tracking compliance after the initial implementation.

There needs to be a clear and consistent message sent to all staff involved. It should be clear to them that in the new program, these are the roles within it, and everyone will be held responsible to perform these tasks from this point forward. It is not uncommon for there to be some resistance to change initially, but offering feedback—both on opportunities for improvement and on successes—will keep the program moving forward and make the transition easier.

Tracking Outcomes

Once a wound care program is in place, there needs to be a way to assess the success of the program. As discussed earlier, looking for and assessing trends within the facility is one way to internally monitor the program. There are also methods available that allow for benchmarking against other similar facilities in the area, region, and country.

Formalized outcomes tools are available, such as the Pressure Ulcer Scale for Healing (PUSH) tool for pressure ulcers and the Bates-Jensen Wound Assessment Tool (BWAT), which can assess wounds of various etiologies.[7,8] Many vendors now offer prevalence and incidence studies that can assist a facility in benchmarking not only against other like facilities, but also against itself from year to year. State and federal agencies may require facilities to track their wound infections or nosocomial pressure ulcers. Beyond that, there are limitless possibilities for tracking outcomes based on the specific patients a facility treats. Outcomes may also be reflected in wound volume measurements from admission to discharge, time to healing, and number of times a patient receives a specific treatment intervention.

The key to outcomes tracking is to pick indicators that are meaningful for the patient population being seen. Tracking data for data's sake does not often translate into improving outcomes for patients. When the data collected have a real application to those being treated, that data can help drive practice and be used to market the strengths and unique characteristics of the program.

▶ **PEARL 34•4** Outcomes tracking needs to contribute to a bigger picture—think process improvement.

Outpatient Wound Care Program

Patient treatment components of an outpatient wound care program will be fairly similar to that of its inpatient counterpart. Pulling the right team of clinicians together remains extremely important, and the same opportunities for standardization exist. Outpatient reimbursement and marketing have their own unique challenges and will be explored below. An overview of the challenges and general work flow involved in new construction will also be discussed.

Market Assessment

There are several factors that need to be considered as part of a comprehensive market analysis for an outpatient wound care program. The potential patients are just one small piece. One must also take into account physicians (as a source of referrals), managed care companies, and third-party payer systems, as well as regulating bodies.[9] All interact and have effects on the ultimate feasibility of the program.

Investigate the demographics of the program area. An area with a large Native American and Hispanic population would probably be very well served by a limb salvage center or a diabetic foot clinic as there is a high prevalence of diabetes among both of these groups. An area in which the primary occupations are factory or machine work may have a higher incidence of crush or traumatic injuries.

Have the core physicians that are part of the wound care program network with their peers. This is important not only in generating referrals to the program, but also in recruiting additional specialists who may be needed at some point. Consultants are much easier to find in an inpatient setting where they are already on staff. An outpatient program requires an in-depth assessment of the types of interventions to be performed and negotiation of specialist contracts based on the findings. Is there a plastic surgeon as a core member of the outpatient wound care team who plans on performing extensive wound débridements on-site? If so, has a contract been obtained for anesthesiology services?

Become very familiar with the FI or MAC and any managed care companies in the area. Most managed care companies require providers to be in-network before they will reimburse for services. These contracts should be negotiated well in advance of opening an outpatient clinic to ensure a sufficient revenue stream to maintain operations. One of the team members should register to receive regulatory updates so the program stays current with any reimbursement changes. These changes pertain not only to specific billing codes or physician fees, but also to products and supplies themselves. This can be a full-time job itself, and it is one that requires expertise in the area of billing and reimbursement. Some programs find it easier to outsource this piece to an experienced vendor.

It is also vital to have someone very familiar with the state and federal guidelines that govern outpatient services. Requirements will vary if you have an outpatient wound care program that offers hyperbaric oxygen services or surgical services as part of the treatment continuum. Knowledge of the regulations will not only impact reimbursement once the program is up and running, but can also affect the speed with which state inspections are passed during the construction process.

Services to Be Offered

Once a comprehensive market assessment has been done and the decision has been made to move forward with building an outpatient wound program, the scope of services needs to be defined. There are numerous biophysical technologies and adjunctive treatments that can be used to treat all types of wounds and any number of specialties that could be involved. The information gathered from the market analysis should help narrow down the scope of these services. Offering too narrow a scope could limit opportunities to capture patients, whereas too broad a scope could lead to a program that is mediocre at just about everything, but truly excels at nothing.

> **▶ PEARL 34•5** An objective assessment of the market and scope of services must be completed before moving forward with an outpatient wound care program.

A helpful tool in making some of these decisions is a SWOT analysis. SWOT is an acronym for *strengths, weaknesses, opportunities,* and *threats.* Strengths and weaknesses in this model are attributes internal to the program, whereas opportunities and threats are external factors that also need to be considered. To truly appreciate the full benefit of such an exercise, the analysis must be done with complete honesty and without bias. The hope is that this evaluation leads to an *informed* decision about program viability. If threats that are present can be turned into opportunities, the program has a strong likelihood of success. If the weaknesses or threats present are insurmountable, the entire program can be re-evaluated before huge expenses have been incurred.[10] Table 34.2 gives a sample SWOT analysis as it may relate to beginning an outpatient wound program. In this example one of the threats present is the fact that there are two other programs in the vicinity that already offer hyperbaric services. This could be handled in one of two ways, depending on the specifics of the program. Perhaps the decision is made that the new program will not offer hyperbaric services, so there is no competition for that specific patient population. Or, the decision may be made that the strength of the physician and transdisciplinary team makes the new program much more comprehensive than either of the competitors, and the program proceeds as planned.

Project Management

The following portion of this chapter assumes creation of a new outpatient wound program and will discuss construction details to consider. Due to all of the variables involved, it is not possible to discuss every possible scenario. Key questions are raised for the reader to consider. Once the market assessment and SWOT analysis confirm a sound foundation for an outpatient wound program, build-out or conversion of the clinic space begins. There are three important overall concepts to consider for adequate management of the project: time, cost, and resource availability.[10]

Table 34•2 Sample SWOT Analysis

Strengths	Weaknesses	Opportunities	Threats
Corporate backing for build-out of new clinic space	No experience with outpatient billing requirements	Only program in the area with a fully transdisciplinary team	Two other programs in 15-mile radius with hyperbaric chambers
Dedicated wound care and hyperbaric physician to staff clinic 5 days a week	Currently no physician contract in place for vascular surgeons	Recent acquisition of a fourth generation ultrasonic débridement device (only one in a 100-mile radius)	Current managed care contract with insurance company X does not cover outpatient services.
Wound care–trained physical therapist, nurse, and lymphedema therapist already on staff			

SWOT, strengths, weaknesses, opportunities, and threats.

Time

There are a multitude of tasks that need to be completed when redesigning a space or beginning new construction. Many of these tasks are interdependent, and the sequence in which these tasks are performed is just as important as the task itself. Many of these timing issues are handled by the architecture firm and general contractor involved, but the clinicians need to be included in every step of the process to ensure a final product that meets the patient-care needs of the program.

It is helpful for all involved to create a Gantt chart to illustrate the timeline of the project and ensure that clinician input is solicited early enough for it to be included in the plans. The Gantt chart in Table 34.3 gives an example of different tasks involved in construction of a new clinic. For actual use this Gantt chart would be much more detailed and often cover several pages. At each point in the process, clinician input is necessary. Even if the architect and contractor are familiar with health-care construction, the clinicians are the experts in what will occur in the clinic on a daily basis.

Cost

Before any project can really get off the ground, a budget needs to be in place. For the outpatient wound care program, this may be driven by a corporate office or by clinicians who have entered into a business agreement to finance the project. Regardless, there are several variables to be considered. What is the initial capital available for the project? This will determine how much of the necessary equipment is acquired via capital purchase versus an operating purchase once the clinic has opened. It may also impact how much equipment is purchased outright and how much is leased. Leasing allows equipment acquisition early in the process with less up-front cost. The drawback is that the monthly payments of a lease need to be subtracted from monthly revenue. This impacts the bottom line of the program.

Resource Availability

Resources for this type of project include not only money, but also equipment, space, people, etc. From a cost-containment standpoint, only personnel vital to the planning process should be on payroll from the start. Some of the key members

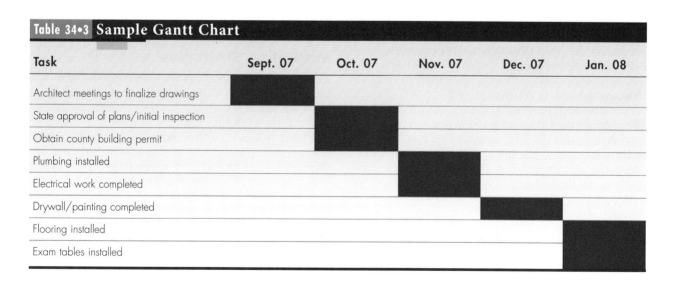

Table 34•3 Sample Gantt Chart

Task	Sept. 07	Oct. 07	Nov. 07	Dec. 07	Jan. 08
Architect meetings to finalize drawings	■				
State approval of plans/initial inspection		■			
Obtain county building permit		■			
Plumbing installed			■		
Electrical work completed			■		
Drywall/painting completed				■	
Flooring installed					■
Exam tables installed					■

may even be willing to act as consultants until the program is open and they are needed full time for patient care. Look for creative ways to control costs. Take advantage of available group purchasing agreements for equipment, and negotiate with vendors for unique lease or rental arrangements.

Project Meetings

Architect meetings are the first step in the process. The initial meeting typically includes the key clinicians involved in the process and representatives from the architecture firm. Likely, there will be many clinicians with ideas for the project, but in the interest of decision making and time management, four to five key members should be selected to attend these meetings and communicate information back and forth. At this meeting there is a lot of discussion about how the space needs to be used: how many treatment rooms, what will be in each of them, how big a waiting area is needed, etc. Right from the start, preferred equipment becomes very important. The architects prefer to get as many "cut-sheets" as possible for the equipment going into the space. Cut-sheets are vendor-provided specifications with space and power requirements, if applicable. Submitting these early helps avoid issues later in the process, such as the examination table selected not fitting in the desired space and an alternative having to be ordered.

At the next meeting, the architects will come back with floor plan options for the space based on the initial discussions. At this point it is still relatively easy to make changes. Clinicians should now assess the proposed layout with regard to patient and clinician flow. Is there easy access for patients to enter the clinic? Does the entrance location make sense, or are patients walking through treatment areas to get to their destination? These are concerns that may or may not have been addressed in the drawings.

Once the final floor plan has been determined there is typically another meeting with the architects and some of the subcontractors for the project, specifically those dealing with electrical, plumbing, information systems, and interiors. Again, clinician input is vital to the eventual function of the space. The electrical contractor will want input on the number and type of power outlets. Where should the outlets be located? How many outlets need to be supplied by emergency power? They also need to know about lighting for the different areas of the clinic. Does there need to be specific "exam" lights in any of the rooms? The clinicians need to be very comfortable with how they will be using the space to make sure these questions can be answered properly.

The other contractors will function in much the same way. The plumbers need to know where sinks are to be placed and what size they are to be. Information systems contractors need to know how many phone and data lines are needed and where they are to be installed. This is a good time to take a step back and think about the big picture. If the ultimate goal for the program is to have an electronic medical record, even though it will not be in place upon opening, a plan for this must be made during initial construction. It is much more cost effective to have additional data lines dropped before any drywall is in place rather than after the building is completed. Interior designers are concerned with the aesthetics of the space. Paint colors, flooring, and room furniture need to be discussed. Areas that will be exposed to bodily fluids on a regular basis may be better served from an infection-control standpoint by having sheet vinyl flooring rather than composite tile flooring.

Following this meeting the architect typically issues another set of plans with all contractor details specified for approval. These plans should be carefully studied. Once they are approved and sent to the state for review, any changes affect the timeline of the project and result in change costs from the architect. The amount of time the state has to review and approve these plans varies, as will the requirements for county and city approval. The state will send an inspector to the site. The outcome of this site inspection determines how quickly an actual building permit can be obtained and true construction can begin.

It is important for clinicians, or at the minimum, the project manager for the outpatient wound program to inspect construction on a regular basis. Often there may be many different architect plans issued before the final version, and it is much easier to have a given contractor correct oversights right away. This construction phase is also the ideal time to ensure that the inner workings of the program are in place. Policies and procedures should be developed and approved, product formularies established, and algorithms for patient care formalized.

As construction nears completion, the state inspector will again visit the site and determine occupancy. Once occupancy is obtained, staff can begin to inhabit the space. This means that offices can be moved into and equipment training can begin. This is an ideal time to have vendors train staff on the use of and preventative maintenance necessary for all equipment. A biomedical testing service needs to certify safety of all electrical equipment before it can be used on patients. During this occupancy phase, all staff need to become experts of the life safety codes associated with the new space. This includes smoke compartments, evacuation routes, and emergency procedures. When the state inspector returns for final inspection, staff will be questioned about the actions they need to take in these situations. This plays a large role in when the clinic opens to patients.

Marketing Strategies

As the outpatient wound care program is gearing up to take patients and the final touches are being made, a strong marketing push to raise awareness and generate referrals is necessary. It is hoped that the clinicians involved in the program have been networking with peers and vendors on an ongoing basis during the project. The demographic research that was done initially and the services the program provides can help target additional promotion of the program.

There are four components to consider when deciding on a promotional mix. They are advertising, personal selling, sales promotion, and public relations. Advertising can occur in a variety of different media types, from billboards to newspapers to television. The cost of these different options needs to be considered as well as which medium will effectively capture the target audience. Personal selling helps to make one-on-one contact with potential patients or referral sources, but it tends to be much more expensive as a result. This can be an effective strategy but needs to be balanced with some of the more cost-effective marketing strategies. Sales promotion also tends to be fairly expensive. This strategy would include purchasing space in a vendor hall during a national conference and having staff available to answer questions and recruit. Public relations typically involves some form of community involvement. A common example of this would be a "grand opening" event for the new outpatient wound care program. The guest list should include potential referral sources, potential payers, and community leaders. This is a great opportunity to showcase the program and the clinicians involved. It may also lead to additional public relations opportunities that will help raise awareness of the new program. Perhaps there are volunteer activities available in the community in which staff members could be involved.[9]

One of the most effective marketing strategies is one that is very hard for the program itself to control: positive patient experience. Patients who have a good experience or achieve a good outcome will spread that news to family, friends, and their regular physicians. All of these contacts can open new referral streams. The power of this type of marketing should not be underestimated, especially because a negative experience has an equal ability to decrease referrals.

There will always be some patients who are not able to realize the outcome that the wound program staff or the patient hoped for. The key to mitigating the negative response often goes back to communicating with patients on a regular basis and involving them in their own care. If patients have been active participants in their care from the beginning and understand the multitude of interventions that were attempted, they are more likely to understand an outcome that differs from the initial plan.

Summary

From clinical aspects to the business aspects, there are a multitude of processes to consider when developing a wound care program. Both inpatient and outpatient programs have unique challenges, but there is significant overlap as well. The main goal of a wound care program is to provide excellent care with excellent outcomes to patients with wounds. Establishing the right processes and having the right clinicians in place can help attain that goal for those involved in the program and their patients.

▶ **Case Study 34•1** ▏ **Planning a Wound Care Team**

History

A rural community hospital wants to develop a more comprehensive inpatient wound program. Currently, there is one physical therapist and one nurse with wound care experience on staff. The two are located on different floors and rarely see each other during the workday. Care delivered by the floor staff varies, depending on who is working that day. Last month 10 nosocomial pressure ulcers were reported in the facility.

Team Members

Assuming the physical therapist and nurse that currently have wound experience are interested, they could be the cornerstones of the team to be developed. Other team members to be recruited include physicians (someone to head the team, as well as consultants), dietitians, staff nurses, nursing assistants, orthotists, pedorthists, podiatrists, case managers, social workers, reimbursement specialists, pharmacists, and materials managers. The roles need to be delineated for each of these new members. If the staff nurses will be expected to perform daily dressing changes, they will need continuing education to ensure they are competent in carrying out these duties.

Process Standardization and Outcomes Tracking

The team needs to choose a risk assessment appropriate for the patient population, educate staff on how to use it, and then make sure every patient's risk is assessed on a regular basis. Based on that assessment, further prevention/treatment interventions will be initiated.

The team needs to decide which vendors and products they will use for dressing supplies, topical treatments, and support surfaces. Once these decision have been objectively made, further education on the chosen products should be implemented.

The wound team should decide which basic treatment options will be offered and put a process in place for consulting the wound team further if the interventions fail to show improvement. Patient progress should be continually monitored and treatments adjusted as needed. Wound team meetings may be a good place to discuss specific patient cases and problem-solve when obstacles are present.

References

1. Lyder, C, van-Rijswijk, L: Pressure ulcer prevention and care: Preventing and managing pressure ulcers in long-term care: An overview of the revised federal regulation. Ostomy Wound Manage 2005; 4(suppl):1–19.

2. Sanderson, B, Askew, C, Stewart, I, et al: Short-term effects of cycle and treadmill training on exercise tolerance in peripheral arterial disease. J Vasc Surg 2006; 44:119–127.

3. Yang, D, Vandongen, YK, Stacey MC, et al: Effect of exercise on calf muscle pump function in patients with chronic venous disease. Br J Surg 1999; 86:338–341.

4. National Pressure Ulcer Advisory Panel Website. Available at: http://www.npuap.org/s3i.htm. Accessed 10/15/07.

5. Healthcare Purchasing News Website. Available at: http://www.hpnonline.com/inside/2006-07/HPNonline.com%20-%20 what%20works%20-%20kaleida%20-%200607.html. Accessed 10/15/07.

6. Institute for Healthcare Improvement Website. Available at: http://www.ihi.org/IHI/Programs/Campaign/PressureUlcers.html. Accessed 10/15/07.

7. National Pressure Ulcer Advisory Panel Website. Available at: http://www.npuap.org/PDF/push3.pdf. Accessed 10/15/07.

8. Borun Center for Gerontological Research Website. Available at: http://www. borun.medsch.ucla.edu/modules/Pressure_ulcer_prevention/puBWAT.pdf. Accessed 10/15/07.

9. Kovacek, PR: Business Skills in Physical Therapy: Strategic Marketing. American Physical Therapy Association, Alexandria, VA, 2003, pp 15, 52.

10. Hack, L, Hillyer, RW, Kovacek, PR, et al: Business Skills in Physical Therapy: Defining Your Business. American Physical Therapy Association, Alexandria, VA, 2003, pp 25–27.

chapter 35

Legal Concepts and Their Impact on Health-Care Providers

Joyce Stamp Lilly, RN, JD, PC

Introduction

This chapter is meant to be a practical guide for health-care providers who may be unfamiliar with our civil legal system and its terminology, structure, and procedures. Practitioners should always be aware that their practice involves legal issues and that the delivery of appropriate health care and sound medical treatment that meets the standard of care are goals to strive for not only for the patient, but for each practitioner who may at some point be forced to look back at and justify judgments, decisions, and interventions.

This book contains discussion and current peer reviewed references that encourage and mandate appropriate evaluation, interventions, and treatment of wounds, both acute and chronic. While no one decision or intervention may be absolute or correct, what is offered in this text is information and knowledge that affords practitioners the ability to use this information in scientifically acceptable ways to deliver the best care and treatment possible under the various and uncountable circumstances that exist in health care today.

The standard of care for all areas of health-care delivery is developed from many sources, including clinical practice guidelines that may be published by various specialties,[1,1a] policies and procedures developed by health-care providers or specialty groups, peer-reviewed literature, and sometimes

case law. Health-care providers should be held to the standard of care by those within the health-care delivery system as well as the general public. The issues to be determined in medical negligence legal cases are the duty to the patient and the standard of care, if it has been violated, and if that violation has caused particular damages to the complaining party or parties.

This chapter will look at general legal concepts and terms that apply to civil litigation, specifically medical negligence, with a goal of assisting those who deliver care to understand how the system works and how their behavior and care management can impact not only the physical, mental, and social outcome for the patient and family, but also upon issues that may be litigated if persons or agencies are involved in a lawsuit.

Civil Law and Health-Care Providers

This section will familiarize health-care providers with general legal concepts and terms. The law is ever changing and, like medicine, is not exact. Lawyers are advocates and are trained to argue various sides of issues depending on circumstances. Often, there is no clear-cut correct answer, only shades of gray.

Advocacy skills, knowledge of human behavior, and how the "system" works are often the keys to victory when issues present themselves in a legal atmosphere.

Medical Negligence

Medical negligence law has, in the past 5 to 10 years, swung on the pendulum of change to its current state of extreme conservatism in many states. Tort reform has brought changes to the medical negligence arena, some onerous and resulting in many persons, often the elderly and disabled, having no legal redress for damages suffered. The National Association of Mutual Insurance Companies published a study documenting that as of 2004, 23 states had enacted laws affecting noneconomic damages,[2,3] a calculation usually left to the province of juries, a power most often given to them by the respective state constitutions. A May 17, 2005, study conducted by the Economic Policy Institute claims that the tort crisis was overblown[4] and was based on figures that had no relation to the legal system.[5] With whichever side of the tort reform equation one is aligned, the reality is that today there are far fewer lawsuits involving medical negligence. The reasons are many, including increased expense of pursuing the cases, more conservative jury pools, and, perhaps most significant, caps on noneconomic damages often limiting recovery to $250,000 for a person who may have no economic losses such as wage loss or future medical expenses.[6] While this amount of money may seem large at first glance, one must realize that these cases take years to resolve, costing tens of thousands of dollars for experts, discovery, medical records, and court appearances, all costs that are not recoverable as damages.

Definitions

Plaintiff

The plaintiff is the person or entity that has suffered damages as a result of another's (the defendant) negligent act or failure to act. A lawsuit can have one plaintiff or many; a plaintiff may be a business entity or a person. The plaintiff hires an attorney to represent him or her in going forward with the lawsuit. Personal injury plaintiff attorneys usually represent plaintiff/clients under a power of attorney agreement that provides for a contingency fee arrangement. This arrangement means that, generally, the client pays no expenses for the prosecution of the lawsuit, the attorney supports the case financially and receives no compensation or expense reimbursement unless and until the case is resolved, either by settlement prior to trial or at the trial level, or beyond if the case is appealed. After the case is resolved, and if monies are collected on behalf of the client, the attorney will collect a fee that was indicated in the power of attorney agreement that was signed at the outset by the client and attorney. The attorney's expenses will also be reimbursed from the proceeds. Additionally, medical expenses may have to be reimbursed to third-party payers and must be reimbursed to Medicare and Medicaid, again from the proceeds of the settlement or jury trial.

Negligence

Negligence in the broadest sense is doing something that a reasonable person would not do under the same or similar circumstances or not doing something that a reasonable person would do under the same or similar circumstances. Negligent acts are not intentional. In a medical negligence case, the reasonable person standard usually is defined in terms of the behavior of a like-qualified medical care provider, for example, a reasonable nurse, a reasonable physical therapist, a reasonable orthopedic surgeon.

Burden of Proof

In all lawsuits, the moving party, or the party bringing the action, must prove certain elements of the case to the judge or jury, also called the fact finder. In a civil case, as opposed to a criminal case, the complaining party must prove by what is usually defined as a "preponderance of the evidence" that a particular thing occurred. Unlike criminal cases where the burden for the prosecutor is "beyond a reasonable doubt," the burden in a civil case is less, also defined as "more likely than not," or more than 50%. There may be doubt in a civil case, but the evidence presented should lead the jury to conclude that the weight of the evidence points to victory for the complaining party, or, conversely, to the other side if the burden is not met by the complaining party. It is important to understand that the defendant does not have to prove anything; he or she has no burden to prove anything to anyone.

Standard of Care

How practitioners of similar specialties would have managed the patient's care under the same or similar circumstances is referred to as the standard of care. The burden of proof is on the complaining party, the plaintiff, to establish with reasonable medical probability that the defendant(s) failed to meet the appropriate standard of care. The plaintiff must also demonstrate that the standard of care was breached or violated and resulted in harm or damages to the plaintiff. To be successful in this goal, the plaintiff must have expert testimony from a health-care practitioner in the same or similar specialty. States may vary in the requirements for experts. Generally, the expert should be of the same type of specialty so that there will be no challenge to his or her qualifications or testimony. For example, if the defendant is a family practitioner, the expert should also be in that area of medicine, or if the defendant is a radiologist, the expert must be a radiologist in order to comment convincingly on the actions of the radiologist's practice.

Duty

Health-care providers have a duty to provide health care within the standard of care to patients. This duty, or responsibility, is a concept found in all realms of life. Police have a duty to protect the public, accountants have a duty to clients to practice their specialty in compliance with certain standard accounting practices, nurses have a duty to their patients to practice within the rules and regulations of their respective nursing practice acts and other standards that may apply.

Defendant

The defendant is the party in the lawsuit who allegedly caused the plaintiff harm, resulting in damages. There can be one or many defendants in any one lawsuit. In medical negligence claims, the defendant usually has liability insurance, and the insurance company hires the defense lawyer to represent the defendant. Depending upon the circumstances, the defendant may wish to hire his or her own personal attorney to oversee the case and to attend various hearings or depositions. Often, some defendants will be included in a suit initially and be dismissed in the future once more facts are uncovered, shedding light on those who are liable for the damages to the plaintiff.

Damages

Damages may be economic, such as lost wages, loss of particular services, or medical or living expenses incurred in the past or to be incurred in the future as a result of the alleged negligent act. Noneconomic damages are intangible, such as loss of enjoyment of life, pain and suffering, loss of consortium, and disfigurement. Damages may be computed from the date of the alleged negligent act into the future.

Depending on the statutory or case law of the particular state, damages may be found to be above and beyond those stemming from general negligence. The behavior causing these damages is often defined as intentional, malicious, or in reckless disregard of the plaintiff's safety or rights. In these instances, the damages may rise to what is referred to as gross or punitive damages and are calculated by the judge or jury above and beyond those compensatory damages or general negligence damages. Punitive damages are meant to punish the defendant(s) and to deter similar behavior in the future.

Statute of Limitations

Every state has a statute of limitations that essentially closes off the possibility of filing a lawsuit for particular acts after a certain amount of time has passed. Most states have a 2- or 3-year time period during which the potential plaintiff must file his or her lawsuit or be forever barred from doing so.[7]

In some states there is a legal concept called the discovery rule, which generally tolls or postpones the statute of limitations from running until the plaintiff discovers the harm. This allows a plaintiff additional time if the problem could not have been discovered during the statutory time period. The discovery rule has been eliminated by statute or recent case law, eliminating this opportunity to extend the statutory time period in certain states. Many argue that this results in giving protection to those who can hide the wrongful act and thus avoid liability.

Discovery

Discovery is a formal process by which the attorneys for the parties gather information to be used as evidence in preparation for eventual trial. The purpose of discovery is to allow each side to gather evidence that may be used by the other side so that they may prepare responsive evidence. Discovery includes interrogatories, requests for production, requests for admissions, depositions, and, depending on the state civil procedure rules, may include other procedures.

Interrogatories

Written questions submitted by the attorneys from both sides to the opposing party are referred to as interrogatories. Interrogatories are to be answered by the respective clients within a set time period, usually 30 days or longer by agreement. Frequently, parties receive these requests from the attorneys and are confused by the myriad of questions that often seem irrelevant, elementary, or not in any way pertinent to the claims brought or defenses made. Attorneys should always let clients know that they will work with them in answering these discovery requests and that the final product will be sent from the attorney's office after reviewing the answers as they pertain to the civil procedure requirements of the particular state. Often there are objections that will be filed by the attorneys for particular questions that, in the opinion of the attorney, do not have to be answered. The opposing lawyers will then either agree or will have to file motions and responses and go to court to argue their respective opinions to the judge who will decide whether the interrogatory will be answered or if the question may be limited in some way.

Requests for Production

Requests for production are also written requests sent by attorneys for the parties to the opposing parties. These requests ask for items to be produced within a set time period. Documents or items requested may be medical records, billing records, correspondence, statements, expert opinions, references used in formulating any expert opinions, medical equipment, and many other items that any attorney representing any party in the case may believe is pertinent to the issues being brought forward. As with interrogatories, any attorney may have objections to producing or answering a particular request and may advise the client that a particular thing does not have to be produced. The issue will have to be agreed to among the attorneys, or again, the attorneys will be obliged to file motions and responses and appear in court so that the judge may intervene.

Requests for Admissions

Requests for admissions are written statements sent by an attorney to the other side that the answering party must admit or deny as being true. For example, "Admit or deny that Northwest Health Concepts is a health-care facility that offers hyperbaric oxygen therapy to patients." Again, objections may be made to particular requests using the same process as noted above for interrogatories or requests for production.

Deposition

The out-of-court sworn testimony of a person who may be a party, either plaintiff or defendant, an expert, or a fact witness, is called a deposition. The deposition of a party, plaintiff or defendant, is usually taken at the office of the attorney who represents the person being deposed, referred to as the deponent. Frequently, if the deposition is for fact witnesses employed by a health-care facility, the deposition will be held at the health-care facility for the convenience of the deponents. The attorneys for both parties attend the deposition, and the parties are all allowed but not obligated to attend any deposition in the case. The nonparty deponent is allowed to have his or her own attorney attend if they have hired one. Other persons present at a deposition will be a court reporter to record the testimony, a videographer if the deposition is to be videoed, and other persons, if the parties' attorneys agree beforehand.

Mediation

Mediation is a process that is used in almost all cases today in an effort to allow the parties to settle their differences before going to trial. The mediator is usually an attorney or former judge with experience in civil litigation who functions as an impartial intermediary with no alliances to either party. Generally, mediation takes place after discovery has been completed or nearly completed. The lawyers prepare a mediation statement setting out the case facts, the status of discovery, the issues remaining to be decided, and the demands and counteroffers, if any. The parties attend mediation, usually after mutually agreeing upon a mediator, although sometimes he or she may be appointed by the court. Anything that occurs in mediation is confidential and cannot be used outside the mediation process.

Mediation can take anywhere from half a day to many days or weeks, depending on the complexity of the case and the parties involved. The mediator meets with all of the parties, the lawyers, and anyone who has responsibility for the monies that may be necessary to settle the dispute. Usually, the mediator makes a statement to the group as a whole, explaining the process and how the day will proceed. The respective sides may proceed to different rooms, and the mediator will go from room to room delivering messages, discussing the issues, case law, potential jury reaction to the case, and any other issues that are relevant in attempts to have the sides compromise and come to an agreement.

The mediator's goal is to educate the parties about the process as a whole. The mediator will discuss the issues and how a jury in a particular venue is likely to view the evidence. He or she will discuss recent, similar cases that may have been decided by a jury; the mediator may have knowledge of a particular judge and how trials proceed in that court. They will ask questions about the evidence from the perspective of one who has not "lived with" the case and who has no emotional attachment to the arguments.

The mediator stresses that, with mediation, the parties have some control over the outcome of the case, as opposed to appearing at a trial where there is no control. Once the jury is seated, the trial begins; the parties sit and listen, hoping that their lawyer can show the jury the error of the other side's ways and ultimately find for their side.

▶ Case Study 35•1[8] ▐ Hospital Cannot Escape Liability Even When the Basics Are Ignored

James Doe was a 37-year-old single male with spina bifida who was admitted to Houston East Lake Hospital with end-stage renal failure and pneumonia on August 30, 1996. Mr. Doe's history included multiple orthopedic surgeries, neurogenic bladder with self catheterization, pyelonephritis, cholecystitis, and diabetes. On admission he was vomiting blood, noted to have pulmonary edema, and was diaphoretic, lethargic, and pale. He had an elevated white blood count (WBC) and was anemic. He was intubated on admission and started on dopamine and dialysis. Although paraplegic, Mr. Doe had no history of pressure ulcers despite being wheelchair bound for 17 years prior to admission. Despite his presentation, the admission nursing assessment done on the intensive care unit (ICU) completed by a licensed vocational nurse (LVN) noted that his physical condition was good, his nutritional status was good, and this same nurse also noted that he had strong movement to his lower extremities.

Mr. Doe was noted to be at high risk for pressure ulcers, yet, despite the hospital policy of RN assessment on admission and daily (Fig. 35.1) mandatory consultation with the Skin Resource Team (Fig. 35.2) when a person at high risk is admitted to the hospital, no assessment was done by an RN, no consultation was called, and no evidence of any orders for particular intervention for skin care is found in the record until September 26, 1996, 4 weeks following admission.

The admission assessment documented that his lower extremities displayed positive and strong reflexes and strength. (Fig. 35.3) This assessment of strength in the lower extremities was repeated by various staff for the first 5 days of admission. On September 1, Mr. Doe was restrained due to agitation. Rashes were noted by nursing to be "all over back" on September 3, four days after admission, yet there was no call to the physician or the Skin Resource Team. By September 6, he was noted to be itching and scratching, and a sacral skin tear was noted; Duoderm was placed. By September 7 he was noted to be confused, agitated, and was placed in wrist restraints; he extubated himself and was reintubated. The initial wound care flow sheet was initiated on September 6 (Fig. 35.4), however, no call was made to the Skin Resource Team.

There was a notation by a nurse that the Duoderm was changed on the coccyx on September 9, 1996, but no additional notation as to the location, size, appearance, drainage, etc was made. No call was made to the Skin Resource Team and no notation was made with regard to reporting this skin breakdown to a charge nurse or nurse manager. The dressing was changed on September 11, 1996, and the area was noted to be "raw"; however, once again, no call to either the skin team, the physician, or nurse manager was documented. Finally, on September 15, 1996, at 4:10 a.m., a nurse notes that Mr. Doe's "sacral area . . . draining on draw sheet." When the Duoderm was removed, she documented the wound as being 8 cm by 3 cm in size. At this time, the nurse noted that the wound had "worsened"; however, no call was made at this time to the skin team, the physician, or any charge nurse or unit manager. The next day, the sacral area was noted to have slough tissue and inflammation; however, the nurse noted that it was "improved." Despite the appearance of slough tissue, once again there was no call to any of the persons, who, according to the policy and procedures at Houston East Lake, would be more knowledgeable about pressure ulcers.

▶ **Case Study 35•1[8]** **Hospital Cannot Escape Liability Even When the Basics Are Ignored—cont'd**

The wound progressed to a much larger size, although the measurements were inconsistent, transitioning from inches to centimeters without explanation. (Figs. 35.5, 35.6). The care plan (Fig. 35.7) noted for the first time the presence of a skin problem on September 22, 1996, more than 3 weeks following admission and more than 2 weeks after the first notation of a skin tear.

Finally, on September 19, 1996, a nurse changed the dressing and noted that she soaked 4 × 4s and covered it with ABD pad (there was no order for this particular treatment). At that time, the attending physician, Dr. Holly, ordered a consultation with Dr. Monte, a plastic surgeon. This order was given as a verbal order from Dr. Holly to the nurse, and Dr. Holly at the same time ordered moist saline dressing to the site twice daily.

Nursing Service
POLICY/PROCEDURE

Effective Date: 8/96
Supersedes: new
Page 1 of 9

TITLE: SKIN/WOUND MANAGEMENT

PURPOSE: To provide a standard guideline for the prevention and management of alterations in skin integrity.

TYPE: Independent

RELATED TO: "Documentation on the Patient Admission Assessment/Discharge Record"

REPLACES: "Pressure Ulcer Record"

RULES:

1. The patient's risk for alteration in skin integrity is assessed by an RN on admission and at least every 24 hours during hospital stay.

2. A numerical score according to the Admission Skin Risk Data Collection Guidelines (Addendum A) will be assigned on Admission and daily thereafter.

3. If patient is at risk (numerical score of 10 or above), the Guidelines for Skin Care (Addendum A and B) will be initiated.

4. Wound Measurement
   a) There will be separate measuring device used for each wound. The same measuring device is never used on more than one patient.
   b) The measuring device is cleaned with alcohol swab after use and stored in a small plastic bag marked with the location of the wound (e.g., "sacrum, " "Left heel,". etc.) and patient's name.

5. Wound Documentation Record:
   a) A Wound Documentation Record (Addendum B) will be initiated by the licensed nurse who first identifies an alteration in skin integrity.
   b) There will be one Wound Documentation Record completed for each wound present in order to mark progression of wound.

Figure 35•1 *The East Lake policy clearly calls for RN assessment of skin integrity on admission and at least every 24 hours.*

Continued

▶ **Case Study 35•1⁸** | **Hospital Cannot Escape Liability Even When the Basics Are Ignored—cont'd**

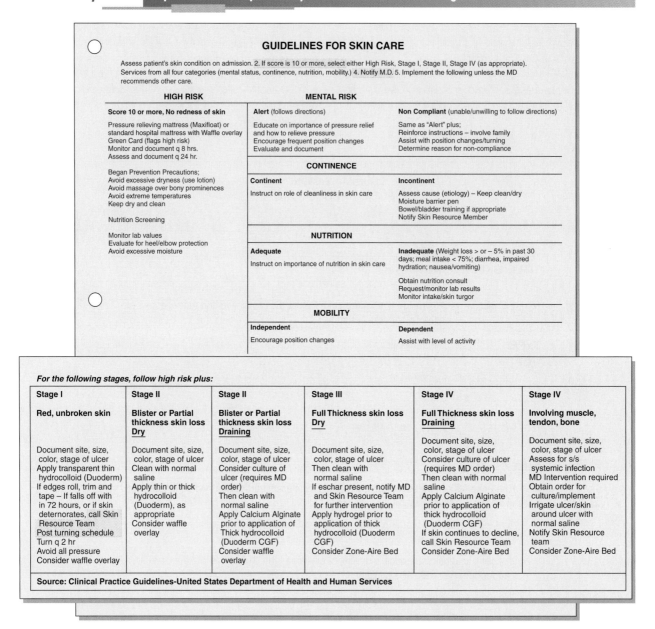

GUIDELINES FOR SKIN CARE

Assess patient's skin condition on admission. 2. If score is 10 or more, select either High Risk, Stage I, Stage II, Stage IV (as appropriate). Services from all four categories (mental status, continence, nutrition, mobility.) 4. Notify M.D. 5. Implement the following unless the MD recommends other care.

HIGH RISK	MENTAL RISK	
Score 10 or more, No redness of skin	**Alert** (follows directions)	**Non Compliant** (unable/unwilling to follow directions)
Pressure relieving mattress (Maxifloat) or standard hospital mattress with Waffle overlay Green Card (flags high risk) Monitor and document q 8 hrs. Assess and document q 24 hr.	Educate on importance of pressure relief and how to relieve pressure Encourage frequent position changes Evaluate and document	Same as "Alert" plus; Reinforce instructions – involve family Assist with position changes/turning Determine reason for non-compliance
Began Prevention Precautions; Avoid excessive dryness (use lotion) Avoid massage over bony prominences Avoid extreme temperatures Keep dry and clean	**CONTINENCE**	
	Continent	**Incontinent**
Nutrition Screening	Instruct on role of cleanliness in skin care	Assess cause (etiology) – Keep clean/dry Moisture barrier pen Bowel/bladder training if appropriate Notify Skin Resource Member
Monitor lab values Evaluate for heel/elbow protection Avoid excessive moisture	**NUTRITION**	
	Adequate	**Inadequate** (Weight loss > or – 5% in past 30 days; meal intake < 75%; diarrhea, impaired hydration; nausea/vomiting)
	Instruct on importance of nutrition in skin care	Obtain nutrition consult Request/monitor lab results Monitor intake/skin turgor
	MOBILITY	
	Independent	**Dependent**
	Encourage position changes	Assist with level of activity

For the following stages, follow high risk plus:

Stage I	Stage II	Stage II	Stage III	Stage IV	Stage IV
Red, unbroken skin	**Blister or Partial thickness skin loss Dry**	**Blister or Partial thickness skin loss Draining**	**Full Thickness skin loss Dry**	**Full Thickness skin loss Draining**	**Involving muscle, tendon, bone**
Document site, size, color, stage of ulcer Apply transparent thin hydrocolloid (Duoderm) If edges roll, trim and tape – If falls off with in 72 hours, or if skin deternorates, call Skin Resource Team Post turning schedule Turn q 2 hr Avoid all pressure Consider waffle overlay	Document site, size, color, stage of ulcer Clean with normal saline Apply thin or thick hydrocolloid (Duoderm), as appropriate Consider waffle overlay	Document site, size, color, stage of ulcer Consider culture of ulcer (requires MD order) Then clean with normal saline Apply Calcium Alginate prior to application of Thick hydrocolloid (Duoderm CGF) Consider waffle overlay	Document site, size, color, stage of ulcer Then clean with normal saline If eschar present, notify MD and Skin Resource Team for further intervention Apply hydrogel prior to application of thick hydrocolloid (Duoderm CGF) Consider Zone-Aire Bed	Document site, size, color, stage of ulcer Consider culture of ulcer (requires MD order) Then clean with normal saline Apply Calcium Alginate prior to application of thick hydrocolloid (Duoderm CGF) If skin continues to decline, call Skin Resource Team Consider Zone-Aire Bed	Document site, size, color, stage of ulcer Assess for s/s systemic infection MD Intervention required Obtain order for culture/implement Irrigate ulcer/skin around ulcer with normal saline Notify Skin Resource team Consider Zone-Aire Bed

Source: Clinical Practice Guidelines-United States Department of Health and Human Services

Figure 35•2 *Upon notation of high risk for a Stage I pressure ulcer, the policy calls for consultation with the Skin Resource Team and other interventions.*

Dr. Monte did not see Mr. Doe until 4 days later, on September 23, 1996. At that time he noted that the pressure area was "contaminated with feces." He noted that the right and left heel had some redness with blisters that had ruptured, and he noted that Mr. Doe had an additional ulcer on his left hip, which had not been noted by nursing staff. Dr. Monte noted that the pressure ulcer had developed during Mr. Doe's time on the intensive care unit. At that time Dr. Monte ordered an airflow bed, heel protectors, turning of the patient right to left to decrease pressure on the sacrum,

and additionally asked the staff to "maintain the area free of feces."

Dr. Monte débrided the wound on September 25, 1996. He noted that the wound "was going very close to the anus, and there was full-thickness of the skin with necrosis." At that time the wound was documented by nursing as a stage III with no tunneling or undermining, no drainage, and no depth. (Fig. 35.5)

Mr. Doe eventually developed two stage IV necrotic ulcers on his sacrum and hip and required flap surgery. He was transferred to a rehabilitation hospital in January of 1997 and went

▶ **Case Study 35•1**[8] **Hospital Cannot Escape Liability Even When the Basics Are Ignored—cont'd**

DATE: 8/31/96	CODES	+ = PRESENT 0 = ABSENT – = REFER TO NARRATIVE NOTES	EDEMA SCALE	PUPILS: = Reactive = Sluggish = Non-reactive	PUPILS 2 3 4 5 6 7 8 9

		TIME	23	24	01	02	03	04	05	06	07	08	09	10	11	12	13	14	15	16	17	18	19	20	21	22	GLASGOW COMA SCALE
NEUROLOGICAL		INITIALS	JR		JR		JR		JR			JR		JR		JR		JR		JR		JR		JR		JR	GCS RECORD BEST RESPON
	GCS	EYES	4		4		4		4			4		4		4		4		4		4		4		4	EYES OPEN 4 Spontaneously 3 To verbal common 2 To pain 1 No response
		MOTOR	6		6		6		6			6		6		6		6		6		6		6		6	BEST MOTOR RESPON 6 Obeys 5 Locates pain
		VERBAL	ETT		ETT		ETT		ETT			ETT		ETT		ETT		ETT		ETT		ETT		ETT		ETT	4 Flexion – withdraw 3 Flexion to pain
	PUPILS SIZE REACTION	R	+									2+		+2				+2		2+		2+		2+		2+	2 Extension to pain 1 No response
		L	+									2+		+2				+2		2+		2+		2+		2+	BEST VERBAL RESPON 5 ?
	EXTREMITIES	RU	+	+	+	+						+		+		+		+		+		+		+		+	4 Disoriented 3 Inappropriate work
		RL	+	+	+	+						+		+		+		+		+		+		+		+	
		LU	+	+	+	+						+		+		+		+		+		+		+		+	
		LL	+	+	+	+						+		+		+		+		+		+		+		+	

DATE: 8/31/96	CODES	+ = PRESENT 0 = ABSENT – = REFER TO NARRATIVE NOTES	EDEMA SCALE	PUPILS: = Reactive = Sluggish = Non-reactive	PUPILS 2 3 4 5 6 7 8 9

		TIME	23	24	01	02	03	04	05	06	07	08	09	10	11	12	13	14	15	16	17	18	19	20	21	22	GLASGOW COMA SCALE
NEUROLOGICAL		INITIALS	JR		JR		JR		JR			JR		JR		JR		JR		JR		JR		JR		JR	GCS RECORD BEST RESPON
	GCS	EYES	4		4		4		4			4		4		4		4		4		4		4		4	EYES OPEN 4 Spontaneously 3 To verbal common 2 To pain 1 No response
		MOTOR	6		6		6		6			6		6		6		6		6		6		6		6	BEST MOTOR RESPON 6 Obeys 5 Locates pain
		VERBAL	ETT		ETT		ETT		ETT			ETT		ETT		ETT		ETT		ETT		ETT		ETT		ETT	4 Flexion – withdraw 3 Flexion to pain
	PUPILS SIZE REACTION	R	+									2+		+2				+2		2+		2+		2+		2+	2 Extension to pain 1 No response
		L	+									2+		+2				+2		2+		2+		2+		2+	BEST VERBAL RESPON 5 ?
	EXTREMITIES	RU	+	+	+	+						+		+		+		+		+		+		+		+	4 Disoriented 3 Inappropriate work
		RL	+	+	+	+						+		+		+		+		+		+		+		+	
		LU	+	+	+	+						+		+		+		+		+		+		+		+	
		LL	+	+	+	+						+		+		+		+		+		+		+		+	

Figure 35•3 *Admission assessment to ICU completed by LVN. (Note: Documentation of strong lower extremities for the first 5 days following admission.)*

home in March with a release to return to work. Although he had worked full time for many years in a sedentary position, he was not able to return to work because he was unable to sit for any length of time. He lost his job and was not able to find other employment.

This case was filed in 1997, and discovery was undertaken, experts retained, depositions taken of plaintiff and many nurses, administrators of the hospital, Dr. Holly, and other doctors involved in Mr. Doe's treatment. The plaintiff had eight experts, some of whom were from outside Texas, and defense had seven experts, all from Houston. This case finally went to mediation and was settled in 2001, 5 years after the initial hospitalization. As a result of the settlement, Mr. Doe was able to have an income for his costs of living, make some changes to his home environment, purchase some items that made his life more comfortable, and secure a van with the necessary equipment that allowed him to drive. Mr. Doe died of complications of kidney disease in 2003.

A medical chronology is included in this chapter to allow for a detailed review of systems failures and how attorneys may document care rendered and persons involved with the care

and treatment. Specific examples of medical record documentation are illustrated in Figures 35.1 through Figure 35.7.

Medical Summary on James Doe—Houston East Lake

Name: Doe, James

DOB: 9/14/58

Social: Smoking history: (96: 3HEL-226, 297)* 2 packs/ cigarettes a day (3HEL-297); Secular: *; Phone dispatcher: (97: 3HEL-3)

Significant medical history: Cholecystitis: (96: 3HEL-226, 228)
Diabetes (3HEL-304)
Neurogenic bladder (96: 3HEL-59, 70, 226)
Pneumonia (96: 3HEL-59)
Pyelonephritis (96: 3HEL-226, 228)
Spina bifida (96: 3HEL-59, 70)
Urinary tract infections, recurrent/cystitis (96: 3HEL-59, 226, 228)
Significant surgical history: Multiple orthopedic surgeries (96: 3HEL-59)

Continued

▸ **Case Study 35•1**[8] **Hospital Cannot Escape Liability Even When the Basics Are Ignored—cont'd**

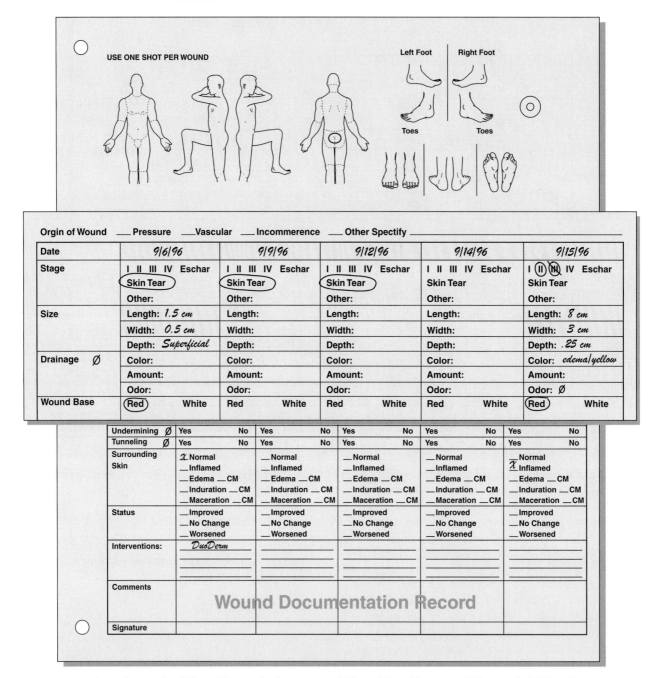

Figure **35•4** *According to Guidelines (Fig. 35.2), physician and Wound Care Team should be notified. Note: Progression in size of ulcer from 9/6/96 to 9/15/96.*

‣ **Case Study 35•1**[8] **Hospital Cannot Escape Liability Even When the Basics Are Ignored—cont'd**

USE ONE SHOT PER WOUND

Left Foot   Right Foot

Toes   Toes

Orgin of Wound ✓ Pressure ___ Vascular ___ Incommerence ___ Other Specifty_____

Date	9/25/96	9/25/96	9/26/96	9/26/96	9/27/96
Stage	I II (III) IV Eschar Skin Tear Other:	I II III IV Eschar Skin Tear Other:	I II (III) IV Eschar Skin Tear Other:	I II III IV Eschar Skin Tear Other:	I II (III) IV Eschar Skin Tear Other:
Size	Length: 10" Width: 6.5" Depth:	Length: 10" Width: 6.5" Depth: *Green*	Length: 10" Width: 6.5" Depth:	Length: Width: Depth:	Length: Width: Depth:
Drainage	Color: *Green* Amount: *Small* Odor: Ø	Color: Amount: *Mod* Odor:	Color: *Greenish* Amount: *Mod* Odor:	Color: Amount: Odor:	Color: Amount: Odor:
Wound Base	Red White Yellow (Black)	Red White Yellow (Black)	Red White Yellow (Black)	Red White Yellow Black	Red White Yellow (Black)
Necrosis	(Eschar) Slough	Eschar Slough	(Eschar) Slough	Eschar Slough	(Eschar) Slough
Granulation	Yes (No)	Yes No	Yes (No)	Yes No	Yes (No)
Undermining	Yes (No)	Yes No	Yes (No)	Yes No	Yes (No)
Tunneling	Yes (No)	Yes No	Yes (No)	Yes No	Yes (No)
Surrounding Skin	___Normal _X_Inflamed ___Edema ___CM ___Induration ___CM ___Maceration ___CM	___Normal _X_Inflamed ___Edema ___CM ___Induration ___CM ___Maceration ___CM	___Normal _X_Inflamed ___Edema ___CM ___Induration ___CM ___Maceration ___CM	___Normal ___Inflamed ___Edema ___CM ___Induration ___CM ___Maceration ___CM	___Normal _X_Inflamed ___Edema ___CM ___Induration ___CM ___Maceration ___CM
Status	___Improved ___No Change ___Worsened	___Improved ___No Change ___Worsened	___Improved ___No Change ___Worsened	___Improved ___No Change ___Worsened	___Improved ___No Change ___Worsened
Interventions:	*Change dressing.* *q4h. NS 4 x 4* *Turn q2h*	*Dressing NS 4 x 4*	*Turn of 2h* *Dressing x2* *NS 4 x 4*		*Duo Derm*
Comments					
Signature					

Figure 35•5 *Note progression of pressure ulcer to 10 inches by 6.5 inches.*

Continued

▸ Case Study 35•1[8] Hospital Cannot Escape Liability Even When the Basics Are Ignored—cont'd

USE ONE SHOT PER WOUND

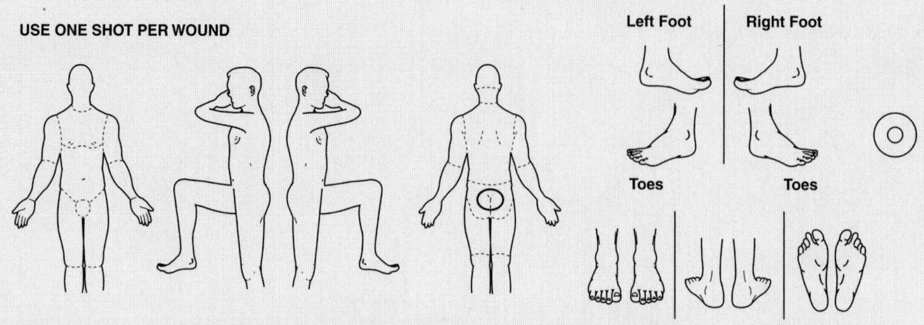

Left Foot Right Foot

Toes Toes

Orgin of Wound ___ Pressure ___ Vascular ___ Incommerence ___ Other Specityt _____

Date	9/28/96	9/29/96	9/29/96 gb 7-3	9/29/96 (3-11)	9/29/96 (4-7)
Stage	I II III (IV) Eschar Skin Tear Other:	I II III IV Eschar Skin Tear Other:	I II III (IV) Eschar Skin Tear Other:	I II III (IV) Eschar Skin Tear Other:	I II III (IV) Eschar Skin Tear Other:
Size	Length:	Length:	Length: 10 cm	Length: 10 cm	Length: 10 cm
	Width:	Width:	Width: 12 cm	Width: 12 cm	Width: 12 cm
	Depth:	Depth:	Depth: 10 cm	Depth: 10 cm	Depth: 10 cm
Drainage	Color: Yellow/green	Color:	Color:	Color: White/black	Color:
	Amount:	Amount:	Amount:	Amount:	Amount:
	Odor:	Odor:	Odor: Yes	Odor:	Odor:
Wound Base	Red White	Red White	Red White	Red (White)	Red (White)
	Yellow Black	Yellow Black	Yellow (Black)	Yellow (Black)	Yellow (Black)
Necrosis	(Eschar) Slough	Eschar Slough	(Eschar) Slough	Eschar (Slough)	Eschar (Slough)
Granulation	(Yes) No	Yes No	Yes No	Yes (No)	Yes (No)
Undermining	Yes (No)	Yes No	Yes No	Yes (No)	Yes (No)
Tunneling	Yes (No)	Yes No	Yes No	Yes (No)	Yes (No)
Surrounding Skin	__Normal __Inflamed __Edema __CM __Induration __CM X Maceration __CM	__Normal __Inflamed __Edema __CM __Induration __CM __Maceration __CM	__Normal __Inflamed __Edema __CM __Induration __CM X Maceration __CM	__Normal __Inflamed __Edema __CM __Induration __CM X Maceration __CM	__Normal __Inflamed __Edema __CM __Induration __CM X Maceration __CM
Status	__Improved X No Change __Worsened	__Improved __No Change __Worsened	__Improved X No Change __Worsened	__Improved X No Change __Worsened	__Improved X No Change __Worsened
Interventions:				W/D dress with NS and Santyl ointment	
Comments		Duo Derm in piecce			
Signature					

Figure 35•6 *Note documentation of infant Duoderm that measurements have changed from inches to centimeters and stage has changed from III to IV.*

▸ **Case Study 35•1**[8] **Hospital Cannot Escape Liability Even When the Basics Are Ignored—cont'd**

Patient Name _____ Patient Number _____ Date _____

PLANNING

__ Patient __ Family __ Significant Other __ None, involved in Assessment/Planning Process

Admission Assessment **NOTE:** _*Admitted via stretcher from ER, alert, oriented, follows commands, intubated,*_
*skin warm and moist*

Assessment Completed by Surgeon _____ *(LPN)* _____ R.N. Time/Date _____

DATE INITIATED	NURSES INITIALS	PROBLEM	DESCRIPTION	RELATED OR DUE TO	DATE RESOLVED	NURSES INITIALS
8/30/96	JA	2.1	Pain, anxiety	Chest pain, back pain	No Data	
8/30/96		3.1	Anxiety	Hospitalization icu, intubation		
8/30/96		5.3	Knowledge deficit	Hospitalization ESRD, Dialysis		
8/30/96		10.4	Gas exchange	SOB, Pulmonery edema		
8/31/96	JR	9.1	Tissue perfusion	Low BP + low H/H		
8/31/96	TW	9.4	Hyperthermia	Disease process		
9/3/96		10.1	Airway problems	Intubation		
9-18-96	CC	Routine	Chaplain visit patient couldn't talk receiving breathing TX			
9/22/96	CC	6.2	Skin integrity	Ulcer sacrum		
10/8/96	D	8.1	Activity deficit	Paraplegics		
10/16/96	DW			SNF Transfer	↓	

MULTIONSCIPLINARY/DISCHARGE ROUNDS (Initial Appropriate Boxes)

DATE	ATTENDED BY:	DSCG. PL.	CH	NUTR.	O.T.	S.P.	P.T.	H.H.	NSG	OTHER
DATE	ATTENDED BY: ☐	DSCG. PL. ☐	CH ☐	NUTR. ☐	O.T. ☐	S.P. ☐	P.T. ☐	H.H. ☐	NSG ☐	OTHER ☐
DATE	ATTENDED BY: ☐	DSCG. PL. ☐	CH ☐	NUTR. ☐	O.T. ☐	S.P. ☐	P.T. ☐	H.H. ☐	NSG ☐	OTHER ☐
DATE	ATTENDED BY: ☐	DSCG. PL. ☐	CH ☐	NUTR. ☐	O.T. ☐	S.P. ☐	P.T. ☐	H.H. ☐	NSG ☐	OTHER ☐
DATE	ATTENDED BY: ☐	DSCG. PL. ☐	CH ☐	NUTR. ☐	O.T. ☐	S.P. ☐	P.T. ☐	H.H. ☐	NSG ☐	OTHER ☐

Figure 35•7 *Note first notation of skin problems on 9/22/96. This document was the entire care plan. No additional pages followed.*

Continued

▶ Case Study 35•1[8]

Table 35-1 Medical Chronology on James Doe

Hospital Cannot Escape Liability Even When the Basics Are Ignored—cont'd

Date	Status	Nursing & Nurses' Notes/ Signs & Symptoms	MD Orders/ Progress Notes	Skin Assessments/Treatments	Therapies/Procedures/ Tests/Care Plans
8/30/96	* Production database. Dx: - Failure - Acute pulmonary edema - End stage renal disease - Spina bifida with neurogenic bladder (3HEL-70, 72, 73, 313-320, 472, 536, 937-942) - Social service: Discharge planning: Sister to initiate social security disability application. (3HEL-536) * Presents to Houston East Lake emergency room with 2-week history of shortness of breath, hemoptysis, and occasional fever. Presents today vomiting blood and becoming progressively short of breath. Intubated and admitted to Houston East Lake ICU. (3HEL-70, 226, 228, 229,	* Nursing: - Turn/position schedule (3HEL-594) - Weight: 103 kg (3HEL-918); 250 pounds (3HEL-939) - Patient admission/assessment/ discharge record: (May be completed by NA, LVN, RN, or Tech) Gaymar pressure ulcer risk assessment is done: chair-bound, immobile. (3HEL-1045) * Nurses' Notes: - Dr H to ICU (p. 88) (3HEL-600) * Signs & Symptoms: - Skin moist & warm - Diaphoretic - Lethargic/sleepy (3HEL-600)	* Doctor's orders: - MD orders begin p. 185/ 3HEL-408. No orders for skin care, specialty bed, turning patient, passive PT activities, bed rest. (p. 185) (3HEL-408-411) - Consult: pulmonary: Dr. HA (p. 76) - Consult Dr. K (p. 78) (3HEL-408) - Consult: Social services: "Medicaid" (3HEL-409) * Progress notes: - 3HEL-230-232. Initial observations (ie, renal/pulmonary physicians).	* Skin Assessment: - ER Report: Dr. D: Integumentary system: "No rash or skin sores" (p. 88, 89) (3HEL-310) - EC Treatment Summary: ER Nurse (PG, RN): Clammy, diaphoretic, cool, color pale, pasty. No integumentary exam included (3HEL-317) - Production database: Integumentary: Clammy, diaphoretic cool, pale, pasty (3HEL-937) - Care plan: "Skin warm & dry without discoloration, deformities, edema, lesions, or decubiti." (3HEL-1042)	* Therapy: Dialysis initiated at 1130 a.m.-ish (3HEL-600, 889) Respiratory therapy: Put on ventilator. (3HEL-939) * Procedures: Intubation by ER physician (3HEL-70, 232, 311, 939) Dr. K: Placement of Quintin catheter through right subclavian artery (3HEL-70, 232, 299, 937) * Lab: Blood Culture:)Preliminary report= STRMTS/BACLOE (p. 372) (3HEL-494). Final report of 9/10/96, (3HEL-1119) Chemistry: Lyte, metabolic, enzyme, and liver function abnormalities (3HEL-1095) Hematology: Low H&H, high white blood count, etc. (3HEL-1112) * Care Plan: — "Skin warm & dry without discoloration, deformities, edema, lesions, or decubiti." Only "mobility, impaired physical" is circled. (3HEL-1042)

309, 319), ER report: Impression:
● Acute pulmonary edema
● End stage renal failure, question exact cause
● Spina bifida with neurogenic bladder (3HEl-310-312)

Date		
9/14/96	* Production database (3HEl-975)	* Nursing: - Turn/position schedule. Bedrest. Regarded as having pressure ulcer risk. (3HEl-718) - Weight: 102.2 kg (3HEl-919) * Nurses' notes: (no mention of skin) - 4:00 p.m.: Patient continues to sit upright (3HEl-724) * Signs & symptoms: - Skin warm and dry - Itching (3HEl-717, 724) * Progress notes: - 3HEl-259. * Skin Assessment: - Wound documentation record: ● Skin tear: Sacral area: "Duoderm intact" (3HEl-1038) * Treatments: Sacral/coccyx: - Duoderm to coccyx (3HEl-1038)	* Therapy: - Respiratory therapy: (3HEl-975) * Lab: - Chemistry abnormalities: (ie, BUN, creatinine) (3HEl-1091) - Hematology: Low H&H, low platelets, etc. (3HEl-1107, 1108) * X-ray: - CT/chest: empyemas with questionable bronchopleural fistula to the left empyema, left basilar consolidation, adenopathy, small lesion in the liver. (3HEl-563)
9/15/96	* Production database (3HEl-976-978) * Blood transfusion given (3HEl-505)	* Nursing: - Turn/position schedule. Bedrest. Regarded as having pressure ulcer risk (3HEl-727) * Nurses' notes: - 4:10 a.m.: "Patient's sacral area draining on draw sheet. Duoderm removed. Area cleaned and documented on wound documentation record." (3HEl-732) * Signs & symptoms: - Skin warm and dry - Itching (3HEl-726, 32) * Doctor's orders: - Consult Dr. K: pleural effusion. - D/C TPN tomorrow. (3HEl-437) * Progress notes: - 3HEl-260-261. Highlights: ● Chest tube inserted (3HEl-261) * Skin assessment: - Nurses' Notes: Sacral wound draining (3HEl-732) - Wound documentation record: ● Sacral area: Stage II, 8 cm × 3-5 cm × 0.25 cm, clear/yellow drainage, no odor, red/yellow wound base, slough tissue, + inflammation. "Worsened." (3HEl-1038) * Treatments: Sacral: - "Area cleaned." (3HEl-1038) - "Cleaned with normal saline . . . Duoderm applied." (3HEl-1039)	* Therapy: - Respiratory therapy: (3HEl-976, 977) * Procedure: - Left chest tube insertion by Dr. K (3HEl-344, 733) * Lab: - Chemistry abnormalities: (ie, BUN, creatinine) (3HEl-1091) - Hematology: Low H&H, low platelets, etc. (3HEl-1107, 1108)

Continued

⟩ Case Study 35•1[8]

Table 35-1 Medical Chronology on James Doe—cont'd

Hospital Cannot Escape Liability Even When the Basics Are Ignored—cont'd

Date	Status	Nursing & Nurses' Notes/ Signs & Symptoms	MD Orders/ Progress Notes	Skin Assessments/Treatments	Therapies/Procedures/ Tests/Care Plans
9/20/96	* Production database (3HEL-70, 71, 74, 473, 985) * Consult with Dr. M re: decubitus ulcer (p. 220) (3HEL-70, 472)	* Nursing: - Flow sheet: decubitus is noted. (3HEL-765) - Turn schedule: "turns self" "turns with assistance." Dressing changes noted at 8:00 a.m. and 9:00 p.m. (3HEL-766) * Nurses' notes: - 12 mn: "Assessed skin (dry, flaky) stage 3 decubitus of sacral area. Waffle mattress ordered. Turned q 2 hours." (3HEL-768) * Signs & symptoms: - Dry, flaky skin; skin integrity interrupted (3HEL-765) - Constipation (3HEL-768)	* Doctor's orders: - Waffle mattress - Consult Dr. M re: decubitus ulcer - Up in chair ×1 per day - Wound culture, sacral decubitus (p. 220) (3HEL-446, 472, 473) * Progress notes: - 3HEL-266-267. Highlights: Renal: • "Back-decubitus . . . . Decubitus ulcer: Wet to dry normal saline. Plastic surgery consult." • Anemic: Transfuse blood. (3HEL-266)	* Skin assessment: - Wound documentation record: • Coccyx: Stage III/eschar, 10 cm × 6 cm × 1-2 cm, moderate-scant/ greenish/odorous drainage, black wound base, eschar necrosis. + maceration, + inflammation (3HEL-1041) • Right buttock/hip: Stage II, width: 2 cm × 2 cm, white drainage, white wound base, slough tissue, dry surrounding skin. "Worsened." (3HEL-1040) * Treatments: Sacral/coccyx: - Moist dressing applied to area (normal saline); covered with ABD. (3HEL-1041) Right buttock/hip: - Duoderm applied/Turn q 2 hours. (3HEL-1040)	* Therapy: Dialysis (3HEL-901) * Lab: - Chemistry abnormalities: (ie, BUN, creatinine) (3HEL-1088, 1089) - Hematology: low H&H, low platelets, low white blood count, etc. (3HEL-1106, 1107)
9/21/96	* Production data-base (3HEL-70, 986, 987) * Consult Dr. S re: Hematology/rash (3HEL-70, 269, 472) * Blood transfusions given (3HEL-504)	* Nursing: - Flow sheet: decubitus is noted. (3HEL-770) - Turn schedule: "turns self" No dressing changes are noted. Much of 3-11: no documentation. (3HEL-771) * Nurses' notes: - 4:30 p.m.: "Turned q 2 hours. Dressing change done." (3HEL-773) * Signs & symptoms: - Edema (3HEL-770)	* Doctor's orders: - Consult Dr. S - Transfuse 2 units PRBCs (3HEL-447, 472) * Progress notes: - 3HEL-268. Highlights: - Anemic: Transfuse 2 units blood (3HEL-268)	* Skin assessment: - Wound documentation record: • Coccyx: 10cm × 6 cm × 1-2 cm, black wound base, eschar necrosis. (3HEL-1041) • Right buttock/hip: White wound base, slough tissue, dry/scaly surrounding skin. "Duoderm to area" (3HEL-1040) * Treatments: Sacral/coccyx - Moist dressing applied to area (normal saline); covered with ABD. (3HEL-1041)	* Therapy: - Dialysis (3HEL-901) - Respiratory therapy: Pulse oximeter. Chest PT. (3HEL-986, 987) * Lab: - Chemistry abnormalities: (ie, BUN, creatinine) (3HEL-1089) - Hematology: low H&H, low white blood count, etc. (3HEL-1105, 1106)

| 9/25/96 | * Production database (3HEL-70, 994, 995)
* Débridement of pressure sore by Dr. M: (3HEL-351)
* Consult with Dr. K re: air leak (3HEL-70, 453, 472)
* Social Services Notes: Discharge planning. (3HEL-995) | * Nursing:
- Perioperative record: Pressure sores sacrum, right hip, both heels. (p. 133) (3HEL-353)
- Discharge criteria met. (p. 135) (3HEL-357)
- Flow sheet: decubitus is not noted. "See skin sheet." (3HEL-787)
- Turn schedule: Bedrest, turn q 2 hours. Dressing changes are not noted here. (3HEL-788)
* Nurses' notes:
- Outpatient Nursing Care Record: Narrative nurses' notes: Instructed pt. to turn from side to side, try to keep pressure off of sacrum. Client verbalized understanding (p. 135) (3HEL-356)
- 2:00 a.m.: "Assessed skin breaks current. Turned patient q 2 hours. No further breakdown noted, however skin is increasingly flaky on upper extremities." (3HEL-790)
- No other skin references are made (3HEL-790)
* Signs & symptoms:
- Skin dry & flaky (3HEL-787) | * Doctor's orders:
- Pack sacral area with 4×4 gauze with normal saline, change Q6hrs (p. 225) (3HEL-450)
- Consult Dr. Kodak: persistent air leak (3HEL-453)
* Progress notes:
- 3HEL-273-274. Highlights:
● Dr. M: **Débridement of the pressure sacral area under local with MAC.** (3HEL-273)
● Pulmonary: Low grade temp. Chest tube air leak persists. Will ask Dr. K to evaluate. (3HEL-274)
● Renal: Broncho-pleural fistula. Dr. K to evaluate (3HEL-274) | * Skin Assessment:
- Operative report: The sore was going very close to the anus and there was full thickness of the skin with necrosis (3HEL-351)
- Wound documentation record:
● Sacral area: Pressure wound: Stage III, 10 cm × 6.5 cm, small/green/odorous drainage, black wound base, + eschar, + inflammation. (3HEL-1048)
● Right hip/buttock: Pressure wound: Stage II, 2 cm × 2 cm, no drainage, white wound base, + inflammation. (3HEL-1047)
<u>Left hip:</u>
1. + Rash in left hip area (3HEL-1052, 1053)
2. Pressure wound: Stage II, 1.5-2 cm × 2 cm, whitish drainage, white wound base, + slough, + inflammation. (3HEL-1046, 1054).
● Left heel: 2 cm × 2cm × 2 cm, red wound base, inflamed. (3HEL-1062)
● Right heel: Stage III, 3cm × 2 cm, red wound base, + eschar, + granulation, + inflammation. "Worsened." (3HEL-1070) | Right buttock/hip:
- Duoderm to area/turn q 2 hours. (3HEL-1040)

* Therapy:
- Dialysis (3HEL-904)
- Respiratory therapy: Chest PT. (3HEL-994, 997)
* Procedure:
- Débridement of full thickness of skin through skin and subcutaneous tissue and necrotic tissue completely excised. Area irrigated with bacitracin, Kantrex, and saline and packed with gauze with the same. Operative report: (p. 131) (3HEL-351)
* Lab:
- Pathology: Sacral decubitus: 6.2 × 2.7 cm. Skin w/totally ulcerated surface w/extension necrosis. (p. 132) (3HEL-352)
- Chemistry abnormalities: (ie, BUN, creatinine, uric acid, liver enzymes, etc.). (3HEL-1088)
- Hematology: low H&H, low white blood count, etc (3HEL-1104, 1105) |

Continued

▷ **Case Study 35·1**[8]

Table 35-1 **Medical Chronology on James Doe—cont'd**

Date	Status	Nursing & Nurses' Notes/Signs & Symptoms	MD Orders/Progress Notes	Skin Assessments/Treatments	Therapies/Procedures/Tests/Care Plans
9/27/96	* Production database (3HEL-70, 71, 73, 74, 75, 472, 473, 474, 998-1000) (SNF 466/67) * Zoneair bed started (3HEL-75) * Remains in ICU. Weaned off ventilator. Extubated. Tolerated well. (3HEL-810, 811)	* Nursing: - Turn schedule. Bedrest. Heel protectors on. (3HEL-805) * Nurses' notes: - 12 mn: "Encouraged to turn to increase healing-decubitus." - 400 a.m.: "Decubitus on coccyx. Reddened with some purulent drainage. Dressing change. Continue to assess." - 11:00 a.m.: "Dr. M on round(s). Decubitus examined. Orders written." - 12:00 p.m.: "Placed on Advance Aerial Air Bed." - 3:30 p.m.: "Skin sheet notations to chart . . . heel protectors . . . Zoneair bed . . ." - 7:35 p.m.: "Prepared to turn patient. Patient refused. 'When my sister gets back.' Instructed patient that it could not wait too long. Will reattempt in 30 minutes if family member not returned." - 8:05 p.m.: "Entered room behind sister. Patient ready to turn." (3HEL-810-812) * Signs & symptoms: - Skin warm, dry, pale. No edema. (3HEL-804) - Itching. Benadryl given. (3HEL-812)	* Doctor's orders: - Start débridement with Santyl. Apply to the sacral area × 2 per day, rinse with normal saline, pack with 4x4 gauze. Place patient on an air bed. (p. 234) (3HEL-459, 472, 473) * Nursing order: Santyl BID rinse w/NS & pack w/4x4 gauze Santyl ointment, Collagenase ointment. Apply to sacral area bid. (3HEL-71, 73, 74) - Zoneair bed (3HEL-72, 472) * Progress notes: - 3HEL-276-277. Highlights: ● Pulmonary: Low grade temp. Wean off vent. (3HEL-276) ● Dr. M: "Dressing changed. Sacral area with necrotic tissue. Will start débridement with Santyl and change his bed to air bed." (3HEL-277) ● Renal: Rash with itching. (3HEL-277) ● Hematology: Recovering well. (3HEL-277)	* Skin Assessment: - Wound documentation record: ● Sacral area: Pressure wound: Stage III, black wound base, + eschar, + inflammation. (3HEL-1048) ● Left hip: Rash?/inflamed area. Duoderm intact. (3HEL-1052) ● Left heel: Stage I. (3HEL-1062) ● Right heel: Stage III, 3cm × 2 cm, red wound base (3HEL-1070) * Treatments: Sacral: - Production Database: Apply Santyl ointment and collagenase ointment to sacral area. ● 3:30 p.m.: Sheryl Capo, RN (3HEL-998, 1048) Left hip: - Duoderm (3HEL-1052) Left heel: - Duoderm. Heel protectors. (3HEL-1062) Right heel: - Duoderm. Heel protectors. (3HEL-1070)	* Therapy: - Respiratory therapy: (3HEL-999) * Procedure: - Dr. M: Sacral dressing changed. (3HEL-277) * Lab: - Chemistry abnormalities: (ie, BUN, creatinine, uric acid, etc.) (3HEL-1088) - Hematology: low H&H, high white blood count, etc. (3HEL-1104, 1105) * Other: - Abnormal ABGs (3HEL-529-531)

10/1/96

* Production database (3HEL-72, 75, 473, 1007, 1008)
* Quinton catheter clogs (3HEL-838)
* Right chest tube removed by Dr. K (3HEL-838)

* Nursing:
- Flow sheet: decubitus is noted. (3HEL-835)
- Turn schedule: Turns self, bedrest, turn q 2 hours. Dressing changes are noted at 9:00 a.m. (3HEL-836)
* Nurses' notes:
- 9:25 a.m.: "Turned to side with pillow. Skin nurse paged re: pad for bed."
- 4:00 p.m.: "Turn q 2 hours . . . Patient on special bed." (3HEL-838)
* Signs & symptoms:
- Skin dry & flaky.
- Pedal edema. (3HEL-835)

* Progress notes:
- 3HEL-281-283. Highlights:
- Right chest tube discontinued (3HEL-281)
- **Dr. M: Dressing changed. Still with some necrotic tissue, not ready for flap repair.** (3HEL-282)
- Plan placement of Permacath in AM since having difficulties (3HEL-283)
- Anesthesia pre-op (3HEL-283)

* Skin Assessment:
- Wound documentation record:
- Sacral: Stage IV Eschar, 10 cm × 18 cm × 5 cm, yellow-white/red-white scant-moderate drainage, red/yellow/black wound base, + eschar. "Notified Dr. H of appearance." (3HEL-1056). Nurses' notes: "Still with black, firm 4 × 4 × 2 cm eschar, fresh breakdown with yellowish moderate drainage. No odor . . . Skin nurse paged re: pad for bed." (3HEL-838)
- Left hip/buttock: No status. (3HEL-1065)
- Left heel: (3HEL-1060)
- Right heel: No status given. (3HEL-1068)

* Treatments:
Sacral:
- Production Database: Apply Santyl ointment and collagenase ointment to sacral area.
- 9:00 a.m.: Jeeni Grayson, RN
- 5:00 p.m.: Angel Opthera, RN (3HEL-838, 1007, 1056)
Left hip/buttock:
- Duoderm (3HEL-1065)
Left heel:
- Duoderm. Heel protectors (3HEL-1060)
Right heel:
- Duoderm. Heel protectors. (3HEL-1068)

* Therapy:
- Respiratory therapy: Pulse oximeter spot check. Chest PT. (3HEL-1007)
* Procedure:
- Dr. M: Dressing changed. (3HEL-281)
- Dr. K: Removes right chest tube at bedside (3HEL-838)
* Lab:
- Chemistry abnormalities: (i.e., BUN, creatinine) (3HEL-1087)
- Hematology: low H&H, high white blood count, etc. (3HEL-1103, 1104)

Continued

» Case Study 35•1[8] Hospital Cannot Escape Liability Even When the Basics Are Ignored—cont'd

Table 35-1 Medical Chronology on James Doe—cont'd

Date	Status	Nursing & Nurses' Notes/Signs & Symptoms	MD Orders/Progress Notes	Skin Assessments/Treatments	Therapies/Procedures/Tests/Care Plans
10/9/96	* Production database (3HEL-1024, 1025) * Home health notes re: rental of wheel chair (p. 415) (3HEL-888, 1025)	* Nursing: - Flow sheet: sacral decubitus is not noted. (3HEL-870) - Turn schedule: Out of bed in chair 4 p.m.-6 p.m. Turns self. Dressing changes are not noted. (3HEL-871) * Nurses' notes: - Skin integrity not addressed. - 3-11 shift: Out of bed to chair. (3HEL-873) * Signs & symptoms: - Skin dry & flaky. (3HEL-870)	* Doctor's orders: - Bicarb bath - Consent for sacral débridement to be done under spinal. (3HEL-479) * Progress notes: - 3HEL-289-290. Highlights: • Dr. M: Dressing changed . . . . "Necrotic tissue. Will need another débridement. Will schedule when possible." (3HEL-290)	* Skin Assessment: - Wound documentation record: • Sacral area: Pressure wound: 10 cm × 18 cm × deep, dark yellow odorous drainage, red/yellow/black/white wound base, + maceration, "Necrosis." (3HEL-605) • Left hip: No status given_(3HEL-604) • Left heel: No status given_(3HEL-604) • Right heel: No status given_(3HEL-604) * Treatments: Sacral: - Production Database: Apply Santyl ointment and collagenase ointment to sacral area. • 9:00 a.m.: Femma Jayne Robinson, LVN • 5:00 p.m.: Marsha Robbins, LVN (3HEL-1024) Left hip: Duoderm intact (3HEL-604) Left heel: Duoderm intact (3HEL-604) Right heel Duoderm intact (3HEL-604)	* Therapy: - Dialysis (3HEL-911) - Respiratory therapy: Pulse oximeter spot check. Chest PT. (3HEL-1024, 1025) * Procedure: - Dr. M. Dressing changed. (3HEL-290) * Lab: - Chemistry: electrolyte/liver enzyme abnormalities (i.e., BUN, creatinine, CK, SGOT, Alk phos) (3HEL-585) - Hematology: low H&H, etc. (3HEL-1101)
10/21/96	* Production database: (3HEL-121, 122)	* Nursing: - Flow sheet: decubitus acknowledged. (3HEL-175) - Turn schedule: Chair with assistance 4:00 p.m.-6:00 p.m. Dressing change is noted at 9:00 p.m. (3HEL-176) - wt. 213 [where is this?] * Nurses' Notes: Topics - Skin integrity is addressed. (3HEL-174)	Progress Notes: - 3HEL-62. • Renal: Wound infection (3HEL-62)	* Skin Assessment: - Wound documentation record: • Sacral area: Pressure wound: Stage IV. 10 cm × 6 cm × 4 cm. Purulent/large/odorous drainage. Wound base = red & yellow. Maceration, + slough, + granulation, + undermining, + tunneling (3HEL-145) * Treatments: Sacral: - Production Database: Nursing:	* Therapies: - Respiratory therapy. Pulse oximeter. Chest PT. (3HEL-122) * Lab: - Some electrolyte abnormalities (high BUN, creatinine) (3HEL-91) Shelly Sowetho PTA SNF496 Spvr Arnold Hines PT SNF 495

Apply Santyl ointment and collagenase ointment to sacral area.

- 9:00 a.m.: Maria G. Ponds, LVN
- 9:00 p.m.: Valencia Burnetta, LVN (3HEL-121)

- Nurses' notes: "Up in chair for meals. Turn and assist in positioning q 2 hours." (3HEL-174)

Left heel:
- Duoderm to left heel :

- 5:00 p.m.: MP, LVN. Not given; site pink

Left hip:
- Duoderm to left hip

- 8:00 p.m.: MP, LVN. Not given; site pink

| 10/27/96 | * Production database: (3HEL-134, 135) |

* Nursing:
- Flow sheet: decubitus acknowledged. (3HEL-201)
- Turn schedule. Chair with assistance: 11:00 a.m., 1:00 p.m., 3:00 p.m., 5:00 p.m. Sacral dressing changed: 10:00 a.m. and 7:30 p.m. (3HEL-202)

* Nurses' Notes:

Topics
- Skin integrity is addressed. Encourage to turn. Up in chair with assist. Statements of interest:

- "Patient refuses to most repositioning. No further skin breakdown."
- "Wound granulating well. NO odor noted on sacral decubitus." (3HEL-200)

* Progress notes:
- 3HEL- 65. Stable for transfer to Braden Port. Renal function improving.

* Skin Assessment:
- Wound documentation record:

- Sacral area: Pressure wound: Stage IV. 11 cm × 8 cm × 6 cm. No drainage. Wound base = red, + granulation, + undermining, "Improved." (3HEL-146)
- Right thigh: No status given (3HEL-147, 200)

* Treatments:
-Production Database: Nursing: (3HEL-134)

Sacral:
Apply Santyl ointment and collagenase ointment to sacral area.

- 9:00 a.m.: CL, RN
- 7:30 p.m.: DL, RN

Right thigh:
- Duoderm. "Change q 3" (3HEL-147)

Left hip:
- Duoderm, left hip:

- 9:00 a.m.: Cyril Emkata Lolaro, RN

* Therapies:
- Respiratory therapy. Pulse oximeter. Chest PT. (3HEL-134)

* Lab:
- Some electrolyte abnormalities (high BUN, creatinine) (3HEL-90)

The Lawsuit—James Doe vs Houston East Lake Hospital and Dr. Veronica Holly

Elements of the lawsuit are to be proved by the plaintiff Mr. Doe by a preponderance of the evidence.

Duty

Mr. Doe's lawyers had to prove by a preponderance of the evidence that the defendants East Lake Hospital, the nursing staff, and Dr. Veronica Holly had a duty to the plaintiff, Mr. James Doe. On admission, the nursing staff owed a duty to properly assess Mr. Doe for risks associated with development pressure ulcers. They had a duty to follow the policy of the hospital and the rules and regulations of the state Nursing Practice Act and to act within the standards of care for a patient such as Mr. Doe. The hospital had a duty to see that the staff followed the policy and that the staff was properly trained and educated to understand the risks and potential complications and dangers faced by patients in Mr. Doe's circumstance.

The hospital and the nursing staff had a duty to report properly to the physician and appropriate members of the team on admission, and once the ulcers were discovered, the nursing staff had a duty to the patient to report to the physician and to work with the Skin Resource Team to properly assess, intervene, and evaluate the treatment and to prevent progression of the ulcer and formation of additional ulcers.

The nursing staff had a duty to properly evaluate using clear and consistent documentation, following standards of care and hospital policy regarding the wound documentation record, and again, the hospital had a duty to see that the policy was being followed appropriately. The hospital and nursing staff had a duty to be familiar with current skin care treatment, readily found in the literature and easily accessible from the National Pressure Ulcer Advisory Panel and many other sources.

Dr. Holly had a duty to the patient to properly address his risks associated with his various medical problems. She wrote no orders for consultation with the Skin Resource Team or with physical therapy or physical medicine regarding interventions that may be appropriate for a patient with Mr. Doe's complicated medical problems. Of note, Dr. Holly stated in her deposition that this was not her duty, as "I am a nephrologist." It was pointed out to her that she in fact was the admitting physician and so could not ignore the realm of problems faced by the patient as a whole.

Breach

Mr. Doe's lawyers had to prove by the same preponderance of the evidence that the defendants breached the duty they had to Mr. Doe. For example, that the nurses did not properly assess the plaintiff for risks of pressure ulcer and then did not intervene, treat, and evaluate in accordance with the standard of care. In this case, the admission assessment was completed by a LVN, despite the fact that the policy of the hospital clearly stated that the intensive care unit admission assessment was to be completed by an registered nurse who would also complete a care plan. Mr. Doe's lawyers had to prove that Dr. Holly, as a reasonable nephrologist who admitted a patient with many medical problems, had a duty to call the appropriate consultations so that the issues could be addressed. Although her area of specialty was nephrology, as an admitting physician she was responsible for the overall care of the patient. She did not have to be expert in all areas, but she had a duty to understand that as admitting physician, she was the one who must order consults, or she must take charge of the problem herself.

Damages

Mr. Doe's lawyers had to prove that the breach of the duty by the defendant's hospital and nursing staff, whose actions are vicariously those of the hospital, and Dr. Holly caused Mr. Doe to suffer damages, both economic and noneconomic. For example, they had to prove by a preponderance of the evidence that Mr. Doe developed stage IV pressure ulcers on his sacrum and hip, required flap surgery, eventually leading to septic arthritis in the knee on the same side of the body as the hip ulcer. They had to prove that the defendants caused him to suffer both economic losses and pain and suffering in the past and present and in all likelihood would continue to have associated economic and noneconomic damages into the future.

In addition to the obvious pain and suffering (at the time of this case there was no cap on economic damages[9]), Mr. Doe incurred medical expenses of over $800,000. Following discharge, he had to hire additional household help to care for him at a cost of $2890 per month. He had permanent disfigurement and risk for developing additional ulcers over the sites; the inability to sit for extended periods of time, causing him to lose his job; and physical impairment beyond that which he had prior to admission.

Causation

The lawyers for Mr. Doe had to prove by a preponderance of the evidence that the damages listed above were in fact caused by the negligence of the hospital, the nurses, and Dr. Holly, and that, but for that negligence, the pressure ulcers and the damages that flowed from them would not have developed.

Defense Arguments

If one looks carefully at the list of the elements above, one can imagine all types of arguments that can be and were used by the attorneys defending the hospital and Dr. Holly. It is important to understand that for the vast majority of cases, even if the plaintiff's allegations clearly point to liability on the part of the defendant(s), they will be vigorously defended in attempts to limit damages or, even better from the perspective of the defendant(s), to make the case go away.

Defense attorneys for the hospital and nursing staff would usually readily agree that, yes, there was a duty to the patient, but their argument in this case would and did focus on the fact that Mr. Doe was a patient who would have developed the ulcers anyway. Thus, the fact that the assessment was done by an LVN or that the wound documentation sheet was inconsistent did not, in fact, cause his damages. The argument was that the LVN assessed Mr. Doe, perhaps ineptly, but it did not matter because he would have gotten the ulcers anyway. Thus the negligence, if it did occur, was not the cause of the damage. The defense called in experts from the hospital who opined that, because of Mr. Doe's many medical problems, he would inevitably have developed the ulcers. He was poorly nourished, hypoxic, diabetic, agitated, paraplegic, in kidney failure, and at times noncompliant with turning: all impediments to optimal functioning of the body's systems to prevent "skin failure."

An additional argument from the hospital's perspective was that Dr. Holly saw the patient and did not order the interventions that would have allegedly been appropriate. Since she was the doctor, and nurses follow the doctor's orders, the liability is not there for the nurses; hence, the hospital is not liable.

Additionally, they argued that since an assessment was done, nursing did not breach the duty because the LVN did assess Mr. Doe. The argument is always advanced that the risk assessment tools,[10] policies and procedures of the hospital, and the AHCPR (Agency for Healthcare Policy and Research) guidelines[11] are just guidelines, not strict parameters.

The damages, in any case, are usually argued to be inflated, speculative, and, in this case, not a result of the lack of assessment or violations in the standard of care for assessment and treatment of pressure ulcers because Mr. Doe would have gotten the ulcers anyway. Finally, there is the argument that the patient is at least partially responsible for his damages because even if the nurse was negligent in her assessment, the patient was periodically noncompliant with turning, occasionally did not want to go to therapy, and was not eating adequately.

Expert Testimony

In order to prove the case and counter the defense arguments, the lawyers for Mr. Doe must have experts in the appropriate specialty who can testify about the duty, the standard of care, the violation of those standards, and the causative component that leads to the damages suffered by the plaintiff.

In this case, the experts used by Mr. Doe's lawyers were an internationally known and well-respected Wound Ostomy and Continence Nurses Society nurse, another nurse with rehabilitation background, an ICU nurse, a nephrologist, an internal medicine physician, a rehabilitation specialist, a physical medicine physician, and a life-care planner to establish future expenses. Plaintiff attorneys, not surprisingly, usually have to go outside of the city, and often outside the state, to find experts willing to testify against health-care providers. In this case, the plaintiff's experts came from Illinois, Virginia, Florida, and Austin and Dallas, Texas.

Mr. Doe's lawyers used the experts to point out that despite the obvious fact that Mr. Doe had many medical problems placing him at high risk for the development of pressure ulcers, the hospital cannot use that as a defense if they do not undertake the recognized interventions that can and do prevent ulcers from starting or progressing. The experts all reviewed the entire medical file and testified that the hospital and Dr. Holly breached the standard of care during Mr. Doe's hospitalization. They all agreed that despite the medical problems that were compounded by very large ulcers requiring invasive surgical intervention, Mr. Doe recovered, went to rehabilitation, and eventually went home. They were able to state that within reasonable

medical probability, had he been treated according to the standard of care with the correct preventive measures put in place initially, he would not have developed the ulcers. His body had the resources to overcome the severe stressors placed upon him, as evidenced by his eventual wound closure and discharge home.

The defense experts, all from Houston, testified that no one who cared for Mr. Doe breached any standard of care, that the policies and procedures, protocols, and literature are all just guidelines for treatment and not to be taken as exact parameters, and, as stated above, that Mr. Doe would have developed the ulcers even with the best of care, given his many medical issues.

The lawyers on both sides must be sure that the experts are well spoken and will be clear in their opinions and testimony. If an expert offers an opinion, he or she must stand by what is said. Experts are not to be advocates for the case itself, or for the side for which they are testifying, but they must be able to stand by and support their opinions by the facts of the case and accepted science. Not surprisingly, medical literature can be used to support various sides of an argument, many times only when taken somewhat out of context. An experienced expert is aware of this and will be knowledgeable about all of the literature; the expert will know better than to stretch the science to fit what he or she thinks the lawyer wants to hear. The lawyer should endeavor to be familiar with the literature so that he or she will know if the expert, or an opposing expert, is using portions of literature to support his or her opinions and ignoring other pertinent portions of the same articles or literature in the same subject matter.

Expert Witness Responsibilities

As discussed above, an expert witness is a person who is retained by either side in a lawsuit to give expert opinions in a case. State law may vary on qualifications of experts and who may be retained, but generally the expert will be in the area or field of practice that is the focus of a particular issue in the case. A medical negligence case may require 1 or 20 experts, depending on the facts of the case. The best scenario for the plaintiff is when the treating physician(s) will agree to offer expert testimony for the plaintiff and will agree to write a report and be deposed.

Many times treating physicians are confused by the term *expert witness*. Frequently, the plaintiff lawyer will contact treating physicians who will naively say that they "don't want to be involved." Health-care providers must understand that if they are treating a person, they are involved. They may or may not be cooperative (that is a different issue), but they cannot become uninvolved. In medical malpractice litigation, treaters in the same locale as a defendant are usually hesitant to testify against persons in the same geographical area. Many health-care providers will never give opinion testimony about the breach of the standard of care, no matter where the case is located. Frequently, the plaintiff's lawyer may ask the treater to testify not about the standard of care, but as to damages, and sometimes treaters will agree to this as long as they do not have to point a finger regarding liability or breach of the standard of care. The ethical obligation of health-care providers to testify on behalf of a patient who has legitimately been harmed by negligent care is often a topic of heated debate.[12]

If treating physicians are asked by the plaintiff's lawyers to testify as treaters, the lawyers hope they will be willing to offer expert opinions that support the theories of the case regarding liability or damages, or both. Sometimes an additional expert in the specialty will be retained to support the treater's testimony, especially if the treater is not board certified, or if he or she does not have the credentials that the plaintiff attorney may believe is necessary to overcome the defense experts' opposing opinions.

States differ as to rules allowing defense attorney contact with treating health-care providers. Experts should check with the attorney with whom they are working to be clear on what rules apply in the jurisdiction of the particular case.

Whether experts are retained as outside experts or as treating physicians, they will usually be paid by the attorney who plans to use their testimony. Experts should review all medical records in a case to ensure that they are forming an opinion based on all of the data. It is uncomfortable to be in a deposition and to be asked about an incident or a medical issue that one is not familiar with. Opposing counsel will take advantage of any situation that may imply that the expert has been less than complete in the medical review and evaluation before arriving at an opinion.

Experts should have a fee agreement in writing that sets out hourly charges and addresses the issue of travel expenses. It is considered unethical to be reimbursed based upon the outcome of the case, therefore an hourly fee arrangement should be developed. Opposing counsel will ask for and be allowed to review any fee agreements, billing invoices, or correspondence sent or received by the expert, as well as all other documents that the expert has reviewed and/or generated regarding the case.

In *Doe vs Houston East Lake*, none of the treating physicians at Houston East Lake Hospital were experts for the plaintiff; they were all named as experts for the defense. However, two physical medicine physicians who treated Mr. Doe after his discharge from Houston East Lake were named as experts for Mr. Doe and willingly testified about his damages and the standard of care as it related to skin care and prevention of pressure ulcers for a person such as Mr. Doe.

If one agrees to be an expert, either as a treating physician or a nontreating retained expert, there is responsibility involved. All of the records must be reviewed, including all deposition testimony and other related documents, and the expert must be very familiar with the scientific literature involved with the issues in the case. Many times physicians will recall negative experiences when serving as an expert, often because they have not had the opportunity to become, or did not realize the importance of being, exquisitely prepared. If an expert offers opinion testimony, it must be supported with literature; an opinion will not be considered true just because he or she says so. An expert treads on dangerous ground if unprepared for questioning from the other side and if his or her opinions cannot be supported.

If one agrees to be an expert, one should expect to be paid for time spent and expect that the retaining attorney will send all the relevant documents in a timely manner. Documents to be reviewed may include medical records, expert reports from the other side, literature relied upon by the opposing expert, employment and/or school documents, employment records, and any other materials that may have been produced by the opposing party and by the side for which the expert is retained. If the documents are not received in time for adequate review, the expert must insist on additional time for preparation.

The expert must understand that this is an adversarial process and that the other side will also have an expert who will review the case and the literature and most likely have a different opinion. Most medical societies have statements regarding the responsibilities of an expert witness, generally calling for truthfulness and a willingness to assist in the process so as to reach the appropriate outcome for the patient and society.[13]

Trial

A trial is time consuming, stressful, expensive, and has an outcome that often is unexpected.

As mentioned above, mediation is a process that is frequently used in civil litigation and often leads to settlement of the claims. If a case cannot be settled, the parties move on to trial. The trial may be held before a judge and jury, or just a judge.

If the trial is to be before a jury, a process called *voir dire* is undertaken, during which both sides' lawyers introduce the case to the potential jury panel and ask questions designed to determine those on the panel who may have a bias that would prevent them from being fair in the particular case. The lawyers get a certain amount of time for these questions, and sometimes a panel member may be questioned by the judge as well. After the questioning, the lawyers choose whom they wish to excuse, and eventually a jury is picked. Courts, judges, and states have differing rules about voir dire in terms of time taken, questions that may be asked, and how many jurors each side may disqualify.

Once a jury is picked and the trial is started, the parties lose control of what happens. The lawyers often are constrained by rules of procedure that may not be understood by or explained to the clients, and many motions may be heard by the court outside the presence of the jury and the parties.

Opening statements are presented by plaintiff, then by the defense attorneys. The plaintiff lawyer then presents his or her client's side first, followed by the defense. After the case is presented, closing statements are made by plaintiff and defense lawyers. The jury then receives instructions from the judge regarding the law and their responsibility and returns to the jury room for deliberations. Everyone involved in the trial then waits until the jury reaches a decision.

A case may still be settled among the parties at any time prior to trial, during trial, or during jury deliberations. Settlement can also be achieved after a jury verdict if the losing party decides to appeal the verdict, forcing both sides to face the prospect of a lengthy and expensive appeals process. If the jury decides in favor of the plaintiff and awards damages, the plaintiff may wish to settle for an amount less than the jury awarded rather than take the chance of the case being overturned or sent back by the higher court for a new trial if the defendant plans to appeal.

All of these decisions are impacted by variables that exist in the reality of the particular venue—the timing, the judges, the appellate courts, the politics.

Avoiding Litigation

Perhaps the best advice that can be given, other than to deliver care that meets the proper standard, is to communicate with patients and families. Many inquiries are received by medical malpractice attorneys from patients and families who have been left in the dark and ultimately feel that something has been hidden from them. This is dangerous for health-care providers. Of course, outcomes are not always positive, and certainly not all negative outcomes are the result of negligence. However, if no one will communicate with patients and families, or if they feel that the physician is trying to avoid discussing issues, they understandably feel that someone is trying to "pull the wool over their eyes."

Whether or not to apologize in the health-care arena is a question that is being discussed in medical and legal settings.[14,15] In 1987 the Lexington, Kentucky, VA Hospital instituted a new policy calling for assuming responsibility for errors in treatment and care. Their litigation costs went from among the highest legal costs to one of the lowest in the VA system.[16] According to the Gerlin article, the policy "requires giving information as soon as possible by aggressively seeking out patients and families, even after discharge if necessary."

Some states have passed legislation that shields comments expressing apologies made from being used as evidence of wrongdoing in civil matters. Whether this can be successfully legislated remains to be seen. It is true, however that all plaintiff lawyers have heard some variation of the comment, "If they had only talked with us, we probably would have understood, it's not about the money, it's that they lied to us."

Documentation and Consistency

Nothing looks worse than poor and inconsistent documentation, as seen in the *Doe vs Houston East Lake* case history. In health care today many different specialties offer consultations, the consultants often write orders without referencing progress notes or orders written by others, and nursing staff is often stretched beyond capacities to keep track of the details involved in caring for patients.

With specific regard to wound care, subjective observations can make documentation appear to be inconsistent. When it is inconsistent, and treaters use different parameters to describe the same thing, problems are compounded, and invariably the patient suffers.

It is imperative that facilities have policies and procedures in place, and it is just as important to ensure that the policies and procedures are taught to the staff and that ongoing educational programs keep up with changes in staff, new developments in science, and best treatment practices.

Proper Assessment and Documentation Facilitates Intervention, Evaluation, and Treatment

If the assessment policy exists regarding who, what, when, and where, follow it—if there is no policy, there should be.

Upon admission of a patient, nursing staff must be aware of the risk assessment tools that should be used: the Braden scale,[17] Norton scale,[18] or Gosnell scale.[19] Presumably, if the risk assessed is of a certain level, the wound care clinician will be consulted. If there is no wound care consultant, other options should be available, unless all the staff caring for the patient can be considered experts in delivering care to this particular wound.

The above suggestions are seen over and over in the literature. It is no secret that proper assessment of risks, a pertinent and complete history, and a physical examination, taking into account nutrition and other medications or medical problems, is of paramount importance in treating patients with skin or wound problems. If care is not delivered following the appropriate standards and documented clearly, and if the case develops into a medical negligence lawsuit, the depositions of those providers delivering substandard care will be difficult, at best.

The Wound Care Team

The wound care team must institute procedures that will prevent patients from falling through the cracks. They must develop education modules for staff and be sure that all staff take part in the education offered. The wound care team should use educational materials from organizations such as the National Pressure Ulcer Advisory Panel (NPUAP) or Wound Ostomy and Continence Nurses Association (WOCN). Because documentation facilitates communication among health-care team members, the educational materials should be for all members of the team, not just for nursing. Dr. Holly should have called the team together to discuss issues with other health-care providers and clinicians who may supplement interventions, that is, medical staff, physical therapists, pain management specialists, nutritionists, and social services staff.

If the documentation is faulty, and if team members rely on it, the system fails, outcomes are impacted negatively, and the patient suffers the result. If the documentation is inconsistent, not only is it a failure for the patient, it is embarrassing (or should be) for the team and the facility.

Documentation Facilitates Reimbursement

According to a report from the Office of Inspector General (OIG), "64% of surgical débridement services in 2004 did not meet Medicare program requirements, resulting in approximately $64 million in improper payments. Medicare allowed approximately $188 million in 2004 for surgical débridement services. An estimated 64% of these services did not meet one or more Medicare program requirements. As a result, Medicare allowed an estimated $64 million in improper payments in 2004."[20] The OIG report recommended improved education with regard to what constitutes appropriate débridement but also suggested that improved documentation was needed so as to adequately support the medical necessity of the procedures and equipment submitted for payment.

Clearly, documentation is extremely important, from the initial assessment at the bedside or office, not only for communication in the record and among health-care team members so as to facilitate the best care, but to allow for correct billing practices and to avoid Medicare calling back monies that they may allege were paid out incorrectly following an audit.

New Medicare Rules Published in Federal Register August 22, 2007

Medicare will not reimburse for "preventable events" effective October 1, 2008. Medicare has recently instituted changes to the Hospital Inpatient Prospective Payment Systems and Fiscal Year 2008 Rates.[21] At this point what Medicare defines as serious preventable events are as follows:

Object left in surgery
Air embolism
Blood incompatibility
Catheter-associated urinary tract infections
Pressure ulcers
Vascular catheter-associated infection
Surgical site infection-mediastinitis after coronary artery bypass graft surgery (CABG)
Hospital-acquired injuries—fractures, dislocations, intracranial injury, crushing injury, burn, and other unspecified effects of external causes
Medicare is looking at more events to include such as deep vein thrombosis.

Discussion

One can only anticipate what these new rules for payment may mean to providers and practitioners. If the hospital does not get paid, will they not reimburse specific departments that may share care and fiscal responsibility? Who decides if a urinary tract infection (UTI) is a result of negligent care (is that the parameter?), or just one of the things that can happen to a medically compromised individual, whether in a hospital setting or not?

Hospitals now are communicating to their staff that documentation will be key: Present on admission, or POA, may be the term used to refer to potential preventable events that are present when the patient arrives. But if a UTI is not present on admission, what should be done when it turns up 4 days later? No doubt hospitals will require staff to aggressively assess incoming patients so that the hospital will not incur the liability for a UTI or ulcer that may have been present on admission.

Do these rules mean that Medicare considers all these things absolutely preventable? Does that mean they are caused by negligence? Will health-care facilities develop checklists similar to Informed Consent forms and list every conceivable potential event as being not present on admission, not present yet, but an expected consequence of the medical status of the patient, therefore not preventable?

What about the patient who is admitted to a wound care facility for treatment, but their medical status is very precarious and they could be considered at risk for developing more ulcers. Do they bypass the treatment and just go to hospice? Does the wound care facility take the risk of treatment and risk not being paid if other ulcers develop or if the ulcers present on admission do not improve?

These are questions that will be faced by practitioners and facilities alike. Those who deliver the immediate care, the nurses, nurse practitioners, and therapists, may not be reimbursed and may have no recourse. Large hospitals and corporations may not be reimbursed, but no doubt will develop some avenue to gather the money through another vehicle—tax discounts or some other incentives given by the government for the larger players in the health-care arena. (Box 35.1)

Summary

When one understands basic terms, concepts, and procedures involved in the civil legal system, it is easier to see how medical practice and delivery of health care can be impacted. No one wants to be in the midst of a lawsuit as a party-plaintiff or defendant. Being involved on either side is extremely stressful for different reasons, but stressful nonetheless. It is never a

---

▶ **Box 35•1** | **Key Points**

- Practitioners should always be aware that their practice involves legal issues.
- The issues to be determined in medical negligence cases are:
  determining if there was a duty to the patient,
  determining what the standard of care is and if it has been violated, and
  if that violation has caused damages to the complaining party or parties.
- The plaintiff is the person or entity that has suffered damages as a result of another's (the defendant) negligent act or failure to act.
- Negligence in the broadest sense is doing something that a reasonable person would not do under the same or similar circumstances or not doing something that a reasonable person would do under the same or similar circumstances.

- How practitioners of similar specialties would have managed the patient's care under the same or similar circumstances is referred to as the standard of care.
- Damages may be economic and/or noneconomic.
- Discovery is a formal process by which the attorneys for the parties gather information to be used as evidence in preparation for an eventual trial.
- Mediation is a process that is used in almost all cases today in an effort to allow the parties to settle their differences before going to trial.
- An expert witness is a person who is retained by either side in a lawsuit to give expert opinions in a case.
- To avoid becoming a defendant, health-care providers must deliver care that meets the proper standard; it is also important is to communicate with patients and families.

good option to endeavor to discover reasons why things went terribly wrong by filing a lawsuit. This is not the purpose of the legal system.

It is hoped that practitioners can be convinced to talk about difficult outcomes or bad results with patients and families. To be honest about errors made and being forthright regarding fair compensation should be a realistic goal. Health-care providers cannot ask patients to take more responsibility for their own health if those who give care refuse to take responsibility for the care they deliver.

References

1. Wound Ostomy and Continence Nurses Society (WOCN). Guideline for Prevention and Management of Pressure Ulcers, WOCN Clinical Practice Guideline Series. Glenview, IL, WOCN, 2003.

1a. Association of Women's Health, Obstetric and Neonatal Nurses (AWHONN). Neonatal Skin Care Evidence-Based Clinical Practice Guideline. Washington, DC, AWHONN, 2001.

2. National Association of Mutual Insurance Companies (NAMIC). Available at: http://www.namic.org/reports/tortReform/default.asp. Accessed 2004.

3. Damages incurred by a person that may not have an easily ascertainable value or are intangible such as pain and suffering, loss of enjoyment of life.

4. Chimerine, L, Eisenbrey, R: The Frivolous Case for Tort Law Change. Economic Policy Institute, Washington, DC, May 2005.

5. Available at: http://www.epi.org/policy/200505_response_to_ttp-policy_memo.pdf. Accessed July 6, 2007.

6. Available at: http://www.namic.org/reports/tortReform/NoneconomicDamage.asp. Accessed July 7, 2007.

7. Available at: http://www.law.freeadvice.com/resources/personal_injury_statute_of_limitations.htm. Accessed July 9, 2007.

8. All names and locations have been altered.

9. In 2003 the Texas Legislature passed House Bill 4, which capped non-economic damages at $250,000.00. Tex. Civ. Prac. & Rem. Code § 74.301.

10. Braden, B, Bergstrom, N: Clinical utility of the Braden scale for predicting pressure sore risk. Decubitus 1989; 2:44.

11. U. S. Department of Health and Human Services. Clinical Practice Guideline. Pressure Ulcers in Adults: Treatment of Pressure Ulcers. No. 15, Pub. No. 95-0652. Rockville, MD, U.S. Department of Health and Human Services, Public Health Service, Agency for Health Care Policy and Research, 1994.

12. American Medical Association: Principles of Medical Ethics. AMA. E-9.07 Medical Testimony. Available at: http://www.ama-assn.org. Accessed July 14, 2007 per phone conf with Joyce Lilly.

13. Brody, B: Medical Ethics: Analysis of the Issues Raised by the Codes, Opinions, and Statements. Bureau of National Affairs, Inc. Washington, DC, 2001, pp. 508–511.

14. Cohen, JR: Apology and Organizations: Exploring an Example from Medical Practice. Fordham Urban Law Journal, 2000; 27:1447–1482.Kraman, S, Hamm, G: Risk management: Extreme honesty may be the best policy. Annals Internal Med 1999; 12:963.

16. Gerlin, A: Accepting responsibility, by policy. Philadelphia Inquirer, Sept. 14, 1999, p. A18.

17. Braden, BJ, Bergstrom, N: Clinical utility of the Braden scale for predicting pressure sore risk. Decubitus 1989; 2:44.

18. Norton, D: Calculating the risk: Reflections on the Norton scale. Adv Wound Care 1996; 9:38.

19. Gosnell, DJ: Pressure sore risk assessment, a critique, Part I: The Gosnell scale. Decubitus 1989; 2:32(pt 1).

20. Medicare Payments for Surgical Debridement Services in 2004. Report by Department of Health and Human Services, Office of Inspector General, May, 2007. Available at: http://www.oig.hhs.gov/oei/reports/oei-02-05-00390.pdf. Accessed July 14, 2007 per phone conference with Joyce Lilly.

21. Medicare Program; Changes to the Hospital Inpatient Prospective Payment Systems and Fiscal Year 2008 Rates; Correction; Final Rule.

Appendix 1: Braden Scale for Predicting Pressure Sore Risk

Patient's Name: _____   Evaluator's Name: _____   Date of Assessment: _____

	1	2	3	4
SENSORY PERCEPTION Ability to respond meaningfully to pressure-related discomfort	**1. Completely Limited:** Unresponsive (does not moan, flinch or gasp) to painful stimuli due to diminished level of consciousness or sedation OR Limited ability to feel pain over most of body surface.	**2. Very Limited:** Responds only to painful stimuli. Cannot communicate discomfort except by moaning or restlessness. OR Has a sensory impairment that limits the ability to feel pain or discomfort over half of body.	**3. Slightly Limited:** Responds to verbal commands but cannot always communicate discomfort or need to be turned. OR Has some sensory impairment that limits ability to feel pain or discomfort in one or two extremities.	**4. No Impairment:** Responds to verbal commands. Has no sensory deficit that would limit ability to feel or voice pain or discomfort.
MOISTURE Degree to which skin is exposed to moisture	**1. Constantly Moist:** Skin is kept moist almost constantly by perspiration, urine, etc. Dampness is detected every time patient is moved or turned.	**2. Very Moist:** Skin is often but not always moist. Linen must be changed at least once a shift.	**3. Occasionally Moist:** Skin is occasionally moist requiring an extra linen change approximately once a day.	**4. Rarely Moist:** Skin is usually dry. Linen only requires changing at routine intervals.
ACTIVITY Degree of physical activity	**1. Bedfast:** Confined to bed.	**2. Chairfast:** Ability to walk severely limited or non-existent. Cannot bear own weight and/or must be assisted into chair or wheelchair.	**3. Walks Occasionally:** Walks occasionally during day but for very short distances with or without assistance. Spends majority of each shift in bed or chair.	**4. Walks Frequently:** Walks outside the room at least twice a day and inside room at least once every two hours during waking hours.
MOBILITY Ability to change and control body position	**1. Completely Immobile:** Does not make an even slight change in body or extremity position without assistance.	**2. Very Limited:** Makes occasional slight changes in body or extremity position but unable to make frequent or significant changes independently.	**3. Slightly Limited:** Makes frequent, though slight changes in body or extremity position independently.	**4. No Limitations:** Makes major and frequent changes in position without assistance.
NUTRITION *Usual* food intake pattern	**1. Very Poor:** Never eats a complete meal. Rarely eats more than one-third of any food offered. Eats two servings or less of protein (meat or dairy products) per day. Takes fluids poorly. Does not take a liquid dietary supplement. OR Is NPO and/or maintained on clear liquids or IVs for more than five days.	**2. Probably Inadequate:** Rarely eats a complete meal and generally eats only about half of any food offered. Protein intake includes only three servings of meat or dairy products per day. Occasionally will take a dietary supplement. OR Receives less than optimum amount of liquid diet or tube feeding.	**3. Adequate:** Eats over half of most meals. Eats a total of four servings of protein (meat, dairy products) each day. Occasionally will refuse a meal, but will usually take a supplement if offered. OR Is on a tube feeding or TPN regimen that probably meets most of nutritional needs.	**4. Excellent:** Eats most of every meal. Never refuses a meal. Usually eats a total of four or more servings of meat and dairy products. Occasionally eats between meals. Does not require supplementation.
FRICTION AND SHEAR	**1. Problem:** Requires moderate to maximum assistance in moving. Complete lifting without sliding against sheets is impossible. Frequently slides down in bed or chair requiring frequent repositioning with maximum assistance. Spasticity, contractures or agitation leads to almost constant friction.	**2. Potential Problem:** Moves feebly or requires minimum assistance. During a move skin probably slides to some extent against sheets, chair, restraints or other devices. Maintains relatively good position in chair or bed most of the time but occasionally slides down.	**3. No Apparent Problem:** Moves in bed and in chair independently and has sufficient muscle strength to lift up completely during move. Maintains good position in bed or chair at all times.	

Appendix 2: Norton Risk Assessment Scale

		PHYSICAL CONDITION		MENTAL CONDITION		ACTIVITY		MOBILITY		INCONTINENT		TOTAL SCORE
Name	Date	Good 4 Fair 3 Poor 2 V. Bad 1		Alert 4 Apathetic 3 Confused 2 Stupor 1		Ambulant 4 Walk/help 3 Chairbound 2 Bed 1		Full 4 Sl. limited 3 V. limited 2 Immobile 1		Not 4 Occasional 3 Usually/Urine 2 Doubly 1		

Appendix 3: History and Physical Information

ADMISSION INFORMATION **DATE** _____ **TIME** _____

Reason For Visit: _____

Primary Language: _____ Interpreter Needed: ☐ Yes ☐ No

Psycho/Social: _____

Do you have: ☐ Contacts ☐ Glasses ☐ Hearing Aid ☐ Dentures/Partial Plate

Have you had: ☐ Hepatitis ☐ MRSA ☐ HIV Positive ☐ Other _____

Prior Surgeries: _____ Vital Signs: P_____ R_____ BP_____/_____

CURRENT MEDICATIONS (INCLUDE OTC)			
Drug	Dose	Freq	Last Dose

ALLERGIES

DRUGS? ☐ Yes ☐ No
Describe: _____
_____
_____
OTHER? _____
_____
_____
FOOD? _____
_____
_____
Known latex allergy or
sensitivity? ☐ Yes ☐ No
Describe reaction: _____
_____

HISTORY OF SUBSTANCE ABUSE

TOBACCO? ☐ Yes ☐ No
Types & Amount/Day:_____

ALCOHOL? Type & Amount/Day: Time of last alcohol intake: _____	☐ Yes ☐ No
Non prescribed/Non OTC drugs?	☐ Yes ☐ No ☐ N/A
In drug treatment? If yes, where?_____	☐ Yes ☐ No ☐ N/A
Seeking drug treatment?	☐ Yes ☐ No ☐ N/A

CARDIOVASCULAR

☐ Angina
☐ MI
☐ Hypertension
☐ CHF
☐ Coronary Disease
☐ Orthopnea
☐ Rest Pain
☐ Claudication
☐ Varicose Veins
☐ DVT
☐ Other _____
☐ None

NEUROLOGIC

☐ Dizziness
☐ Seizures
☐ Paralysis _____
☐ CVA _____
☐ Other _____
☐ None

ENDOCRINE

☐ _____ Neuropathy
☐ Diabetic since _____
Control: ☐ Insulin ☐ Oral ☐ Diet
• Test blood sugar freq. _____
  Meter used: _____
• Recent reading _____
• Recent HbA1C _____
• Diabetic Teaching _____
  When? _____
• Indications for Diabetes Ed. Referral

PULMONARY

☐ Emphysema
☐ Asthma
☐ Pneumonia
☐ Dyspnea _____
☐ Other _____
☐ None

GENITOURINARY/RENAL

☐ Fecal Incontinence
☐ Urinary Incontinence
☐ Hemodialysis
☐ Peritoneal Dialysis
☐ Other _____
☐ None

FUNCTIONAL MOBILITY

☐ Wheelchair
☐ Ambulate
• Level of Assist _____
• Assistive Device _____

GASTROINTESTINAL

☐ Nausea
☐ Emesis
☐ Bleeding
☐ Cirrhosis
☐ Other _____
☐ None

MUSCULOSKELETAL

☐ Amputation _____
☐ Osteoarthritis
☐ Rheumatoid Arthritis
☐ Endoprosthesis
☐ Contractures _____
_____
☐ History of Falls
☐ Other _____
☐ None

OTHER

(continued)

Appendix 3: History and Physical Information (Continued)

	YES
Do you have an illness that made you change the kind and/or amount of food you eat?	2
Do you eat fewer than two meals per day?	3
Do you eat fewer than two fruits or vegetables or milk products per day?	2
Do you have three or more drinks of beer, liquor or wine almost every day?	2
Do you have tooth or mouth problems that make it hard for you to eat?	2
Do you always have enough money to buy the food you need?	4
Do you eat alone most of the time?	1
Do you take three or more different prescribed or over-the-counter drugs a day?	1
Have you had any unintentional weight loss or gain in the last six months?	2
Are you always physically able to shop and cook for yourself?	2
TOTAL	

TOTAL SCORE

0-2 → Good!
3-5 → Moderate nutritional risk
6 or more → high nutritional risk
More than 3 → refer to Dietitian

WOUND HISTORY

Length of time wound present: _____
Current wound treatment: _____
Provider of wound treatment: _____
Most recent labs: _____
Most recent x-rays: _____
Most recent vascular studies: _____

PERIPHERAL PULSES (Present/Absent)

Dorsalis Pedis	R _____	L _____
Posterior Tibial	R _____	L _____
Popliteal	R _____	L _____
Femoral	R _____	L _____

DOPPLER (None/Mono/Biphasic)

Dorsalis Pedis	R _____	L _____
Posterior Tibial	R _____	L _____
Popliteal	R _____	L _____
Femoral	R _____	L _____

ABI

Ankle Pressure	R _____	L _____
Brachial Pressure	R _____	L _____
$\frac{\text{Ankle}}{\text{Brachial}}$ Index	R _____	L _____

MONOFILAMENT TESTING
(Present/Impaired/Absent)

Foot	R _____	L _____

COMMENTS

_____

_____

_____

_____

_____

_____

_____

Signature/Title _____ Date _____

Appendix 4: Wound Evaluation/Assessment Tool

Date	Site #	Size (cm)				Tissue (%)				Exudate (Amount/Color)				Peri-Wound						Edema (cm)						Tracing/Photo	Pain*	Culture	Sharp Débridement	Treatment Pain	Clinician Initials
		Length x Width	Depth	Tunnel/Sinus	Undermining	Slough	Eschar	Granulation	Serous	Sanguinous	Serosanguinous	Purulent	Intact	Macerated	Hyperpigmented	Hard/Indurated	Dry/Scaly	Weeping	Right MTPs	Right Superior Malleolus	Right 4" Below Tibial Tuberosity	Left MTPs	Left Superior Malleolus	Left 4" Below Tibial Tuberosity		Other Other Other Other				

*Visual Analog Scale (0-10)

Site #	Site Location	Wound Type	Wound Classification		Date	Type of Pain	Pain Threshold

Patient/Caregiver Education

Name/Title	Signature/Title	Initials

Addressograph

Appendix 5: Weekly Measurement Tool

Patient Name: _____ **Date:** _____

Location: _____ Tunnel: _____ o'clock _____ cm
Size (length x width): _____ cm _____ o'clock _____ cm
Depth: _____ cm _____ o'clock _____ cm

Wound base: _____ % red _____ % yellow _____ % black

Odor: _____ present _____ absent

Exudate: _____ color _____ amount

Dressing Type: _____

Frequency Change: _____

Pertinent Labs: _____

Nutritional Supplements: _____

Pressure-Relieving Program/Devices: _____

Clinician Signature/Title: _____

Appendix 6: Wound Care Evaluation

Patient   **Room #:**   **Age:**
Name: _____   _____   _____
Past Medical History: _____
_____
_____

Precautions: _____
_____

For Wound Tracing—See Attached Diagram

Pressure Sore Status Tool
Complete the rating sheet to assess pressure sore status. Evaluate each item by picking the response that best describes the wound and entering the score in the item score column for the appropriate date.

Location: Anatomic Site. Circle, identify right (R) or left (L) and use **"X"** to mark site on body diagrams:

_____ Sacrum & Coccyx   _____ Lateral Ankle
_____ Trochanter   _____ Medial Ankle
_____ Ischial Tuberosity   _____ Heel   Other site _____

Shape: Overall wound pattern: assess by observing perimeter and depth. Circle and date appropriate description:

_____ Irregular   _____ Linear or elongated
_____ Round/Oval   _____ Bowl/Boat
_____ Square/Rectangle   _____ Butterfly   Other site _____

Item	Assessment	#1 Score	#2 Score	#3 Score
1. Size	1 = Length x width < 4 sq cm 2 = Length x width 4-16 sq cm 3 = Length x width 16.1-36 sq cm 4 = Length x width 36.1-80 sq cm 5 = Length x width > 80 sq cm			
2. Depth	1 = Non-blanchable erythema on intact skin 2 = Partial thickness skin loss involving epidermis and/or dermis 3 = Full thickness skin loss involving damage or necrosis of subcutaneous tissue; may extend down to but not through underlying fascia; and/or mixed partial and full thickness and/or tissue layers obscured by granulation tissue. 4 = Obscured by necrosis 5 = Full thickness skin loss with extensive destruction, tissue necrosis or damage to muscle, bone or supporting structures			
3. Edges	1 = Indistinct, diffuse, none clearly visible 2 = Distinct, outline clearly visible, attached, even with wound base 3 = Well-defined, not attached to wound base 4 = Well-defined, not attached to wound base, rolled under, thickened 5 = Well-defined, fibrotic, scarred or hyperkeratotic			
4. Undermining	1 = Undermining < 2 cm in any area 2 = Undermining 2-4 cm involving < 50% wound margins 3 = Undermining 2-4 cm involving > 50% wound margins 4 = Undermining > 4 cm in any area 5 = Tunneling and/or sinus tract formation			
5. Necrotic Tissue Type	1 = Non visible 2 = White/gray non-viable tissue and/or non-adherent yellow 3 = Loosely adherent yellow slough 4 = Adherent, soft, black eschar 5 = Firmly adherent, soft, black eschar			

(continued)

Appendix 6: Wound Care Evaluation (Continued)

Item	Assessment	#1 Score	#2 Score	#3 Score
6. Necrotic Tissue Amount	1 = Non visible 2 = < 25% of wound bed covered 3 = 25% to 50% of wound covered 4 = > 50% and < 75% of wound covered 5 = 75% to 100% of wound covered			
7. Exudate Type	1 = None or bloody 2 = Serosanguineous: thin, watery, pale red/pink 3 = Serous: thin, watery, clear 4 = Purulent: thin or thick, opaque, tan/yellow 5 = Foul purulent: thick, opaque, yellow/green with odor			
8. Exudate Amount	1 = None 2 = Scant 3 = Small 4 = Moderate 5 = Large			
9. Skin Color Surrounding Wound	1 = Pink or normal for ethnic group 2 = Bright red and/or blanches to touch 3 = White or gray pallor or hypopigmented 4 = Dark red or purple and/or non-blanchable 5 = Black or hyperpigmented			
10. Peripheral Tissue Edema	1 = Minimal swelling around wound 2 = Non-pitting edema extends < 4 cm around wound 3 = Non-pitting edema extends ≥ 4 cm around wound 4 = Pitting edema extends < 4 cm around wound 5 = Crepitus and/or pitting edema extends ≥ 4 cm			
11. Peripheral Tissue	1 = Minimal firmness around wound 2 = Induration < 2 cm around wound 3 = Induration 2-4 cm extending < 50% around wound 4 = Induration 2-4 cm extending ≥ 50% around wound 5 = Induration > 4 cm in any area			
12. Granulation Tissue	1 = Skin intact or partial thickness wound 2 = Bright, beefy red; 75% to 100% of wound filled and/or tissue overgrowth 3 = Bright, beefy red; < 75% and > 25% of wound filled 4 = Pink and/or dull, dusky red and/or fills ≤ 25% around wound 5 = No granulation tissue present			
13. Epithelialization	1 = 100% wound covered, surface intact 2 = 75% to <100% wound covered and/or epithelial tissue extends > 0.5 cm into wound bed 3 = 50% to < 75% wound covered and/or epithelial tissue extends to < 0.5 cm into wound bed 4 = 25% to < 50% wound covered 5 = < 25% wound covered			
	TOTAL SCORE			

Pressure Sore Status Continuum

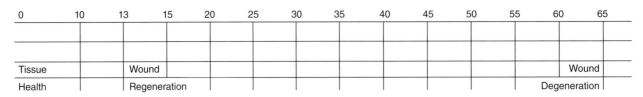

Plot the total score on the Pressure Sore Status Continuum by putting an "**X**" on the line and the date beneath the line. Plot multiple scores with their dates to see-at-a-glance regeneration or degeneration of the wound.

Short Term Treatment Goals:

1. Decrease wound size by _____ cm or decrease total surface area of wound by _____ cm.

2. Promote granulation by _____%.

3. Decrease necrotic tissue by _____% or decrease total surface of necrotic tissue by _____%.

4. Decrease edema to grade _____. (Grades 1-4)

5. Decrease amount of drainage to _____ (small, moderate, large).

6. Decrease odor to _____ (minimum, moderate, strong).

7. Decrease erythema to _____ (minimum, moderate, severe).

8. Decrease tunneling by _____ cm.

9. Educate staff/family/patient. Teach staff/family/patient _____. (Be specific.)

10. Assess pressure-relieving devices, splinting, equipment modification, positioning, etc.

Long Term Treatment Goals:

1. Reduce wound from stage _____ to stage _____.

2. Patient is maintaining proper nutritional status.

3. Staff/family/patient safe and competent in protecting and preventing reoccurrence.

Plan: _____

_____

_____

_____

_____

_____

_____

_____

_____

_____

See Dietary Consult for nutritional status

Nursing Signature: _____ Date: _____

Therapist Signature: _____ Date: _____

Appendix 7: Weekly Wound Care Progress Note

Patient
Name: _____   Room #: _____   Age: _____

For Wound Tracing—See Attached Diagram

Pressure Sore Status Tool
Complete the rating sheet to assess pressure sore status. Evaluate each item by picking the response that best describes the wound and entering the score in the item score column for the appropriate date.

Location: Anatomic Site. Circle, identify right (R) or left (L) and use "**X**" to mark site on body diagrams:

_____ Sacrum & Coccyx	_____ Lateral Ankle	
_____ Trochanter	_____ Medial Ankle	
_____ Ischial Tuberosity	_____ Heel	Other site _____

Shape: Overall wound pattern: assess by observing perimeter and depth. Circle and date appropriate description:

_____ Irregular	_____ Linear or elongated	
_____ Round/Oval	_____ Bowl/Boat	
_____ Square/Rectangle	_____ Butterfly	Other site _____

Item	Assessment	#1 Score	#2 Score	#3 Score
1. Size	1 = Length x width < 4 sq cm 2 = Length x width 4-16 sq cm 3 = Length x width 16.1-36 sq cm 4 = Length x width 36.1-80 sq cm 5 = Length x width > 80 sq cm			
2. Depth	1 = Non-blanchable erythema on intact skin 2 = Partial thickness skin loss involving epidermis and/or dermis 3 = Full thickness skin loss involving damage or necrosis of subcutaneous tissue; may extend down to but not through underlying fascia; and/or mixed partial and full thickness and/or tissue layers obscured by granulation tissue. 4 = Obscured by necrosis 5 = Full thickness skin loss with extensive destruction, tissue necrosis or damage to muscle, bone or supporting structures			
3. Edges	1 = Indistinct, diffuse, none clearly visible 2 = Distinct, outline clearly visible, attached, even with wound base 3 = Well-defined, not attached to wound base 4 = Well-defined, not attached to wound base, rolled under, thickened 5 = Well-defined, fibrotic, scarred or hyperkeratotic			
4. Undermining	1 = Undermining < 2 cm in any area 2 = Undermining 2-4 cm involving < 50% wound margins 3 = Undermining 2-4 cm involving > 50% wound margins 4 = Undermining > 4 cm in any area 5 = Tunneling and/or sinus tract formation			
5. Necrotic Tissue Type	1 = Non visible 2 = White/gray non-viable tissue and/or non-adherent yellow 3 = Loosely adherent yellow slough 4 = Adherent, soft, black eschar 5 = Firmly adherent, soft, black eschar			
6. Necrotic Tissue Amount	1 = Non visible 2 = < 25% of wound bed covered 3 = 25% to 50% of wound covered 4 = > 50% and < 75% of wound covered 5 = 75% to 100% of wound covered			

Item	Assessment	#1	#2	#3
		Score	Score	Score
7. Exudate Type	1 = None or bloody 2 = Serosanguineous: thin, watery, pale red/pink 3 = Serous: thin, watery, clear 4 = Purulent: thin or thick, opaque, tan/yellow 5 = Foul purulent: thick, opaque, yellow/green with odor			
8. Exudate Amount	1 = None 2 = Scant 3 = Small 4 = Moderate 5 = Large			
9. Skin Color Surrounding Wound	1 = Pink or normal for ethnic group 2 = Bright red and/or blanches to touch 3 = White or gray pallor or hypopigmented 4 = Dark red or purple and/or non-blanchable 5 = Black or hyperpigmented			
10. Peripheral Tissue Edema	1 = Minimal swelling around wound 2 = Non-pitting edema extends < 4 cm around wound 3 = Non-pitting edema extends ≥ 4 cm around wound 4 = Pitting edema extends < 4 cm around wound 5 = Crepitus and/or pitting edema extends ≥ 4 cm			
11. Peripheral Tissue	1 = Minimal firmness around wound 2 = Induration < 2 cm around wound 3 = Induration 2-4 cm extending < 50% around wound 4 = Induration 2-4 cm extending ≥ 50% around wound 5 = Induration > 4 cm in any area			
12. Granulation Tissue	1 = Skin intact or partial thickness wound 2 = Bright, beefy red; 75% to 100% of wound filled and/or tissue overgrowth 3 = Bright, beefy red; < 75% and > 25% of wound filled 4 = Pink and/or dull, dusky red and/or fills ≤ 25% around wound 5 = No granulation tissue present			
13. Epithelialization	1 = 100% wound covered, surface intact 2 = 75% to <100% wound covered and/or epithelial tissue extends > 0.5 cm into wound bed 3 = 50% to < 75% wound covered and/or epithelial tissue extends to < 0.5 cm into wound bed 4 = 25% to < 50% wound covered 5 = < 25% wound covered			
	TOTAL SCORE			

Pressure Sore Status Continuum

0	10	13	15	20	25	30	35	40	45	50	55	60	65
Tissue Health		Wound Regeneration										Wound Degeneration	

Plot the total score on the Pressure Sore Status Continuum by putting an "**X**" on the line and the date beneath the line. Plot multiple scores with their dates to see-at-a-glance regeneration or degeneration of the wound.

(continued)

Appendix 7: Weekly Wound Care Progress Note (Continued)

Short Term Treatment Goals:

1. Decrease wound size by _____ cm or decrease total surface area of wound by _____ cm.

2. Promote granulation by _____%.

3. Decrease necrotic tissue by _____% or decrease total surface of necrotic tissue by _____%.

4. Decrease edema to grade _____. (Grades 1-4)

5. Decrease amount of drainage to _____ (small, moderate, large).

6. Decrease odor to _____ (minimum, moderate, strong).

7. Decrease erythema to _____ (minimum, moderate, severe).

8. Decrease tunneling by _____ cm.

9. Educate staff/family/patient. Teach staff/family/patient _____. (Be specific.)

10. Assess pressure-relieving devices, splinting, equipment modification, positioning, etc.

Plan: _____

_____

_____

_____

_____

_____

_____

_____

_____

_____

_____

_____

_____

_____

See Dietary Consult for nutritional status

Nursing Signature: _____ Date: _____

Therapist Signature: _____ Date: _____

Appendix 8: Initial Wound Assessment and Treatment Plan

Patient Name:	**Date of Evaluation:**

Location:

Type:

Measurements (Length x Width x Depth):

Wound Base:

Signs/Symptoms of Infection (Yes/No):

Girth Measures:

Sensation:

Peripheral Pulses:

Other Tests (TCPO$_2$, Vascular Studies, X-Rays, Labs, etc.):

Consultations (MD, Rehab, Social Services, Home Health, Diabetes Education, etc.):

Treatment Plan (include plan, DME, home dressing supplies):

1.

2.

3.

4.

5.

6.

Appendix 9: Annotated Multiple Choice Questions

Chapter 1

1. The two major layers of the skin are:
   a. Epidermis and subdermis
   b. Epidermis and dermis
   c. Dermis and subcutaneous
   d. Dermal and fatty layer

ANSWER: B The skin is classically subdivided into two major components, the epidermis and the dermis.

2. How frequently does the epidermis typically regenerate?
   a. 1–3 weeks
   b. 4–6 weeks
   c. 7–9 weeks
   d. 10–12 weeks

ANSWER: B The epidermis is a thin outer layer of skin. It is an avascular layer that regenerates itself every 4 to 6 weeks.

3. Up to 75% of the skin's total dry weight is composed of
   a. elastin.
   b. collagen.
   c. keratin.
   d. sebum.

ANSWER: B Collagen is the most abundant structural protein in the body and accounts for upward to 75% of the skin's total dry weight.

4. The outermost layer of the epidermis is termed the stratum
   a. corneum.
   b. granulosum.
   c. spinosum.
   d. basale.

ANSWER: A The outermost layer of the epidermis is the stratum corneum and is composed of dead keratinocytes.

Chapter 2

1. Which of the following is the correct sequential order of the phases of healing?
   a. Remodeling, inflammation, hemostasis, and repair
   b. Inflammation, hemostasis, proliferation, and maturation
   c. Hemostasis, inflammation, repair, and remodeling
   d. Inflammation, maturation, proliferation, and hemostasis

ANSWER: C Each phase of wound healing serves as a prerequisite for the following stage. During hemostasis, bleeding ceases and a fibrin clot develops to serve as a provisional matrix for infiltrating inflammatory and repair cells. Inflammation is a necessary next step to clear bacteria and debris before repair cells begin to proliferate in the wound bed. The proliferative (repair) phase follows inflammation with the capacity to fill in the defect with neovascular structures, fibroblasts, and new matrix proteins. The remodeling (maturation) phase is last and longest and consists of normalization of vascularity and collagen composition and strength over time.

2. Which of the following leukocytes is responsible for the initial attack on bacteria at the wound site?
   a. B lymphocyte
   b. T lymphocyte
   c. Macrophage
   d. Neutrophil

ANSWER: D Neutrophils are the first line of defense against bacteria and are filled with antibacterial and bactericidal agents in their granules. Macrophages appear on the scene next to clear the debris left in the wake of neutrophils. Lymphocytes are recruited during the later stages of inflammation and repair and have directed activity against specific bacterial antigens.

3. Contraction of the wound margin is the hallmark sign of:
   a. keratinocyte migration.
   b. keloid formation.
   c. myofibroblast differentiation.
   d. the repair phase.

ANSWER: C When fibroblasts sense tension in the extracellular matrix, they differentiate into myofibroblasts, marked by their expression of α-SMA, which gives them contractile properties. These contractile myofibroblasts adhere to the collagen matrix and have the capacity to pull the wound margins toward themselves. Keloid formation is thought to be the result of persistent myofibroblast activity due to overexpression of TGF-β and α-SMA, adding to tension and additional contracture and scarring. The hallmarks of the repair phase include granulation tissue in early repair and keratinocyte coverage in late repair phase.

4. Which of the following coupled molecules participate in the firm adhesion of leukocytes to the vessel wall prior to diapedesis?
   a. CD44 and hyaluronan
   b. E-selectin and surface carbohydrate
   c. Integrins and ICAM/VCAM
   d. P-selectin and surface carbohydrate

ANSWER: C Activated integrins on the leukocyte surface bind ICAM and VCAM on the endothelial surface to produce shear-resistant, high-affinity interactions that arrest the leukocyte on the vessel's luminal surface. These interactions are called firm adhesions. The other three choices (CD44 and hyaluronan, surface carbohydrates and E-selectin/P-selectin) are involved in the initial phase of "rolling." These interactions are transient with low-affinity binding capacity so they serve to slow the leukocyte down in the bloodstream but are not firm enough to arrest.

Chapter 3

1. Which matrix protein provides mechanical strength to the wound site?
a. Fibrin
b. Collagen
c. Fibronectin
d. Proteoglycan

ANSWER: B Collagen is elaborated by fibroblasts and provides the principal source of mechanical strength in the wound.

2. The basement membrane serves to:
a. provide a protective layer over the wound surface.
b. prevent cell migration.
c. separate epithelial and connective tissue cells.
d. anchor subcutaneous fat to underlying structures.

ANSWER: C The basement membrane is a specialized layer of extracellular matrix that defines the boundary between the epithelial sheet and the underlying connective tissue.

3. What is a key activity of fibroblast growth factor-2?
a. Inflammation
b. Extracellular matrix formation
c. Angiogenesis
d. Cell enlargement

ANSWER: C Fibroblast growth factor can stimulate fibroblast growth, but one of its most prominent actions is to stimulate the growth and movement of vascular endothelial cells, leading to the formation of new microcirculation through the process of angiogenesis.

4. Which of the following growth factors is unique in that some of it may reach the wound site from the liver?
a. IGF
b. PDGF
c. HGF
d. EGF

ANSWER: C HGF, which stands for hepatocyte growth factor, can reach the wound in an inactive form from the liver. It may be particularly useful in transforming sedentary epidermal keratinocytes cells into migratory ones.

Chapter 4

1. Which of the following is associated with the initial stages of starvation?
a. There is an increase in metabolic rate.
b. Glycogen stores in the liver are exhausted.
c. Muscle mass decreases.
d. Ketone bodies provide a small amount of the needed energy.

ANSWER: B In starvation there is a general decrease in metabolic rate within 24 hours after the onset of starvation. During these first 24 hours, glycogen stores in the liver are exhausted as an early form of nutrition. The body knows to increase mobilization of fatty acids from fat stores to preserve overall muscle mass.

In the process of starvation, the brain, which normally uses glucose, can actually use products from fatty acid metabolism known as ketone bodies. In the presence of starvation, ketone bodies mobilized from fatty acids can provide up to 70% of the body's normal energy requirements.

2. Which of the following occurs in response to stress?
a. There is increased vascular resistance.
b. Cardiac output decreases.
c. Hyperglycemia frequently develops.
d. Muscle starts to be sacrificed.

ANSWER: C In the stress response, which usually follows an injury or severe stress such as a septic event, there is an overall change in the cardiac and vascular physiology with a decreased systemic vascular resistance that causes lower blood pressures. This, in turn, causes elevated cardiac output, increasing the metabolic demands of the heart. This is usually accompanied by fever and overall inability to use glucose normally, which leads to hyperglycemia. Additionally, muscle is sacrificed to power the body in this time of stress.

3. The condition in infants younger than 1 year of age manifested by severe muscle wasting caused by protein-energy malnutrition is known as
a. marasmus.
b. kwashiorkor.
c. avitaminosis.
d. mineral deficiency.

ANSWER: A Severe calorie deprivation in infants leads to wasting known as marasmus. These patients often have concomitant vitamin and mineral deficiencies and may sometimes have normal visceral protein levels but have had significant weight loss. Common causes of marasmus include cancer and chronic obstructive pulmonary disease (COPD). Kwashiorkor is a similar condition that occurs after the age of 18 months.

4. Which laboratory test is most cost effective and gives a fairly good representation of the current state of protein nutrition?
a. Albumin
b. Prealbumin
c. Transferrin
d. Retinal-binding protein

ANSWER: B The classic visceral protein measurement is albumin. Unfortunately, albumin has a long half-life, upward of 20 days, and can be very sensitive to hydration status, which may be problematic in hepatic or renal disease. Other, more accurate measures of visceral protein are transferrin and retinal-binding protein. These are not widely available, however, and are expensive to use. Prealbumin has been the most widely used measure of protein over the last 10 to 15 years. It has a short, reasonable half-life of 48 to 72 hours, which, when monitored twice weekly, will allow for intervention and follow-up to be made in the same week. Prealbumin is not affected by dehydration or overall hydration status, has a relatively small body pool, and in modern tests is not affected by renal failure.

5. Alternative ways of assessing nutritional status include all of the following *except*:
   a. evaluation of dentures (fix, use, etc.).
   b. social status.
   c. cultural eating habits and food choices.
   d. skin turgor.

ANSWER: D Classic ways of assessing a patient's nutritional status include questionnaires and visceral proteins, but alternative methods can also be used. Alternative methods can include anything that affects a patients eating ability or affects their food choices, such as economic status, ability to obtain and cook food, and any cultural or religious factors that affect food intake. Skin turgor is a sign of hydration status. It is not a sign of food intake, or considered a nutritional assessment tool.

6. Using an alternative assessment for nutrition, which of the following is considered a risk for possible malnourishment?
   a. Vegetarian diet with proper supplements
   b. Good fitting and properly maintained dentures
   c. Elderly widowed patient who lives alone
   d. Elderly widower who lives in a retirement community

ANSWER: C Vegetarians do lack some nutrients that are important in many bodily activates and functions. These deficiencies can easily be overcome with standard supplements. Well-fitting dentures are an important part of mastication, which is the first part of food intake via the gastrointestinal tract. Older individuals are at higher risk for malnutrition than younger persons, but this can be over come by close social contact or by ensuring a person has food delivery or someone who prepares their meals on a regular basis.

7. When treating patients for protein energy malnutrition, one must provide calories to sustain normal body function in the form of what?
   a. Carbohydrates and fats
   b. Complex proteins
   c. Collagen
   d. Fibronectin

ANSWER: A Calories to provide energy to the body are different from those used for rebuilding tissue. Wound healing requires protein to form collagen and other building blocks, such as fibronectin, a protein used in the matrix substance. Calories to provide energy should be provided as carbohydrates and fats, otherwise the body must use its own store of protein.

8. In treating malnutrition one must provide energy and substrates for healing. Interventions can be complex to very simple. Which of the following are simple ways to intervene?
   a. Total parenteral nutrition (IV food)
   b. Eating one large meal per day
   c. Instant breakfast powder and milk
   d. mRNA-enhanced formulas

ANSWER: C Many complex supplements and interventions are available to assist in providing a patient with nutritional support.

Unfortunately, most health-care providers fail to start any intervention, even something as simple as instant breakfast and whole milk.

Chapter 5

1. Which of the following statements is correct concerning the microcirculation?
   a. The microcirculation can be assessed using a detailed physical exam.
   b. The presence of a palpable pulse on physical exam will always result in adequate tissue perfusion and healing.
   c. Hyperspectral analysis, transcutaneous oxygen monitoring, and laser Doppler imaging can help the clinician assess the macrocirculation.
   d. The microcirculation should be measured in addition to the macrocirculation when working up a patient with a nonhealing wound.

ANSWER: D A patient with a non-healing wound should be assessed on both the macrovascular and micro-vascular levels. They may have compromised macrovascular flow but due to compensatory mechanisms such as the development of collateral flow be able to heal a wound.

2. All of the following has a known negative effect on healing *except*:
   a. history of diabetes.
   b. patient depression.
   c. low level bacterial colonization.
   d. obesity.

ANSWER: C Many bacteria are present in the norma flora of our skin and may appear in the wound bed. The simple presence of low level bacterial colonization has not been demonstrated to delay wound healing.

3. The following medications have a potential negative impact on wound healing, *except*:
   a. steroids.
   b. vitamin A.
   c. cox 2 inhibitors.
   d. ace inhibitors.

ANSWER: B Several studies have suggested that Vitamin A has been demonstrated to reverse the negative effects of steroids on healing. Though this has been challenged by some, vitamin A has not been noted to impede healing.

Chapter 6

1. Which of the following are the common areas of assessment in the Braden, Norton, Gosnell, and Waterlow scales/scores?
   a. Patient mobility/activity and moisture/incontinence
   b. Mental status and moisture/incontinence
   c. Sensation and friction/shear
   d. Age and nutrition/appetite

ANSWER: A All four of the tools listed have in common the assessment of patient mobility/activity and moisture/continence.

2. You are assessing a patient with a pressure ulcer. The wound bed is 80% slough and 20% black eschar. Which of the following is the accurate stage for this wound?
   a. Stage II
   b. Stage III
   c. Stage IV
   d. Unstageable

ANSWER: D If the wound base is covered with slough and/or eschar, then the clinician cannot stage the ulcer.

3. The clinician removes the wound dressings and finds there is a minimal amount of wound exudate that is pink or reddish in color. Which of the following is the accurate assessment of this wound exudate?
   a. The color and amount of exudate are a concern, since the wound is probably infected.
   b. This is serous drainage; it is normal exudate for a wound in the proliferative stage.
   c. Wounds should not be exhibiting drainage, thus this wound must be left open to dry.
   d. Minimal serosanguinous exudate is a normal for an inflamed or proliferating wound.

ANSWER: D Minimal serosanguinous exudate, which is pinkish/reddish, is a normal finding for a wound in inflammation or proliferation. Exudate in an infected wound will most likely be yellow, green, tan, and blue and have an odor. Serous drainage is clear in color, not pink/reddish. Wounds should not be left open to dry. Wounds need moisture to heal.

4. Which of the following appear to be plausible predictors of positive wound healing?
   a. Younger patient with good vascular status and normal limb girth
   b. Adherence to recommended interventions and wound exudate
   c. Small initial size, wound dimensions decrease, and shorter wound duration
   d. If no comorbidities, good nutrition and the dressings appropriate

ANSWER: C Venous, neuropathic, and pressure ulcer prognostic literature is pointing toward smaller, shorter-duration wounds being more likely to heal. Wounds that decrease in size in the first 2 to 4 weeks of interventions are more likely to heal.

Chapter 7

1. Which vascular test involves an assessment of color changes on the plantar surface of the foot?
   a. Venous filling time
   b. Trendelenburg
   c. Rubor of dependency
   d. Capillary refill

ANSWER: C In the rubor of dependency test, a patient's leg is elevated to drain venous blood and is then lowered to the bed and an assessment made of how long it takes for arterial blood to refill the capillaries on the bottom of the foot. In arterial disease, filling is slowed, and when capillaries finally fill, the foot turns a bright red. This is reported as a positive rubor of dependency test.

2. Which of the following could cause a false negative when performing a venous filling time test?
   a. Valvular incompetence
   b. Atherosclerosis
   c. Hypertension
   d. Bradycardia

ANSWER: A In the venous filling time test, the examiner evaluates arterial blood flow by measuring the speed with which superficial veins refill through the arterial pathway following emptying. If venous valvular incompetence is present, blood can retroflow in the venous system and refill the foot veins, thereby giving the appearance that arterial flow is adequate.

3. In performing an ankle-brachial index (ABI) test the examiner notes a brachial pressure of 120 mm Hg and an ankle pressure of 130 mm Hg. This should be reported as an ABI of:
   a. 120 mm Hg
   b. 12:13
   c. 1.08
   d. 10

ANSWER: C The ABI represents a measurement obtained by dividing the systolic pressure in the lower extremity by the systolic pressure in the upper extremity, which in this case would give a value of 1.08.

4. When performing a Semmes-Weinstein monofilament test, a patient is noted to have lost protective sensation when he first cannot feel a monofilament that applies how many grams of force?
   a. 5
   b. 10
   c. 15
   d. 20

ANSWER: B The 5.07 monofilament takes 10 grams of force to bend. If patients cannot perceive this degree of pressure, studies have indicated that they have lost their protective sensation and are at an increased risk of developing a plantar ulcer.

Chapter 8

1. Which of the following is true regarding bacteria found within biofilms?
   a. They are described as planktonic.
   b. They may be multiple species and reside in a protective polysaccharide matrix.
   c. They are the easiest to target with antimicrobials.
   d. They are easily visualized on the surface of the wound.

ANSWER: B Biofilms are complex communities of bacteria and other microorganisms that adhere to solid surfaces. These communities are embedded in an extracellular polysaccharide matrix or glycocalyx, which protects the bacteria from human immune cells, phagocytic cells, and antimicrobial agents. Under the right conditions, all bacteria can grow a biofilm.

2. Levine's technique for obtaining a culture specimen involves:
   a. swabbing the entire wound from the top to the bottom in a sweeping motion.
   b. obtaining a specimen from the residual exudate from the previous dressing.
   c. cleansing the wound and identifying the area clean and free from necrotic tissue.
   d. cutting a piece of tissue from the deepest section of the wound.

ANSWER: C The Levine technique involves thoroughly cleansing the wound surface and identifying a 1-cm area of the wound that is free from necrotic tissue. The swab is rotated while applying pressure sufficient to express fluid from the wound tissue. This technique is thought to yield the most accurate results, compared to the Z-stroke or, most certainly, swabbing residual exudate at the time of dressing removal.

3. The foundation for wound bed preparation includes all of the following *except*:
   a. cleansing of the wound.
   b. management of bioburden and infection.
   c. débridement of nonviable tissue with attention to edges.
   d. use of an advanced or biological dressing to enhance the wound bed.

ANSWER: D The concept of wound bed preparation implies preliminary care to prepare a wound to heal. The foundation for wound bed preparation—cleansing, débridement of necrotic or nonviable tissue with attention to wound edges, and management and prevention of infection—must be part of every wound encounter and integrated into routine care.

Chapter 9

1. When imaging the deep tissues in a child, consideration should be given to ultrasound because:
   a. MRI uses ionizing radiation.
   b. CT does not use ionizing radiation.
   c. ultrasound does not use ionizing radiation.
   d. children's tissue is not radiosensitive.

ANSWER: C Children are particularly vulnerable to the long-term and cumulative tissue effects of ionizing radiation ("d" is incorrect), and for this reason consideration should first be given to nonionizing modalities when soft tissue imaging is needed. Ultrasound does not use ionizing radiation ("c" is correct), can be performed portably, and is widely available. MRI does not use ionizing radiation ("a" is incorrect), and can be used

for deep soft tissue and bone marrow imaging in appropriate circumstances.

2. Safety in the magnetic resonance environment includes all of the following *except*:
   a. using only items specially designed for or compatible with a strong magnetic field.
   b. allowing the patient to enter the MR area in his or her own wheelchair.
   c. screening patients for implantable devices and foreign bodies such as pacemakers and shrapnel.
   d. restricting access to the area.

ANSWER: B The magnetic resonance (MR) scanner consists of a large superconducting magnet that produces a static strong magnetic field, and the surrounding area is restricted. Patients, personnel, and equipment must be screened before entry into the MR environment, and only specially designed wheelchairs and medical equipment are accommodated. Items "a," "c," and "d" are all performed to ensure safety. The correct answer is "b."

3. The oral antihyperglycemic metformin needs to be temporarily discontinued when obtaining:
   a. ultrasound.
   b. MR without contrast.
   c. CT with intravenous contrast.
   d. nuclear medicine procedures.

ANSWER: C Intravenous contrast studies with iodinated materials can lead to acute alteration of renal function and have been associated with lactic acidosis in patients receiving metformin ("c" is correct). Oral diabetes medications have no adverse effect on MR without contrast or ultrasound and would not need to be discontinued for nuclear medicine studies.

4. Diagnostic Ultrasound:
   a. is not a useful imaging modality for venous evaluation of the extremities.
   b. can be performed portably at the bedside of critically ill patients.
   c. employs a focused beam of x-rays.
   d. uses gadolinium contrast agents.

ANSWER: B Ultrasound uses pulsed focused sound, not an x-ray beam ("c" is incorrect), and is the procedure of choice for extremity venous evaluation ("a" is incorrect). Lack of ionizing radiation and the ability to be performed portably at the bedside of ill patients ("b" is correct) are advantages of this modality. Gadolinium chelate contrast agents are widely used in magnetic resonance imaging, not ultrasound ("d" is incorrect).

5. The most helpful imaging in the *early* detection of clinically suspected osteomyelitis is:
   a. ultrasound.
   b. CT.
   c. catheter angiography.
   d. nuclear medicine bone scan.

ANSWER: D CT is excellent for depiction of bone destruction and periosteal reaction, but initial findings of bone infection are in the marrow and not well depicted by CT early in the process ("b" is incorrect). Magnetic resonance imaging and nuclear medicine bone scans play a greater role in detecting the edema and hyperemia of inflammation before osseous changes ensue ("d" is correct), and three-phase bone scans may be abnormal as early as 24 to 72 hours after initial infection. Ultrasound is insensitive to marrow changes, as the sound beam cannot penetrate cortical bone ("a" is incorrect), and catheter angiography allows study of the vasculature, rather than the bone marrow ("c" is incorrect).

Chapter 10

1. Which of the following diseases demonstrates pathergy?
   a. Vasculitis
   b. Mycetoma
   c. Pyoderma gangrenosum
   d. Necrotizing fasciitis

ANSWER: C Mechanistically in susceptible patients, pathergy plays a role in pyoderma gangrenosum PG lesion development. Pathergy is described when lesions are induced to develop in areas of known trauma or injury. It is estimated that approximately 25% of PG patients experience the pathergy phenomenon.

2. Twenty-five percent magnesium sulphate should be applied to which of the following types of chemical burns?
   a. Squaric acid
   b. Hydrofluoric acid
   c. Chromic acid
   d. Phenol

ANSWER: B Copious irrigation with saline for at least 30 minutes to all areas exposed to the chemical agent is the initial standard of care for chemical burn victims. Certain chemicals require additional therapy because of their unique properties. If burned by hydrofluoric acid, one should apply 25% magnesium sulphate. If chromic acid is the culprit, it is best to excise the affected area if possible, and if exposed to phenol, one should apply a 2:1 mixture of polyethylene glycol and ethanol.

3. Marjolin ulcer refers to which type of cancer?
   a. Melanoma
   b. Lymphoma
   c. Basal cell carcinoma
   d. Squamous cell carcinoma

ANSWER: D Malignant degeneration of a wound into a squamous cell carcinoma, the so-called Marjolin ulcer, chiefly affects middle-aged to elderly males who have had a preexisting condition for a chronic period of time, such as 20 to 50 years.

4. Which of the following conditions is also called rose gardener's disease?
   a. Sporotrichosis
   b. Chromomycosis
   c. *Mycobacterium marinum*
   d. Paracoccidioidomycosis

ANSWER: A Sporotrichosis, also known as rose gardener's disease, is a subcutaneous mycosis caused by the dimorphic fungal organism *Sporothrix schenckii*. The disease is a consequence of traumatic inoculation of the fungus deep into the skin, most commonly acquired via a prick by a contaminated rose thorn.

Chapter 11

1. The fastest, most efficacious means to remove necrotic tissue is by:
   a. maggot débridement therapy.
   b. autolytic débridement.
   c. enzymatic débridement.
   d. surgical/sharp débridement.

ANSWER: D The other methods are more conservative and require as much as a few days to weeks to liquefy the necrotic tissue. Although they may be tolerated better by some patients, surgical or sharp débridement is still considered the fastest means and should always be the method of choice in light of serious infection.

2. Which mechanical débridement method has been shown to be least detrimental to granulation tissue, while still effectively removing surface bacteria and loose necrotic tissue?
   a. Whirlpool
   b. Water Pik
   c. Pulsed lavage with suction
   d. Wet-to-dry dressings

ANSWER: C Pulsed lavage with suction, using an impact pressure between 4 and 15 psi, has been recommended to effectively reduce surface bacteria and remove necrotic tissue. Haynes et al showed an increase in granulation tissue formation while using PLWS, when compared with those receiving whirlpool treatment. There is insufficient research to show that whirlpool effectively débrides while not harming granulation tissue. The impact pressure of whirlpool is not consistent or known. Water Pik impact pressure can easily exceed 15 psi, and there is no suction associated with it to aid in removal of necrotic tissue. Wet-to-dry dressing has been shown to be traumatic to granulation tissue, as evidenced by pain, bleeding, and adherence of the dressing to the wound bed.

3. Which of the following statements is *incorrect* concerning débridement?
   a. Enzymatic débridement requires a physician order/prescription for the topical agent.
   b. Physical therapists performing sharp débridement should progress until a bleeding base is observed.
   c. The active wound care management CPT® code of 97598 should be billed if PLWS is performed on a wound with a surface area measuring greater than 24 cm².
   d. PLWS treatment must be performed in a private room with walls and a door that shuts.

ANSWER: B Sharp débridement involves the removal of only nonviable tissue. There should not be any bleeding associated with sharp débridement. Although a bleeding base is thought to stimulate growth factor release, only surgical débridement involves wide excision of both viable and nonviable tissue. Surgical débridement is not within the scope of practice of physical therapists or nurses.

4. The framework for wound bed preparation includes all of the following concepts *except*:
   a. Selecting appropriate dressings to achieve moisture balance within the wound bed.
   b. Aggressively débriding wounds on a patient who exhibits poor vascular supply or clotting deficiencies.
   c. Considering all comorbidities and assessing the patient for wound "healability."
   d. Including patient participation and education in the treatment plan.

ANSWER: B Wound bed preparation contains several principles. In addition to débridement, bacterial control, and adequate moisture balance, the concept of wound bed preparation includes a comprehensive template for patient and wound examination with targeted interventions and specific clinical outcomes. Although débridement is an important component, extreme precaution must be taken when attempting to remove necrotic tissue on a nonhealable wound (patient who is medically unstable, lacks adequate vascular supply, or is on anticoagulant medications). Patients with these conditions should never be débrided aggressively.

Chapter 12

1. In present-day management of wounds, the primary role of dressings would best be described as one of:
   a. controlling bioburden.
   b. managing tissue hydration.
   c. facilitating débridement.
   d. modulating enzyme levels.

ANSWER: B The primary role of a dressing in the wound environment is to manage tissue moisture levels. This is a relatively new expectation in terms of wound-dressing history since in the past many dressings were intended to promote tissue desiccation. Cells function best in a moist environment and not in one that is overly wet or dry.

2. Which of the following types of dressings would most impede moisture vapor loss from a wound?
   a. Hydrocolloid
   b. Alginate
   c. Foam
   d. Hydrofiber

ANSWER: A Hydrocolloid and transparent film dressings are the two types of advanced dressings that best control evaporative moisture loss from a wound. Alginate and hydrofiber dressings require a secondary cover and as such would take on the moisture vapor characteristics of the secondary. Foam dressings vary in thickness from thin foams that allow a moderate degree of evaporation to thicker foams that allow less evaporation but still allow more than a hydrocolloid dressing.

3. One of the potential undesirable effects associated with some alginate dressings is:
   a. increased infections.
   b. delayed epithelialization.
   c. poor patient acceptance.
   d. drying and adherence to wound bed.

ANSWER: D Despite the gelling properties of alginate dressings, they can dry out in the wound bed and adhere to underlying tissue. This can make them as uncomfortable as wet-to-dry gauze dressings. One way to prevent this trauma is to rehydrate the dressing prior to removal or to use a more occlusive secondary dressing.

4. Skin substitutes that come from another species are termed
   a. xenogeneic.
   b. autologous.
   c. allogeneic.
   d. homogeneic.

ANSWER: A Xenogeneic skin substitutes typically come from animals such as pigs. They serve as temporary coverings and are not incorporated by the body.

Chapter 13

1. Clinical Scenario: A 35-year-old female presents with a history of Crohn's disease. She developed a painful ulcer on her right lower leg that also drains copious amount of greenish exudate. She was diagnosed with pyoderma gangrenosum at a wound care clinic. Which of the following signs and symptoms is **_not_** consistent with deep wound infection?
   a. Presence of copious greenish exudate
   b. Persistence of the usual but ongoing pain
   c. Increased in local wound temperature
   d. New breakdown areas

ANSWER: B (a) Increased exudate is a sign of deep infection; (b) although pain is common in inflammatory disease, it is a sudden increase in pain that suggests the presence of infection; (c, and d) all are signs of deep infection.

2. In a wound where bacterial burden is more important than cytotoxicity, which topical antiseptic could be considered for a short-term use?
   a. EUSOL (Edinburgh University solution of lime)
   b. EMLA (eutectic mixture of local anesthetics)
   c. Acetic acid 9%
   d. Chlorhexidine hydrochloride

ANSWER: D (a) High toxicity index and not necessary; (b) no antimicrobial property; (c) very high concentration of acetic acid can induce tissue injury; (d) less toxic to tissue and possesses broad antimicrobial property.

3. The bacterial swab of the wound base grew *Pseudomonas* on culture. Which antimicrobial agent would you use?
   a. Clindamycin dressing
   b. Metronidazole cream
   c. Silver-impregnated alginate
   d. Mupirocin ointment

ANSWER: C (a) Clindamycin is not active against *Pseudomonas*; (b) no activity against *Pseudomonas*; (c) ionized silver has a board-spectrum antimicrobial activity, including *Pseudomonas*; (d) only sensitive against gram-positive bacteria.

4. Which of the following factors is not likely to be related to pain in chronic wounds?
   a. Persistent inflammation
   b. The use of strong adhesive dressing
   c. Anxiety
   d. Autolytic débridement

ANSWER: D (a) Pain is associated with inflammation; (b) strong adhesive dressing can be traumatic upon removal, inducing pain; (c) pain and anxiety are correlated; (d) this is usually painless.

5. Chronic wounds are characterized by all the following *except*:
   a. Increased MMPs levels.
   b. Decreased TIMPS levels.
   c. Decreased growth factor concentration.
   d. Increased mitogenic activity.

ANSWER: D (a) Increased MMP levels in chronic wounds; (b) decreased TIMPS in chronic wounds; (c) decreased growth factor; (d) increased mitogenic activity

Chapter 14

1. Which of the following statements is most accurate regarding peripheral neuropathy associated with diabetes?
   a. It extends from proximal to distal in the extremities.
   b. It is referred to as a stocking and glove distribution.
   c. Neuropathy develops along dermatomal patterns.
   d. It affects sensory and motor nerves, but spares autonomic nerves.

ANSWER: B Neuropathy associated with diabetes is referred to as polyneuropathy because it affects sensory, motor, and autonomic nerves. The neuropathy begins distally and progresses proximally in a stocking and glove distribution. It typically begins in the feet, but it also affects the hands.

2. The gold standard for diagnosing osteomyelitis in the foot of a diabetic individual is a:
   a. probe-to-bone test.
   b. magnetic resonance image.
   c. bone biopsy.
   d. physical examination.

ANSWER: C Only a bone biopsy can definitively diagnose osteomyelitis in the early stages. MRI and other imaging modalities can be used, but they often are inconclusive in the early stages. The probe-to-bone test is not as accurate as a bone biopsy, but it is fast and inexpensive and is commonly used in the clinic. Physical examination may not be remarkable due to the blunted immune response associated with diabetes.

3. Which device has been shown to be the most effective for off-loading a forefoot ulcer in a patient with diabetes?
   a. Extra-depth diabetic footwear with custom orthotics
   b. Adhesive felt padding applied directly to the foot
   c. Removable cast walker with modifiable insoles
   d. Total contact cast

ANSWER: D Pressure reduction on the plantar aspect of the forefoot can be achieved by increasing the total weight-bearing area or decreasing the force going through the foot. The total contact cast increases the total weight-bearing surface and also reduces the force on the wound by transferring weight up the leg, as well as through the relief area at the wound site. The rigidity of the cast prevents dorsiflexion during gait, which helps to reduce forefoot pressure. Finally, the cast is also advantageous because it cannot be removed by the patient, and thus leads to off-loading 100% of the time.

4. Which of the following would be the most likely presentation of an acute Charcot arthropathy?
   a. Patient does not recall injuring foot; loss of protective sensation; edema present
   b. Loss of protective sensation; bounding pulse; skin temperature unchanged
   c. Erythema resolves with antibiotics; fracture apparent on x-ray; intact sensation
   d. Edema and erythema present; systemic fever; loss of protective sensation

ANSWER: A The mechanism of injury for a Charcot foot is often not known, primarily due to loss of protective sensation, which is a prerequisite for the development of a Charcot joint. The foot often presents swollen, erythematous, and warm to touch compared to the contralateral foot. Bounding pulses are common in the acute stage as the arteries remain vasodilated due to autonomic dysfunction. Because the Charcot arthropathy is not an infection, it does not lead to systemic fever and will not respond to antibiotic therapy. Fractures may not be initially apparent on radiographs, depending on the nature of the injury.

5. What is considered to be the most important factor in the development of a foot ulceration in an individual with diabetes?
   a. Autonomic neuropathy
   b. Motor neuropathy
   c. Sensory neuropathy
   d. Vascular impairment

ANSWER: C Although all contribute to the development of ulceration, sensory neuropathy is the most crucial. Motor neuropathy can lead to deformities and muscle imbalances that make areas susceptible to injury, and autonomic neuropathy can make the skin less resilient to stress and vascular compromise may lead to problems with wound healing. All three of these typically require some outside stress that leads to ulceration. With sensory neuropathy, that stress, whether it be poor-fitting shoes or stepping on a nail, goes unchecked and ultimately results in a wound. Some studies show sensory neuropathy to be present in over 80% of diabetic foot wounds.

Chapter 15

1. All of the following result from hyperglycemia in people with diabetes **except**:
   a. Intracellular dehydration.
   b. Extracellular dehydration.
   c. Decreased blood volume.
   d. Increasing cellular function.

ANSWER: D Hyperglycemia impairs glucose diffusion through cell membranes, creating a dehydrating effect. This dehydration is from both an intracellular and extracellular perspective leaving the person with an overall decrease in blood volume.

2. What is the term for the molecules that are formed in the "reversible" stage of protein glycation before formation of advanced glycation of end products?
   a. Plaque
   b. Arteriosclerosis
   c. Amadori products
   d. Hypercoagulation

ANSWER: C In the early stages of nonenzymatic glycation, glucose chemically attaches to the amine group of proteins, creating a stable molecule that accumulates over the surface of cell membranes and structural and circulating proteins. At this stage, these molecules are called Amadori products, they are stable and reversible.

3. Pre-diabetes is defined as a fasting blood glucose of:
   a. 88–100 mg/dL
   b. 100–126 mg/dL
   c. 126–140 mg/dL
   d. 140–152 mg/dL

ANSWER: B Pre-diabetes has been officially recognized and is considered to be a fasting blood glucose of between 100–126 mg/dL.

4. The test that best identifies whether a patient's diabetes management program is functional is:
   a. Fasting capillary blood glucose
   b. HbA1c
   c. Fructosamine
   d. Oral glucose tolerance test

ANSWER: B The hemoglobin A1c test provides the "average" blood glucose over the previous 2–3 months. This test is recognized by the ADA and other authorities as the best laboratory value for determining whether the overall diabetes management program a patient has in place is successful.

Chapter 16

1. Venous pressure measured in the foot of a normal individual in the standing position is generally in the range of:
   a. 30 to 60 mm Hg
   b. 60 to 90 mm Hg
   c. 90 to 120 mm Hg
   d. 120 to 150 mm Hg

ANSWER: B Venous pressure, measured in the foot vein of a person in the upright position, is proportional to the height of the column of blood between the foot and the right side of the heart. Typically, this pressure ranges from 60 to 90 mm Hg.

2. While many factors contribute to the development of a venous ulcer, which of the following is felt to be the primary cause?
   a. Leukocyte trapping
   b. Fibrin cuff
   c. Venous stasis
   d. Ambulatory venous hypertension

ANSWER: D As the individual ambulates, muscle pumps in the feet and legs push venous blood from the lower extremities, thereby reducing ambulatory venous pressure. As the calf pump fails, pressure begins to rise in the veins and ulcerations may result. Ambulatory venous hypertension is widely accepted as the primary cause of venous ulcerations.

3. Skin pigment changes seen in venous insufficiency are a result of:
   a. Hemosiderin deposits
   b. Cellulitis
   c. Leukocyte trapping
   d. Leakage of fibrinogen

ANSWER: A Hemosiderosis occurs when red blood cells leak from the capillaries, become trapped in the pericapillary tissue, and undergo lysis, causing the release of the pigment hemosiderin from the hemoglobin.

4. Which of the following statements is most accurate concerning venous insufficiency ulcers?
   a. They are predominantly found in the area of the medial malleolus.
   b. Ulcer borders tend to be ill defined.
   c. The ulcer has a punched-out appearance.
   d. Patients complain of pain out of proportion to ulcer size.

ANSWER: A The classic presentation of a venous ulcer is one involving the medial leg (gaiter region), irregular in shape, with well-defined borders. The pain associated with a venous ulcer is much less than would be seen with a much smaller ischemic ulcer.

Chapter 17

1. The most influential of the controllable risk factors for arterial occlusive disease is:
   a. diet.
   b. family history.
   c. smoking.
   d. age.

ANSWER: C Smoking. Smoking has been linked to severity of peripheral arterial disease and to poor healing prognosis. Diet is an indirect variable since it may influence hypertension (HTN), diabetes risk, and cholesterol, which are additional risk factors linked to peripheral arterial disease (PAD).

2. Claudication pain is hypothesized to occur in patients with arterial insufficiency due to:
   a. metabolic imbalance of O_2 supply and demand.
   b. damage to muscle fibers from activity.
   c. neuropathic changes in conduction velocity.
   d. eating within a half an hour of activity.

ANSWER: A Claudication pain is thought to be associated with metabolic muscle needs exceeding the O_2 delivery in the presence of obstruction or occlusion.

3. You receive a referral for bedside débridement of a (L) heel ulcer in a 73-year-old male. Upon chart review and examination in the ICU, you learn he has sustained a recent myocardial infarct, has end-stage renal disease and is receiving dialysis, and is a type 2 diabetic.

   The heel appears with a dry intact eschar measuring 3×1.6 cm; periwound is nonerythematous; dorsal pedal pulse = 1+; limb is pale, cool, and thin. Your treatment priority should be:
   a. bedside sharp débridement.
   b. vascular surgery referral.
   c. pressure relief with protective boot along with close monitoring.
   d. enzymatic débridement with daily dressing changes.

ANSWER: C Pressure relief and monitoring are appropriate in this case of a closed stable eschar. Vascular referral may still be indicated for full work-up, but the main priority in a medically complex patient in the intensive care unit (ICU) will be protection of this site while it is not causing additional complication for the patient.

4. The same patient in question 3 presents with a soft brown eschar measuring 2 cm × 2.4 cm. He has 2+ pedal edema and 4 cm of surrounding erythema. He is afebrile. Your treatment priority should be:
   a. bedside sharp débridement.
   b. vascular surgery referral.
   c. antimicrobial occlusive dressings.
   d. pressure relief with protective boot along with close monitoring.

ANSWER: B Vascular referral is indicated in this high-risk patient. Given his confounding variables, surgery may not be feasible immediately, and bedside débridement is likewise not a wise choice until the vascular system has been evaluated further. Collaborative risk assessment is necessary, and pressure relief will clearly be a component of care.

5. Which of the following treatment modalities has shown the greatest efficacy in increasing ambulation distance in patients with claudication?
   a. Clopidogrel
   b. Supervised exercise
   c. High-voltage pulsed current
   d. Intermittent pneumatic foot compression

ANSWER: B Supervised exercise has been proven in many randomized controlled trials to reduce claudication pain in patients with PAD. It has been shown to be superior to pharmacological interventions.

6. Which of the following diagnostic tests has demonstrated independent predictive validity for presence of PAD?
   a. ABI
   b. Pulse palpation
   c. $TcPo_2$
   d. Rubor of dependency

ANSWER: A ABI has been shown to be an independent predictor of PAD. T_cPo_2 has been shown to have linear relationship to PAD. Pulse palpation alone is not sufficient for diagnosis.

Chapter 18

1. A 24-year-old female noticed her right lower extremity appears larger than her left. She states this has been an insidious and ongoing problem for the past 2 years. She does not recall injuring her right lower extremity and reports her leg just "feels heavy." Assuming this is lymphedema, which best describes her presentation?
   a. Primary lymphedema, lymphedema precox
   b. Primary lymphedema, lymphedema tardum
   c. Secondary lymphedema, lymphedema precox
   d. Secondary lymphedema, lymphedema tardum

ANSWER: A Primary lymphedema and lymphedema precox. She does not have any precipitating factors that could have contributed to her developing lymphedema (such as surgery, trauma, or radiation); therefore, her lymphedema is more likely related to a congenital issue. Because she developed lymphedema before the age of 35, it is considered lymphedema precox.

2. Currently, the only clinical test that has been shown to be a reliable and valid method to diagnose lymphedema is:
   a. two-point discrimination.
   b. circumferential limb measurement.
   c. Stemmer sign.
   d. venous duplex.

ANSWER: C Stemmer sign. A positive Stemmer sign is the inability to "tent" or pick up the skin over the proximal phalanges of the toes or fingers of the involved extremity. If positive, it is a definite indication of lymphedema; if negative, its absence is not certain.

3. What makes lymphedema unique compared to virtually all other types of edema?
a. Predisposition for cellulitis
b. High content of protein in the interstitial fluid
c. Bilateral, symmetrical involvement
d. Greater proximal involvement compared to distal

ANSWER: B High content of protein in the interstitial fluid. Lymphedema is caused by mechanical insufficiency, or low-volume insufficiency of the lymphatic system. The transport capacity drops below the physiological level of the lymphatic loads. This means the lymphatic system is not able to clear the interstitial tissues, and an accumulation of high-protein fluid is the result.

4. Complete decongestive therapy involves which of the following?
a. Skin and nail care, manual lymph drainage, bandaging/compression, and the use of diuretics
b. Skin and nail care, manual lymph drainage, pneumatic compression, and exercise
c. Skin and nail care, massage, bandaging/compression, and exercise
d. Skin and nail care, manual lymph drainage, bandaging/compression, and exercise

ANSWER: D Skin and nail care, manual lymph drainage, bandaging/compression, and exercise. Diuretics solely to manage lymphedema should not be considered. Diuretics mobilize fluid, but not protein. In the case of lymphedema, the proteins in the interstitial tissues would draw in more water, ultimately leading to more fibrosis. Pneumatic compression should not be used in place of bandaging and compression as the pump cannot maintain the benefits achieved with complete decongestive therapy (CDT). The pump should not be used to decongest, but to maintain the benefits of CDT. Traditional massage should not be used to manage lymphedema as the techniques can cause a spasm in the lymphatic vessels exacerbating the condition. Manual lymphatic drainage (MLD) is designed specifically to cause a slight stretch of lymphatic vessel walls, increasing lymph angiomotoricity.

5. Short-stretch bandages are the best choice for lymphedema management because these bandages have a:
a. high working pressure and low resting pressure.
b. low working pressure and high resting pressure.
c. moderate working pressure and low resting pressure.
d. high working pressure and moderate resting pressure.

ANSWER: A High working pressure and low resting pressure. Resting pressure is pressure exerted by elastic when put on stretch, whether or not the patient is moving or activating a muscle pump. Working pressure is pressure produced by the muscles when they are active and push against a compression bandage. Short-stretch bandages supply a comfortable degree of support (without a tourniquet effect), but the total pressure increases significantly when the muscles contract against fixed resistance.

Chapter 19

1. Which of the following is an appropriate use of interface pressure measurements?
a. determine capillary closing pressure
b. determine which mattress should be used for all patients
c. educate the client in positioning and in effective pressure-relief movements
d. alert client when to change positions during sleep

ANSWER: C Interface pressure measurements are an excellent educational tool for patients but would obviously not be a device that would alarm all through the night while the patient was sleeping. A surface pressure measurement would also not tell you if the capillaries were closed and would also have drawbacks in determining proper mattress purchases for certain patients.

2. Pressure ulcers are treated with all of the following *except*:
a. compression.
b. positioning.
c. individualized support surface and seat cushion prescription.
d. individual evaluation and reevaluation.

ANSWER: A Adding compression to an area already at risk for pressure ulcer development would only worsen the situation. All other choices provide common sense approaches to the management of any person at risk for pressure ulcer development.

3. The sacrum can be protected from pressure and shearing in bed by doing any of the following *except*:
a. tilting the pelvis so that the sacral spinous processes are unweighted.
b. limiting the head-of-bed elevation degree and time.
c. positioning the patient in supine with head slightly elevated.
d. using any low-air-loss mattress or foam pad.

ANSWER: C A patient at risk for a sacral pressure ulcer would be complicated by remaining in the supine position without some type of positional adjustment. Efforts should be taken to relieve pressure from this area by some of the other techniques mentioned.

Chapter 20

1. Which of the following is a potential toxic side effect of silver sulfadiazine (Silvadene®)?
a. Neutropenia
b. Thrombocytopenia
c. Anemia
d. Metabolic acidosis

ANSWER: A Cleansing of wounds and topical antimicrobial dressings are the mainstay of treatment for partial-thickness wounds. These topical agents decrease bacterial populations to allow the best environment for healing. One potential side effect of the use of silver sulfadiazine is the development of neutropenia. The other common finding seen with topical agents is metabolic acidosis, which occurs at times with the use of mafenide acetate.

2. Which of the following is a potential toxic side effect of mafenide acetate (Sulfamylon®) when used on large surface areas?
a. Neutropenia
b. Thrombocytopenia
c. Anemia
d. Metabolic acidosis

ANSWER: D While neutropenia is also seen with the use of topical antimicrobial agents in large surface burns, this is most frequently seen with silver sulfadiazine. Mafenide acetate (Sulfamylon) is most frequently associated with metabolic acidosis.

3. The Parkland formula used in burn volume resuscitation is:
a. 3 cc/kg/% total body surface area (TBSA) of lactated Ringers
b. 3 cc/kg/% TBSA of normal saline
c. 4 cc/kg/% TBSA of lactated Ringers
d. 4 cc/kg/%TBSA of normal saline

ANSWER: C The Parkland formula is the most common guideline for fluid resuscitation of second- and third-degree burn injuries. Resuscitation involves the delivery of lactated Ringers. The volume to be given is 4 cc/kg/TBSA. As a starting point, half of this calculated volume is given in the first 8 hours, and the remainder is given over the next 16 hours.

4. First aid in chemical burn injury is to:
a. find a appropriate neutralizing agent.
b. irrigate with water.
c. use detergents to wash the burn.
d. apply calcium gluconate topically or by injection.

ANSWER: B For chemical burn injuries, all contaminated clothing should be removed. Water is used in large volumes to dilute and remove the chemical. Usually, the area is irrigated for at least 20 to 45 minutes or to neutral pH (pH of 7). Adding an acid to a base (or conversely a base to an acid) can be an exothermic reaction and lead to further injury. Hydrofluoric acid burns are treated with intra-arterial infusion of calcium gluconate to bind with fluoride to convert it to a soluble salt.

5. Adequate urine output in an adult is:
a. 0.5 cc/kg/hr.
b. 1.5 cc/kg/hr.
c. 2.0 cc/kg/hr.
d. 2.5 cc/kg/hr.

ANSWER: A As intravascular volume begins to decline, the body begins to divert blood to critical organs (brain, heart, kidney) at the expense of other organs (skin/extremities and gut). Urine output is the best indicator of

volume status. Tachycardia and decreased blood pressure are not apparent until the volume status is even lower. A child's kidney cannot concentrate urine as well as an adult's, so they will make more urine. Adequate urine output in an adult is 0.5 cc/kg/hr and in a child 1 cc/kg/hr.

6. Most fatalities from house fires are due to:
a. cutaneous burn injury.
b. carbon monoxide poisoning.
c. other trauma.
d. electrical burns.

ANSWER: B Carbon monoxide is a competitive inhibitor of oxygen for binding to hemoglobin. Carbon monoxide has a greater affinity for hemoglobin than does oxygen. If in sufficient quantity, this can lead to hypoxia and asphyxia. When compared to the magnitude of burn injury (total body surface area), and possibly other injuries, hypoxia/anoxia is more rapidly fatal.

Chapter 21

1. Which of the following joints is the most frequently involved in contracture development?
a. Knee
b. Elbow
c. Shoulder
d. Hip

ANSWER: C Contractures after a burn injury have a reported incidence of 28% to 42%. The shoulder is the most frequently contracted joint, followed by the elbow, hand, and knee.

2. Which of the following has been recommended for use when traditional splints have failed or when patients are nonadherent to instructions?
a. Sedation
b. Antianxiety medication
c. Postoperative joint immobilizers
d. Casts

ANSWER: D Cast indications include patients nonadherence with traditional splinting, failure of gains with traditional splinting, or with children. Casts have been found to be effective in increasing range of motion.

3. Which of the following sets of factors is thought to most affect hypertrophic scar formation?
a. Depth of burn, race, location, and time of injury to complete closure
b. Nonadherent skin grafts, infection, race, size of burn wound
c. Infection, depth of burn, race, gender
d. Persistent necrotic tissue, age, location, and mechanism of burn injury

ANSWER: A Gender, age, size of the burn wound or the mechanism of injury *are not* factors found to influence hypertrophic scar development.

4. A deep partial-thickness burn is classified by which of the following characteristics?
   a. Waxy white in color, dry, rigid, nonpainful
   b. Mottled white, pink to cherry red in color, wet surface, edematous
   c. Blistered skin, erythema, very painful
   d. Large areas require skin grafting, decreased elasticity, decreased sweating

ANSWER: B A deep partial-thickness burn damages the tissue that extends into the reticular layers of the dermis and may include fat domes of the subcutaneous layer. It may be mottled white (pale) or bright pink to cherry red. There is a very wet surface with marked edema. Healing is slow (21 to 35 days) if there is no infection; however, it may convert to full thickness if infection occurs.

Chapter 22

1. Secondary hyperalgesia (pain outside the area of tissue injury) is likely due to which of the following?
   a. Central sensitization
   b. Referred pain
   c. Peripheral sensitization
   d. Neurogenic inflammation

ANSWER: A Central sensitization. Secondary hyperalgesia is thought to occur due to changes in the central nervous system, whereas primary hyperalgesia is due to changes in the peripheral nervous system.

2. Which pain assessment tool would be appropriate to assess the influence of pain on a patient's function?
   a. McGill Pain Questionnaire
   b. Brief Pain Inventory
   c. Numerical rating scale
   d. Krasner's Wound Model of wound pain

ANSWER: B Brief Pain Inventory. Only the Brief Pain Inventory assesses the relation between pain and function.

3. Individuals with venous insufficiency present with lower extremity edema and pain that is exacerbated by:
   a. rest.
   b. elevation.
   c. dependent positioning.
   d. walking.

ANSWER: C Dependent position. If the limb is placed in a dependent position, the venous system has an increased workload that it is not able to manage, thus causing pain.

4. Individuals with second-degree burns frequently describe their pain as:
   a. minimal.
   b. severe.
   c. nonexistent.
   d. nonexistent or severe.

ANSWER: D Nonexistent or severe. Second-degree burns cause tissue damage to both the epidermis and dermis. If the tissue damage is severe, the nociceptors are destroyed, and pain is not reported. If the tissue damage is severe, but the nociceptors are still intact, then pain reports are quite severe.

5. Electrical stimulation decreases pain through what process?
   a. Activation of the opioid system
   b. Absorption of infrared energy
   c. Decrease in swelling
   d. Decrease in inflammation

ANSWER: A Activation of the opioid system. Low-frequency TENS activates μ-opioid receptors, whereas high frequency TENS activates δ-opioid receptors.

Chapter 23

1. The diagnosis of osteomyelitis is best confirmed by:
   a. MRI.
   b. bone scan.
   c. plain film radiograph.
   d. bone biopsy.

ANSWER: D Osteomyelitis is *best* confirmed by bone biopsy. Culturing a single microorganism is the most accurate modality to confirm and identify a bone infection. The patient should be off antibiotics for at least 48 hours before biopsy to minimize a false-negative result. While the other choices are reasonable, biopsy is most accurate.

2. The most efficient and effective form of débridement is:
   a. sharp.
   b. enzymatic.
   c. hydrotherapy.
   d. mechanical wet to dry.

ANSWER: A The best form of débridement of a wound is sharp débridement. This not only removes the devitalized tissue but also stimulates ingrowth of fibroblasts and other desirable cells. While enzymatic débridement may be useful, it is slow to show results. Hydrotherapy débridement can only remove loosely attached devitalize tissue. Mechanical wet to dry is painful and of limited benefit.

3. Which of the following would be most important to check on a patient prior to performing sharp débridement on a lower-extremity wound?
   a. Hba$_{1c}$
   b. Anticoagulation status
   c. Ability to use crutches
   d. Serum glucose

ANSWER: B Prior to performing a débridement procedure that could result in bleeding, the clinician should be aware of whether the patient is using any blood thinners. While other tests could provide useful information on the patient's general health and postdébridement management, coagulation status would be most important.

4. In general, when can sutures be removed from an uncomplicated wound of the abdomen?
  a. 3 to 5 days
  b. 5 to 7 days
  c. 7 to 10 days
  d. 10 to15 days

ANSWER: C According to the times for various wounds listed in Table 23.2, sutures can generally be removed from uncomplicated abdominal wounds in 7 to 10 days. Sutures can be removed from an uncomplicated facial wound earlier, and complicated wounds often require more than 10 days.

Chapter 24

1. What is the upper limit of the ankle-brachial index (ABI) above which measurements are considered unreliable?
  a. 0.9
  b. 1.0
  c. 1.15
  d. 1.20

ANSWER: C The International Consensus on the Diabetic Foot (ICDF) guidelines suggest that an ABI of 1.15 represents the upper limit above which measurements are deemed unreliable.

2. What is the primary predictor of initial healing and freedom from major amputation in patients requiring toe or partial amputations?
  a. Maintaining an optimal blood sugar between 100 and 120
  b. Off-loading the surgical site to remove trophic pressure
  c. Intraoperative culture and sensitivity showing no bacterial growth
  d. Revascularization of the operative site to ensure adequate blood flow.

ANSWER: D In patients requiring toe or partial amputation, a prospective study involving 162 patients found that success of revascularization was the primary predictor of initial healing and freedom from major amputation.

3. What is the most common location in the foot affected by Charcot disease?
  a. Metatarsal phalangeal joints
  b. Subtalar (talocalcaneal) joint
  c. Chopar's joint (joint between the talus and calcaneus posteriorly and the navicular and cuboid bones anteriorly)
  d. The Lisfranc's (tarsometatarsal) joint

ANSWER: D The most common location in the foot affected by Charcot joint affliction is the tarsometatarsal joints. Instability to these joints leads to a rocker-bottom foot deformity.

4. What is one of the central tenets of healing neuropathic diabetic foot wounds?
  a. Provide aggressive surgical débridement and off-loading.
  b. Administer appropriate antibiotic therapy immediately.
  c. Restore proper neurological function.
  d. Aggressively control the patients' HbA_{1c} below 7%.

ANSWER: A One of the central tenets of healing neuropathic diabetic foot wounds is appropriate aggressive surgical débridement and off-loading. Débridement should include removal of all necrotic and devitalized tissue from the wound. The goal is to convert a chronic wound into an acute one.

5. Persons with diabetes:
  a. incur 1.7 times the health-care expenditures than those without diabetes.
  b. incur the same health-care expenditures as those without diabetes.
  c. account for only a small portion of the direct Medicare expenditures.
  d. account for less time spent in the hospital, saving Medicare money.

ANSWER: A Persons with diabetes incur 1.7 times the health-care expenditure than those without diabetes because they often require more extensive care and hospital admissions.

6. Which of the following statements is correct regarding neurovascular status in the lower extremity?
  a. Good functional recovery after major amputation does not argue for foot-sparing surgery.
  b. 20% of 100 million persons in the United States will develop a neuropathic ulcer.
  c. Detecting significant arterial compromise is important to the prevention of further limb loss and to the success of surgical procedures.
  d. The palpation of pulses is sufficient to determine the available blood flow to the foot.

ANSWER: C Detecting significant arterial compromise is important to the prevention of further limb loss and to the success of surgical procedures. Palpation of peripheral arterial pulses is not enough, and further studies must be performed to establish the available blood flow to the extremity.

7. In individuals with neuropathic feet, lengthening of the Achilles tendon is performed to:
  a. increase forefoot pressure and increase foot purchase.
  b. increase ankle dorsiflexion, thus reducing forefoot pressure.
  c. strengthen the posterior muscle group and increase push-off strength.
  d. produce a calcaneus gait and redirect pressure to the posterior heel.

ANSWER: B By lengthening the Achilles tendon, ankle dorsiflexion is increased, reducing forefoot pressure and redistributing pressure across the foot more evenly. The ankle is often in an equinus position and cannot reach a neutral position.

8. With respect to limb salvage and reconstruction, identify the statement that is true.
   a. The selection of a surgeon for the procedure is multifactorial and includes the patient preference as well as the pattern and extent of infection.
   b. As a wound remains open for a greater duration of time, there is less probability of an infection spreading and devastating the limb.
   c. Local antibiotic therapy such as PMMA beads is less effective than systemic antibiotic therapy.
   d. Deep-space infection within the foot is one that rapidly spreads along the long flexor tendons, placing the foot at greater risk for more proximal amputation.

ANSWER: D A deep-space infection spreads along the long flexor tendons reaching the leg from the foot, providing the infection with a means of quickly migrating proximally along a conduit and placing the entire limb at risk.

Chapter 25

1. Neonatal skin becomes structurally similar to the adult at:
   a. 27 weeks.
   b. 29 weeks.
   c. 33 weeks.
   d. 36 weeks.

ANSWER: D Once neonates reach full term (36 weeks), the skin becomes structurally similar to that of the adult.

2. Skin protective measures that should be implemented in the presence of epidermolysis bullosa include:
   a. adhesive dressings.
   b. increased environmental humidity and heat.
   c. securing of dressings with nonstretchy, non-latex tubular gauze netting.
   d. flat-seamed clothing turned inside out.

ANSWER: D Adhesives, increased humidity, increased heat, and nonstretchy tubular gauze should be avoided.

3. When selecting a common wound dressing for a child, the clinician should consider all of the following *except*:
   a. goals of therapy.
   b. integumentary maturity.
   c. basal metabolic rate.
   d. manufacturer's recommended use.

ANSWER: C The goals of therapy, integumentary maturity, and the manufacturer's recommended use statement are all important to consider when selecting products for children.

4. Wound débridement interventions available for neonates include all of the following *except*:
   a. autolytic.
   b. enzymatic.
   c. surgical.
   d. sharp.

ANSWER: B The safety and efficacy of topical enzymes in the pediatric population has not been studied. The manufacturer's recommended use of topical enzymes is only for those over the age of 18 years.

Chapter 26

1. Which statement best describes how electric fields influence cell migration?
   a. They increase dermal $TcPO_2$, causing cells to migrate to a higher oxygen concentration.
   b. They stimulate the formation of chemical gradients that cause cells to migrate to higher chemical concentrations.
   c. Positively and negatively charged live cells behave like ions and migrate to an EF of opposite polarity.
   d. In general, cells migrate in the direction of the EF, but not all cell types migrate in the same direction.

ANSWER: D Electrotaxis is not explained by simple physics that live organic cells behave as positively or negatively charged inorganic particles (eg, ions) and therefore move toward an EF of opposite polarity. Rather, cells such as human epithelial cells from skin, as well as neutrophils, macrophages, fibroblast, and endothelial cells, respond to applied EFs of physiological strength by directional cell migration, meaning they migrate in the direction of the EF.

2. Investigators have objectively determined that angio-genesis or improved perfusion had occurred in clinical studies by all of the following mechanisms **except**?
   a. Laser Doppler imaging (LDI) or flowmetry (LDF)
   b. $TcPO_2$, oximetry
   c. Intravital video microscopy (IVM)
   d. Rubor of dependency

ANSWER: D Numerous clinical studies have demonstrated that ES improves perfusion in intact skin of subjects with spinal cord injuries or diabetes measured by $TcPO_2$ and wounds and periwound skin as measured by LDI and/or IVM and by $TcPO_2$ and LDF. Rubor of dependency is a subjective clinical test that is used to time capillary refilling in the presence of ischemia.

3. An advantage of high-voltage monophasic pulsed current (HVMPC) over traditional direct current (DC) or charged unbalanced low-voltage biphasic pulsed current (LVBPC) is that:
   a. HVMPC treatment is easier to set up.
   b. HVMPC does not cause pH changes.
   c. only HVMPC mimics the endogenous wound EF.
   d. only HVMPC has been shown to enhance wound healing.

ANSWER: B Human subject research has shown that HVMPC does not cause harmful pH changes on the skin.

4. An FDA-cleared antimicrobial wound dressing that contains 25 microbatteries per square inch and a silver formulary has been shown to:
   a. deliver 20 μA to the wound surface for up to 3 days.
   b. kill microbes through the synergistic action of the bioelectric field and silver.
   c. kill bacteria and viruses but not fungi.
   d. have antimicrobial effects only in postsurgical wounds.

ANSWER: B Electrically generated silver ions have been shown to be a potent antibacterial agent with an exceptionally broad spectrum.

Chapter 27

1. Which statement best describes how signals from PRF devices are delivered to wound and periwound tissues?
   a. A 27-MHz electromagnetic field transmitted from one or two coils positioned over the target tissue area induces an electric field in the wound and periwound tissues.
   b. 60-Hz electrical impulses from electrodes contacting the skin and wound conduct an electric field into the wound and periwound tissues.
   c. A 2.7-MHz electromagnetic field transmitted from electrodes contacting the skin and wound induces an electric field in the wound and periwound tissues.
   d. 100-MHz electrical impulses from a coil positioned over the target tissue area induces an electric field in the wound and periwound tissues.

ANSWER: A For soft tissue wound healing a 27-MHz electromagnetic field is transmitted from one or two treatment coils placed over the wound and periwound area.

2. Which of the following is the primary radio frequency (RF) or "carrier" frequency from which pulsed electromagnetic field (PEMF), pulsed radio frequency (PRF), and pulsed shortwave diathermy (PSWD) signals are derived?
   a. 27 Hz
   b. 27 kHz
   c. 27 MHz
   d. 27 GHz

ANSWER: C All PEMF, PRF, and PSWD devices emit signals that are modulated from the primary PRF frequency of 27 MHz.

3. The strength of the induced voltage per centimeter produced by a PEMF device used for bone healing is not the same as the strength of the induced voltage per centimeter used by PRF devices that are used for soft tissue wound healing. Which of the following represents the voltage strength for wound healing with a PRF signal?
   a. pV/cm
   b. μV/cm
   c. mV/cm
   d. V/cm

ANSWER: D A weaker voltage (mV/cm) is used for bone healing versus the stronger voltage (V/cm) that is use for soft tissue wound healing.

4. A patient has a Stage IV sacral pressure ulcer with a saline-moist gauze dressing in the wound. Depending on duty cycle, which of the following interventions could be contraindicated?
   a. Pulsed electromagnetic field stimulation
   b. Pulsed shortwave diathermy stimulation
   c. Pulsed radio frequency stimulation
   d. Pulsed high-voltage electrical stimulation

ANSWER: B Pulsed shortwave diathermy set at a duty cycle that produces significant thermal energy could excessively heat the saline-moist dressing, resulting in a local wound tissue burn.

Chapter 28

1. Ultrasound (US) wound débridement provides the following benefit that is not realized with other forms of débridement:
   a. Removal of necrotic tissue
   b. Decreased bioburden
   c. Cavitation
   d. Ultrasonic interface

ANSWER: C In unstable cavitation with kilohertz US, tiny shock waves produced by bubble implosions cause preferential and rapid liquefaction and fragmentation (débridement) of necrotic fibrin and microorganisms on wound surfaces.

2. Microcavitation is achieved in tissues treated with US and directly results in the following:
   a. Decreased bioburden
   b. Release of growth factors
   c. Angiogenesis
   d. Fibroblast stimulation

ANSWER: A Several in vitro and in vivo studies have shown that kilohertz US can destroy bacteria and biofilms, thereby reducing the risk of wound infection.

3. US at 22.5-, 25-, and 35-kHz frequencies can achieve immediate tissue débridement with results similar to sharp techniques when used in which of the following modes?
   a. Surgical
   b. Contact
   c. Noncontact
   d. Dissection

ANSWER: B Contact US at the three mentioned kilohertz frequencies has been reported to rapidly emulsify necrotic, fibrinous slough on the surface of chronic wounds.

4. Of the four kilohertz US frequencies, which one has the most research evidence that supports using that frequency to enhance wound healing?
a. 22.5
b. 25
c. 35
d. 40

ANSWER: D Numerous clinical studies of different designs (retrospective, randomized controlled trials, case studies) have reported enhanced wound healing outcomes following treatment with 40 kHz US.

Chapter 29

1. Which of the following wavelengths of electromagnetic energy would penetrate the deepest into the skin?
a. 660 nm
b. 700 nm
c. 800 nm
d. 850 nm

ANSWER: D The longer the wavelength, the greater electromagnetic energy penetrates into the skin.

2. Which of the following UV energy bands is more commonly associated with skin cancer and late cutaneous skin responses such as elastosis?
a. UVA
b. UVB
c. UVC
d. All are equally associated

ANSWER: B UVB is most closely associated with damage due to sunburns and the resulting changes in the epidermis and dermis that lead to late cutaneous responses such as elastosis.

3. Which of the following UV energy bands is effective in killing methicillin-resistant *Staphylococcus aureus* (MRSA)?
a. UVA
b. UVB
c. UVC
d. All are equally effective

ANSWER: C UVC has been shown to effectively kill MRSA in laboratory studies and to reduce MRSA numbers in animal and human tissues.

Chapter 30

1. According to Laplace's law, when applying a compression bandage, which of the following changes in physical factors would result in an increase in sub-bandage pressure if all other factors remained constant?
a. A decrease in bandage tension
b. A decrease in the width of the bandage
c. A decrease in the number of layers applied
d. An increase in the circumference of the limb

ANSWER: B Sub-bandage pressure is inversely proportional to bandage width; as the width of a bandage increases, pressure is spread over a larger surface area. Conversely, as bandage width is decreased, pressure becomes more focal.

2. An Unna's boot would most closely fall into which of the following bandage types?
a. Long stretch
b. Short stretch
c. Multicomponent system
d. Hosiery

ANSWER: B An Unna's boot consists of a woven cotton gauze that is impregnated with various substances such as zinc oxide, calamine, and gelatin. It by nature has very low elastic properties and would therefore be best classified as a short-stretch bandage.

3. When performing a spiral wrap of an extremity using a long-stretch bandage, how should the bandage be stretched and overlapped?
a. 25% stretch, 50% overlap
b. 25% stretch, 75% overlap
c. 50% stretch, 50% overlap
d. 50% stretch, 75% overlap

ANSWER: C Studies have shown that when long-stretch bandages are elongated to 50% of their elastic tension and then overlapped by 50% with each successive layer of bandage, a sub-bandage pressure is generated that is in the range of 40 to 50 mm Hg. Providing less stretch will result in decreased pressure, while overlapping the bandage at 75% may increase the sub-bandage pressure.

4. What class of stocking would most effectively provide 40 to 50 mm Hg pressure at the ankle?
a. I
b. II
c. III
d. IV

ANSWER: C Class III stockings provide between 40 and 50 mmHg of pressure. Class I provides 0 to 30 mm Hg; Class II, 30 to 40 mm Hg; and Class IV stockings provide greater than 50 mm Hg of pressure.

Chapter 31

1. Which of the following wounds would be indicated for treatment with negative-pressure wound therapy (NPWT)?
a. Wagner grade 5 diabetic foot ulcer
b. Unstageable sacral pressure ulcer
c. Lower extremity ulcer on patient with 0.5 ABI bilaterally
d. Postdébridement wound on patient with necrotizing fasciitis

ANSWER: D NPWT is ideal for treatment of clean, granulating wounds with adequate perfusion. Answer "D" is the best choice, assuming the infection has been eradicated following the radical soft tissue débridement.

2. Which of the following is believed to be the primary cellular level mechanism responsible for the increase in granulation tissue during NPWT?
   a. Microdeformation
   b. Protease reduction
   c. Pressure gradient
   d. Improved bioburden

ANSWER: A While all four answers are proposed mechanisms of action for NPWT, answer "A" is correct because microdeformation is the mechanical stretching of cells known to stimulate cell mitosis, cell proliferation, and angiogenesis. Microdeformation is the cellular level mechanism believed to be responsible for the proliferative changes seen following NPWT.

3. Which of the following is considered a *contraindication* for the use of NPWT?
   a. Tendon exposure
   b. Untreated osteomyelitis
   c. Enterocutaneous fistula
   d. Sternal dehiscence

ANSWER: B Untreated osteomyelitis is a contraindication for NPWT. Negative-pressure wound therapy can be initiated following appropriate antibiotic treatment and/or débridement of affected bone. The other conditions listed are not contraindicated; however, caution should be exercised to protect tendons, explore fistulas, and ensure vital organs are not exposed before initiating NPWT. Follow manufacturer's guidelines for clinical treatment guidelines and protocols.

4. Which of the following should occur *first* when preparing a wound for NPWT?
   a. Débride necrotic tissue
   b. Assess patient's pain level
   c. Prepare periwound skin
   d. Educate caregivers

ANSWER: B Accurate pain assessments and management, if indicated, should be a top priority in the treatment of all patients with wounds before initiating or continuing wound care.

5. Which of the following should be performed *first* before applying NPWT as a postoperative graft bolster?
   a. Place a nonadherent contact layer over graft.
   b. Lower negative pressure settings.
   c. Ensure airtight seal along periwound.
   d. Avoid excessive pressure to graft.

ANSWER: A A nonadherent contact layer is recommended to place on top of a skin or skin substitute graft to avoid displacement of the graft. All the other answers are also appropriate

considerations but are performed subsequent to placement of the contact layer.

Chapter 32

1. HBOT is indicated by Medicare for patients with which of the following classifications of diabetic foot ulcers?
   a. Wagner 1 and 2
   b. Wagner 2 and 3
   c. Wagner 1, 2, and 3
   d. Wagner 3, 4, and 5

ANSWER: D The Centers for Medicare and Medicaid Services (CMS) have approved the use of HPOT for the management of diabetic foot ulcers of a Wagner stage 3 or higher.

2. In addition to Wagner stage classification, CMS has approved the use of HBOT in the management of the DFU if which of the following criteria have been met?
   a. The patient is nutritionally compromised.
   b. Wound must have failed standard wound care.
   c. Patient is nondiabetic.
   d. Amputation is inevitable.

ANSWER: B CMS requires that the patient must have diabetes and a lower extremity wound that has not responded to standard wound care demonstrated by no measurable signs of healing in 30 days. Standard therapy must include assessment of vascular status, optimization of nutrition/glucose control, débridement, moist dressings, offloading, and treatment of infection.

Chapter 33

1. Which wound characteristic ***is not*** appropriate to represent the severity of a chronic wound?
   a. Dimensions
   b. Odor
   c. Amount of necrotic tissue
   d. Quantity of exudate

ANSWER: B Various odors may be associated with a wound and caused by maceration of tissue, mild colonization or dressing by products. Wound odor alone tells us little about severity.

2. The reimbursement of wound care services is defined in either local coverage determinations (LCDs) or national coverage decisions (NCDs). Which of the following ***does not*** presently have a NCD?
   a. Electrical stimulation
   b. Débridement
   c. Electromagnetic therapy
   d. Whirlpool

ANSWER: B Decisions on whether or not to reimburse for débridement are made at the local level as there is not currently a national policy.

3. Which of the following **_is not_** appropriate for documentation in the medical record?
   a. Previous medical history/onset of the wound
   b. Placing blame for the ulcer occurrence
   c. Patient education
   d. Wound measurements

ANSWER: B It would be considered very inappropriate and unprofessional to note blame in a patient note. Certainly issues of patient/caregiver understanding and compliance issues should be addressed and documented.

4. What is the most appropriate interval for wound assessments following the initial evaluation and examination?
   a. Daily
   b. Weekly
   c. Monthly
   d. Each visit/patient encounter

ANSWER: B Most standards of documentation indicate that a note be written everytime there is a change in patient status and at least on a weekly basis.

Chapter 34

1. Which of the following would be the most helpful in determining the types of services to offer as part of a new outpatient wound program?
   a. Algorithm
   b. Sales promotion
   c. SWOT analysis
   d. Gantt chart

ANSWER: C A SWOT analysis examines strengths, weaknesses, opportunities, and threats as they pertain to the program and can help objectively determine what services may be viable. An algorithm is a clinical decision-making tool, sales promotion is a type of marketing strategy, and a Gantt chart illustrates project timelines.

2. What is a benefit of process standardization?
   a. It allows every patient to be treated exactly the same way.
   b. It ensures that all areas affecting the treatment plan have been addressed.
   c. It gives staff a "cookbook" for treating patients with wounds.
   d. It does not allow for any product variation.

ANSWER: B Process standardization makes sure all the bases are covered, *but* still allows for care to be individualized for each patient. To that end, there will be product variation from time to time based on what a specific patient needs.

3. What would be a useful outcomes measure for a facility with a large population of patients with pressure ulcers?
   a. Norton scale
   b. Braden scale
   c. Wagner scale
   d. PUSH tool

ANSWER: D The PUSH tool is an outcomes measure that looks specifically at pressure ulcers. The Norton scale and Braden scale are risk assessment tools, *not* outcomes tools, and the Wagner scale categorizes the severity of neuropathic foot ulcers.

Chapter 35

1. The standard of care for all areas of health-care delivery is developed from many sources including which of the following:
   a. Clinical Practice Guidelines, which may be published by various specialties, Policies and Procedures developed by health-care providers or specialty groups, peer-reviewed literature, and, sometimes, case law
   b. Textbooks and current literature only
   c. Periodicals, *Gray's Anatomy*, and the Internet
   d. WebMD, Policies and Procedures, and the *New England Journal of Medicine*

ANSWER: A Standard of care is derived from a broad variety of settings as indicated in answer A. Highly technical textbooks, journals and postings on the Internet are not reliable sources.

2. The four elements that must be present in a medical negligence case and must be proved by a preponderance of the evidence are:
   a. relationship, poor communication, poor care, death.
   b. duty, breach, damages, causation.
   c. duty, poor communication, death, damages.
   d. procedure, policies, pain and suffering, loss.

ANSWER: B A plaintiff must establish that a legal duty existed for the provider to undertake care of the patient, that the standard of care was breached and that it resulted in damages and that the breach of duty was a proximate cause of the injury that resulted.

3. Doing something that a reasonable person would not do under the same set of circumstances would be an example of
   a. negligence.
   b. proximate cause.
   c. liability.
   d. punitive damages.

ANSWER: A Negligence in the broadest sense is doing something that a reasonable person would not do under the same or similar circumstances; or not doing something that a reasonable person would do under the same or similar circumstances.

4. Noneconomic damages are:
   a. not subject to an economics theory.
   b. lost wages if you work as a contract worker.
   c. pain and suffering, loss of enjoyment of life.
   d. damages for which you cannot ask.

ANSWER: C Non-economic damages are those damages that are for pain, suffering, and loss of companionship. These are opposed to economic losses such as a loss of wages, medical bills, and damage to property.

5. An expert witness:
  a. must be a treating health-care provider in the case.
  b. can be from any specialty if he or she knows what he or she is talking about.
  c. may be a treating health-care provider or may be retained, not as a treater, but to give expert opinion testimony.
  d. shouldn't look at every medical record involving the case in which he or she is an expert.

ANSWER: C It is not required that an expert witness be an actively treating health-care provider, but that they actually have documented evidence of expertise in the matter at hand.

6. In a criminal case, the burden of proof is "beyond a reasonable doubt." In a civil case, the burden of proof is:
  a. beyond an unreasonable doubt.
  b. a preponderance of the evidence.
  c. 100%.
  d. 90%.

ANSWER: B The highest level of proof, "beyond a reasonable doubt" is typically what is required for conviction in a criminal case. In civil cases, the requirement is typically "a preponderance of evidence."

Index

An "f" following a page number indicates a figure; a "t" following a page number indicates a table; a "b" following a page number indicates a box.

A

Abduction brace, for burn patient, 368
ABI (ankle-brachial index), in arterial perfusion assessment, 96–97, 97f, 97t
Abrasions, 340
Accommodative felt padding, 225
ACE® bandages, for compression therapy, 379
Acetic acid, in burn wound management, 344
Achilles tendon, lengthening of, in neuropathic foot, 424–425
Acid burns, 337–338
Acoustic microstreaming, from ultrasound, 551–552, 551f
Acrocyanosis, 262
Adenosine triphosphate (ATP) synthesis, laser therapy effects on, 588
Adhesive proteins, in extracellular matrix, 37–38
Advanced glycation end products (AGEs), in diabetes, healing and, 234
Age
    leg ulcers and, 248
    wound healing and, 58–59, 413
Aging
    diabetes and, 238
    effects of, on basement membrane zone, 3, 3f
    of skin, 6–7, 58–59, 58t
Air-fluidized beds, 327–328
Air plethysmography, in arterial and venous function assessment, 100–101
Airplane splint, thermoplastic conformer, for burn patient, 367
Airway management, for burn patient, 343, 343f
Alcohol use, in patient history, 67
Alcohols, as topical antiseptics, 203t
Alginate dressings, 184
    in wound care in pediatrics, 445
Alkali burns, 337
Allergies, in patient history, 67
AlloDerm, for burn wounds, 351
Allodynia, 394
    definition of, 391
    in second degree burns, 401
Allografts, cadaveric
    for burn wounds, 350–351, 350f
    for wound coverage in neuropathic foot, 425
Alternating current (AC), 464–465, 465f
Alternobaric vertigo, 626
Ambulation, of burn patient, 363, 370–371
Ambulatory Payment Classifications (APCs), 638–639
Amelogenin dressings, 190
Amino acids, in nutrition therapy, 48
Amorphous aqueous gel, as coupling medium for ultrasound, 549
Amputation(s)
    for chronic vascular insufficiency, 417
    in diabetic patients, 421
    in neuropathic foot
        digital, 423
        midfoot, 426–427
        transmetatarsal, 424, 426
    for PAD, 273
    transmetatarsal, stabilization of, Achilles tendon lengthening for, 424–425

Anabolic steroids, to increase recovery, 48
Analgesics, topical, for wound pain, 402
Anchoring fibrils, in basement membranes, 38
Anchoring filaments, of lymphatic system, 279, 280f
Anesthetics, topical, impacting healing, 59
Angiogenesis
    definition of, 20
    endogenous currents stimulating, 459, 459f
    in neovascularization, 20–21
    wound, electrical stimulation enhancing, 473–474
Angiogenic growth factors, 40–41
Angiograms, catheter, 122, 122f, 123f
Angiography
    computed tomography, in arterial evaluation, 124–125, 125f
    magnetic resonance, in arterial evaluation, 125, 125f
Animal electricity, brief history of, 451–452
Ankle
    burn injuries of, splints for, 368, 368f
    limb salvage at, 428, 429f
        reconstructive procedures for, 430–431, 431f
Ankle-brachial index (ABI), in arterial perfusion assessment, 96–97, 96t, 97f
Anterior chest, of burn patient, splints for, 367, 368f
Anthropometric characteristics, in lymphedema, 284
Anthropometric measurements, in nutritional assessment, 46
Anti-inflammatory agents
    nonsteroidal
        impacting healing, 59
        for wound pain, 402
    topical, 210
Antibacterial effects. *See* Antimicrobial effects
Antibiotics. *See* Antimicrobials
Antimicrobial effects. *See also* Bactericidal effects
    of electrical stimulation, 467–469, 468t, 469f, 470f
    of kilohertz ultrasound, 558–560, 558f, 559f
Antimicrobials
    in burn wound management, 343–344, 344f, 345f
    in controlling bioburden, 114
    in dressings, 188
    effectiveness of, against biofilm and cancer cells, electrical stimulation and, 470
    impacting healing, 59
    topical, 206–210, 209t
        in controlling bioburden, 115
Antiphospholipid antibody syndrome (APS), 143, 143f
Antiseptics
    in controlling bioburden, 114
    in dressings, 188
    in wound care, 203t
Antitorticollis strap and neck splint, dynamic, for burn patient, 366
Aplasia cutis congenital, in pediatric patients, 441
Apligraf®, for wound coverage in neuropathic foot, 425

Apocrine sweat glands, 4, 359, 359f
APS (antiphospholipid antibody syndrome), 143, 143f
Aptiva™ Move HVPC device, 500, 500f
Aqueous gel, as coupling medium for ultrasound, 549, 549f
Arginine, in nutrition therapy, 48
Arterial insufficiency. *See also* Peripheral arterial disease (PAD)
    case study on, 274–275
    classification of, 257, 257t
    guideline recommendations on, 87t
    impeding healing, 57, 57t
    pain related to, 400
    pathophysiology and etiology of, 256–262
    wound healing compromised by, surgery for, 417
Arterial occlusive disease, thromboangiitis obliterans as, 259–260
Arterial perfusion, assessing, 94–99
    ankle-brachial index in, 96–97, 96t, 97f
    capillary refill test in, 96
    claudication onset time in, 96
    invasive techniques in, 99
    pulse volume recordings in, 97, 99f
    pulses in, 94–95
    rubor of dependency, 95, 95f
    segmental pressure in, 97, 97t, 98f
    skin perfusion pressure in, 99
    transcutaneous partial pressure of oxygen in, 97, 98t
    venous filling time in, 95, 95f
Arterial ulceration(s)
    appearance of, 263–264, 264f
    clinical features of, 262, 266t
    conservative management of, 256–278
    examination of, 264, 264f
        findings in, 263–267
    history of, 262–263
    infection in, management and prevention of, 269–273
        electrical stimulation in, 270
        hyperbaric oxygen therapy in, 271
        limb protection in, 271–272
        medical and pharmacological, 272–273
        negative pressure wound therapy in, 271
        pneumatic compression devices in, 271
        risk factor reduction in, 272
        surgical, 273
        ultrasound in, 271
    lower extremity, pulsed electromagnetic field stimulation for, 523–524, 524b
    tests and measures of, 264, 266–267, 266b, 266t
    treatment of, 267–269
        local care in, 267–269
    viable *versus* necrotic tissues in, 264, 265t
Arteries, evaluation of, 122–126
Arteriograms
    catheter, 122, 122f, 123f
    physical basis of, 120
Arteriosclerosis obliterans, 257–258
Arteritis, Takayasu's, 261
Arthropathy, Charcot. *See* Charcot arthropathy
Ascorbic acid, in nutrition therapy, 49